William G. Shafer, B.S., D.D.S., M.S.

Distinguished Professor and Chairman,
Department of Oral Pathology,
Indiana University School of Dentistry

Maynard K. Hine, D.D.S., M.S.

Chancellor Emeritus
Indiana University-Purdue University
at Indianapolis

Barnet M. Levy, D.D.S., M.S.

Professor of Pathology
The University of Texas Dental Branch and
Graduate School of Biomedical Sciences
at Houston

With contributions by

Charles E. Tomich, D.D.S., M.S.D.

Professor of Oral Pathology,
Indiana University School of Dentistry

A Textbook of Oral Pathology

FOURTH EDITION/ILLUSTRATED

1983

W.B. Saunders Company

Philadelphia / London / Toronto / Mexico City / Rio de Janeiro / Sydney / Tokyo

W. B. Saunders Company: West Washington Square
Philadelphia, PA 19105

1 St. Anne's Road
Eastbourne, East Sussex BN21 3UN, England

1 Goldthorne Avenue
Toronto, Ontario M8Z 5T9, Canada

Apartado 26370—Cedro 512
Mexico 4, D.F., Mexico

Rua Coronel Cabrita, 8
Sao Cristovao Caixa Postal 21176
Rio de Janeiro, Brazil

9 Waltham Street
Artarmon, N.S.W. 2064, Australia

Ichibancho, Central Bldg., 22-1 Ichibancho
Chiyoda-Ku, Tokyo 102, Japan

Library of Congress Cataloging in Publication Data

Shafer, William G.

A textbook of oral pathology.

Includes bibliographical references.

1. Teeth—Diseases.   2. Mouth—Diseases.   I. Hine,
Maynard Kiplinger, 1907– .   II. Levy, Barnet M.   III.
Title.   IV. Title: Oral pathology. [DNLM: 1. Mouth dis-
eases—Pathology. WU 140 S525t]

RK307.S44 1983   617'.522   82-40349
ISBN 0–7216–8128–X

Listed here is the latest translated edition of this book together with
the language of the translation and the publisher.

Spanish (*1st Edition*)—Nueva Editorial Interamericana S.A. de C.V.
          Mexico 4 E.F., Mexico

Portuguese (*3rd Edition*)—Editora Interamericana Ltda.
          Rio de Janeiro, Brazil

A Textbook of Oral Pathology   ISBN 0-7216-8128-X

Last digit is the print number: 9   8   7   6   5   4   3   2   1

Dedication

*This book is dedicated
to the student of dentistry,
for with him lies the future of our profession.*

PREFACE
to the
Fourth Edition

The explosion of scientific knowledge and technology which occurred within the past few decades has reached out to leave its impact on all branches of the healing disciplines, including dentistry. Thus the practice of dentistry today is as different from its practice 30 years ago as the microcomputer today is from the abacus centuries ago. Furthermore, the practice of dentistry in the year 2000 will be as unlike practice today as the computer of today will be unlike that instrument of the next century.

Oral pathology was in its infancy when the first edition of this textbook was published in 1958, having been recognized as a specialty of dentistry by the American Dental Association for only about 10 years. Our knowledge in this area was limited and patchy, and had incredible voids. What knowledge we did possess was due largely to the determined efforts of a very few pioneers, often working alone, who tried to assemble our meager knowledge into some semblance of scientific order. On this foundation, our comprehension of oral disease has been accumulating at a nearly logarithmic pace. This has been achieved through the efforts of an increasing number of individuals who have devoted their professional careers to this field. Their research, utilizing and applying the burgeoning advances made possible in other fields and ranging from cytogenetics and molecular biology to ultrastructural physiology and immunohistochemistry, has contributed significantly to recent knowledge in oral pathology.

As has been pointed out previously, although the dentist is still dependent upon technical skills, the increasing emphasis on a biologic orientation in dental practice has underscored the necessity for both the general practitioner and the specialist to have a working knowledge of oral pathology. The broadening parameters of prevention of oral disease and maintenance of oral health make it no longer sufficient or acceptable for the dentist to be concerned with only the repair of past dental problems. He now needs a sufficiently thorough scientific background as well as the knowledge to permit him to examine the patient, evaluate the various findings, draw a definitive diagnostic conclusion and institute proper treatment. The authors' intention here is to provide the reader with an appreciation of the importance of understanding the etiology and pathogenesis of oral diseases as well as to supply the knowledge itself. We have attempted to stress those disease processes which are encountered most frequently in clinical practice or which illustrate an important pathologic concept. Space limitation has necessitated omitting or treating briefly some areas of oral pathology that might be considered important. Some relatively rare entities have been included because of fundamental concepts which they may illuminate. Decisions have been made conscientiously but will obviously differ from those that might have been made by others.

To those familiar with the previous edition of this book, an increase in content will be apparent. This is a necessity because of the advances discussed. In addition, there are many alterations in ideas and concepts consistent with changes conceived since the last edition. We have attempted to deal with current knowledge in a broad, encompassing yet succinct fashion, the principal consideration being the needs of the student and also of the dental practitioner.

THE AUTHORS

ACKNOWLEDGMENTS

Many persons have contributed unselfishly their time, special talents, knowledge and illustrative material to aid in the completion of this book. Those allowing free use of their illustrations have been credited in the legends for the particular figures, and grateful acknowledgment is once again made here. In addition, special acknowledgment must be made to numerous individuals for use of their excellent material in the preparation of the color plates. Of many hundreds of clinical color photographs reviewed, very few were of a quality sufficient to warrant their duplication in color. The authors expressly wish to thank the following individuals for permission to use their material: Dr. George G. Blozis, one illustration in Plate VII; Dr. Stephen F. Dachi, eleven illustrations in Plates II, III, IV, V and VI; Dr. Warren B. Davis, one illustration in Plate IV; Dr. Thomas B. Fast, one illustration in Plate IV; Dr. John R. Mink, one illustration in Plate IV; Dr. David F. Mitchell, four illustrations in Plates I, II and III; Dr. Wilbur C. Moorman, one illustration in Plate VII; Dr. Gil Small, one illustration in Plate II; Dr. S. Miles Standish, two illustrations in Plates I and IV; and Dr. Henry M. Swenson, two illustrations in Plate VII.

Various chapters and sections of the text have been read, criticized and corrected by persons with a particular interest in certain areas of pathology, and to them are extended sincere thanks. These include Drs. Sumter S. Arnim, David Bixler, Manuel G. Bloom, Boynton H. Booth, Charles Burstone, Samuel Dreizen, Harris Keene, Martin Lunin, Irwin Mandel, David F. Mitchell, S. Miles Standish, Harold Stanley and Merrill Wheatcroft. A special vote of thanks to Dennis Lynch for his careful critique of the chapter on Oral Aspects of Metabolic Diseases. Hours of consultation also were devoted to this project by many members of the staffs of Indiana University School of Dentistry and School of Medicine, including Drs. J. William Adams, Charles W. Gish, G. Thaddeus Gregory, Victor C. Hackney, J. Frank Hall, Harry J. Healey, Charles E. Hutton, Ralph E. McDonald, Chris H. Miller, Wilbur C. Moorman, Timothy J. O'Leary, Ralph W. Phillips, Ronald S. Ping, Robert J. Rohn, Lawrence M. Roth, Henry M. Swenson, George K. Stookey, Grant Van Huysen and Frank Vellios.

Our deep appreciation is due to a number of persons with whom, over a period of years, we have held lengthy discussions of the technical and philosophical aspects of oral pathology which have resulted in the authors' arrival at many of their conclusions and beliefs. This list must include Dr. S. Miles Standish, whose inestimable aid and calm wisdom can never be properly or sufficiently acknowledged; Drs. Donald A. Kerr and Robert J. Gorlin, particularly for their critical reading and suggestions; Drs. William G. Sprague and Charles A. Waldron for their continued inspiration through constant discussions, agreement and disagreement; Drs. Charles E. Tomich and Lawrence I. Goldblatt for so willingly sharing the burdens; Dr. Frank Vellios, for his willing help and advice; and, finally, the many stimulating graduate students with whom it has been our privilege to be associated over the years.

The photographs have been prepared largely by Mr. Richard Scott, Mrs. Gloria Spray, Mrs. Alana Fears and Mr. Michael Halloran of the Illustration Department of Indiana University School of Dentistry. The drawings were made by Drs. Peter Kesling and Rolando DeCastro. Assistance for the preparation of illustrative material, an important part of any book, is gratefully acknowledged.

The many rough drafts and the final copy of the manuscript were typed by Mrs. Sondra Hawkins, Mrs. Dorothy Lincoln, Miss Margaret Herron, Miss Sharon Hendricks and Miss Vicki Taylor, to whom special thanks are due. Mrs. Ruth Chilton also aided in typing some sections.

The tissue laboratory of the Department of Oral Pathology was in the charge of Mrs. Patricia G. Clark, who had responsibility for the excellent histologic material used in most of the photomicrographs.

A special debt of gratitude is owed to Sylvia Levy for her part in this undertaking. For all editions of the text, she painstakingly read and reread not only rough and final copies of the manuscript, but also all galley and page proofs, correcting errors in punctuation, spelling, grammar and syntax with an unselfish devotion. The undertaking of this book would have been impossible also without the sacrifices made by the authors' wives in tolerating the long hours spent in writing. To them, special recognition is offered.

THE AUTHORS

PREFACE
to the
First Edition

ORAL PATHOLOGY represents the confluence of the basic sciences and clinical dentistry. Since it has no methods of its own, knowledge in this field is acquired through the adaptation of methods and disciplines of those sciences basic to dental practice, such as gross and microscopic anatomy, chemistry, microbiology and physiology, and through information obtained by clinical histories and observation of patients. Through the science of oral pathology, an attempt is made to correlate human biology with the signs and symptoms of human disease. The oral pathologist attempts to understand oral disease so that it can be properly diagnosed and adequately treated.

In this text we have attempted to bring the reader to an understanding of the patient and his problems through applied basic science. We have tried to explain clinical signs and symptoms in the light of known histologic, chemical and physiologic alterations. Where possible, the prognosis of each disease is considered as a reflection of the underlying tissue changes and what we know can be done about them today.

In numerous sections of the text we have attempted to integrate information from many of the basic sciences for adequate diagnosis of oral disease. This approach is a departure from that of the usual textbook of oral pathology, representing an effort to place more emphasis on the physiologic and chemical aspects of oral disease.

The references at the end of each chapter are extensive enough to be of value to those interested in additional reading. Only those papers which constitute good review articles or exceptional discussions or which are of historical importance are included. Because the field of oral pathology is large, much of the bibliographic material has had to be curtailed or omitted. The highlights alone have been stressed. It is our hope that this book will prove to be a stimulus to study as well as a guide for undergraduate and graduate students and practitioners of both dentistry and medicine.

THE AUTHORS

CONTENTS

SECTION III   INJURIES AND REPAIR

SECTION IV   DISTURBANCES OF METABOLISM

SECTION V   DISEASES OF SPECIFIC SYSTEMS

APPENDIX

SECTION I

DISTURBANCES OF DEVELOPMENT AND GROWTH

CHAPTER 1

Developmental Disturbances of Oral and Paraoral Structures

An understanding of the many disturbances of development and growth that involve the oral and paraoral structures is predicated upon a thorough understanding of the embryology and histology of these structures. Some of the conditions to be discussed here develop *in utero,* are present at birth, and persist throughout life. Others may not manifest themselves for many years. The recognition that some abnormalities follow the traditional patterns of inheritance has been of great help to the scientist in explaining many unusual pathologic conditions which affect the living organism. Great care must be taken, however, to distinguish between hereditary and congenital conditions. A congenital disease is one which is present at or before birth but is not necessarily inherited, i.e., transmitted through the genes. In contrast, many hereditary conditions are apparent at birth, whereas others do not become evident for a number of years after birth.

The explanation for the tendency of a person to inherit certain features or characteristics from his parents is based upon the monumental observations of Gregor Mendel, who did much to establish the laws of heredity. From his painstaking and carefully recorded work arose the science of genetics.

One of Mendel's most important discoveries was that of the principle of dominance, which was based upon experiments showing that if the two members of a given pair of individuals with contrasting characters are brought together in a cross, there is a decided difference in the ability of these characters to be expressed in the resulting offspring. Thus one of the characters, but not the other, may manifest itself. Of great importance, however, is the fact that the unexpressed character is not eliminated, for it may be manifested in subsequent generations. The terms "dominant" and "recessive" have been applied, respectively, to those features which do and which do not appear in the first filial generation following the cross. The subsequent separation and reappearance of characters in the offspring of hybrid persons are known as the principle of segregation and are a feature of inheritance.

It is well established that the many characteristics of a person are represented in the genes of the gametes, or reproductive cells. In speaking of or comparing only two characteristics, the possibilities of assortment are relatively limited, but as the number of characteristics increases, it is obvious that the possibilities of combinations become infinitely more complex.

Another important principle of inheritance, discovered by T. H. Morgan, is that of linkage between factors, which offers an explanation for the early observation that two or more characters may remain linked in their passage from one generation to another. An offshoot of this principle was the discovery of sex linkage, or the linkage of certain characters with the factors that determine sex. For example, a man may transmit a sex-linked trait to his grandsons through his daughters, but not to or through his sons. Such a transmission depends on the paired sex chromosomes of an individual.

Many of the developmental and growth disturbances of the oral and paraoral structures, as well as other oral diseases to be discussed, have a definite hereditary background. Other diseases in which the evidence for inheritance is suggestive but not conclusive are sometimes said to present "familial tendencies." Dentistry has much to offer in helping to determine the true etiologic factors in the many disturbances

2

of development and growth of the teeth, bones, and various soft tissues. Very valuable texts on the role of genetics in dentistry have been written by Witkop and by Stewart and Prescott, to which the reader is referred for in-depth discussions of many of these diseases. Witkop has stressed the fact that in some dental diseases, inherited factors can be either decisive or only contributory to the production of a specific illness. As examples of hereditary oral diseases, he has presented the compilation shown in Table 1–1.

Genetic factors are undoubtedly of importance in the development of many human congenital malformations, although it has been estimated that only about 10 per cent of such malformations can be explained on a genetic basis. In his broad discussion of teratology, Smith has listed the possible genetic dysmorphogenic influences, shown in Table 1–2. A

Table 1–1. Hereditary Oral Diseases

ORAL DISEASE	MODE OF INHERITANCE D—DOMINANT R—RECESSIVE S—SEX-LINKED IS—INTERMEDIATE SEX-LINKED	ACCURACY OF GENETIC PROGNOSIS ...—ACCURATE ..—APPROXIMATE .—QUESTIONABLE
Heritable defects in dentition without generalized defects:		
Hypoplasia of enamel	SD	..
Hypocalcification of enamel	D	...
Hypomaturation of enamel	SR	...
Pigmented hypomaturation of enamel	R	.
Local hypoplasia of enamel	D (with incomp. penetrance)	..
Dentin dysplasia	D	...
Dentinogenesis imperfecta	D	...
Missing or peg laterals	D	...
Missing maxillary incisors and cuspids	D or R	..
Missing premolars	D	..
Missing third molars	D	..
Gigantism of maxillary central incisors	D	..
Fused primary mandibular incisors	D?	..
Familial dentigerous cysts	D	..
Heritable defects in dentition with generalized defects:		
Dentinogenesis imperfecta with osteogenesis imperfecta	D	..
Enamel hypoplasia in vitamin D-resistant rickets	D (irregular)	..
Enamel hypoplasia with epidermolysis bullosa dystrophia	R	..
Local hypoplasia of enamel with Fanconi syndrome	R?	.
Missing teeth with ectodermal dysplasia	IS or D	..
Missing premolars with premature whitening of hair	D	...
Missing lateral incisors with ptosis of eyelid	D	..
Retarded eruption with cleidocranial dysostosis	D	..
Heritable defects of oral structures without generalized defects:		
Ankyloglossia	D	..
Elephantiasis gingivae	D	..
Harelip and harelip with cleft palate	R?	.
Heritable defects of oral structures with generalized diseases:		
Gangrenous stomatitis with acatalasemia	R	..
Periodontitis with agammaglobulinemia	SR	..
Periodontitis and osteoporosis of jaw bones with thalassemia major	R	...
Alveolar bone changes in sickle cell disease	R	..
Gingival and postoperative hemorrhage in hemophilia and Christmas disease	SR	...
Mucosal telangiectasia in hemorrhagic telangiectasia (Osler)	D	..
Facial angiomatosis with Sturge-Weber disease	D (irregular)	.

(Table continued on following page.)

Table 1–1. Hereditary Oral Diseases—*Continued.*

ORAL DISEASE	MODE OF INHERITANCE D—DOMINANT R—RECESSIVE S—SEX-LINKED IS—INTERMEDIATE SEX-LINKED	ACCURACY OF GENETIC PROGNOSIS ...—ACCURATE ..—APPROXIMATE .—QUESTIONABLE
Oral hematomas with Ehlers-Danlos syndrome	D	..
Facial deformity in gargoylism	R (RS)	..
Facial deformity with mandibulofacial dysostosis (Franceschetti)	D (irregular)	..
Facial deformity with craniofacial dysostosis (Crouzon)	D (irregular)	..
Micrognathia with Pierre Robin syndrome	R (incomp. dom.)	.
Hypoplasia of maxilla with achondroplasia	D	..
Multilocular cystic fibrous dysplasia of the jaws and face (Jones)	D	...
Osteosclerosis in Albers-Schönberg disease	D (irregular)	..
Hyperostosis of jaws in generalized hyperostotic bone disease (Witkop)	R	...
Hypercementosis and bone changes in osteitis deformans (Paget)	D (incomp.)	.
Neurofibroma and pigmentation in neurofibromatosis (von Recklinghausen)	D	..
Circumoral pigmentation with gastrointestinal polyposis (Peutz-Jeghers)	D	..
Facial pigmentation and carcinomas of lip in xeroderma pigmentosum	ISR or R	..
Gingival and lingual amyloid deposits in familial amyloidosis	D	..
White spongy nevus of mucous membranes	D	...

From C. J. Witkop, Jr.: Genetics and Dentistry. Eugenics Q., 5:15, 1958.

Table 1 is a partial classification of hereditary oral diseases listing the common mode of inheritance and the accuracy of prognosis based on the oral findings. Some traits, such as dentinogenesis imperfecta, are known to be inherited only in the manner listed, while others, such as peg or missing laterals, may be associated with a number of genetic entities or may be phenocopies; that is, due to a non-genetic cause. If good evidence exists that a trait does occur in a hereditary form, then that trait has been included. Thus, a specific trait such as premature whitening of the hair and missing premolars is known to be inherited in an autosomal dominant manner in some kindreds. This does not mean that all cases of premature whitening of the hair will be associated with missing premolars or that all cases of missing premolars will be inherited with premature whitening of the hair.

A single trait may show two forms of inheritance. Thus, missing teeth may be found in two forms of ectodermal dysplasia. One form shows an autosomal dominant mode of inheritance in some families, while in other families the gene apparently is passed on the X-chromosome. In this latter form, males are severely affected, but females with the gene may show only a few missing teeth.

This list should be used as a guide only and should not be relied upon as the sole evidence for making a genetic prognosis in any individual case. A genetic prognosis in any individual case should be made on the basis of a complete family history of how the trait in question is inherited in that particular family.—Carl J. Witkop, Jr.

Table 1–2. Possible Genetic Dysmorphogenic Influences

1. Single mutant gene
   a. Autosomal dominant
   b. X-linked dominant
   c. X-linked recessive in XY individual
2. Pair of mutant alleles
   a. Autosomal recessive
   b. X-linked recessive in an XX individual
3. Polygenic: The combined effects of more than one gene acting in concert
4. Gross chromosomal abnormality causing a genetic imbalance
   a. Altered number of chromosomes due to faulty chromosomal distribution at cell division
   b. Chromosomal breakage ± rearrangement of the pieces ultimately resulting in genetic imbalance

From D. W. Smith: Dysmorphology (teratology). J. Pediatr., 69:1150, 1966.

second important factor in the development of such disturbances is that of pathologic environmental conditions, and these have been estimated to account for an additional 10 per cent of developmental anomalies. The remaining 80 per cent are, in light of present knowledge, idiopathic.

A remarkable scientific interest has developed in the possible environmental causes of congenital malformations, and a vast number of both clinical and experimental animal studies have been carried out to clarify this relationship.

Haring and Lewis have reviewed the scientific literature on known etiologic factors in both spontaneous and experimental congenital developmental anomalies and have tabulated all currently known teratogenic factors. These are listed in Table 1–3. In considering the problem of congenital malformations, Haring and Lewis

Table 1–3. Experimental and Clinical Causes of Congenital Developmental Anomalies

Genetic factors ...Inherited	6-Mercaptopurine
Mutagenetic	Azaserine
Environmental factors:	5-Fluorodeoxyuridine
1. Infections ...Rubella	6-Aminonicotinamide
Influenza A	Thiadiazole
2. Physical	6-Chloropurine
injuries .....Pressure	Thioguanine
Temperature changes	2-6-Diamonopurine
Radiation	Polyfunctional alkylating
3. Hormones ...Diabetes mellitus	agents:
Alloxan diabetes	HN_2
Hyperthyroidism	CB 1348
Hypothyroidism	TEM
Antuitrin G	ThioTEPA
ACTH	Myleran and others
Cortisone	Triazene
Androgens	Quinine
Estrogens	Urethane
Oral progestins	Colchicine
Insulin	Trypan blue
4. Nutrition ....Deficiencies of	Pilocarpine
Vitamin A	Eserine
Vitamin B_1	Boric acid
Vitamin B_2	Thallium
Vitamin B_6	Selenium
Niacin	Nicotine
Folic acid	Sulfonamides
Vitamin B_{12}	Tetracyclines
Vitamin D	Chloroquine
Vitamin E	Thalidomide
Vitamin K	Salicylates
Proteins	Malachite green
Amino acids	7. Maternal
Unsaturated fatty acids	diseases and
Potassium	defects ......Uterine tumors
Excess of vitamin A	Uterine inflammation
5. Respiration ..Hypoxia	Uterine malformation
Carbon dioxide excess	Defects in implantation
Carbon monoxide	Age
Anesthesia with ether-gas-	Emotional disturbances
oxygen	Stress
6. Miscellaneous drugs and chemicals	Multiple pregnancies
Antimetabolites	Phenylpyruvic
Aminopterin	oligophrenia
Amethopterin	8. Embryonic
	defects ......Abnormalities of the ovum
	Abnormalities of the semen
	Antigen-antibody reactions

Courtesy of Drs. Olga M. Haring and F. John Lewis: Surg., Gynecol. Obstet., *113*:1, 1961, modified.

evolved certain principles, based on scientific evidence, applicable to both animal and human teratogenesis. These principles are as follows: (1) experimentally induced malformations in animals are similar to those occurring spontaneously and sporadically in the animal population, i.e., phenocopies; (2) many different agents can induce the same type of defect; (3) the same agent applied at different stages of development produces different types of defects; (4) the same defect can be induced regularly and at will if a teratogenic agent is applied at the same and proper time during the development in the same strain; (5) specific defects can be induced with greater ease in certain strains of a species than in others; (6) teratogenic agents do not necessarily alter the mother's condition of health.

It is of considerable interest to the dental profession that experimental studies of teratogenic agents have almost invariably revealed a variety of head, neck, and oral malformations, many of which have a human counterpart. Conway and Wagner have compiled a list of the most common malformations of the head and neck, as shown in Table 1–4.

DEVELOPMENTAL DISTURBANCES OF THE JAWS

AGNATHIA

Agnathia is an extremely rare congenital defect characterized by absence of the maxilla or mandible. More commonly, only a portion of one jaw is missing. In the case of the maxilla, this may be one maxillary process or even the premaxilla. Partial absence of the mandible is even more common. The entire mandible on one side may be missing or, more frequently, only the condyle or the entire ramus, although bilateral agenesis of the condyles and of the rami also has been reported. In cases of unilateral absence of the mandibular ramus, it is not unusual for the ear to be deformed or absent as well.

MICROGNATHIA

Micrognathia literally means a small jaw, and either the maxilla or the mandible may be affected. Many cases of apparent micrognathia are due not to an abnormally small jaw in terms of absolute size, but rather to an abnormal positioning or an abnormal relation of one jaw to the other or to the skull, which produces the illusion of micrognathia.

True micrognathia may be classified as either (1) congenital, or (2) acquired. The etiology of the *congenital* type is unknown, although in many instances it is associated with other congenital abnormalities, including particularly congenital heart disease and the Pierre Robin syndrome (q.v.). This form of the disease has been discussed by Monroe and Ogo. It occasionally follows a hereditary pattern. Micrognathia of the maxilla is frequently due to a

Table 1–4.   Fifteen Most Common Malformations of the Head and Neck*

MALFORMATION	MALE	FEMALE	TOTAL
Cleft lip and palate	325	202	527
Anencephalus	207	267	474
Cleft palate	227	240	467
Cleft lip	295	168	463
Hemangioma or nevus	160	170	330
Malformation of ear (increasing agenesis)	193	119	312
Preauricular cysts, tabs, sinus	151	116	267
Ankyloglossia	95	58	153
Encephalocoele	31	58	89
Microcephalus	36	36	72
Klippel-Feil syndrome	23	28	51
Branchial cyst	27	19	46
Torticollis	22	23	45
Cystic hygroma	20	23	43
Defect skull bone	24	18	42
Total	1836	1545	3381

From H. Conway and K. J. Wagner: Congenital anomalies of the head and neck. Plast. Reconstr. Surg., 36:71, 1965.

*Figures are taken from the records of the New York City Department of Health, 1952 to 1962.

deficiency in the premaxillary area, and patients with this deformity appear to have the middle third of the face retracted. Although it has been suggested that mouth-breathing is a cause of maxillary micrognathia, it is more likely that the micrognathia may be one of the predisposing factors in the mouth-breathing, owing to associated maldevelopment of the nasal and nasopharyngeal structures.

True mandibular micrognathia of the congenital type is often difficult to explain. Some patients appear clinically to have a severe retrusion of the chin, but, by actual measurements, the mandible may be found to be within the normal limits of variation. Such cases may be due to a posterior positioning of the mandible with regard to the skull or to a steep mandibular angle resulting in an apparent retrusion of the jaw. Agenesis of the condyles also results in a true mandibular micrognathia.

The *acquired* type of micrognathia is of postnatal origin and usually results from a disturbance in the area of the temporomandibular joint. Ankylosis of the joint, for example, may be caused by trauma or by infection of the mastoid, of the middle ear, or of the joint itself. Since the normal growth of the mandible depends to a considerable extent on normally developing condyles as well as on muscle function, it is not difficult to understand how condylar ankylosis may result in a deficient mandible.

The clinical appearance of mandibular micrognathia is characterized by severe retrusion of the chin, a steep mandibular angle, and a deficient chin button (Fig. 1–1).

MACROGNATHIA

Macrognathia refers to the condition of abnormally large jaws. An increase in size of both jaws is frequently proportional to a generalized increase in size of the entire skeleton, e.g., in pituitary gigantism. More commonly only the jaws are affected, but macrognathia may be associated with certain other conditions, such as (1) Paget's disease of bone, in which overgrowth of the cranium and maxilla or occasionally the mandible occurs; (2) acromegaly, in which there is progressive enlargement of the mandible owing to hyperpituitarism in the adult; or (3) leontiasis ossea, a form of fibrous dysplasia in which there is enlargement of the maxilla.

Cases of mandibular protrusion or prognathism, uncomplicated by any systemic condition, are a rather common clinical occurrence (Fig. 1–2). The etiology of this protrusion is unknown, although some cases follow hereditary patterns. In many instances the prognathism is due to a disparity in the size of the maxilla in relation to the mandible. In other cases the mandible is measurably larger than normal. The angle between the ramus and the body also appears to influence the relation of the mandible to the maxilla, as does the actual height of the ramus. Thus prognathic patients tend to have long rami which form a less steep angle with the body of the mandible. The length of the ramus, in turn, may be associated with the growth of the condyle. It may be reasoned, therefore, that excessive condylar growth predisposes to mandibular prognathism.

General factors which conceivably would influence and tend to favor mandibular prognathism are as follows: (1) increased height of the ramus, (2) increased mandibular body length, (3) increased gonial angle, (4) anterior positioning of the glenoid fossa, (5) decreased maxillary length, (6) posterior positioning of the maxilla in relation to the cranium, (7) prominent chin button, and (8) varying soft-tissue contours.

Surgical correction of such cases is feasible. Ostectomy, or resection of a portion of the mandible to decrease its length, is now an

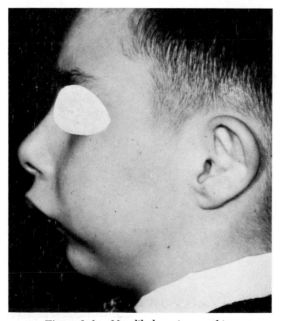

Figure 1–1. *Mandibular micrognathia.*
(Courtesy of Drs. G. Thaddeus Gregory and J. William Adams.)

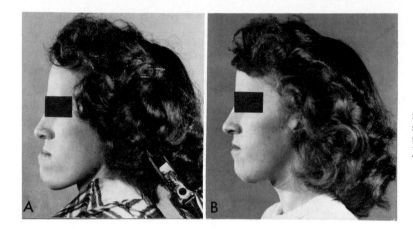

Figure 1–2. *Macrognathia (prognathia) of the mandible.* A, The protrusion of the mandible is obvious. B, The same patient after surgical correction (ostectomy). (Courtesy of Drs. G. Thaddeus Gregory and J. William Adams.)

established procedure, and the results are usually excellent from both a functional and a cosmetic standpoint.

FACIAL HEMIHYPERTROPHY

A very mild degree of facial asymmetry is present in nearly all persons, and this is often imperceptible to even close observation. Occasionally, however, a congenital hemihypertrophy may occur, involving (1) the entire half of the body, (2) one or both limbs, or (3) the face, head, and associated structures. Although the unilateral facial hypertrophy is the most striking feature in patients with this disturbance, the unusual hemihypertrophy of the jaws and teeth is the most significant finding to the dentist.

Etiology. The cause is unknown, but the condition has been variously ascribed to (1) hormonal imbalance, (2) incomplete twinning, (3) chromosomal abnormalities, (4) localized alteration of intrauterine development, (5) lymphatic abnormalities, (6) vascular abnormalities, and (7) neurogenic abnormalities. Of all of these, the last two, vascular and neural abnormalities, seem the most plausible to explain the clinical findings.

Clinical Features. Patients affected by facial hemihypertrophy exhibit enlargement of one half of the head (Fig. 1–3). In some cases this is obvious even at birth. The enlarged side grows at a rate proportional to the uninvolved side, so that the disproportion is maintained throughout life, although growth of the entire face generally ceases by the age of 20 years. Familial occurrence has been reported on a few occasions, according to the excellent review of the condition by Rowe, who described four additional cases. A wide variety of associated

abnormalities have been recorded by Ringrose and his associates in a review of 129 cases of hypertrophy; the most common of these are listed in Table 1–5. Fraumeni and his co-workers have also stressed that there appears to be some relationship between hemihypertrophy and neoplasms of the kidney, liver, and adrenal cortex in children. At the time of their review, there had been 26 cases of children with Wilms' tumor of the kidney and congenital hemihypertrophy, as well as six cases of adrenocortical

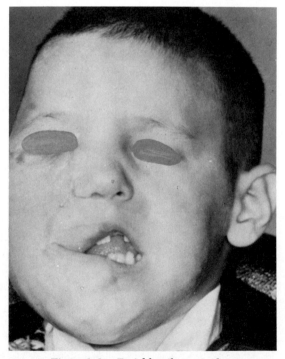

Figure 1–3. *Facial hemihypertrophy.* The asymmetric disfigurement is obvious despite several attempts at surgical correction.

Table 1–5. Incidence of Associated Abnormalities in Hemihypertrophy

ASSOCIATED ABNORMALITIES	INCIDENCE (%)
Mental deficiency	28
Skin abnormalities	47
Nevi	19
Telangiectasia	11
Hair thicker on involved side	7
Hemangioma	6
Skin coarser on involved side	5
Compensatory scoliosis	17
Varicose veins	7
Umbilical hernia	5

From R. E. Ringrose, J. T. Jabbour, and D. K. Keele: Hemihypertrophy. Pediatrics, 36:434, 1965.

tumor and four of hepatoblastoma associated with the malformation.

Of all reported cases, females are affected somewhat more frequently than males (63 per cent versus 37 per cent), according to the review by Ringrose. There is almost equal involvement of the right and left sides.

Oral Manifestations. The dentition of the hypertrophic side, according to Rowe, is abnormal in three respects: (1) crown size, (2) root size and shape, and (3) rate of development. Rowe has also pointed out that not all teeth in the enlarged area are necessarily affected in a similar fashion. There is little information about the effects on the deciduous dentition, but the permanent teeth on the affected side are often enlarged, although not exceeding a 50 per cent increase in size. This enlargement may involve any tooth, but seems to occur most frequently in the cuspid, premolars, and first molar. The roots of the teeth are sometimes proportionately enlarged but may be short.

Characteristically, the permanent teeth on the affected side develop more rapidly and erupt before their counterparts on the uninvolved side (Fig. 1–4). Coincident to this phenomenon is premature shedding of the deciduous teeth. The bone of the maxilla and mandible is also enlarged, being wider and thicker, sometimes with an altered trabecular pattern.

The tongue is commonly involved by the hemihypertrophy and may show a bizarre picture of enlargement of lingual papillae in addition to the general unilateral enlargement and contralateral displacement. In addition, the buccal mucosa frequently appears velvety and may seem to hang in soft, pendulous folds on the affected side.

Histologic Features. Tissue examination has been infrequently reported but is generally uninformative. In those cases reported, true muscular hypertrophy was not found.

Treatment and Prognosis. There is no specific treatment for this condition other than attempts at cosmetic repair. Its exact effect on life expectancy is not certain, but in some cases the patients have lived a normal life span.

Differential Diagnosis. There are certain diseases of the jaws, such as neurofibromatosis and fibrous dysplasia of the jaws, that may give the clinical appearance of facial hemihypertrophy, but these can usually be differentiated readily by the lack of effect on tooth size and rate of eruption.

FACIAL HEMIATROPHY

(Parry-Romberg Syndrome; Romberg Syndrome; Hemifacial Atrophy)

Facial hemiatrophy is a progressive atrophy of some or all of the tissues on one side of the face, occasionally extending to other parts of the body.

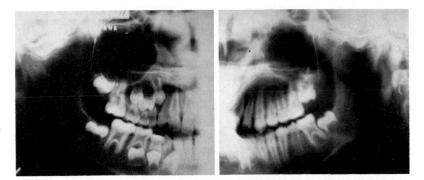

Figure 1–4. *Facial hemihypertrophy.* The difference in the eruption pattern of the teeth on each side is apparent. The teeth on the affected side, where all deciduous teeth have already been lost, are not appreciably larger than those on the unaffected side. (Courtesy of Dr. John B. Wittgen.)

Etiology. The cause of the condition is unknown, although suggested factors have included (1) a trophic malfunction of the cervical sympathetic nervous system, (2) trauma, (3) infection, (4) heredity, (5) peripheral trigeminal neuritis, and (6) a form of localized scleroderma.

Clinical Features. The onset of the condition is usually noticed in the first or second decade of life as a white line, furrow, or mark on one side of the face or brow near the midline. Presence at birth as well as onset in middle age has also been observed, however. This initial lesion extends progressively to include atrophy of the skin, subcutaneous tissue, muscle, and bone, resulting in facial deformity of varying degree depending upon severity of the atrophy. There may be hollowing of the cheek, and the eye may appear depressed in the orbit. The response of the atrophic facial muscle to faradic stimulation may be unaltered. The cartilage of the nose, ear, larynx, and palpebral tarsus also may become involved. In addition, contralateral Jacksonian epilepsy, trigeminal neuralgia, and changes in the eyes and hair commonly occur. Affected skin often becomes darkly pigmented, although vitiligo sometimes develops. Loss of facial hair is common. There is a marked predilection reported for involvement of the left side of the face.

Oral Manifestations. Hemiatrophy of the lips and the tongue is reported, as are dental effects. Foster has reported that growth of the teeth may be affected just as other tissues are involved. The roots of the teeth may exhibit deficiency of root development and reduced growth of the jaws on the affected side. Eruption of teeth on the affected side may also be retarded.

Treatment and Prognosis. There is no specific treatment for the condition. It has been found that typically the disease will be progressive for a period of several years and then remain unchanged for the remainder of the patient's life.

ABNORMALITIES OF DENTAL ARCH RELATIONS

In the preceding sections the conditions discussed are those in which there is an actual or apparent abnormal variation in size of one or both jaws. Of far greater importance than a simple disparity in size are the disparity in relation of one jaw to the other and the difficulties in occlusion and function that result.

A great many different types of malocclusion exist, and many classifications have been evolved in an attempt to unify methods of treatment. The classification of Angle, proposed in 1899, is the most universally known and used. That classification, with the approximate percentage occurrence as determined by Angle in a large group of orthodontic patients, is as follows:

Class	**I.**	Arches in normal mesiodistal relations	69.0%
Class	**II.**	Mandibular arch distal to normal in its relation to the maxillary arch	
	Division 1.	Bilaterally distal, protruding maxillary incisors	9.0
	SUBDIVISION.	Unilaterally distal, protruding maxillary incisors	3.5
	Division 2.	Bilaterally distal, retruding maxillary incisors	4.0
	SUBDIVISION.	Unilaterally distal, retruding maxillary incisors	10.0
Class	**III.**	Mandibular arch mesial to normal in its relation to the maxillary arch	
	Division.	Bilaterally mesial	3.5
	SUBDIVISION.	Unilaterally mesial	1.0

Since these abnormal jaw relations constitute a separate course of study, no further allusion to this subject will be made here.

DEVELOPMENTAL DISTURBANCES OF THE LIPS AND PALATE

CONGENITAL LIP AND COMMISSURAL PITS AND FISTULAS

Congenital lip pits and fistulas are malformations of the lips, often following a hereditary pattern, that may occur alone or in association with other developmental anomalies such as various oral clefts. Both Taylor and Lane and McConnel and his associates have emphasized that in 75 to 80 per cent of all cases of congenital labial fistulas, there is an associated cleft lip or cleft palate or both. The association of pits of the lower lip and cleft lip and/or cleft palate, termed van der Woude's syndrome, has been reviewed by Cervenka and his associates.

Commissural pits are an entity probably very closely related to lip pits, but occur at the lip commissures, lateral to the typical lip pits. Everett and Wescott have described this entity and noted that it is also frequently hereditary, possibly a dominant characteristic following a mendelian pattern, and may be associated with other congenital defects.

Etiology. Many theories of the etiology of congenital lip pits have been offered, but none has been universally accepted. Pits may result from notching of the lip at an early stage of development, with fixation of the tissue at the base of the notch, or from failure of complete union of the embryonic lateral sulci of the lip, which persist and ultimately develop into the typical pits.

Commissural pits are also difficult to explain, but they occur at the site of the horizontal facial cleft and may represent defective development of this embryonic fissure.

Clinical Features. The lip pit or fistula is a unilateral or bilateral depression or pit that occurs on the vermilion surface of either lip but far more commonly on the lower lip (Fig. 1–5, A). In some cases a sparse mucous secretion may exude from the base of this pit. The lip sometimes appears swollen, accentuating the appearance of the pits.

Commissural pits appear as unilateral or bilateral pits at the corners of the mouth on the vermilion surface (Fig. 1–5, B). An actual fistula

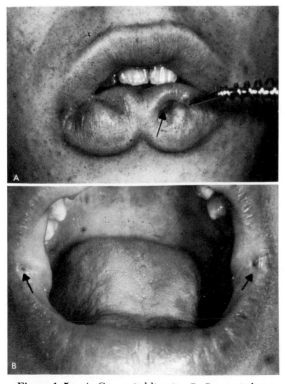

Figure 1–5. *A*, Congenital lip pits. *B*, Congenital commissural pits. (Courtesy of Drs. Robert J. Gorlin and Cesar Lopez.)

may be present from which fluid may be expressed. Whether this tract, either in lip or commissural fistulas, represents a true duct is not clear. Interestingly, in several cases preauricular pits have been reported in association with commissural pits.

Treatment. Surgical excision of these various pits has been recommended but primarily for academic information, since the pits are harmless and seldom manifest complications.

DOUBLE LIP

Double lip is an anomaly characterized by a fold of excess tissue on the inner mucosal aspect of the lip. It may be congenital or acquired as a result of trauma to the lip.

Clinical Features. This redundant mass of tissue usually occurs on the upper lip, although the lower lip and, on rare occasions, both upper and lower lips are involved. When the upper lip is tensed, the double lip resembles a "cupid's bow." The double lip usually cannot be seen when the lips are at rest. There is no information available concerning familial, sex, or racial predilection. Occasionally, it occurs in random association with other oral anomalies. The condition has been reviewed by Barnett and his associates.

The occurrence of acquired double lip in association with blepharochalasis and nontoxic thyroid enlargement is known as *Ascher's syndrome*. Blepharochalasis is a drooping of the tissue between the eyebrow and the edge of the upper eyelid so that it hangs loosely over the margin of the lid. It is caused by relaxation of the supratarsal fold as a result of atrophy and thinning of the skin of the eyelid. In these cases, the eye and lip abnormalities usually develop abruptly. The thyroid enlargement is not constant and, as pointed out by Papanayotou and Hatziotis, many cases exhibit only lip and eyelid involvement. However, it was emphasized by Ascher that the thyroid enlargement may not appear until several years after the eyelid involvement.

Treatment. No treatment is necessary except for cosmetic purposes or functions involving speech and mastication. The excess tissue is easily excised surgically.

CLEFT LIP AND CLEFT PALATE

Facial clefts occur along many planes of the face as a result of faults or defects in develop-

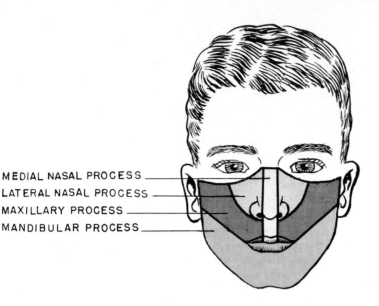

MEDIAL NASAL PROCESS
LATERAL NASAL PROCESS
MAXILLARY PROCESS
MANDIBULAR PROCESS

Figure 1–6. *Developmental processes of the face.*

ment or maturation of embryonic processes (Fig. 1–6). Thus, we may recognize such anomalies as the oblique and transverse facial clefts, which extend from the upper lip or ala of the nose to the eye and from the angle of the mouth to the ear, respectively. By far the most important of the facial clefts, however, is the cleft lip, mandibular or maxillary.

The *mandibular cleft lip* is an extremely rare condition that occurs in the midline of the lower lip; its development is due either to failure of the copula to give rise to the mandibular arch or to persistence of the central groove of the mandibular process. Only the lip or, occasionally, both the lip and the jaw may be involved. This latter type of midline mandibular cleft has been reviewed by Weinberg and his associates.

The *maxillary cleft lip* is the more common and important of the lip clefts; the literature dealing with this subject and with the cleft palate is voluminous. Inasmuch as the cleft lip and cleft palate are so intimately related genetically, embryologically, and functionally, they will be discussed here together.

The usual maxillary cleft lip at one time was thought to be due to failure of the globular portion of the median nasal process to unite properly with the lateral nasal and maxillary process. More recently, it has been suggested that this cleft is due not to an actual lack of union of the processes but rather to a failure of mesodermal penetration and the obliteration of the ectodermal grooves separating these mesodermal masses that actually constitute the facial processes. Either the absence or deficiency of these mesodermal masses or their failure to

penetrate the ectodermal grooves leads to breakdown of the ectoderm, causing cleft formation. Since penetration occurs between either of the paired lateral mesodermal masses and the single central mesodermal mass, it is obvious that the maxillary cleft may be a unilateral or bilateral defect, but not a midline one. Occasionally, however, a portion of the central process is defective or absent, and the resulting cleft does appear in the midline. This median cleft of the upper lip has been discussed by Sharma.

The *cleft palate* appears to represent a disturbance in the normal fusion of the palatal shelves: failure to unite due to lack of force, interference by the tongue, or a disparity in the size of the parts involved. The soft palate and uvula do not appear to be formed as a result of fusion of parts but rather as a posterior extension of the palatal processes; thus a cleft of these structures is basically an extension of a cleft of the hard palate. This mechanism of cleft palate formation has been discussed by Fraser and more recently by Smiley.

Etiology.   It has been clearly established by Fogh-Andersen and confirmed by numerous other investigators that two separate and distinct entities exist: (1) cleft lip with or without associated cleft palate, and (2) isolated cleft palate. Heredity is undoubtedly one of the most important factors to be considered in the etiology of these malformations. However, there is increasing evidence that environmental factors are important as well. According to Fogh-Andersen, slightly less than 40 per cent of the cases of cleft lip with or without cleft palate are genetic in origin, whereas slightly less than 20 per cent of the cases of isolated cleft palate appear to be genetically derived. Most investigations indicate that the inheritance pattern in cleft lip with or without cleft palate is different from that in isolated cleft palate. The mode of transmission of the defect is uncertain. This has been discussed by Bhatia, who pointed out that the possible main modes of transmission are either by a single mutant gene, producing a large effect, or by a number of genes (polygenic inheritance), each producing a small effect which together create this condition. It should be pointed out that cytogenetic studies have failed to reveal visible alterations in chromosomal morphology of the affected individuals.

Bixler more recently has expanded upon this concept and reiterated that there are two forms of clefts. The most common is hereditary, its nature being most probably *polygenic* (determined by several different genes acting together). In other words, when the total genetic liability of an individual reaches a certain minimum level, the threshold for expression is reached and a cleft occurs. Actually, it is presumed that every individual carries some genetic liability for clefting, but if this is less than the threshold level, there is no cleft. When the individual liabilities of two parents are added together in their offspring, a cleft occurs if the threshold value is exceeded. However, even though this is the most common form of cleft, the threshold value is sufficiently high that it is a low-risk type. The second form of cleft is *monogenic* or *syndromic* and is associated with a variety of other congenital anomalies. Since these are monogenic, they are of a high-risk type. Bixler has pointed out that, fortunately, the clefting syndromes are rare and probably make up only 5 per cent of all cleft cases even though, according to Cohen, there are now over 150 clefting syndromes reported in the literature.

Although there is insufficient evidence that nutritional disturbances cause cleft palates in human beings, abnormal dietary regimens have caused developmental clefts in animals. Cleft palate has been experimentally produced in newborn rats by feeding diets either deficient or excessive in vitamin A to maternal rats during pregnancy. Riboflavin-deficient diets fed to pregnant rats also have produced offspring with a high incidence of cleft palate. The administration of cortisone to pregnant rabbits has induced similar clefts in their young. A complete tabulation of teratogenic agents, a great many of which have induced cleft palate, is shown in Table 1–3.

Strean and Peer reported that physiologic, emotional, or traumatic stress may play a significant role in the etiology of human cleft palate, since stress induces increased function of the adrenal cortex and secretion of hydrocortisone. Their study, based on histories of 228 mothers of children with cleft palate, confirms the experimental findings of cleft palate in animals due to the action of stressor agents or the administration of cortisone. However, Fraser and Warburton have reported data which indicate that neither maternal emotional stress nor the lack of a prenatal nutritional supplement was causally related to the occurrence of cleft lip or cleft palate.

Other factors that have been suggested as possible causes of cleft palate include: (1) a defective vascular supply to the area involved; (2) a mechanical disturbance in which the size of the tongue may prevent the union of parts; (3) circulating substances, such as alcohol and certain drugs and toxins; (4) infections; and (5) lack of inherent developmental force.

Despite the numerous clinical and experimental investigations, the etiology of cleft palate in the human being is still largely unknown. It must be concluded, however, that heredity is probably the most important single factor.

Incidence. There have been a great many statistical studies dealing with the incidence and relative frequency of cleft lip and cleft palate. One of these is shown in Table 1–6. An

Table 1–6. Relative Frequency of Cleft Lip and Cleft Palate

	MALES		FEMALES		SEXES COMBINED	
	NO. OF CASES	PER CENT	NO. OF CASES	PER CENT	NO. OF CASES	PER CENT
Cleft lip (alone)	90	65.2	48	34.8	138	22.1
Cleft lip and palate	257	71.4	103	28.6	360	57.6
Cleft palate (alone)	43	33.9	84	66.1	127	20.3
Total	390	62.4	235	37.6	625	100.0

Modified from P. Fogh-Andersen: Inheritance of Harelip and Cleft Palate. Copenhagen, Nyt Nordisk Forlag, Arnold Busck, 1942.

extensive study in Pennsylvania by Grace showed that one infant in every 800 was born with a cleft lip or cleft palate and that the highest percentage of these deformities occurred in babies born to women between the ages of 21 and 25. This is in contradistinction to other types of anomalies which occur more often in the offspring of women at the late childbearing ages. MacMahon and McKeown, however, reported that the incidence of cleft lip, with or without cleft palate, increases with maternal age and concluded that this is independent of association with other malformations. There are numerous similar contradictory studies. The genetic and nongenetic variables have been reviewed by Woolf and his associates. Other studies in this country, such as that by Davis, have reported a ratio of one affected child in approximately every 1200 births, while the statistical study of Fogh-Andersen in Denmark reported a frequency ratio of one in 665. These malformations, separated into cleft lip with or without cleft palate and isolated cleft palate, and their incidence in various countries have been compiled by Bhatia (Table 1–7). Thus, although there is some variation in reported incidence in the different studies, the condition is common enough to cause concern.

Clinical Features. The *maxillary cleft lip* may present a varied clinical picture, depending on the severity of the condition (Fig. 1–7). A classification of such clefts according to appearance, with the percentage of occurrence, is shown in Table 1–8.

As the names would indicate, the unilateral cleft lip involves only one side of the lip; the bilateral, both sides of the lip. The latter type has given rise to the term "harelip," which is now frequently applied to all cleft lips. The

Table 1–8. Classification of Cleft Lip

TYPE	OCCURRENCE (%)
Unilateral incomplete	33
Unilateral complete	48
Bilateral incomplete	7
Bilateral complete	12

From V. Veau: Division palatine; anatomie, chirurgie, phonetique. Paris, Masson et Cie, 1931.

incomplete cleft extends for a varying distance toward the nostril and frequently involves the palate as well. The complete cleft extends into the nostril and even more commonly involves the palate.

The cleft lip and cleft palate are somewhat more common in boys than in girls, and the lip cleft occurs about three times more frequently on the left side than on the right. Boys are more apt to have the more severe defects. In contrast, isolated cleft palate is more common in girls.

The *cleft palate* may exhibit wide variation in the degree of severity and the involvement of tissue. There may be a cleft of both the hard and the soft palates (Fig. 1–8) or, in some cases, a cleft of the soft palate only (Fig. 1–9). In many instances, the cleft of the hard palate extends anteriorly through the alveolar ridge and lip, producing a complete cleft in the lip, ridge, and palate. Occasionally a patient is seen with only a cleft or bifid uvula (Fig. 1–10), which is probably the mildest form of cleft palate.

The typical patient with cleft palate and cleft ridge exhibits a large defect in the roof of the palate, with a direct opening into the nasal

Table 1–7. Incidence of Clefts of Lip and Palate Estimated in Various Countries

COUNTRY	AUTHORS	INCIDENCE PER 1000 BIRTHS	
		Cleft Lip With or Without Cleft Palate	*Isolated Cleft Palate*
United States			
Los Angeles	Lutz and Moor	0.65	0.32
California	Loretz et al.	1.02	0.36
New York City	Wallace et al.	0.52	0.29
England	MacMahon and McKeown	0.81	0.49
	Knox and Braithwaite	0.96	0.46
Denmark	Fogh-Andersen	1.04	0.43
Sweden	Böök	1.34	0.36
Tasmania	Rank and Thompson	1.10	0.56

From S. N. Bhatia: Genetics of cleft lip and palate. Br. Dent. J., *132*:95, 1972.

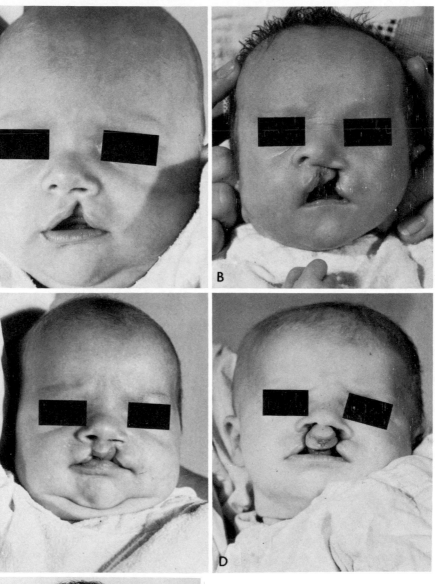

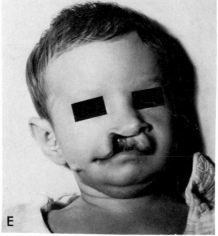

Figure 1-7. *Cleft lip.*
A, Unilateral partial cleft lip. *B,* Unilateral complete cleft lip. *C,* Bilateral partial cleft lip. *D,* Bilateral complete cleft lip. *E,* Unilateral complete cleft lip associated with macrostomia. (Courtesy of Drs. John M. Tondra and Harold M. Trusler.)

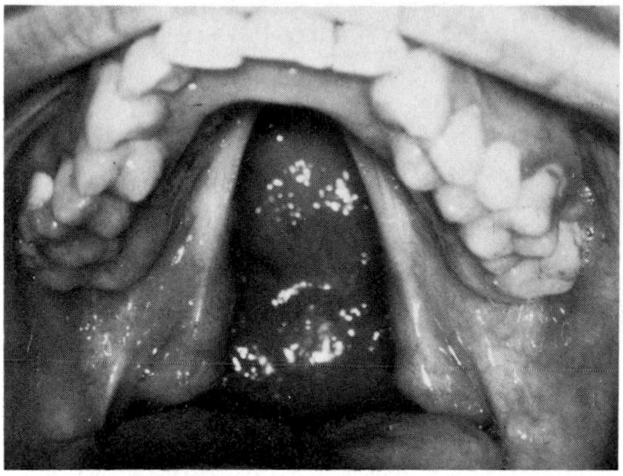

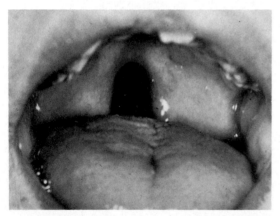

Figure 1–8. *Cleft involving both the hard and the soft palates.*
(Courtesy of Drs. John M. Tondra and Harold M. Trusler.)

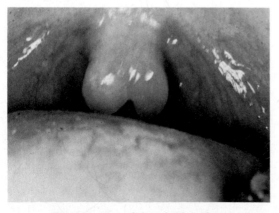

Figure 1–9. *Cleft involving the soft palate only.*
(Courtesy of Drs. John M. Tondra and Harold M. Trusler.)

Figure 1–10. *Cleft or bifid uvula.*
(Courtesy of Dr. Everett R. Amos.)

cavity. This midline defect continues anteriorly to the premaxilla, where it then deviates to either the right or the left. Occasionally, the entire premaxillary portion of bone will be missing and, in such instances, the cleft may appear to be an entirely midline defect. The usual cleft ridge, however, appears in the region between the lateral incisor and cuspid teeth, or it may occur between the maxillary central and lateral incisors. There is frequently a disturbance in the dental structures in this region, so that teeth may be missing, deformed, displaced, or divided, thus producing supernumerary teeth.

The isolated cleft palate is associated with other developmental abnormalities in about 50 per cent of the cases, according to Ingalls and his associates. Among those abnormalities reported are congenital heart disease, polydactylism and syndactylism, hydrocephalus, microcephalus, clubfoot, supernumerary ear, hypospadias, spina bifida, hypertelorism, and mental deficiency. Similar anomalies may occur with cleft lip with or without cleft palate but are less common, occurring in less than 20 per cent of the cases.

A *median maxillary anterior alveolar cleft* is a relatively common defect, occurring in approximately 1 per cent of the population, according to Stout and Collett, but this is unrelated to cleft lip or cleft palate. This type of cleft has been discussed by Gier and Fast, who suggested that it might be due to precocious limitation of the growth of the primary ossification centers on either side of the midline at the primary palate, or to their subsequent failure to fuse. In addition, Miller and his coworkers have suggested that at least some cases may represent an incomplete manifestation of the *median cleft-face syndrome* (hypertelorism, median cleft of the premaxilla and palate, and cranium bifidum occultum). This syndrome has no clinical manifestations and is usually detected only on routine intraoral roentgenographic examination (Fig. 1–11).

Clinical Significance and Treatment. Most cases of cleft lip can be surgically repaired with excellent cosmetic and functional results. It is customary to operate before the patient is one month old or when he has regained his original birth weight and is still gaining.

Both the physical and psychologic effects of cleft palate on the patient are of considerable concern. Eating and drinking are difficult because of regurgitation of food and liquid through the nose. The speech problem is also serious

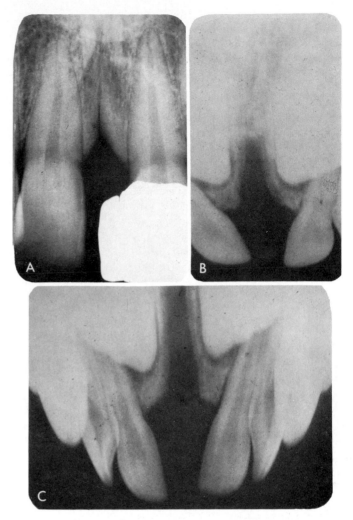

Figure 1–11. *Median maxillary anterior alveolar cleft.*
All degrees of severity of the cleft may occur. (Copyright by the American Dental Association. Reprinted by permission and by courtesy of Dr. Arthur S. Miller. From A. S. Miller, J. N. Greeley, and D. L. Catena: Median maxillary anterior alveolar cleft: report of three cases. J. Am. Dent. Assoc., 79:896, 1969.)

and tends to increase the mental trauma suffered by the patient.

Surgery can correct the cleft palate in the majority of cases. The operation to close the cleft is not usually carried out until the patient is about 18 months old. Definitive speech habits have not been established by this time, yet sufficient maturation has occurred so that the danger of seriously interfering with important growth centers is at least minimized.

CHEILITIS GLANDULARIS

In cheilitis glandularis, an uncommon condition occurring most frequently in adult males, the lower lip becomes enlarged, firm, and finally everted.

Etiology. The cause of cheilitis glandularis is unknown, although it has been suggested that chronic exposure to sun, wind and dust, as well as the use of tobacco, may be important factors. In several cases, emotional disturbance, as well as familial occurrence, suggesting hereditary factors, has also been cited. As pointed out by Doku and his co-workers, this condition has many of the features of a glandular hyperplasia with a superimposed bacterial infection of long duration.

Clinical Features. The labial salivary glands become enlarged and sometimes nodular, while the orifices of the secretory ducts are inflamed and dilated, appearing as small red macules on the mucosa. A viscid mucous secretion may seep from these openings of the everted, hypertrophic-appearing lip.

Three basic types of cheilitis glandularis have been described: (1) the simple type, (2) the superficial suppurative type, and (3) the deep suppurative type. The simple type, the most common, is characterized by multiple painless, pinhead-sized lesions, with central depressions and dilated canals. This type may be transformed into either of the other two types. The superficial suppurative type (Baelz's disease) is characterized by painless swelling, induration, crusting, and superficial and deep ulcerations of the lip. The deep suppurative type (cheilitis glandularis apostematosa, myxadenitis labialis) is basically a deep-seated infection, with abscesses and fistulous tracts that eventually form scars.

Treatment and Prognosis. There is no definitive treatment, although some authorities consider this lesion premalignant, as cases have been reported in which the patient subsequently had carcinoma of the lip. Thus, epidermoid carcinoma of the lip has been associated with cheilitis glandularis in 18 to 35 per cent of the reported cases, according to Weir and Johnson. Because of this relatively high incidence of associated malignancy, a vermilionectomy or surgical stripping of the lip has been recommended in a recent review of the disease by Oliver and Pickett, since in most cases this has been shown to eliminate the disease while providing acceptable esthetic results.

CHEILITIS GRANULOMATOSA

(Miescher's Syndrome)

Cheilitis granulomatosa is a condition of unknown etiology that is not related to cheilitis glandularis except by the similarity in the clinical appearance of the two diseases, which has caused them to be frequently confused.

Clinical Features. In cheilitis granulomatosa there is diffuse swelling of the lips, especially the lower lip. This swelling is usually soft and exhibits no pitting upon pressure. The skin and adjacent mucosa may be of normal color or erythematous. In some cases scaling, fissuring, and vesicles or pustules have been reported on the vermilion border. Pain is generally absent.

Cheilitis granulomatosa has been reported in both children and adults and is almost invariably a chronic disease. Once appearing, it may persist for many years.

Excellent reviews of this disease have been given by Rhodes and Stirling and by Laymon, who also drew attention to its relation to the *Melkersson-Rosenthal syndrome*. Although cheilitis granulomatosa may occur without any other manifestations of a disease process, it sometimes appears in association with facial paralysis and scrotal tongue. This unusual triad has been referred to as the Melkersson-Rosenthal syndrome. According to Alexander and James, in some cases of this syndrome the lip lesions are edematous rather than granulomatous, so that the Melkersson-Rosenthal syndrome is often subdivided into the sarcoid and the lymphedematous types.

This syndrome has been discussed in detail by Worsaae and Pindborg, who have pointed out that recurrent facial swellings, often at more than one site, are characteristic and that oral swellings, including gingival enlargements, are sometimes seen as a manifestation.

Histologic Features. The histologic features of cheilitis granulomatosa and the swellings of the syndrome are rather characteristic, consisting of a chronic inflammatory cell infiltrate—particularly peri- and paravascular aggregations of lymphocytes, plasma cells, and histiocytes—and focal noncaseating granuloma formation with epithelioid cells and Langhans type giant cells. The microscopic findings are suggestive of sarcoidosis, but as yet there is insufficient evidence to relate cheilitis granulomatosa with sarcoid.

Treatment. Many forms of therapy have been tested, but all were found unsatisfactory in this disease.

HEREDITARY INTESTINAL POLYPOSIS SYNDROME

(Peutz-Jeghers Syndrome; Intestinal Polyposis with Melanin Pigmentation)

The hereditary intestinal polyposis syndrome is an unusual condition which is of interest to the dentist because of the oral findings. Essentially, the syndrome as described by Jeghers consists of familial generalized intestinal polyposis and pigmented spots on the face, oral cavity, and sometimes the hands and feet (Fig. 1–12).

Clinical Features. The melanin pigmentation of the lips and oral mucosa is usually present from birth and appears as small brown macules measuring 1 to 5 mm. in diameter. Intraorally, the buccal mucosa is most frequently involved, with the gingiva and hard palate next (Fig. 1–13). Seldom does the tongue show this pigmentation. On the face the spots tend to be grouped around the eyes, nostrils, and lips (Fig. 1–12). The mucosal surface of the lips, particularly the lower lip, is almost invariably involved. Interestingly, the facial pigmen-

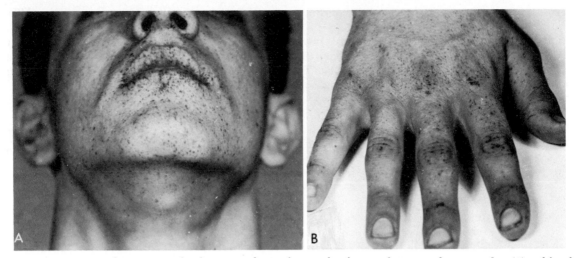

Figure 1–12. Hereditary intestinal polyposis syndrome showing distribution of pigmented spots on face (A) and hand (B). (Courtesy of Drs. Hyman Goldberg and Paul Goldhaber: Oral Surg., 7:378, 1954.)

tation tends to fade later in life, although the mucosal pigmentation persists.

Oromucosal pigmentation, including melanin pigmentation, occurs with considerable frequency in a variety of other situations such as: (1) local and ethnic pigmentation, (2) oral pigmentary manifestations of systemic diseases, (3) pigmentary disturbances associated with pharmaceuticals and other chemicals, and (4) benign and malignant pigmented neoplasms. These have been reviewed in detail by Dummett and Barens.

The intestinal polyps are usually distributed through the entire intestine but manifest themselves clinically in the small intestine. Thus many patients with this syndrome have frequent episodes of abdominal pain and signs of minor obstruction, often terminating in intussusception. It is significant that a strong tendency exists for multiple polyposis of the colon to undergo malignant change. However, this does not seem to hold true for polyposis incident to the Jeghers syndrome, and most authorities such as Bartholomew and his co-workers now consider the polyps in this syndrome to be simply hamartomatous intestinal excrescences with very low malignant potential. Still, there are at least 28 documented cases in the literature of patients with the syndrome who developed gastrointestinal carcinoma, according to Wesley and his associates in an excellent discussion of the disease. It has been reported by Burdick and his co-workers that the histologic picture of the Peutz-Jeghers polyp is specific,

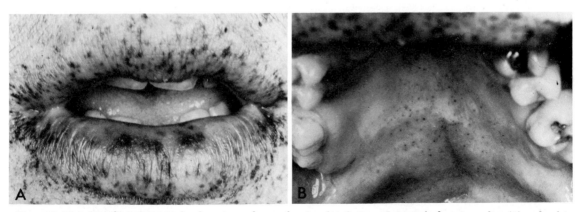

Figure 1–13. Hereditary intestinal polyposis syndrome showing distribution of pigmented spots on lips (A) and palate (B). (Courtesy of Drs. Hyman Goldberg and Paul Goldhaber: Oral Surg., 7:378, 1954.)

permitting these polyps to be distinguished from other forms of gastrointestinal polyps.

Generalized intestinal polyposis with oral pigmentation is inherited as a simple mendelian dominant characteristic. It is not sex-linked, since both males and females carry the factor and both are affected about equally. The polyposis and pigmentation appear to be due to a single pleiotropic gene and not to linked genes. Only about 50 per cent of reported patients have a familial history of the syndrome; the remainder are isolated cases resulting from sporadic mutations.

The role of the dentist in detecting this syndrome is important, since the intestinal condition may be recognized early through a tentative diagnosis based on the oral and paraoral manifestations.

LABIAL AND ORAL MELANOTIC MACULE

(Ephelis, Focal Melanosis, Solitary Labial Lentigo)

The *labial* melanotic macule is a melanotic lesion of the lips first described under this name by Weathers and associates, whereas the *oral* melanotic macule is a similar intraoral lesion described by Page and his co-workers.

Clinical Features. The *labial* melanotic macule may occur at any age and presents as a single or multiple small, flat, brown or brown-black asymptomatic lesion of the lip, almost invariably near the midline. The lower lip was involved in approximately 85 per cent of the series of 55 cases reported by Weathers and his associates. The vast majority of macules measured 5 mm. or less in diameter. These appear to represent three distinct entities: (1) postinflammatory or posttraumatic pigmentation, (2) true ephelides, and (3) a unique lesion for which there is no cutaneous counterpart.

The *oral* melanotic macule may also occur at any age, according to the series of 80 cases reported by Page and his co-workers. The clinical appearance of the lesion is similar to that of the labial lesions. Nearly all were under 1 cm. in diameter. They occurred with nearly equal frequency on the gingiva, buccal mucosa, and palate (totaling 94 per cent of the cases), with occasional lesions on mucobuccal fold and tongue. The term "oral melanotic macule" was suggested by Page and his co-workers to be reserved for those oral lesions without an identifiable etiologic factor, since similar lesions are known to result from racial pigmentation, endocrine disturbance, antimalarial therapy,

Peutz-Jeghers syndrome, trauma, hemachromatosis, and chronic pulmonary disease.

A series of 105 melanotic macules—32 labial and 73 oral—has been reported by Buchner and Hansen, and their data coincide very closely with those cited by Page.

Histologic Features. The microscopic features of the labial and the oral melanotic macules are quite similar. The overall thickness of the epithelium is variable, depending upon location. However, there are always increased amounts of melanin in the basal cell layer. Sometimes, clear cells and dendritic cells are found, but they are not usually prominent characteristics. Where there is clear cell activity (melanocytic hyperplasia), the melanocytes do not show atypia. Finally, there may be variable amounts of melanin incontinence in the lamina propria, although melanophages are relatively uncommon. Chronic inflammatory cells may also be found.

Treatment. Those melanotic macules with a relatively short history should be excised to establish a definitive diagnosis and to rule out the possibility of malignant melanoma. Lesions present for five years or more without change in size or color may be followed unless the patient requests removal. Occasionally, a melanotic macule does show an increase in size or change in color and this is a positive indication for immediate removal. However, all information currently available suggests that the melanotic macule is benign and does not have malignant potential.

DEVELOPMENTAL DISTURBANCES OF THE ORAL MUCOSA

FORDYCE'S GRANULES

(Fordyce's Disease)

This is not a disease of the oral mucosa, as the name might indicate, but rather a developmental anomaly characterized by heterotopic collections of sebaceous glands at various sites in the oral cavity. It has been postulated that the occurrence of sebaceous glands in the mouth may result from inclusion in the oral cavity of ectoderm having some of the potentialities of skin in the course of development of the maxillary and mandibular processes during embryonic life. A complete review of Fordyce's granules was published by Miles, and a superb investigation of the sebaceous glands of the lips and oral cavity was carried out by Sewerin.

PLATE I

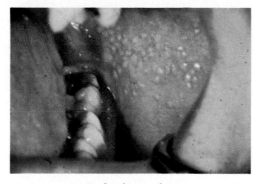
Fordyce's granules

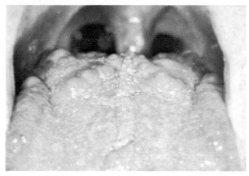
Circumvallate papillae

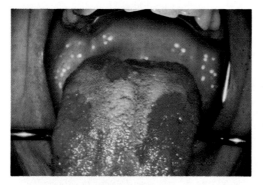
Geographic tongue

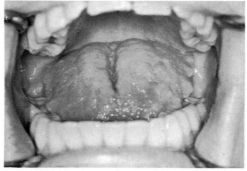
Cleft and lobulated tongue

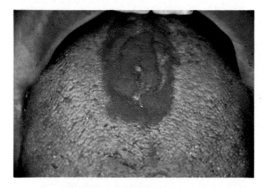
Median rhomboid glossitis

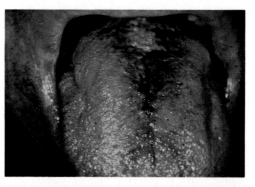
Hairy tongue

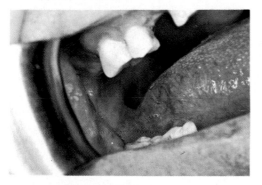
Lingual tonsil

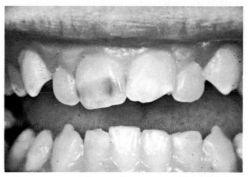
Mottled enamel (dental fluorosis)

Clinical Features. Fordyce's granules appear as small yellow spots, either discretely separated or forming relatively large plaques, often projecting slightly above the surface of the tissue (see Plate I). They are found most frequently in a bilaterally symmetrical pattern on the mucosa of the cheeks opposite the molar teeth but also occur on the inner surfaces of the lips, in the retromolar region lateral to the anterior faucial pillar, and occasionally on the tongue, gingiva, frenum, and palate. Ectopic sebaceous glands have been discussed in an excellent review by Guiducci and Hyman and are recognized to occur, besides in the oral cavity, in the esophagus, the female genitalia including the cervix uteri, the male genitalia, the nipples, the palms and soles, the parotid gland, the larynx, and the orbit.

Studies by Halperin and co-workers, confirmed by Miles, have indicated that the oral condition is present in approximately 80 per cent of the population, with apparently no significant differences in occurrence between the sexes or races. Fewer children than adults exhibit Fordyce's granules, probably because the sebaceous glands and hair system do not reach maximal development until puberty. Nevertheless, Miles has reported that large numbers of sebaceous glands in the cheeks and lips may sometimes be found in children long before the age of puberty. Because of the high incidence of these glands in the oral cavity, Knapp has suggested that they be regarded as sebaceous nevi rather than ectopic glandular tissue.

Histologic Features. These heterotopic collections of sebaceous glands are identical with those seen normally in the skin, but are unassociated with hair follicles, although a single hair follicle and hair shaft growing from the gingiva—an extremely rare occurrence—has been reported recently by Baughman (Fig. 1–14; see also Plate I). The glands are usually superficial and may consist of only a few or a great many lobules, all grouped around one or more ducts which open on the surface of the mucosa. These ducts may show keratin plugging.

Treatment. These glands are innocuous, have no clinical or functional significance, and require no treatment. However, very rarely a benign sebaceous gland adenoma may develop from these intraoral structures, such as in the case involving the buccal mucosa reported by Miller and McCrea. Sewerin has also reported the occasional development of keratin-filled pseudocysts from the ducts of these sebaceous glands.

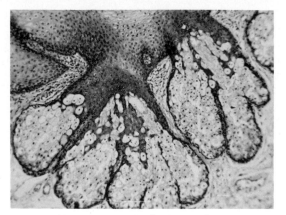

Figure 1–14. *Fordyce's granules.*
Heterotopic collections of sebaceous glands.

FOCAL EPITHELIAL HYPERPLASIA
(Heck's Disease)

The term "focal epithelial hyperplasia" was used by Archard, Heck, and Stanley in 1965 to designate a type of lesion first observed by Heck on the oral mucosa of a group of Navajo Indian children. Praetorius-Clausen and his co-workers have reviewed this condition, which has now been reported also to occur in Colombia, Ecuador, Venezuela, Brazil, El Salvador, Guatemala, Paraguay, Israel, and Egypt, and in Greenlandic Eskimos and Alaskan Eskimos.

Clinical Features. Focal epithelial hyperplasia presents as multiple nodular lesions, usually with a sessile base, occurring most commonly on the lower lip but also seen on the buccal mucosa, commissures, upper lip, and tongue. The gingivae and anterior faucial pillars are infrequently involved and lesions do not appear to occur on the floor of the mouth or palate. These nodular lesions, usually 1 to 5 mm. in diameter, are soft and have the same color as the adjacent mucosa.

This condition appears to occur predominantly in children between the ages of 3 and 18 years, although adults have been described with these lesions. They often appear to undergo spontaneous regression after 4 to 6 months, although in some cases they have persisted for a year or more. Occasionally, the lesions recur.

Praetorius-Clausen and Willis have reported finding virus-like particles in the lesions of focal epithelial hyperplasia occurring in Greenlandic Eskimos. These viral particles were similar in size and morphologic appearance to those described in human oral papillomas, in human verruca, and in human condylomas. Thus, Praetorius-Clausen and Willis have suggested that the particles represent a virus of the papova virus group. Whether this is the etiologic agent in focal epithelial hyperplasia is still uncertain.

Histologic Features. The lesions appear as nodular elevations in which there is acanthosis or thickening of the spinous layer, with thickening, elongation, and fusion of the rete pegs. Mild hyperparakeratosis is usually present over the surface. The underlying supportive fibrous connective tissue shows occasional clumps of lymphocytes as well as occasional collections of polymorphonuclear leukocytes. Some focal areas of liquefaction degeneration of the basal layer may be found. No significant epithelial dysplasia is present and there is no evidence of inclusion bodies.

Treatment. No treatment is necessary, since these are harmless lesions, many of which regress spontaneously.

DEVELOPMENTAL DISTURBANCES OF THE GINGIVA

FIBROMATOSIS GINGIVAE

(Elephantiasis Gingivae; Hereditary Gingival Fibromatosis; Congenital Macrogingivae)

Fibromatosis gingivae is a diffuse fibrous overgrowth of the gingival tissues, described for many years under a variety of terms. In the majority of reported cases the condition was hereditary, being transmitted through a dominant autosomal gene. Zackin and Weisberger have reviewed this condition and presented a family of 11 affected children and 10 normal children from six marriages over four generations, while Emerson has reported the pedigree of a family over four generations in which nine marriages between affected and unaffected persons resulted in seven affected and 11 normal offspring. But many cases have appeared to be sporadic, with no familial background. Occasionally other abnormalities have been reported in association with fibromatosis gingivae, but of these, only hypertrichosis has been noted more than a few times. Even this association, in terms of total number of reported cases, is rare.

Clinical Features. This condition is manifested as a dense, diffuse, smooth, or nodular overgrowth of the gingival tissues of one or both arches, usually appearing about the time of eruption of the permanent incisors. It has been reported, however, in even very young children and, in a few instances, at birth (Fig. 1–15,A). The tissue is usually not inflamed, but is of normal or even pale color, and it is often so firm and dense that it may prevent the normal eruption of teeth. It is not painful and shows no tendency for hemorrhage. The extent of the tissue overgrowth may be such that the crowns of the teeth are nearly hidden even though they are fully erupted with respect to the alveolar bone (Fig. 1–16).

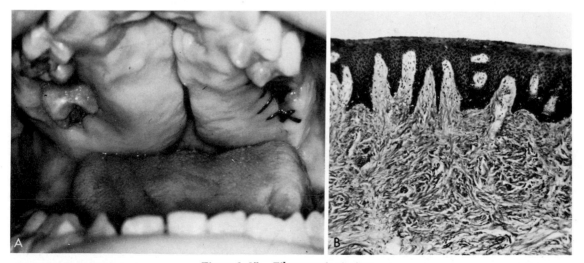

Figure 1–15. *Fibromatosis gingivae.*
A, The palatal vault is nearly filled with a dense fibrous mass of tissue. The apparent midline cleft extends only to the bone and is not a true cleft. The maxillary gingiva is also involved. *B,* The photomicrograph reveals that the mass is made up only of a dense mass of fibrous connective tissue covered by normal epithelium.

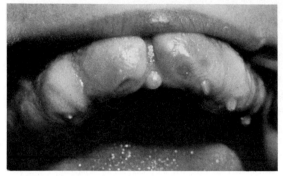

Figure 1–16. *Fibromatosis gingivae.*
The firm fibrous tissue mass has covered all but the incisal edges and the tips of the cusps of the maxillary teeth.

Histologic Features. The microscopic picture of the tissue in fibromatosis gingivae is similar to that of any fibrous hyperplasia. The epithelium may be somewhat thickened with elongated rete pegs, although the bulk of the tissue is composed of dense fibrous connective tissue. The bundles of collagen fibers are coarse and show few interspersed fibroblasts or blood vessels. Inflammation is an unrelated and variable finding (Fig. 1–15,*B*).

Treatment and Prognosis. When tooth eruption is impeded, surgical removal of the excessive tissue and exposure of the teeth are indicated. The cosmetic appearance may also require surgical excision. The tissue sometimes recurs. It has been reported that tooth extraction alone will cause the tissues to shrink almost to normal and that recurrences can be prevented by this means.

RETROCUSPID PAPILLA

The retrocuspid papilla, first described by Hirshfeld in 1933 but not reported until 1957, is a small, elevated nodule located on the lingual mucosa of the mandibular cuspids.

Clinical Features. This soft, well-circumscribed, sessile, mucosal nodule, commonly bilateral, is located lingual to the mandibular cuspid, between the free gingival margin and the mucogingival junction.

It is exceedingly common in children, occurring in 99 per cent of those between the ages of 8 and 16 years, according to the original report of Hirshfeld, but decreases in incidence with age, occurring in 38 per cent of those between the ages of 25 and 39 years and in 19 per cent of those between the ages of 60 and

80 years. Thus there appears to be regression of the structure with maturity. In addition, most studies have found a greater occurrence bilaterally than unilaterally. A study by Berman and Fay, who have reviewed the studies dealing with the retrocuspid papilla, reported from their own data that the structure was consistently more common in females than in males.

Histologic Features. The structure appears as an elevated mucosal tag often showing mild hyperorthokeratosis or hyperparakeratosis, with or without acanthosis. The underlying connective tissue is sometimes highly vascularized and may exhibit large stellate fibroblasts as well as occasional epithelial rests.

Treatment. Because of its frequency of occurrence, the retrocuspid papilla is often considered to be a "normal" anatomic structure which regresses with age and requires no treatment.

DEVELOPMENTAL DISTURBANCES OF THE TONGUE

MICROGLOSSIA

Microglossia is a rare congenital anomaly manifested by the presence of a small or rudimentary tongue. At least one case has been recorded of the tongue being completely absent at birth, a condition known as *aglossia*. The difficulties in eating and talking that would be encountered by patients with aglossia or microglossia are obvious.

MACROGLOSSIA

An enlarged tongue, a somewhat more common condition than microglossia, may be either congenital or secondary in type. *Congenital* macroglossia is due to an over-development of the musculature, which may or may not be associated with generalized muscular hypertrophy or hemihypertrophy.

Secondary macroglossia may occur as a result of a tumor of the tongue, such as a diffuse lymphangioma or hemangioma, from neurofibromatosis, or occasionally from blockage of the efferent lymphatic vessels in cases of malignant neoplasms of the tongue. In cases of acromegaly due to hyperpituitarism in the adult, an enlarged tongue is also a common finding and probably occurs as a result of relaxation of the muscles concomitant with the growth of the mandible. In addition, macroglossia may occur in cretinism or congenital hypothyroidism, but its pathogenesis in these cases is somewhat more obscure.

Macroglossia of either type may produce displacement of teeth and malocclusion because of the strength of the muscles involved and the pressure exerted by the tongue on the teeth. It is not uncommon to see crenation or scalloping of the lateral borders of the tongue in this condition, the tips of the scallops fitting into the interproximal spaces between the teeth.

Macroglossia is also a prominent feature of *Beckwith's hypoglycemic syndrome*, which additionally includes neonatal hypoglycemia, mild microcephaly, umbilical hernia, fetal viscero-megaly, and postnatal somatic giantism. This syndrome has been discussed by Arons and his associates.

There is no particular treatment for macroglossia except removal of the primary cause, although in some instances surgical trimming has been used to reduce the bulk of tissue present.

ANKYLOGLOSSIA

Complete ankyloglossia occurs as a result of fusion between the tongue and the floor of the mouth. Partial ankyloglossia, or the common "tongue-tie," is a much more frequent condition and is usually a result of a short lingual frenum or one which is attached too near the tip of the tongue (Fig. 1–17). Because of the restricted movement of the tongue, patients with this defect exhibit speech difficulties, chiefly in the pronunciation of certain consonants and diphthongs. Although some cases of partial ankylo-

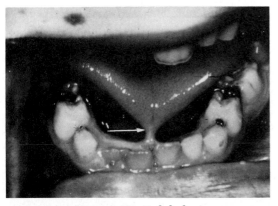

Figure 1–17. *Ankyloglossia.*
The lingual frenum is short and attached near the tip of the tongue.

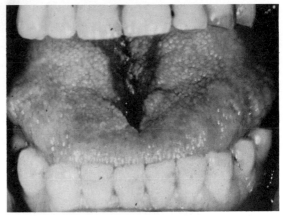

Figure 1–18. *Cleft tongue.*
A deep cleft is present in the midline of the dorsum of the tongue.

glossia are self-corrective, the majority are treated surgically by clipping the frenum. This condition has been reviewed by Mathewson and his co-workers.

CLEFT TONGUE

A completely cleft or bifid tongue is a rare condition that is apparently due to lack of merging of the lateral lingual swellings of this organ. A partially cleft tongue is considerably more common and is manifested simply as a deep groove in the midline of the dorsal surface (Fig. 1–18; see also Plate I). The partial cleft results because of incomplete merging and failure of groove obliteration by underlying mesenchymal proliferation. Interestingly, it is often found as one feature of the oral-facial-digital syndrome in association with thick, fibrous bands in the lower anterior mucobuccal fold eliminating the sulcus and with clefting of the hypoplastic mandibular alveolar process. It is of little clinical significance except that food debris and microorganisms may collect in the base of the cleft and cause irritation.

FISSURED TONGUE
("Scrotal" Tongue)

The fissured tongue is a malformation manifested clinically by numerous small furrows or grooves on the dorsal surface, often radiating out from a central groove along the midline of the tongue (Fig. 1–19). Although the clinical appearance has been the basis of a classification of fissured tongue (i.e., foliaceous, cerebriform,

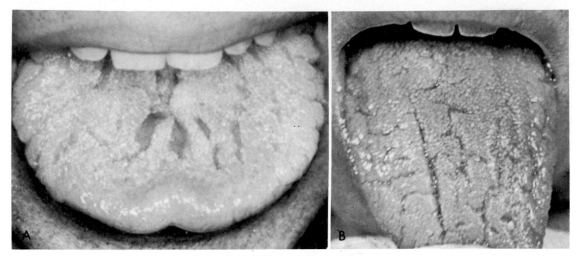

Figure 1–19. *Fissured ("scrotal") tongue.*
Two examples of the mild form in which numerous small fissures of varying depth traverse the surface of the tongue.

or transverse), the appearance has been reported to vary so remarkably as to make the classification unsatisfactory for use. It has been reported to develop simultaneously with, or as a sequel to, geographic tongue or benign migratory glossitis (q.v.), although this association is quite uncommon.

A study by Halperin and co-workers has shown that since the incidence of this condition apparently increases with age, it is probably not a developmental malformation. More likely it is associated with some extrinsic factor such as chronic trauma or vitamin deficiencies. There appear to be no significant differences in its sex or racial distribution. Considerable variation exists in the reported occurrence of fissured tongue, the studies of Prinz and Greenbaum showing a 0.5 per cent incidence without regard to age, but Fitzwilliams reporting a 60 per cent incidence in persons reaching the age of 40. The study of Halperin and associates reported an over-all incidence of approximately 5 per cent. Redman has reported a prevalence of 1.08 per cent in a group of children between 5 and 18 years of age. The disparity in reported incidence in the different studies may be due, in part at least, to lack of agreement as to what constitutes a fissured tongue.

Fissured tongue is usually painless except in occasional cases in which food debris tends to collect in the grooves and produce irritation. Here the material may be removed by stretching and flattening the fissures and using a toothbrush or gauze sponge to cleanse the surface.

MEDIAN RHOMBOID GLOSSITIS
(*Central Papillary Atrophy of the Tongue*)

Median rhomboid glossitis has been described classically as a congenital abnormality of the tongue, which is presumably due to failure of the tuberculum impar to retract or withdraw before fusion of the lateral halves of the tongue, so that a structure devoid of papillae is interposed between them. However, considerable doubt has arisen recently concerning this theory of origin. Baughman has provided an excellent review of the literature on this condition, especially concerning its etiology and occurrence, and also has questioned whether it is actually a developmental disturbance, since he found no cases of median rhomboid glossitis in over 10,000 school children whom he examined. If this lesion were truly of developmental origin, it should be found with equal frequency in children and adults. Although it is recognized that nearly all cases reported in the literature have occurred in adults, Redman has reported three cases in children under ten years of age.

Most current evidence strongly suggests an etiologic relationship between median rhomboid glossitis and a localized chronic fungal infection, specifically *Candida albicans*. For example, Cooke has demonstrated the presence of fungal hyphae in histologic sections of biopsies of all ten cases of median rhomboid glossitis that he studied. Wright also studied this problem and was able to demonstrate the presence of fungal hyphae in histologic sections of 85 per cent of a series of 28 cases of median rhomboid glossitis. Farman and his associates and van der Waal and his co-workers demonstrated some support for this idea in their studies. Farman, incidentally, also pointed out that this condition is particularly common among diabetics.

Thus, while the prevailing evidence is highly suggestive of a close association between this tongue lesion and a chronic fungal infection, a direct cause-and-effect relationship has not yet been established unequivocally.

Clinical Features. Median rhomboid glossitis appears clinically as an ovoid-, diamond-, or rhomboid-shaped reddish patch or plaque on the dorsal surface of the tongue immediately anterior to the circumvallate papillae. A flat or slightly raised area (Fig. 1–20), sometimes mamelonated, it stands out distinctly from the rest of the tongue because it has no filiform papillae. It is most obvious clinically when the rest of the tongue appears coated or the papillae are heavy and matted.

The incidence, as determined by the clinical studies of Halperin and co-workers, is less than 1 per cent (approximately three cases per 1000 population), with other reported series in the same general range. The condition is reported to occur about three times more frequently in men than in women, although in at least one reported series, that of Wright, women outnumbered men by a ratio of about 4:1.

Histologic Features. These lesions have been described by Sammet as showing the following characteristic features: (1) a loss of papillae with varying degrees of hyperparakeratosis, (2) a proliferation of the spinous layer with elongation of the rete ridges, which may branch and anastomose, (3) a lymphocytic infiltrate within the connective tissue, (4) numerous blood vessels and lymphatics, and (5) degeneration and hyalin formation within the underlying muscle (Fig. 1–20). Nearly all cases will exhibit these features. In addition, when present, the fungal hyphae are usually found in the parakeratin or in the very superficial spinous layer of epithelium or in both. They are best visualized by a periodic acid-Schiff (PAS) stain.

Treatment. There is no specific treatment for this lesion. Farman and his associates treated a group of patients with antifungal agents, either nystatin or amphotericin B, and found that the lesions regressed in some instances but not in others. Sometimes these lesions will regress spontaneously without treatment. In general, they appear to be relatively innocuous.

BENIGN MIGRATORY GLOSSITIS

(Geographic Tongue; Wandering Rash of the Tongue; Glossitis Areata Exfoliativa; Erythema Migrans)

Benign migratory glossitis is an interesting lesion of unknown etiology, although it has been suggested that it may be related to emotional stress.

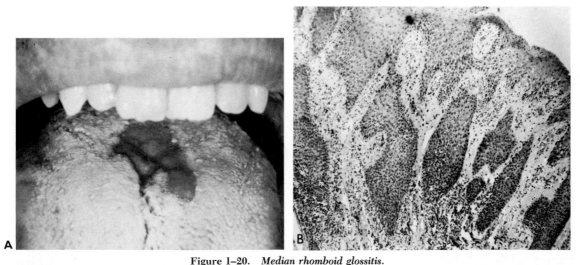

Figure 1–20. *Median rhomboid glossitis.*
The lesion is particularly prominent because of the heavy coating of the tongue (A). The area microscopically shows a typical mild epithelial proliferation and lymphocytic infiltrate (B). (B, Courtesy of Dr. David F. Mitchell.)

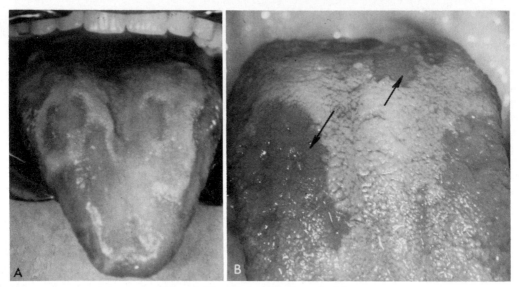

Figure 1–21. *Benign migratory glossitis.*
Extensive desquamated areas appear more prominent, owing to the coating on the tongue.

Clinical Features. The condition consists usually of multiple areas of desquamation of the filiform papillae of the tongue in an irregular circinate pattern (Fig. 1–21; see also Plate I). The central portion of the lesion sometimes appears inflamed, while the border may be outlined by a thin, yellowish-white line or band. The fungiform papillae persist in the desquamated areas as small, elevated red dots.

The areas of desquamation remain for a short time in one location and then heal and appear in another location, thus giving rise to the idea of migration. It is not unusual for smaller lesions to coalesce. The condition may persist for weeks or months and then regress spontaneously, only to recur at a later date. It is said to occur frequently in association with fissured tongue, although this may be coincidental.

In two clinical studies the incidence of benign migratory glossitis has been reported as 2.4 per cent of all patients examined by McCarthy and 1.4 per cent by Halperin and collaborators. In the latter study the male to female ratio of affected patients was 1:2, with no racial differences noted. It occurs with similar frequency in children, Redman reporting a prevalence of 1.4 per cent in a group of over 3600 school children between the ages of 5 and 18 years. However, he found no sex predilection. Other epidemiologic studies, such as those of Richardson and of Meskin and his co-workers, have shown similar data on incidence.

There have also been a number of cases reported under the term "ectopic geographic tongue," or erythema circinata, in which the patients have had similar reddish lesions usually with well-defined borders that appear clinically similar to the lesions of geographic tongue but are located at other sites in the oral cavity, e.g., buccal mucosa, gingiva, palate, lips, and floor of the mouth. These may or may not occur in a given patient in association with typical tongue lesions. Histologically, these ectopic lesions are very similar to the lesions of the tongue. This condition has been reviewed and discussed by Weathers and his associates.

It is of related interest that there is absence of the fungiform and circumvallate papillae in persons with familial dysautonomia. The taste buds located in these papillae are also presumably absent, thus explaining the taste deficit in patients with this disease. Smith and his co-workers have described the tongue in these patients as being so characteristically uniform and smooth that the diagnosis of familial dysautonomia may be made at birth.

Histologic Features. The filiform papillae are lost, and at the margin of the lesion there is usually hyperparakeratosis and some acanthosis. Closer to the center of the lesion, corresponding to the clinical red area, the parakeratin is often desquamated, with marked migration of polymorphonuclear leukocytes and lymphocytes into the epithelium, producing degeneration of epithelial cells and microabscess formation near the surface, which is sometimes termed subcorneal pustular mucositis. There is also inflammatory cell infiltration of the underlying connective tissue, chiefly neutrophils, lymphocytes, and plasma cells.

The histologic picture is very reminiscent of psoriasis and has often been described as a psoriasiform appearance. In fact, it has even been questioned whether this might not represent a part of the spectrum of skin psoriasis. This concept has been discussed by Weathers and his co-workers.

Treatment and Prognosis. Since the etiology is unknown, the treatment is empirical. Because the condition is a benign one, there should be no need for concern other than to reassure the patient. Heavy therapeutic doses of vitamins have been used, but in general all types of treatment have been unsuccessful. Banoczy and her associates have reported an excellent ten-year study of 70 patients with geographic tongue treated in a variety of ways and have concluded that treatment did not influence either the lesions or the subjective complaints of the patients.

HAIRY TONGUE

Hairy tongue is an unusual condition that is not specifically a developmental disturbance but is best considered with the other tongue lesions of this group.

Clinical Features. This condition is characterized by hypertrophy of the filiform papillae of the tongue, with lack of normal desquamation which may be extensive and form a thick matted layer on the dorsal surface (Fig. 1–22; see also Plate I). The color of the papillae may vary from yellowish white to brown or even black, depending upon their staining by such extrinsic factors as tobacco, certain foods, medicines, or chromogenic organisms of the oral cavity. The papillae, which may be of considerable length, occasionally will brush the palate of the patient and produce gagging.

Etiology. Although the etiology is unknown, it has been suggested that microorganisms, particularly fungi, might be the exciting factor. It is true that many different types of organisms, including *Candida albicans*, may be cultured from scrapings of the papillae, but there is no proof of a cause-and-effect relation. Some work has indicated that the organisms present are simply saprophytes and that their eradication does not necessarily result in a return of the tongue to normal.

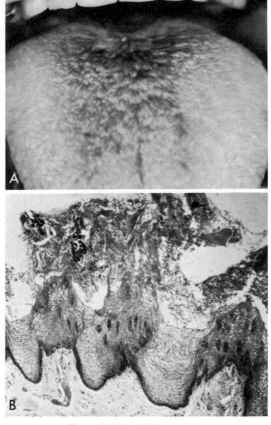

Figure 1–22. *Hairy tongue.*
A, Much of the dorsum is covered by extensive proliferation of the filiform papillae, which form a large matted patch on the tongue. The patch is stained brown by tobacco smoke. *B,* The microscopic section reveals the elongated papillae with large amounts of keratin, bacterial colonies, and debris.

An alternative explanation has been that systemic disturbances (e.g., anemia, gastric upsets) are responsible for hairy tongue. Again, little supportive evidence is available except for occasional cases in which the condition has regressed coincidentally with treatment of the systemic disturbance.

It has even been suggested that the oral use of certain drugs (e.g., sodium perborate, sodium peroxide, and antibiotics such as penicillin and Aureomycin) may incite this condition. In the case of antibiotics, it is reasoned, there is suppression of growth of the normal oral bacterial population and a concomitant unrestrained growth of fungi. There is no clear-cut evidence to support these ideas, however. Most studies agree that the majority of patients with hairy tongue are heavy smokers, although the prevalence of this habit may render questionable its apparent significance.

The development of hairy tongue is rather frequently seen in patients who have had extensive x-ray radiation about the head and neck for the treatment of a tumor. Almost invariably it has been found that the radiation was directed through some or all of the salivary glands, thereby undoubtedly altering their function to some extent. The ensuing hairy tongue is probably due to some change in the local oral environment, although it is not known whether this is a physical or chemical change in the saliva itself or a change in the microbial flora.

Treatment. This is a benign condition. Treatment is empirical because the etiology is still unknown. Food debris often collects deep between the papillae and produces irritation of the tongue. In such cases the tongue may be brushed with a toothbrush to promote desquamation and remove the debris.

LINGUAL VARICES

(Lingual or Sublingual Varicosities)

A varix is a dilated, tortuous vein, most commonly a vein which is subjected to increased hydrostatic pressure but poorly supported by surrounding tissue. Varices involving the lingual ranine veins are relatively common, appearing as red or purple shotlike clusters of vessels on the ventral surface and lateral borders of the tongue as well as in the floor of the mouth. However, varices also do occur in other oral sites such as the upper and lower lip, buccal mucosa, and buccal commissure.

There has been no direct association established between these varicosities and other specific organic diseases. However, Kleinman has concluded that these varicosities represent an aging process and that, when they occur prior to 50 years of age, they may indicate premature aging. In his study, lingual varicosities were not related to cardiac pulmonary disease. In an investigation of 1751 persons (755 males and 996 females) ranging in age from 7 to 99 years, Ettinger and Manderson found that 68 per cent of the persons over 60 years of age had sublingual varices. In this study, there appeared to be a significant relationship between the presence of leg varicosities and sublingual varices.

Thrombosis of any of these varices is a relatively frequent occurrence, as indicated in a report of 12 such cases by Weathers and Fine, but is apparently of little clinical significance.

LINGUAL THYROID NODULE

The thyroid gland develops in the embryo from the ventral floor of the pharynx by means of an entodermal invagination or diverticulum. The tongue forms at the same time from this pharyngeal floor and is anatomically associated with the thyroid gland by connection through the thyroglossal tract, the lingual remnant of which is known as the foramen caecum.

The lingual thyroid is an anomalous condition in which follicles of thyroid tissue are found in the substance of the tongue, possibly arising from a thyroid anlage that failed to "migrate" to its predestined position or from anlage remnants that became detached and were left behind. Baughman has reviewed and discussed in detail the various theories on the development of lingual thyroglossal remnants and the lingual thyroid nodule.

Etiology. The benign enlargement of lingual thyroid tissue is thought to be due in some cases to functional insufficiency of the chief thyroid gland in the neck, since some patients with such a lingual lesion are without a demonstrable main thyroid gland. Other cases of lingual thyroid nodules occur in patients residing in goitrous areas, but it is not certain that the condition is a form of goiter. In addition, it has been suggested that the failure of the primitive thyroid anlage to descend is the cause of the majority of cases of nongoitrous sporadic cretinism.

Clinical Features. The incidence of this benign condition is not known, since a routine autopsy seldom includes an examination of the base of the tongue. Montgomery, in an exceptionally complete and thorough review of the entire subject of the lingual thyroid, analyzed 144 acceptable previously reported cases, pointing out that these represented only cases showing hypertrophy of the lingual thyroid tissue. Though information is inadequate about racial and geographic distribution of lingual thyroid nodules, a difference in sex incidence does appear to be significant. Of 135 cases in which the sex was recorded, 118 patients were female and only 17 were male. The majority of patients had their onset of symptoms relatively early in life, chiefly during puberty, adolescence, and early maturity, though cases have been recorded as early as birth and as late as the seventh decade.

In contrast, Sauk carried out a study to determine the frequency with which ectopic thyroid tissue occurred in the tongue of "normal"

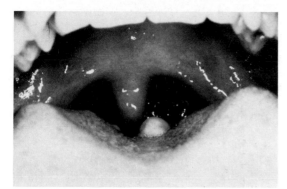

Figure 1–23. *Lingual thyroid nodule.*
(Courtesy of Dr. Ronald A. Baughman.)

persons—i.e., those without a definite symptomatic mass for which treatment was sought. In a series of 200 consecutive necropsies, ectopic thyroid tissue was found in 10 per cent of the cases, with an equal distribution between the sexes. Nearly identical data have been reported by Baughman in his own investigation of 184 tongues from human cadavers. Since the condition is more often clinically apparent in females, Sauk suggested that hormonal factors may be involved in the genesis of symptoms. Most cases appear to arise in females during puberty, adolescence, pregnancy, or menopause.

The lingual thyroid may be manifested clinically as a nodular mass in or near the base of the tongue in the general vicinity of the foramen caecum and often, but not always, in the midline (Fig. 1–23). This mass, which more commonly appears deeply situated rather than as a superficial exophytic lesion, tends to have a smooth surface. In some cases it may appear vascular, while in others the color of the mucosa is not atypical. The size of the lesion in many of the reported cases has approximated 2 to 3 cm. in diameter. The chief symptoms of the condition may vary, but the presenting complaint is often dysphagia, dysphonia, dyspnea, hemorrhage with pain, or a feeling of tightness or fullness in the throat.

Histologic Features. The benign lingual thyroid nodules may present a variety of microscopic patterns, but in the majority of cases they resemble either normal thyroid tissue or thyroid tissue of an embryonal or fetal type. In some instances the nodules exhibit colloid degeneration or goiter.

Great care must be taken to distinguish these lesions from lesions derived from accessory salivary glands in the same location. Both the lingual thyroid and these salivary glands may give rise to adenomas and adenocarcinomas in the tongue.

Treatment. Care must be exercised in handling the lingual thyroid lesion. It has been emphasized by Hung and his associates that a careful physical examination should be performed to demonstrate the presence of a normally located thyroid gland in patients presenting with midline masses in the lingual or sublingual area. If the thyroid gland cannot be palpated, a scintiscan with a tracer dose of radioactive iodine, ^{131}I, should be carried out to determine whether there is a normally located thyroid gland and if the lingual mass is ectopic thyroid. It is usually recommended that a patient with an ectopic thyroid gland should have a trial of replacement thyroid hormone therapy before excision is contemplated, since this will often decrease the size of the lesion and make surgery unnecessary. Occasionally, the clinical manifestations of the lesion and its size necessitate surgical excision.

DEVELOPMENTAL DISTURBANCES OF ORAL LYMPHOID TISSUE

Discrete lymphoid aggregates are normally found in many locations in the oral cavity, the chief sites being the posterior portion of the dorsolateral aspect of the tongue ("lingual tonsils"), the ventral tongue, the buccal mucosa, the floor of the mouth, and the soft palate. These collections of lymphoid tissue may be affected by the same pathologic processes that involve discrete lymph nodes elsewhere and, for this reason, it is important that they be recognized. These oral lymphoid aggregates have been discussed in detail by Doyle and his associates, by Knapp, and by Vickers and his colleagues.

REACTIVE LYMPHOID AGGREGATE

(Reactive Lymphoid Hyperplasia)

The lingual tonsil, one of the largest oral lymphoid aggregates, is located on the posterior portion of the tongue on the dorsolateral aspect. It is typically surrounded by a crypt lined by stratified squamous epithelium. It frequently becomes inflamed and enlarged so that it is clinically evident. Such enlargement is usually bilateral but, if unilateral, may easily be mistaken clinically for early carcinoma. This reactive lingual tonsil has often been called "foliate papillitis," referring to the vestigial foliate papilla in this area.

Similar reactive hyperplasia may occur in the lymphoid aggregates in the other locations mentioned previously, the buccal mucosa being especially common. This presents clinically as a firm nodular submucosal mass which may be tender. Since this lymphoid tissue may be the site for the development of lesions of the malignant lymphoma group, early microscopic diagnosis is essential whenever the lesions do not regress in a short period of time.

Hyperplastic lymphoid polyps have also been described as polypoid structures composed entirely of lymphoid tissue. They are reported to occur on the gingiva, buccal mucosa, tongue, and floor of the mouth.

LYMPHOID HAMARTOMA

(Angiofollicular Lymph Node Malformation)

This is a benign proliferative lesion of lymphoid tissue, which may represent either a localized hyperplasia or a hamartoma. It has not been reported to occur within the oral cavity, although the neck is the second most common site of occurrence after the mediastinum. Because of its microscopic similarity to lesions in the malignant lymphoma group, the major importance of this lymphoid hamartoma is its recognition as a benign lesion that requires conservative treatment. The lesion has been described in detail by Abell.

ANGIOLYMPHOID HYPERPLASIA WITH EOSINOPHILS

(Kimura's Disease; Eosinophilic Lymphoid Granuloma; Eosinophilic Folliculosis)

Angiolymphoid hyperplasia with eosinophils or eosinophilia can best be described as a reactive, angioproliferative lesion which is usually found in the subcutaneous tissue of the head and neck, most often in young or middle-aged females. It is of unknown etiology but may be related to some benign, localized form of vasculitis.

Buckerfield and Edwards, as well as Eveson and Lucas, have reported cases involving the oral cavity and the inner surface of the upper lip. They have thoroughly reviewed the disease as well as discussed its relationship and similarity to Kimura's disease. Buchner and his associates have also reported a case on the lower lip.

As indicated by the name, the lesion is characterized by an atypical endothelial proliferation with a chronic inflammatory infiltrate, many eosinophils, and aggregates of lymphoid tissue. Care must be taken to distinguish it from angiosarcoma, since the disease is self-limiting.

LYMPHOEPITHELIAL CYST

(Branchial Cyst; Branchiogenic Cyst; Benign Cystic Lymphoid Aggregate)

The lymphoepithelial cyst of the oral cavity is a relatively uncommon lesion that apparently originates from cystic transformation of glandular epithelium included within the oral lymphoid aggregates during embryogenesis. Thus, these lesions appear to represent the intraoral counterpart of the benign lymphoepithelial cysts of the cervical area which, at one time, were called branchial cleft cysts (q.v.).

Clinical Features. The oral lymphoepithelial cyst appears as a small asymptomatic, well-circumscribed, yellowish elevated nodule, usually on the floor of the mouth or the ventral tongue, although a few cases have been reported on the soft palate, mandibular vestibule, anterior pillar, and retromolar pad (Fig. 1–24). It may be only a few millimeters in diameter or as large as 1.5 to 2.0 cm. It may occur at any age, the mean in Bhaskar's reported series of 24 cases being 36 years, with a range of 15 to 65 years. In the same series, males were affected more frequently than females by a ratio of greater than 2:1. In a series of 38 cases reported by Buchner and Hansen, the male-to-female ratio was approximately 3:2, although among 21 cases reported by Giunta and Cataldo, females were affected more frequently than males by a ratio of 4:3.

Histologic Features. The lesion consists basically of a cystic cavity lined by stratified squamous epithelium, all embedded in a rather well-circumscribed mass of lymphoid tissue, usually showing discrete follicles (Fig. 1–24). The lining epithelium is quite thin, lacking rete pegs, and is usually parakeratotic. Occasionally the lining epithelium is columnar in type, with or without goblet cells. The lumen of the cyst often contains sloughed epithelial cells, lymphocytes, and eosinophilic, amorphous coagulum.

Treatment. Treatment should consist of conservative local surgical excision. The lesion seldom recurs.

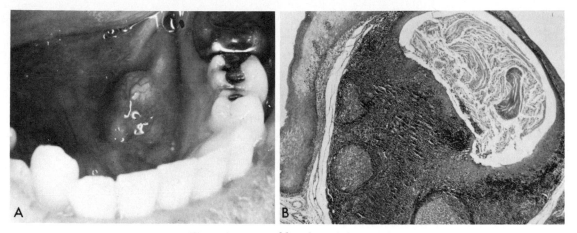

Figure 1–24. *Oral lymphoepithelial cyst.*
An elevated nodule in the floor of the mouth *(A)* histologically exhibited a keratin-filled epithelium-lined cyst in a lymphoid aggregate *(B)*. (Courtesy of Dr. Joseph A. Regezi.)

DEVELOPMENTAL DISTURBANCES OF THE SALIVARY GLANDS

APLASIA

(Agenesis)

Congenital absence of the major salivary glands is an uncommon occurrence. Any one of the glands or groups of glands may be missing, unilaterally or bilaterally. This abnormality is of unknown etiology and is not necessarily associated with other ectodermal dysplasias. Little is known about a possible familial or hereditary pattern. Two such cases, occurring in a father and son, have been reported by Smith and Smith, who also reviewed the literature dealing with this condition. They noted that it was only the second case in which a familial pattern had been demonstrated.

Clinical Features. One of the chief complaints of patients with this defect is the xerostomia, or dry mouth, which may be so severe as to necessitate the constant sipping of water throughout the day and particularly during meal times. Clinically, the oral mucosa appears dry, smooth, or sometimes pebbly, and shows a tendency for the accumulation of debris. Patients also exhibit, characteristically, cracking of the lips and fissuring of the corners of the mouth.

The absence of saliva with the concomitant lack of its washing action permits the collection and stagnation of food debris around the teeth, resulting in rampant dental caries and the early loss of both deciduous and permanent teeth. It is not uncommon in such conditions to see carious destruction of the crowns of the teeth even before eruption is completed. This type of caries is reminiscent of that seen in patients who have had the salivary glands irradiated, purposely or inadvertently, in the treatment of oral or paraoral tumors and in whom xerostomia almost invariably ensues.

Treatment. There is no particular treatment for the condition except the institution of scrupulous oral hygiene in an attempt to decrease dental caries and preserve the teeth as long as possible.

Xerostomia

Xerostomia, or dryness of the mouth, is a clinical manifestation of salivary gland dysfunction, but does not in itself represent a disease entity.

Clinical Features. All degrees of xerostomia exist. In some cases the patient complains of a dry or burning sensation, but the mucosa appears normal. In other cases there is a complete lack of saliva.

When the deficiency of saliva is pronounced, there may be severe alterations in the mucous membranes, and the patient may have extreme discomfort. The mucosa will appear dry and atrophic, sometimes inflamed or, more often, pale and translucent. The tongue may manifest the deficiency by atrophy of the papillae, inflammation, fissuring, and cracking and in severe cases by areas of denudation. Soreness, burning, and pain of the mucous membrane and tongue are common symptoms. Xerostomia, in all its aspects, has been discussed by Bertram.

Etiology. Temporary or transient xerostomia, while quite disconcerting to the patient, seldom produces notable changes in the oral mucosa. Therefore, the xerostomia associated with an emotional reaction, with blockage of the duct by calculus, with acute or chronic infection of the salivary glands, or with administration of various drugs such as atropine or various antihistaminic drugs will not be considered here. It might be pointed out, however, that some persons habitually use antihistaminic drugs as a prophylactic measure against chronic sinusitis, hay fever, and various allergies. Such use may lead to a partial chronic xerostomia to which the patient may become accustomed.

SALIVARY GLAND APLASIA. Lack of development of the salivary glands has already been discussed and the ensuing xerostomia pointed out.

X-RAY RADIATION. Loss of salivary gland function following x-ray radiation either to the glands themselves or to adjacent structures is a well-recognized phenomenon. Radiation, usually administered in the treatment of a tumor in this general area, induces a rather prompt xerostomia, which may be one of the first and chief complaints of the patient. The dryness may be only a temporary phenomenon lasting for a period of weeks or months. In some cases, however, the change is permanent, apparently brought about by atrophy of the glands induced by the x-ray therapy.

VITAMIN DEFICIENCY. A deficiency of vitamin A affects specialized epithelium throughout the body, including the epithelium of the salivary glands. In animals the experimental induction of an avitaminosis A results in squamous metaplasia of the duct epithelium with retention of salivary secretion as well as inflammation with abscess formation. Wolbach reported similar findings in the human being deficient in vitamin A, leading to the suggestion that the sicca syndrome, or keratoconjunctivitis sicca, is caused by a vitamin A deficiency. Little evidence has been found to support this belief, however.

Xerostomia has been reported in patients with riboflavin and nicotinic acid deficiencies. In some cases this condition has responded to administration of the B vitamins. But since salivation has also been associated with these deficiencies, it is questionable whether a true cause-and-effect relation exists.

SJÖGREN'S SYNDROME. One of the characteristic features of this disease (q.v.), also called the sicca syndrome (*siccus*, dry), is the xerostomia which occurs because of the destruction and atrophy of the acinar tissue of the salivary glands.

The relation of xerostomia to an endocrine disturbance has been noted many times, and the apparent predilection for occurrence of Sjögren's syndrome in menopausal women strengthens these observations.

MISCELLANEOUS FACTORS. A variety of other causes of xerostomia may be found in the literature. Pernicious anemia has been reported by Faber to be associated with decreased salivary secretion. He states that dry mouth is common in the iron deficiency anemias also.

Loss of fluid from the body through hemorrhage, excessive sweating, diarrhea, or vomiting may lead to decreased salivary secretion and xerostomia. The polyuria accompanying diabetes mellitus and diabetes insipidus probably accounts for the diminished salivary secretion and consequent thirst in patients with these diseases.

Occasional cases appear to be due to organic lesions of the nervous system which interfere with normal secretory nerve stimulation and thus inhibit secretion.

Clinical Significance. Aside from annoyance to the patient, there is one feature of the condition that is serious. In many cases chronic xerostomia predisposes to rampant dental caries and subsequent loss of teeth. Moreover, patients with xerostomia have difficulty with artificial dentures. Dental appliances are extremely disagreeable against dry mucosa and cannot be tolerated by some patients.

Treatment. The treatment of xerostomia will depend upon the nature of the disease. If the cause can be discovered, obviously it should be corrected. The majority of patients, however, can be offered only symptomatic relief.

HYPERPLASIA OF PALATAL GLANDS

An unusual localized hyperplasia or hypertrophy of minor accessory salivary glands in the palate has been described by Giansanti and his associates, although they have also accepted the view that this lesion may represent a benign adenoma of these glands. The cause of this focal enlargement is unknown although, according to these investigators, the following have been reported to result in salivary gland enlargement: (1) endocrine disorders, (2) gout, (3) diabetes mellitus, (4) menopause, (5) hepatic disease, (6) starvation, (7) alcoholism, (8) inflammation, (9) benign lymphoepithelial lesion, (10) Sjögren's syndrome, (11) the adiposity, hyperthermia, oligomenorrhea, and parotid swelling syndrome, (12) aglossia-adactylia syndrome, (13) Waldenström's macroglobulinemia, (14) uveoparotid fever, (15) Felty's syndrome, (16) certain drugs, and (17) the aging process.

A series of ten cases has been reported recently by Arafat and her associates. They also could find no associated abnormalities and had to consider the cases idiopathic. Interestingly, one of their cases involved the glands of the retromolar area rather than the palate.

Clinical Features. Palatal gland hyperplasia presents as a small localized swelling, measuring from several millimeters to 1 cm. or more in diameter, usually on the hard palate or at the junction of the hard and soft palates. The lesion has an intact surface and is firm, sessile, and normal in color. It is usually asymptomatic and the patient may be unaware of the lesion. Too few cases have been reported to determine whether there is any age or sex predilection.

Histologic Features. The mass appears microscopically as closely packed collections of normal-appearing mucous acini with the usual intermingling of normal ducts. There is no inflammation, no spillage of mucin, and no fibrosis.

Treatment. Because hyperplasia of palatal glands cannot be differentiated clinically from a small salivary gland neoplasm in this area, it is essential that they be excised for microscopic examination. No further treatment is necessary and the condition is not reported to recur.

ATRESIA

Congenital occlusion or absence of one or more of the major salivary gland ducts is an exceedingly rare condition. When it does occur, it may result in the formation of a retention cyst or produce a relatively severe xerostomia. Such a case has been reported by Foretich and his associates.

ABERRANCY

Because of the widespread distribution of normal accessory salivary glands in the oral cavity, it is difficult to define the condition of aberrancy. Since such accessory glands may be found in the lips, palate, buccal mucosa, floor of the mouth, tongue, and retromolar area, aberrancy may be construed as simply that situation in which these glands are found farther than normal from their usual location. In any

event, there is no clinical significance to be attached to aberrant salivary glands other than that they may be the site of development of a retention cyst or neoplasm.

Occasional cases have been reported in the literature of salivary gland tissue present within the body of the mandible. It has been found, in many instances, that this glandular tissue anatomically communicated with the normal submaxillary or sublingual gland, generally through a stalk or pedicle of tissue which perforated the lingual cortical plate. For this reason, this aberrancy of salivary gland tissue probably represents only an extreme example of the condition known as the "developmental lingual mandibular salivary gland depression" described next.

DEVELOPMENTAL LINGUAL MANDIBULAR SALIVARY GLAND DEPRESSION

(Static Bone Cavity or Defect of the Mandible; Lingual Mandibular Bone Cavity; Static Bone Cyst; Latent Bone Cyst; Stafne Cyst or Defect)

One unusual form of slightly aberrant salivary gland tissue is the developmental inclusion of glandular tissue within or, more commonly, adjacent to the lingual surface of the body of the mandible in a deep, well-circumscribed depression. First recognized by Stafne in 1942, numerous cases have since been reported, and the lesion should not be considered rare. In a study of 4963 adult patients subjected to panoramic roentgenograms, 18 cases of salivary gland depression were found by Karmiol and Walsh, an incidence of nearly 0.4 per cent. Similar studies of the frequency of such depressions range from 0.1 per cent in 10,000 cases investigated by Oikarinen and Julku to 1.3 per cent in a group of 469 dried specimens examined by Langlais and his associates. A study of a series of 2693 panoramic radiographs by Correll and his associates revealed a total of 13 cases of lingual cortical defects, an incidence of 0.48 per cent. Most authorities now agree that this entity is a congenital defect, although it has rarely been observed in children and its precise anatomic nature is still uncertain. Also unexplained is the fact that far more cases have been reported in men than in women. For example, in the series reported by Correll and his coworkers, every case was found in a male; the same held true in the series of Oikarinen and Julku.

Roentgenographic Features. The lesion, usually asymptomatic and discovered during

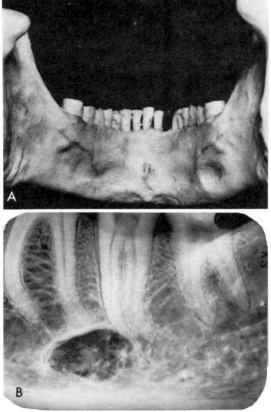

Figure 1–25. *Developmental lingual mandibular salivary gland depression.*
    The obvious anatomic depression on the lingual surface of the mandible (*A*) is demonstrated by a roentgenogram of this area as a well-circumscribed radiolucency just above the inferior cortex (*B*). (Courtesy of Drs. David F. Mitchell and Grant Van Huysen.)

routine roentgenographic examination, appears as an ovoid radiolucency generally situated between the mandibular canal and the inferior border of the mandible, commonly in the second or third molar area or just anterior to the angle. It is occasionally bilateral. Boerger and his associates and Harvey and Noble have recently reviewed the literature on this condition, adding cases of their own, and have pointed out that the radiolucent defect may represent either actual enclavement of salivary gland tissue within the mandible during embryonic development or, more frequently, an indentation on the lingual surface of the mandible with a portion of the submaxillary gland lying within the defect (Figs. 1–25, 1–26).

The lesion may be regarded properly as a developmental defect rather than a pathologic lesion and, once diagnosed, needs no treatment. It can and should be differentiated from the "traumatic" or hemorrhagic bone cyst (q.v.), since the traumatic bone cyst almost invariably lies above the mandibular canal on the intraoral periapical roentgenogram, while the salivary gland depression lies below the canal. Nevertheless, definitive differential diagnosis from other lesions sometimes cannot be made without surgical exploration.

ANTERIOR LINGUAL DEPRESSION. It has also been recognized that a similar asymptomatic round or ovoid radiolucency may occur in the anterior segment of the mandible, generally appearing as a rather poorly circumscribed lesion somewhere between the central incisor and the first premolar area. This anterior radiolucency also represents a cavity or depres-

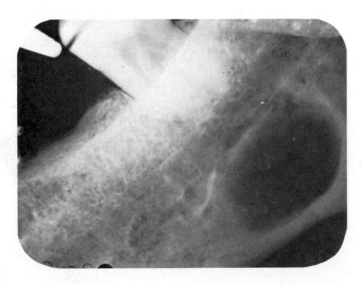

Figure 1–26. *Developmental lingual mandibular salivary gland depression.*
    Note the position of the radiolucency below the mandibular canal.

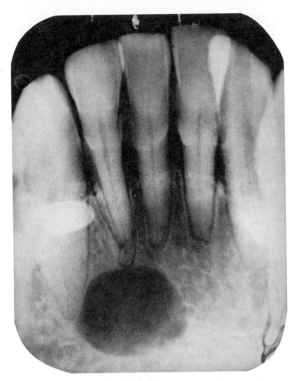

Figure 1–27.   *Developmental lingual mandibular salivary gland depression of sublingual gland.*
(Courtesy of Dr. Michael J. Freeman.)

sion on the lingual surface of the mandible. It has been reviewed by Miller and Winnick and more recently by Connor. Langlais and his co-workers examined 12 dried mandibles with such anterior depressions and concluded that these might represent either anatomic variants re-

lated to the digastric or sublingual fossa or developmental anomalies caused by impingement of the sublingual gland. These are far less common than the posterior lesion (Fig. 1–27).

Complications.   A complication, occasionally reported in the literature, is the development of a true central salivary gland neoplasm from the included salivary gland tissue, but this is rare. This has been discussed in Chapter 3 on tumors of the salivary gland (q.v.) in the section on mucoepidermoid carcinoma.

DEVELOPMENTAL DISTURBANCES IN SIZE OF TEETH

MICRODONTIA

This term is used to describe teeth which are smaller than normal, i.e., outside the usual limits of variation. Three types of microdontia are recognized: (1) true generalized microdontia, (2) relative generalized microdontia, and (3) microdontia involving a single tooth.

In *true generalized microdontia*, all the teeth are smaller than normal. Aside from its occurrence in some cases of pituitary dwarfism, this condition is exceedingly rare. The teeth are reportedly well formed, merely small.

In *relative generalized microdontia*, normal or slightly smaller than normal teeth are present in jaws that are somewhat larger than normal, and there is an illusion of true microdontia. Since it is well recognized that a person may inherit the jaw size from one parent and the

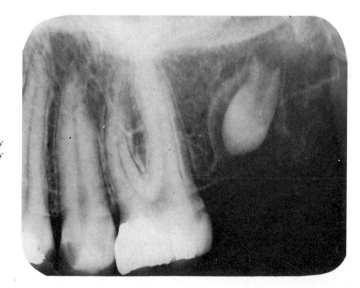

Figure 1–28.   *Microdontia.*
The third molar is small and incompletely formed. The second molar had been previously extracted.

tooth size from the other parent, the role of hereditary factors in producing such a condition is obvious.

Microdontia involving only a single tooth is a rather common condition (Fig. 1–28). It affects most often the maxillary lateral incisor and the third molar. These two teeth are among those most often congenitally missing. It is of interest to note, however, that other teeth often congenitally absent, the maxillary and mandibular second premolars, seldom exhibit microdontia. Supernumerary teeth, however, are frequently small in size.

One of the common forms of localized microdontia is that which affects the maxillary lateral incisor, a condition that has been called the "peg lateral" (Fig. 1–29). Instead of exhibiting parallel or diverging mesial and distal surfaces, the sides converge or taper together incisally, forming a peg-shaped or cone-shaped crown. The root on such a tooth is frequently shorter than usual.

MACRODONTIA

Macrodontia is the opposite of microdontia and refers to teeth that are larger than normal. Such teeth may be classified in the same manner as in microdontia.

True generalized macrodontia, the condition in which all teeth are larger than normal, has been associated with pituitary gigantism, but is extremely rare.

Relative generalized macrodontia is somewhat more common and is a result of the presence of normal or slightly larger than normal teeth in small jaws, the disparity in size

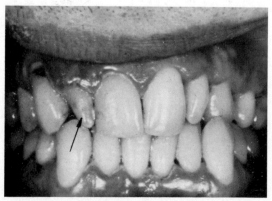

Figure 1–29. *Microdontia.*
Peg-shaped maxillary lateral incisor.

giving the illusion of macrodontia. As in microdontia, the importance of heredity must be considered.

Macrodontia of single teeth is relatively uncommon, but is occasionally seen. It is of unknown etiology. The tooth may appear normal in every respect except for its size. True macrodontia of a single tooth should not be confused with fusion of teeth, in which, early in odontogenesis, the union of two or more teeth results in a single large tooth.

A variant of this localized macrodontia is the type that is occasionally seen in cases of hemihypertrophy of the face, in which the teeth of the involved side may be considerably larger than those of the unaffected side.

DEVELOPMENTAL DISTURBANCES IN SHAPE OF TEETH

GEMINATION

Geminated teeth are anomalies which arise from an attempt at division of a single tooth germ by an invagination, with resultant incomplete formation of two teeth. The structure is usually one with two completely or incompletely separated crowns that have a single root and root canal. It is seen in the deciduous as well as the permanent dentition and in some reported cases appears to exhibit a hereditary tendency. It is not always possible to differentiate between gemination and a case in which there has been fusion between a normal tooth and a supernumerary tooth.

The term "twinning" has sometimes been used to designate the production of equivalent structures by division resulting in one normal and one supernumerary tooth. These terms, as well as "fusion" and "concrescence," have been discussed by Levitas.

FUSION

Fused teeth arise through union of two normally separated tooth germs. Depending upon the stage of development of the teeth at the time of the union, fusion may be either complete or incomplete. It has been thought that some physical force or pressure produces contact of the developing teeth and their subsequent fusion. If this contact occurs early, at least before calcification begins, the two teeth may be completely united to form a single large

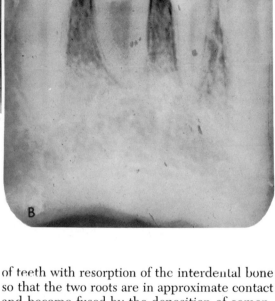

Figure 1–30. *Fusion of teeth.*
A, There has been complete fusion between the mandibular left central and lateral incisors and the right central and lateral incisors. *B*, The intraoral roentgenogram shows a common pulp chamber and root canal in each pair of fused teeth.

tooth (Fig. 1–30). If the contact of teeth occurs later, when a portion of the tooth crown has completed its formation, there may be union of the roots only. The dentin, however, is always confluent in cases of true fusion. The tooth may have separate or fused root canals, and the condition is common in the deciduous as well as in the permanent dentition. In fact, Grahnén and Granath have reported that fusion of teeth is more common in the deciduous than in the permanent dentition.

In addition to affecting two normal teeth, fusion may also occur between a normal tooth and a supernumerary tooth such as the mesiodens or the distomolar (Fig. 1–31). In some cases the condition has been reported to show a hereditary tendency.

The possible clinical problems related to appearance, spacing, and periodontal conditions brought about by fused teeth have been discussed by Mader, who has also reported several illustrative cases.

CONCRESCENCE

Concrescence of teeth is actually a form of fusion which occurs after root formation has been completed. In this condition, the teeth are united by cementum only. It is thought to arise as a result of traumatic injury or crowding of teeth with resorption of the interdental bone so that the two roots are in approximate contact and become fused by the deposition of cementum between them. Concrescence may occur before or after the teeth have erupted, and although it usually involves only two teeth, there is at least one case on record of union of three teeth by cementum.

The diagnosis can frequently be established by roentgenographic examination. Since with fused teeth the extraction of one may result in

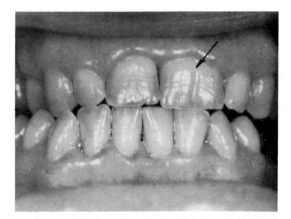

Figure 1–31. *Fusion of teeth.*
There has been nearly complete fusion between both the maxillary right and left central incisors and a supernumerary tooth, probably a bilateral mesiodens.

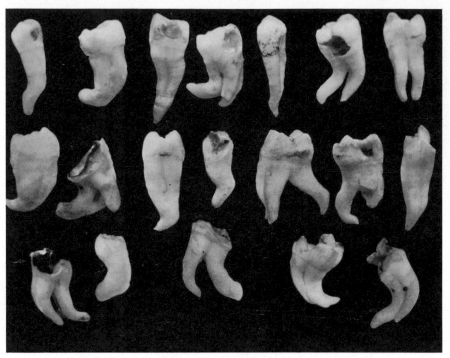

Figure 1–32. *Dilaceration.*
Examples of various types of curves and angles involving roots of teeth.

the extraction of the other, it is desirable that the dentist be forewarned of the condition and advise the patient.

DILACERATION

The term "dilaceration" refers to an angulation, or a sharp bend or curve, in the root or crown of a formed tooth (Fig. 1–32). The condition is thought to be due to trauma during the period in which the tooth is forming, with the result that the position of the calcified portion of the tooth is changed and the remainder of the tooth is formed at an angle. The curve or bend may occur anywhere along the length of the tooth, sometimes at the cervical portion, at other times midway along the root or even just at the apex of the root, depending upon the amount of root formed when the injury occurred. It has been emphasized by van Gool that such an injury to a permanent tooth, resulting in dilaceration, often follows traumatic injury to the deciduous predecessor in which that tooth is driven apically into the jaw. He has discussed this condition in detail, reporting 18 such cases.

Since dilacerated teeth frequently present difficult problems at the time of extraction if

the operator is unaware of the condition, the need for preoperative roentgenograms before any surgical procedures are carried out is self-evident.

TALON CUSP

The talon cusp, an anomalous structure resembling an eagle's talon, projects lingually from the cingulum areas of a maxillary or mandibular permanent incisor. This cusp blends smoothly with the tooth except that there is a deep developmental groove where the cusp blends with the sloping lingual tooth surface (Fig. 1–33). It is composed of normal enamel and dentin and contains a horn of pulp tissue.

This anomaly has been discussed by Mellor and Ripa, who have emphasized the problems it poses for the patient in terms of esthetics, caries control, and occlusal accommodation. They have recommended prophylactically restoring the groove to prevent caries. If there is occlusal interference, it should be removed, but exposure of the pulp horn, necessitating endodontic therapy, is almost certain to occur. Fortunately, this anomaly is quite uncommon among the general population. However, it has been reported by Gardner and Girgis that it

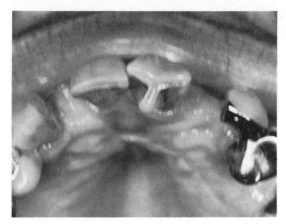

Figure 1–33.   *Talon cusp.*

appears to be more prevalent in persons with the Rubinstein-Taybi syndrome (developmental retardation, broad thumbs and great toes, characteristic facial features, delayed or incomplete descent of testes in males, and stature, head circumference, and bone age below the fiftieth percentile). The talon cusp has not been reported as an integral part of any other syndrome, although Mader, in his thorough review, suggested that it may be associated with other somatic and odontogenic anomalies.

"DENS IN DENTE"

(Dens Invaginatus; Dilated Composite Odontome)

The "dens in dente" is a developmental variation which is thought to arise as a result of an invagination in the surface of a tooth crown before calcification has occurred. Several causes of this condition have been proposed. These include an increased localized external pressure, focal growth retardation, and focal growth stimulation in certain areas of the tooth bud.

The permanent maxillary lateral incisors are the teeth most frequently involved, and in the majority of cases the "dens in dente" appears to represent simply an accentuation in the development of the lingual pit (Fig. 1–34,A). The maxillary central incisors are sometimes involved, and the condition is frequently bilateral. Oehlers has presented an excellent discussion of this condition and emphasized that not only are posterior teeth sometimes affected but also an analogous form of invagination occasionally occurs in the roots of teeth. This radicular variety of "dens in dente" has been discussed by Bhatt and Dholakia, who pointed out that the radicular invagination usually results from an infolding of Hertwig's sheath and takes its origin within the root after development is complete.

The cases that have been reported in the literature indicate that the condition is fairly common and that an extremely wide range in degree of variation can exist. The term "dens in dente," originally applied to a severe invagination that gave the appearance of a tooth within a tooth, is actually a misnomer, but it has continued in usage (Fig. 1–34,B). In the mild form there is a deep invagination in the lingual pit area, which may not be evident clinically. Roentgenographically, it is recognized as a pear-shaped invagination of enamel

Figure 1–34.   "Dens in dente."
A slight invagination may be seen in the lingual pit area of the maxillary lateral incisor on the roentgenogram (A). The ground section of tooth represents a severe form of "dens in dente" and illustrates how the anomaly may resemble a tooth within a tooth (B).

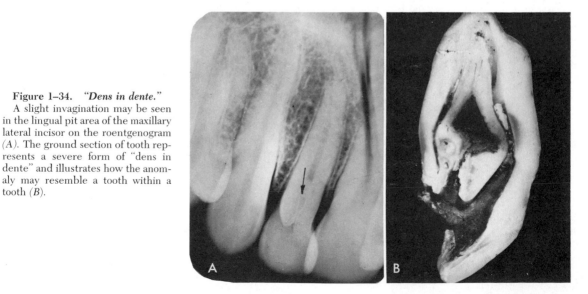

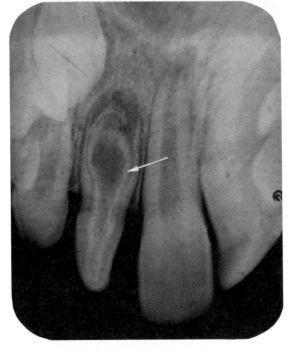

Figure 1–35. *"Dens in dente."*
A nearly complete invagination in a maxillary lateral incisor.

the minor invaginations are included, the incidence may be as high as 5 per cent of all patients examined (Table 1–9). The more severe forms, however, are much less common.

To prevent caries, pulp infection, and premature loss of the tooth, the condition must be recognized early and the tooth prophylactically restored. Fortunately, the defect may be recognized roentgenographically even before the teeth erupt.

DENS EVAGINATUS

(Occlusal Tuberculated Premolar; Leong's Premolar; Evaginated Odontome; Occlusal Enamel Pearl)

The dens evaginatus is a developmental condition that appears clinically as an accessory cusp or a globule of enamel on the occlusal surface between the buccal and lingual cusps of premolars, unilaterally or bilaterally, although it has been reported to occur rarely on molars, cuspids, and incisors (Fig. 1–36). It has been thought to develop only in persons of Mongoloid ancestry: Chinese, Japanese, Filipinos, Eskimos, and American Indians. Its prevalence in a group of 2373 Chinese schoolchildren in Singapore, reported by Yip, was 2.2 per cent. However, Palmer has reported a series of cases in Caucasians in England.

The pathogenesis of the lesion is thought to be the proliferation and evagination of an area of the inner enamel epithelium and subjacent odontogenic mesenchyme into the dental organ during early tooth development. Thus, it has been considered to be the antithesis of the mechanism of development of the dens in dente or dens invaginatus.

The clinical significance of the condition is similar to that of the talon cusp, which it may physically resemble. This "extra" cusp may contribute to incomplete eruption, displacement of teeth and/or pulp exposure with subsequent

and dentin with a narrow constriction at the opening on the surface of the tooth and closely approximating the pulp in its depth. Food debris may become packed in this area with resultant caries and infection of the pulp, occasionally even before the tooth has completely erupted. The more severe forms of "dens in dente" may exhibit an invagination that extends nearly to the apex of the root, and these present a bizarre roentgenographic picture (Fig. 1–35), reflecting a severe disturbance in the normal anatomic and morphologic structure of the teeth.

It is important to realize that this condition, particularly in its mild form, is fairly common. The clinical studies of Amos have shown that if

Table 1–9. Incidence of "Dens in Dente" in Maxillary Lateral Incisors as Diagnosed by Roentgenograms

	TOTAL NUMBER OF PATIENTS	BILATERAL CASES	LEFT LATERAL INCISOR	RIGHT LATERAL INCISOR	TOTAL INCIDENCE (%)
Shafer (1953)	2452	19	5	7	1.26
Amos (1955)	1000	22	17	12	5.10

From (1) W. G. Shafer: Dens in dente. N.Y. Dent. J., *19*:220, 1953; and (2) E. R. Amos: Incidence of the small dens in dente. J. Am. Dent. Assoc., *51*:31, 1955.

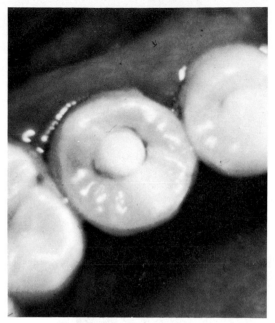

Figure 1–36. *Dens evaginatus.*
(Courtesy of Dr. Charles E. Tomich.)

infection following occlusal wear or fracture. This phenomenon has been discussed by Senia and Regezi, who have reported periapical infection of caries-free premolars affected by dens evaginatus.

TAURODONTISM

The term "taurodontism" was originated by Sir Arthur Keith in 1913 to describe a peculiar dental anomaly in which the body of the tooth is enlarged at the expense of the roots. The term means "bull-like" teeth and its usage is derived from the similarity of these teeth to those of ungulate or cud-chewing animals. Shaw further classified taurodont teeth into hypotaurodont, mesotaurodont, and hypertaurodont forms, with hypertaurodontism being the extreme form in which the bifurcation or trifurcation occurs near the apices of the roots and hypotaurodontism being the mildest form.

A variety of possible causes of taurodontism have been enumerated by Mangion as follows: (1) a specialized or retrograde character, (2) a primitive pattern, (3) a mendelian recessive trait, (4) an atavistic feature, and (5) a mutation resulting from odontoblastic deficiency during dentinogenesis of the roots. Hamner and his associates believe that the taurodont is caused by failure of Hertwig's epithelial sheath to invaginate at the proper horizontal level. The heritability of this condition requires further study, although after finding 11 cases of taurodontism among members of three families, Goldstein and Gottlieb have stated that the condition appears to be genetically controlled and familial in nature.

This condition is of anthropologic interest inasmuch as it has been found commonly in fossil hominids, especially in the Neanderthal man, with a very high prevalence during the neolithic period. At one time it was thought to be confined to these early populations, but it is now known to be widespread in many modern races. Hamner and his associates have discussed these anthropologic aspects in detail, while Blumberg and his co-workers have carried out a biometric study of the condition. A case of taurodontism occurring concomitantly with amelogenesis imperfecta has been reported by Crawford. In addition, it has been reported that many patients with the Klinefelter syndrome (males whose sex chromosome constitution includes one or more extra X chromosomes) exhibit taurodontism, but it is not a constant feature of this syndrome. For this reason, Gardner and Girgis have recommended that male patients exhibiting taurodontism should have chromosomal studies performed, especially if there is any nonspecific diagnosis of mental retardation and if the patient has a tall, thin appearance with long arms and legs and a prognathic jaw.

Clinical Features. Taurodontism may affect either the deciduous or permanent dentition, although permanent tooth involvement is more common. The teeth involved are almost invariably molars, sometimes only a single tooth, at other times several molars in the same quadrant. The condition may be unilateral or bilateral or may exhibit any combination of quadrant involvement. The teeth themselves have no remarkable or unusual morphologic clinical characteristics.

Roentgenographic Features. The unusual nature of this condition is best visualized on the roentgenogram. Involved teeth frequently tend to be rectangular in shape rather than taper toward the roots. The pulp chamber is extremely large with a much greater apico-occlusal height than normal. In addition, the pulp lacks the usual constriction at the cervical of the tooth and the roots are exceedingly short. The bifurcation or trifurcation may be only a few millimeters above the apices of the roots

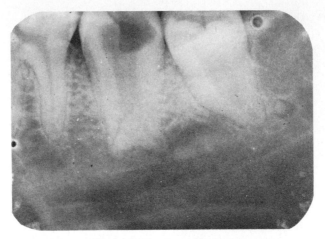

Figure 1–37. *Taurodontism.*

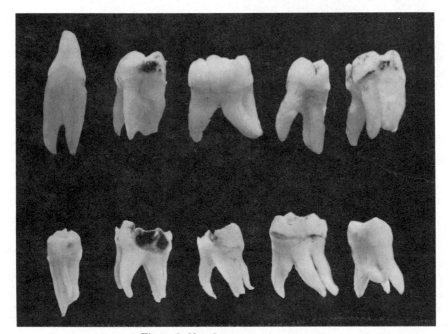

Figure 1–38. *Supernumerary roots.*

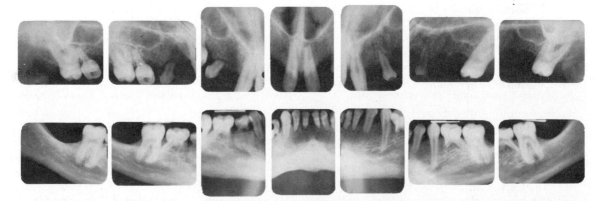

Figure 1–39. *Anodontia.*
There is congenital absence of nearly all permanent teeth with retention of many deciduous teeth.

Table 1-10. Distribution of Congenitally Missing Teeth, Expressed as Percentage of Affected Cases

	CENTRAL INCISOR	LATERAL INCISOR	CUSPID	1ST PRE-MOLAR	2ND PRE-MOLAR	1ST MOLAR	2ND MOLAR	TOTAL
Maxilla	0.0	12.3	1.8	5.5	25.3	0.0	0.8	45.7
Mandible	2.2	1.1	0.0	3.0	47.3	0.0	0.7	54.3

Of 10,000 children (6–15 years of age) examined, 340 exhibited congenital absence of 709 teeth or tooth germs. Third molars were *not* studied.

From E. Dolder: Deficient dentition. Dent. Record, 57:142, 1937.

(Fig. 1–37). This roentgenographic picture is quite striking and characteristic.

Treatment. No special treatment is necessary for this anomaly.

SUPERNUMERARY ROOTS

This developmental condition is not uncommon and may involve any tooth (Fig. 1–38). Teeth that are normally single-rooted, particularly the mandibular bicuspids and cuspids, often have two roots. Both maxillary and mandibular molars, particularly third molars, also may exhibit one or more supernumerary roots. This phenomenon is of considerable significance in exodontia, for one of these roots may be broken off during extraction and, if unrecognized and allowed to remain in the alveolus, may be the source of future infection.

DEVELOPMENTAL DISTURBANCES IN NUMBER OF TEETH

ANODONTIA

True anodontia, or congenital absence of teeth, may be of two types, total and partial.

Total anodontia, in which all teeth are missing, may involve both the deciduous and the permanent dentition (Fig. 1–39). This is a rare condition; when it occurs, it is frequently associated with a more generalized disturbance, hereditary ectodermal dysplasia (q.v.).

Induced or false anodontia occurs as a result of extraction of all teeth, while the term pseudoanodontia is sometimes applied to multiple unerupted teeth. The condition under discussion here is a true failure of odontogenesis and should not be confused with false or pseudoanodontia.

True partial anodontia (hypodontia or oligodontia) involves one or more teeth and is a rather common condition (Fig. 1–40). Although any tooth may be congenitally missing, there is a tendency for certain teeth to be missing more frequently than others (Table 1–10). Studies on the frequency of missing third molars have shown this tooth to be congenitally absent in as many as 35 per cent of all subjects examined, with a frequent absence of all four third molars in the same person (Table 1–11). Other studies have shown that the maxillary lateral incisors and maxillary or mandibular second premolars are commonly missing, often bilaterally (Fig. 1–41). In severe partial anodontia, the bilateral

Table 1-11. Incidence of Congenitally Missing Third Molars

	MALES		FEMALES	
	NO.	%	NO.	%
Total number of patients in study	735	...	314	...
Total number of patients with congenitally missing third molars	201	27.4	110	35.0
Number of missing third molars				
1	64	31.8	30	27.3
2	74	36.8	31	28.2
3	28	13.9	18	16.4
4	35	17.4	31	28.2

From M. Hellman: Our third molar teeth; their eruption, presence and absence. Dent. Cosmos, 78:750, 1936.

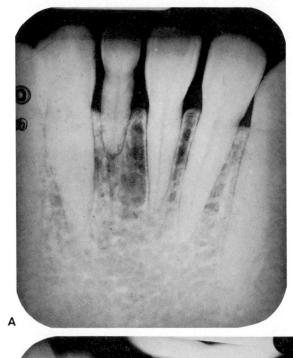

A

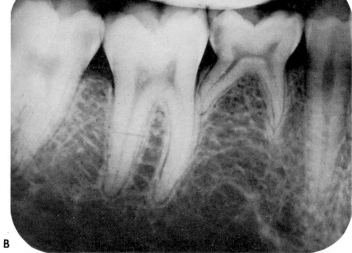

B

Figure 1–40.   *Partial anodontia.*
The mandibular permanent left central incisor is congenitally missing. The deciduous incisor is retained (*A*). There is congenital absence of the mandibular second bicuspid with retention of the deciduous molar (*B*).

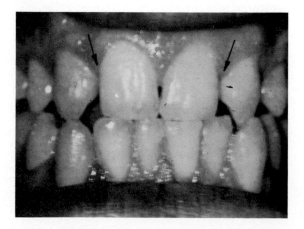

Figure 1–41.   *Partial anodontia.*
Both maxillary lateral incisors are congenitally missing.

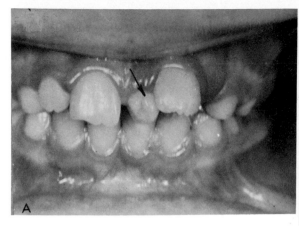

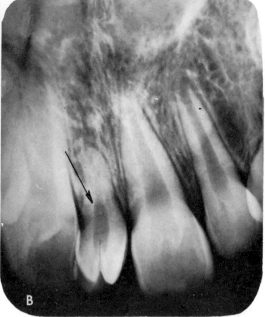

Figure 1–42. *Supernumerary tooth.*
A, The supernumerary tooth between the maxillary permanent central incisors is called a mesiodens. *B,* The intraoral roentgenogram.

absence of corresponding teeth may be striking. An outstanding review of this subject has been reported by Graber, who showed that the overall frequency of patients with congenitally missing teeth (excluding third molars) has ranged from 1.6 to 9.6 per cent in various series of studies in different countries.

Congenitally missing deciduous teeth are uncommon but, when occurring, usually involve the maxillary lateral incisor. Mandibular lateral incisors and mandibular cuspids may also be missing, according to the study of Grahnén and Granath. Their studies also showed a close correlation between congenitally missing deciduous teeth and their permanent successors, suggesting at least in some instances a genetic factor.

Although the etiology of single missing teeth is unknown, a familial tendency for this defect is present in many instances. Graber, in reviewing congenital absence of teeth, reported the accumulating evidence that it is actually the result of one or more point mutations in a closely linked polygenic system, most often transmitted in an autosomal dominant pattern with incomplete penetrance and variable expressivity. Some investigators believe cases of missing third molars to be evidence of an evolutionary trend toward fewer teeth. Hereditary ectodermal dysplasia may be associated with partial anodontia, and in these instances the few teeth that are present may be deformed or misshapen, frequently cone-shaped.

Occasionally one sees children with teeth of one quadrant or both quadrants on the same side missing owing to x-ray radiation of the face at an early age. Tooth buds are extremely sensitive to x-ray radiation and may be destroyed completely by relatively low dosages. Teeth already forming and partially calcified may be stunted by x-ray radiation.

SUPERNUMERARY TEETH

A supernumerary tooth may closely resemble the teeth of the group to which it belongs, i.e., molars, premolars, or anterior teeth, or it may bear little resemblance in size or shape to the teeth with which it is associated. It has been suggested that supernumerary teeth develop from a third tooth bud arising from the dental lamina near the permanent tooth bud, or possibly from splitting of the permanent bud itself. This latter view is somewhat unlikely, since the associated permanent teeth are usually normal in all respects. In some cases there appears to be a hereditary tendency for the development of supernumerary teeth.

Although these teeth may be found in any location, they have an apparent predilection for certain sites (Table 1–12). The most common supernumerary tooth is the "mesiodens," a tooth situated between the maxillary central incisors and occurring singly (Fig. 1–42) or paired, erupted (Fig. 1–43) or impacted and,

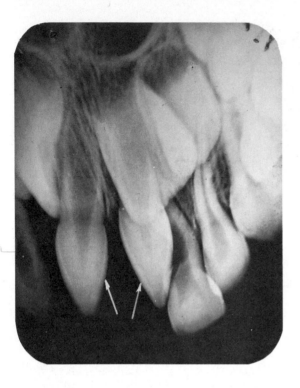

Figure l–43. *Supernumerary teeth.*
An unusual case of bilateral erupting mesiodens. (Courtesy of Dr. Bernard A. Ackerman.)

Table 1–12. Distribution of 500 Supernumerary Teeth

	CENTRAL INCISORS	LATERAL INCISORS	CUSPIDS	PREMOLARS	PARAMOLARS	FOURTH MOLARS	TOTAL
Maxilla	227	19	2	9	58	131	446
Mandible	10	0	1	33	0	10	54

From E. C. Stafne: Supernumerary teeth. Dent. Cosmos, 74:653, 1932.

Figure l–44. *Supernumerary teeth.*
An unusual case of bilateral inverted mesiodens.

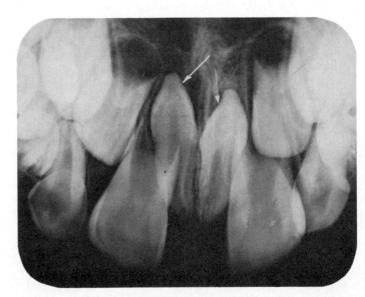

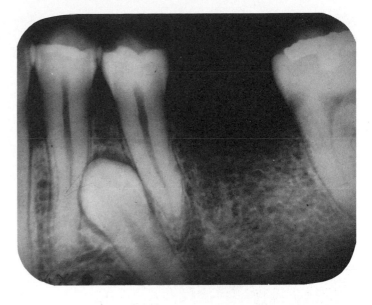

Figure 1–45. *Supernumerary tooth.* The supernumerary mandibular right bicuspid is impacted.

occasionally, even inverted (Fig. 1–44). The "mesiodens" is usually a small tooth with a cone-shaped crown and a short root. Its incidence in Caucasian populations is reported to range between 0.15 and 1.0 per cent with a 2:1 predilection for occurrence in males. Sedano and Gorlin have stated that, on the basis of rather scanty information, it appears that the "mesiodens" is transmitted as an autosomal dominant trait, with lack of penetrance in some generations.

The maxillary fourth molar is the second most common supernumerary tooth and is situated distal to the third molar. It is usually a small rudimentary tooth, but may be of normal size. A mandibular fourth molar also is seen occasionally, but this is much less common than the maxillary molar.

Other supernumerary teeth seen with some frequency are maxillary paramolars, mandibular premolars, and maxillary lateral incisors. Mandibular central incisors and maxillary premolars are found on occasion (Fig. 1–45). The paramolar is a supernumerary molar, usually small and rudimentary, which is situated buccally or lingually to one of the maxillary molars or interproximally between the first and second or second and third maxillary molars. It is of interest, and as yet unexplained, that approximately 90 per cent of all supernumerary teeth occur in the maxilla.

Supernumerary teeth in the deciduous dentition are less common than in the permanent dentition, according to studies of Grahnén and Granath. When this situation does occur in the deciduous dentition, the supernumerary tooth is usually a maxillary lateral incisor, although both supernumerary maxillary and mandibular deciduous cuspids have also been reported.

Any supernumerary tooth may be erupted or impacted. Because of the additional tooth bulk, supernumerary teeth frequently cause malposition of adjacent teeth or prevent their eruption. Multiple supernumerary teeth, many of them impacted, are characteristically found in cleidocranial dysostosis (q.v.).

Gardner's syndrome is an interesting disease complex, reviewed by Fader and his associates and by Duncan and his associates. It is also characterized by the occurrence of multiple impacted supernumerary teeth. This syndrome consists of (1) multiple polyposis of the large intestine, (2) osteomas of the bones, including long bones, skull, and jaws, (3) multiple epidermoid or sebaceous cysts of the skin, particularly on the scalp and back, (4) occasional occurrence of desmoid tumors, and (5) the impacted supernumerary and permanent teeth (Figs. 1–46, 1–47).

It is due to a single pleiotropic gene and has an autosomal dominant pattern of inheritance, with complete penetrance and variable expression. Indicative of its inheritability is a report by Watne and his associates, who studied 280 patients from 11 families with Gardner's syndrome. They found that 126 of the 280, or 45 per cent of the patients at risk, exhibited some part of the syndrome. Significantly, the intestinal polyps in this disease are premalignant, and polyps were found to be present in 85 of

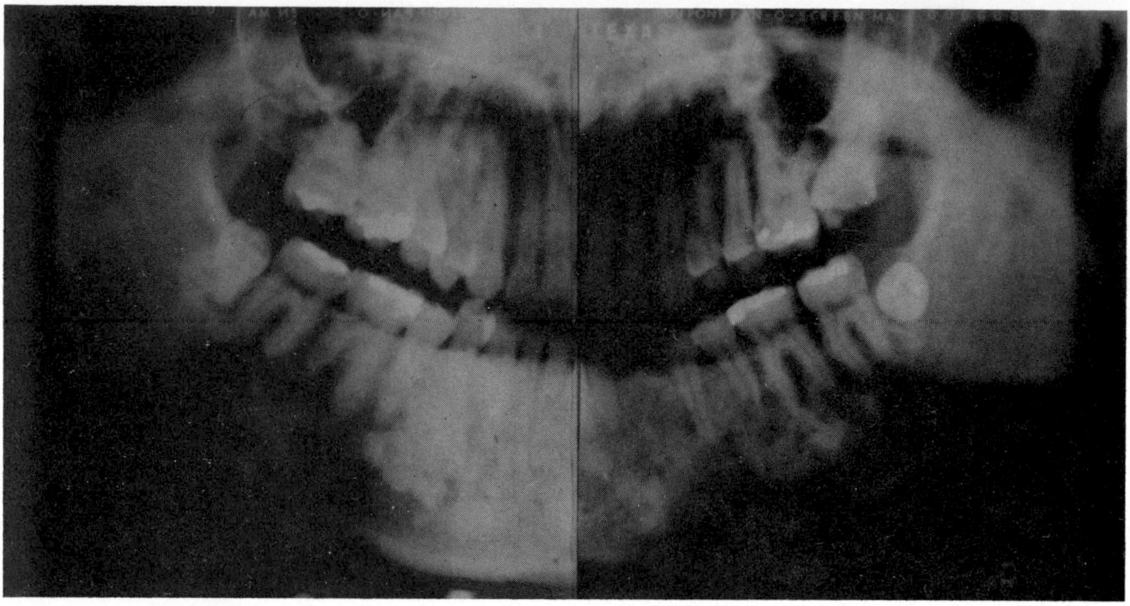

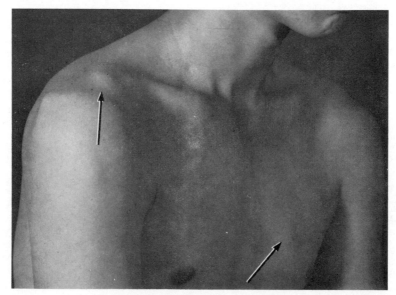

Figure 1–46. *Gardner's syndrome.*
Multiple diffuse osteomas of the maxilla and mandible are present, although the patient does not have supernumerary teeth. (Courtesy of Drs. Wesley P. Titterington and William M. Wade, Jr.)

the 126 patients. In 41 of the patients, carcinoma of the intestine subsequently developed and only 27 per cent survived. This disease is of interest to the dental profession, since the impacted teeth and osteomas of the jaws may lead to early diagnosis of the entire syndrome.

PREDECIDUOUS DENTITION

Infants occasionally are born with structures which appear to be erupted teeth, usually in the mandibular incisor area. These structures must be distinguished from true deciduous

Figure 1–47. *Gardner's syndrome.*
Sebaceous cysts of the skin are present over the shoulder and chest. (Courtesy of Drs. Wesley P. Titterington and William M. Wade, Jr.)

teeth, or the so-called natal teeth described by Massler, which may have erupted by the time of birth. The predeciduous teeth have been described as hornified epithelial structures without roots, occurring on the gingiva over the crest of the ridge, which may be easily removed. Prematurely erupted true deciduous teeth, of course, are not to be extracted. These predeciduous teeth have been thought to arise either from an accessory bud of the dental lamina ahead of the deciduous bud or from the bud of an accessory dental lamina.

The concept of predeciduous teeth has been questioned by Spouge and Feasby, however. They are probably correct in believing that considering predeciduous teeth as an entity is a misinterpretation and that such structures, present at birth, undoubtedly represent only the dental lamina cyst of the newborn (q.v.). This cyst does commonly project above the crest of the ridge, is white in color and is packed with keratin, so that it appears "hornified" and can be easily removed.

POSTPERMANENT DENTITION

A few cases are recorded of persons who have had all their permanent teeth extracted and yet have subsequently erupted several more teeth, particularly after the insertion of a full denture. The majority of such cases are the result of delayed eruption of retained or embedded teeth. A small number of cases, however, do appear to represent examples of a postpermanent or third dentition, although it probably would be better to classify these as simply multiple supernumerary unerupted teeth, since they probably develop from a bud of the dental lamina beyond the permanent tooth germ.

DEVELOPMENTAL DISTURBANCES IN STRUCTURE OF TEETH

AMELOGENESIS IMPERFECTA

(Hereditary Enamel Dysplasia; Hereditary Brown Enamel; Hereditary Brown Opalescent Teeth)

Amelogenesis imperfecta represents a group of hereditary defects of enamel unassociated with any other generalized defects. It is entirely an ectodermal disturbance, since the mesodermal components of the teeth are basically normal.

The development of normal enamel occurs in three stages: (1) the formative stage, during which there is deposition of the organic matrix; (2) the calcification stage, during which this matrix is mineralized; and (3) the maturation stage, during which crystallites enlarge and mature. Accordingly, three basic types of amelogenesis imperfecta are recognized: (1) the hypoplastic type, in which there is defective formation of matrix; (2) the hypocalcification (hypomineralization) type, in which there is defective mineralization of the formed matrix; and (3) the hypomaturation type, in which enamel crystallites remain immature.

A classification of amelogenesis imperfecta based on clinical, histologic, and genetic criteria has been established by Witkop and Sauk as follows:

1. Hypoplastic
   a. Pitted, autosomal dominant
   b. Local, autosomal dominant
   c. Smooth, autosomal dominant
   d. Rough, autosomal dominant
   e. Rough, autosomal recessive
   f. Smooth, X-linked dominant
2. Hypocalcified
   a. Autosomal dominant
   b. Autosomal recessive
3. Hypomaturation
   a. Hypomaturation—hypoplastic with taurodontism, autosomal dominant
   b. X-linked recessive
   c. Pigmented, autosomal recessive
   d. Snow-capped teeth

Clinical Features. As an aid in diagnosis for the clinician, the general clinical features of the three major types of amelogenesis imperfecta have also been established by Witkop and Sauk:

1. Hypoplastic type. The enamel has not formed to full normal thickness on newly erupted developing teeth (Fig. 1–48).

2. Hypocalcified type. The enamel is so soft that it can be removed by a prophylaxis instrument (Fig. 1–49).

3. Hypomaturation type. The enamel can be pierced by an explorer point under firm pressure and can be lost by chipping away from the underlying normal-appearing dentin.

The teeth in these various forms of amelogenesis imperfecta listed in this classification may vary remarkably in clinical appearance from type to type, as the descriptions suggest. In any given case, all teeth of both dentitions are affected to some degree. In some cases, the teeth may appear essentially normal; in others,

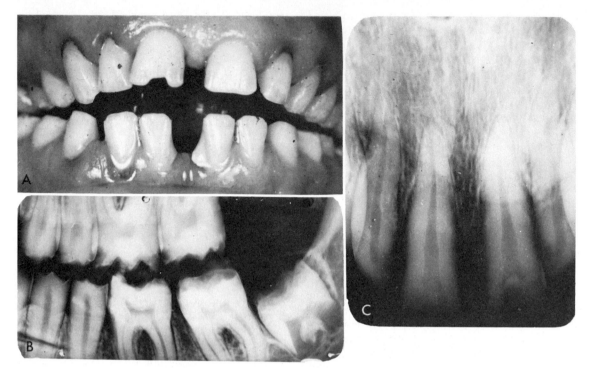

Figure 1–48. *Amelogenesis imperfecta, hypoplastic (aplastic) type.*
A, The patient has complete agenesis of enamel. Note the severe bobby pin abrasion of the exposed dentin. *B,* The enamel is absent except for a thin shell over the tips of the cusps. *C,* The roentgenogram shows complete absence of enamel and marked secondary dentin formation beneath the area of abrasion.

they may be extremely unsightly. In some forms, there is even a difference in the appearance of the teeth between males and females.

The crowns of the teeth may or may not show discoloration. If present, it varies depending upon the type of the disorder, ranging from yellow to dark brown. In some cases, the enamel may be totally absent; in others, it may have a chalky texture or even a cheesy consist-

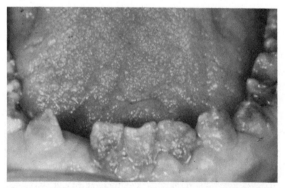

Figure 1–49. *Amelogenesis imperfecta, hypocalcification type.*
The enamel is poorly calcified and irregular.

ency or be relatively hard. Sometimes the enamel is smooth or it may have numerous parallel vertical wrinkles or grooves. It may be chipped or show depressions, in the base of which dentin may be exposed. Contact points between teeth are often open and occlusal surfaces and incisal edges frequently are severely abraded.

Roentgenographic Features. The over-all shape of the tooth may or may not be normal, depending upon the amount of enamel present on the tooth and the amount of occlusal and incisal wear. The enamel may appear totally absent on the roentgenogram or, when present, may appear as a very thin layer, chiefly over the tips of the cusps and on the interproximal surfaces (Fig. 1–48). In other cases the calcification of the enamel may be so affected that it appears to have the same approximate radiodensity as the dentin, making differentiation between the two difficult.

Histologic Features. The general histologic features of the enamel also parallel the general type of amelogenesis imperfecta that has been diagnosed. There is a disturbance in the differentiation or viability of ameloblasts in the hypoplastic type, and this is reflected in defects in matrix formation up to and including total absence of matrix. In the hypocalcification types there are defects of matrix structure and of mineral deposition. Finally, in the hypomaturation types there are alterations in enamel rod and rod sheath structures.

Treatment. There is no treatment except for improvement of cosmetic appearance. However, in some cases, these teeth do not appear markedly abnormal to the casual observer.

ENVIRONMENTAL ENAMEL HYPOPLASIA

Enamel hypoplasia may be defined as an incomplete or defective formation of the organic enamel matrix of teeth. Two basic types of enamel hypoplasia exist: (1) a hereditary type, described previously under amelogenesis imperfecta, and (2) a type caused by environmental factors. In the hereditary type, both the deciduous and permanent dentitions usually are involved and generally only the enamel is affected. In contrast, when the defect is caused by environmental factors, either dentition may be involved and sometimes only a single tooth;

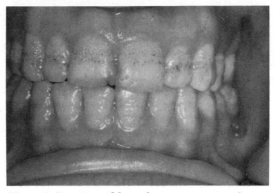

Figure 1–51. *Enamel hypoplasia, environmental type.* Several rows of irregular, stained pits cover much of the labial surfaces of the teeth.

both enamel and dentin are usually affected, at least to some degree.

Many studies, both experimental and clinical, have been carried out in an attempt to determine the cause and nature of environmental enamel hypoplasia. It is known that a number of different factors, each capable of producing injury to the ameloblasts, may give rise to the condition, including: (1) nutritional deficiency (vitamins A, C, and D); (2) exanthematous diseases (e.g., measles, chickenpox, scarlet fever); (3) congenital syphilis; (4) hypocalcemia; (5) birth injury, prematurity, Rh hemolytic disease; (6) local infection or trauma; (7) ingestion of chemicals (chiefly fluoride); and (8) idiopathic causes.

In mild environmental hypoplasia, there may be only a few small grooves, pits, or fissures on the enamel surface (Fig. 1–50). If the condition is more severe, the enamel may exhibit rows of deep pits arranged horizontally across the surface of the tooth (Fig. 1–51). There may be only a single row of such pits or several rows indicating a series of injuries. In the most severe cases, a considerable portion of enamel may be absent, suggesting a prolonged disturbance in the function of the ameloblasts.

Hypoplasia results only if the injury occurs during the time the teeth are developing or, more specifically, during the formative stage of enamel development. Once the enamel has calcified, no such defect can be produced. Thus, knowing the chronologic development of the deciduous and permanent teeth, it is possible to determine from the location of the defect on the teeth the approximate time at which the injury occurred.

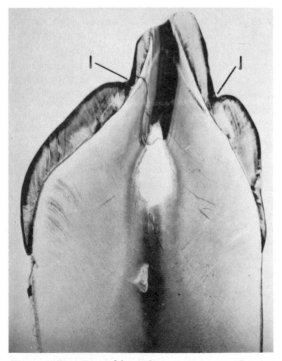

Figure 1–50. *Enamel hypoplasia, environmental type.* The ground section of tooth shows a pitlike defect on both the labial and lingual surfaces *(1)*.

Hypoplasia Due to Nutritional Deficiency and Exanthematous Fevers

Some studies have shown that rickets during the time of tooth formation is the most common known cause of enamel hypoplasia. For example, in a series of rachitic children reported by Shelling and Anderson, 43 per cent of teeth showed hypoplasia. At present, however, rickets is not a prevalent disease. Deficiencies of vitamin A and vitamin C have also been named as causes.

Some studies have indicated that the exanthematous diseases, including measles, chickenpox, and scarlet fever, are etiologic factors, but other investigators have been unable to confirm this finding. In general, it might be stated that any serious nutritional deficiency or systemic disease is potentially capable of producing enamel hypoplasia, since the ameloblasts are one of the most sensitive groups of cells in the body in terms of metabolic function.

The type of hypoplasia occurring from these deficiency or disease states is usually of the pitting variety described above. Since the pits tend to stain, the clinical appearance of the teeth may be very unsightly.

Clinical studies indicate that most cases of enamel hypoplasia involve those teeth that form within the first year after birth, although teeth that form somewhat later may be affected. Thus the teeth most frequently involved are the central and lateral incisors, cuspids, and first molars. Since the tip of the cuspid begins formation before the lateral incisor, some cases involve only the central incisor, cuspid, and first molar. Premolars and second and third molars are seldom affected, since their formation does not begin until about the age of 3 years or later.

There has been considerable controversy as to whether there is any relation between enamel hypoplasia and dental caries experience, and clinical reports have given conflicting results. It is most reasonable to assume that the two are not related, although hypoplastic teeth do appear to decay at a somewhat more rapid rate once caries has been initiated.

Enamel Hypoplasia Due to Congenital Syphilis

The hypoplasia due to congenital syphilis is most frequently not of the pitting variety previously described but instead presents a characteristic, almost pathognomonic, appearance. This hypoplasia involves the maxillary and man-

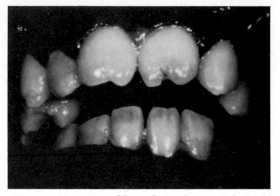

Figure 1–52. *Enamel hypoplasia of congenital syphilis (Hutchinson's incisors).*
There is characteristic notching of the incisal edges of the maxillary central incisors as well as tapering of the mesial and distal surfaces toward the incisal portion.

dibular permanent incisors and the first molars. The anterior teeth affected are sometimes called "Hutchinson's teeth," while the molars have been referred to as "mulberry molars" (Moon's molars, Fournier's molars).

Characteristically, the upper central incisor is "screw-driver" shaped, the mesial and distal surfaces of the crown tapering and converging toward the incisal edge of the tooth rather than toward the cervical margin (Fig. 1–52). In addition, the incisal edge is usually notched. The mandibular central and lateral incisors may be similarly involved, although the maxillary lateral incisor may be normal. The cause of the tapering and notching of the maxillary incisor has been explained on the basis of the absence of the central tubercle or calcification center. The crowns of the first molars in congenital syphilis are irregular and the enamel of the occlusal surface and occlusal third of the tooth appears to be arranged in an agglomerate mass of globules rather than in well-formed cusps (Fig. 1–53). The crown is narrower on the occlusal surface than at the cervical margin.

It has been reported by Fiumara and Lessell that between 1958 and 1969 there has been over a 200 per cent increase in reported cases of primary and secondary syphilis in the United States and that, consequently, congenital syphilis in children under 1 year of age increased 117 per cent during the 10-year period from 1960 to 1969. Investigating 271 patients with congenital syphilis, they found that over 63 per cent had Hutchinson's teeth but they pointed out that this may not be the true incidence, since some of the patients had had their teeth extracted. In addition, approximately 65 per

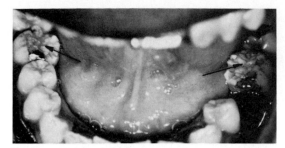

Figure 1–53. *Enamel hypoplasia of congenital syphilis ("mulberry molars").*
The mandibular first molars show many small globular masses of enamel on the occlusal portion of the tooth.

cent of this group of patients with congenital syphilis also had the characteristic "mulberry molars."

Not all patients with congenital syphilis will exhibit these dental findings. Also, occasional patients will appear to have Hutchinson's teeth without having a history of congenital syphilis. Therefore one must not be hasty in making the diagnosis of syphilis, particularly in the absence of the other conditions of Hutchinson's triad (q.v.).

Enamel Hypoplasia Due to Hypocalcemia

Tetany, induced by a decreased level of calcium in the blood, may result from several conditions, the most common being vitamin D deficiency and parathyroid deficiency (parathyroprivic tetany). In tetany the serum calcium level may fall as low as 6 to 8 mg. per 100 ml., and at this level enamel hypoplasia is frequently produced in teeth developing concomitantly. This type of enamel hypoplasia is usually of the pitting variety and thus does not differ from that resulting from a nutritional disturbance or exanthematous disease.

Hypoplasia Due to Birth Injuries

The neonatal line or ring, described by Schour in 1936 and present in deciduous teeth and first permanent molars, may be thought of as a type of hypoplasia because there is produced in the enamel, and in the dentin as well, a disturbance indicative of the trauma or change of environment at the time of birth. In traumatic births the formation of enamel may even cease at this time. In addition, Miller and Forrester have reported a clinical study with evidence that enamel hypoplasia is far more common in

prematurely born children than in normal term infants. In this same study they not only drew attention to the widely recognized staining of teeth in children who had suffered from Rh hemolytic disease at birth (q.v.) but also reported enamel hypoplasia in these cases. Grahnén and Larsson have also shown an increased incidence of enamel hypoplasia in premature children, but interestingly no differences in caries incidence between this group and a control group of children.

Although the literature indicates that most cases of enamel hypoplasia of deciduous teeth involve enamel formed after birth, it is seen also in prenatal enamel. In such instances a gastrointestinal disturbance or some other illness in the mother may be responsible.

Enamel Hypoplasia Due to Local Infection or Trauma

A type of hypoplasia occasionally seen is unusual in that only a single tooth is involved, most commonly one of the permanent maxillary incisors or a maxillary or mandibular premolar. There may be any degree of hypoplasia, ranging from a mild, brownish discoloration of the enamel to a severe pitting and irregularity of the tooth crown (Fig. 1–54). These single teeth are frequently referred to as "Turner's teeth," and the condition is called "Turner's hypoplasia."

If a deciduous tooth becomes carious during the period when the crown of the succeeding permanent tooth is being formed, a bacterial infection involving the periapical tissue of this deciduous tooth may disturb the ameloblastic layer of the permanent tooth and result in a hypoplastic crown. The severity of this hypoplasia will depend upon the severity of the infection, the degree of tissue involvement, and the stage of permanent tooth formation during which the infection occurred.

A similar type of hypoplasia may follow trauma to a deciduous tooth, particularly when the deciduous tooth has been driven into the alveolus and has disturbed the permanent tooth bud. If this permanent tooth crown is still being formed, the resulting injury may be manifested as a yellowish or brownish stain or pigmentation of the enamel, usually on the labial surface, or as a true hypoplastic pitting defect or deformity. This form of dental injury has been discussed by Via, who has pointed out that a disturbance either in matrix formation or in calcification can occur, depending chiefly upon the stage of tooth formation at the time of injury.

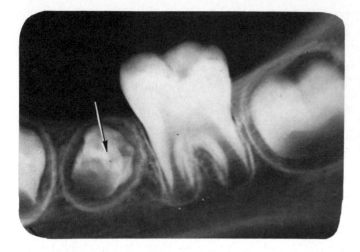

Figure 1–54. *Enamel hypoplasia due to local infection ("Turner's hypoplasia").*
The crown of the unerupted bicuspid is extremely irregular, owing to disruption of the forming tooth by infection through the preceding deciduous tooth. (Courtesy of Dr. Ralph E. McDonald.)

Enamel Hypoplasia Due to Fluoride: Mottled Enamel

Mottled enamel is a type of enamel hypoplasia that was first described under that term in this country by G. V. Black and Frederick S. McKay in 1916. Earlier reference to the condition is known in the foreign literature, however. Black and McKay recognized that this lesion exhibited a geographic distribution and even suggested that it was a result of some substance in the water supply, although it was not until some years later that fluorine was shown to be the causative agent.

Etiology. It is now recognized that the ingestion of fluoride-containing drinking water during the time of tooth formation may result in mottled enamel. The severity of the mottling increases with an increasing amount of fluoride in the water. Thus there is little mottling of any clinical significance at a level below 0.9 to 1.0 part per million of fluoride in the water, whereas it becomes progressively evident above this level.

Pathogenesis. This type of hypoplasia is due to a disturbance of the ameloblasts during the formative stage of tooth development. The exact nature of the injury is not known, but since there is histologic evidence of cell damage, it is likely that the cell product, the enamel matrix, is defective or deficient. It also has been shown that, with somewhat higher levels of fluoride, there is interference with the calcification process of the matrix.

Epidemiologic studies have reported that not all children born and reared in an area of

Table 1–13. Incidence of Dental Fluorosis (Mottled Enamel) as Related to the Fluoride Concentration of the Water Supply

CITY	NO. OF PATIENTS EXAMINED	% AFFECTED	F (PPM)	PERCENTAGE DISTRIBUTION						AGE GROUP OF PATIENTS (YRS.)
				SIGNS ABSENT		WHITE OPAQUE SPOTS		BROWN STAINS AND PITTING		
				NORMAL	QUESTIONABLE	VERY MILD	MILD	MODERATE	SEVERE	
Zanesville, Ohio	459	1.5	0.2	85.4	13.1	1.5	0.0	0.0	0.0	12–14
Marion, Ohio	263	6.1	0.4	57.4	36.5	5.3	0.8	0.0	0.0	12–14
Kewanee, Illinois ...	123	12.2	0.9	52.8	35.0	10.6	1.6	0.0	0.0	12–14
Joliet, Illinois	447	25.3	1.3	40.5	34.2	22.2	3.1	0.0	0.0	12–14
Colorado Springs, Colorado	404	73.8	2.6	6.4	19.8	42.1	21.3	8.9	1.5	12–14
Lubbock, Texas	189	97.8	4.4	1.1	1.1	12.2	21.7	46.0	17.9	9–12
Bauxite, Arkansas ..	26	100.0	14.1	0.0	0.0	3.9	3.9	38.5	53.8	14–19

Modified from H. T. Dean: Epidemiological studies in the United States; in Fluorine and Dental Health. Washington, D.C., American Association for the Advancement of Science, 1942.

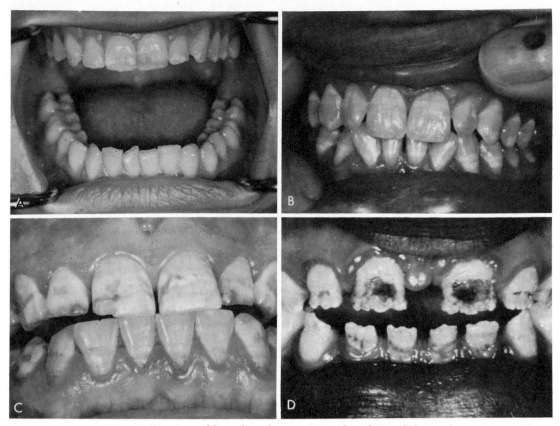

Figure 1–55. *Enamel hypoplasia due to excessive fluoride (mottled enamel).*
There is (A, B) flecking of the enamel surface by white opaque spots, (C) involvement of most of the tooth surface by opaque white areas, and (D) severe pitting and staining of the tooth surface.

endemic fluorosis exhibit the same degree of mottling even though they all have used the same water supply. Furthermore, a few persons may exhibit mild mottling even when exposed to a very low concentration of fluoride (Table 1–13). These findings may be related to individual variation in total water consumption and thus to total fluoride intake.

Clinical Features. Depending upon the level of fluoride in the water supply, there is a wide range of severity in the appearance of mottled teeth, varying from (1) questionable changes characterized by occasional white flecking or spotting of the enamel (Fig. 1–55, A), through (2) mild changes manifested by white opaque areas involving more of the tooth surface area (Fig. 1–55, B), to (3) moderate and severe changes showing pitting and brownish staining of the surface (Fig. 1–55, C), and even (4) a corroded appearance of the teeth (Fig. 1–55, D). Those teeth which are moderately or severely affected may show a tendency for wear and even fracture of the enamel. Early studies

actually noted the difficulty of retaining restorations in such teeth. (See also Plate I.)

Geographic Distribution. Mottled enamel has been reported in many parts of the world, including Europe, Africa, and Asia as well as the United States. In this country, persons in at least 400 areas in 28 states have shown dental evidence of endemic fluorosis, and undoubtedly more communities remain to be reported. Most of the areas affected are west of the Mississippi River, the largest single area being the Texas Panhandle, but there are numerous communities east of the Mississippi River in which fluorosis is present, the most notable being in Illinois.

The well-known relation between mottled enamel (or actually fluoride intake) and dental caries will be discussed in the chapter on dental caries.

Treatment. Mottled enamel frequently becomes stained an unsightly brown color. For cosmetic reasons, it has become the practice to bleach the affected teeth with an agent such as hydrogen peroxide. This is frequently effective, but the procedure must be carried out periodically, since the teeth continue to stain.

Hypoplasia Due to Idiopathic Factors

Although numerous factors have been reported as being possibly responsible for causing enamel hypoplasia, clinical studies have shown that, even with careful histories, the majority of cases are of unknown origin. Since the ameloblast is a sensitive type of cell and easily damaged, it is likely that in those cases in which the etiology cannot be determined, the causative agent may have been some illness or systemic disturbance so mild that it made no impression on the patient and was not remembered. Even relatively severe cases of enamel hypoplasia arise with no pertinent past medical history to account for their occurrence.

Dentinogenesis Imperfecta

(Hereditary Opalescent Dentin)

Cases representative of dentinogenesis imperfecta have been reported under a variety of terms, the most common being "hereditary opalescent dentin" and "odontogenesis imperfecta." This latter term is incorrect, however, since only the mesodermal portion of the odontogenic apparatus is disturbed. This abnormality differs from amelogenesis imperfecta, as the name would indicate, in that the dentin rather than the enamel is defective. Yet the two conditions have been frequently confused.

Among the earliest reported cases were those of Wilson and Steinbrecher, who traced this condition through four generations of one family. Excellent studies of the chemical, physical, histologic, roentgenographic, and clinical aspects of dentinogenesis imperfecta were made by Finn in 1938 and by Hodge and his coworkers in 1939 and 1940. A racially isolated inbred group of persons with an unusually high incidence of dentinogenesis imperfecta was investigated by Hursey and his associates, who reported wide variation in the manifestations of the dentinal disturbance among the cases studied. Heys and her co-workers have described the clinical and genetic factors in 18 families afflicted with dentinogenesis imperfecta occurring in association with osteogenesis imperfecta (q.v.). This association between dentinogenesis

imperfecta and osteogenesis imperfecta, both hereditary mesodermal defects, is well recognized, although each condition may occur independently.

The variability in expression of various cases of dentinogenesis imperfecta has made it clear that several forms of the disease apparently exist. In order to separate these for clarity, Shields and his co-workers have suggested the following classification:

Type I. Dentinogenesis imperfecta (DI) that always occurs in families with osteogenesis imperfecta (OI), although the latter may occur without dentinogenesis imperfecta. Type I DI segregates as an autosomal dominant trait with variable expressivity but can be recessive if the accompanying osteogenesis imperfecta is recessive (usually the severe OI congenita type).

Type II. Dentinogenesis imperfecta that never occurs in association with osteogenesis imperfecta unless by chance. This type is the one most frequently referred to as hereditary opalescent dentin. It is inherited as an autosomal dominant trait and in fact is one of the most common dominantly inherited disorders in humans, affecting approximately one in every 8000 persons. Sporadic cases are virtually unreported.

Type III. Dentinogenesis imperfecta of the "Brandywine type." This is a racial isolate in Maryland with this unusual form of DI characterized by the same clinical appearance of the teeth as types I and II but also by multiple pulp exposures in deciduous teeth, a characteristic not seen in types I or II. Type III is an autosomal dominant trait.

Clinical Features. The clinical appearance of the teeth in all three types of this condition

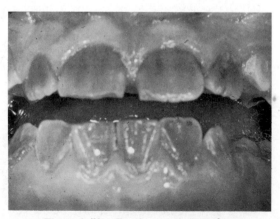

Figure 1–56. *Dentinogenesis imperfecta.*

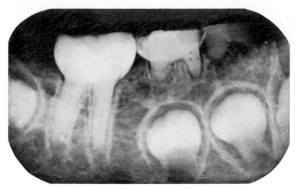

Figure 1–57. *Dentinogenesis imperfecta.*
The roentgenogram illustrates obliteration of the pulp chambers and root canals not only of the permanent teeth but also of the primary teeth. The primary teeth also show severe attrition.

varies greatly. In general, the deciduous teeth are more severely affected than the permanent teeth in type I, whereas in type II the dentitions are equally affected. Both dentitions are affected in type III, but information on relative severity is sketchy.

The color of the teeth may range from a gray to brownish violet or yellowish brown, but they exhibit a characteristic unusual translucent or opalescent hue (Fig. 1–56). The enamel may be lost early through fracturing away, especially on the incisal and occlusal surfaces of the teeth, presumably because of an abnormal dentinoenamel junction. The usual scalloping of this junction, which tends to form an interlocking union between the enamel and dentin, is reportedly absent, although this finding has been refuted in other reports. With the early loss of enamel, the dentin undergoes rapid attrition, and the occlusal surfaces of deciduous and permanent molars are often severely flattened. The teeth do not appear to be more susceptible to dental caries than normal teeth.

Roentgenographic Features. The teeth in types I and II present an unusual and pathognomonic appearance on the dental roentgenogram. The most striking feature is the partial or total precocious obliteration of the pulp chambers and root canals by continued formation of dentin (Figs. 1–57, 1–58). This is seen in both the deciduous and the permanent teeth. Although the roots may be short and blunted, the cementum, periodontal membrane, and supporting bone appear normal.

In type III, there is a great variability in the

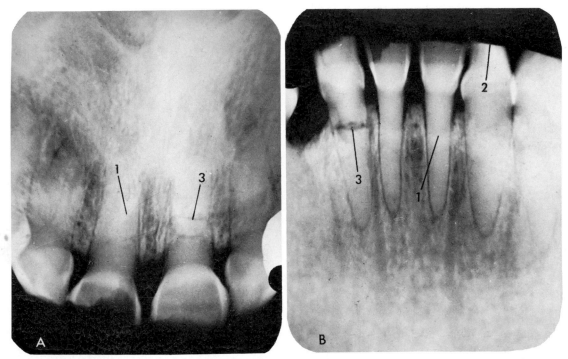

Figure 1–58. *Dentinogenesis imperfecta.*
The roentgenograms illustrate the obliteration of the pulp chambers and root canals *(1)*, attrition *(2)*, and root fractures *(3)*.

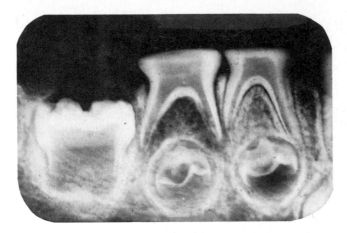

Figure 1–59. *Dentinogenesis imperfecta, type III with enamel aplasia.*
(From C. B. Schimmelpfennig and R. E. McDonald: Oral Surg., 6:1444, 1953.)

deciduous teeth, ranging from normal to those changes just described in types I and II. However, the affected patients in the Brandywine population reported by Witkop had features characterized as "shell teeth." This condition was originally described by Rushton under that name and represents a dentinal disturbance in which the enamel of the tooth appears essentially normal, while the dentin is extremely thin, and the pulp chambers are enormous. The large size of the pulp chambers is due not to resorption but rather to insufficient and defective dentin formation. In addition, the roots of the teeth are extremely short. On the roentgenogram, all of the teeth appear as "shells" of enamel and dentin surrounding extremely large pulp chambers and root canals. While most of the teeth exhibit short roots, there is no evidence of root resorption. One other similar case has been reported by Schimmelpfennig and McDonald under the term "enamel and dentin aplasia" (Fig. 1–59). Essentially the report described a family with "shell teeth" of type III in combination with enamel aplasia. This family was subsequently found to be related to the Brandywine group.

Histologic Features. The histologic appearance of the teeth in types I and II emphasizes the fact that this is purely a mesodermal disturbance. The appearance of the enamel is essentially normal except for its peculiar shade, which is actually a manifestation of the dentinal disturbance. The dentin, on the other hand, is composed of irregular tubules, often with large areas of uncalcified matrix (Fig. 1–60). The tubules tend to be larger in diameter and thus less numerous than normal in a given volume of dentin (Fig. 1–61). In some areas there may be complete absence of tubules. Cellular inclusions, probably odontoblasts, in the dentin are

not uncommon and, as pointed out previously, the pulp chamber is usually almost obliterated by the continued deposition of dentin. The odontoblasts have only limited ability to form well-organized dentinal matrix, and they appear to degenerate readily, becoming entrapped in this matrix.

The histopathology of the teeth in type III has not been adequately documented.

Chemical and Physical Features. Chemical analysis explains many of the abnormal features of the teeth of types I and II of dentinogenesis

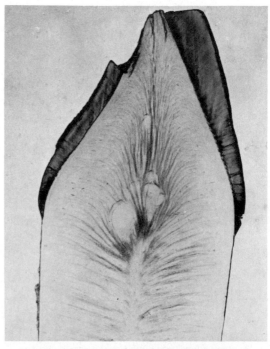

Figure 1–60. *Dentinogenesis imperfecta.*
Ground section of tooth.

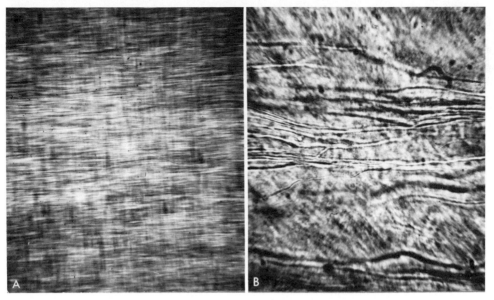

Figure 1–61. *Dentinogenesis imperfecta.*
A, Normal dentin showing regular dentinal tubules. *B,* Large irregular dentinal tubules in dentinogenesis imperfecta.
Both photomicrographs taken at same magnification.

imperfecta. Their water content is greatly increased, as much as 60 per cent above normal, while the inorganic content is less than that of normal dentin. As might be expected, the density, x-ray absorption, and hardness of the dentin are also low. In fact, the micro-hardness of the dentin closely approximates that of cementum, thus explaining the rapid attrition of affected teeth. There is no significant information available on teeth in type III.

Treatment. The treatment of patients with dentinogenesis imperfecta is directed primarily toward preventing the loss of enamel and subsequent loss of dentin through attrition. Cast metal crowns on the posterior teeth and jacket crowns on the anterior teeth have been used with considerable success, although care must be taken in the preparation of the teeth for such restorations. Caution must also be exercised in the use of partial appliances which exert stress on the teeth, because the roots are easily fractured. Experience has further shown that fillings are not usually permanent because of the softness of the dentin.

DENTIN DYSPLASIA

("Rootless Teeth")

Dentin dysplasia is a rare disturbance of dentin formation characterized by normal en-amel but atypical dentin formation with abnormal pulpal morphology.

At one time this was thought to be a single disease entity, but it now has been separated by Shields and his associates into type I (dentin dysplasia) and type II (anomalous dysplasia of dentin). However, Witkop has suggested that as a guide to the clinician, these conditions be referred to as *radicular dentin dysplasia (type I)* and *coronal dentin dysplasia (type II)*. It has been found that type I is by far the more common.

The first description of the disease was that of Ballschmiede, who in 1920 reported the spontaneous exfoliation of multiple teeth in seven children of one family and called this phenomenon "rootless teeth." The first concise description of the disease was published in 1939 by Rushton, who was also the first to designate it as "dentin dysplasia."

Etiology. Dentin dysplasia, both type I and type II, appears to be a hereditary disease, transmitted as an autosomal dominant characteristic. Nothing is known of the mutation rate, but it must be extremely low.

Clinical Features. *Type I (radicular).* Both dentitions are affected, although the teeth appear clinically normal in morphologic appearance and color. On occasion, there may be a slight amber translucency. The teeth generally exhibit a normal eruption pattern, although delayed eruption has been reported in a few

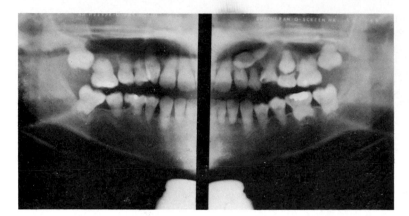

Figure 1–62. *Dentinal dysplasia, type I (radicular).*
The exceptionally short roots and obliteration of pulp chambers and root canals are clearly evident. (Courtesy of Dr. Arthur S. Miller; from A. S. Miller and K. Brookreson: Pa. Dent. J., 37:134, 1970.)

cases. However, the teeth characteristically exhibit extreme mobility and are commonly exfoliated prematurely or after only minor trauma as a result of their abnormally short roots.

Type II (coronal). Both dentitions are also affected in this form of dentin dysplasia, although the involvement of each dentition is different clinically, radiographically, and histologically. The deciduous teeth have the same yellow, brown, or bluish-grey opalescent appearance as seen in dentinogenesis imperfecta. However, the clinical appearance of the permanent dentition is normal.

Roentgenographic Features. *Type I (radicular).* In both dentitions, the roots are short, blunt, conical, or similarly malformed (Fig. 1–62). In the deciduous teeth, the pulp chambers and root canals are usually completely obliterated, while in the permanent dentition, a crescent-shaped pulpal remnant may still be seen in the pulp chamber. This obliteration in the permanent teeth commonly occurs pre-eruptively. Of significant interest is the discovery of periapical radiolucencies representing granulomas, cysts, or abscesses involving apparently otherwise intact teeth.

Type II (coronal). The pulp chambers of the deciduous teeth become obliterated as in type I and in dentinogenesis imperfecta. This does not occur before eruption. The permanent teeth, however, exhibit an abnormally large pulp chamber in the coronal portion of the tooth, often described as "thistle-tube" in shape, and within such areas radiopaque foci resembling pulp stones may be found. Periapical radiolucencies do not occur unless for an obvious reason.

Histologic Features. *Type I (radicular).* A portion of the coronal dentin is usually normal. Apical to this may be areas of tubular dentin,

but most of that which obliterates the pulp is calcified tubular dentin, osteodentin, and fused denticles. Normal dentinal tubule formation appears to have been blocked so that new dentin forms around obstacles and takes on the characteristic appearance described as "lava flowing around boulders" (Fig. 1–63). Electron microscope studies by Sauk and his co-workers

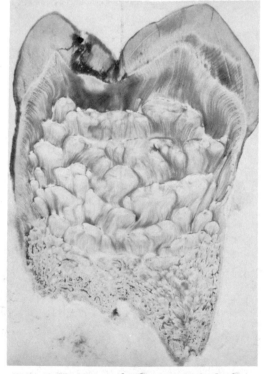

Figure 1–63. *Dentin dysplasia, type I (radicular).*
The atypicality of root dentin and dentin filling the pulp chamber is seen in this ground section of tooth. (Courtesy of Drs. Richard K. Wesley and George Wysocki. From Oral Surg., 41:516, 1976.)

have suggested that this pattern of "cascades of dentin" results from repetitive attempts to form root structure. Interestingly, the dentin itself is histologically normal but is simply disoriented.

Type II (coronal). The deciduous teeth exhibit amorphous and atubular dentin in the radicular portion, while coronal dentin is relatively normal. The permanent teeth also show relatively normal coronal dentin, but the pulp has multiple pulp stones or denticles.

Excellent scanning electron microscope studies of both types I and II dentin dysplasia have been reported by Melnick and his associates, and these have added appreciably to our knowledge of the atypical structure of this dentin.

Treatment and Prognosis. There is no treatment for the disease, and its prognosis depends upon the occurrence of periapical lesions necessitating tooth extraction as well as upon the exfoliation of teeth due to increased mobility.

REGIONAL ODONTODYSPLASIA

(Odontodysplasia; Odontogenic Dysplasia; Odontogenesis Imperfecta; "Ghost Teeth")

This is an unusual dental anomaly in which one or several teeth in a localized area are affected in an unusual manner. Apparently the maxillary teeth are involved more frequently than the mandibular, the most frequently affected teeth being the maxillary permanent central incisor, lateral incisor, and cuspid. In

the mandible, the same three anterior teeth are most often affected. The deciduous teeth as well as the permanent may be involved.

The etiology of this disease is unknown inasmuch as there is no history of trauma or systemic illness. It has been suggested that the condition may represent a somatic mutation, although the possibility has also been raised that it could be due to a latent virus residing in the odontogenic epithelium, which subsequently becomes active during the development of the tooth. In an excellent review of cases in the literature and a discussion of the condition, Walton and his co-workers observed that in three cases of regional odontodysplasia that they reported, all three patients had had vascular nevi of the overlying facial skin as infants. They reported similar involvement in three additional cases in the literature, and these findings suggested to them that local vascular defects are involved in the pathogenesis of the condition. An early comprehensive account was also reported by Rushton.

Clinical Features. The teeth affected by odontodysplasia exhibit either a delay or a total failure in eruption. Their shape is markedly altered, being generally very irregular in appearance, often with evidence of defective mineralization.

Roentgenographic Features. The roentgenograms are uniquely characteristic, showing a marked reduction in radiodensity so that the teeth assume a "ghost" appearance (Fig. 1–64,

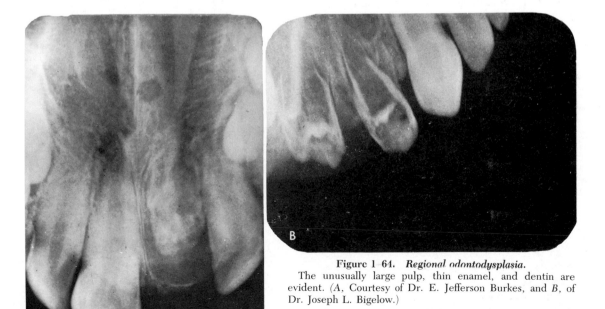

Figure 1–64. *Regional odontodysplasia.*
The unusually large pulp, thin enamel, and dentin are evident. (*A*, Courtesy of Dr. E. Jefferson Burkes, and *B*, of Dr. Joseph L. Bigelow.)

A, B). Both the enamel and dentin appear very thin and the pulp chamber is exceedingly large. The enamel layer often is not evident.

Histologic Features. The most characteristic features of the disease are the marked reduction in the amount of dentin, the widening of the predentin layer, the presence of large areas of interglobular dentin, and an irregular tubular pattern of dentin. Characteristically, the reduced enamel epithelium around nonerupted teeth shows many irregular calcified bodies. Ultrastructural studies by Sapp and Gardner have proved enlightening in detailing some of the fine components of both the soft and calcified tissues in regional odontodysplasia.

Treatment. Because of the poor cosmetic appearance of these teeth, extraction with restoration by a prosthetic appliance is usually indicated.

DENTIN HYPOCALCIFICATION

Normal dentin is calcified by deposition of calcium salts in the organic matrix in the form of globules, which increase in size by further peripheral deposition of salts until all the globules are finally united into a homogeneous structure. In dentinal hypocalcification there is failure of union of many of these globules, leaving interglobular areas of uncalcified matrix. This globular dentin is easily detected in both ground sections and decalcified histologic sections of teeth, but there is no alteration in their clinical appearance.

Many clinicians believe that they can detect areas of globular dentin by the softness of the dental structure. Although this remains to be proved, it is logical that hypocalcified dentin would be softer than well-calcified dentin.

The causes of dentin hypocalcification are similar to those of environmental enamel hypocalcification and enamel hypoplasia. Obviously, any factor which interferes with normal calcification, such as parathyroid deficiency or rickets, could produce hypocalcification.

DISTURBANCES OF GROWTH (ERUPTION) OF TEETH

It is recognized that a broad range of variation exists in the normal eruption times of the deciduous and permanent teeth in different persons. A valuable modification of the usually accepted chronology of the calcification and eruption times of the deciduous teeth has been published by Lunt and Law. Because of this inherent biologic variation, which is particularly notable in the human being, it is difficult to determine when the eruption dates of the teeth of a given person are outside the limits of the normal range. Nevertheless, certain cases do occur in which the eruption time is grossly beyond the extremes of normality and may be considered a pathologic state. The significance of this is frequently not apparent.

PREMATURE ERUPTION

Deciduous teeth that have erupted into the oral cavity are occasionally seen in infants at birth. These are called *natal teeth* in contrast with *neonatal teeth*, which have been defined as those teeth erupting prematurely in the first 30 days of life. Usually only one or two teeth erupt early, most often the deciduous and mandibular central incisors. The etiology of this phenomenon is unknown, although in some instances it follows a familial pattern. It is well recognized in experimental animals that the secretion of several endocrine organs (e.g., thyroid, adrenals, and gonads) may alter the eruption rate of teeth, and it has been suggested that in some cases of early eruption in humans a poorly defined endocrine disturbance may be present. In cases of the adrenogenital syndrome (q.v.) developing early in life, premature eruption of teeth is sometimes seen. Most cases, however, defy explanation.

Spouge and Feasby have pointed out that prematurely erupted teeth are often well formed and normal in all respects except that they may be somewhat mobile. These teeth should be retained even though nursing difficulties may be experienced. A series of 18 cases of natal and neonatal teeth has been studied clinically and histologically by Berman and Silverstone, who reported that these were essentially normal teeth compatible with their chronologic age of development.

The premature eruption of permanent teeth is usually a sequela of the premature loss of deciduous teeth. This is best demonstrated in the situation in which only a single deciduous tooth has been lost, with subsequent eruption of the succedaneous tooth. Occasionally, cases occur involving the entire dentition, and here again the possibility of an endocrine dysfunction (e.g., hyperthyroidism) must be considered.

ERUPTION SEQUESTRUM

The eruption sequestrum, an anomaly associated with the eruption of teeth in children, was first described by Starkey and Shafer.

Clinical Features. The eruption sequestrum is a tiny irregular spicule of bone overlying the crown of an erupting permanent molar, found just prior to or immediately following the emergence of the tips of the cusps through the oral mucosa. The spicule directly overlies the central occlusal fossa but is contained within the soft tissue. As the tooth continues to erupt and the cusps emerge, the fragment of bone completely sequestrates through the mucosa and is lost. For a few days, the fragment of bone may be seen lying on the crest of the ridge in a tiny depression from which it may easily be removed (Fig. 1–65, A).

Roentgenographic Features. It is possible to recognize the eruption sequestrum roentgenographically even before the teeth begin to erupt into the oral cavity or before the bony spicule perforates the mucosa. It appears as a tiny irregular opacity overlying the central occlusal fossa but separated from the tooth itself (Fig. 1–65, B).

Etiology. The explanation of this phenomenon is relatively simple. As the molar teeth erupt through the bone, they will occasionally separate a small osseous fragment from the surrounding contiguous bone, much in the fashion of a corkscrew. In most cases, this fragment probably undergoes total resorption prior to eruption. If the bony spicule is large or eruption is fast, complete resorption cannot occur and the eruption sequestrum is observed.

Clinical Significance and Treatment. The clinical significance associated with this condition is that, occasionally, a child may complain of a slight soreness in the area, probably produced by compression of the soft tissue over the spicule during eating and just prior to its breaking through the mucosa, or by the movement of the spicule in the soft tissue crypt during mastication and following eruption through the mucosa. No treatment is necessary, since the condition corrects itself.

DELAYED ERUPTION

Retarded or delayed eruption of the deciduous teeth is difficult to establish unless the eruption is grossly overdue. In many cases the etiology is unknown, although in some instances it may be associated with certain systemic conditions, including rickets, cretinism, and cleidocranial dysplasia (q.v.). Local factors or circumstances may also delay eruption, as in the case of fibromatosis gingivae, in which the dense connective tissue will not permit eruption.

When the local factors can be established as the cause, their treatment may alleviate the condition. In cases of generalized or systemic disturbances in which the dental problem is of secondary importance, treatment of the primary condition, if possible, will frequently bring about tooth eruption.

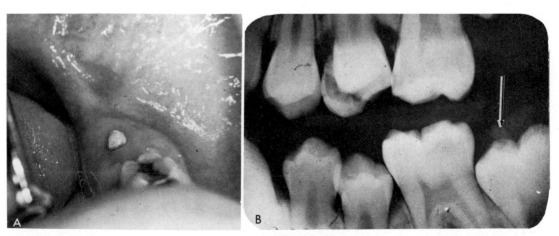

Figure 1–65. *Eruption sequestrum.*
The bony sequestrum is lying on the crest of the ridge (*A*) and may be seen as a small radiopacity (*B*). (From P. E. Starkey and W. G. Shafer: Eruption sequestra in children. J. Dent. Child., *30*:84, 1963.)

Delayed eruption of the permanent dentition as a whole may be associated with the same local or systemic conditions causing the retardation of deciduous tooth eruption. Since there is a wider range of variation in the time of eruption of the permanent teeth, it is frequently difficult to state exactly when a case of retardation exists.

MULTIPLE UNERUPTED TEETH

There is an uncommon condition in which there is a more or less permanently delayed eruption of teeth. The person affected may have retained his deciduous teeth, or, more commonly, the deciduous teeth may have been shed but the permanent teeth have failed to erupt. The term "pseudoanodontia" is sometimes applied to this latter circumstance. In many instances the clinical and roentgenographic examinations reveal apparently normal jaws and teeth. What seems to be lacking is eruptive force.

If this condition is due to an endocrine dysfunction, proper treatment may result in the eruption of teeth; if it is associated with cleidocranial dysplasia (q.v.), there is no known therapy.

EMBEDDED AND IMPACTED TEETH

Embedded teeth are individual teeth which are unerupted usually because of a lack of eruptive force. Impacted teeth are those prevented from erupting by some physical barrier in the eruption path. Some writers do not differentiate between the two terms and call all unerupted teeth impacted.

Lack of space due to crowding of the dental arches or to the premature loss of deciduous teeth with subsequent partial closure of the area they occupied is a common factor in the etiology of partially or completely impacted teeth (Fig. 1–66). Even more common, however, is the rotation of tooth buds resulting in teeth which are "aimed" in the wrong direction because their long axis is not parallel to a normal eruption path.

Any tooth may be impacted, but certain ones are more commonly affected than others. Thus the maxillary and mandibular third molars and the maxillary cuspids are most frequently impacted, followed by the premolars and supernumerary teeth. Of the third molars, the mandibular teeth are more apt to exhibit severe impaction than the maxillary teeth.

Dachi and Howell have published the results of a study of 3874 routine full-mouth roentgenograms of patients over 20 years of age. They found that 17 per cent of these persons had at least one impacted tooth. The incidence of impaction of maxillary and mandibular third molars was 22 per cent and 18 per cent, respectively, while the incidence of impacted maxillary cuspids was 0.9 per cent.

Impacted mandibular third molars may exhibit a great variety of positions (Fig. 1–67). A simple classification of the types of impactions of mandibular third molars, based upon position, has been devised by Winter as follows:

MESIOANGULAR IMPACTION. The third molar lies obliquely in the bone, the crown pointing

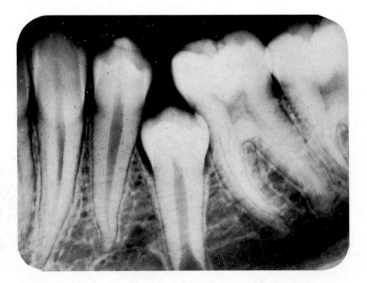

Figure 1–66. *Partial tooth impaction due to premature loss of deciduous molar.*

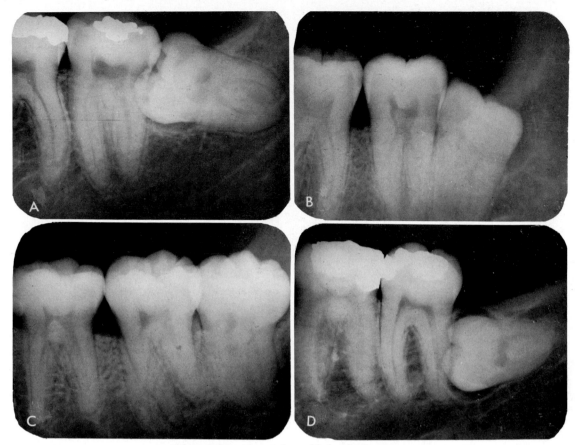

Figure 1–67. *Impacted mandibular third molars.*
A, Mesioangular impaction. *B,* Distoangular impaction. *C,* Vertical impaction. *D,* Horizontal impaction. (Courtesy of Dr. Wilbur C. Moorman.)

in a mesial direction, usually in contact with the distal surface of the root or crown of the second molar. This is the most common type of impaction.

DISTOANGULAR IMPACTION. The third molar lies obliquely in the bone, the crown of the tooth pointing distally toward the ramus, the roots approximating the distal root of the second molar.

VERTICAL IMPACTION. The third molar is in its normal vertical position, but is prevented from erupting by impingement on the distal surface of the second molar or the anterior border of the ramus. Thus, in most cases of this type, there is simply lack of space for eruption.

HORIZONTAL IMPACTION. The third molar is in a horizontal position with respect to the body of the mandible, and the crown may or may not be in contact with the distal surface of the second molar crown or roots. In this type of impaction the third molar may lie at any level within the bone from the crest of the ridge to the inferior border of the mandible.

In addition to these types of impaction in which there is variation of angulation in the sagittal plane, the impacted third molars may also be deflected either buccally or lingually in any case of the foregoing circumstances. Cases also have been recorded of complicated impactions in which the third molar is inverted, the crown pointing toward the inferior border of the mandible, or in which the third molar has been situated completely within the ramus of the mandible.

In the case of impaction of any tooth, but particularly of the mandibular third molar, it is important to determine whether the tooth is completely or only partially impacted. By definition, a completely impacted tooth is one which lies completely within the bone and has no communication with the oral cavity. A partially impacted tooth is not completely encased in bone but lies partially in soft tissue. Although there may be no obvious communication of the tooth with the oral cavity, one may exist (e.g., through a periodontal pocket on the distal of

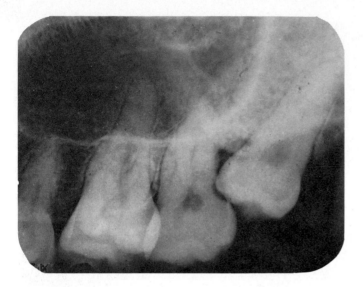

Figure 1–68. *Partially impacted maxillary third molar (mesioangular type).*

the second molar) and create an ideal situation for infection and even dental caries of the impacted tooth crown. A completely embedded or impacted tooth cannot become infected or carious.

Impacted maxillary third molars may be impacted in a manner similar to the mandibular third molar (Fig. 1–68). Thus they may show a mesioangular, distoangular, vertical, or even a horizontal position and may be deflected buccally or lingually.

Impacted maxillary cuspids also assume a variety of positions ranging from horizontal to vertical (Fig. 1–69). In horizontally impacted cuspids the crown usually points in an anterior direction and may impinge on the roots of any of the incisors or premolars. The horizontal tooth may lie either labial or lingual to the associated teeth. The vertically impacted cuspid is usually situated between the roots of the lateral incisor and first premolar and is prevented from eruption simply by lack of space.

The treatment of an impacted tooth depends to a great extent upon the type of tooth involved and the individual circumstances. In some cases, such as the impacted cuspid, it is possible by a suitable orthodontic appliance to bring the tooth into normal occlusion. The majority of impacted teeth, however, must be surgically removed. Because of their location, impacted teeth frequently cause resorption of the roots of adjacent teeth. They may also cause periodic pain and even trismus, particularly when infection occurs around partially impacted teeth. Referred pain from impacted teeth has also been described.

A dentigerous cyst may develop around the

coronal portion of an impacted tooth and may cause displacement of the tooth and destruction of bone. In the study of Dachi and Howell, 37 per cent of impacted mandibular third molars and 15 per cent of impacted maxillary third molars exhibited an area of radiolucency about the crown. About 10 per cent of these radiolucencies were of such a size that they could be considered dentigerous cysts. Furthermore,

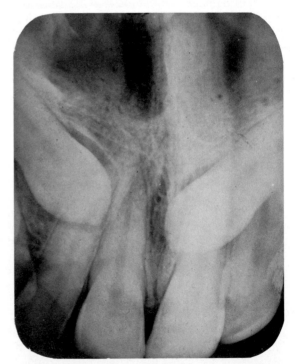

Figure 1–69. *Bilateral impacted maxillary cuspids.*
(Courtesy of Dr. Wilbur C. Moorman.)

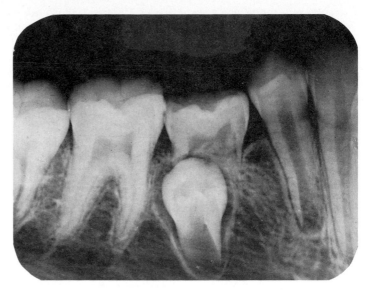

Figure 1–70. *Ankylosed ("submerged") deciduous second molar.* The ankylosed deciduous tooth appears submerged because of the difference in crown height between the deciduous and permanent teeth and continued growth of the alveolar process.

cases of ameloblastoma have been reported developing in the wall of such a cyst. (Dentigerous cysts are discussed in more detail in the chapter on odontogenic cysts and tumors.)

Occasionally, impacted teeth allowed to remain in situ may undergo resorption. The reason that some teeth are resorbed whereas others are not is unknown. The process usually begins on the crown of the tooth and results in destruction of the enamel and dentin, as well as of the cementum, with subsequent replacement by bone. Roentgenographically, early resorption resembles a carious lesion of the crown and has often been mistakenly called caries of an impacted tooth. Obviously, caries is impossible in a tooth that is completely impacted.

ANKYLOSED DECIDUOUS TEETH

("Submerged" Teeth)

"Submerged" teeth are deciduous teeth, most commonly mandibular second molars, that have undergone a variable degree of root resorption and then have become ankylosed to the bone. This process prevents their exfoliation and subsequent replacement by permanent teeth (Fig. 1–70). After the adjacent permanent teeth have erupted, the ankylosed tooth appears to have submerged below the level of occlusion. This illusion is explained by the fact that there has been continued growth of the alveolar process and also that the crown height of the deciduous tooth is less than that of the adjacent permanent teeth, so that the relative level of occlusion has been changed, not the position of the deciduous tooth. This relation between sub-

mersion and ankylosis of human deciduous molars has been studied in detail by Darling and Levers.

The diagnosis of ankylosis of a tooth is usually suspected clinically and confirmed by roentgenographic examination. The teeth affected lack mobility even though root resorption is far advanced. Upon percussion, an ankylosed tooth imparts a characteristic solid sound in contrast to the dull, cushioned sound of a normal tooth. Roentgenographically, at least partial absence of the periodontal ligament is seen, with areas of apparent blending between the tooth root and bone. The process is basically one of resorption of tooth substance and bony repair with the result that the tooth is locked in bone.

The cause of ankylosis is not known, although in some cases trauma, infection, disturbed local metabolism, or a genetic influence has been considered an important etiologic factor. These influences have been discussed by Henderson, who also emphasized that a patient who has had one or two ankylosed teeth is very likely to have other teeth ankylose over a period of time. This condition is usually treated by the surgical removal of the ankylosed tooth to prevent the development of a malocclusion, a local periodontal disturbance, or dental caries.

FISSURAL (INCLUSION, DEVELOPMENTAL) CYSTS OF THE ORAL REGION

A number of different types of fissural (or inclusion) cysts of bone occur in the jaws and have generally been considered arising, as the name would indicate, along lines of fusion of various bones or embryonic processes. These are true cysts (i.e., pathologic cavities lined by epithelium, usually containing fluid or semisolid material), the epithelium being derived from epithelial cells which are entrapped between embryonic processes of bones at union lines. These fissural cysts may be classified as follows: (1) median anterior maxillary cyst, (2) median palatal cyst, (3) globulomaxillary cyst, and (4) median mandibular cyst.

There are several additional developmental cysts derived from embryologic structures or faults which involve the oral or adjacent soft-tissue structures. These may be listed as follows: (1) nasoalveolar cyst, (2) palatal cysts of the neonate, (3) thyroglossal tract cyst, (4) benign cervical lymphoepithelial cyst, (5) epidermoid and dermoid cyst, and (6) heterotopic oral gastrointestinal cyst.

MEDIAN ANTERIOR MAXILLARY CYST

(Nasopalatine Duct Cyst; Incisive Canal Cyst)

The median anterior maxillary cyst, which lies in or near the incisive canal, is the most common type of maxillary developmental cyst. It arises from proliferation of epithelial remnants of the nasopalatine duct, an embryologic structure consisting of a duct or cord of epithelial cells lying within the incisive canal. This canal joins the nasal and oral cavities and is

formed when the palatal processes fuse with the premaxilla, leaving a passageway on each side of the nasal septum. As these paired ducts and the canals approach the oral cavity, they fuse, then exit through a common opening in the palatal bone just posterior to the palatine papilla. Sometimes the incisive canal is subdivided into two separate canals, one for the nasopalatine duct and one for the nasopalatine nerves and vessels. These additional canals have been referred to as the canals of Scarpa and they open onto the hard palate, one behind the other, as the foramina of Scarpa. On rare occasions, the nasopalatine duct may remain patent and appear unilaterally or bilaterally as a tiny slit in the mucosa on either side of the palatine papillae. These structures have been discussed in detail by Goebel.

A rare type of *median alveolar cyst* has been described arising anterior to the incisive canal within the alveolar bone. It is most likely, however, that this type represents a primordial cyst (q.v.) developing from a supernumerary mesiodens tooth bud and, therefore, is not an example of a true fissural cyst but rather a type of odontogenic cyst.

Clinical Features. The studies of Stafne and co-workers concerning the incidence of median anterior maxillary cysts indicate that they may be found in no less than one in every 100 patients and thus cannot be considered rare lesions. According to Abrams and his co-workers, nasopalatine duct cysts can occur at any age, even in the fetus, although their clinical

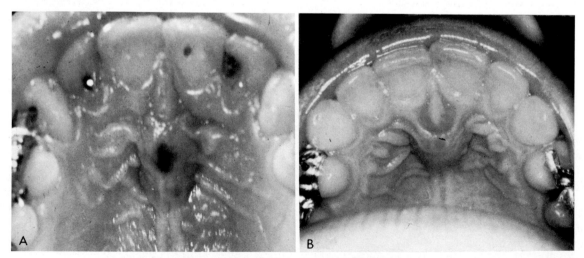

Figure 1–71. *Median anterior maxillary cyst.*
A, An infected cyst has perforated and is draining. B, A cyst of the palatine papilla. (B, Courtesy of Dr. Stephen F. Dachi.)

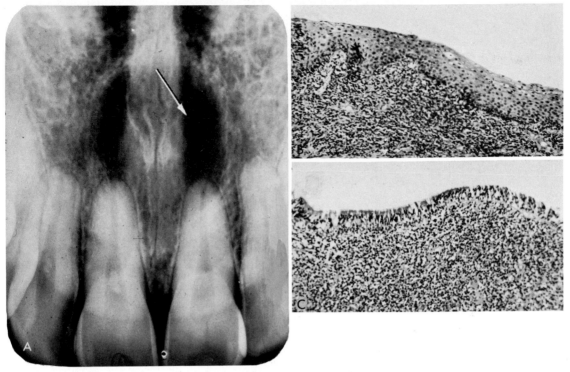

Figure 1–72. *Median anterior maxillary cyst.*

A, The roentgenogram illustrates a relatively large cystic area in the region of the incisive canal. This cyst is lined partially by stratified squamous epithelium *(B)* and partially by ciliated columnar epithelium *(C)*.

discovery is most frequently in the fourth to sixth decades of life.

Many median anterior maxillary cysts give little clinical evidence of their presence. In the series reported by Abrams, nearly 40 per cent of the cases were totally asymptomatic. Sometimes they become infected by some unknown mechanism, producing pain and swelling, and open by a tiny fistula on or near the palatine papilla (Fig. 1–71, *A*). In such cases a tiny drop of watery fluid or pus may be elicited by pressure in the area.

An uncommon variant of these cysts occurs as a swelling within the palatine papilla and has been described as arising from epithelial nests in the incisive foramen rather than in the bone (Fig. 1–71, *B*). It is usually not visible by roentgenographic examination. Lesions of this type are generally called *cysts of the palatine papilla* even though they represent a form of the median anterior maxillary cyst.

Roentgenographic Features. These cysts are often discovered in routine roentgenographic examination of the teeth. A round, ovoid, or heart-shaped radiolucent area, usually bilaterally symmetrical and well outlined, is noted on the roentgenogram (Fig. 1–72, *A*). The area appears to lie in the midline between or above the roots of the maxillary central incisors and may be causing some apparent separation or divergence of the roots. It is not always possible roentgenographically to distinguish between a small cyst and the incisive foramen. Larger cysts usually cause no difficulty in interpretation.

Histologic Features. Median anterior maxillary cysts are lined by stratified squamous epithelium (Fig. 1–72, *B*), pseudostratified ciliated columnar epithelium (Fig. 1–72, *C*), cuboidal epithelium, or any combination of these. The variable type of epithelium emphasizes the origin of the cysts from the nasopalatine duct, this duct itself being composed of the same types of epithelium: respiratory in its nasal portion and squamous in its oral portion. The connective tissue wall of this cyst frequently shows inflammatory cell infiltration. In addition, collections of mucous glands are often present as well as several large blood vessels and nerves. The embryology of the nasopalatine duct, as well as the etiology and pathogenesis of the cyst originating from this structure, have been discussed in detail by Abrams and his co-workers.

Since these cysts are not of odontogenic origin, caution must be exercised to distinguish them from inflammatory cysts associated with a tooth and to thereby avoid the needless extraction of sound teeth.

Treatment. Malignant transformation of the lining epithelium of this cyst has not been reported. Furthermore, these cysts seldom become large or destroy any significant amount of bone. Therefore, surgical excision of asymptomatic nasopalatine duct cysts in dentulous patients may not be necessary. In edentulous patients, failure to remove the cyst prior to construction of a prosthetic appliance not uncommonly leads to acute infection, followed by perforation of the mucosa and suppurative drainage.

MEDIAN PALATAL CYST

The median palatal cyst arises from epithelium entrapped along the line of fusion of the palatal processes of the maxilla.

Clinical Features. The median palatal cyst is located in the midline of the hard palate between the lateral palatal processes. It may become large over a prolonged period of time and produce a definite palatal swelling that is visible clinically (Fig. 1–73, A). The cause of the epithelial proliferation and subsequent cyst formation is unknown.

Roentgenographic Features. On the palatal roentgenogram a well-circumscribed radiolucent area is seen opposite the bicuspid and molar region, frequently bordered by a sclerotic layer of bone (Fig. 1–73, B).

Histologic Features. The lining of such a cyst usually consists of stratified squamous epithelium overlying a relatively dense fibrous connective tissue band which may show chronic inflammatory cell infiltration. However, occasional cases have been reported to be lined by pseudostratified ciliated columnar epithelium or even a "modified" squamous epithelium, as pointed out by Courage and his associates in a review of this lesion.

Treatment. The treatment, as for most of the fissural cysts, is surgical removal and thorough curettage.

GLOBULOMAXILLARY CYST

The globulomaxillary cyst is found within the bone at the junction of the globular portion of the medial nasal process and the maxillary process, the globulomaxillary fissure, usually between the maxillary lateral incisor and cuspid teeth. However, there are reports of evidence

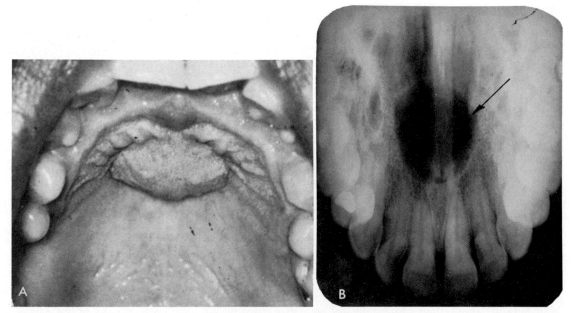

Figure 1–73. *Median palatal cyst.*
A large swelling (*A*) and underlying defect in the bone (*B*) are present in the midline of the palate. This cyst is not associated with the teeth and is posterior to the area of the incisive canal.

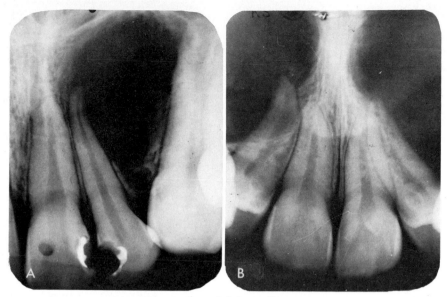

Figure 1–74. *Globulomaxillary cyst.*
There is a large cyst between the maxillary lateral incisor and cuspid teeth with a characteristic inverted pear shape *(A)*. The same type of cyst may occur bilaterally *(B)*. Note the divergence of the roots of these teeth. (Courtesy of Drs. Michael J. Freeman and Richard Oliver.)

that the cyst actually forms in the bone suture between the premaxilla and maxilla, the incisive suture, so that its location may be different from the cleft ridge and palate. Because of this, Ferenczy has suggested the term "premaxilla-maxillary cyst" as more accurately describing its origin. The cause of the proliferation of epithelium entrapped along this line of fusion is unknown. Virtanen and Laine have carried out an extensive review and discussion of the globulomaxillary cyst.

Christ has also thoroughly evaluated the literature dealing with globulomaxillary cysts and has concluded that, embryologically, facial processes per se do not exist and, therefore, ectoderm does not become entrapped in the facial fissures of the nasomaxillary complex. Thus, he believes that this cyst should be removed from the category of orofacial fissural cysts, since modern embryologic concepts do not support such a view. Instead, he suggests that an odontogenic origin for this cyst is far more likely, the clinical and roentgenographic appearance being entirely compatible with a lateral periodontal, lateral dentigerous, or primordial cyst. In addition, numerous reported cases have had the histologic features of the odontogenic keratocyst (q.v.), while nests of odontogenic epithelium in the wall of globulomaxillary cysts are not rare. Furthermore, there is at least one case, reported by Aisenberg and Inman, of an

ameloblastoma developing in a globulomaxillary cyst, which suggests an odontogenic origin.

Clinical Features. The globulomaxillary cyst seldom if ever presents clinical manifestations. Nearly every recorded case has been discovered accidentally during routine roentgenographic examination. Rarely, the cyst does become infected, and the patient may complain of local discomfort or pain in the area.

Roentgenographic Features. This cyst, on the intraoral roentgenogram, characteristically appears as an inverted, pear-shaped radiolucent area between the roots of the lateral incisor and cuspid, usually causing divergence of the roots of these teeth (Fig. 1–74). Interestingly, there are several known cases of bilateral globulomaxillary cyst (Fig. 1–74, *B*).

Care must be exercised not to confuse this lesion with an apical periodontal cyst arising as a result of pulp involvement or trauma to one of the adjacent teeth. The teeth associated with a globulomaxillary cyst are vital unless coincidentally infected.

It has been emphasized recently by Wysocki, reviewing 37 cases of "globulomaxillary radiolucencies," that many different types of lesions may present radiographically with features characteristic of a globulomaxillary cyst and that these must be included in any differential diagnosis of such a radiolucency in this area. He cited as examples such lesions as the periapical granuloma, apical periodontal cyst, lateral periodontal cyst, odontogenic keratocyst, central giant cell granuloma, calcifying odontogenic cyst, and odontogenic myxoma. He also concluded, in agreement with Christ, that cysts in the globulomaxillary region are odontogenic rather than fissural in origin.

Histologic Features. The globulomaxillary cyst classically has been described as being lined by either stratified squamous or ciliated columnar epithelium. However, Christ has emphasized that, in the literature, there is no accepted case of globulomaxillary cyst that is lined by pseudostratified ciliated columnar epithelium. The remainder of the wall is made up of fibrous connective tissue, usually showing inflammatory cell infiltration.

Treatment. This type of cyst should be surgically removed, preserving the adjacent teeth if possible.

MEDIAN MANDIBULAR CYST

The median mandibular developmental cyst is an extremely rare lesion occurring in the midline of the mandible. It is of disputed origin. Some authorities consider it a true developmental condition originating from proliferation of epithelial remnants entrapped in the median mandibular fissure during fusion of the bilateral mandibular arches. The possibility does exist, however, that the lesion may represent some type of odontogenic cyst such as a primordial cyst originating from a supernumerary enamel organ in the anterior mandibular segment, particularly since the bones uniting at the mandibular symphysis originate deep within the mesenchyme and thereby provide little opportunity for inclusion and subsequent proliferation of epithelial rests deep within the bone. It is also conceivable that this lesion represents a lateral periodontal cyst occurring in the midline, although the origin of this latter lesion is also obscure. The pertinent literature about this unusual type of cyst has been reviewed by White and his co-workers.

Clinical Features. Most of the median mandibular developmental cysts are clinically asymptomatic and are discovered only during routine roentgenographic examination. They seldom produce obvious expansion of the cortical plates of bone, and the associated teeth, unless otherwise involved, react normally to pulp vitality tests.

Roentgenographic Features. The roentgenographic appearance of the cyst is generally that

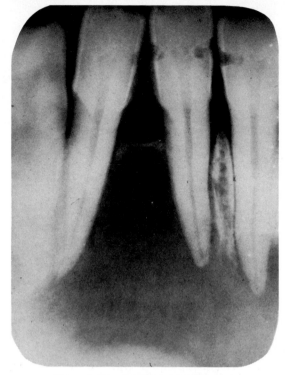

Figure 1–75. *Median mandibular cyst.*
All teeth in the anterior segment were vital. (Courtesy of Dr. Howard H. Morgan.)

of a unilocular, well-circumscribed radiolucency, although it may also appear multilocular (Fig. 1–75).

Histologic Features. Histologic examination of the lesion shows a thin, stratified squamous epithelium, often with many folds and projections, lining a central lumen. But in some reported cases, the cyst has been lined by a pseudostratified ciliated columnar epithelium.

Treatment and Prognosis. Too few cases have been reported to be certain of the prognosis of the median mandibular developmental cyst, but conservative surgical excision with preservation of associated teeth, if possible, is deemed advisable.

NASOALVEOLAR CYST

(Nasolabial Cyst; Klestadt's Cyst)

The nasoalveolar cyst is not found within bone, but is usually described as a rare fissural cyst that may involve bone secondarily. It has been thought to arise at the junction of the globular process, the lateral nasal process, and the maxillary process as a result of proliferation of entrapped epithelium along the fusion line.

Clinical Features. The nasoalveolar cyst may cause a swelling in the mucolabial fold as well as in the floor of the nose, being located near the attachment of the ala over the maxilla. Superficial erosion of the outer surface of the maxilla may be produced by pressure of the nasoalveolar cyst, but it should be noted that they are not primarily central lesions and therefore may not be visible on the roentgenogram. Bilateral cases, such as reported by Brandao and his associates, are very rare.

Roed-Petersen, in a discussion of this lesion, reviewed 160 reported cases and noted that slightly over 75 per cent of cases occurred in women. The mean age of occurrence was between 41 and 46 years, although cases have been reported in persons from 12 to 75 years of age.

Excellent reviews of the nasoalveolar cyst, with recapitulations of its etiology and pathogenesis, have been published by Moeller and Philipsen and by Campbell and Burkes. It has been suggested by Roed-Petersen and emphasized by Christ that this cyst probably originates from the lower anterior part of the nasolacrimal duct rather than from epithelium entrapped in the naso-optic furrow.

Histologic Features. Histologically, the nasoalveolar cyst may be lined by pseudostratified columnar epithelium which is sometimes ciliated, often with goblet cells, or by stratified squamous epithelium.

Treatment. The cyst should be surgically excised, although care must be exercised to prevent perforation and collapse of the lesion.

PALATAL CYSTS OF THE NEONATE

(Epstein's pearls, Bohn's nodules)

Tiny multiple cysts of the palate in fetuses and neonates were first described by Heinrich Bohn in 1866 and by Alois Epstein in 1880. Those described by Bohn were scattered over the hard palate, tended to be most numerous along the junction of the hard and soft palate, and appeared to be derived from epithelial remnants of developing palatal salivary glands. The cysts described by Epstein were collected linearly along the median raphe of the hard palate and appeared to be derived from entrapped epithelial remnants along the line of fusion. A third type of cyst of the neonate is found on the alveolar ridges, is derived from remnants of the dental lamina, and is thus odontogenic in origin. This type is known as the dental lamina cyst of the newborn (q.v.).

Clinical Features. Both types of palatal cysts appear as small, white, raised nodules, usually multiple, measuring a fraction of a millimeter to 2 or 3 mm. in diameter. As just described, they tend to cluster along the junction of the hard and soft palate in a linear fashion or are scattered diffusely over the hard palate.

It has been reported by Cataldo and Berkman that in a clinical examination of 209 full-term infants one to five days old, 80 per cent had cysts of the alveolar or palatal mucosa or both. The most common location was along the median raphe (65 per cent of cases). In the same report, histologic sections of alveolar and palatal mucosa of 31 newborns and infants showed that 11 of 26 cases (42 per cent) with no clinical evidence of cysts did have histologic microcysts of alveolar mucosa. Fromm also reported that of 1367 newborn infants examined clinically, 1028 (75 per cent) had inclusion cysts of the oral cavity in one of these three locations. Those along the midpalatine raphe were the most common. In fact, Monteleone and McLellan concluded that the median palatal nodules appeared to be a normal finding because of their high frequency.

Histologic Features. All cysts of the neonate, both palatal and alveolar, are true cysts, being lined by a thin, compressed layer of stratified squamous epithelium with the lumen generally packed with orthokeratin or parakeratin.

Treatment. No treatment is necessary for any of these lesions, since they undergo healing spontaneously through self-marsupialization as they enlarge and contact the overlying epithelium.

THYROGLOSSAL TRACT CYST

The thyroglossal tract cyst is an uncommon developmental cyst which may form anywhere along the embryonic thyroglossal tract between the foramen caecum of the tongue and the thyroid glands (Fig. 1–76). It apparently arises from remnants of this tract that do not become obliterated. The reason for the appearance of the cyst is unknown, but it may be triggered by infection of the lymphoid tissue in the area of the remnants of the thyroglossal tract through drainage from an upper respiratory tract infection.

Clinical Features. The thyroglossal tract cyst usually occurs in young persons but can develop at any age. It appears clinically as a firm, cystic midline mass, varying in size from a few millimeters to several centimeters (Fig. 1–77, A). It

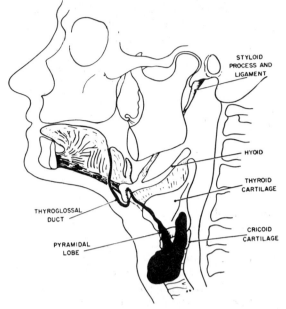

Figure 1–76. *Diagrammatic representation of the course of the thyroglossal tract.*
(From E. J. Brintnall, J. Davies, W. C. Huffman and D. M. Lierle: Arch. Otolaryngol., 59:282, 1954.)

may lie to one side of the midline. The swelling generally develops slowly and is asymptomatic unless it occupies a position high in the tract, near the tongue. In such cases dysphagia may be present. The cyst itself may lie near the foramen caecum, in the floor of the mouth, or inferiorly near the thyroid or cricoid cartilage. Occasionally a fistula will form, leading from the cyst and opening on the skin or mucosal surface.

Histologic Features. The thyroglossal tract cyst may be lined by stratified squamous epithelium, ciliated columnar epithelium, or intermediate transition type, since it is actually derived from cells originating from the embryonic pharyngeal floor (Fig. 1–77, *B, C, D*). With increased intracystic pressure, the cells may become flattened. The connective tissue wall of the cyst will frequently contain small patches of lymphoid tissue, thyroid tissue, and mucous glands. Interestingly, nodular collections of sebaceous glands in association with thyroglossal ductlike structures of the tongue occasionally have been reported. Leider and his associates have described such a case as a sebaceous choristoma of the lingual thyroglossal duct.

Treatment and Prognosis. The treatment for the thyroglossal tract cyst is complete surgical excision. This procedure must be relatively radical if recurrence is to be avoided.

It is of some interest that, although rare, cases have been reported of carcinoma developing from epithelial remnants of the thyroglossal tract or from the epithelial lining of thyroglossal tract cysts. LiVolsi and her associates reported a total of 76 instances of thyroglossal tract carcinoma.

BENIGN CERVICAL LYMPHOEPITHELIAL CYST

(Branchial Cleft Cyst; Lateral Cervical Cyst; Benign Cystic Lymph Node)

The benign cervical lymphoepithelial cyst is a cyst which occurs on the lateral aspect of the neck and has been described classically as originating from remnants of the branchial arches or pharyngeal pouches. There is considerable evidence, however, to indicate that this type of cyst is not related to the branchial arches. It is not a true fissural cyst, but it is best considered here because of its developmental origin.

Bhaskar and Bernier have reported on a series of 468 cases of this form of cyst and have thoroughly discussed the possibilities of the histogenesis of this lesion. Their evidence is convincing that this cyst originates through cystic transformation of epithelium entrapped in cervical lymph nodes. The source of this epithelium is unknown, but it is probably of salivary gland origin, a distinct embryologic possibility. For this reason, Bhaskar and Bernier have suggested substitution of the terms "benign cystic lymph nodes" or "benign lymphoepithelial cysts" for the more classic term. Whether the so-called branchial fistulas, or lateral cervical fistulas, are related to the present lesion has not been clearly determined.

In contrast, Little and Rickles have reported a study of lymph nodes in or adjacent to the parotid gland, submandibular and sublingual glands, and the cervical areas, with respect to salivary gland inclusions. They concluded that when one attempts to correlate the incidence of these cysts with the areas of greatest concentrations of the two types of epithelial remnants that could give rise to the cysts—parotid versus branchial—it appeared that the branchial apparatus was the more likely origin for this unique cyst. On this basis, they have questioned the acceptability of the salivary gland inclusion theory for the histogenesis of this cyst.

Clinical Features. The majority of these cysts occur in young adults, although they may become evident in early childhood. They are slow-growing and may have a duration of weeks to many years.

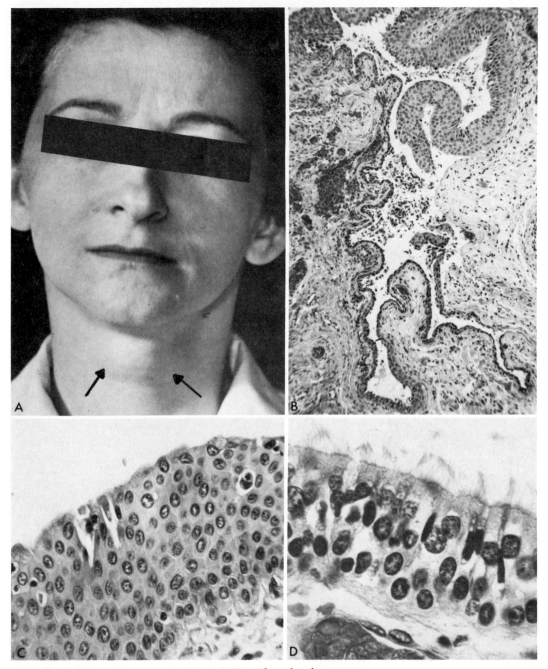

Figure 1–77.   *Thyroglossal tract cyst.*
Patient demonstrates a midline palpable fluctuant lesion *(A)*, which was found to be an epithelium-lined cyst *(B)* composed of both stratified squamous epithelium *(C)* and pseudostratified, ciliated columnar epithelium *(D)*. (Courtesy of Dr. James O. Beck, Jr.)

The lesion presents as an asymptomatic, circumscribed movable mass on the lateral aspect of the upper neck, usually close to the anterior border of the sternocleidomastoid muscle (Fig. 1–78, *A*). Although most of these cysts occur in the neck, many have been reported at the angle of the mandible, in the submandibular area, and even in the preauricular and parotid areas. There have also been 21 cases of this cyst reported occurring in the parotid gland, according to a review by Weitzner.

Histologic Features. This cyst is usually lined by stratified squamous epithelium, but may contain some pseudostratified columnar epithe-

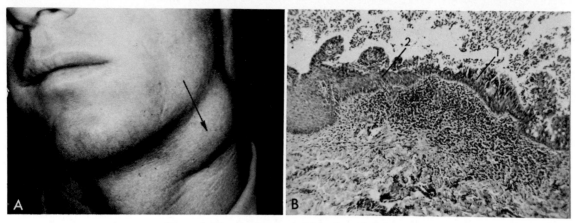

Figure 1–78. *Benign cervical lymphoepithelial cyst.*

A, This type of cyst appears clinically as a swelling in the neck beneath the body of the mandible and associated with the sternocleidomastoid muscle. *B,* The cyst is lined by both pseudostratified columnar epithelium *(1)* and stratified squamous epithelium *(2)*. (Courtesy of Dr. Frank Vellios.)

lium (Fig. 1–78, *B*). The wall of the cyst generally exhibits lymphoid tissue with a typical lymph node pattern. A variable amount of connective tissue is also present in the wall. The cyst itself may contain a thin watery fluid or a thick, gelatinous, mucoid material.

Treatment and Prognosis. This cyst should be treated by thorough surgical removal. Recurrence results if residual remnants arc left or if the lesion is simply aspirated or drained. The development of carcinoma from the epithelium lining the branchial cleft cyst has been reported by Collins and Edgerton, but it is relatively uncommon. Compagno and his associates pointed out that many cases originally thought to represent branchiogenic carcinoma have been shown subsequently to represent cervical metastases from a distant primary carcinoma, often in the oronasopharynx.

EPIDERMOID AND DERMOID CYSTS

The dermoid cyst is a form of cystic teratoma derived principally from embryonic germinal epithelium, but in some instances also containing structures of the other germ layers. New and Erich reported a series of 103 dermoid cysts of the head and neck region and noted that the floor of the mouth and the submaxillary and sublingual areas were common sites of occurrence. These cysts are presumed to be derived from enclavement of epithelial debris in the midline during closure of the mandibular and hyoid branchial arches. Since some of these cells are totipotent blastomeres, the occurrence

of nonepithelial structures can be readily understood.

Clinical Features. Those dermoid cysts arising in the floor of the mouth are seldom present at birth, in contradistinction to dermoids in some other locations. The majority occur in young adulthood and show no sex predilection.

The typical lesion produces a bulge in the floor of the mouth, often causing elevation of the tongue and ensuing difficulty in eating and talking (Fig. 1–79). This is particularly true if the cyst occurs above the geniohyoid muscle, between it and the oral mucosa. If the cyst is situated deeper, between the geniohyoid and mylohyoid muscles, bulging in the submental area is more common. This cyst may also arise below the mylohyoid muscle. The lesions vary

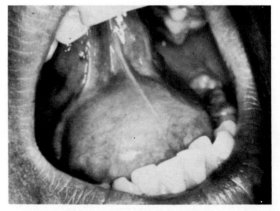

Figure 1–79. *Epidermoid cyst.*
Lesion appears as a symmetrical swelling in the floor of the mouth. (Courtesy of Dr. Cesar Lopez.)

in size but generally approach several centimeters in diameter. The usual cyst has a "doughlike" feel to palpation but may be more fluctuant, depending upon the contents of the cyst.

These cysts sometimes become infected and occasionally develop sinus tracts opening intraorally or on the skin. They have been described as undergoing malignant transformation.

There are a number of lesions which bear strong clinical resemblance to the dermoid cyst, and these have been listed by Meyer as follows: (1) ranula, (2) unilateral or bilateral blockage of Wharton's ducts, (3) thyroglossal tract cyst, (4) cystic hygroma, (5) branchial cleft cyst, (6) acute infection or cellulitis of the floor of the mouth, (7) infections of submaxillary and sublingual glands, (8) benign and malignant tumors of the floor of the mouth and adjacent salivary glands, and (9) normal fat mass in the submental area.

Histologic Features. The histologic appearance of the dermoid cyst is a varied one, depending upon the complexity of the lesion. Certain of these cysts are composed only of a connective tissue wall lined on the inner surface by a thin layer of stratified squamous epithelium, usually showing keratinization. The lumen may actually be filled with keratin. There may be no other specialized structures demonstrable, and the term "epidermoid cyst" is best used to describe this simple lesion. In other cases there may be numerous sebaceous glands and even hair follicles in addition to occasional sweat glands. The lumen contains sebaceous material as well as keratin. This is the dermoid cyst. Finally, some lesions contain structures of a varied nature such as bone, muscle, and gastrointestinal derivatives and thus represent a complex teratoma.

Treatment and Prognosis. The epidermoid or dermoid cyst should be removed surgically; it does not usually recur.

HETEROTOPIC ORAL GASTROINTESTINAL CYST

Heterotopic islands of gastric mucosa have been found in the esophagus, small intestine, thoracic cysts, omphalomesenteric cysts, pancreas, gallbladder, and Meckel's diverticulum, according to the review by Gorlin and Jirasek. In addition, Harris and Courtemanche cited at least 17 cases of cysts lined by gastric or intestinal mucosa occurring in the oral cavity, in the tongue, or in the floor of the mouth, probably from misplaced embryonal rests.

Clinical Features. This choristomatic cyst can be found in patients at any age, although the majority have been infants or young children. It may be significant that the lesion occurs overwhelmingly in males.

The cyst presents as a small nodule entirely within the body of the tongue, either anterior or posterior, or in the floor of the mouth, in the neck, or adjacent to the submaxillary gland. It may be asymptomatic or may cause difficulty in eating or speaking. Some cysts communicate with the surface mucosa by a tube or ductlike structure.

Histologic Features. This cyst is usually lined partly by stratified squamous epithelium and partly by gastric mucosa similar to that found in the body and fundus of the stomach, with both parietal and chief cells. Sometimes intestinal epithelium is found, including Paneth, goblet and argentaffin cells. A muscularis mucosa may or may not be present.

Treatment. Surgical excision is the treatment of choice, although this lesion cannot be diagnosed clinically and is seldom suspected.

REFERENCES

Abell, M. R.: Lymphoid hamartoma. Radiol. Clin. N. Amer., 6:15, 1968.

Abrams, A. M., Howell, F. V., and Bullock, W. K.: Nasopalatine cysts. Oral Surg., 16:306, 1963.

Aisenberg, M. S., and Inman, B. W.: Ameloblastoma arising within a globulomaxillary cyst. Oral Surg., 13:1352, 1960.

Akira, K., and Kitamura, J.: Clinical report of a case of globulomaxillary cyst. Oral Surg., 5:705, 1952.

Alexander, R. W., and James, R. B.: Melkersson-Rosenthal syndrome: review of literature and report of case. J. Oral Surg., 30:599, 1972.

Amos, E. R.: Incidence of the small dens in dente. J. Am. Dent. Assoc., 51:31, 1955.

Angle, E. H.: Classification of malocclusion. Dent. Cosmos., 41:284, 1899.

Arafat, A., Brannon, R. B., and Ellis, G. L.: Adenomatoid hyperplasia of mucous salivary glands. Oral Surg., 52:51, 1981.

Archard, H. O., Heck, J. W., and Stanley, H. R.: Focal epithelial hyperplasia: an unusual oral mucosal lesion found in Indian children. Oral Surg., 20:201, 1965.

Arons, M. S., Solitaire, G. B., and Grunt, J. A.: The macroglossia of Beckwith's syndrome. J. Plast. Reconstr. Surg., 45:341, 1970.

Ascher, K. W.: Das syndrom blepharochalasis, Struma und Doppellippe. Klin. Wochenschr., 1:2287, 1922.

Ballschmiede: Dissertation, Berlin, 1920, Quoted in Herbet, E. H., and Apffelstaedt, M.: Malformations of the Jaws and Teeth. New York, Oxford University Press, 1930.

Bánóczy, J., Szabó, L, and Csiba, A.: Migratory glossitis. Oral Surg., 39:113, 1975.

Bartels, H. A., and Maillard, E. R.: Hairy tongue. Oral Surg., 8:659, 1955.

Bartholomew, L. G., Moore, C. E., Dahlin, D. C., and Waugh, J. M.: Intestinal polyposis associated with mucocutaneous pigmentation. Surg., Gynecol. Obstet., 115:1, 1962.

Baughman, R. A.: Median rhomboid glossitis: a developmental anomaly? Oral Surg., 31:56, 1971.

Idem.: Lingual thyroid and lingual thyroglossal tract remnants. A clinical and histopathologic study with review of the literature. Oral Surg., 34:781, 1972.

Baughman, R. A., and Heidrich, P. D., Jr.: The oral hair: an extremely rare phenomenon. Oral Surg., 49:530, 1980.

Berendt, H. C.: Report of seven cases of anodontia partialis. Oral Surg., 3:1435, 1950.

Berman, D. S., and Silverstone, L. M.: Natal and neonatal teeth. Brit. Dent. J., 139:361, 1975.

Berman, F. R., and Fay, J. T.: The retrocuspid papilla. A clinical survey. Oral Surg., 42:80, 1976.

Bertram, U.: Xerostomia. Acta Odontol. Scand., 25 (Suppl. 4):1967.

Bhaskar, S. N.: Lymphoepithelial cysts of the oral cavity. Oral Surg., 21:120, 1966.

Bhaskar, S. N., and Bernier, J. L.: Histogenesis of branchial cysts. A report of 468 cases. Am. J. Pathol., 35:407, 1959.

Bhatia, S. N.: Genetics of cleft lip and palate. Br. Dent. J., 132:95, 1972.

Bhatt, A. P., and Dholakia, H. M.: Radicular variety of double dens invaginatus. Oral Surg., 39:284, 1975.

Bixler, D.: Heritability of clefts of the lip and palate. J. Prosthet. Dent., 33:100, 1975.

Idem.: Heritable disorders affecting dentin; in R. E. Stewart and J. Prescott (eds.): Oral Facial Genetics. St. Louis, C. V. Mosby Company, 1976.

Black, G. V., and McKay, F. S.: Mottled teeth: an endemic developmental imperfection of the enamel of the teeth heretofore unknown in the literature of dentistry. Dent. Cosmos, 58:129, 1916.

Blattner, R. J., Heys, F., and Robinson, H. B. G.: Osteogenesis imperfecta and odontogenesis imperfecta. J. Dent. Res., 21:325, 1942.

Blumberg, J. E., Hylander, W. L., and Goepp, R. A.: Taurodontism: a biometric study. Am. J. Phys. Anthropol., 34:243, 1971.

Bodecker, C. F.: Enamel hypoplasia. J. Dent. Res., 20:447, 1941.

Boerger, W. G., Waite, D. E., and Carroll, G. W.: Idiopathic bone cavities of the mandible; a review of the literature and report of case. J. Oral Surg., 30:506, 1972.

Bohn, H.: Die Mundkrankheiten der Kinder. Leipzig, W. Engelmann, 1866.

Boone, C. G.: Nasoalveolar cyst. Oral Surg., 8:40, 1955.

Brandao, G. S., Ebling, H., and Faria e Souza, I.: Bilateral nasolabial cyst. Oral Surg., 37:480, 1974.

Brekhus, P. J., Oliver, C. P., and Montelius, G.: A study of the pattern and combinations of congenitally missing teeth in man. J. Dent. Res., 23:117, 1944.

Bronstein, I. P., Abelson, S. M., Jaffe, R. H., and von Bonin, G.: Macroglossia in children. Am. J. Dis. Child., 54:1328, 1937.

Brucker, M.: Studies on the incidence and cause of dental defects in children. II. Hypoplasia. J. Dent. Res., 22:115, 1943.

Buchner, A., and Hansen, L. S.: Melanotic macule of the oral mucosa. Oral Surg., 48:244, 1979.

Idem.: Lymphoepithelial cysts of the oral cavity. Oral Surg., 50:441, 1980.

Buchner, A., Silverman, S., Jr., Wara, W. M., and Hansen, L. S.: Angiolymphoid hyperplasia with eosinophilia (Kimura's disease). Oral Surg., 49:309, 1980.

Buckerfield, J. B., and Edwards, M. B.: Angiolymphoid hyperplasia with eosinophils in oral mucosa. Oral Surg., 47:539, 1979.

Burdick, D., Prior, J. T., and Scanlon, G. T.: Peutz-Jeghers syndrome: a clinical-pathological study of a large family with a 10-year follow-up. Cancer, 16:854, 1963.

Burket, L. W.: Histopathologic studies in congenital syphilis. Int. J. Orthod. Oral Surg., 23:1016, 1937.

Calman, H. I.: Nasoalveolar cyst. N.Y. Dent. J., 20:320, 1954.

Campbell, R. L., and Burkes, E. J., Jr.: Nasolabial cyst: report of case. J. Am. Dent. Assoc., 91:1210, 1975.

Cataldo, E., and Berkman, M. D.: Cysts of the oral mucosa in newborns. Am. J. Dis. Child., 116:44, 1968.

Cervenka, J., Gorlin, R. J., and Anderson, V. E.: The syndrome of pits of the lower lip and/or cleft palate. Am. J. Hum. Genet., 19:416, 1967.

Chaudhry, A. P., Johnson, O. N., Mitchell, D. F., Gorlin, R. J., and Bartholdi, W. L.: Hereditary enamel dysplasia. J. Pediatr., 54:776, 1959.

Christ, T. F.: The globulomaxillary cyst: an embryologic misconception. Oral Surg., 30:515, 1970.

Cohen, M. M., Jr.: Syndromes with cleft lip and cleft palate. Cleft Palate J., 15:306, 1978.

Cohlon, S. Q.: Excessive intake of vitamin A as a cause of congenital anomalies in the rat. Science, 117:535, 1953.

Collins, N. P., and Edgerton, M. T.: Primary branchiogenic carcinoma. Cancer, 12:235, 1959.

Compagno, J., Hyams, V. J., and Safavian, M.: Does branchiogenic carcinoma really exist? Arch. Pathol. Lab. Med., 100:311, 1976.

Connor, M. S.: Anterior lingual mandibular bone concavity. Oral Surg., 48:413, 1979.

Conway, H., and Jerome, A. P.: The surgical treatment of branchial cysts and fistulas. Surg. Gynecol. Obstet., 101:621, 1955.

Conway, H. C., and Wagner, K. J.: Congenital anomalies of the head and neck. Plast. Reconstr. Surg., 36:71, 1965.

Cooke, B. E. D.: Median rhomboid glossitis and benign glossitis migrans (geographical tongue). Br. Dent. J., 112:389, 1962.

Idem.: Median rhomboid glossitis, Candidiasis and not a developmental anomaly. Br. J. Dermatol., 93:399, 1975.

Correll, R. W., Jensen, J. L., and Rhyne, R. R.: Lingual cortical mandibular defects. Oral Surg., 50:287, 1980.

Courage, G. R., North, A. F., and Hansen, L. S.: Median palatine cysts. Oral Surg., 37:745, 1974.

Crawford, J. L.: Concomitant taurodontism and amelogenesis imperfecta in the American caucasian. J. Dent. Child., 37:171, 1970.

Dachi, S. F., and Howell, F. V.: A survey of 3,874 routine full-mouth radiographs. II. A study of impacted teeth. Oral Surg., 14:1165, 1961.

Darling, A. I.: Some observations on amelogenesis imperfecta and calcification of the dental enamel. Proc. R. Soc. Med., 49:759, 1956.

Darling, A. I., and Levers, B. G. H.: Submerged human deciduous molars and ankylosis. Arch. Oral Biol., 18:1021, 1973.

Davis, W. B.: Congenital deformities of the face. Surg., Gynecol. Obstet., 61:201, 1935.

Dean, H. T.: Chronic endemic dental fluorosis. J.A.M.A., 107:1269, 1936.

Diamond, M., and Weinmann, J. P.: The Enamel of Human Teeth. New York, Columbia University Press, 1940.

Dinnerman, M.: Vitamin A deficiency in unerupted teeth of infants. Oral Surg., 4:1024, 1951.

Doku, H. C., Shklar, G., and McCarthy, P. L.: Cheilitis glandularis. Oral Surg., 20:563, 1965.

Dolder, E.: Deficient dentition. Dent. Record, 57:142, 1937.

Downs, W. G.: Studies in the causes of dental anomalies. J. Dent. Res., 8:367, 1928.

Doyle, J. L., Weisinger, E., and Manhold, J. H., Jr.: Benign lymphoid lesions of the oral mucosa. Oral Surg., 29:31, 1970.

Dummett, C. O., and Barens, G.: Oromucosal pigmentation: an updated literary review. J. Periodontol., 42:726, 1971.

Duncan, B. R., Dohner, V. A., and Priest, J. H.: The Gardner syndrome: need for early diagnosis. J. Pediatr., 72:497, 1968.

Emerson, T. G.: Hereditary gingival hyperplasia. A family pedigree of four generations. Oral Surg., 19:1, 1965.

Epstein, A.: Ueber Epithelperlen in der Mundhöhle Neugeborener Kinder. Ztsch. für Heilkunde 1:59, 1880.

Ettinger, R. L., and Manderson, R. D.: A clinical study of sublingual varices. Oral Surg., 38:540, 1974.

Eveson, J. W., and Lucas, R. B.: Angiolymphoid hyperplasia with eosinophilia. J. Oral Path., 8:103, 1979.

Everett, F. G., and Holder, T. D.: Cheilitis glandularis apostematosa. Oral Surg., 8:405, 1955.

Everett, F. G., and Wescott, W. B.: Commissural lip pits. Oral Surg., 14:202, 1961.

Fader, M, Kline, S. N., Spatz, S. S., and Zubrow, H. J.: Gardner's syndrome (intestinal polyposis, osteomas, sebaceous cysts) and a new dental discovery. Oral Surg., 15:153, 1962.

Fainstat, T.: Cortisone-induced congenital cleft palate in rabbits. Endocrinology, 55:502, 1954.

Farman, A. G.: Atrophic lesions of the tongue: a prevalence study among 175 diabetic patients. J. Oral Path., 5:255, 1976.

Idem.: Cellular changes and Candida in diabetic outpatients having glossal central papillary atrophy. Tydskr. Tandheelkd. Ver. S. Afr. 33:425, 1978.

Farman, A. G., van Wyk, C. W., Staz, J., Hugo, M., and Dreyer, W. P.: Central papillary atrophy of the tongue. Oral Surg., 43:48, 1977.

Ferenczy, K.: The relationship of globulomaxillary cysts to the fusion of embryonal processes and to cleft palate. Oral Surg., 11:1388, 1958.

Finn, S. B.: Hereditary opalescent dentin. I. An analysis of literature of hereditary anomalies of tooth color. J. Am. Dent. Assoc., 25:1240, 1938.

Fitzwilliams, C. D. L.: The Tongue and Its Diseases. New York, Oxford University Press, 1927.

Fiumara, N. J., and Lessell, S.: Manifestations of late congenital syphilis. Arch. Dermatol., 102:78, 1970.

Fogh-Andersen, P.: Inheritance of Harelip and Cleft Palate. Copenhagen, Nyt. Nordisk Forlag. Arnold Busck, 1942.

Foretich, E. A., Cardo, V. A., Jr., and Zambito, R. F.: Bilateral congenital absence of the submandibular duct orifices. J. Oral Surg., 31:556, 1973.

Foster, T. D.: The effects of hemifacial atrophy on dental growth. Br. Dent. J., 146:148, 1979.

Fraser, F. .: Workshop on embryology of cleft lip and cleft palate. Teratology, 1:353, 1968.

Fraser, F. C., and Warburton, D.: No association of emotional stress or vitamin supplement during pregnancy to cleft lip or palate in man. Plast. Reconstr. Surg., 33:395, 1964.

Fraumeni, J. F., Jr., Geiser, C. F., and Manning, M. D.: Wilms' tumor and congenital hemihypertrophy: report of 5 new cases and review of literature. Pediatrics, 40:886, 1967.

Frerichs, D. W., and Spooner, S. W.: Median palatine cyst. Oral Surg., 6:1181, 1953.

Fromm, A.: Epstein's pearls, Bohn's nodule and inclusion cysts of the oral cavity. J. Dent. Child., 34:275, 1967.

Gardner, D. G.: The dentinal changes in regional odontodysplasia. Oral Surg., 38:887, 1974.

Gardner, D. G., and Girgis, S. S.: Taurodontism, shovel-shaped incisors and the Klinefelter syndrome. J. Can. Dent. Assoc., 8:372, 1978.

Idem.: Talon cusps: a dental anomaly in the Rubinstein-Taybi syndrome. Oral Surg., 47:519, 1979.

Gardner, D. G., and Sapp, J. P.: Ultrastructural, electron-probe, and microhardness studies of the controversial amorphous areas in the dentin of regional odontodysplasia. Oral Surg., 44:549, 1977.

Giansanti, J. S., and Allen, J. D.: Dentin dysplasia, type II, or dentin dysplasia, coronal type. Oral Surg., 38:911, 1974.

Giansanti, J. S., Baker, G. O., and Waldron, C. A.: Intraoral mucinous, minor salivary gland lesions presenting clinically as tumors. Oral Surg., 32:918, 1971.

Gier, R. E., and Fast, T. B.: Median maxillary anterior alveolar cleft. Oral Surg., 24:496, 1967.

Giunta, J., and Cataldo, E.: Lymphoepithelial cysts of the oral mucosa. Oral Surg., 35:77, 1973.

Goebel, W. M.: Bilateral patent nasopalatine ducts. J. Oral Med., 30:96, 1975.

Goetsch, E.: Lingual goiter; report of three cases. Ann. Surg., 127:291, 1948.

Goldberg, H., and Goldhaber, P.: Hereditary intestinal polyposis with oral pigmentation (Jeghers' syndrome). Oral Surg., 7:378, 1954.

Goldstein, E., and Gottlieb, M. A.: Taurodontism: familial tendencies demonstrated in eleven of fourteen case reports. Oral Surg., 36:131, 1973.

Gorlin, R. J., and Goldman, H. M. (eds.): Thoma's Oral Pathology. 6th ed. St. Louis, C. V. Mosby Company, 1970.

Gorlin, R. J., and Jirasek, J. E.: Oral cysts containing gastric or intestinal mucosa: unusual embryologic accident or heterotopia. J. Oral Surg., 28:9, 1970.

Gorlin, R. J., Pindborg, J. J., and Cohen, M. M.: Syndromes of the Head and Neck, 2nd ed. New York, McGraw-Hill, Inc., 1976.

Gorlin, R. J., Meskin, L. H., and St. Geme, J. W.: Oculodentodigital dysplasia. J. Pediatr., 63:69, 1963.

Graber, L. W.: Congenital absence of teeth: a review with emphasis on inheritance patterns. J. Am. Dent. Assoc., 96:266, 1978.

Grace, L. G.: Frequency of occurrence of cleft palates and harelips. J. Dent. Res., 22:495, 1943.

Grahnén, H., and Granath, L. E.: Numerical variations in primary dentition and their correlation with the permanent dentition. Odontol. Revy., 12:348, 1961.

Grahnén, H., and Larsson, P. G.: Enamel defects in deciduous dentition of prematurely born children. Odontol. Revy., 9:143, 1958.

Guiducci, A. A., and Hyman, A. B.: Ectopic sebaceous glands. Dermatologica, 125:44, 1962.

Gunter, G. S.: Nasomaxillary cleft. Plast. Reconstr. Surg., 32:637, 1963.

Halperin, V., Kolas, S., Jefferis, K. R., Huddleston, S. D., and Robinson, H. B. G.: The occurrence of Fordyce spots, benign migratory glossitis, median rhomboid glossitis, and fissured tongue in 2,478 dental patients. Oral Surg., 6:1072, 1953.

Hamner, J. E., III, Witkop, C. J., and Metro, P. S.: Taurodontism. Report of a case. Oral Surg., 18:409, 1964.

Haring, O. M., and Lewis, F. J.: The etiology of congenital developmental anomalies. Surg., Gynecol. Obstet. (Int. Abst. Surg.), 113:1, 1961.

Harris, C. N., and Courtemanche, A. D.: Gastric mucosal cyst of the tongue. Plast. Reconstr. Surg., 54:612, 1974.

Harvey, W., and Noble, H. W.: Defects on the lingual surface of the mandible near the angle. Br. J. Oral Surg., 6:75, 1968.

Hellman, M.: Our third molar teeth: their eruption, presence and absence. Dent. Cosmos, 78:750, 1936.

Henderson, H. Z.: Ankylosis of primary molars: a clinical, radiographic, and histolgic study. J. Dent. Child., 46:117, 1979.

Henzel, J. H., Pories, W. J., and DeWeese, M. S.: Etiology of lateral cervical cysts. Surg. Gynecol. Obstet., 125:87, 1967.

Heys, F. M., Blattner, R. J., and Robinson, H. B. G.: Osteogenesis imperfecta and odontogenesis imperfecta: clinical and genetic aspects in eighteen families. J. Pediatr., 56:234, 1960.

Hirshfeld, I.: The retrocuspid papilla. Am. J. Orthod., 33:447, 1947.

Hodge, H. C., Finn, S. B., Lose, G. B., Gachet, F. S., and Bassett, S. H.: Hereditary opalescent dentin. II. General and oral clinical studies. J. Am. Dent. Assoc., 26:1663, 1939.

Hodge, H. C., Finn, S. B., Robinson, H. B. G., Manly, R. S., Manly, M. L., Van Huysen, G., and Bale, W. F.: Hereditary opalescent dentin. III. Histological, chemical and physical studies. J. Dent. Res., 19:521, 1940.

Hung, W., Randolph, J. G., Sabatini, D., and Winship, T.: Lingual and sublingual thyroid glands in euthyroid children. Pediatrics, 38:647, 1966.

Hursey, R. J., Jr., Witkop, C. J., Jr., Miklashek, D., and Sackett, L. M.: Dentinogenesis imperfecta in a racial isolate with multiple hereditary defects. Oral Surg., 9:641, 1956.

Ingalls, T. H., Taube, I. E., and Klingberg, M. A.: Cleft lip and cleft palate: epidemiologic considerations. Plast. Reconstr. Surg., 34:1, 1964.

Jeghers, H., McKusick, V. A., and Katz, K. H.: Generalized intestinal polyposis and melanin spots of the oral mucosa, lips and digits. N. Engl. J. Med., 241:993, 1031, 1949.

Karmiol, M., and Walsh, R. F.: Incidence of static bone defect of the mandible. Oral Surg., 26:225, 1968.

Kennedy, J. M., and Thompson, E. C.: Hypoplasia of the mandible (Pierre Robin syndrome) with complete cleft palate: report of a case. Oral Surg., 3:421, 1950.

Kleinman, H. Z.: Lingual varicosities. Oral Surg., 23:546, 1967.

Knapp, M. J.: Lingual sebaceous glands and a possible thyroglossal duct. Oral Surg., 31:70, 1971.

Idem: Oral tonsils: location distribution and histology. Oral Surg., 29:155, 1970.

Idem: Pathology of oral tonsils. Oral Surg., 29:295, 1970.

Kreshover, S. J.: The pathogenesis of enamel hypoplasia: an experimental study. J. Dent. Res., 23:231, 1944.

Langlais, R. P., Cottone, J., and Kasle, M. J.: Anterior and posterior lingual depressions of the mandible. J. Oral Surg., 34:502, 1976.

Lapage, C. P.: Micrognathia in the new-born. Lancet, 1:323, 1937.

Laymon, C. W.: Cheilitis granulomatosa and Melkersson-Rosenthal syndrome. Arch. Dermatol., 83:112, 1961.

Leider, A. S., Lucas, J. W., and Eversole, L. R.: Sebaceous choristoma of the thyroglossal duct. Oral Surg., 44:261, 1977.

Levitas, T. C.: Gemination, fusion, twinning, and concrescence. J. Dent. Child., 32:93, 1965.

Little, J. W., and Rickles, N. H.: The histogenesis of the branchial cyst. Am. J. Pathol., 50:533, 1967.

LiVolsi, V. A., Perzin, K. H., and Savetsky, L.: Carcinoma arising in median ectopic thyroid (including thyroglossal duct tissue). Cancer, 34:1303, 1974.

Logan, J., Becks, H., Silverman, S., Jr., and Pindborg, J. J.: Dentinal dysplasia. Oral Surg., 15:317, 1962.

Lunt, R. C., and Law, D. B.: A review of the chronology of calcification of deciduous teeth. J. Am. Dent. Assoc., 89:599, 1974.

Idem.: A review of the chronology of eruption of deciduous teeth. J. Am. Dent. Assoc., 89:872, 1974.

Lyons, D. C.: Biochemical factors in the possible developments of malformations of the oral tissues, especially cleft palate and harelip. Oral Surg., 3:12, 1950.

MacMahon, B., and McKeown, T.: The incidence of harelip and cleft palate related to birth rank and maternal age. Am. J. Hum. Genet., 5:176, 1953.

Mader, C. L.: Fusion of teeth. J. Am. Dent. Assoc. 98:62, 1979.

Idem.: Talon cusp. J. Am. Dent. Assoc., 103:244, 1981.

Mandel, L., and Baurmash, H.: Thyroglossal tract abnormalities. Oral Surg., Path., 10:113, 1957.

Mangion, J. J.: Two cases of taurodontism in modern human jaws. Br. Dent. J., 113:309, 1962.

Martin, H. E., and Howe, M. E.: Glossitis rhombica mediana. Ann. Surg., 107:39, 1938.

Maskow, B. S.: Bilateral congenital nasopalatine communication. Oral Surg., 53:458, 1982.

Massler, M., and Savara, B. S.: Natal and neonatal teeth. J. Pediatr., 36:349, 1950.

Mathewson, R. J., Siegel, M. J., and McCanna, D. L.: Ankyloglossia: a review of the literature and a case report. J. Dent. Child., 33:238, 1966.

McCarthy, F..P.: A clinical and pathologic study of oral disease. J.A.M.A., 116:16, 1941.

McConnel, F. M. S., Zellweger, H., and Lawrence, R. A.: Labial pits: cleft lip and/or palate syndrome. Arch. Otolaryngol., 91:407, 1970.

McEvitt, W. G.: Cleft lip and palate and parental age: a statistical study of etiology. Plast. Reconstr. Surg., 10:77, 1952.

McKay, F. S.: Investigation of mottled enamel and brown stain. J. Natl. Dent. Assoc., 4:273, 1917.

Idem: A brief statement of the case against fluorine in water as the cause of mottled enamel. J. Dent. Res., 13:133, 1933.

McKay, F. S., and Black, G. V.: An investigation of mottled teeth. Dent. Cosmos, 58:477, 627, 781, 894, 1916.

Mellor, J. K., and Ripa, L. W.: Talon cusp: a clinically significant anomaly. Oral Surg., 29:224, 1970.

Melnick, M., Eastman, J. R., Goldblatt, L. I., Michaud, M., and Bixler, D.: Dentin dysplasia, type II: a rare autosomal dominant disorder. Oral Surg., 44:592, 1977.

Melnick, M., Levin, L. S., and Brady, J.: Dentin dysplasia, type I: a scanning electron microscopic analysis of the primary dentition. Oral Surg., 50:335, 1980.

Meskin, L. H., Redman, R. S., and Gorlin, R. J.: Incidence of geographic tongue among 3,668 students at the University of Minnesota. J. Dent. Res., 42:895, 1963.

Meyer, A. W.: Median anterior maxillary cysts. J. Am. Dent. Assoc., 18:1851, 1931.

Meyer, I.: Dermoid cysts (dermoids) of the floor of the mouth. Oral Surg., 8:1149, 1955.

Miles, A. E. W.: Sebaceous glands in the lip and cheek mucosa of man. Br. Dent. J., 105:235, 1958.

Miller, A. S., and McCrea, M. W.: Sebaceous gland adenoma of the buccal mucosa. J. Oral Surg., 26:593, 1968.

Miller, A. S., and Winnick, M.: Salivary gland inclusion in the anterior mandible. Oral Surg., 31:790, 1971.

Miller, A. S., Greeley, J. N., and Catena, D. L.: Median maxillary anterior alveolar cleft: report of three cases. J. Am. Dent. Assoc., 79:896, 1969.

Miller, J., and Forrester, R. M.: Neonatal enamel hypoplasia associated with haemolytic disease and with prematurity. Br. Dent. J., 106:93, 1959.

Miller, J. B., and Moore, P. M., Jr.: Nasoalveolar cysts. Ann. Otol. Rhinol. Laryngol., 58:200, 1949.

Miller, W. A., and Seymour, R. H.: Odontodysplasia. Br. Dent. J., 125:56, 1968.

Moeller, J. F., and Philipsen, H. P.: A case of nasoalveolar cyst (Klestadt's cyst). Tandlaegebladet, 62:659, 1958.

Monroe, C. W., and Ogo, K.: Treatment of micrognathia in the neonatal period. Report of 65 cases. Plast. Reconstr. Surg., 50:317, 1972.

Monteleone, L., and McLellan, M. S.: Epstein's pearls and Bohn's nodules of the palate. J. Oral Surg., 22:301, 1964.

Montgomery, M. L.: Lingual thyroid: a comprehensive review. West J. Surg. Obstet. Gynecol., 43:661, 1935; 44:54, 122, 189, 237, 303, 373, 442, 1936.

Moulton, F. R. (ed.): Fluorine and Dental Health. Washington, D.C., American Association for the Advancement of Science, 1942.

Idem: Dental Caries and Fluorine. Washington, D.C., American Association for the Advancement of Science, 1946.

Nathanson, I.: Macroglossia. Oral Surg., 1:547, 1948.

New, E. B., and Erich, J. B.: Dermoid cysts of the head and neck. Surg. Gynecol. Obstet., 65:48, 1937.

Oehlers, F. A. C.: A case of multiple supernumerary teeth. Br. Dent. J., 90:211, 1951.

Idem: Dens invaginatus (dilated composite odontome). I. Variations of the invagination process and associated anterior or crown forms. II. Associated posterior crown forms and pathogenesis. Oral Surg., 10:1204, 1302, 1957.

Idem: The radicular variety of dens invaginatus. Oral Surg., 11:1251, 1958.

Oikarinen, V. J., and Julku, M.: An orthopantomographic study of developmental mandibular bone defects. Int. J. Oral Surg., 3:71, 1974.

Oliver, I. D., and Pickett, A. B.: Cheilitis glandularis. Oral Surg., 49:526, 1980.

Page, L. R., Corio, R. L., Crawford, B. E., Giansanti, J. S., and Weathers, D. R.: The oral melanotic macule. Oral Surg., 44:219, 1977.

Palmer, M. E.: Case reports of evaginated odontomes in Caucasians. Oral Surg., 35:772, 1973.

Papanayotou, P. H., and Hatziotis, J. CH.: Ascher's syndrome. Oral Surg., 35:467, 1973.

Pindborg, J. J.: Pathology of the Dental Hard Tissues. Philadelphia, W. B. Saunders Company, 1970.

Praetorius-Clausen, F.: Geographical aspects of oral focal epithelial hyperplasia. Path. Microbiol., 39:204, 1973.

Praetorius-Clausen, F., and Willis, J. M.: Papova virus-like particles in focal epithelial hyperplasia. Scand. J. Dent. Res., 79:362, 1971.

Praetorius-Clausen, F., Møgeltoft, M., Roed-Petersen, B., and Pindborg, J. J.: Focal epithelial hyperplasia of the oral mucosa in a south-west Greenlandic population. Scand. J. Dent. Res., 78:287, 1970.

Prinz, H., and Greenbaum, S. S.: Diseases of the Mouth and Their Treatment. 2nd ed. Philadelphia, Lea & Febiger, 1939.

Prowler, J. R., and Glassman, S.: Agenesis of the mandibular condyles. Oral Surg., 7:133, 1954.

Rao, R., Venkata: Naso-labial cyst. J. Laryngol. Otol., 69:352, 1955.

Ray, G. E.: Congenital absence of permanent teeth. Br. Dent. J., 90:213, 1951.

Redman, R. S.: Prevalence of geographic tongue, fissured tongue, median rhomboid glossitis, and hairy tongue among 3,611 Minnesota school children. Oral Surg., 30:390, 1970.

Rhodes, E. L., and Stirling, G. A.: Granulomatous cheilitis. Arch. Dermatol., 92:40, 1965.

Richardson, E. R.: Incidence of geographic tongue and median rhomboid glossitis in 3,319 Negro college students. Oral Surg., 26:623, 1968.

Ringrose, R. E., Jabbour, J. T., and Keele, D. K.: Hemihypertrophy. Pediatrics, 36:434, 1965.

Robinson, H. B. G.: Classification of cysts of the jaws. Am. J. Orthod. Oral Surg., 31:370, 1945.

Robinson, H. B. G., and Koch, W. E.: Diagnosis of cysts of the jaw. J. Mo. Dent. Assoc., 21:187, 1941.

Robinson, H. B. G., Koch, W. E., Jr., and Jasper, L. H.: Infected globulomaxillary cyst. Am. J. Orthod. Oral Surg., 29:608, 1943.

Roed-Petersen, B.: Nasolabial cysts: a presentation of five patients with a review of the literature. Br. J. Oral Surg., 7:84, 1969.

Rowe, N. H.: Hemifacial hypertrophy. Review of the literature and addition of four cases. Oral Surg., 15:572, 1962.

Royer, R. W., and Bruce, K. W.: Median rhomboid glossitis: report of a case. Oral Surg., 5:1287, 1952.

Rushton, M. A.: A case of dentinal dysplasia. Guys Hosp. Rep., 89:369, 1939.

Idem: A new form of dentinal dysplasia: shell teeth. Oral Surg., 7:543, 1954.

Idem: Odontodysplasia. "Ghost Teeth." Br. Dent. J., 119:109, 1965.

Saarenmaa, L.: The origin of supernumerary teeth. Acta Odontol. Scand., 9:293, 1951.

Sammett, J. F.: Median rhomboid glossitis. Radiology, 32:215, 1939.

Sapp, J. P., and Gardner, D. G.: Regional odontodysplasia: an ultrastructural and histochemical study of the soft-tissue calcifications. Oral Surg., 36:383, 1973.

Sarnat, B. G., and Schour, I.: Enamel hypoplasia (chronologic enamel aplasia) in relation to systemic disease: a chronologic, morphologic and etiologic classification. J. Am. Dent. Assoc., 28:1989, 1941; 29:67, 1942.

Sarnat, B. G., and Shaw, N. G.: Dental development in congenital syphilis. Am. J. Dis. Child., 64:771, 1942; Am. J. Orthod. Oral Surg., 29:270, 1943.

Sauk, J. J., Jr.: Ectopic lingual thyroid. J. Pathol., 102:239, 1970.

Sauk, J. J., Trowbridge, H. O., and Witkop, C. J.: An electron optic analysis and explanation for the etiology of dentin dysplasia. Oral Surg., 33:763, 1972.

Schimmelpfennig, C. B., and McDonald, R. E.: Enamel and dentine aplasia. Oral Surg., 6:1444, 1953.

Schneider, W., and Reiter, E. H.: Median cleft lip: report of a case. J. Oral Surg., 9:329, 1951.

Schour, I.: The neonatal line in the enamel and dentin of the human deciduous teeth and first permanent molar. J. Am. Dent. Assoc., 23:1946, 1936.

Schour, I., and Smith, M. C.: Mottled teeth: an experimental and histologic analysis. J. Am. Dent. Assoc., 22:796, 1935.

Schroff, J.: Unusual cysts in the maxilla; cysts of nasopalatine duct and fissural cysts. Dent. Items Interest, 51:107, 1929.

Sedano, H. O., and Gorlin, R. J.: Familial occurrence of mesiodens. Oral Surg., 27:360, 1969.

Sedano, H. O., Sauk, J. J., and Gorlin, R. J.: Oral Manifestations of Inherited Disorders. Woburn, Mass., Butterworth (Publishers) Inc., 1977.

Senia, E. S., and Regezi, J. A.: Dens evaginatus in the etiology of bilateral periapical pathologic involvement in caries-free premolars. Oral Surg., 38:465, 1974.

Sewerin, I.: The sebaceous glands in the vermilion border of the lips and in the oral mucosa of man. Acta Odontol. Scand., 33(Suppl. 68):1975.

Sewerin, I., and Praetorius-Clausen, F.: Keratin-filled pseudocysts of ducts of sebaceous glands of the vermilion border of the lip. J. Oral Path., 3:279, 1975.

Shafer, W. G.: Dens in dente. N.Y. Dent. J., 19:220, 1953.

Sharma, L. K.: Median cleft of the upper lip. Plast. Reconstr. Surg., 53:155, 1974.

Shear, M.: Hereditary hypocalcification of enamel. J. Dent. Assoc. S. Afr., 9:262, 1954.

Shelling, D. H., and Anderson, G. M.: Relation of rickets and vitamin D to the incidence of dental caries, enamel hypoplasia and malocclusion in children. J. Am. Dent. Assoc., 23:840, 1936.

Shields, E. D., Bixler, D., and El-Kafrawy, A. M.: A proposed classification for heritable human dentine defects with a description of a new entity. Arch. Oral Biol., 18:543, 1973.

Smiley, G. R.: A possible genesis for cleft palate formation. Plast. Reconstr. Surg., 50:390, 1972.

Smith, A. A., Farbman, A., and Dancis, J.: Tongue in familial dysautonomia: a diagnostic sign. Am. J. Dis. Child., 110:152, 1965.

Smith, D. W.: Dysmorphology (teratology). J. Pediatr., 69:1150, 1966.

Smith, M. C., Lanz, E., and Smith, H. V.: The cause of mottled enamel. J. Dent. Res., 12:149,1932.

Smith, M. C., and Smith, H. V.: Mottled enamel of deciduous teeth. J. Am. Dent. Assoc., 22:814, 1935.

Smith, N. J. D., and Smith, P. B.: Congenital absence of major salivary glands. Br. Dent. J., 142:259, 1977.

Spouge, J. D., and Feasby, W. H.: Erupted teeth in the newborn. Oral Surg., 22:198, 1966.

Spriestersbach, D. C., Spriestersbach, B. R., and Moll, K. L.: Incidence of clefts of the lip and palate in families with children with clefts and families with children without clefts. Plast. Reconstr. Surg., 29:392, 1962.

Stafne, E. C.: Supernumerary teeth. Dent. Cosmos, 74:653, 1932.

Idem: Bone cavities situated near the angle of the mandible. J. Am. Dent. Assoc., 29:1969, 1942.

Stafne, E. C., Austin, L. T., and Gardner, B.: Median anterior maxillary cysts. J. Am. Dent. Assoc., 23:801, 1936.

Starkey, P. E., and Shafer, W. G.: Eruption sequestra in children. J. Dent. Child., 30:84, 1963.

Stein, G.: Enamel damage of systemic origin in premature birth and disease of early infancy. Am. J. Orthod. Oral Surg., 33:831, 1947.

Stewart, R. E., and Prescott, G. H. (eds.): Oral Facial Genetics. St. Louis, C. V. Mosby Company, 1976.

Stout, F. W., and Collett, W. K.: Etiology and incidence

of the median maxillary anterior alveolar cleft. Oral Surg., 28:66, 1969.

Strean, L. P., and Peer, L. A.: Stress as an etiologic factor in the development of cleft palate. Plastic Reconstr. Surg., 18:1, 1956.

Taylor, W. B., and Lane, D. J.: Congenital fistulas of the lower lip. Arch. Dermatol., 94:421, 1966.

Thoma, K. H.: Facial cleft or fissural cysts. J. Orthod. Oral Surg., 23:83, 1937.

Idem: Principal factors controlling development of mandible and maxilla. Am. J. Orthod. Oral Surg., 24:171, 1938.

Tobias, N.: Inheritance of scrotal tongue. Arch. Dermatol. Syph., 52:266, 1946.

Toller, P. A.: A clinical report on six cases of amelogenesis imperfecta. Oral Surg., 12:325, 1959.

van der Waal, I., Beemster, G., and van der Kwast, A. M.: Median rhomboid glossitis caused by Candida? Oral Surg., 47:31, 1979.

van Gool, A. V.: Injury to the permanent tooth germ after trauma to the deciduous predecessor. Oral Surg., 35:2, 1973.

Veau, V.: Division palatine; anatomie, chirurgie, phonetique. Paris, Masson et Cie, 1931.

Via, W. F., Jr.: Enamel defects induced by trauma during tooth formation. Oral Surg., 25:49, 1968.

Vickers, R. A., Gorlin, R. J., and Smark, E. A.: Lymphoepithelial lesions of the oral cavity. Report of four cases. Oral Surg., 16:1214, 1963.

Virtanen, I., and Laine, P.: A study on the relative frequency of the globulomaxillary cyst. Suom. Hammaslaak. Toim., 57:191, 1961.

Vorheis, J. M., Gregory, G. T., and McDonald, R. E.: Ankylosed deciduous molars. J. Am. Dent. Assoc., 44:68, 1952.

Walton, J. L., Witkop, C. J., Jr., and Walker, P. O.: Odontodysplasia. Oral Surg., 46:676, 1978.

Ward, G. E., Hendrick, J. W., and Chambers, R. G.: Thyroglossal tract abnormalities: cysts and fistulas. Surg. Gynecol. Obstet., 89:727, 1949.

Warkany, J., and Deuschle, F. M.: Congenital malformations induced in rats by maternal riboflavin deficiency: dentofacial changes. J. Am. Dent. Assoc., 51:139, 1955.

Watne, A. L., Core, S. K., and Carrier, J. M.: Gardner's syndrome. Surg. Gynecol. Obstet., 141:53, 1975.

Weathers, D. R., Baker, G., Archard, H. O., and Burkes, E. J., Jr.: Psoriasiform lesions of the oral mucosa (with emphasis on "ectopic geographic tongue"). Oral Surg., 37:872, 1974.

Weathers, D. R., Corio, R. L., Crawford, B. E., Giansanti, J. S., and Page, L. R.: The labial melanotic macule. Oral Surg., 42:196, 1976.

Weathers, D. R., and Fine, R. M.: Thrombosed varix of oral cavity. Arch. Dermatol., 104:427, 1971.

Webster, R. C.: Cleft palate. Oral Surg., 1:647, 943, 1948; 2:99, 485, 1949.

Weinberg, S., Moncarz, V., and Van de Mark, T. B.: Midline cleft of the mandible: review of literature and report of case. J. Oral Surg., 30:143, 1972.

Weinmann, J. P., Svoboda, J. F., and Woods, R. W.: Hereditary disturbances of enamel formation and calcification. J. Am. Dent. Assoc., 32:397, 1945.

Weir, T. W., and Johnson, W. C.: Cheilitis glandularis. Arch. Dermatol., 103:433, 1971.

Weitzner, S.: Lymphoepithelial (branchial) cyst of parotid gland. Oral Surg., 35:85, 1973.

Wesley, R. K., Delaney, J. R., and Pensler, L.: Mucocutaneous melanosis and gastrointestinal polyposis

(Peutz-Jeghers syndrome): clinical considerations and report of a case. J. Dent. Child., *44*:131, 1977.

Wesley, R. K., Wysocki, G. P., Mintz, S. M., and Jackson, J.: Dentin dysplasia type I. Oral Surg., *41*:516, 1976.

White, D. K., Lucas, R. M., and Miller, A. S.: Median mandibular cyst: review of the literature and report of two cases. J. Oral Surg., *33*:372, 1975.

Wilson, G. W., and Steinbrecher, M.: Hereditary hypoplasia of the dentin. J. Am. Dent. Assoc., *16*:866, 1929.

Winter, G. B.: Principles of Exodontia as Applied to the Impacted Mandibular Third Molar. St. Louis, American Medical Book Company, 1926.

Winter, G. R., and Maiocco, P. D.: Osteogenesis imperfecta and odontogensis imperfecta. Oral Surg., *2*:782, 1949.

Witkop, C. J., Jr., (ed.): Genetics and Dental Health. New York, McGraw-Hill Book Company, 1962.

Idem: Genetics and dentistry. Eugenics Quart., 5:15, 1958.

Idem: Hereditary defects of dentin. Dent. Clin. North Am., *19*:3, 1975.

Witkop, C. J., Jr., MacLean, C. J., Schmidt, P. J. and Henry, J. L.: Medical and dental finding in the Brandywine isolate. Ala. J. Med. Sci., 3:382, 1966.

Witkop, C. J., Jr., and Niswander, J. D.: Focal epithelial hyperplasia in Central and South American Indians and Ladinos. Oral Surg., *20*:213, 1965.

Witkop, C. J., Jr., and Sauk, J. J., Jr.: Heritable defects of enamel; in R. E. Stewart and G. H. Prescott (eds.): Oral Facial Genetics. St. Louis, The C. V. Mosby Company, 1976.

Woodbourne, A. R., and Philpott, O. S.: Cheilitis glandularis: a manifestation of emotional disturbance. Arch. Dermatol. Syph., *62*:820, 1950.

Woolf, C. M., Woolf, R. M., and Broadbent, T. R.: Genetic and nongenetic variables related to cleft lip and palate. Plast. Reconstr. Surg., *32*:65, 1963.

Worsaae, N., and Pindborg, J.: Granulomatous gingival manifestations of Melkersson-Rosenthal syndrome. Oral Surg., *49*:131, 1980.

Wright, B. A.: Median rhomboid glossitis: not a misnomer. Oral Surg., *46*:806, 1978.

Wysocki, G. P.: The differential diagnosis of globulomaxillary radiolucencies. Oral Surg., *51*:281, 1981.

Yip, W. K.: The prevalence of dens evaginatus. Oral Surg., *38*:80, 1974.

Zackin, S. J., and Weisberger, D.: Hereditary gingival fibromatosis. Oral Surg., *14*:828, 1961.

Zaus, E., and Teuscher, G. W.: Report on three cases of congenital dysfunction of the major salivary glands. J. Dent. Res., *19*:326, 1940.

Zegarelli, E. V., Kesten, B. M., and Kutscher, A. H.: Melanin spots of the oral mucosa and skin associated with polyps. Oral Surg., *7*:972, 1954.

CHAPTER 2

Benign and Malignant Tumors of the Oral Cavity

The study of tumors of the oral cavity and adjacent structures constitutes an important phase of dentistry because of the role which the dentist plays in the diagnosis and treatment of these lesions. Although tumors constitute only a small minority of the pathologic conditions seen by the dentist, they are of great significance since they have the potential ability to jeopardize the health and longevity of the patient. Many of the great variety of oral tumors will seldom be seen by the general practitioner of dentistry. Yet it is of utmost importance that he be familiar with them so that when one does present itself, he may either institute appropriate treatment or refer the patient to the proper therapist.

A tumor, by definition, is simply a swelling of the tissue; in the strict sense, the word does not imply a neoplastic process. Many of the lesions to be discussed in this section are called tumors only because they are manifested as swellings; they are in no way actually related to true neoplasms.

Neoplasia is a poorly understood biologic phenomenon which, in some instances, cannot be clearly differentiated from other processes or tissue reactions. Although no precise definition of a neoplasm exists, particularly one without exception, a neoplasm is often considered an independent, uncoordinated new growth of tissue which is potentially capable of unlimited proliferation and which does not regress after removal of the stimulus which produced the lesion.

BENIGN TUMORS OF EPITHELIAL TISSUE ORIGIN

PAPILLOMA

The papilloma is a common benign neoplasm originating from surface epithelium. It is frequently confused clinically with other benign intraoral neoplasms, particularly the fibroma. In most cases, however, the astute observer will encounter no difficulty in distinguishing the papilloma from the fibroma, since each has certain definite characteristics.

Clinical Features. The papilloma is an exophytic growth made up of numerous, small finger-like projections which result in a lesion with a roughened, verrucous or "cauliflower-like" surface. It is nearly always a well circumscribed pedunculated tumor, occasionally sessile, and intraorally is found most commonly on the tongue, lips, buccal mucosa, gingiva and palate, particularly that area adjacent to the uvula (Fig. 2–1). The majority of papillomas are only a few millimeters in diameter, but lesions may be encountered which measure several centimeters. These growths occur at any age and are seen even in young children. A series of 110 cases has been reported by Greer and Goldman, while a series of 464 cases has been studied by Abbey and his co-workers; this is somewhat indicative of the prevalent nature of the lesion.

The common wart, or *verruca vulgaris,* is a frequent tumor of the skin analogous to the oral

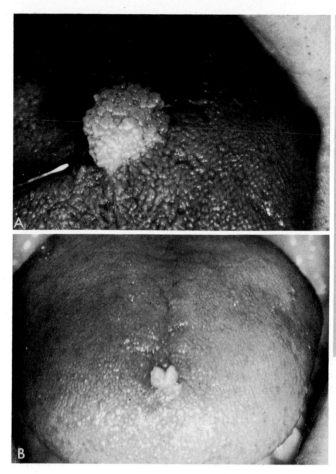

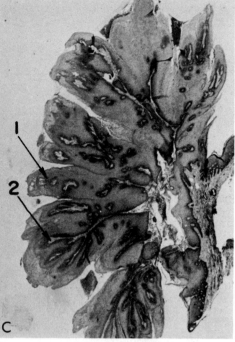

Figure 2–1. *Papilloma*.
Large (A) and small (B) papillomas of the tongue
illustrate the variation in clinical appearance of the
lesion. The photomicrograph (C) illustrates the
many finger-like projections (1), each containing a
thin, central connective tissue core (2), of which
the lesion is composed.

papilloma. Although it has been established that
in at least a considerable percentage of cases
the skin wart is caused by a virus known as the
papillomavirus, there is considerable question
whether this is true of the human oral papilloma. For example, an investigation has been
reported by Jenson and his associates involving
67 proliferative squamous epithelial lesions of
the oral cavity examined for the papillomavirus
antigen by a peroxidase-antiperoxidase immu-
nocytochemical technique against known controls. They found 18 of 29 verrucae of the lips
virus-antigen positive, 3 of 5 condylomata positive, but only 2 of 5 multiple papillomas positive. Twenty-eight keratoacanthomas tested
were also all negative. Actually, multiple oral
papillomas are quite uncommon, except in certain situations such as the *focal dermal hypoplasia syndrome* (q.v.), the usual lesion being a
solitary papilloma so that it might be questioned
whether those reported by Jenson and associates as viral-positive oral papillomas might represent only intraoral verrucae. In a related
study, Wysocki and Hardie have demonstrated

typical intranuclear viral inclusions in 6 of 10
lesions diagnosed histopathologically as verruca
vulgaris but in none of 10 lesions diagnosed as
papillomas. Oral papillomas of viral origin do
exist in several other species of animals, however, such as the dog and rabbit. At present
there has been no case of papilloma in the
human being induced by the injection of a cell-
free extract of an oral papilloma from another
person.

Lesions that are histologically identical to the
verruca vulgaris of the skin are frequently found
on the lips and occasionally intraorally (Fig. 2–
2). These are often seen in patients with verrucae on the hands or fingers, and the oral
lesions appear to arise through autoinoculation
by finger sucking or fingernail biting.

Papilloma-like or papillomatous lesions as
well as "pebbly" lesions and fibromas of various
sites in the oral cavity are recognized as one of
the many manifestations of the *multiple hamartoma and neoplasia syndrome* (Cowden's syndrome). This is an autosomal dominant disease
characterized by facial trichilemmomas associ-

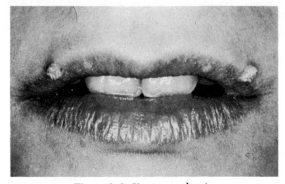

Figure 2–2. *Verruca vulgaris.*
These verrucae of the lips occurred in a girl, with similar lesions on the fingers, who habitually bit her fingernails. (Courtesy of Dr. Paul E. Starkey.)

ated with gastrointestinal tract, thyroid, CNS and musculoskeletal abnormalities as well as the oral lesions. It is also considered a cutaneous marker of breast cancer.

Histologic Features. The microscopic appearance of the papilloma is characteristic and consists of many long, thin, finger-like projections extending above the surface of the mucosa, each made up of a continuous layer of stratified squamous epithelium and containing a thin, central connective tissue core which supports the nutrient blood vessels (Fig. 2–1, *C*). Some papillomas exhibit hyperkeratosis, although this finding is probably secondary to the location of the lesion and the amount of trauma or frictional irritation to which it has been subjected. The essential feature is a proliferation of the spinous cells in a papillary pattern; the connective tissue present is supportive stroma only and is not considered a part of the neoplastic element. Mitotic activity in the epithelial cells is sometimes disturbingly prevalent. The presence of chronic inflammatory cells may be variably noted in the connective tissue.

Treatment and Prognosis. Treatment of the papilloma consists of excision, including the base of the mucosa into which the pedicle or stalk inserts. Removal should never be accomplished by an incision *through* the pedicle. If the tumor is properly excised, recurrence is rare. The possibility of malignant degeneration in the oral papilloma is quite unlikely, although fixation of the base or induration of the deeper tissues should always be viewed with some suspicion.

SQUAMOUS ACANTHOMA

The squamous acanthoma is an uncommon lesion which probably represents a reactive phenomenon of epithelium rather than a true neoplasm. It bears no known relationship to the *clear cell acanthoma*, which occurs with considerable frequency on the skin and may also be found on the lips, as in the two cases reported by Weitzner.

The squamous acanthoma has no distinctive clinical appearance by which it may be identified or even suspected, and may occur at virtually any site on the oral mucosa, usually in older adults. It is generally described as a small flat or elevated, white, sessile or pedunculated lesion on the mucosa. The lesion is histologically distinctive and consists of a well-demarcated elevated and/or umbilicated epithelial proliferation with a markedly thickened layer of orthokeratin and underlying spinous layer of cells. Tomich and Shafer, who originally described this lesion, postulated that it was caused by trauma and developed its characteristic morphology through a series of epithelial alterations beginning with a localized pseudoepitheliomatous hyperplasia. It is not known to recur after excision.

KERATOACANTHOMA

(Self-healing Carcinoma; Molluscum Pseudocarcinomatosum; Molluscum Sebaceum; Verrucoma)

The keratoacanthoma is a lesion which both clinically and histologically resembles epidermoid carcinoma so closely that it is frequently mistaken for cancer, but it is nevertheless a benign epithelial lesion. The etiology is unknown, although both genetic and viral factors have been considered. Furthermore, it has been demonstrated that the keratoacanthoma can be readily induced on the skin in a wide variety of experimental animals by the action of chemical carcinogens, so these also may play some role in the production of the lesion in man.

Clinical Features. The keratoacanthoma occurs about twice as frequently in men as in women and the majority of cases occur between the ages of 50 and 70 years, according to a study of 238 cases reported by Ghadially and his associates. However, it can occur even in the second decade. In this series, about 90 per cent of the tumors occurred on the exposed skin, with the cheeks, nose and dorsum of the hands being most often involved. The lesion occurred on the lips in 8.1 per cent of the cases. Intraoral lesions are quite uncommon, a total of four cases being reviewed by Freedman and his associates. The more common keratoacan-

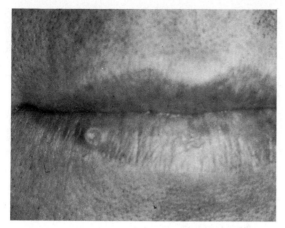

Figure 2–3. Keratoacanthoma.
This small keratoacanthoma of the lip illustrates the typical elevated, umbilicated appearance of the lesion. (Courtesy of Dr. Charles E. Hutton.)

thoma of the lip has been discussed by Silberberg and his co-workers, who cited 41 cases, approximately equally distributed between the upper and lower lips, and by Kohn and Eversole.

The lesion appears as an elevated umbilicated or crateriform one with a depressed central core or plug (Fig. 2–3). It is seldom over 1.0 to 1.5 cm. in diameter. The lesion is often painful and regional lymphadenopathy may be present.

The clinical course of the lesion is one of its unusual aspects. It begins as a small, firm nodule that develops to full size over a period of four to eight weeks, persists as a static lesion for another four to eight weeks, then undergoes spontaneous regression over the next six- to eight-week period by expulsion of the keratin core with resorption of the mass. However, lesions with an overall duration of as long as two years have been reported. Recurrence is rare.

Histologic Features. The lesion consists of hyperplastic squamous epithelium growing into the underlying connective tissue. The surface is covered by a thickened layer of parakeratin or orthokeratin with central plugging. The epithelial cells do not usually show atypia but occasionally dysplastic features are found. At the deep leading margin of the tumor, islands of epithelium often appear to be invading and frequently this area cannot be differentiated from epidermoid carcinoma. Lapins and Helwig, among others, have also reported that the keratoacanthoma on occasion may invade perineural spaces, but this does not adversely affect the biologic behavior of the lesion; neither can it be used as a distinguishing characteristic

between keratoacanthoma and epidermoid carcinoma. The connective tissue in the area shows chronic inflammatory cell infiltration. The most characteristic feature of the lesion is found at the margins where the normal adjacent epithelium is elevated toward the central portion of the crater; then an abrupt change in the normal epithelium occurs as the hyperplastic acanthotic epithelium is reached. For this reason, the diagnosis may be impossible if the adjacent border of the specimen is not included in the biopsy.

Treatment. The lesion is usually treated by surgical excision inasmuch as one cannot be absolutely certain of the nature of the lesion from the clinical appearance. Spontaneous regression does not occur in every case; where it has occurred, residual scar may be present. The various modalities of treatment of keratoacanthoma of the lip have been discussed specifically by Hardman.

PIGMENTED CELLULAR NEVUS

(Pigmented Mole; Benign Melanocytic Nevus)

A nevus is defined as a congenital, developmental tumor-like malformation of the skin or mucous membrane. Although this term has been used also to describe such growths as the hemangioma, it is applied most frequently to a skin lesion containing melanin pigment: the common mole. This pigmented nevus is a superficial lesion composed of so-called nevus cells; hence the term "cellular" nevus. It is seen occasionally in the oral cavity, but occurs far more frequently on the skin. Buchner and Hansen have reviewed the reported cases of oral mucosal nevi as well as adding 32 new cases to the literature. A number of different types of nevi are recognized, and these may be classified as congenital and acquired nevi. The acquired nevi may be further subdivided as follows: (1) intradermal nevus (common mole), (2) junctional nevus, (3) compound nevus, (4) spindle cell and/or epithelioid cell nevus, and (5) blue (Jadassohn-Tieche) nevus. In addition, variants of these nevi have been described.

Clinical Features. Ainsworth and her colleagues separate the congenital nevi of the skin into "small" and "garment" nevi. The "small" nevi are greater than 1 cm. in diameter and usually 3 to 5 cm. The "garment" nevi are greater than 10 cm. in diameter and can cover large areas of the skin. The congenital nevi occur in 1 to 2.5 per cent of neonates and, with the passage of time, may change from flat, pale

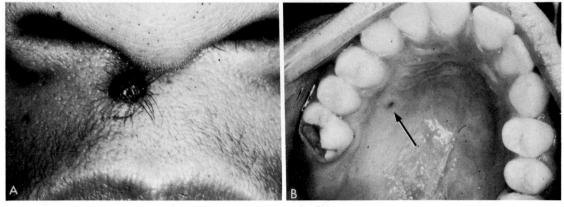

Figure 2–4. *Pigmented cellular nevus.*
Typical examples of nevi of the skin (A) and palate (B) are illustrated.

tan macules to elevated, verrucous, hairy lesions. Approximately 15 per cent occur on the skin of the head and neck. Intraoral occurrence is extremely rare.

Acquired nevi are extremely common. They appear about the eighth month of life and increase in number with age, apparently reaching their peak numerically in the late third decade of life. Clark has stated that the number of nevi which a person has is genetically determined. Interestingly, the number of nevi begin to decrease as one ages, so that elderly persons average far fewer nevi than younger adults.

The *intradermal nevus* is one of the most common lesions of the skin, most persons exhibiting several, often dozens, scattered over the body. The common mole may be a smooth flat lesion or may be elevated above the surface; it may or may not exhibit brown pigmentation, and it often shows strands of hair growing from its surface (Fig. 2–4, *A*). This form of mole seldom occurs on the soles of the feet, the palms of the hands or the genitalia.

The *junctional nevus* may appear clinically similar to the intradermal nevus, the distinction being chiefly histologic. It is extremely important, however, that a distinction be drawn, since the prognosis of the two lesions is different, as will be pointed out later.

The *compound nevus* is a lesion composed of two elements: an intradermal nevus and an overlying junctional nevus.

The *spindle cell and/or epithelioid cell nevus* occurs chiefly in children, only about 15 per cent appearing in adults, and may appear histologically similar to malignant melanoma in the adult. Seldom, however, does this lesion exhibit clinically malignant features. Essentially, this lesion is clinically benign, but histologically

malignant. Weedon and Little have reviewed 211 cases of spindle cell and epithelioid cell nevi while Allen has reviewed 262 cases, and none of these authors have found any nevus of this type on a mucous membrane surface, including the oral cavity.

The *blue nevus* is a true mesodermal structure composed of dermal melanocytes which only rarely undergo malignant transformation. It occurs chiefly on the buttocks, on the dorsum of the feet and hands, on the face and occasionally on other areas. The majority of blue nevi are present at birth or appear in early childhood and persist unchanged throughout life. The lesion is smooth, exhibits hairs growing from its surface and varies in color from brown to blue or bluish black. Scofield reviewed this lesion in 1959 and reported two intraoral cases, the first recorded occurrences of the lesion in the mouth. Since then, numerous intraoral cases have been reported, such as the eight instances in the study by Buchner and Hansen.

Histologic variants of acquired nevi such as neural, balloon cell and halo nevi occur. Only the halo nevus is clinicopathologically distinctive. The neural and balloon cell nevi are histologic variants of intradermal or compound nevi.

Oral Manifestations. Acquired pigmented nevi of all types, with the exception of the spindle cell and/or epithelioid cell nevus, occasionally occur on the oral mucosa. There is no epidemiologic data available on the actual frequency of intraoral lesions. All information available is based upon retrospective analyses of excised intraoral nevi. Based upon such data, Buchner and Hansen found that intramucosal nevi (the mucosal counterpart of intradermal nevi) accounted for slightly more than 55 per cent of 107 reported nevi. The blue nevus accounted for 36 per cent, the compound nevus nearly six per cent and the junctional nevus slightly less than three per cent. Of some interest is the fact that the blue nevus accounts for such a high percentage of intraoral nevi. This cannot be dismissed solely as a function of reporting.

Intraoral nevi occur in all decades of life except the first and are twice as common in females as in males. The nevus may occur at any site, but the hard palate, buccal mucosa, lip and gingiva account for the majority of cases (Fig. 2-4, *B*). Most nevi present as raised, pigmented lesions but 20 per cent are flat, macular lesions which must be distinguished histologically from other pigmented lesions of the oral mucosa, such as the melanotic macule, premalignant melanosis and amalgam tattoo. Occasional lesions lack pigmentation and may appear as excrescences of normal color.

Histologic Features. Theories about the origin of the nevus cell are controversial. However, most authorities believe that nevus cells are derived from the neural crest.

The nevus cells themselves are large discrete cells, each with an ovoid, vesicular nucleus and pale cytoplasm. They tend to be grouped in sheets or cords and may contain granules of melanin pigment in their cytoplasm (Fig. 2-5, *C*). The arrangement of these cells in an alveolar pattern is referred to as thèques. Multinucleated giant nevus cells are sometimes seen, but are of little prognostic significance. Mitotic figures are not common.

In the *intradermal nevus*, the nevus cells are situated within the connective tissue and are separated from the overlying epithelium by a well defined band of connective tissue. Thus, in the intradermal nevus, the nevus cells are not in contact with the surface epithelium (Fig. 2-5, *A*).

In the *junctional nevus*, this zone of demarcation is absent and the nevus cells contact and seem to blend into the surface epithelium. This overlying epithelium is usually thin and irregular and shows cells apparently crossing the junction and growing down into the connective tissue—the so-called *abtropfung* or "dropping-off" effect. This "junctional activity" has serious implications because junctional nevi have been known to undergo transformation into malignant melanomas.

The *compound nevus* shows features of both

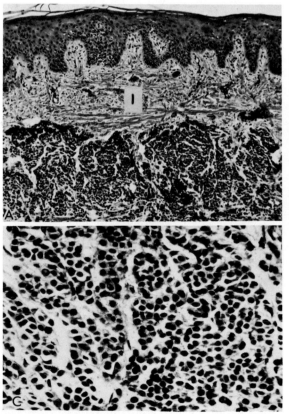

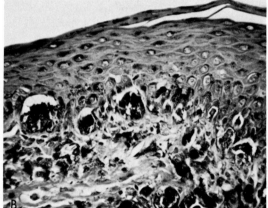

Figure 2-5. *Pigmented cellular nevus.*
The intradermal nevus (*A*) demonstrates a thick band of connective tissue (*1*) separating the nevus cells from the overlying epithelium. In the compound nevus (*B*), the nevus cells are in contact with the overlying epithelium and are in the underlying connective tissue. The nevus cells are shown under high magnification (*C*).

the junctional and intradermal nevus. Nests of nevus cells are dropping off from the epidermis, while large nests of nevus cells are also present in the dermis (Fig. 2–5, B).

The *spindle cell and/or epithelioid cell nevus* is commonly composed of pleomorphic cells of three basic types: spindle cells, oval or "epithelioid" cells, and both mononuclear and multinucleated giant cells. These are arranged in well-circumscribed sheets and there is generally considerable junctional activity.

The *blue nevus* is of two types: the common blue nevus and the cellular blue nevus. In the common blue nevus, elongated melanocytes with long branching dendritic processes lie in bundles, usually oriented parallel to the epidermis, in the middle and lower third of the dermis. There is no junctional activity. The melanocytes are typically packed with melanin granules, sometimes obscuring the nucleus, and these granules may extend into the dendritic processes. In the cellular blue nevus, an additional cell type is present: a large, round or spindle cell with a pale vacuolated cytoplasm. These cells commonly are arranged in an alveolar pattern.

Treatment and Prognosis. Because the acquired pigmented nevus is of such common occurrence, it would obviously be impossible to attempt to eradicate all such lesions. It has become customary to recommend removal of pigmented moles if they occur in areas which are irritated by clothing, such as at the belt or collar line, or if they suddenly begin to increase in size, deepen in color, or become ulcerated. Allen and Spitz have stated that it is fairly certain that trauma to an intradermal nevus will not induce malignancy. Whether simple trauma to a junctional nevus will produce malignancy is not known.

On the other hand, it is now well recognized that the congenital nevi have a great risk for transformation to malignant melanoma. Kaplan reported seven cases which were seen at the Stanford University Hospital and discussed 49 other cases. It is estimated that 14 per cent of the large congenital nevi may undergo malignant transformation. Of particular interest is the occurrence of the *B–K mole syndrome* described by Clark and co-workers. This autosomal dominant condition is characterized by large pigmented nevi and a high risk for the development of melanoma. Its occurrence, however, has not been documented intraorally.

Surgical excision of all intraoral pigmented nevi is recommended as a prophylactic measure because of the constant chronic irritation of the mucosa in nearly all intraoral sites occasioned by eating, toothbrushing, etc.

"PREMALIGNANT" LESIONS OF EPITHELIAL TISSUE ORIGIN

LEUKOPLAKIA

Leukoplakia is a term that has been used for many years to indicate a white patch or plaque occurring on the surface of a mucous membrane, not only that of the oral cavity, but also that of the vulva, uterine cervix, urinary bladder, renal pelvis and upper respiratory tract. Actually, a variety of lesions, including certain very specific disease entities, may manifest themselves clinically as white patches on the oral mucosa. Unfortunately, there has been lack of agreement among some clinicians and pathologists as to the exact meaning of the term "leukoplakia." In some instances the term has been used to describe a white patch on the mucosa which will not rub or strip off. At the opposite extreme, the diagnosis of leukoplakia has been based on strict histologic criteria, and such a diagnosis has often been made even though clinically the lesion does not appear as a white patch.

Thus, the scientific literature includes a range of histologic terminology used to designate clinical leukoplakia. This includes keratosis, leukokeratosis, hyperkeratosis, hyperkeratosis simplex, hyperkeratosis complex, nonspecific focal keratosis, pachyderma oralis, leukoplakia and intraepithelial carcinoma. Numerous authors have required the presence of epithelial dysplasia or dyskeratosis for a microscopic diagnosis of leukoplakia. Their writings have implied that a microscopic diagnosis of leukoplakia by this criterion carries a possibility of malignant transformation. In the absence of dysplasia, these authors used terms such as "focal keratosis" and "hyperkeratosis" for the clinical white patch.

To eliminate such confusion, there has been an increasing tendency to use the word "leukoplakia" as a rather loose clinical term having no histologic connotation. Accordingly, the term "leukoplakia" as used here will imply only the clinical feature of a white plaque on the mucosa (specifically excluding all definite entities also manifesting as white lesions, such as lichen planus, syphilitic mucous patches, white sponge nevus, moniliasis, lupus erythematosus, chemical burns and other stomatitides) and will carry absolutely no histologic connotation, although it is characterized inevitably by some form of disturbance of the surface epithelium. This is basically the same definition that has been proffered by the World Health Organization (WHO) Collaborating Center for Oral Precancerous Lesions, which was established in 1967 "to characterize and define those lesions that should be considered in a study of oral precancer and to determine, if possible, their relative risk of becoming malignant."

Extensive reviews of the literature on oral leukoplakia have been published by Waldron and Shafer, and these have included citation of the various controversial aspects of the disease as well as a résumé of the current concepts. In addition, an in-depth overview of the subject of oral premalignancy, including leukoplakia, has been the subject of a symposium edited by Mackenzie and his associates. The WHO Collaborating Center for Oral Precancerous Lesions has also published a report of its studies on oral precancer.

Etiology. The etiology of leukoplakia is conceded by most investigators to be a varied one. Some workers believe that the initiation of the condition may depend not only upon extrinsic local factors, but also upon intrinsic predisposing factors. Factors most frequently blamed have been tobacco, alcohol, oral sepsis, local irritation, syphilis, vitamin deficiency, endocrine disturbances, galvanism, and actinic radiation in the case of leukoplakia of the lips.

TOBACCO. Tobacco has been cited most frequently as the offending agent, and there is considerable evidence for this assumption. Many of the chemical constituents of tobacco and its combustion end-products, such as tobacco tars and resins, are irritating substances which are capable of producing leukoplakic alterations of the oral mucosa. It is generally accepted that important sources of irritation of the mucous membrane are not only the combustion products brought about by the burning tobacco and the heat, but also the materials which leach out of the tobacco when it is chewed or, in the case of snuff, allowed to rest against moist mucosa.

Some investigators believe that pipe smoking is most harmful. A specific lesion of the palate which is called *stomatitis nicotina* (or "pipe-smoker's palate") is seen frequently in persons who are heavy pipesmokers. This condition, recognizable both clinically and microscopically, is first manifested by redness and inflammation of the palate. Soon the palate develops a diffuse, grayish-white, thickened, multinodular or papular appearance with a small red spot in the center of each tiny nodule, representing the dilated and sometimes partially occluded orifice of an accessory palatal salivary gland duct around which inflammatory cell infiltration is prominent (Fig. 2–6). Fissures and cracks may appear, producing a wrinkled, irregular surface. The epithelium around the ducts shows excessive thickening and keratinization. Many investigators regard this as simply an anatomic variant of leukoplakia.

The experimental studies of Roffo showed that when either nicotine or tobacco extract was applied to the gingiva of rabbits, no lesions were produced. But when tobacco smoke was blown onto the gingiva, white spots similar to leukoplakia developed within a short time. Of possible significance is the study by Kreshover and Salley, who showed that exposing the mouse ear to tobacco smoke produced no marked histologically demonstrable effects in the epithelium unless the animals were deficient in vitamin B complex. In such animals alterations occurred in the epithelium which could be interpreted as potentially malignant changes. Similar alterations in oral mucosa could not be produced, however. The regression of certain of these lesions after discontinuance of the use of tobacco is further evidence of a cause-and-effect relation. In 36 cases of leukoplakia reported by Cooke, 13 were considered to be related to smoking; 18 were considered caused by frictional irritation, and three were associated with syphilis. Renstrup found the probable etiology of 90 cases of leukoplakia to be tobacco in 23 instances, local irritation in 19 instances and syphilis in three instances. In 45 cases no etiologic factor could be elicited.

In more recent years, even greater attention has focused on the use of tobacco and its role in the etiology of leukoplakia as well as oral cancer, probably in large part because of tobacco's recognized role in the increasing incidence of lung cancer. Unfortunately, data relating the use of smoking tobacco, in the form of cigarettes, cigars and pipes, appear far more difficult to relate to the etiology of leukoplakia than the use of smokeless tobacco, i.e., snuff and chewing tobacco. This difficulty is related to the widespread use of smoking tobacco and the fact that the smoke is dispersed throughout the entire oral cavity although leukoplakia most frequently develops at only one or a few localized sites. In comparison, the use of snuff or chewing tobacco is relatively uncommon and

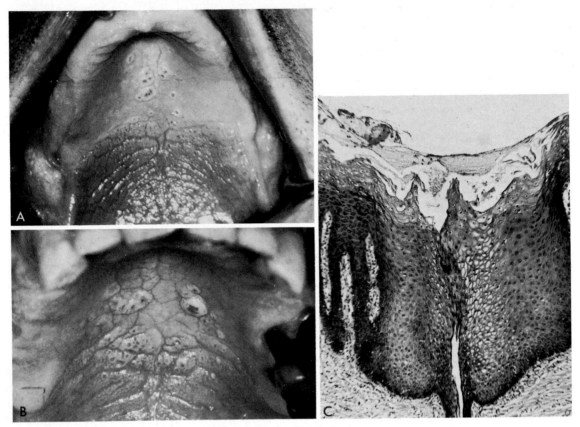

Figure 2–6. *Stomatitis nicotina.*
The nodular thickened areas on the palate demonstrate the tiny gland orifices (*A, B*). There is thickening of the epithelium adjacent to the orifice seen in the photomicrograph (*C*).

the tobacco itself is typically held at a given site on the mucosa so that if a lesion of leukoplakia were to develop at that site, this would be fairly convincing evidence of a cause-and-effect relation. Nevertheless, there are still few studies that are based on more than simply clinical observation and conjecture. Pindborg and his co-workers have described tobacco-induced changes in oral leukoplakic epithelium in groups of Danish and Indian leukoplakia patients, but these appeared to be associated chiefly with the use of pipes, snuff and hooklis (a short-stemmed clay pipe used in India). Several other studies from Scandinavia and India, where the tobacco problem is somewhat different than that in the United States, have also been published but there are actually few controlled studies dealing with this agent in the United States.

One interesting lesion, described as the "cigarette smoker's lip lesion," has been described by Berry and Landwerlen in a large segment of hospital patients smoking chiefly nonfiltered cigarettes. These lesions have a variety of clinical appearances but are generally flat or slightly elevated, nodular white lesions on one or both lips corresponding to the site at which the cigarette is held and apparently smoked down to an extremely short length. The majority of the patients exhibited associated characteristic finger-burns. No malignancy was found developing in any of these lesions.

ALCOHOL. The use of alcohol has also been suggested as being of etiologic importance because it may be irritating to the mucosa. But persons who habitually consume considerable quantities of alcohol are usually also inveterate smokers, so that it is difficult to establish the effects of alcohol alone.

A number of workers, such as Wynder et al., have suggested that the same factors that are important in the etiology of oral cancer are operable in the etiology of leukoplakia. The role of multiple, coexistent predisposing factors such as liver damage, and use of tobacco and alcohol, and the like, has been emphasized by Trieger and his co-workers.

CHRONIC IRRITATION. Trauma or local chronic irritation is considered by some investigators to be extremely important in the etiology of leukoplakia, and any chronic irritating factor in the oral cavity, such as malocclusion producing chronic cheek-biting, ill-fitting dentures, or sharp, broken-down teeth which constantly irritate the mucosa, should be suspected. Hot spicy foods are also frequently mentioned as an etiologic factor, and it is at least conceivable that with continued use they may be of some importance.

SYPHILIS. Although the older literature stressed the importance of syphilis in the development of leukoplakia, reports of Hobaek, Cooke and Renstrup would indicate that it plays a relatively minor role, although there is considerable evidence to indicate that there is a somewhat higher incidence of leukoplakia among patients who have had syphilitic glossitis than among those with a non-syphilitic background.

VITAMIN DEFICIENCY. It is well recognized that a deficiency of vitamin A will induce metaplasia and keratinization of certain epithelial structures, particularly of glands and respiratory mucosa. Hence it has been suggested that a deficiency of this vitamin is related to the development of leukoplakia. Vitamin B complex deficiency has also been suggested as a predisposing factor in the development of leukoplakia. The mechanism for this is unknown, but might be related to alteration in the oxidation patterns of the epithelium, making it more susceptible to irritation. On this basis, treatment with brewer's yeast is classic.

HORMONES. The keratogenic effect of both male and female sex hormones also has been demonstrated under certain situations. Current literature gives little clinical support, however, to the role of endocrine dysfunction and vitamin deficiency, and there has been a general lack of recent investigations of these factors, making their significance in the etiology of leukoplakia difficult to evaluate.

GALVANISM. Galvanism was at one time considered to be of etiologic importance, although recent authors have tended to discount this mechanism as a significant etiologic factor.

CANDIDOSIS. The presence of *Candida albicans*, a relatively common oral fungus, has been reported as occurring very frequently in association with leukoplakia. For example, in a study of 226 patients with leukoplakia, Roed-Petersen and colleagues found that 31 per cent of the biopsy tissue specimens contained *Candida*. However, at the present time, it is not known whether the organisms bear any responsibility for initial development of the leukoplakia or whether they are only secondary invaders.

Furthermore, in a series of 235 patients with leukoplakia, Renstrup has reported finding epithelial atypia in 56 per cent of those which showed candidal invasion, particularly the "speckled" type of leukoplakia. She has suggested the possibility that invading *Candida* hyphae may be responsible for a disorderly maturation of the epithelium. However, the WHO leukoplakia report (1978) states that the interrelationship between candidal infection, epithelial dysplasia and the risk of future malignancy remains uncertain.

Clinical Features. The lesions of oral leukoplakia show considerable variation in size, location and clinical appearance. Most reports indicate that leukoplakia is more common in men than in women, and that it is seen chiefly in the older age group. Renstrup noted that 90 per cent of the 90 patients in one study were over the age of 40, while Hobaek reported an average age of 60.1 years for his 246 patients. Shafer and Waldron studied 332 tissue specimens from 286 patients with clinical leukoplakia and reported an occurrence in females that was considerably higher than generally reported: males, 69 per cent; females, 31 per cent. Pindborg and his group reported very similar findings in a series of 214 patients. Although occasional cases occurred in the second decade of life, most were seen in the fifth to seventh decades. Approximately 81 per cent of the patients in the study of Shafer and Waldron were over 40 years of age. It was interesting that there appeared to be a slight trend for earlier occurrence of leukoplakia in females.

In a subsequent and much larger study of 3256 patients, Waldron and Shafer found an even closer sex distribution of 54 per cent males and 46 per cent females. This may indicate an increase in the incidence of leukoplakia in women in more recent years. While the majority of their large series of cases occurred in the fifth, sixth and seventh decades of life, approximately 5 per cent of the patients were under the age of 30 years (Fig. 2–7).

Although leukoplakic patches may be found anywhere in the oral cavity, certain sites of predilection have been noted. Renstrup reported that the buccal mucosa and commissures were most frequently involved, followed in descending order by the alveolar mucosa, tongue, lip, hard and soft palates, floor of the mouth and gingiva. In Hobaek's cases the tongue and

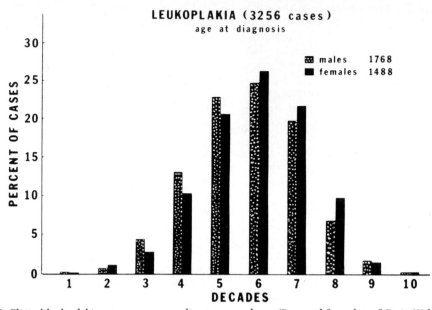

Figure 2–7. Clinical leukoplakia, occurrence according to age and sex. (Prepared from data of C. A. Waldron and W. G. Shafer. Cancer, 36:1386, 1975. By courtesy of Dr. Charles A. Waldron.)

floor of the mouth were most frequently involved, followed in order by the lower lip, buccal mucosa, palate and gingiva. Multiple areas of involvement were common. The extent of involvement may vary from small, well localized, irregular patches to diffuse lesions covering a considerable portion of the oral mucosa. In the study of Waldron and Shafer, the greatest number of cases of leukoplakia occurred on the

mandibular alveolar ridge, gingiva or mucobuccal fold (25.1 per cent). There was a greater frequency of occurrence in these locations among females than among males, however. This finding was accounted for, in a small part at least, by the use of snuff among women in their study and its habitual placement in the mandibular mucobuccal fold. The next most common site was buccal mucosa (21.9 per cent),

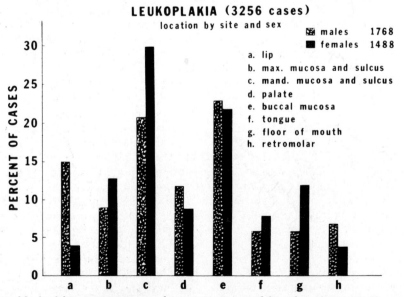

Figure 2–8. Clinical leukoplakia, occurrence according to site. (Prepared from data of C. A. Waldron and W. G. Shafer. Cancer, 36:1386, 1975. By courtesy of Dr. Charles A. Waldron.)

so that this, with the previous sites, accounted for nearly half of all cases. Of considerable interest also was the relatively low frequency of occurrence of lesions on the lower lip in females (4.0 per cent) as contrasted to males (15.6 per cent). The tongue generally has been believed to be a common site of occurrence of leukoplakia. In both males and females, however, this was one of the least frequent sites of occurrence in the study of Waldron and Shafer (Fig. 2–8). It was also of interest that no lesions on the upper lip in either sex were found in their early study.

On clinical examination, patches of leukoplakia may vary from a nonpalpable, faintly translucent white area to thick, fissured, papillomatous, indurated lesions (Fig. 2–9; see also Plate III). The surface of the lesion is often finely wrinkled or shriveled in appearance and may feel rough on palpation. The lesions are white, gray or yellowish-white but, with heavy use of tobacco, may assume a brownish-yellow color.

Sharp described three stages of leukoplakia, the earliest lesion being a non-palpable, faintly translucent, white discoloration. Later, localized or diffuse, slightly elevated plaques of irregular outline develop. These are opaque white and may have a fine granular texture. In some instances the lesions progress to thickened, white lesions, showing induration, fissuring and ulcer formation.

There is little doubt that a certain percentage of cases of leukoplakia will undergo transformation into epidermoid carcinoma. This will be discussed in detail subsequently. The possibility of clinical distinction between the innocuous white patch and the potentially malignant one is a matter of considerable interest and importance. This problem has been discussed exten-

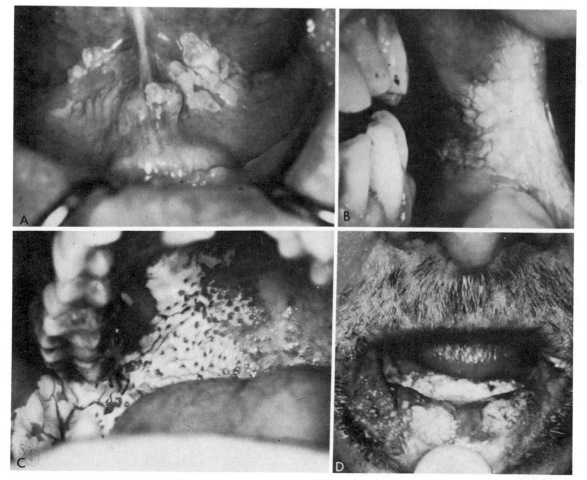

Figure 2–9. *Leukoplakia of oral mucous membrane.*
The lesion in the floor of the mouth *(A)* is a relatively early one. Those in the angle of the mouth *(B)*, the palate *(C)* and the lip and alveolar ridge *(D)* are advanced cases of leukoplakia.

sively in a number of papers. Renstrup studied biopsy material on 80 patients with clinical leukoplakia and concluded that it was not possible to demonstrate histologic changes that correlate with the clinical concept of leukoplakia. Cooke also reported that he found little correlation between the various clinical pictures and the histopathology in his series of cases. Shira pointed out that although some keratotic lesions in the mouth ("leukoplakia") are dangerous, most are innocuous and merely represent a benign thickening of the oral mucosa which has developed as a protective mechanism against local stimulation or irritation. He further emphasized that the clinician cannot distinguish between the potentially dangerous and the innocuous lesion and stressed the importance of biopsy. Kollar et al. also emphasized this point and reported five cases which illustrated the danger of inadequate patient management on the basis of "leukoplakia" as a diagnosis. Although some authors indicate that the verrucous, fissured and thickened types of leukoplakia are most likely to become malignant, others have demonstrated that small, granular, gray, pinkish-gray or red areas with indefinite margins and without induration may represent carcinoma in situ or even invasive cancer. By some authors, this lesion has been referred to as erythroplakia (q.v.).

In summary, it has been stressed by Shafer and Waldron, as well as Pindborg and many others, that there is no correlation between the clinical appearance of leukoplakia and the histologic findings. Some of the most severe-looking cases of leukoplakia clinically are found to be only severe keratosis with no cellular atypia. In contrast, some very small and very mild leukoplakias clinically have proved to be invasive cancer. Thus, biopsy is mandatory.

Histologic Features. Most authorities, regardless of their criteria for microscopic diagnosis of leukoplakia, agree that this lesion represents a dysplasia of the surface epithelium. For this reason a definition of certain microscopic terms is necessary here:

1. HYPERORTHOKERATOSIS. There is a moderate amount of orthokeratin present on the surface of normal oral epithelium, and this will vary slightly in amount from area to area in the oral cavity, depending upon frictional irritation, such as toothbrushing and mastication. Hyperorthokeratosis refers to an abnormal increase in thickness of this orthokeratin layer or stratum corneum in a particular location (Fig. 2–10). Although an orthokeratin layer of a certain thickness may be normal for that area, a layer of the same thickness may be decidedly abnormal for another area.

2. HYPERPARAKERATOSIS. Parakeratin differs from orthokeratin in the persistence of nuclei or nuclear remnants in the keratin layer. This is also a normal finding in certain areas of the oral cavity. The presence of parakeratin in areas where it is not usually found or, more particularly, a thickening of the parakeratin layer is referred to as hyperparakeratosis (Fig. 2–10). It is not unusual in the oral cavity to observe alternating areas of orthokeratin and parakeratin or hyperorthokeratosis and hyperparakeratosis in the same histologic section. The significance of this finding is not known.

Considerable importance is often attached to differentiation between hyperorthokeratosis and hyperparakeratosis in dermatologic pathology with respect to diagnostic significance. In oral lesions, however, the significance of such differentiation, if any, is still obscure. It has been noted that the presence of a granular layer or stratum granulosum is obvious only in orthokeratinized oral epithelium. The granular layer is often thickened and extremely prominent in cases of hyperorthokeratosis, but is seldom seen even in severe cases of hyperparakeratosis.

3. ACANTHOSIS. The thickness of the spinous layer (the stratum spinosum or prickle cell layer) also varies considerably between different areas of the oral cavity. Thus a certain thickness may be normal for one area, but abnormal for another. Acanthosis refers to the abnormal thickening of the spinous layer for a particular location. This may be severe with elongation, thickening, blunting, and confluence of the rete pegs or may consist only of their elongation (Fig. 2–10). Acanthosis may or may not be associated with hyperorthokeratosis or hyperparakeratosis, sometimes occurring independently of changes in the overlying layer.

4. DYSPLASIA. Numerous criteria exist for the diagnosis of epithelial dysplasia, and there is not always a clear-cut distinction between what represents a mild dysplasia consisting only of a focal atypia, a moderate dysplasia, and a severe dysplasia which may represent carcinoma in situ. Neither do we have knowledge that dysplasia represented by focal atypia will inevitably, or even usually, progress to obvious carcinoma in situ and thence to invasive carcinoma, although this has generally been conceded to be the case. Criteria which have often been used for the diagnosis of epithelial dyspla-

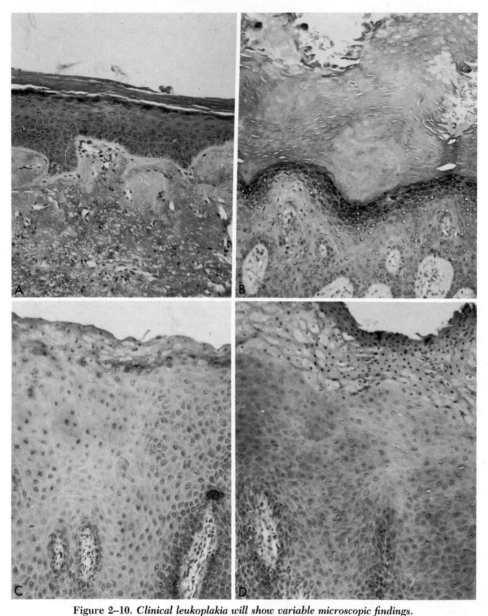

Figure 2–10. *Clinical leukoplakia will show variable microscopic findings.*
A, Mild hyperorthokeratosis, no acanthosis; *B*, severe hyperorthokeratosis, mild acanthosis; *C*, mild parakeratosis, marked acanthosis; *D*, severe hyperparakeratosis, marked acanthosis. Each illustration was photographed at the same magnification for comparative purposes.

sia include (a) increased, and particularly abnormal, mitoses, (b) individual cell keratinization, (c) epithelial pearls within the spinous layer, (d) alterations in the nuclear-cytoplasmic ratio, (e) loss of polarity and disorientation of cells, (f) hyperchromatism of cells, (g) large, prominent nucleoli, (h) dyskaryosis or nuclear atypism, including giant nuclei, (i) poikilocarynosis or division of nuclei without division of cytoplasm, and (j) basilar hyperplasia (Fig. 2–11). Distinction must be made between malig-nant dysplasia, sometimes referred to as dyskeratosis and characterized by these features, and so-called benign dyskeratosis such as is seen in Darier's disease and molluscum contagiosum.

5. CARCINOMA IN SITU, OR INTRAEPITHELIAL CARCINOMA. A definitive distinction cannot always be drawn between dysplasia and carcinoma in situ. Certain of the criteria listed for dysplasia when encompassing an even greater area than could be considered focal, when ex-

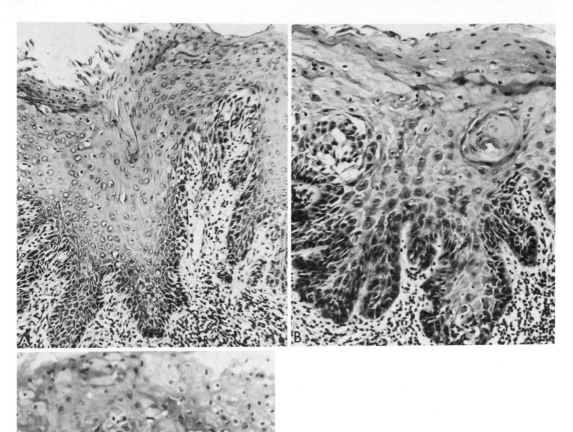

Figure 2–11. *Epithelial dysplasia.*
The dysplastic epithelial changes may be relatively mild
(A), moderate (B), or very severe, bordering on carcinoma
in situ (C).

tremely severe in degree or when exhibiting "top to bottom" change, particularly with respect to basilar hyperplasia, must undoubtedly be diagnosed as carcinoma in situ, provided of course that it has not progressed to the point of true invasion of the connective tissue (Fig. 2–11, C).

It is of considerable interest that some intraoral lesions exhibit "top to bottom" basilar hyperplasia, loss of polarity, increased mitosis,

hyperchromatism, dyskaryosis, and alterations in nuclear-cytoplasmic ratio without any evidence of thickening of the epithelial layer or, more significantly, without any evidence of a disturbance of the keratinization process. Thus, in approximately half of all lesions in the series of Shafer and Waldron diagnosed as carcinoma in situ, there was no individual cell keratinization, no epithelial pearl formation, and no hyperkeratosis. Invariably these lesions were described clinically as being flat, red, velvety, and granular in appearance. Their experience suggested that intraoral carcinoma in situ did not inevitably present as a clinically hyperkeratotic or leukoplakic lesion. In some specimens, however, areas of flat, thin, red carcinoma in situ alternated with areas showing hyperortho- or parakeratosis, with or without acanthosis and focal atypia. This corresponds to the "speckled leukoplakia" of Pindborg or the "speckled erythroplakia" of Shear.

Malignant Potential. There are remarkably few significant studies demonstrating a clinicopathologic correlation of leukoplakia. The majority of authors have dealt with either the clinical features of the disease or the microscopic appearance of various white patches, but few have presented the microscopic findings of any sizable group of patients with lesions diagnosed clinically as leukoplakia. For this reason it is only within very recent years that any significant information has been made available on the incidence of ominous histologic changes in any given series of patients with clinical leukoplakia.

One such large series has been that of Shafer and Waldron, who studied 332 cases of routine biopsy specimens from patients with leukoplakia. It was found that most of the cases in this study consisted of benign and innocuous lesions characterized by hyperorthokeratosis and acanthosis, hyperparakeratosis and acanthosis or hyperorthokeratosis alone. (Percentages could not be calculated throughout because there was overlap in some cases; e.g., certain lesions presented areas of both hyperorthokeratosis and hyperparakeratosis.) A few lesions showed only acanthosis or only hyperparakeratosis. It was of interest that hyperparakeratosis alone was relatively uncommon in contrast to hyperorthokeratosis alone, whereas hyperparakeratosis in association with acanthosis was seen more frequently than hyperorthokeratosis with acanthosis.

There appeared to be no real differences in the occurrence of the different forms of epithelial dysplasia between men and women except for the greater preponderance of carcinoma in men, a well-recognized clinical phenomenon.

In 26 cases in the Shafer-Waldron series of 332 specimens (approximately 7.8 per cent) epithelial dysplasia was found to be associated with any one or more of these conditions. Six cases of carcinoma in situ and 27 cases of invasive carcinoma, all clinically diagnosed as leukoplakia, were found in their series. Together these represented 17.7 per cent of all

white lesions biopsied excluding lichen planus and all other specific entities (Fig. 2–12).

An even more significant study on 3256 patients with oral leukoplakia has been reported by Waldron and Shafer. The biopsies from the lesions in these patients represented approximately 6.2 per cent of all tissue specimens processed between 1960 and 1973 by Emory University and Indiana University Schools of Dentistry, thus giving some indication of the frequency of this disease. Histologically, 80.1 per cent of leukoplakias were varying combinations of hyperorthokeratosis, hyperparakeratosis and acanthosis without evidence of epithelial dysplasia or more serious alterations. Mild to moderate epithelial dysplasia was found in 12.2 per cent of cases and severe epithelial dysplasia or carcinoma in situ was found in 4.5 per cent. Invasive epidermoid carcinoma was found in 3.1 per cent of cases which had been biopsied with a clinical diagnosis of leukoplakia. There was considerable range in the risk of epithelial dysplasia, carcinoma in situ or invasive carcinoma, depending upon the anatomic location of the lesion in the oral cavity (Fig. 2–12, A, B). The site at highest risk was the floor of the mouth, where 42.9 per cent of all leukoplakic lesions were epithelial dysplasia, carcinoma in situ or invasive carcinoma. This was followed by the tongue, with 24.2 per cent of these serious lesions, and 24.0 per cent for lip leukoplakias (Table 2–1). For all oral sites combined, 20.0 per cent of all of these leukoplakias were serious or potentially serious lesions. The high risk of malignant transformation in this disease in the floor of the mouth has been confirmed by Kramer and his associates.

The results of a similar but smaller study by Sovadina in 1955, by Pindborg and his coworkers in 1963 and by Banoczy in 1977 are shown in Table 2–2. While there is some difference in the manner of recording the "premalignant" lesions, it is apparent that between 3.2 and 8.1 per cent of the cases of clinical leukoplakia represented invasive carcinoma at the time they were initially biopsied. Furthermore, serious microscopic alterations variously recorded as epithelial atypia, dysplasia or carcinoma in situ were found in an additional 7.3 to 17.1 per cent of the cases of clinical leukoplakia at the time they were initially biopsied. Thus, in these studies, the percentage of cases of clinical leukoplakia which had malignant or "premalignant" microscopic features present at the time of initial biopsy of the lesions varied between 14.6 and 23.1 per cent.

Since between 76.9 and 85.4 per cent of

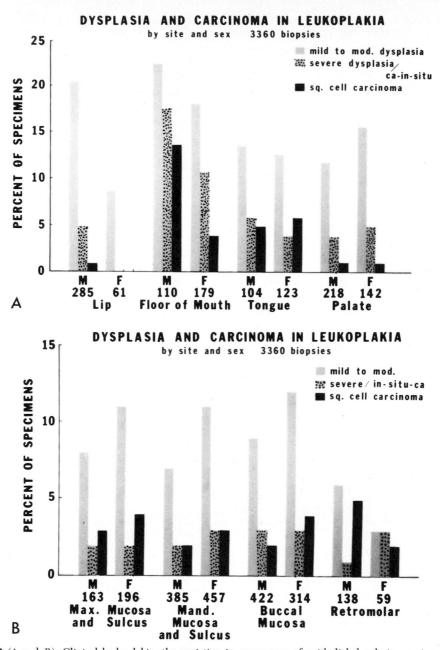

Figure 2–12 (*A* and *B*). Clinical leukoplakia, the variation in occurrence of epithelial dysplasia, carcinoma-in-situ and invasive carcinoma by anatomic site and sex. (Prepared from data of C. A. Waldron and W. G. Shafer. Cancer, 36:1386, 1975. By courtesy of Dr. Charles A. Waldron.)

these cases of clinical leukoplakia were histologically benign lesions at the time of initial biopsy, it becomes most important to ascertain follow-up of this group of patients. In Table 2–3, a series of studies, all reported since 1959, are shown dealing with follow-up investigations of patients with clinical leukoplakia of the benign form to determine the frequency of malignant transformation. Again, with the exception of data from India which may represent a special problem in itself, there is rather amazing agreement in the percentage of cases of leukoplakia which undergo malignant transformation, despite the marked variation in follow-up periods. It can be seen that the percentage of cases of leukoplakia which ultimately show malignant

Table 2–1.   Leukoplakia—Site and Pathology

SITE	% OF CASES AT SITE	EPITHELIAL DYSPLASIA, CARCINOMA IN SITU OR INVASIVE CANCER	
		NO. OF AFFECTED CASES/NO. OF CASES AT SITE	% OF AFFECTED CASES AT SITE
Lips	10	83/346	24.0
Maxillary mucosa and sulcus	11	53/359	14.8
Mandibular mucosa and sulcus	25	123/845	14.6
Palate	11	68/361	18.8
Buccal mucosa	22	121/736	16.5
Tongue	7	55/227	24.2
Floor of mouth	9	124/289	42.9
Retromolar	6	23/197	11.7
Total		650/3256	20.0

From Waldron, C. A., and Shafer, W. G.: Leukoplakia revisited. A clinicopathologic study of 3256 oral leukoplakias. Cancer, *36*:1386, 1975.

transformation ranges between 1.4 and 6.0 per cent, averaging slightly over 4.0 per cent.

These data have been interpreted as meaning that if approximately 6.0 per cent of clinical leukoplakias represent invasive carcinoma at the time of initial biopsy, and approximately 4.0 per cent of the remaining group (a minimal figure, since it cannot be determined from reports whether patients who were followed included *untreated* patients with various forms of epithelial dysplasia) undergo subsequent malignant transformation, then approximately 10 per cent of patients who develop leukoplakia

have invasive carcinoma in their lesion or will develop carcinoma at some time in the future.

Treatment.   The treatment of leukoplakia over the years has included such modalities as the administration of vitamin A, vitamin B complex and estrogens, x-ray therapy, fulguration, surgical excision and topical chemotherapy.

Generally speaking, the treatment of the disease is aimed at the elimination of any recognizable irritating factors. Discontinuance of the use of tobacco or alcohol, correction of any possible malocclusion, replacement of ill-fitting

Table 2–2.   Histologic Character of Oral Leukoplakia

AUTHOR (COUNTRY)	YEAR	NO. OF PATIENTS	INCIDENCE OF ALTERATION (%)
Bánóczy (Hungary)	1977	670	17.1 Dysplasia 6.0 Carcinoma 23.1
Waldron and Shafer (United States)	1975	3256	12.2 Mild to moderate dysplasia 4.5 Severe dysplasia—Carcinoma in situ 3.1 Carcinoma 19.8
Pindborg et al. (Denmark)	1963	185	12.4 Atypia 3.2 Carcinoma 15.6
Shafer and Waldron (United States)	1961	332	7.8 Atypia 1.8 Carcinoma in situ 8.1 Carcinoma 17.7
Sovadina (Czechoslovakia)	1955	53	7.3 Premalignant 7.3 Malignant 14.6

Table 2–3.   Malignant Transformation of Oral Leukoplakia

AUTHOR (COUNTRY)	YEAR	NO. OF PATIENTS	OBSERVATION PERIOD	MALIGNANT CHANGE (%)
Bánóczy (Hungary)	1977	670	1–30 years	6.0
Pindborg (Denmark)	1975	170	7 years	3.5
Roed-Petersen (Denmark)	1971	331	4.3 years (median)	3.6
Pindborg et al. (Denmark)	1968	248	3 months– 9 years	4.4
Silverman and Rozen (United States)	1968	117	1–5 years	6.0
Einhorn and Wersall (Sweden)	1967	782	1–44 years	4.0
Mela and Mongini (Italy)	1966	141	3–11 years	3.5
Skach et al. (Czechoslovakia)	1960	71	3–6 years	1.4
Sugar and Bánóczy (Hungary)	1959	86	0 to 11 years	5.8

dentures, and so forth, are recommended. The correction of local factors is probably of greater benefit than treatment of possible systemic factors. In one investigation of a group of patients with leukoplakia which had regressed, Bánóczy and Sugár reported a high incidence of smokers who had stopped smoking completely.

Relatively small lesions may be totally excised or cauterized, although the possibility of "field cancerization" must always be considered. Extensive lesions are often treated by multiple-stage stripping procedures, with or without skin grafting. A stripping procedure, without grafting, for lip leukoplakia is especially common and successful. X-ray radiation should be discouraged.

Differential Diagnosis. From a clinical standpoint, lichen planus (q.v.) is probably the most important lesion to consider in the differential diagnosis of leukoplakia. Although in most instances lesions of lichen planus can be identified from clinical findings, biopsy in some cases is necessary. Other white lesions of the oral mucosa to be differentiated from leukoplakia include chemical burns, syphilitic mucous patches, mycotic infections (chiefly candidosis), psoriasis, lupus erythematosus, and white sponge nevus or white folded gingivostomatitis (q.v.).

The occurrence of tylosis, or palmar-plantar keratosis, with esophageal carcinoma and its transmission as an autosomal dominant characteristic has been recognized since the description by Clarke and his associates in 1957. More recently, oral lesions in these patients have been described by Tyldesley and his co-workers as "preleukoplakia" in childhood and leukoplakia in adulthood. It is not known whether these oral lesions have neoplastic potential or represent some other disease process.

Many cases of leukoplakia cannot be differentiated from other specific white oral lesions without biopsy, and there should be no hesitation in establishing the diagnosis by this means.

LEUKOEDEMA

Leukoedema is an abnormality of the buccal mucosa which clinically resembles early leukoplakia, but appears to differ from it in certain respects.

Clinical Features. The gross appearance of leukoedema varies from a filmy opalescence of the mucosa in the early stages to a more definite grayish-white cast with a coarsely wrinkled surface in the later stages (Fig. 2–13, A). Lesions occur bilaterally in the majority of cases and frequently involve most of the buccal mucosa,

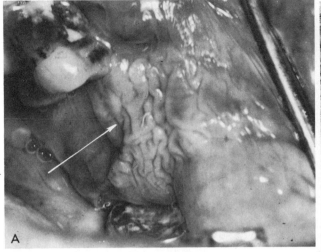

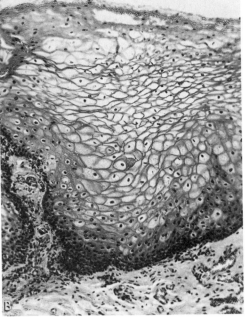

Figure 2–13. *Leukoedema.*
The opaque appearance of the buccal mucosa (A) is somewhat different from that in leukoplakia. The photomicrograph (B) shows only acanthosis with intracellular edema of the spinous cells.

extending onto the oral surface of the lips. Leukoedema is most noticeable along the occlusal line in the bicuspid and molar region. In some cases, desquamation occurs, leaving the surface eroded.

The etiology of leukoedema is unknown. An extensive study of this condition was carried out in the United States by Sandstead and Lowe, who found no apparent correlation between the incidence of the condition and the use of tobacco, the pH of the saliva, oral bacterial infection, syphilis or galvanic irritation. In their study the incidence of leukoedema was approximately 45 per cent in Caucasian men and 40 per cent in Caucasian women, while it was 94 per cent in Negro men and 86 per cent in Negro women, all adults with an average age of 45 years.

It has now been identified in many countries around the world with a remarkable variation in prevalence that suggests some ethnic association. The different reported epidemiologic studies have been reviewed by Axéll and Henricsson, who also noted an incidence of occurrence of nearly 50 per cent in a survey of over 20,000 persons aged 15 years and over in Sweden. Their data suggested to them that tobacco smoking was closely correlated with the occurrence of the leukoedema, although studies from India, where tobacco use is extremely prevalent, have shown a very low incidence of leukoedema.

Histologic Features. The microscopic features of leukoedema consist of an increase in thickness of the epithelium, intracellular edema of the spinous or malpighian layer, a superficial parakeratotic layer several cells in thickness, and broad rete pegs which appear irregularly elongated (Fig. 2–13, B). The characteristic edematous cells appear extremely large and pale, and they present a reticular pattern. The cytoplasm appears lost, and the nuclei appear absent, clear or pyknotic. Inflammatory cell infiltration of the subjacent connective tissue is not a common finding.

In a review and discussion of leukoedema, Archard and his co-workers have concluded that the clinical appearance of the lesion is due to a retained superficial layer of parakeratotic cells.

Clinical Significance. It has been suggested that leukoedema may represent a lesion of the oral mucosa in which leukoplakia is more apt to develop than in normal epithelium. This conclusion is based upon the fact that nearly all patients examined who manifested leukoplakia also exhibited leukoedema in the adjacent mucosa. However, Archard and his co-workers have concluded, on the basis of their studies, that there is no evidence to support this contention. Furthermore, they concluded that there is no evidence that this lesion is premalignant or in any way associated with potential malignant alteration.

Since leukoedema appears to be simply a variant of normal mucosa, no treatment is necessary.

INTRAEPITHELIAL CARCINOMA
(Carcinoma in Situ)

Intraepithelial carcinoma is a condition which arises frequently on the skin, but occurs also on mucous membranes, including those of the oral cavity. Some authorities believe that this disease represents a precancerous dyskeratotic process, but others say that it is a laterally spreading, intraepithelial type of superficial epithelioma or carcinoma. As Chandler Smith has expressed it in a discussion of the concept of the term carcinoma in situ, it "does not reveal whether the lesion is a cancer now but has not yet become invasive, or whether it is not a cancer now but will become a cancer at some later time." Nevertheless, in this stage it does not exhibit invasive malignant properties. Since metastasis cannot occur without infiltration of tumor cells into connective tissue and consequent accessibility to lymphatic or blood vessels, metastasis is impossible in intraepithelial carcinoma.

Bowen's disease is a special form of intraepithelial carcinoma occurring with some frequency on the skin, particularly in patients who have had arsenical therapy, and is often associated with the development of internal or extracutaneous cancer. On rare occasions, as reported by Gorlin, Bowen's disease may occur in the oral cavity.

Clinical Features. In a study of 82 lesions of carcinoma in situ in 77 patients reported by Shafer, he found that the clinical appearance was that of a leukoplakia in 45 per cent of the lesions, an erythroplakia in 16 per cent of the lesions, a combination leukoplakia and erythroplakia in 9 per cent , an ulcerated lesion in 13 per cent, a white and ulcerated lesion in 5 per cent, a red and ulcerated lesion in 1 per cent and not stated in 11 per cent.

These lesions have been reported to occur at all intraoral sites but the most common in the study of Shafer were floor of mouth (23 per cent), tongue (22 per cent) and lips in males (20 per cent). This distribution is roughly comparable to that found in a series of 158 lesions of asymptomatic early oral epidermoid carcinoma reported by Mashberg and his associates. They appear to be somewhat more common in men than in women (1.8:1) and tend to occur principally in elderly persons.

Histologic Features. Intraepithelial carcinoma is characterized by a remarkable range of variation in histologic appearance. Keratin may or may not be found on the surface of the lesion

but, if present, is more apt to be parakeratin rather than orthokeratin. Individual cell keratinization and epithelial or keratin pearl formation are exceedingly rare. In fact, these appear to be a hallmark of transformation of carcinoma in situ into invasive carcinoma, so that if these are found, a further search should be made for carcinomatous invasion. In some instances, there appears to be hyperplasia of the altered epithelium, while in others there is atrophy.

Certain cytologic alterations may also occur. An increased nuclear/cytoplasmic ratio and nuclear hyperchromatism are sometimes seen, but many cases do not show these. Cellular pleomorphism is quite uncommon. One of the most conspicuous and consistent alterations is loss of orientation of cells and loss of their normal polarity. Mitotic activity is extremely variable and of little significance unless overwhelming (Fig. 2–14).

It has also been found that sometimes a sharp line of division between normal and altered epithelium extends from the surface down to the connective tissue rather than a blending of epithelial changes. It is also not unusual to find multiple areas of carcinoma in situ interspersed by essentially normal-appearing epithelium, producing multifocal carcinoma in situ.

All of the above changes occur within the surface epithelium, which remains confined by the basement membrane.

Treatment and Prognosis. There is no uniformly accepted treatment for intraepithelial carcinoma. The lesions have been surgically excised, irradiated, cauterized and even exposed to solid carbon dioxide. If the condition is left untreated, carcinomatous invasion is thought to occur eventually. Spontaneous regression of carcinoma in situ without treatment is known to occur in certain sites, chiefly the uterine cervix, in a significant percentage of cases. However, it is doubtful that this happens in the oral cavity; although progression into invasive carcinoma may take years in some instances, in others it apparently develops within months.

ERYTHROPLAKIA
(Erythroplasia of Queyrat)

Erythroplakia is a disease originally described under the name "erythroplasia" by Queyrat in 1911 as a lesion occurring on the glans penis of an elderly syphilitic person. Since then, similar lesions have been described as occurring on the

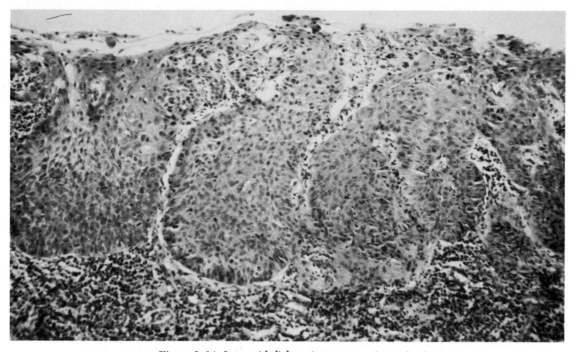

Figure 2–14. *Intraepithelial carcinoma or carcinoma in situ.*
The epithelial cells exhibit all the features of malignant cells, but invasion of the connective tissue has not begun.

vulva and oral mucosa. The syphilis present in the original cases is now known to have been purely an incidental finding and was not related to the condition.

Investigators now recognize that erythroplakia is a clinical entity and represents a lesion of mucous membrane which, histologically, in a large percentage of cases, exhibits epithelial changes ranging from mild dysplasia to carcinoma in situ and even invasive carcinoma. While earlier workers believed that erythroplakia and Bowen's disease of the mucous membrane were the same disease, current evidence indicates that they are different diseases with different clinical characteristics and a different clinical course.

Erythroplakia has been reviewed by Williamson, by Shear and by Shafer and Waldron. It has been pointed out that there are many other types of oral lesions which are clinically indistinguishable from the dysplastic one, thus emphasizing the importance of biopsy of all such red lesions. Such clinically similar lesions include candidosis, tuberculosis and histoplasmosis, as well as other relatively nonspecific conditions such as denture irritation.

Clinical Features. There appear to be three different clinical manifestations of erythroplakia in the oral cavity. These have been described by Shear as: (1) the homogeneous form which appears as a bright red, soft velvety lesion, with straight or scalloped well-demarcated margins, often quite extensive in size, commonly found on the buccal mucosa and sometimes on the soft palate, more rarely on the tongue and floor of the mouth; (2) erythroplakia interspersed with patches of leukoplakia in which the erythematous areas are irregular and often not as bright red as the homogeneous form, most frequently seen on the tongue and floor of the mouth; and (3) soft, red lesions that are slightly elevated with an irregular outline and a granular or finely nodular surface speckled with tiny white plaques, often referred to as "speckled leukoplakia" or, more properly, "speckled erythroplakia." This latter form may occur anywhere in the oral cavity and, in a study by Pindborg, 14 per cent of 35 lesions in a series of 29 patients histologically showed invasive carcinoma, while 51 per cent revealed epithelial dysplasia. In a related study of 158 cases of early, asymptomatic oral epidermoid carcinoma, Mashberg and his associates found that 143 or 91 per cent had an erythroplastic component, but that only 98 or 62 per cent had a white component. They concluded that an asymptomatic erythroplastic lesion was the earliest visible sign of oral epidermoid carcinoma—invasive or in situ.

Oral erythroplakia is an uncommon disease

in contrast with leukoplakia. For example, Shafer and Waldron have reported a series of 58 cases of erythroplakia that were the total retrieved from a group of 65,354 consecutively accessioned biopsy-surgical specimens (0.09 per cent) in contrast to 3256 cases of leukoplakia retrieved from 52,145 similarly accessioned specimens (6.2 per cent). According to this series of Shafer and Waldron, oral erythroplakia has no apparent significant sex predilection (31 males, 27 females) and it occurs most frequently in the sixth and seventh decades of life. While some differences existed in predilection for sites of occurrence between sexes, the most frequent site was floor of mouth, then retromolar area, followed by tongue, palate and mandibular mucosa and sulcus.

Histologic Features. The vast majority of cases of erythroplakia are histologically either invasive epidermoid carcinoma, carcinoma in situ or epithelial dysplasia at the time of biopsy. The histologic findings in 65 biopsies of the 58 cases of erythroplakia have been reported by Shafer and Waldron. They found that 33 specimens (51 per cent) were invasive carcinoma, 26 (40 per cent) were either carcinoma in situ or severe epithelial dysplasia and 6 (9 per cent) were mild or moderate epithelial dysplasia. They found no significant differences between males and females in the distribution of these various epithelial alterations.

The epidermoid carcinoma may show any degree of differentiation—from poorly to well differentiated. Even though the carcinoma may involve a relatively large surface area, it is usually a fairly shallow lesion. It often appears to be multicentric in origin.

The carcinoma in situ lesion shows epithelial dysplasia throughout the entire thickness of the epithelium without invasion into the underlying connective tissue (Fig. 2–15, A, B). These various cytologic alterations have been discussed under intraepithelial carcinoma (q.v.). Because the dysplastic or neoplastic cells extend to the very surface of the lesion, a careful cytologic smear will usually reveal these atypical cells.

The reason for the red appearance of the lesion clinically becomes apparent when these lesions are studied histologically. It will be found that the connective tissue pegs extend very high into the epithelium and that the epithelium over the tips of these pegs is often very thin. Furthermore, the capillaries in these superficial pegs are frequently quite dilated. Finally, the absence of any significant amount of surface orthokeratin or parakeratin, or at the most only a very thin layer, also contributes to the red hue of the lesion.

Treatment. The treatment is the same as that for any invasive epidermoid carcinoma or carcinoma in situ. Erythroplasia of the penis has been treated with some success by topical 5-fluorouracil but its use in the oral cavity has been only experimental.

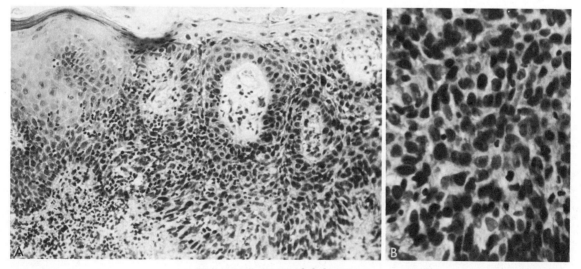

Figure 2–15. *Intraepithelial carcinoma.*
This lesion, which clinically was erythroplakia, shows normal epithelium on the left and an abrupt transition into dysplastic epithelium on the right *(A)*. Under high magnification *(B)*, the dysplastic cells show basilar hyperplasia with top-to-bottom change, loss of orientation of cells, increased mitoses, and hyperchromatic nuclei, but only mild pleomorphism.

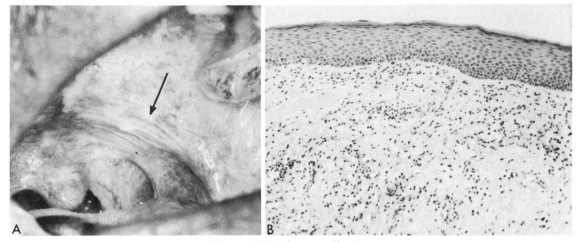

Figure 2–16. *Submucous fibrosis.*
The typical fibrotic bands are noted on the soft palate *(A)*, while the photomicrograph reveals the epithelial atrophy and fibrosis *(B)*. (Courtesy of Dr. Jens J. Pindborg.)

ORAL SUBMUCOUS FIBROSIS

Oral submucous fibrosis is a peculiar disease which is considered to be a precancerous condition. It occurs chiefly in southeast Asia, but has been reported on rare occasions in other countries around the world, including the United States. It was first reported in a group of East Indian women by Schwartz, but has been most extensively studied by Pindborg and his associates. These investigators define the disease as "an insidious chronic disease affecting any part of the oral cavity and sometimes the pharynx. Although occasionally preceded by and/or associated with vesicle formation, it is always associated with a juxta-epithelial inflammatory reaction followed by a fibroelastic change of the lamina propria, with epithelial atrophy leading to stiffness of the oral mucosa and causing trismus and inability to eat."

The etiology of the disease is obscure, although there is some evidence to suggest that it may be related to a peculiar dietary component, chillies, a strongly irritating spice commonly used in India. Other possible etiologic agents have been reviewed by Paissat, and these have included vitamin B deficiency, protein deficiency, and betel nut chewing.

Clinical Features. The disease is characterized by a burning sensation of the mouth, particularly when eating spicy foods. This is accompanied or followed by the formation of vesicles (often on the palate), ulcerations or recurrent stomatitis, with excessive salivation or xerostomia and defective gustatory sensation.

Ultimately, the patients develop stiffening of certain areas of the oral mucosa with difficulty in opening the mouth and swallowing, thus simulating systemic sclerosis or scleroderma.

The mucosa eventually becomes blanched and opaque (although erythroplakic areas are sometimes seen), and fibrotic bands appear, usually involving the buccal mucosa, soft palate, lips and tongue (Fig. 2–16, *A*).

It is most common between 20 and 40 years of age but can occur in any decade of life. Studies are contradictory concerning a sex predilection.

Histologic Features. In the advanced cases of submucous fibrosis, the oral epithelium is almost invariably extremely atrophic with complete loss of rete pegs (Fig. 2–16, *B*). Epithelial atypia may also be present. The underlying connective tissue shows severe hyalinization with homogenization of collagen bundles. Fibroblasts are markedly diminished in number and the blood vessels are completely obliterated or narrowed. Some chronic inflammatory cell infiltrate may be present. It has been reported that special stains and electron microscope studies of the collagen show severe alterations from the normal.

Treatment and Prognosis. A variety of therapeutic modalities have been tried, generally without success. Systemic corticosteroids and local hydrocortisone have appeared to offer some temporary remissions.

The facts that a high percentage of patients with oral cancer had coexisting submucous fibrosis (40 per cent in one study by Pindborg and Zachariah), that epithelial atypia is present in 13 to 14 per cent of all cases, and that histologic carcinoma is found in 5 to 6 per cent of cases without clinical signs of cancer suggest that the disease is a precancerous condition.

MALIGNANT TUMORS OF EPITHELIAL TISSUE ORIGIN

BASAL CELL CARCINOMA

(Basal Cell Epithelioma; Rodent Ulcer)

Basal cell carcinoma develops most frequently on the exposed surfaces of the skin, the face and the scalp in middle-aged or elderly persons. Blond people of fair complexion who have spent much of their lives out of doors are often victims of this lesion, but it is by no means confined to such persons. It is probably the most common type of carcinoma in men.

Basal cell carcinoma exhibits practically no tendency for metastasis, and for this reason has often been called a "benign" carcinoma. The term implies a misconception, since the lesion may kill by direct invasion. Occasionally, this form of carcinoma does metastasize to lymph nodes or distant viscera, and this situation has been reviewed by Costanza and her associates, who found less than 100 metastatic basal cell carcinomas reported between 1894 and 1973. The head and neck is the site of the primary tumor in 85 per cent of the cases. In his series of over 9000 cases of basal cell carcinoma of skin, the incidence of metastasis was found by Cotran to be 0.1 per cent.

Etiology. The relation between prolonged exposure to sunlight and skin cancer has been recognized for many years. The protective role of skin pigmentation has also been shown to account for the relative rarity of skin cancer in blacks. The specific factor in sunlight responsible for skin carcinogenesis appears to be the ultraviolet radiation, and experimental skin tumors of animals have been produced by exposure to ultraviolet light. An extremely thorough and erudite review of the current concepts of ultraviolet carcinogenesis, with particular regard to nonmelanoma skin cancer, has been published by Granstein and Sober.

Epidemiologic studies have shown that skin cancer is far more common in areas of the United States that receive a great deal of sunshine than in those areas that receive less sunshine. Thus, according to figures of the United States Public Health Service, the reported incidence of skin cancer in Dallas, Texas, is 140 cases per 100,000 population, while that in Pittsburgh, Pennsylvania, is only 37 cases per 100,000.

It should not be inferred that ultraviolet radiation is the only important etiologic factor in the development of basal cell carcinoma. Certainly the exposure to both recognized and unknown carcinogenic agents of other types must be considered, and these include ionizing radiation, burn scars as well as other scars, and many different types of chemicals. In addition, it is possible that the general atrophy associated with the aging process at least predisposes to the development of skin cancer.

Clinical Features. Basal cell carcinoma occurs most frequently in persons in the fourth decade of life or later, but it has been reported as occurring in younger persons, even children. It is much more common in men than in women, probably because men are exposed to the environmental elements more than women.

The basal cell carcinoma usually begins as a small, slightly elevated papule which ulcerates, heals over and then breaks down again (Fig. 2–17; see also Plate II). It enlarges, but still evidences periods of attempted healing. Eventually the crusting ulcer, which appears superficial, develops a smooth, rolled border representing tumor cells spreading laterally beneath the skin. Untreated lesions continue to enlarge, infiltrate adjacent and deeper tissues and may even erode deeply into cartilage or bone (Fig. 2–18).

The basal cell carcinoma is most frequently seen in the middle third of the face, but may occur anywhere on the skin. It is important to realize that this form of carcinoma does not arise from oral mucosa and thus is never seen in the oral cavity unless it arrives there by invasion and infiltration from a skin surface.

Histologic Features. A variety of histologic types of basal cell carcinoma are recognized, but in general the disease is characterized by the appearance of nests, islands or sheets of cells showing indistinct cell membranes with large, deeply staining nuclei and variable numbers of mitotic figures. The individual cells exhibit little variation in appearance. The periphery of the cell nests is composed of a layer of cells, usually well polarized, that are strongly suggestive of cells of the basal layer of skin (Fig. 2–19).

The basal cell is a pluripotential cell which

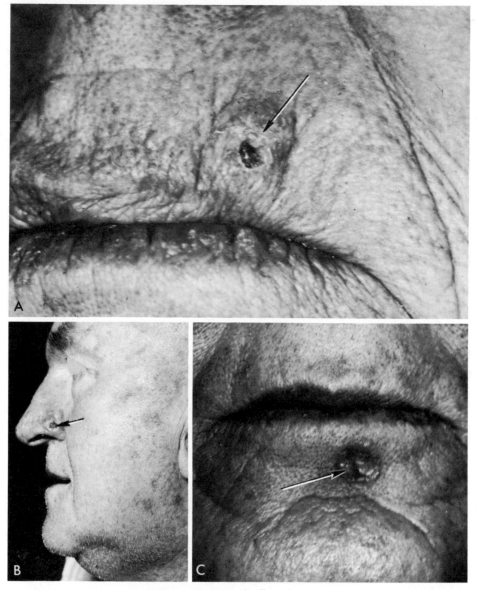

Figure 2–17. *Basal cell carcinoma.*
The tumor of the upper lip *(A)* is a small crusted lesion with an obvious surrounding border of induration. The lesion of the nose *(B)* is a superficial ulcer, while the basal cell carcinoma of the lower lip *(C)* is also a crusted ulcer.

may develop in several directions. It may form hair, sebaceous glands, sweat glands or squamous epithelium and eventually keratin. For this reason the basal cell carcinoma may be expected to make at least abortive attempts to form these structures. The *adenoid basal cell carcinoma* represents that neoplasm which mimics glandular formation. The presence of many cysts in the lesion has given rise to the term *"cystic basal cell carcinoma."* Keratotic *basal cell carcinoma* refers to formation of parakeratotic cells and horn cysts and attempted formation of hair structures similar to the tri-

choepithelioma. In typical *solid* or *primordial basal cell carcinoma*, however, the cells have little tendency to differentiate.

Treatment and Prognosis. Each lesion must be considered separately when contemplating the choice of therapy. In general, equally good results may be expected from surgical excision of the tumor or from x-ray radiation. There is probably an equal number of failures or recurrences subsequent to each type of treatment. Some lesions stubbornly resist treatment and exhibit great propensity for recurrence and subsequent destruction of tissue.

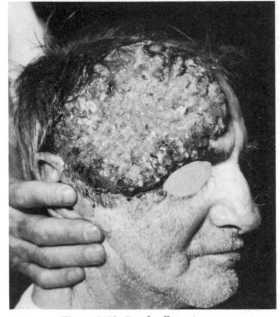

Figure 2–18. *Basal cell carcinoma.*
This neoplasm may become extensive if left untreated and, though it does not metastasize, may invade tissues locally. This particular lesion, neglected by the patient, had been present for many years. (Courtesy of Dr. John Tondra.)

occurrence in the development of many cases of intraoral epidermoid carcinoma.

Multiple basal cell carcinomas of the skin are also one of the characteristic features of the "jaw cyst-bifid rib-basal cell nevus" syndrome (q.v.). In this hereditary syndrome, the skin lesions may develop at an early age.

The prognosis of basal cell lesions is good, since the neoplasm grows slowly, does not tend to metastasize and responds well to treatment. Most difficulties, which may lead to death by local invasion, are due to neglect on the part of the patient who fails to seek medical aid until his lesion is in a far-advanced state.

EPIDERMOID CARCINOMA

(Squamous Cell Carcinoma)

The epidermoid carcinoma is the most common malignant neoplasm of the oral cavity. Although it may occur at any intraoral site, certain sites are more frequently involved than others (Table 2–4). Because of the differences in clinical appearance, the nature of the lesion and particularly the prognosis, it is well to describe the tumors individually, as they may arise in these various areas.

Etiology. The study of general etiologic factors in carcinoma of the oral cavity is an extremely difficult problem, but is best approached by the application of epidemiologic techniques utilizing incidence patterns. One of the best such investigations has been that of Wynder and his associates, from which considerable valuable information may be drawn.

Some patients over a period of years may have multiple basal cell lesions, separate and distinct from each other. This tendency undoubtedly represents "field cancerization" or the "preparation" of a considerable area of tissue by a carcinogenic agent and the development of separate, individual foci of cancer at varying times. Such a phenomenon is also a recognized

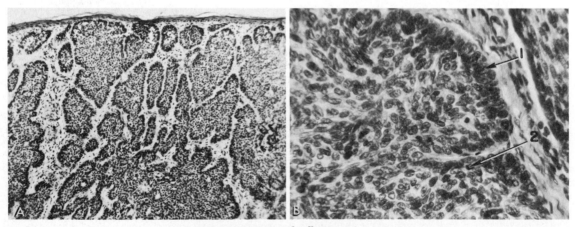

Figure 2–19. *Basal cell carcinoma.*
The low-power photomicrograph *(A)* is taken from the indurated periphery of a lesion, away from the ulceration, and illustrates the sheets and nests of cells resembling those of the basal layer. Under higher magnification *(B)* this similarity becomes more apparent. In addition, the peripheral polarization of the cells *(1)* and mitotic figures *(2)* are obvious.

Table 2–4. Anatomic Distribution of Oral Carcinoma

PRIMARY SITE	NO. IN GROUP	% OF TOTAL IN GROUP	% OF TOTAL IN GROUP (EXCLUDING LIPS)
Lower lip	5,399	38	=
Tongue	3,117	22	38
Floor of mouth	2,479	17	30
Gingiva	923	6	11
Palate	786	5.5	9
Tonsil	673	5	8
Upper lip	553	4	=
Buccal mucosa	245	2	3
Uvula	78	0.5	1
Total	14,253	100	100
			(8,301 cases)

Modified from Krolls, S. O., and Hoffman, S.: Squamous cell carcinoma of the oral soft tissues: a statistical analysis of 14,253 cases by age, sex, and race of patients. J. Am. Dent. Assoc., 92:571, 1976.

As a general indication of the seriousness of this disease, Wynder and his group pointed out that in 1954 in the United States 4210 men and 1172 women died from oral cancer. This mortality rate has increased in more recent years. For example, the American Cancer Society has estimated the death rate from oral cancer in 1981 to be 6300 men and 2850 women. Wynder also reported that a United States Public Health Service study showed that the incidence of oral cancer in a 10-city survey was 19.4 per 100,000 population for men and 5.2 per 100,000 population for women. This confirms most other studies that the morbidity and mortality rates of oral cancer are approximately three to four times greater in men. However, in very recent years there appears to be a trend developing for the increasing incidence of oral cancer in females, thus decreasing the long-recognized overwhelming male to female ratio of this disease in a fashion similar to that well-documented decreased ratio now recognized for lung cancer, presumed to result from increased cigarette smoking in women. There is great variation, however, in sex incidence between various sites in the oral cavity. Great variation in geographic distribution also occurs, and as an extreme example, it was cited that oral cancer is the most common type of cancer of men in India and actually accounted for 40 per cent of all forms of cancer in one hospital in Bombay.

The age of occurrence of epidermoid carcinoma of the oral cavity is usually in the later decades of life. However, cases have been reported at nearly every age, including children. It is of interest that in the series of 9775 cases of oral cancer reported by Krolls and Hoffman, about 32 per cent of the patients were in the seventh decade of life, while the vast majority, nearly 87 per cent, were between the ages of 40 and 80 years (Table 2–5). Significantly, 326 patients, or 3.5 per cent, were under the age of 30. These authors have also pointed out that since 1970, in all anatomic locations except the lower lip and the buccal mucosa, the largest number of carcinomas occurred in patients a decade earlier in life than in patients whose neoplasms were diagnosed before 1970. For the lower lip, the patients were two decades younger than before 1970. This trend for earlier occurrence in life of oral cancer in recent years has been confirmed by the studies of White and his co-workers as well as others, although its cause is unknown.

The most commonly suspected environmental etiologic factors in the development of oral cancer are (1) tobacco, (2) alcohol, (3) syphilis, (4) nutritional deficiencies, (5) sunlight (in the case of lip cancer), and (6) miscellaneous factors, including heat (particularly heat from a pipe stem in cases of lip cancer), trauma, sepsis and

Table 2–5. Age Distribution of Oral Carcinoma

AGE	NO. IN GROUP	% OF TOTAL IN GROUP
0–14	3	0.03
15–19	16	0.2
20–29	307	3.2
30–39	713	7.3
40–49	1,746	17.9
50–59	2,427	24.8
60–69	3,113	31.8
70–79	1,204	12.3
80–89	194	2.0
90–99	52	0.5
Total	9,775	100

Modified from Krolls, S. O., and Hoffman, S.: Squamous cell carcinoma of the oral soft tissues: a statistical analysis of 14,253 cases by age, sex, and race of patients. J. Am. Dent. Assoc., 92:571, 1976.

irritation from sharp teeth and dentures. These factors were investigated in the statistical study of 659 patients with oral cancer reported by Wynder and his group, and their findings will be summarized here. In addition, (7) viruses have become increasingly suspect as a carcinogenic agent.

1. SMOKING was found to be an important factor in the development of oral cancer. Only 3 per cent of patients with oral cancer had never smoked, contrasted to 10 per cent of the control patients without oral cancer. Furthermore, 29 per cent of oral cancer patients were heavy smokers, as contrasted to only 17 per cent of the control group. In this study cigar and pipe smoking increased the risk for oral cancer more than cigarette smoking, in distinct contrast to similar studies on lung cancer. Tobacco chewing was also found to be of etiologic importance, but not as important as smoking.

The findings in a study by Peacock and his co-workers, investigating this same problem, have been interpreted as indicating that the use of tobacco and snuff is a promoting influence but not specifically an initiating factor in the development of oral cancer, although a highly significant relation was found between the use of tobacco and snuff and the development of oral "leukoplakia."

Moore has also reported data relating smoking and oral cancer. In a group of 102 smokers, all of whom had been "cured" of mouth or throat cancer, 65 continued smoking while 37 stopped. Within six years, 21 of the 65 (32 per cent) who continued smoking acquired a second "tobacco area" cancer; only 2 of the 35 (5 per cent) who had stopped smoking developed a second cancer within the same period. Virtually identical findings have been reported by Silverman and Griffith in a series of 174 patients.

2. ALCOHOL also appeared in the study of Wynder to be an important factor in the development of oral cancer, particularly in patients who drank over 7 ounces of whiskey a day. Only 12 per cent of control patients drank this amount of alcohol, while 33 per cent of male patients with oral cancer drank this quantity.

In an investigation on the epidemiology of oral cancer, Graham and his co-workers stated that, based on data from 584 males with oral cancer and 1222 control patients with nonneoplastic diseases, the oral cancer risk for males with the traits of heavy alcohol use, heavy smoking and poor dentition combined was 7.7 times that of men with none of these traits.

3. SYPHILIS was found to be important in cases of cancer of the lip and anterior two thirds of the tongue. But whether the cancer was a result of the syphilitic glossitis or of the arsenic therapy which the majority of the patients had received could not be determined.

4. NUTRITIONAL DEFICIENCIES were difficult to evaluate, but there appeared to be no dramatic relation between oral cancer and nutritional or other medical problems. Nevertheless the unquestionable relation between oral cancer and Plummer-Vinson syndrome (q.v.) must be remembered. Furthermore, Trieger and his associates have reported that liver dysfunction may be of some significance, since, in a study of 152 patients with oral cancer, cirrhotic patients had a 19 per cent 5-year survival rate, while the noncirrhotic patients had a 40 per cent 5-year survival rate. This relationship has been confirmed in a series of 408 patients reported by Keller.

5. SUNLIGHT, in cases of lip cancer, appeared to be of only minor etiologic significance. However, this has not been the consensus of most workers who have studied this problem. For example, a conference on cancer of the lip based on a series of 3166 cases was reported by Stoddart, and it was concluded that the same factors that affect the skin to produce cancer affect the lip in an identical fashion. This is the generally accepted reason for its occurrence preponderantly in fair-skinned outdoor male workers who are affected by exposure of the lower lip to the sun, whereas the upper lip is partially protected. The marked predilection for occurrence in males can also be explained by the females' generally lessened exposure to sunlight and the partial protection of their lips by lipstick. Most recent investigators are in accord with this widely accepted concept.

6. TRAUMA AND DENTAL IRRITATION were not found to be significant etiologic factors in oral cancer. In this regard, Monkman and his associates also have carried out a thorough review of the literature relating cancer to trauma and found no evidence to suggest that single uncomplicated trauma can cause cancer. They also found it debatable whether trauma can aggravate or accelerate existing malignancies. However, they concluded that trauma, in combination with other factors, may act as a cocarcinogen and that there was adequate evidence suggesting that metastatic spread of malignant tumors can be affected by trauma.

7. VIRUSES. In recent years, there has been increasing attention drawn to the possibility of a causal relationship between viruses and var-

ious forms of cancer in humans. Much of this is due to the known causal role of viruses in animal cancers, a fact that has been well recognized for over 50 years. The search for human oncogenic viruses is proceeding with marked rapidity and, while proof is still lacking, quantities of circumstantial evidence have accumulated, suggesting that a variety of human cancers are caused by viruses. These include: carcinoma of the nasopharynx, breast, uterus, and lymphoid tissues including the African jaw lymphoma, as well as some forms of leukemia and certain sarcomas. While a number of different viruses have been implicated, one of the most frequently suspected groups is that of the herpes viruses. There are four herpes viruses that are known to cause human disease: 1) the Epstein-Barr virus (EBV), 2) the cytomegalovirus (CMV), 3) the herpes simplex virus (HSV), and 4) the varicella-zoster virus (VZV). Each of these is the cause of an acute infection in the human: (1) EBV—infectious mononucleosis, (2) CMV—cytomegalic inclusion disease, (3) HSV—herpes simplex infection in a number of different clinical forms, and (4) VZV—chicken pox–herpes zoster or shingles. It is significant that the first three of these viruses have also been implicated in certain malignant diseases in the human as well: (1) EBV—the African jaw (Burkitt's) lymphoma and nasopharyngeal carcinoma, (2) CMV—Kaposi's sarcoma, and (3) HSV type II—carcinoma of the uterine cervix. To date, VZV has not been linked to any human malignant neoplasms.

The type II herpes simplex virus, which at one time was most commonly associated with herpes genitalis, is very similar in many biologic characteristics to type I herpes simplex virus, which at one time was most commonly associated with herpes labialis. For this reason, it is only logical that the possible relationship of type I herpes simplex infection to oral cancer be suggested. In addition, since oral infections with type II herpes simplex and genital infections with type I are becoming exceedingly common, because of liberal sexual habits, the possibility of the type II virus, already implicated in cervical cancer, being implicated in oral cancer when translocated becomes a question of great practical significance. Shillitoe and his associates, who have reviewed this subject, have reported investigations on neutralizing antibodies to herpes simplex type I, type II and the measles virus (a virus not linked to cancer) in patients with oral cancer, in patients with oral leukoplakia and in controls (both smokers and nonsmokers). They concluded that their data were consistent with a positive role for both herpes simplex type I and for smoking in the pathogenesis of oral cancer. It is most likely that great strides will be made in the field of viral oncology within the next decade.

The problem of multiple lesions of oral carcinoma must also be considered when evaluating etiologic factors, since if one area in the oral cavity is predisposed to the development of a malignancy, multiple areas might be predisposed as well. There is now sufficient evidence to indicate that "field cancerization" actually does occur, and many patients with oral cancer do have multiple, anatomically separated lesions at the same time or at intervals.

The literature on multiple malignant oral tumors has been extensively reviewed by Meyer and Shklar, quoting one worker who demonstrated that the occurrence of multiple oral malignancies was approximately 15 times as common as would be expected if occurring by chance alone. There is an increased tendency not only for the development of multiple oral cancers, but also for the development of malignancies throughout the gastrointestinal tract. Meyer and Shklar reported 48 cases of multiple primary oral malignancies in a series of 768 cases of oral cancer (6.3 per cent), while Moertel and Foss reported 64 cases in 732 patients (8.7 per cent), and Wynder and his group reported 59 cases in 543 male patients (11 per cent). A group of 377 patients with epidermoid carcinoma of the floor of the mouth which had been treated was recently reviewed by Tepperman and Fitzpatrick, and it was found that 123 new cancers (not recurrences) developed in 101 (27 per cent) of the patients. Of this total, 82 (67 per cent) were epidermoid carcinomas of the respiratory and upper digestive tracts, one third of these being in the mouth.

Histologic Features. Considerable histologic variation is presented in intraoral epidermoid carcinomas, although in general they tend to be moderately well-differentiated neoplasms with some evidence of keratinization (Fig. 2–20). Highly anaplastic lesions do occur, but are uncommon; such lesions tend to metastasize early and widely and cause death quickly. The well-differentiated epidermoid carcinoma consists of sheets and nests of cells with obvious origin from squamous epithelium. These cells are generally large and show a distinct cell membrane, although intercellular bridges or tonofibrils often cannot be demonstrated. The nuclei of the neoplastic cells are large and may

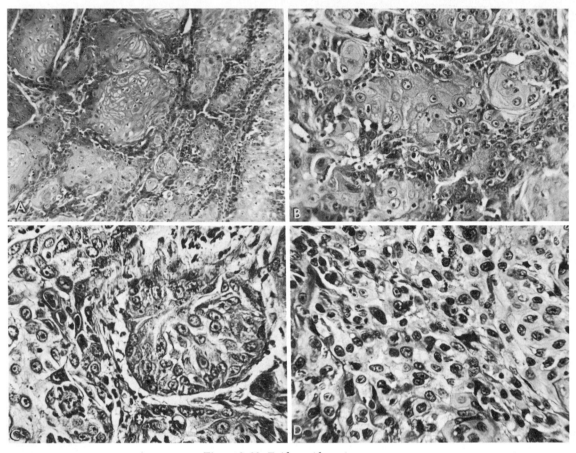

Figure 2–20. *Epidermoid carcinoma.*

Photomicrographs of various cases of epidermoid carcinoma illustrate *(A)* a highly differentiated carcinoma, *(B)* a well-differentiated carcinoma, *(C)* a moderately differentiated carcinoma, and *(D)* a poorly differentiated carcinoma.

demonstrate a good deal of variability in the intensity of the staining reaction. Nuclei which stain heavily with hematoxylin are referred to as hyperchromatic. In the well-differentiated lesions mitotic figures may be found, but they often do not appear to be especially numerous. Many of these mitotic figures are atypical, although this may be obvious only to an experienced histopathologist. One of the most prominent features of the well-differentiated epidermoid carcinoma is the presence of individual cell keratinization and the formation of numerous epithelial, or keratin, pearls of varying size. In a typical lesion, groups of these malignant cells can be found actively invading the connective tissue in a vagarious pattern.

Less well-differentiated epidermoid carcinomas lose certain features, so that their resemblance to squamous epithelium is less pronounced. The characteristic shape of the cells may be altered as well as their typical arrangement one to the other. The growth rate of the individual cells is more rapid, and this is re-

flected in the greater numbers of mitotic figures, the even greater variation in size, shape and tinctorial reaction and the failure to carry out the function of a differentiated squamous cell: the formation of keratin.

The poorly differentiated carcinomas bear little resemblance to their cell of origin and often will present diagnostic difficulties because of the primitive and uncharacteristic histologic appearance of the malignant, rapidly dividing cells. These cells show an even greater lack of cohesiveness and are extremely vagarious.

The recognition that different degrees of differentiation occur in the epidermoid carcinoma prompted Broders to suggest a system of grading tumors in which a grade I lesion was highly differentiated (its cells were producing much keratin), while grade IV was very poorly differentiated (the cells were highly anaplastic and showed practically no keratin formation). The fact that the same tumor may show different degrees of differentiation in varying areas has prompted the discontinuance of the grading

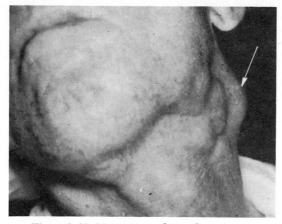

Figure 2–21. *Metastatic epidermoid carcinoma.*
There is massive involvement of the cervical lymph nodes, which are firm, fixed and matted. (Courtesy of Dr. Wilbur C. Moorman.)

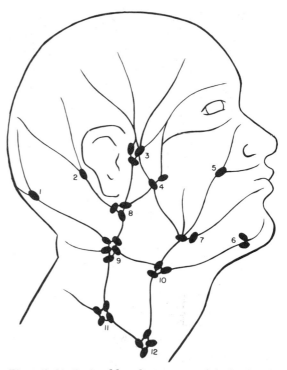

Figure 2–22. *Regional lymphatic system of the head and neck, showing the various groups of lymph nodes.*
1, Occipital nodes. *2*, Posterior auricular nodes. *3*, Anterior auricular (preauricular) nodes. *4*, Parotid nodes. *5*, Facial nodes. *6*, Submental nodes. *7*, Submaxillary nodes. *8*, Inferior auricular nodes. *9*, Lateral upper deep cervical nodes. *10*, Medial upper deep cervical nodes. *11*, Lateral lower deep cervical nodes. *12*, Medial lower deep cervical nodes.

system. Instead, most pathologists now modify the diagnosis of the neoplasm by a descriptive adjective indicative of its differentiation. The one advantage of grading a tumor is that the grade reflects the anaplasticity of the lesion, which in turn indicates the general rapidity of growth, the rapidity of metastatic spread, the general reaction to be expected after x-ray radiation and the prognosis. This great advantage is still retained in the descriptive grading which is replacing the numerical grading system.

Metastases from intraoral carcinoma of different sites involve chiefly the submaxillary and superficial and deep cervical lymph nodes (Figs. 2–21, 2–22, 2–23; see also Plate II). Occasionally, other nodes such as the submental, preauricular and postauricular nodes and supraclavicular nodes may be involved, but blood stream metastasis from oral cancer is uncommon. However, Gowen and de Suto-Nagy have reported on a series of 59 patients who died of carcinoma of the head and neck and were autopsied, with distant metastases being specifically sought. Surprisingly, 57 per cent of these patients did have distant metastases: in the lung in 82 per cent of the cases, in the liver in 45 per cent, and in the bones in 23 per cent.

Mustard and Rosen have reported on the influence of lymph node metastasis on the survival rate of patients with oral cancer. In a series of 1177 patients who did not have regional lymph node involvement at the time of diagnosis of their lesion, 64 per cent lived for 5 years. However, of the group who did have lymph node involvement at the time of admission, only 15 per cent survived for the same period.

Clinical Staging of Oral Cancer. In recent

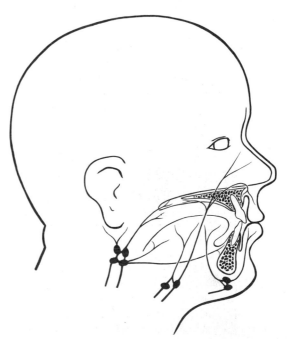

Figure 2–23. *Regional lymphatic drainage of the oral structures.*

PLATE II

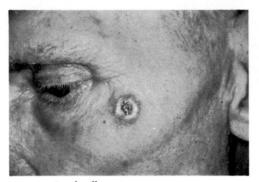

Basal cell carcinoma

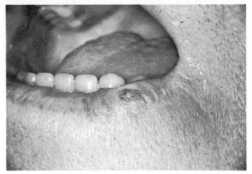

Epidermoid carcinoma of lip

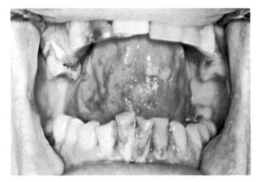

Epidermoid carcinoma of tongue (ventral)

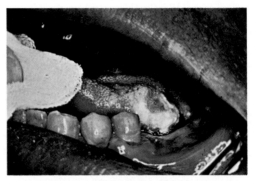

Epidermoid carcinoma of tongue (lateral)

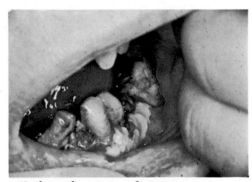

Epidermoid carcinoma of gingiva

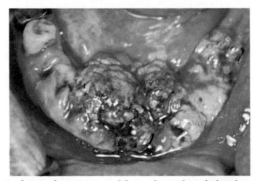

Epidermoid carcinoma of floor of mouth and alveolar ridge

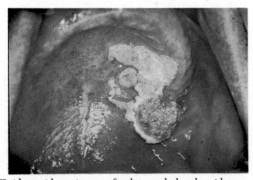

Epidermoid carcinoma of palate and alveolar ridge

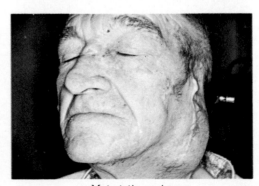

Metastatic carcinoma

Table 2–6. Definition of the TNM Categories of Malignant Tumors about the Oral Cavity

T—Primary Tumor
    T1S—Carcinoma in situ.
    T1—Tumor 2 cm. or less in greatest diameter.
    T2—Tumor greater than 2 cm. but not greater than 4 cm. in greatest diameter.
    T3—Tumor greater than 4 cm. in greatest diameter.
N—Regional Lymph Nodes
    N0—No clinically palpable cervical lymph node(s); or palpable node(s) but metastasis not suspected.
    N1—Clinically palpable homolateral cervical lymph node(s) that are not fixed; metastasis suspected.
    N2—Clinically palpable contralateral or bilateral cervical lymph node(s) that are not fixed; metastasis suspected.
    N3—Clinically palpable lymph node(s) that are fixed; metastasis suspected.
M—Distant Metastasis
    M0—No distant metastasis
    M1—Clinical and/or radiographic evidence of metastasis other than to cervical lymph nodes.

years, the clinical staging of cancer in various sites of the body has assumed an important role in dealing with the cancer patient. Clinical staging refers to an assessment of the extent of the disease before undertaking treatment and has as its purpose: (1) selection of the most appropriate treatment, and (2) meaningful comparison of the end results reported from different sources. The staging system used here is the most widely known and is that developed by the American Joint Committee for Cancer Staging and End Results Reporting (AJCCS) sponsored by the United States Public Health Service, the American College of Surgeons, American College of Physicians, College of American Pathologists, and the American Cancer Society, among others.

The system is known as the TNM system (T–primary tumor; N–regional lymph nodes; M–distant metastases) and was adopted for use in carcinoma of the oral cavity in 1967. The definition of the TNM categories for carcinoma of the oral cavity is shown in Table 2–6, while the clinical stage-grouping of oral cancer is presented in Table 2–7. It should be recognized that specific criteria modify the application of the TNM system according to anatomic site, and that histopathologic classification or grading of the cancer is not involved in clinical staging.

Table 2–7. Clinical Stage-Grouping of Carcinoma of the Oral Cavity

Stage I:	T1 N0 M0	
Stage II:	T2 N0 M0	
Stage III:	T3 N0 M0	
	T1 N1 M0	
	T2 N1 M0	
	T3 N1 M0	
Stage IV:	T1 N2 M0	T1 N3 M0
	T2 N2 M0	T2 N3 M0
	T3 N2 M0	T3 N3 M0
	Or any T or N category with M1.	

Carcinoma of the Lip

Epidermoid carcinoma of the lip is a disease that occurs chiefly in elderly men. Furthermore, the lower lip is involved by this neoplasm far more commonly than the upper lip. Great numbers of cases have been reported in the literature, and the data of Cross, Guralnick and Daland on 563 patients with lip cancer may be cited to illustrate certain typical characteristics. In this large series it was found that 98 per cent of the patients were men and that the age of these patients at the onset of the disease ranged from 25 to 91 years, with the greatest incidence between 55 and 75 years and a mean of 62 years of age. Of the total group of lip cancers, 88.3 per cent occurred on the lower lip, 3.3 per cent on the upper lip and 8.3 per cent on the labial commissures. The right and left sides were affected with equal frequency. In 636 cases reviewed by Schreiner, similar findings were reported. In his series 97 per cent of the lesions occurred in men, and 96 per cent were found on the lower lip. Nearly one third of his cases occurred between the ages of 60 and 70 years.

Etiology. A number of possible etiologic factors have been suggested by the review of the records of many patients. One of the most common of these has been the use of tobacco, chiefly through pipe smoking. The data of Cross and his co-workers indicate that 64 per cent of their patients with lip cancer were pipe smokers, while a total of 94 per cent habitually used tobacco in some form. These observations are in agreement with the data of Widmann, who, in a review of 363 cases of lip cancer, estimated an incidence of approximately 40 per cent pipe smokers. Schreiner reported that 87 per cent of his lip cancer patients were tobacco users. Although no conclusions may be drawn from such data because of the widespread use of tobacco in the general population, it appears suggestive that the heat, the trauma of the pipe stem and possibly the combustion end-products of tobacco may be of some significance in the etiology of lip cancer.

Syphilis is probably not as significant an etiologic factor in lip cancer as in certain other oral sites, since the incidence of lip cancer has been found to be low in syphilitic patients: 7.2 per cent by Cross and his associates, 8 per cent by Widmann and 3.6 per cent by Schreiner. As indicated previously, however, the data of Wynder and his group indicated that syphilis was of etiologic significance in lip cancer.

Sunlight is generally considered to be important, as discussed previously, because the alterations which occur in skin and lips as a result of prolonged exposure to sun are characterized as preneoplastic. Ju has discussed this problem and constructed a profile of the lip cancer patient.

Poor oral hygiene is an almost universal finding in patients with lip cancer. Cross and his group pointed out that only approximately 8 per cent of their entire series of patients had good or even fair oral hygiene. In addition, some patients indicate a history of trauma before the appearance of a lesion. They report not only a single traumatic experience, such as a cigarette burn or a cut, but also chronic trauma from jagged teeth and so forth. Unfortunately, it is difficult to assess scientifically the role of such factors in the etiology of cancer.

Leukoplakia has often been associated with the development of carcinoma. Since clinical leukoplakia is a fairly common lesion of the lip, it was only natural that the relationship should be investigated. Schreiner found leukoplakia present in only 2.4 per cent of his 636 cases of lip cancer, while Cross and co-workers found leukoplakia associated with carcinoma in 14.5 per cent of the cases in their series. This would indicate that the simultaneous occurrence of the two conditions is probably due to chance and that leukoplakia is not a common predecessor of lip cancer. However, in light of more recent studies dealing with the frequency of preneoplastic and neoplastic transformation in lesions of leukoplakia of the lip (q.v.), the interpretation of the above findings is uncertain.

Clinical Features.   There is considerable variation in the clinical appearance of lip cancer, depending chiefly upon the duration of the lesion and the nature of the growth. The tumor usually begins on the vermilion border of the lip to one side of the midline. It often commences as a small area of thickening, induration and ulceration or irregularity of the surface (Plate II). As the lesion becomes larger it may

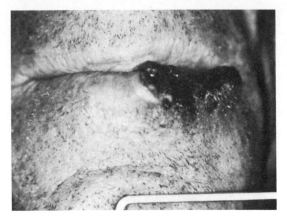

Figure 2–24. *Epidermoid carcinoma of lip.*

create a small crater-like defect (Fig. 2–24) or produce an exophytic, proliferative growth of tumor tissue. Some patients have large fungating masses in a relatively short time, while in other patients the lesion may be only slowly progressive.

Carcinoma of the lip is generally slow to metastasize, and a massive lesion may develop before there is evidence of regional lymph node involvement. Some lesions, however, particularly the more anaplastic ones, may metastasize early. When metastasis does occur, it is usually ipsilateral and involves the submental or submaxillary nodes. Contralateral metastasis may occur, especially if the lesion is near the midline of the lip where there is a cross drainage of the lymphatic vessels.

Histologic Features.   Most lip carcinomas are well-differentiated lesions, often classified as grade I carcinoma. This type of cancer tends to metastasize late in the course of the disease. In the series of Widmann the following approximate distribution of graded lesions was found: grade I, 60 per cent; grade II, 26 per cent; grade III, 13 per cent; grade IV, 2 per cent.

Treatment and Prognosis.   Carcinoma of the lip has been treated by either surgical excision or x-ray radiation with approximately equal success, depending to some degree upon the duration and extent of the lesion and the presence of metastases. Interestingly, in the series of Cross the over-all cure rate of patients with lip cancer treated by surgery was approximately 81 per cent, while in the series of Widmann the cure rate of patients with the same type of neoplasm treated by x-ray radiation was approximately 83 per cent. This would indicate that either form of therapy, in *skilled hands*, will produce equally good results.

Many factors may influence the success or

failure of treatment of lip carcinoma. The size of the lesion, its duration, the presence or absence of metastatic lymph nodes and the histologic grade of the lesion must all be considered carefully by the therapist in planning his approach to the neoplastic problem.

Carcinoma of the Tongue

Cancer of the tongue comprises between 25 and 50 per cent of all intraoral cancer. It is less common in women than in men except in certain geographic localities, chiefly the Scandinavian countries, where the incidence of all intraoral carcinoma in women is high because of the high incidence of a pre-existing Plummer-Vinson syndrome. In a series of 441 cases of tongue cancer reported by Ash and Millar, 25 per cent occurred in women and 75 per cent in men, with an average age of 63 years. In a series of 330 cases of cancer of the tongue reported by Gibbel, Cross and Ariel the average age of the patient was 53 years, with a range of 32 to 87 years. Thus it is essentially a disease of the elderly, but it may occur in relatively young persons. To exemplify this latter point, a series of 11 patients less than 30 years of age, four of them less than 20 years, with carcinoma of the tongue has been reported by Byers. This group of patients represented approximately 3 per cent of all patients seen at M. D. Anderson Hospital with epidermoid carcinoma of the tongue between 1956 and 1973 (418 cases).

Etiology. A number of causes of cancer of the tongue have been suggested, but in our present state of knowledge no precise statements can be made. A definite relation does appear to exist, however, between tongue cancer and certain other disorders. Many investigators have found syphilis, either an active case or at least a past history of it, coexistent with carcinoma of the tongue. In the series of Gibbel et al., 22 per cent of patients with lingual cancer demonstrated a positive complement fixation or Kahn reaction, while in the general admission at their hospital only 5 per cent of the patients had a positive reaction for syphilis. Martin reported that 33 per cent of his patients with cancer of the tongue also had syphilis. The relationship can be explained on the basis of a chronic glossitis produced by the syphilis, chronic irritation long being recognized as carcinogenic under certain circumstances. This explanation implies a local effect of syphilis rather than a generalized or systemic effect. It should be pointed out that some studies do not confirm the theory of a relationship between syphilis

and tongue cancer. Wynder has confirmed this relationship, but questioned whether the neoplasm might be related to the arsenic therapy, the treatment of choice before the advent of antibiotics, rather than to the syphilis itself. Meyer and Abbey have also questioned this relationship since they found only 15 patients (6 per cent) who showed positive evidence of a history of syphilis in a survey of 243 cases of primary carcinoma of the tongue.

Leukoplakia is a common lesion of the tongue which has been observed many times to be associated with tongue cancer. Martin noted that 46 per cent of his series of cancer patients had leukoplakia of the tongue, while Gibbel et al. found only a 10 per cent incidence of leukoplakia in his series. It is not unusual to see typical lesions of carcinoma in leukoplakic areas; on the other hand, many lesions of leukoplakia appear to persist for years without malignant transformation, and many cases of carcinoma of the tongue develop without evidence of pre-existing leukoplakia.

Other factors which have been thought to contribute to the development of carcinoma of the tongue include poor oral hygiene, chronic trauma and the use of alcohol and tobacco. Poor hygiene and the use of alcohol and tobacco are so prevalent as nearly to preclude the possibility of drawing conclusions about a possible cause and effect relation. A considerable number of cases have been observed in which cancer of the tongue developed at a site exactly corresponding to a source of chronic irritation such as a carious or broken tooth or an ill-fitting denture. The work of Wynder and his group, however, suggests that these findings may be fortuitous.

Clinical Features. The most common presenting sign of carcinoma of the tongue is a painless mass or ulcer, although in most patients the lesion ultimately becomes painful, especially when it becomes secondarily infected. The tumor may begin as a superficially indurated ulcer with slightly raised borders and may proceed either to develop a fungating, exophytic mass or to infiltrate the deep layers of the tongue, producing fixation and induration without much surface change (Fig. 2–25, A, B, C; see also Plate II).

The typical lesion develops on the lateral border or ventral surface of the tongue. When in rare cases carcinoma occurs on the dorsum of the tongue, it is usually in a patient with a past or present history of syphilitic glossitis. In a series of 1554 cases of carcinoma of the tongue reported by Frazell and Lucas, only 4 per cent

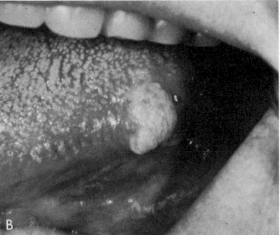

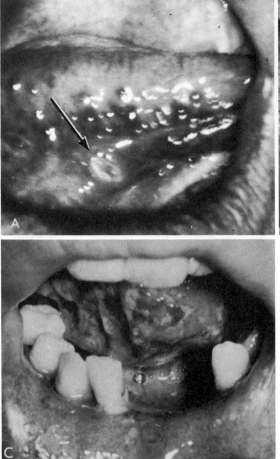

Figure 2–25. *Epidermoid carcinoma of tongue, early to advanced.*

occurred on the dorsum. The lesions on the lateral border are rather equally distributed between the base of the tongue, the anterior third and the mid-portion, although in the above series 45 per cent of cases occurred on the middle third. Lesions near the base of the tongue are particularly insidious, since they may be asymptomatic until far advanced. Even then the only presenting manifestations may be a sore throat and dysphagia. The specific site of development of these tumors is of great significance, since the lesions on the posterior portion of the tongue are usually of a higher grade of malignancy, metastasize earlier and offer a poorer prognosis, especially because of their inaccessibility for treatment.

Metastases occur with great frequency in cases of tongue cancer. In 302 patients on whom information was available, Gibbel and his group reported that cervical metastases from tongue lesions were present in 69 per cent at the time of admission to the hospital. The metastatic lesions may be ipsilateral, bilateral or, because of the cross lymphatic drainage, contralateral in respect to the tongue lesion.

Treatment and Prognosis. The treatment of cancer of the tongue is a difficult problem, and even now no specific statements can be made about the efficacy of surgery in comparison to that of x-ray radiation. As in other areas, it will probably be found that the judicious combination of surgery and x-ray will be of greatest benefit to the patient. Many radiotherapists prefer the use of radium needles or radon seeds to x-ray radiation because they are able with these devices to limit the radiation to the tumor, sparing adjacent normal tissue. Metastatic nodes are highly complicating factors, but treating them without controlling the primary lesion is useless.

The prognosis of cancer in this location is not good. Although statistics vary between series, the 5-year cure rate is generally conceded to be below 25 per cent. Martin reported a 22 per cent survival in 556 patients with tongue cancer, while Gibbel et al. found only a 14 per cent survival among 213 patients. Frazell and Lucas reported an over-all 5-year cure rate of 35 per cent on a series of 1321 patients with tongue cancer.

The most significant factor affecting prognosis of these patients is the presence or absence of cervical metastases. Thus the studies of Gibbel and his associates showed an 81 per cent survival rate if no metastases ever developed, 43 per cent if no metastases were present at the time of hospital admission, and only 4 per cent if metastases were present at the time of admission or developed subsequent to admission. The necessity for early diagnosis thus becomes obvious, and the role of the dentist in recognizing cancerous lesions is, of course, of paramount importance.

Carcinoma of the Floor of the Mouth

Carcinoma of the floor of the mouth represents approximately 15 per cent of all cases of intraoral cancer and occurs in the same age group as other oral cancers. The average age of the patient was 57 years in the series of Tiecke and Bernier, 67 years in the series of 110 cases reported by Ash and Millar and 63 years in the group of 100 cases reported by Ballard and his associates. In the latter report, 81 per cent of the lesions occurred in men, while 93 per cent of the patients were men in the series of Ash and Millar.

Smoking, especially a pipe or cigar, has been considered by some investigators to be important in the etiology of cancer in this location. In the series of Ballard and his co-workers, 50 per cent of the patients were classified as heavy smokers, 33 per cent as heavy drinkers and 28 per cent as heavy smokers and heavy drinkers. Nevertheless little evidence has been gathered to suggest an obvious cause-and-effect relation with regard to tobacco or other factors such as alcohol, poor oral hygiene or dental irritation. Leukoplakia does occur in this location and there is evidence to indicate that epithelial dysplasia and malignant transformation in the leukoplakia occur here with greater frequency than in other oral sites.

Clinical Features. The typical carcinoma in the floor of the mouth is an indurated ulcer of varying size situated on one side of the midline. It may or may not be painful. This neoplasm occurs far more frequently in the anterior portion of the floor than in the posterior area. Because of its location, early extension into the lingual mucosa of the mandible and into the

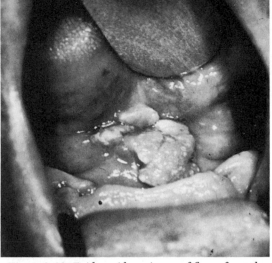

Figure 2–26. *Epidermoid carcinoma of floor of mouth.*

mandible proper as well as into the tongue occurs with considerable frequency (Fig. 2–26; see also Plate II). Carcinoma of the floor of the mouth may invade the deeper tissues and may even extend into the submaxillary and sublingual glands. The proximity of this tumor to the tongue, producing some limitation of motion of that organ, often induces a peculiar thickening or slurring of the speech.

Metastases from the floor of the mouth are found most commonly in the submaxillary group of lymph nodes, and since the primary lesion frequently occurs near the midline where a lymphatic cross drainage exists, contralateral metastases are often present. Of 95 cases of carcinoma of the floor of the mouth reviewed by Ash and Millar, 21 per cent presented lymph node involvement at the time of admission, while an additional 23 per cent subsequently developed lymphadenopathy. Thus the total incidence of metastasis was 44 per cent. This corresponds to the incidence of 42 per cent metastatic lymph node involvement in the series reported by Tiecke and Bernier and 58 per cent by Martin and Sugarbaker. Fortunately, distant metastases are rare.

Treatment and Prognosis. The treatment of cancer of the floor of the mouth is difficult and all too frequently unsuccessful. Large lesions, because of the anatomy of the region, usually are not a surgical problem. Even small tumors are apt to recur after surgical excision. For this reason, x-ray radiation and the use of radium often give far better results than surgery. The problem is complicated, however, if there is concomitant involvement of the mandible.

The prognosis for patients with carcinoma of the floor of the mouth is fair. The net 5-year survival of 86 patients with cancer in this location reviewed by Ash and Millar was 43 per cent. All patients in this series were treated by some form of radiation. Martin and Sugarbaker reported a 5-year survival rate of 21 per cent in their series of 103 patients.

Carcinoma of the Buccal Mucosa

Reported studies of carcinoma of the buccal mucosa reveal exceptional variation in incidence, the widest differences being accounted for by studies from countries other than the United States. In the series of Krolls and Hoffman, cancer of the buccal mucosa comprised 3 per cent of the total cases of intraoral carcinoma. Like most cancers of the oral cavity, cancer of the buccal mucosa is approximately ten times more common in men than in women and occurs chiefly in elderly persons. In the study of Tiecke and Bernier the average age at occurrence of carcinoma of the buccal mucosa was 58 years.

Etiology. The etiology of carcinoma of the buccal mucosa is no better understood than that of carcinoma of other areas of the oral cavity. Several factors appear to be of indisputable significance, however; these include the use of chewing tobacco and the habit of chewing betel nut, which is widespread in many countries in the Far East. It is a fairly common clinical observation that carcinoma of the buccal mucosa develops in the area against which a person has habitually carried a quid of chewing tobacco for years while the opposite cheek may be normal, the patient never having rested the tobacco there. Although this is only presumptive evidence of a cause-and-effect relation, it has been recognized so frequently that it appears to be more than a coincidental finding. A special form of neoplasm known as "verrucous carcinoma" (q.v.) occurs almost exclusively in elderly patients with a history of tobacco chewing. Since the betel nut quid contains tobacco as well as other substances, including slaked lime, the high incidence of cancer in persons addicted to its use may be explained on a similar basis.

Leukoplakia is a common predecessor of carcinoma of the buccal mucosa. It is usually of extremely long duration and may or may not necessarily be associated with the use of tobacco. Chronic trauma in the form of cheek-biting and dental irritation such as that from jagged teeth does not appear to be associated with the development of carcinoma, although focal areas of leukoplakia sometimes occur when these conditions exist.

Clinical Features. There is considerable variation in the clinical appearance of carcinoma of the buccal mucosa. The lesions develop most frequently along or inferior to a line opposite the plane of occlusion. The anteroposterior position is variable, some cases occurring near the third molar area, others forward toward the commissure.

The lesion is often a painful ulcerative one in which induration and infiltration of deeper tissues are common. Some cases, however, are superficial and appear to be growing outward from the surface rather than invading the tissues. Tumors of this latter type are sometimes called exophytic or verrucous growths.

The incidence of metastases from the usual epidermoid carcinoma of the buccal mucosa varies considerably, but is relatively high. Tiecke and Bernier reported that 45 per cent of the patients in their study exhibited metastases at the time of presentation for treatment. This is similar to the incidence of approximately 50 per cent reported by Richards. The most common sites of metastases are the submaxillary lymph nodes.

Treatment and Prognosis. The treatment of carcinoma of the buccal mucosa is just as much of a problem as that of cancer in other areas of the oral cavity. In early cases it is probable that similar results may be obtained by either surgery or x-ray radiation. The combined use of these two forms of treatment undoubtedly also has a place in the therapy of this tumor.

The prognosis of this neoplasm depends upon the presence or absence of metastases. The findings of Modlin and Johnson indicate that the 5-year survival rate for patients with cancer of the buccal mucosa approximates 50 per cent, but in another series Martin reported only a 28 per cent survival.

Carcinoma of the Gingiva

Carcinoma of the gingiva constitutes an extremely important group of neoplasms. The similarity of early cancerous lesions of the gingiva to common dental infections has frequently led to delay in diagnosis or even to misdiagnosis. Hence institution of treatment has been delayed, and the ultimate prognosis of the patient is poorer.

Martin reported that approximately 10 per cent of all malignant tumors of the oral cavity occur on the gingiva. In the study of Krolls and Hoffman, 11 per cent of the intraoral carcinomas occurred on the gingiva, while Tiecke and Bernier found a similar incidence of 12 per cent in their series. In the group reported by Martin, one patient was only 22 years old, but the average age of the patients was 61 years. This is essentially a disease of elderly persons, since only 2 per cent of the tumors occurred in patients under the age of 40 years. In the same group of patients 82 per cent were men and only 18 per cent were women. This is similar to the sex distribution found in oral cancer in other locations.

Etiology. The etiology of carcinoma of the gingiva appears to be no more specific or defined than that in other areas of the oral cavity. Syphilis does not appear to be as significant a factor here as it is in carcinoma of the tongue, and the relation to the use of tobacco is indefinite. Since the gingiva, because of calculus formation and collection of microorganisms, is in nearly all persons the site of a chronic irritation and inflammation lasting over a period of many years, one may speculate on the possible role of chronic irritation in the development of cancer of the gingiva. Occasionally, cases of gingival carcinoma appear to arise after extraction of a tooth. If such cases are carefully examined, however, it may usually be ascertained that the tooth was extracted because of a gingival lesion or disease or because the tooth was loose. In fact, the tooth was extracted *because* of the tumor, which, at the time of surgery, went unrecognized or undiagnosed.

An unusual situation arises in some instances after extraction of a tooth in that a carcinoma appears to develop rapidly and proliferate up out of the socket. Those cases which appear to represent such a phenomenon probably are due to carcinoma of the gingiva growing down along the periodontal ligament and then proliferating suddenly after the dental extraction.

Clinical Features. It is generally agreed that carcinoma of the mandibular gingiva is more common than involvement of the maxillary gingiva, although the distribution of cases varies considerably between different series. In 47 cases reported by Tiecke and Bernier, 81 per cent of the tumors were found on the mandibular gingiva and only 19 per cent on the maxillary gingiva. Martin, however, reported a more equal distribution of 54 per cent on the mandibular gingiva and 46 per cent on the

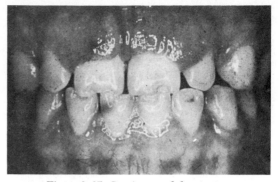

Figure 2–27. *Carcinoma of the gingiva.*
The mild overgrowth of the gingiva over the maxillary central incisors in this 25-year-old girl resembled inflammatory gingival hyperplasia. Microscopic examination of the gingivectomy specimen revealed epidermoid carcinoma. This is an unusual clinical appearance, age and location for this neoplasm, but many early cases are difficult to recognize. (Courtesy of Drs. Harold R. Schreiber and Charles A. Waldron: J. Periodontol., 29:196, 1958.)

maxillary gingiva. The data on the exact position in the dental arch at which carcinoma is most apt to develop are insufficient to draw valid conclusions.

Carcinoma of the gingiva usually is manifested initially as an area of ulceration which may be a purely erosive lesion or may exhibit an exophytic, granular or verrucous type of growth (Fig. 2–27; see also Plate II). Many times, carcinoma of the gingiva does not have the clinical appearance of a malignant neoplasm. It may or may not be painful. The tumor arises more commonly in edentulous areas, although it may develop in a site in which teeth are present. The fixed gingiva is more frequently involved primarily than the free gingiva.

The proximity of the underlying periosteum and bone usually invites early invasion of these structures. Although many cases exhibit irregular invasion and infiltration of the bone, superficial erosion arising apparently as a pressure phenomenon sometimes occurs. In the maxilla, gingival carcinoma often invades into the maxillary sinus, or it may extend onto the palate or into the tonsillar pillar. In the mandible, extension into the floor of the mouth or laterally into the cheek as well as deep into the bone is rather common. Pathologic fracture sometimes occurs in the latter instance (Fig. 2–28).

Metastasis is a common sequela of gingival carcinoma. Cancer of the mandibular gingiva metastasizes more frequently than cancer of the maxillary gingiva. In most series of cases, metastases to either the submaxillary or the cerv-

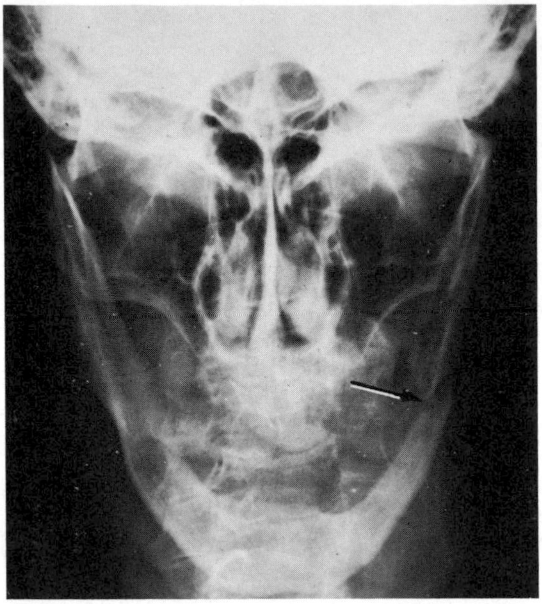

Figure 2–28. *Pathologic fracture of mandible caused by invasion of epidermoid carcinoma arising on alveolar ridge.*

ical nodes eventually occur in over 50 per cent of the patients regardless of whether the involvement is maxillary or mandibular.

Treatment and Prognosis. The use of x-ray radiation of carcinoma of the gingiva is fraught with hazards because of the well-known damaging effect of the x-rays on bone. In general, treatment of carcinoma in this location is a surgical problem.

The prognosis of cancer of the gingiva is not particularly good. In the series of 105 cases reported by Martin, only 26 per cent of the patients were alive and free of the disease 5 years after treatment. It is of great significance that in this same series there were no 5-year survivals if the patient presented lymph node metastases at the time of admission. This again illustrates the great need for early diagnosis of these neoplasms.

CARCINOMA OF THE PALATE

Epidermoid carcinoma of the palate is not a particularly common lesion of the oral cavity. It exhibits approximately the same percentage of occurrence as carcinoma of the buccal mucosa, floor of the mouth and gingiva. The palate was the primary site of 9 per cent of the intraoral epidermoid carcinomas reported by Krolls and Hoffman. In a study by Tiecke and Bernier, of 38 palatal tumors in which the site was specific, 53 per cent occurred on the soft palate, 34 per cent on the hard palate and 13 per cent on both. Ackerman, however, stated that epidermoid carcinoma of the hard palate is a rare finding. New and Hallberg found an incidence of only 0.5 per cent of cases of epidermoid carcinoma of the hard palate among approximately 5000 cases of intraoral carcinoma. (Accessory salivary gland tumors of the hard palate appear to be three to four times more common than epidermoid carcinoma.)

Clinical Features. Palatal cancer usually manifests itself as a poorly defined, ulcerated, painful lesion on one side of the midline (Fig. 2–29; see also Plate II). It frequently crosses the midline, however, and may extend laterally to include the lingual gingiva or posteriorly to involve the tonsillar pillar or even the uvula. The tumor on the hard palate may invade into the bone or occasionally into the nasal cavity, while infiltrating lesions of the soft palate may extend into the nasopharynx.

The epidermoid carcinoma is almost invariably an ulcerated lesion, whereas the tumors of accessory salivary gland origin, even the malignant lesions, are often not ulcerated, but are covered with an intact mucosa. This fact may be of some aid in helping to distinguish clinically between these two types of neoplasms.

Metastases to regional lymph nodes occur in a considerable percentage of cases, but there is little evidence to indicate whether such metastases are more common in carcinoma of the soft palate or in that of the hard palate.

Treatment and Prognosis. Both surgery and

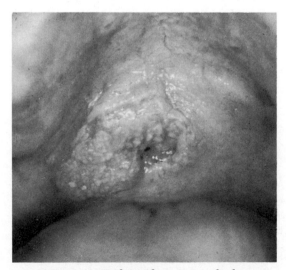

Figure 2–29. *Epidermoid carcinoma of palate.*

x-ray radiation have been used in the treatment of epidermoid carcinoma of the palate. Few large series of cases are available for analysis to aid in determining which form of therapy may be expected to give the greatest survival. Nor are any significant series of purely palatal carcinomas available to aid in the determinations of over-all survival rate of patients with this lesion. It does appear that the prognosis is somewhat comparable to that of carcinoma of the gingiva.

Carcinoma of the Maxillary Sinus

Antral carcinoma is an exceedingly dangerous disease. Although the actual incidence of the disease in respect to intraoral carcinoma cannot be determined, it does appear to be considerably less frequent than any other form of oral cancer. Seelig presented an excellent 10-year survey of the literature and described the chief findings in 624 cases of antral carcinoma; a review of this disease has also been reported by Chaudhry and his associates. Although nothing is known of the etiology of this particular neoplasm, Ackerman stated that chronic sinusitis does not seem to predispose to the development of carcinoma of the maxillary sinus. It might be pointed out here that, although most cases of carcinoma of the maxillary sinus are of the epidermoid type, occasional cases of adenocarcinoma occur, apparently originating from the glands in the wall of the sinus.

Clinical Features. One of the features which contribute to the deadly nature of this disease is that it is often hopelessly advanced before the patient is conscious of its presence. The dentist must be fully aware of the potentialities of this neoplasm and the various ways in which it may manifest itself clinically.

Available studies indicate that carcinoma of the antrum is somewhat more common in men and that, though it is chiefly a disease of elderly persons, occasional cases occur in young adults.

The first clinical sign of antral carcinoma is frequently a swelling or bulging of the maxillary alveolar ridge, palate or mucobuccal fold, loosening or elongation of the maxillary molars or swelling of the face inferior and lateral to the eye (Fig. 2–30). Unilateral nasal stuffiness or discharge is sometimes a primary complaint. In edentulous patients wearing maxillary dentures, loosening of or inability to tolerate the prosthetic appliance may occur before there is any visible clinical evidence of the disease.

The actual spread of the neoplasm which determines the clinical manifestations of the disease is reflected by the extent of involvement of the various walls of the antrum. In some cases only the floor of the sinus is invaded, so that the manifestations of the disease are associated solely with oral structures. If the medial wall of the sinus is involved, nasal obstruction may result. Involvement of the superior wall or roof produces displacement of the eye, while invasion of the lateral wall produces bulging of the cheek. Ulceration either into the oral cavity or on the skin surface may occur, but only late in the course of the disease.

Metastases usually do not occur until the tumor is far advanced, but when they appear they involve the submaxillary and cervical lymph nodes. The lack of metastasis does not indicate a favorable course, since many patients with the disease die from local infiltration alone.

Treatment and Prognosis. Both surgery and x-ray radiation have been used to treat this form of neoplastic disease. If the cancer is confined to the antrum and inferior structures, hemimaxillectomy gives favorable clinical results in some cases. Radiation treatment is frequently in the form of radium needles inserted into the antrum or the tumor mass. This has proved effective in some cases, even though considerable invasion of adjacent structures has occurred.

The over-all prognosis of patients with antral carcinoma is not good. In the series of Chaudhry and his associates, only 10 per cent of 49 patients with carcinoma of the antrum lived for more than 5 years.

VERRUCOUS CARCINOMA

Verrucous carcinoma is a form of epidermoid carcinoma of the oral cavity which was defined as an entity by Ackerman, who reported 31 cases in 1948. Since this original description, it has also been reported to occur in the larynx, esophagus, nasal fossae and paranasal sinuses, external auditory meatus, lacrimal duct, skin, scrotum, penis, vulva, vagina, uterine cervix, perineum, leg and odontogenic cyst lining. The typical oral lesion differs from the usual oral epidermoid carcinoma in that it is generally slow-growing, chiefly exophytic and only superficially invasive at least until late in the course of the disease, has a low metastatic potential, and is often amenable to simple local excision because of its relatively nonaggressive and protracted course. This oral lesion has been re-

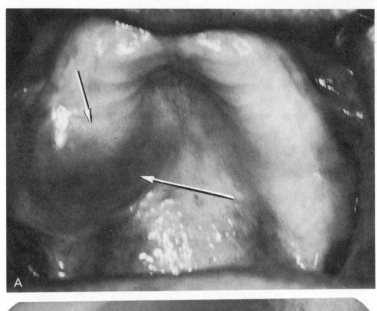

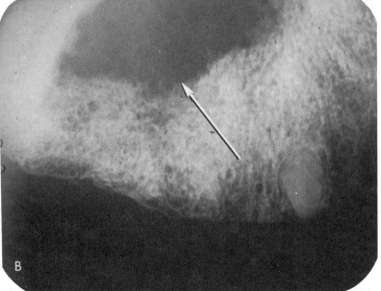

Figure 2–30. *Epidermoid carcinoma of the maxillary sinus.* A, The alveolar ridge shows thickening, reddening and deformity, although there is no ulceration of the mucosa. B, The roentgenogram reveals raggedness of the maxillary sinus and obvious bony alteration.

viewed and discussed by Shafer and more recently by McCoy and Waldron, while Ferlito and Recher have reported 77 cases of the larynx and discussed the lesion in this location.

Clinical Features. Verrucous carcinoma is generally seen in elderly patients, the mean age of occurrence being 60 to 70 years, with nearly 75 per cent of the lesions developing in males, according to a review by Shafer of nearly 300 reported cases. The vast majority of cases occur on the buccal mucosa and gingiva or alveolar ridge, although the palate and floor of the mouth are occasionally involved.

The neoplasm is chiefly exophytic and appears papillary in nature, with a pebbly surface which is sometimes covered by a white leukoplakic film. The lesions commonly have rugae-like folds with deep clefts between them. Lesions of the buccal mucosa may become quite extensive before involvement of deeper contiguous structures. Lesions on the mandibular ridge or gingiva grow into the overlying soft tissue and rapidly become fixed to the periosteum, gradually invading and destroying the mandible (Fig. 2–31, A, B, C). Regional lymph nodes are often tender and enlarged, simulating metastatic tumor, but this node involvement is usually inflammatory. Pain and difficulty in mastication are common complaints, but bleeding is rare.

The term *oral florid papillomatosis* has been used by dermatologists to describe a lesion with not only a clinical and microscopic appearance similar to verrucous carcinoma but also a similar biologic behavior. For this reason, many authorities now believe that oral florid papillomatosis and verrucous carcinoma represent one and the same disease with no justification for continued use of the former term, since it fails to imply the neoplastic nature of the disease.

It is consistently reported that a very high percentage of patients with this disease are tobacco chewers. A small number of patients give no such history but, instead, relate the use of snuff or heavy tobacco smoking. Occasional patients deny the use of tobacco and these usually have ill-fitting dentures.

Histologic Features. The histologic features may be extremely deceptive, and many cases have been diagnosed originally as simple papillomas or benign epithelial hyperplasia because of the orderly and harmless appearance of the specimen. There is generally marked epithelial proliferation with downgrowth of epithelium into the connective tissue but usually without a pattern of true invasion. The epithelium is well differentiated and shows little mitotic activity, pleomorphism or hyperchromatism. Characteristically, cleftlike spaces lined by a thick layer of parakeratin extend from the surface deeply into the lesion. Parakeratin plugging also occurs extending into the epithelium. The parakeratin lining the clefts with the parakeratin plugging is the hallmark of verrucous carcinoma. Even though the lesion may be very extensive, the basement membrane will often appear intact. When the lesions become infected, focal intraepithelial abscesses are often seen. Significant chronic inflammatory cell infiltration in the underlying connective tissue may or may not be present (Fig. 2–32).

Unfortunately, the diagnosis of verrucous carcinoma is often difficult even when the biopsy specimen is generous, and the pathologist will sometimes request a second biopsy.

Treatment and Prognosis. Verrucous carcinoma has been treated in several ways in the past, usually by surgery, x-ray radiation or a combination of the two. However, there have been some reports of anaplastic transformation

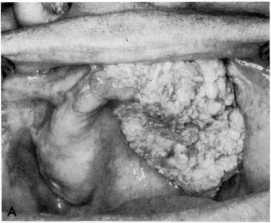
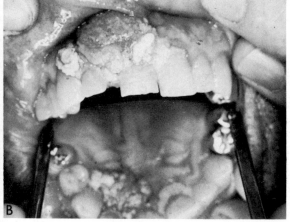
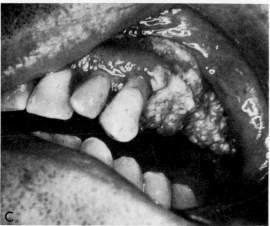

Figure 2–31. *Verrucous carcinoma.*
The exophytic, verrucous nature of the lesion is evident. (*A* and *B*, Courtesy of Dr. Charles A. Waldron, and *C*, of Drs. George G. Blozis and Mirdza E. Neiders.)

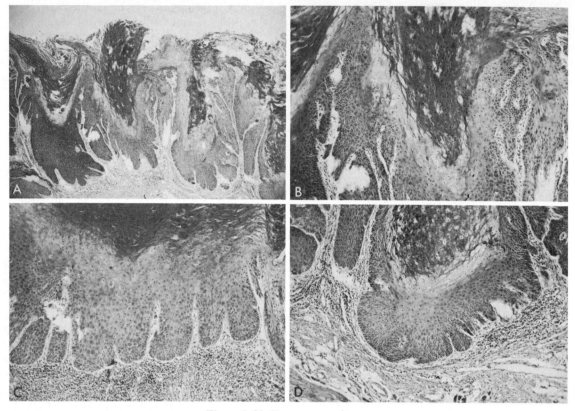

Figure 2–32. *Verrucous carcinoma.*

of lesions occurring in patients treated by ionizing radiation. While the radiation appears to be the triggering mechanism, other factors contributing to or related to the transformation are unknown. Even though such an occurrence is uncommon, many investigators believe the treatment should be entirely surgical. Since the lesion is so slow-growing and late to metastasize, many cases can be treated by relatively conservative excision without a mutilating procedure. The prognosis is much better than for the usual type of oral epidermoid carcinoma.

SPINDLE CELL CARCINOMA

("Carcinosarcoma"; "Pseudosarcoma"; Polypoid Squamous Cell Carcinoma; Lane Tumor)

This is an interesting, unusual and controversial tumor which occurs chiefly in the upper respiratory and alimentary tracts. The controversy has centered around the histogenesis of the malignant spindle cell, some investigators believing the tumor to be either a squamous cell carcinoma associated with an atypical, benign, reactive connective tissue process (pseu-

dosarcoma), a combination of collision growth of a carcinoma and a sarcoma (carcinosarcoma), or a squamous cell carcinoma with spindle cell anaplasia (spindle cell carcinoma). However, the majority today believe that it is epithelial and the tumor a variant of squamous cell carcinoma.

Clinical Features. A series of 59 cases of the oral cavity has been reported by Ellis and Corio, who noted a predilection for occurrence in males, although this finding was somewhat biased because of the number of military cases involved. The mean age of occurrence of the lesion was 57 years, with a range of 29 to 93 years. The lesions developed with greatest frequency on the lower lip (42 per cent), tongue (20 per cent) and alveolar ridge or gingiva (19 per cent) with the remainder scattered at other sites.

The most common presenting findings were swelling, pain and the presence of a nonhealing ulcer. The initial lesion appeared either with a polypoid, exophytic or endophytic configuration. It is perhaps significant that 13 patients in this series were known to have a history of prior therapeutic radiation to the region where the tumor subsequently developed. The time interval from radiation to diagnosis of the tumor ranged from 1.5 to 10 years with a mean of about 7 years.

Histologic Features. Spindle cell carcinoma is a bimorphic or biphasic tumor which, although almost always ulcerated, will show foci of surface epidermoid carcinoma or epithelial dysplasia of surface mucosa, usually just at the periphery and often quite limited. Proliferation and "dropping-off" of basal cells to spindle cell elements is a common phenomenon. The tissue patterns making up the bulk of the tumor have been categorized as either fasciculated, myxomatous or streaming. The cells, particularly in the fasciculated form, are elongated with elliptical nuclei, although pleomorphic cells are also common. The number of mitoses may vary from few to many. Giant cells, both benign appearing of the foreign body type and the bizarre, pleomorphic, atypical cells may be found. Finally, an inflammatory cell infiltrate is often present. Osteoid formation within the tumor component is sometimes seen. Microscopic invasion of subjacent structures is evident, as it is with most epidermoid carcinomas of the oral cavity.

Numerous ultrastructural studies of the spindle cell carcinoma, such as those of Leifer and his associates, have been carried out in clarification of the histogenesis and pathogenesis of this lesion.

Treatment and Prognosis. Surgical removal of the tumor, with and without radical neck dissection, alone or in combination with radiation, or radiation therapy alone all have been used in the treatment of this disease. In the series reported by Ellis and Corio, those treated by surgery had the best survival rate although only 9 of 18 patients treated in this fashion were alive and well. Radiation therapy appears ineffective. The presence of metastasis signals a poor prognosis, since 81 per cent of the patients with recorded metastases in this study died of their disease. The value of chemotherapy is not known.

ADENOID SQUAMOUS CELL CARCINOMA

(Adenoacanthoma; Pseudoglandular Squamous Cell Carcinoma)

This is an interesting tumor of the skin which also occurs with considerable frequency on the lips. It was originally described by Lever in 1947, and Johnson and Helwig reported a comprehensive study of 213 lesions in 155 patients in 1966.

There is considerable evidence that the tumor originates from the pilosebaceous structures, although it also appears likely to arise in areas of senile keratosis with acantholysis. Since there are no pilosebaceous structures on the lips and since senile keratosis is common here, this latter explanation seems quite reasonable.

Clinical Features. The adenoid squamous cell carcinoma is reported to occur as early as 20 years of age, although in the series of Johnson and Helwig, nearly 75 per cent of the patients were 50 years of age or older. In their series, only 2 per cent of the patients were females. Significantly, they found that 93 per cent of the lesions were in the head and neck region.

The lesions on the skin appear as simply elevated nodules that may show crusting, scaling or ulceration. Sometimes there is an elevated or rolled border to the lesion.

A series of 15 cases of adenoid squamous cell carcinoma of the lips (11 lower, 3 upper, 1 unstated) has been reported by Jacoway and his associates, while Tomich and Hutton have reported two cases and discussed the lesion in detail. These lip lesions often appear clinically similar to epidermoid carcinoma, being described frequently as ulcerated, hyperkeratotic or exophytic.

There have been three cases of this lesion reported intraorally, two on the tongue and one on the gingiva, which have borne remarkable histologic similarity to the adenoid squamous cell carcinoma of the skin and lips. However, all three of these lesions behaved in a very aggressive fashion, metastasized in at least two instances and the patient died in all three cases as a result of the tumor. Because of the aggressive nature of the lesions, these intraoral cases may not be identical to those of the skin and lips.

Histologic Features. There is a proliferation of surface dysplastic epithelium into the connective tissue as in the typical epidermoid carcinoma. However, the lateral or deep extensions of this epithelium show the characteristic solid and tubular ductal structures which typify the lesion. These ductlike structures are lined by a layer of cuboidal cells and often contain or enclose acantholytic or dyskeratotic cells.

Treatment and Prognosis. The adenoid squamous cell carcinoma is generally treated by surgical excision. On only rare occasions does it metastasize or cause death of the patient. However, recurrence is relatively common (38 per cent in the series of lip lesions reported by Jacoway and his co-workers, although it is possible that some of these may have been second lesions, since multiple adenoid squamous cell carcinomas in the same patient often occur).

LYMPHOEPITHELIOMA AND TRANSITIONAL CELL CARCINOMA

There is an unusual group of malignant neoplasms exhibiting many features in common which involves the nasopharynx, oropharynx, tongue, tonsil and anatomically associated structures such as the nasal chamber and paranasal sinuses. These tumors arise from the mucosa of these areas, exhibit a relatively specific histologic pattern and react in a rather atypical fashion to x-ray radiation. This group of neoplasms consists of the lymphoepithelioma, transitional cell carcinoma and undifferentiated squamous cell carcinoma.

Regaud, and later Schminke as well as Ewing, described the lymphoepithelioma as a lesion occurring chiefly in the nasopharynx of young or middle-aged persons. It was found to be usually a small lesion which often did not manifest itself clinically before regional lymphadenopathy was apparent. Death of the patient was the frequent outcome of the disease even though the lesion was found to be radiosensitive.

Under the term "transitional cell epidermoid carcinoma," Quick and Cutler reported a series of cases in which the lesions arose chiefly from the tonsil, base of the tongue and nasopharynx. It is in these areas that a transitional type of stratified epithelium is found, the schneiderian membrane. These tumors, then, occurred in areas similar to the sites of the lymphoepithelioma. It was noted, however, that this transitional cell carcinoma was extremely malignant, running a rapid clinical course, metastasizing widely and causing very early death.

Clinical Features. The primary lesion of the lymphoepithelioma or transitional cell carcinoma is usually very small, often completely hidden, usually slightly elevated and either frankly ulcerated or presenting a granular, eroded surface. The tumor is indurated and in some instances appears as an exophytic or fungating growth. Since the primary lesion usually remains small, the patient may not seek advice until metastasis to the regional lymph nodes has already occurred.

Scofield carried out an excellent study of 214 cases of malignant nasopharyngeal lesions, comprising transitional cell carcinoma, lymphoepithelioma and undifferentiated squamous cell carcinoma. He found that swelling of the regional lymph nodes was the most common presenting symptom of the observed patients, followed by sore throat, nasal obstruction, defective hearing or ear pain, headache, dysphagia, epistaxis and ocular symptoms. Differences in the median age of the patients were found, patients with transitional cell carcinoma averaging 44 years of age, those with lymphoepithelioma averaging only 26 years and those with undifferentiated squamous cell carcinoma, 56 years. Bloom published a review of cancer of the nasopharynx with particular reference to the significance of the histopathology of the lesions.

Histologic Features. The diagnosis of these neoplasms and their differentiation depend solely upon their microscopic structure.

The transitional cell epidermoid carcinoma consists of cells growing in solid sheets or in cords and nests. The individual cells are moderately large, round or polyhedral, and exhibit a lightly basophilic cytoplasm and indistinct cell outlines. The nuclei appear large and round, and they exhibit varying degrees of mitotic activity. Although a slight degree of intercellular bridging may be present, keratinization and pearl formation are completely lacking. The stroma exhibits little or no lymphocytic infiltration.

The lymphoepithelioma is made up of cells growing in a syncytial pattern with the stroma infiltrated by varying numbers of lymphocytes. The individual cells are large and polyhedral with indistinct outlines. The cytoplasm stains lightly eosinophilic. The nuclei appear large, oval and vesicular, and characteristically contain one or two large eosinophilic nucleoli.

Treatment and Prognosis. Because of the general inaccessibility of the majority of these lesions and their unusual property of being highly radiosensitive, x-ray radiation has been the most commonly accepted treatment. The response of this tumor to radiation is different from that of the epidermoid carcinoma found in these locations. The regional lymph node metastases also respond well to x-ray radiation. The complicating factor lies in the relative inability to treat the widespread metastases in the various organs.

The outlook for patients with these forms of neoplastic disease is poor. Since widespread metastases frequently occur before there is any clinical manifestation of disease, the unfavorable prognosis can be readily understood. In the series of Scofield the probability of 5-year survival was calculated. He found that, after onset of symptoms, only 30 per cent of treated patients suffering from transitional cell carcinoma or lymphoepithelioma would be alive in 5 years, while only 11 per cent with squamous cell carcinoma in these areas would survive.

MALIGNANT MELANOMA

Malignant melanoma is a neoplasm of epidermal melanocytes. It is one of the more biologically unpredictable and deadly of all human neoplasms. Although it is the third most common cancer of skin (basal and squamous cell carcinomas are more prevalent), it accounts for only 3 per cent of all such malignancies. However, it results in over 83 per cent of all deaths due to skin cancer in the United States.

Cutaneous melanoma is increasing in incidence. Studies by Elwood and Lee have shown a five-fold increase in the incidence of melanoma from 1935–1939 to 1976–1977. Schreiber and his colleagues reported nearly a five-fold increased incidence rate in southern Arizona over a nine-year study period. As of 1978, the crude incidence rate was 28.57 cases per 100,000 in Arizona as compared with nearly 5 cases per 100,000 in the United States as a whole. This is the highest incidence rate in the United States and it is exceeded only by the incidence of the disease in Queensland, Australia. These epidemiologic studies have supported the belief that sunlight is an important etiologic factor in cutaneous melanoma.

For many years, it was believed that many melanomas developed in pre-existing pigmented nevi, particularly junctional nevi. However, Clark and his colleagues are of the opinion that junctional nevi are not histogenetically related to melanomas. It is quite possible that lesions which were interpreted as junctional nevi were, in fact, premalignant melanocytic dysplasias of some type, thus leading to the erroneous concept of malignant transformation of nevi. In support of this is a study by Jones and his colleagues in which 169 cases diagnosed as junctional nevi were studied retrospectively. Only 74 were actually junctional nevi, whereas 41 were actually melanomas in various phases of growth. The remainder were nevoid and nonnevoid pigmented lesions of various types.

In 1975, Clark and his co-workers presented an interesting concept regarding the developmental biology of cutaneous melanoma. They documented two phases in the growth of melanoma: the *radial-growth phase* and the *vertical-growth phase*. The radial-growth phase is the initial phase of growth of the tumor. During this period, which may last many years, the neoplastic process is confined to the epidermis. Neoplastic cells are shed with normally maturing epithelial cells and although some neoplastic cells may actually penetrate the basement membrane, they are destroyed by a host-cell immunologic response. The vertical-growth phase begins when neoplastic cells populate the underlying dermis. This takes place because of increased virulence of the neoplastic cells, a decreased host-cell response, or a combination of both. Metastasis is possible once the melanoma enters the vertical-growth phase. It is recognized that not all melanomas have both radial- and vertical-growth phases. Nodular melanoma (q.v.) exists only in the vertical-growth phase.

Cutaneous melanoma has been classified into a number of types. However, three types constitute nearly 90 per cent of the tumors. These are (1) superficial spreading melanoma, (2) nodular melanoma, and (3) lentigo maligna melanoma.

Clinical Features. Superficial spreading melanoma is the most common cutaneous melanoma in Caucasians. It accounts for nearly 65 per cent of cutaneous melanomas. It exists in a radial-growth phase which has been called *premalignant melanosis* or *pagetoid melanoma in situ*. The lesion presents as a tan, brown, black or admixed lesion on sun-exposed skin, especially the back. It also occurs on skin of the head and neck, chest and abdomen and the extremities. The radial-growth phase may last for several months to several years. The vertical-growth phase is characterized by increase in size, change in color, nodularity and, at times, ulceration.

Nodular melanoma accounts for approximately 13 per cent of cutaneous melanomas. It apparently has no clinically recognizable radial-growth phase, existing solely in a vertical-growth phase. It presents as a sharply delineated nodule with degrees of pigmentation. They may be pink (amelanotic melanoma) or black. They have predilection for occurrence on the back and head and neck skin of men. In other cutaneous sites, there is an even sex distribution.

Lentigo maligna melanoma accounts for approximately 10 per cent of cutaneous melanomas. It exists in a radial-growth phase which is known as *lentigo maligna* or *melanotic freckle of Hutchinson.* The melanotic freckle has been recognized as a clinicopathologic entity for nearly 100 years. However, the concept that it represents a melanoma in a radial-growth phase is much more recent. The lesion occurs characteristically as a macular lesion on the malar skin of middle-aged and elderly Caucasians. It occurs more often in women than in men. In an extensive series of 85 cases, Wayte and Helwig found an average age of 58 years in men and 55 in women. In a series studied by Clark and his colleagues, the median age was 70 years. Both studies showed a female sex predilection. The lesion can remain in the radial-growth phase for years. In Wayte and Helwig's study, the average duration in which an accurate history was possible was 14 years. Clark and Mihm have documented a lentigo maligna for 50 years prior to the development of a vertical-growth phase. Nearly 53 per cent of the lesions evolved into lentigo maligna melanoma, the vertical-growth phase of this form of melanoma.

Melanoma may occur as a primary lesion not only on the skin but also in the eye and on mucous membranes. It has also been reported as a primary lesion in the parotid gland, although melanomas in this site are usually metastatic to lymph nodes in the parotid region.

Oral Manifestations. Malignant melanoma is an uncommon neoplasm of the oral mucosa. Pliskin reviewed the literature on oral melanoma and found that they accounted for 1.6 per cent of over 7500 reported melanomas. Other authors have reported rates of 0.2 to 8 per cent. Conley and Pack reported 26 cases of primary oral melanoma and McCaffrey, Neel and Gaffey reported on the 10 cases treated at the Mayo Clinic. Of epidemiologic interest is the fact that melanoma of the oral mucosa is one of the most common sites for the neoplasm in Japanese. Melanomas in blacks are seldom found in skin yet occur on mucous membranes and on the plantar skin.

Primary oral melanoma is nearly twice as common in men as in women. The over-all age of occurrence is approximately 55 years, with most cases occurring between 40 and 70 years.

The oral melanoma exhibits a definite predilection for the palate and maxillary gingiva/alveolar ridge. Seventy-seven per cent of the cases in Pliskin's review occurred in these two sites. Cases are also recorded on the buccal mucosa, mandibular gingiva, tongue, lips and floor of the mouth. The lesion usually appears as a deeply pigmented area, at times ulcerated and hemorrhagic, which tends to increase progressively in size (Fig. 2–33, *A, B, C*). Significantly, focal pigmentation preceding the development of the actual neoplasm frequently occurred several months to several years before clinical symptoms appeared. For this reason it has been suggested that the appearance of melanin pigmentation in the mouth and its increase in size and in depth of color should be viewed seriously.

Although clinicopathologic correlation is well established for cutaneous melanomas, it is unfortunate that such correlation does not exist for oral melanomas. It is now apparent that melanomas of the oral mucosa can exist in radial- and vertical-growth phases but only a few such cases have been reported. Takagi and his co-workers were able to document a pre-existing or concurrent melanosis in 62 of 94 cases of oral melanomas which they studied. Regezi, Hayward and Pickens evaluated three cases of oral melanoma in accordance with the established clinicopathologic parameters of cutaneous melanomas. They were able to classify one as a superficial spreading melanoma which had a pre-existing melanosis for 11 years. The other two had histologic features consistent with lentigo maligna melanoma. However, since these lesions behaved much more aggressively, they were termed *acral-lentiginous melanomas* as suggested by Clark and his colleagues and by Reed.

Most dermatopathologists recognize the existence of lentigo maligna (melanotic freckle of Hutchinson) only on sun-damaged skin and do not accept its occurrence intraorally. It follows that lentigo maligna melanoma (melanoma arising in melanotic freckle of Hutchinson) cannot occur on oral mucosa, although such a case has been reported by Robinson and Hukill. In light of present knowledge, such a case would be called acral-lentiginous melanoma because of the clinicopathologic similarity of the oral lesion to those on palmar and plantar skin.

Thus, oral melanomas may be expected to exist in superficial spreading, acral-lentiginous and nodular types. Batsakis and his associates and Hansen and Buchner have recently discussed the current concepts of oral mucosal melanomas relative to their cutaneous counterparts.

Histologic   Features. The   intraepithelial component (radial-growth phase) of superficial spreading melanoma is characterized by the presence of large, epithelioid melanocytes distributed in a so-called "pagetoid" manner (Fig. 2–34, *A*). As long as the malignant cells are

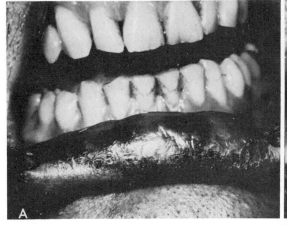

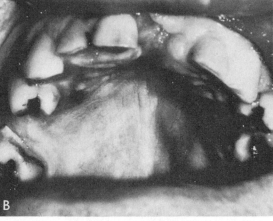

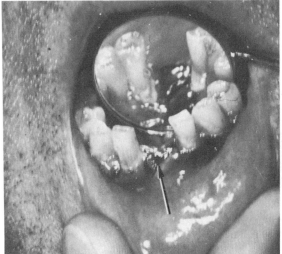

Figure 2–33. *Malignant melanoma.*
Typical lesions involve the lip (*A*), palate (*B*), and the alveolar ridge (*C*). (*C* courtesy of Dr. Wilbur C. Moorman.)

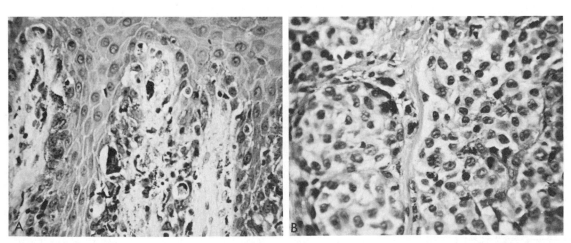

Figure 2–34. *Malignant melanoma.*
(*A*) The radial growth phase or premalignant melanosis is characterized by atypical melanocytes within the epithelium. (*B*) The vertical growth phase is characterized by malignant epithelioid melanocytes invading the underlying connective tissue.

confined to the epithelium, there is no host-cell response in the underlying connective tissue. When melanocytes penetrate basement membrane, a florid host-cell response of lymphocytes develops. Macrophages and melanophages may be present. The tumor cells are often destroyed by this cellular response. The vertical-growth phase is characterized by the proliferation of malignant epithelioid melanocytes in the underlying connective tissues (Fig. 2–34, *B*). The cells may be arranged singly or in clusters. Melanin pigment is usually scanty.

Nodular melanoma also is characterized by large, epithelioid melanocytes within the connective tissue. However, small ovoid and spindle-shaped cells may be present. Melanin pigment is usually but not invariably present. The tumor cells may invade and ulcerate the overlying epithelium and penetrate the deep soft tissues.

Lentigo maligna (melanotic freckle of Hutchinson) has well-defined histologic features which have been discussed by Wayte and Helwig and by Clark and Mihm. The lesion is characterized by increased numbers of atypical melanocytes within the basal epithelial layer. The epithelium is generally atrophic and the dermal collagen shows the effects of sun-damage (basophilic degeneration). If skin appendages are present, they are often involved with atypical melanocytes as well. In time, cords and nests of atypical melanocytes may be evident. Lentigo maligna melanoma is characterized by invasive spindle-shaped cells into the underlying dermis. A lymphohistiocytic infiltrate is usually present.

The acral-lentiginous melanoma is histologically similar to lentigo maligna melanoma. Coleman and his co-workers have studied 35 cases and have pointed out the salient histologic features. These are (1) a lentiginous radial-growth phase, (2) a deep vertical-growth phase composed predominantly of spindle-shaped cells, (3) psoriasiform epidermal hyperplasia, (4) an intense host-cell response, and (5) a prominent desmoplasia associated with the vertical-growth phase.

Although the majority of melanomas are diagnosed by routine light microscopy, ultrastructural study can be of value in diagnosing and distinguishing between various types of melanoma. As pointed out by Klug and Gunther, the three main types of cutaneous melanoma differ ultrastructurally in the number and size of melanosomes. Regezi, Hayward and Pickens studied an oral acral-lentiginous melanoma ultrastructurally and found premelanosomes and melanosomes similar to those found in normal melanocytes and nevus cells.

Less common histologic variants of melanoma such as desmoplastic, neurotropic, spindle cell and balloon cell melanomas exist. These have been discussed by Ainsworth and her colleagues.

Treatment and Prognosis. The treatment of cutaneous malignant melanoma is surgical excision. Although regional lymph node dissection is indicated when nodes are involved, prophylactic lymph node dissection is very controversial. The decision of the surgeon relative to elective node dissection should be based upon the thickness of the lesion and its specific anatomic location. In this regard, tumors greater than 0.75 millimeters in thickness and located in the so-called BANS (back, arm, neck and scalp) sites have a greater tendency to metastasize.

Chemotherapy, immunotherapy and radiation therapy have been used in the treatment of cutaneous melanoma. The role of these modalities is discussed in the monograph on melanoma edited by Clark, Goldman and Mastrangelo.

The treatment of oral melanoma has been and still is surgical excision. Jaw resection and lymph node dissection is indicated in cases involving bone and regional lymph nodes. Other forms of therapy such as cryosurgery, radiation, chemotherapy and immunotherapy have been employed on occasion but none have significantly improved the dismal prognosis of melanoma in the oral cavity.

There are both clinical and histologic factors which are of great prognostic significance in cutaneous melanomas. According to McGovern, clinical features with prognostic significance are the sex and age of the patient and the site of the lesion. Women have a much better survival rate up to the age of 50 years and then the rate declines. Melanomas of the upper back, posterolateral arm, neck and posterior scalp (BANS) tend to have the highest tendency to metastasize and have poor survival rates. On the other hand, melanomas of the skin of the face have a much more favorable prognosis.

Histologic features which are of prognostic significance are histologic type and depth of invasion. Nodular melanoma and superficial spreading melanoma have much poorer prognoses than lentigo maligna melanoma. In fact, McGovern believes that lentigo maligna melanoma should be considered as a separate entity because of its better prognosis. In 1969, Clark and his colleagues related prognosis to the anatomic level of invasion at the time of diagnosis. In 1970, Breslow proposed that the actual thickness of the tumor as measured in millimeters by an ocular micrometer correlated well with prognosis. It is now recognized that tumors less than 0.75 mm in thickness rarely metastasize or cause death, regardless of the location on skin.

Unfortunately, oral mucosal melanomas have a far worse prognosis than cutaneous melanomas. According to Pliskin, the 5-year survival rate for such tumors is approximately 7 per cent. Batsakis and his colleagues have pointed out that establishment of prognostic indicators for oral mucous membrane melanomas has not kept pace with those which have been established for cutaneous melanomas.

BENIGN TUMORS OF CONNECTIVE TISSUE ORIGIN

FIBROMA

This connective tissue tumor is the most common benign soft tissue neoplasm occurring in the oral cavity. It is intimately related to fibrous hyperplasia and, in many instances, is histologically indistinguishable from it. A central fibroma of bone, either maxilla or mandible, has been reported occasionally, but since it has never been clearly separated from the odontogenic fibroma, these fibromas of bone are discussed together in the section on odontogenic tumors (q.v.).

Clinical Features. The fibroma appears as an elevated lesion of normal color with a smooth

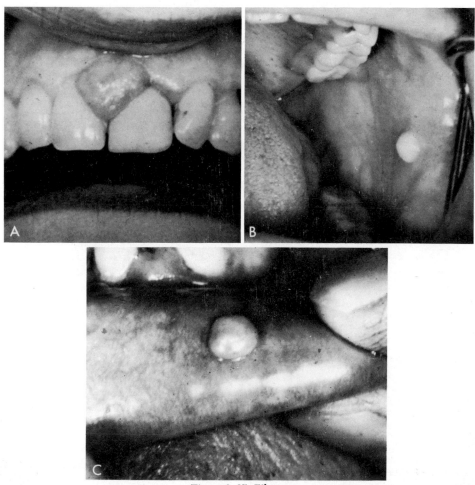

Figure 2–35. Fibroma.
The fibroma of the gingiva (A) arose in a location which might have been irritated by the poorly fitting jacket crown on the central incisor. The fibroma of the buccal mucosa (B) originated at a site corresponding to the plane of occlusion. The fibroma of the lip (C) was in an area that could have been irritated by chronic lip chewing.

PLATE III

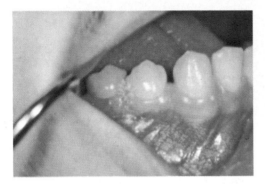

Papilloma

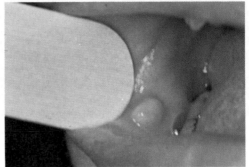

Fibroma

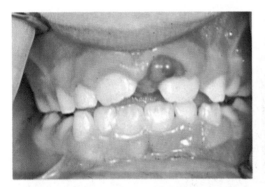

Peripheral giant cell granuloma

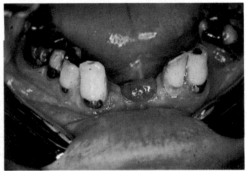

Peripheral giant cell granuloma

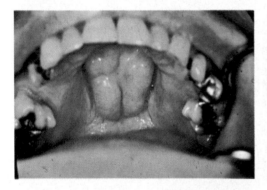

Torus palatinus

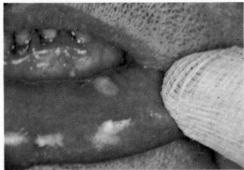

Traumatic neuroma

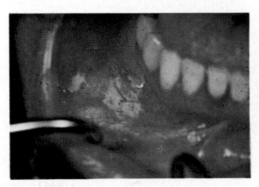

Leukoplakia (snuff patch)

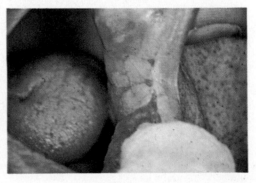

Leukoplakia

surface and a sessile or, occasionally, pedunculated base (Fig. 2–35; see also Plate III). The tumor may be small or, in rare instances, may range up to several centimeters in diameter. Projecting above the surface, the tumor sometimes becomes irritated and inflamed and may even show superficial ulceration. It is nearly always a well-defined, slowly growing lesion that occurs at any age, but is most common in the third, fourth and fifth decades. Although arising in a variety of locations, it most frequently originates on the gingiva, buccal mucosa, tongue, lips and palate.

Because the consistency of the fibroma may be either firm and resilient or soft and spongy, the clinical terms "hard fibroma" and "soft fibroma" are occasionally used. Such terms are of no significance, since there is often little correlation between the consistency and the histologic appearance of the lesion.

Histologic Features. The fibroma consists of bundles of interlacing collagenous fibers interspersed with varying numbers of fibroblasts or fibrocytes and small blood vessels. The surface of the lesion is covered by a layer of stratified squamous epithelium which frequently appears stretched and shows shortening and flattening of the rete pegs (Fig. 2–36). If trauma to the tissue has occurred, vasodilatation, edema and inflammatory cell infiltration are variably present. Areas of diffuse or focal calcification or even ossification are found in some fibromas, chiefly those occurring on the gingiva, and these lesions have sometimes been called "peripheral ossifying fibroma," "ossifying fibroid epulis,"

"peripheral cementifying fibroma" or "peripheral odontogenic fibroma" (q.v.).

It is interesting to note that the fibroma, a true neoplasm of connective tissue origin, is microscopically similar to the condition known as inflammatory hyperplasia, an increased bulk of connective tissue which forms as part of an inflammatory reaction. In few situations is the distinction between the two general processes, hyperplasia and neoplasia, as poorly defined as it is here. Hyperplasia is usually considered to be a self-limiting process which is not etiologically related to neoplasia. Both processes, however, are typified by an increase in the number of cells brought about by increased mitotic activity. Hyperplastic tissue sometimes, but not invariably, regresses after removal of the stimulus or irritant. Neoplastic tissue shows no such regression.

This distinction between hyperplasia and neoplasia is not clear-cut, and cases occur intraorally in which there is focal or diffuse proliferation of tissue obviously due to irritation which does not regress after removal of the irritant. The tissue appears identical with that in other cases which do regress when the irritant is removed. This suggests that the processes of hyperplasia and neoplasia may not be as completely dissociated as previously considered and that a true oral neoplasm may result from chronic irritation.

Many persons think, however, that a great number of the lesions of the oral cavity diagnosed as fibromas are, in reality, simply examples of focal or localized hyperplasia, resulting

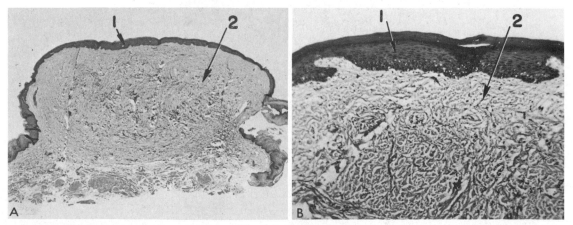

Figure 2–36. *Fibroma.*
A, The lower-power photomicrograph illustrates the typical sessile base, the thin surface epithelium (*1*) and coarse bundles of collagen (2) comprising the bulk of the tumor. *B,* The high-power photomicrograph shows the relative acellularity of the connective tissue.

from inflammation, and that the true fibroma is much rarer than is presently believed. There is no doubt that the pyogenic granuloma (q.v.), if left untreated, will undergo eventual healing by sclerosis and will then microscopically resemble the fibroma.

Treatment and Prognosis. The treatment for the fibroma, or focal inflammatory hyperplasia as the case may be, is conservative surgical excision. Seldom does the lesion recur.

Giant Cell Fibroma

The giant cell fibroma is an oral tumor first described in 1974 by Weathers and Callihan as a distinctive entity. Because of the similarity in terminology, care must be taken not to confuse it with the giant cell granuloma, peripheral or central (q.v.), with which it is totally unrelated.

Clinical Features. The giant cell fibroma may occur at any age. However, in the series of 464 cases reported by Houston, nearly 60 per cent of the patients were under 30 years of age, an age distribution virtually identical to that noted in the 108 cases reported by Weathers and Callihan. There is no remarkable sex predilection. The most common site of occurrence is gingiva followed by tongue, palate, buccal mucosa and lips (Fig. 2–37, A).

The clinical appearance of the lesion is usually that of a small, raised, pedunculated, papillary lesion less than 1 cm. in diameter. It is asymptomatic and may be present for several years.

Histologic Features. The characteristic feature of this lesion is the presence of numerous large stellate and multinucleated giant fibroblasts in the connective tissue which makes up the bulk of the lesion. These stellate cells have large vesicular nuclei, while the cytoplasm is well demarcated and frequently the cells have dendritic-like processes. The multinucleated cells have a similar morphology and occasionally resemble Langhans' giant cells. Some cells may contain melanin granules (Fig. 2–37, B, C, D).

A variety of cutaneous lesions containing similar stellate and multinucleated giant cells occur such as the fibrous papule of the nose, ungual fibroma, acral fibrokeratoma and the fibroblastoma, a virus-induced tumor of the deer. Two other similar mucous membrane lesions also occur: the retrocuspid papilla (q.v.) and the pearly penile papule of the glans penis.

Electron microscope studies of the oral giant cell fibroma by Weathers and Campbell have suggested that the distinctive cells are atypical fibroblasts. They were not able to detect evidence of viral particles in the lesions.

Treatment and Prognosis. These are usually

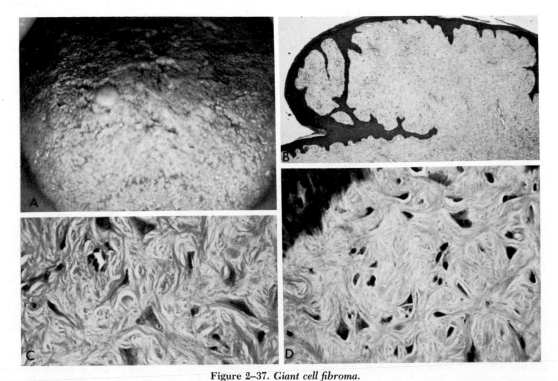

Figure 2–37. *Giant cell fibroma.*
The nodular lesion of the tongue (A) is a fibrous mass (B) containing large, stellate and occasional multinucleated fibroblasts (C,D).

treated by surgical excision and recurrence is very rare.

PERIPHERAL OSSIFYING FIBROMA

(Peripheral Odontogenic Fibroma; Peripheral Cementifying Fibroma; Calcifying or Ossifying Fibroid Epulis; Peripheral Fibroma with Calcification)

There are numerous histologically different types of focal overgrowths which may occur on the gingiva, such as the peripheral giant cell granuloma, the giant cell fibroma, the pyogenic granuloma, the simple fibroma (which may be simply a healed pyogenic granuloma in many cases) and the present lesion, which in the past has been known by a variety of names indicated above. The terms most frequently used have been the "peripheral ossifying fibroma" and the "peripheral odontogenic fibroma." Inasmuch as the latter term has been used for a lesion described by the World Health Organization in their classification of odontogenic tumors as a totally different entity, the term peripheral ossifying fibroma will be used here for that relatively common gingival lesion characterized by a high degree of cellularity usually exhibiting bone formation, although occasionally cementum-like material or rarely dystrophic calcification may be found instead. Some investigators believe that the lesion is nevertheless odontogenic in origin, being derived from the periodontal ligament, especially since it only occurs on the gingiva and may contain oxytalan fibers. At the present time, however, its exact derivation is still uncertain. Despite the similarity in terminology, it is not considered to be the extraosseous counterpart of the central ossifying fibroma. An attempt at clarification of the terms "peripheral ossifying fibroma" and "peripheral odontogenic fibroma" has been published recently by Gardner.

Clinical Features. The peripheral ossifying fibroma can occur at any age, although it appears to be somewhat more common in children and young adults. In a study of 365 cases by Cundiff, 50 per cent of the lesions occurred between the ages of 5 and 25 years with the peak incidence at 13 years, while the mean age was 29 years. Most reported series of cases show a predilection for occurrence in females by a ratio ranging from 2:1 to 3:2. In addition, the lesions are approximately equally divided between the maxilla and the mandible. In the series reported by Cundiff, over 80 per cent of

the lesions in both jaws occurred anterior to the molar area. A series of 185 cases of "peripheral fibroma with calcification" were also reported by Bhaskar and Jacoway with very similar clinical data.

The clinical appearance of the lesion is characteristic but not pathognomonic. It is a well-demarcated focal mass of tissue on the gingiva, with a sessile or pedunculated base (Fig. 2–38A). It is of the same color as normal mucosa or slightly reddened. The surface may be intact or ulcerated. It most commonly appears to originate from an interdental papilla.

Roentgenographic Features. In the vast majority of cases, there is no apparent underlying bone involvement visible on the roentgenogram. However, on rare occasions, there does appear to be superficial erosion of bone.

Histologic Features. The surface of the peripheral ossifying fibroma exhibits either an intact or, more frequently, an ulcerated layer of stratified squamous epithelium. The bulk of the lesion is composed of an exceedingly cellular mass of connective tissue comprising large numbers of plump proliferating fibroblasts intermingled throughout a very delicate fibrillar stroma. The lesion is quite characteristic in its high degree of cellularity in contrast to the usual simple fibroma. In addition, vascularity is not nearly as prominent a feature of this lesion as in the pyogenic granuloma. Several forms of calcification occur in this particular lesion and will vary in amount from case to case. The calcification may be in the form of single or multiple interconnecting trabeculae of bone or osteoid (either mature lamellar bone or immature cellular bone), although less commonly globules of calcified material closely resembling acellular cementum, or a diffuse granular dystrophic calcification may be found (Fig. 2–38, B, C, D, E). Significantly, the degree of cellularity of the lesions is usually greatest in the areas of the bone, cementum or calcification.

On occasion, areas will be found containing multinucleated giant cells which, with the surrounding tissue, bear considerable resemblance to some areas of the peripheral giant cell granuloma.

Treatment and Prognosis. The lesions should be surgically excised and submitted for microscopic examination for confirmation of diagnosis. The extraction of adjacent teeth is seldom necessary or justified. However, the lesions do recur with some frequency and, in fact, repeated recurrences are not uncommon. In the series of Cundiff, 16 per cent of the cases

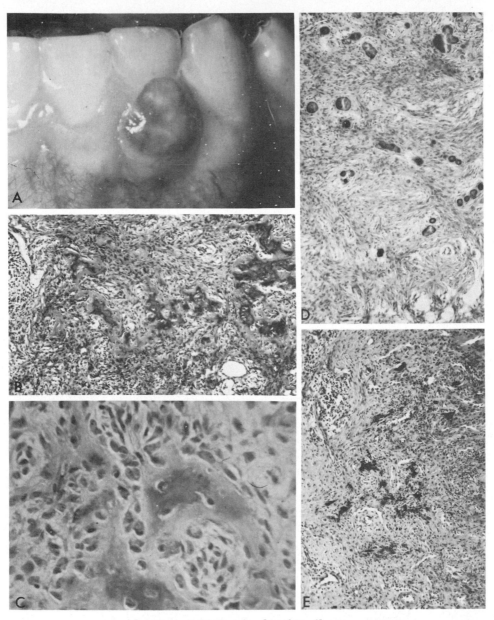

Figure 2–38. *Peripheral ossifying fibroma.*
The sessile lesion on the gingiva (*A*) is histologically a very cellular lesion which also exhibits most frequently irregular trabeculae of osteoid or bone (*B* is low power, *C* high power), but occasionally presents cementum-like droplets (*D*) or even dystrophic calcification (*E*).

recurred, while in a series of 50 cases reported by Eversole and Rovin, the recurrence rate was 20 per cent.

CENTRAL OSSIFYING FIBROMA OF BONE

(Central Fibro-osteoma)

The ossifying fibroma of bone is a central neoplasm of bone which has caused considera-

ble controversy because of confusion of terminology and criteria of diagnosis. It now appears that this represents a definite entity which should be separated from fibrous dysplasia of bone and the other fibro-osseous lesions which do not represent true neoplasms. This concept has been discussed by Pindborg, by Waldron and by many others.

There is a remarkable similarity in clinical features between this lesion and the central cementifying fibroma, a tumor accepted by most investigators as being odontogenic in origin. There is also considerable similarity and even overlap in the histologic features of these two lesions. For these reasons, it has been suggested that: (1) these are two separate benign tumors, identical in nature except for the cell undergoing proliferation, the osteoblast with bone formation in one case, or the cementoblast with cementum formation in the other case; or (2) these represent simply two facets of the same basic tumor. Further investigation will be necessary to clarify the relationship, or lack of it, between the central ossifying fibroma and the central cementifying fibroma.

Clinical Features. The central ossifying fibroma may occur at any age, but is far more common in young adults. The age range of occurrence in a series of 31 cases presented by Shafer was 9 to 52, with a mean of 33 years of age. Langdon and his associates reported similar findings. Either jaw may be involved, but there appears to be a predilection for the mandible. In the series of Shafer, there were 26 cases in the mandible but only 5 in the maxilla. A marked predilection for occurrence in females was also noted: 26 cases compared to only 5 in males. In addition, there was an unusually high incidence of lesions in blacks: 13 cases contrasted to 18 cases in white patients.

The lesion is generally asymptomatic until the growth produces a noticeable swelling and mild deformity; displacement of teeth may be an early clinical feature. It is a relatively slow-growing tumor and may be present for some years before discovery. Because of the slow growth, the cortical plates of bone and overlying mucosa or skin are almost invariably intact.

Roentgenographic Features. The neoplasm presents an extremely variable roentgenographic appearance depending upon its stage of development. Yet despite the stage of development, the lesion is always well circumscribed and demarcated from surrounding bone, in contrast to fibrous dysplasia.

In its early stages the central ossifying fibroma paradoxically appears as a radiolucent area with no evidence of internal radiopacities (Fig. 2–39, A). As the tumor bone apparently matures, there is increasing calcification, so that the radiolucent area becomes flecked with opacities until, ultimately, the lesion appears as a relatively uniform radiopaque mass. Displacement of adjacent teeth is common, as well as impingement upon other adjacent structures.

Histologic Features. The lesion is composed basically of many delicate interlacing collagen fibers, seldom arranged in discrete bundles, interspersed by large numbers of active, proliferating fibroblasts. Although mitotic figures may be present in small numbers, there is seldom any remarkable cellular pleomorphism. This connective tissue characteristically presents many small foci of irregular bony trabe-

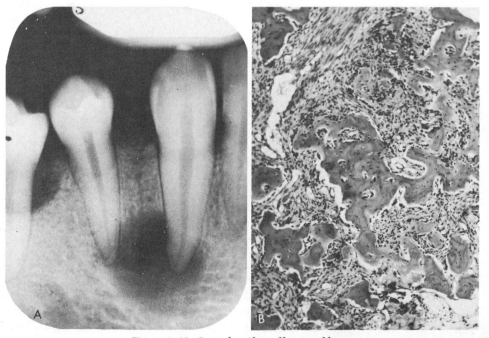

Figure 2–39. *Central ossifying fibroma of bone.*

culae (Fig. 2–39, *B*) which may bear some similarity to the bizarre Chinese-character shape of the bony trabeculae in fibrous dysplasia of bone (q.v.).

As the lesion matures, the islands of ossification increase in number, enlarge and ultimately coalesce. This, with the probable increase in degree of calcification, accounts for increasing radiopaqueness of the lesion on the roentgenogram.

Treatment and Prognosis. The lesion should be excised conservatively, and recurrence is rare.

Peripheral Giant Cell Granuloma

(Peripheral Giant Cell Reparative Granuloma; Peripheral Giant Cell Tumor; Giant Cell Epulis; Osteoclastoma)

The peripheral giant cell granuloma has been described for many years under a great variety of terms in the dental and medical literature. This is indicative of the confusion which it has generally evoked, and even today there is no universal agreement on the true nature of the lesion. Since it is histologically similar to a central lesion of bone containing giant cells, it was only logical that a relationship between the two be suggested. The earlier workers believed that the peripheral giant cell granuloma was a true neoplasm, although the majority of modern investigators support the view that it is an unusual proliferative response of the tissues to injury. Since the lesion does not appear to be truly a "reparative" one, this term has been deleted from the name in the past few years.

Recently the role of trauma has been re-emphasized by some investigators who believe it to be of considerable importance in the etiology of these lesions. The trauma is caused chiefly by tooth extraction, although other factors such as denture irritation or simply chronic infection also may be significant.

The use of the term "epulis" in connection with this or any other oral tumor is to be deplored. By definition, the word means only a growth on the gingiva and is entirely nonspecific. Since it gives no hint as to the true nature of a lesion, the term should be discarded.

Clinical Features. The peripheral giant cell granuloma may vary considerably in clinical appearance. It always occurs on the gingiva or alveolar process, most frequently anterior to the molars, and presents itself as a pedunculated or sessile lesion that seems to be arising from deeper in the tissue than many other superficial lesions of this area such as the fibroma or pyogenic granuloma, either of which it may resemble clinically (Fig. 2–40, *A*; see also Plate III). Thus it seems to originate from either periodontal ligament or mucoperiosteum. The lesion also varies widely in size, but usually is between 0.5 and 1.5 cm. in diameter. It is most often dark red, vascular or hemorrhagic in appearance, and it commonly exhibits surface ulceration.

In the edentulous patient the lesion may appear sometimes as a vascular, ovoid or fusiform swelling of the crest of the ridge, seldom over 1 to 2 cm. in diameter (Fig. 2–41, *A*). Or there may be a granular mass of tissue which seems to be growing from the tissue covering the slope of the ridge. The color of these lesions

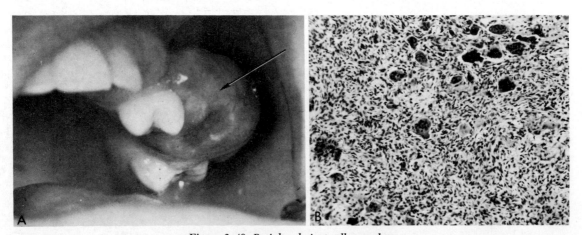

Figure 2–40. *Peripheral giant cell granuloma.*
The growth on the gingiva may be relatively small or quite large (*A*). The photomicrograph reveals many multinucleated giant cells in a granulomatous stroma (*B*).

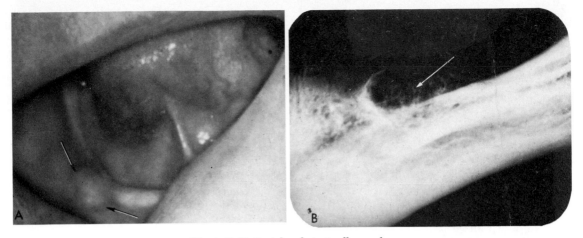

Figure 2–41. *Peripheral giant cell granuloma.*
The lesion in edentulous patients produces a circumscribed growth, causing expansion of the alveolar ridge (A). The roentgenogram shows ragged loss of bone with peripheral "cuffing" (B).

varies, but is usually similar to that of lesions in dentulous patients. Ulceration is less common in the edentulous situation, however.

Giansanti and Waldron have reviewed the literature and added their own series of patients for a total of 720 cases of peripheral giant cell granuloma. In this large series, there was a slight predilection for occurrence in the mandible over the maxilla—55 per cent compared to 45 per cent. In addition, it was found that females were affected almost twice as frequently as males—65 per cent compared to 35 per cent. A similar sex predilection has been found for the central giant cell granuloma. Their analysis of reported cases indicates that the giant cell lesion occurs on the average by about age 30 years, although the lesion may be found in very young children as well as in dentulous or edentulous elderly persons. A marked accumulation of cases in the group between five and 15 years of age was reported by Andersen and his associates in their series of 97 patients with peripheral giant cell granuloma.

Histologic Features. The microscopic appearance of the giant cell lesion is unique. It consists of a nonencapsulated mass of tissue composed of a delicate reticular and fibrillar connective tissue stroma containing large numbers of ovoid or spindle-shaped young connective tissue cells and multinucleated giant cells. The giant cells in some instances resemble osteoclasts and in other cases are considerably larger than the typical osteoclast. Capillaries are numerous, particularly around the periphery of the lesion, and the giant cells sometimes may be found within the lumina of these vessels. Foci of hemorrhage, with liberation of

hemosiderin pigment and its subsequent ingestion by mononuclear phagocytes, as well as inflammatory cell infiltration, are also characteristic features. Spicules of newly formed osteoid or bone are often found scattered throughout the vascular and cellular fibrous lesion (Fig. 2–40, B).

A histochemical study of this lesion has been reported by Shklar and Cataldo with distinct differences observed in different multinucleated giant cells with respect to the distribution of tyrosine and sulfhydryl groups.

The origin of the giant cells has never been established. Although their resemblance to osteoclasts is sometimes striking, seldom are they seen carrying out the ascribed normal resorptive function of such cells. Geschickter and Copeland suggested that the giant cells might be derived from proliferating giant cells associated with the resorption of deciduous tooth roots. Thus they suppose the lesion to be concerned with the transition from the deciduous to the permanent dentition. Unfortunately, such association of lesions is present in only a few cases even though the tumor is a rather common one in youngsters. Such a theory would account for the predominance of the lesions anterior to the permanent molars.

There has been considerable support for another theory of origin from endothelial cells of capillaries. There is some basis in fact for such an idea, the chief being the common occurrence of the giant cells within vascular channels, suggesting that they arise here through fusion of endothelial cells. This suggested to earlier workers that the tumor was a malignant metastasizing one, and they applied to it the term "giant cell sarcoma" or, in some cases, "myeloid sarcoma."

A recent study of the giant cells in the peripheral giant cell granuloma by electron microscopy has been reported by Sapp. He found that these giant cells ultrastructurally contained a sufficient number of features in common with osteoclasts to conclude that they represent a slightly modified form of that cell. In addition, he reported that the stromal cells were structurally compatible with the various stages of differentiating osteoprogenitor cells.

Roentgenographic Features. The intraoral roentgenogram may or may not exhibit evidence of involvement of the bone underlying the lesion. In edentulous areas the peripheral giant cell granuloma characteristically exhibits superficial erosion of the bone with pathognomonic peripheral "cuffing" of the bone as seen on the roentgenogram (Fig. 2–41, *B*). When the tumor occurs in areas in which teeth are present, the roentgenogram may reveal superficial destruction of the alveolar margin or crest of the interdental bone, but this is by no means invariably present.

Treatment and Prognosis. The treatment of the peripheral giant cell granuloma is surgical excision, care being taken to remove the entire base of the lesion. If only superficial excision is carried out, recurrence is seen in some cases. In the past it was common practice to remove the adjacent tooth at the time of excision of the lesion to prevent possible recurrence. This is contraindicated, at least initially, since the recurrence rate is not nearly as high as was once thought. Furthermore, the removal of a tooth associated with a lesion *assumed* to be a giant cell granuloma might prove to be embarrassing if the lesion were found to be of another type. The removal of the growth in an edentulous jaw should be followed by careful smoothing of the bone before closing the incision, since the lesions in this circumstance tend to infiltrate and are not well demarcated.

CENTRAL GIANT CELL GRANULOMA AND GIANT CELL TUMOR OF BONE

Few lesions of bone have provoked greater controversy in recent years than the central giant cell tumor and central giant cell granuloma and their relationship, if any. There has been a general renaissance of interest in the histophysiology and pathology of bone as well as numerous recent scholarly attempts to classify and explain many of the unusual changes, both neoplastic and reactive, which occur in bone. In past years the diagnosis of central giant cell tumor of bone was a common one and was applied generally to any lesion of bone which contained giant cells. Confusion was compounded by the recognition that patients suffering from hyperparathyroidism often present lesions of bone (i.e., von Recklinghausen's disease of bone) which are sometimes characterized by the presence of numerous, multinucleated giant cells and so are histologically similar to, if not identical with, unrelated nonendocrine lesions. Thus it is apparent that, in spite of concerted efforts to study central giant cell lesions from an etiologic and pathogenetic point of view, considerable uncertainty still exists about these jaw lesions.

Re-evaluation of lesions previously classified as central giant cell tumors of the jaws has placed many of these in other now recognized categories of diseases. One such type of lesion has been interpreted as a response to injury and has been designated by Jaffe as a central giant cell reparative granuloma. In recent years, the word "reparative" has been deleted from the term, since it is realized that many of these lesions are more "destructive" than "reparative."

When those giant cell-containing lesions of bone such as hyperparathyroidism, fibrous dysplasia, the giant cell granuloma and a related lesion, the aneurysmal bone cyst, are properly categorized, there still remains a very aggressive group of lesions, and it is these which have been classified as true giant cell tumors (neoplasms) of bone, with both a benign and malignant form being recognized. Many reviews and analyses of cases of the "true" giant cell tumor have been published in recent years, such as those of Schajowicz (85 cases), Hutter and his associates (76 cases), Mnaymneh and his associates (41 cases), Dahlin and his associates (195 cases), Goldenberg and his associates (218 cases) and McGrath (52 cases). With the exception of the series of Schajowicz, it seems most unusual that not a single case of "giant cell tumor" of the jaws was reported in the other series totaling 582 cases. It also seems most unusual that a "giant cell granuloma" has never been reported in any bone of the skeleton other than the jaws, although Hirschl and Katz have reported a possible case in the temporal bone. In other words, although many other reactive and neoplastic diseases of bone occur in many bones of the skeleton and in the jaws as well, it would appear that in this instance there is a nonodontogenic lesion of jaw bones (giant cell granuloma) not found in other bones of the skeleton and, conversely, there is a rather common tumor of other bones of the skeleton (giant cell tumor) that is rarely found in the jaws, a very strange situation at the least. It is on this basis that some controversy still exists as to whether the benign giant cell tumor of bone and the giant cell granuloma of the jaws represents the same disease or two different disease processes.

Occasional lesions described as giant cell tumors (benign) have been reported in the jaws such as those by Shklar and Meyer. However, too few cases are known to be able to adequately characterize the clinical and radiographic features. In most instances, the microscopic findings have guided the investigators into a diagnosis of giant cell tumor rather than giant cell granuloma. These findings have included larger giant cells with more nuclei and the fact that the giant cells were more uniformly dispersed. These reported differences in the giant cells between granuloma and tumor have prompted Abrams and Shear to compare the over-all size and number of nuclei of the giant cells in a series of cases of giant cell granulomas and of giant cell tumors of long bones. They found that the giant cells of the long bone tumors were larger than those of the jaw granulomas and that the giant cells of the jaw lesions contained fewer nuclei. However, they found considerable overlap and concluded that morphologically the cells in the two locations were indistinguishable. Franklin and his associates were able to confirm only a portion of these findings but, utilizing stereological techniques, did confirm significant differences between giant cells of jaw lesions and of long bone tumors in both nuclear numerical density and mean absolute cell volume.

As an incidental note, it might be pointed out here that the giant cell tumor of long bones has been recognized recently as an infrequent complication of osteitis deformans (Paget's disease of bone). Such a case in the maxilla has been reported by Goldstein and Laskin, who also reviewed the literature on this association.

The malignant giant cell tumor of bone behaves in a malignant fashion, and there is generally no difficulty in distinguishing between a benign and malignant lesion. However, the criteria for establishment of this diagnosis according to modern interpretation are quite rigorous, so that no large series of cases based on these criteria is extant. While a number of cases of so-called malignant giant cell tumor of bone in the jaws have been reported, the first documented primary malignant case diagnosed according to the criteria established by Dahlin and his associates has been reported by Mintz and his co-investigators.

Thus, the rarity of both benign and malignant giant cell tumors of the jaws, if one were to concede their occurrence, is such as to preclude their further consideration here. The following discussion, therefore, will concern the relatively common central giant cell granuloma of the jaws.

Clinical Features   The central giant cell granuloma occurs predominantly in children or young adults and, according to nearly all reported series, is somewhat more common in females than in males. Either jaw may be involved, but the mandible is affected more often. A study of 34 cases by Austin and his associates has supported these findings. In this study, over 60 per cent of the cases occurred before the age of 30 years. The sex distribution of 38 cases reported by Waldron and Shafer was approximately 2 to 1, females over males. Furthermore, 60 per cent of their cases were under the age of 20 years. Two-thirds of their cases occurred in the mandible, and only one-third in the maxilla. The lesions are more common in the anterior segments of the jaws and, not uncommonly, cross the midline (Figs. 2–42 and 2–43). Comparable data have been reported in a series of 32 cases by Andersen and his co-workers.

Pain is not a prominent feature of this lesion, although some local discomfort is usually noted. Slight to moderate bulging of the jaw due to expansion of the cortical plates occurs in the involved area, depending upon the extent of bone involvement. The lesion may present no signs or symptoms and may be discovered accidentally. A history of trauma is seldom found.

Roentgenographic Features.   The central giant cell granuloma is essentially a destructive lesion, producing a radiolucent area with either a relatively smooth or a ragged border, and sometimes showing faint trabeculae. Definite loculations are often present, particularly in larger lesions. The cortical plates of bone are often thin and expanded and may become perforated by the mass. Displacement of the teeth by the lesion is seen with some frequency. The appearance of the giant cell granuloma is not pathognomonic and may be confused with that of many other lesions of the jaw, both neoplastic and non-neoplastic (Fig. 2–44, *A* to *F*).

Histologic Features.   The central giant cell granuloma is made up of a loose fibrillar connective tissue stroma with many interspersed proliferating fibroblasts and small capillaries.

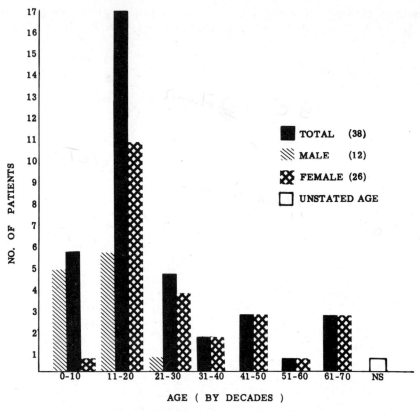

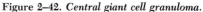

Figure 2–42. *Central giant cell granuloma.*
Age and sex distribution. (From C. A. Waldron and W. G. Shafer: The central giant cell reparative granuloma of the jaws. Am. J. Clin. Pathol., *45*:437, 1966.)

The collagen fibers are not usually collected into bundles; however, groups of fibers will often present a whorled appearance. Multinucleated giant cells are prominent throughout the connective tissue, but not necessarily abundant (Fig. 2–45). These giant cells vary in size from case to case and may contain only a few or several dozen nuclei. In addition, there are

usually numerous foci of old extravasated blood and associated hemosiderin pigment, some of it phagocytized by macrophages. Foci of new trabeculae of osteoid or bone also are often seen, particularly around the periphery of the lesion.

Treatment and Prognosis. The treatment of the giant cell granuloma is curettage or surgical excision. The lesions so treated almost invaria-

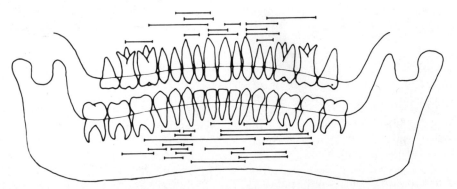

Figure 2–43. *Central giant cell granuloma.*
Distribution of sites of lesions. (From C. A. Waldron and W. G. Shafer: The central giant cell reparative granuloma of the jaws. Am. J. Clin. Pathol., *45*:437, 1966.)

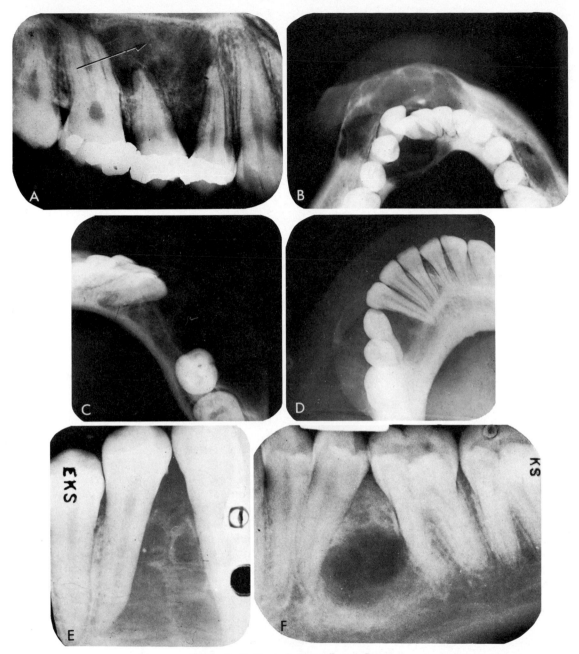

Figure 2–44. *Central giant cell granuloma.*
Various cases all show the radiolucent, expansile, multilocular nature of the lesion.

bly fill in with new bone and heal with no difficulty. Occasional lesions recur, but this is seldom sufficient cause for more radical procedures. X-ray radiation is contraindicated.

ANEURYSMAL BONE CYST

The aneurysmal bone cyst is an interesting solitary lesion of bone which was separated as a distinct entity in 1942 by Jaffe and Lichtenstein. Since their original account, many cases have been reported in the literature, although the first cases occurring in the jaws were not described until 1958.

Clinical Features. The aneurysmal bone cyst is generally a lesion of young persons, predominantly occurring under the age of 20 years, with no significant predilection for either sex.

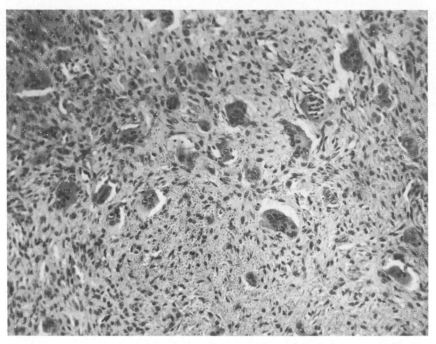

Figure 2–45. *Central giant cell granuloma.*

The lesion is encountered in adults, however, according to reviews of 50 cases by Lichtenstein, 95 cases by Tillman and his associates and 66 cases by Biesecker and his associates. A history of traumatic injury preceding development of the lesion may often be obtained.

Cases of aneurysmal bone cyst have been observed in nearly every part of the skeleton, although over 50 per cent of all cases occur in the long bones and vertebral column. Lesions are also seen frequently in the clavicle, rib, innominate bone, skull and bones of the hands and feet as well as other sites.

The lesions are usually tender or painful, particularly upon motion, and this soreness may limit movement of the affected bone. Swelling over the area of bone involvement is also common.

Gross findings at the time of operation are characteristic. Upon entering the lesion, excessive bleeding is encountered, the blood "welling up" from the tissue. The tissue has been described as resembling a blood-soaked sponge with large pores representing the cavernous spaces of the lesion. In manometric studies by Biesecker and his associates, some of the cysts had elevated vascular pressures as high as arteriolar levels.

Oral Manifestations. The aneurysmal bone cyst occurs with some frequency in the jaws, although many probably are misdiagnosed as some other bone lesion (Fig. 2–46, A). In a review of the literature, Neumann-Jensen and Praetorius found 26 reported cases in the jaws, 17 in the mandible and 9 in the maxilla. Of these, the average age of occurrence was 18 years with a range of 6 to 69 years, although only two patients were over 22 years of age. There was a slight predilection for occurrence in females, 14 to 9, where the sex was known.

Roentgenographic Features. The roentgenographic picture of the lesion is often distinctive. The bone is expanded, appears cystic with a honeycomb or soap bubble appearance in many cases, and is eccentrically ballooned (Fig. 2–46, B). The cortical bone may be destroyed, and a periosteal reaction may be evident.

Histologic Features. The aneurysmal bone cyst consists of a fibrous connective tissue stroma containing many cavernous or sinusoidal blood-filled spaces. These spaces may or may not show thrombosis. Young fibroblasts are numerous in the connective tissue stroma, as well as multinucleated giant cells with a patchy distribution similar to that in the giant cell granuloma. But in the latter lesion the cavernous spaces are not found. Varying amounts of hemosiderin are present and, invariably, new osteoid and bone formation (Fig. 2–47, A to D).

Pathogenesis. The nature of this lesion is still controversial despite the many cases that have been studied and reported. Lichtenstein has proposed that the aneurysmal bone cyst arises as a result of a persistent local alteration

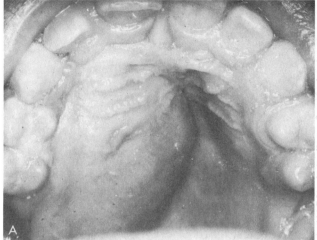

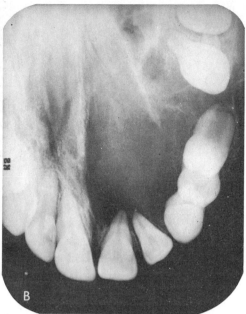

Figure 2–46. *Aneurysmal bone cyst.*
The large palatal swelling is a result of the underlying destructive, expansile mass. (Courtesy of Dr. Jack Todd.)

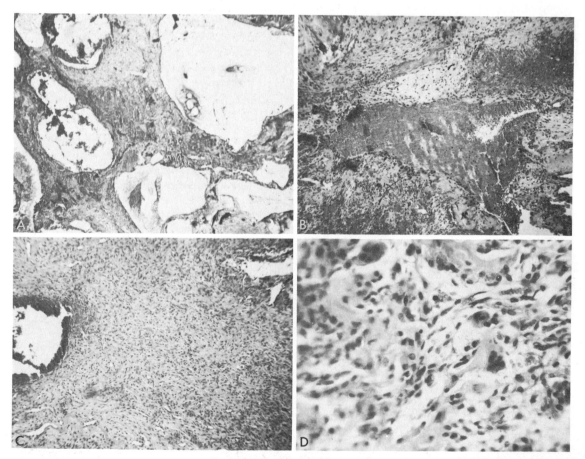

Figure 2–47. *Aneurysmal bone cyst.*
The photomicrograph illustrates the sinusoidal blood spaces, connective tissue, osteoid and giant cells.

in hemodynamics, leading to increased venous pressure and subsequent development of a dilated and engorged vascular bed in the transformed bone area. Resorption of bone then occurs, to which the giant cells are related, and this is replaced by connective tissue, osteoid and new bone.

An alternative explanation of the lesion is that it represents an exuberant attempt at repair of a hematoma of bone, similar to the central giant cell granuloma. But in the case of the aneurysmal bone cyst it is postulated that the hematoma maintains a circulatory connection with the damaged vessel. This would produce a slow flow of blood through the lesion and account for the clinical "welling" of blood when the lesion is entered. Thus the only real difference between this aneurysmal cyst and the giant cell granuloma is that in the latter lesion the damaged blood vessels fail to retain a circulatory connection with the lesion.

It is most significant that Biesecker and his associates have reported that 32 per cent of their series of aneurysmal bone cysts had an accompanying benign primary lesion of bone. On this basis, they have proposed a new hypothesis for the etiology and pathogenesis of this lesion—namely, that a primary lesion of bone initiates an osseous, arteriovenous fistula and thereby creates, via its hemodynamic forces, the secondary reactive lesion of bone: the aneurysmal bone cyst.

This occurrence of aneurysmal bone cyst secondary to or in association with other osseous lesions has been confirmed by other investigators. For example, Levy and his associates reported 57 cases of aneurysmal bone cyst with which the most commonly associated lesion was the solitary or unicameral bone cyst (16 cases), the osteoclastoma or benign giant cell tumor (14 cases) and osteosarcoma (12 cases). Other associated lesions included the nonosteogenic fibroma, benign osteoblastoma, hemangioendothelioma and hemangioma of bone. Five aneurysmal bone cysts were secondary to fracture or other bone trauma.

Hillerup and Hjørting-Hansen have summarized the different theories on the etiology and pathogenesis of the aneurysmal bone cyst, simple bone cyst and central giant cell granuloma of the jaws. They suggested that these three lesions have a common dysvascular etiology and that local environmental factors within the bone may differentiate the pathogenesis.

Treatment and Prognosis. Surgical curettement or excision is the treatment of choice, although low doses of radiation have also been used. The possibility of radiation sarcoma is always a potential hazard, however, and the propriety of treatment of benign lesions by radiation has been seriously questioned on this basis. Recurrence in bones other than the jaws has been reported variously in between 21 and 59 per cent of cases. However, no lesion in the jaws is known to have recurred.

LIPOMA

The lipoma is a relatively rare intraoral tumor, although it occurs with considerable frequency in other areas, particularly in the subcutaneous tissues of the neck.

This is a benign, slow-growing neoplasm composed of mature fat cells. It appears that the cells of the lipoma differ metabolically from normal fat cells even though they are histologically similar. Thus a person on a starvation diet will lose fat from normal fat depots in the body, but not from the lipoma. Furthermore, fatty acid precursors are incorporated at a more rapid rate into lipoma fat than into normal fat while lipoprotein lipase activity is reduced.

Clinical Features. The tumor has been reported to occur in a variety of locations, including the tongue, floor of the mouth, buccal mucosa, gingiva, and mucobuccal or labial folds. It is usually found in adults. It appears as a single or lobulated, painless lesion attached by either a sessile or a pedunculated base (Fig. 2–48, A). The epithelium is usually thin, and the superficial blood vessels are readily visible over the surface. The lipoma is yellowish, and relatively soft to palpation. Some lesions occur deeper in the tissues and produce only a slight surface elevation. These tend to be more diffuse than the superficial type of lipoma. When palpated, the diffuse form feels like fluid, sometimes leading to a mistaken tentative diagnosis of "cyst." Since this diffuse form often occurs in areas in which some fat is normally present, the diagnosis of lipoma depends upon the recognition of simply an overabundance of this tissue. Thus the diagnosis is essentially a clinical one. A series of 26 cases of oral lipoma has been reported by Seldin and his associates and 16 cases with a discussion of the lesion by Greer and Richardson.

Occasional cases of intraosseous lipoma of the jaws are reported, but these are difficult to verify and separate from normal fatty marrow.

Lipoblastomatosis is a rare related lesion originally described by Vellios and his associates in 1958. It is probably not a true neoplasm but rather a continuation of the normal process of

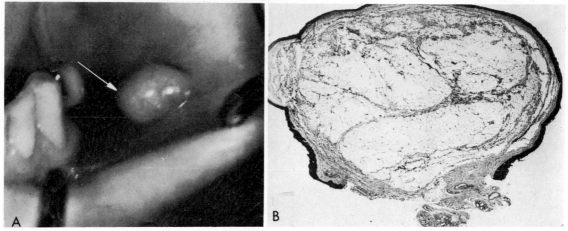

Figure 2–48. *Lipoma.*
The circumscribed mass on the buccal mucosa (A) is composed chiefly of adult fat cells with occasional connective tissue septa coursing through the lesion (B).

fetal fat development carried into postnatal life. It is characterized clinically by the occurrence in infants of solitary or multiple soft-tissue masses developing at various sites such as the buttock, chest, axilla or neck. The lesions are benign but may recur if inadequately excised. A series of 35 cases has been reported and the condition discussed in detail by Chung and Enzinger. A case of oral lipoblastomatosis involving the cheek of an 18-month-old male has been reported by Shear.

Hibernoma is another rare related soft-tissue tumor occurring in a few selected sites in humans, presumably derived from multivacuolated fat that is analogous to the "brown fat" of hibernating animals. Lesions in the oral cavity have not been reported.

Histologic Features. The lipoma is made up of a circumscribed mass of mature fat cells which may exhibit varying numbers of collagen strands coursing through the lesion and supporting occasional small blood vessels (Fig. 2–48, *B*). When this fibrous connective tissue forms a more significant part of the tumor, the term "fibrolipoma" is often used to designate the lesion.

Treatment and Prognosis. The treatment of the lipoma is surgical excision. Recurrence is uncommon.

VERRUCIFORM XANTHOMA

(Histiocytosis "Y")

The verruciform xanthoma is a lesion of the oral cavity of unknown etiology and uncertain nature, first described as an entity by Shafer in 1971. Over 50 cases have now been reported

in the literature, including two on the vulva, one on the penis and one on the skin of the thigh. Neville and Weathers have reviewed the reported cases, adding 21 to those previously described.

Clinical Features. This occurs as a solitary lesion, either normal or reddish in color but sometimes pale or "hyperkeratotic," with a rough, pebbly surface and either a sessile or pedunculated base. It may be as small as 2 mm. or as large as 1.5 cm. in diameter, and is invariably asymptomatic.

There is no sex predilection for occurrence and it appears to develop chiefly in adults over the age of 40 years. The verruciform xanthoma may occur at any site but is most frequently found on the alveolar ridge, or gingiva, followed by the buccal mucosa and then the palate, floor of the mouth, lip and lower mucobuccal fold with equal frequency.

Histologic Features. The lesion has a verrucous, hyperparakeratotic surface showing severe parakeratin plugging. This surface parakeratin is often shaggy with superimposed bacterial colonies. The rete pegs are extremely elongated but very uniformly so, although no increased mitoses or pseudoepitheliomatous hyperplasia are found. The characteristic feature of the lesion is the presence of large, swollen "foam" cells or xanthoma cells, presumably histiocytes, which fill the connective tissue papillae between the epithelial pegs. These are confined to the papillae and do not extend into the dermis beneath the pegs. The nature of this intracellular material is unknown but is presumably lipid material, since fat stains by Zegarelli and his co-workers were positive for the pres-

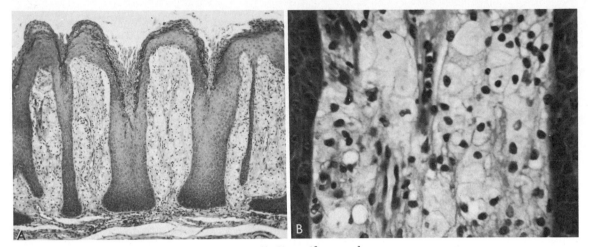

Figure 2–49. *Verruciform xanthoma.*

ence of lipid within these cells (Fig. 2–49, *A*, *B*). Neville and Weathers also found that these cells, in 15 cases tested, contained PAS-positive diastase-resistant granules. Electron microscope study of these lesions by Zegarelli and his group, as well as by Cobb and his associates, have not been particularly enlightening.

Treatment and Prognosis. Since the significance and/or the association of the verruciform xanthoma with any systemic condition is unknown, simple surgical excision is recommended. There are no reported recurrences.

HEMANGIOMA

(Vascular Nevus)

The hemangioma is a common tumor characterized by the proliferation of blood vessels. It is often congenital in nature and usually but not invariably follows a benign course. Some authorities believe that this lesion, particularly the congenital form, is not a true neoplasm, but rather a developmental anomaly or hamartoma, i.e., an abnormal proliferation of tissues of structures native to the part. These tumors seldom actually invade surrounding tissues.

A variety of classifications have been suggested for categorizing the different forms of hemangioma, but since the intraoral group is a limited one, not all the various forms will be considered in detail. A simple classification is that proposed by Watson and McCarthy based upon a series of 1308 blood vessel tumors, and is as follows: (1) capillary hemangioma, (2) cavernous hemangioma, (3) angioblastic or hypertrophic hemangioma, (4) racemose hemangioma, (5) diffuse systemic hemangioma, (6) metastasizing hemangioma, (7) nevus vinosus, or port-wine stain, and (8) hereditary hemorrhagic telangiectasis.

Clinical Features. Most cases of hemangioma are present at birth or arise at an early age. In the study reported by Watson and McCarthy, 85 per cent of the 1308 lesions had developed by the end of the first year of age. An unexplained sex difference was present, the female-to-male ratio being 65 per cent to 35 per cent. The head and neck regions were involved in 56 per cent of the cases, while the remaining six-sevenths of the total body surface area accounted for only 44 per cent of the cases.

Oral Manifestations. The hemangioma of the oral soft tissue is similar to the hemangioma of the skin and appears as a flat or raised lesion of the mucosa, usually deep red or bluish red and seldom well circumscribed. The most common sites of occurrence are the lips, tongue, buccal mucosa and palate (Fig. 2–50). The tumor often is traumatized and undergoes ulceration and secondary infection.

Certain tiny vascular formations of lip vessels called "microcherry," "glomerulus" and "venous lake" have been described by Gius and his associates as lesions encountered with increasing frequency in the later decades of life and occurring with greater frequency in patients with gastric and duodenal ulcers.

The *intramuscular hemangioma* is one special form of hemangioma which is quite rare in the head and neck region. It arises within normal skeletal muscle, comprises less than 1 per cent of all hemangiomas and is important chiefly because of the problem in differential diagnosis and of treatment of the lesion. It has been reviewed in detail by Ivey and his co-workers.

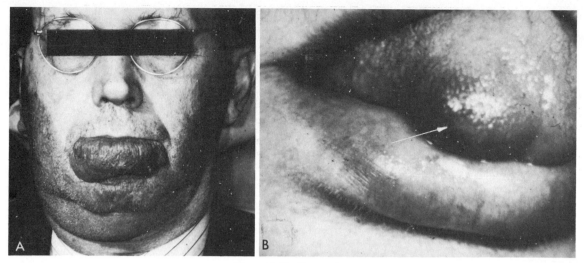

Figure 2–50. *Hemangioma.*

A, Congenital bilateral hemangioma of the face and lip. The lesion follows the distribution of the beard. *B,* The hemangioma of the tongue is superficial but diffuse.

Central hemangiomas of the maxilla or mandible occasionally occur and frequently present difficulty in differential diagnosis. In a review of 56 cases of hemangioma of bone by Unni and his associates, there were five cases in the maxilla and four in the mandible. Lund and Dahlin reviewed 35 cases of hemangioma of the jaws and found that over 50 per cent of the cases occurred in the first two decades of life and that two-thirds of the lesions were located in the mandible. Here the tumor is a bone-destructive lesion which may be of varying size and appearance, but is often suggestive of a cyst (Fig. 2–51). Some central hemangiomas present a honeycombed appearance on the roentgenogram, sometimes with radiating spic-

ules at the expanded periphery forming a "sunburst" appearance reminiscent of that effect seen in osteosarcoma. This has been described by James and by Dorfman and his associates.

The attempt at rash surgical excision of such central lesions has often resulted in severe loss of blood, which occasionally has led to exsanguination of the patient to the point of death. In such bony lesions it is always advisable to attempt to aspirate fluid contents through a needle before surgically opening the area. When the hemangioma is entirely central within bone, Gamez-Araujo and his associates have stated that the prognosis is excellent with adequate surgical intervention, in contrast to those lesions where soft tissue is also involved

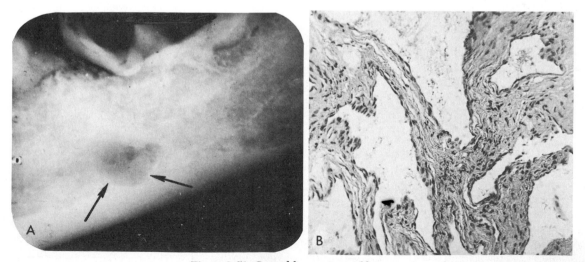

Figure 2–51. *Central hemangioma of bone.*

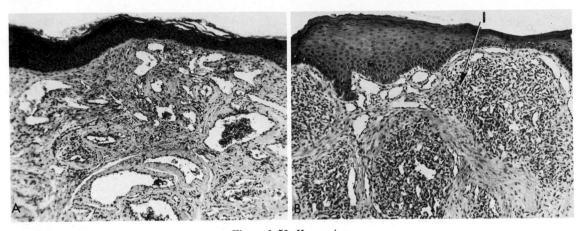

Figure 2–52. *Hemangioma.*
Some lesions (A) are characterized by the presence of many small dilated capillaries and a minimum of endothelial cells, while others (B) show large numbers of proliferating endothelial cells (1), but only moderate numbers of patent capillaries.

by capillary hemangioma. In these latter instances, the lesions become aggressive, invade locally and often recur if not totally eradicated.

The *arteriovenous aneurysm*, or arteriovenous fistula, is an uncommon lesion which often has been mistaken clinically for a hemangioma. It represents a direct communication between an artery and a vein through which the blood bypasses the capillary circulation. The arteriovenous aneurysm may be congenital or acquired, the latter usually being traumatic in origin. It may occur either in the soft tissues, such as in the case of the palate reported by Ingram and Coker, and on the alveolar ridge as reported by McComb and Trott, or central in the jaw as reported by Cook and Zbar. These aneurysms typically are classified as follows: (1) a cirsoid aneurysm which is a tortuous mass of small arteries and veins linking a larger artery and vein; (2) a varicose aneurysm which consists of an endothelium-lined sac connecting an artery and a vein; and (3) an aneurysmal varix representing a direct connection between an artery and a dilated vein. The arteriovenous aneurysm has been reviewed in detail by Gomes and Bernatz, while Orbach has discussed the entire gamut of congenital arteriovenous malformations of the head and neck. He has emphasized the histogenesis and pathogenesis of these abnormalities, stressing the fact that they range from the most trivial angioma to the large-bore arteriovenous fistula.

Histologic Features. The usual hemangioma is composed of many small capillaries lined by a single layer of endothelial cells supported by a connective tissue stroma of varying density. It bears considerable resemblance to young granulation tissue and is nearly identical with some cases of pyogenic granuloma. Some cases show rather remarkable endothelial cell proliferation (Fig. 2–52). In fact, one common form is referred to as a juvenile hemangioendothelioma because it occurs in very early life and is characterized by an extremely cellular pattern. It is generally believed that this lesion is an immature stage of a capillary hemangioma and that, in time, it will either develop into a simple hemangioma or regress.

The cavernous form of hemangioma consists of large dilated blood sinuses with thin walls, each showing an endothelial lining. The sinusoidal spaces usually are filled with blood, although an admixture with occasional lymphatic vessels occurs in some instances.

Intravascular angiomatosis, also referred to in the literature most commonly under the terms hemangioendotheliome vegetant intravasculaire of Masson, Masson's pseudoangiosarcoma, and intravascular papillary endothelial hyperplasia, is actually an unusual form of an organizing thrombus, although it is often mistaken for a vascular tumor, especially a malignant one such as angiosarcoma. This lesion has been discussed by McClatchey and his associates, who described perioral cases, including two on the lips which clinically resembled mucoceles, and emphasized that angiosarcoma could best be excluded as a diagnosis by the intravascular localization, the absent to rare mitoses and necrosis, and the rare solid cellular areas without vascular differentiation.

Treatment and Prognosis. Many congenital hemangiomas have been found to undergo spontaneous regression at a relatively early age.

Cases which do not show such remission or those which arise in older persons have been treated in a variety of ways, including (1) surgery, (2) radiation therapy (external radiation or radium), (3) sclerosing agents, such as sodium morrhuate or psylliate, injected into the lesion, (4) carbon dioxide snow, (5) cryotherapy, and (6) compression. Each form of treatment has its proponents and antagonists, but it appears that in skilled hands each has its proper place.

The prognosis of the hemangioma is excellent, since it does not become malignant or recur after adequate removal or destruction.

HEREDITARY HEMORRHAGIC TELANGIECTASIA

(Rendu-Osler-Weber Disease)

Hereditary hemorrhagic telangiectasia, a form of hemangioma, is a congenital, hereditary disease characterized by numerous telangiectatic or angiomatous areas which are widely distributed on the skin and mucosa of the oral cavity and which tend to undergo repeated hemorrhage. The disease affects both males and females and is transmitted by both sexes as a simple mendelian dominant. Typical cases involving the oral cavity have been reported by Scopp and Quart and by Oliver, who also discussed the disease in detail.

Clinical Features. The spider-like telangiectases are occasionally present at or shortly after birth, although in the majority of cases they do not become conspicuous until after puberty. They appear to increase in number and prominence as the patient ages. The skin lesions are most common on the face, neck, and chest, although any area may be involved (Fig. 2–53). Involvement of the oral mucous membrane constitutes an important feature of the disease,

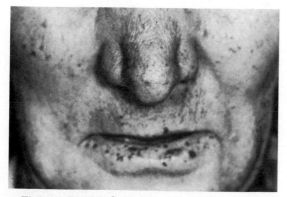

Figure 2–53. *Hereditary hemorrhagic telangiectasia.* (Courtesy of Dr. Theodore Century.)

the most commonly affected areas being the lips, gingiva, buccal mucosa and palate, as well as the floor of the mouth and the tongue.

One of the earliest signs of the disease, often occurring in childhood and preceding the appearance of telangiectasia, is epistaxis, as well as bleeding from the oral cavity, both of which may be difficult to control. The diagnosis may be established if a history of epistaxis dating from childhood, the presence of the telangiectatic areas and the familial history are ascertained.

Similar telangiectases of skin and oral mucous membranes may occur in a variety of other situations, however, and these include progressive systemic sclerosis (scleroderma) and the CREST syndrome (Calcinosis cutis, Raynaud's phenomenon, Esophageal dysfunction, Sclerodactyly and Telangiectasia), lupus erythematosus, sarcoid and other rarer diseases. The differential diagnoses are important and have been discussed by Donaldson and Myall.

Histologic Features. The disease is due primarily to defects in the small blood vessels of the skin and mucosa. Hashimoto and Pritzker have shown, in an electron microscope investigation, that the actual cause of the hemorrhage is either a primary intrinsic defect of the endothelial cells permitting their detachment, or a defect in the perivascular supportive tissue bed which weakens the vessels, rather than a lack of elastic fibers as was thought at one time. Both clotting and bleeding times are normal, as are the blood elements, although with severe bleeding mild anemia and thrombocytopenia may result.

Treatment and Prognosis. The treatment of the disease is varied, depending upon its severity. The spontaneous hemorrhages may be controlled by pressure packs, particularly the nasal bleeding. The angiomatous or telangiectatic areas are sometimes cauterized, treated with x-ray radiation or surgically excised.

The disease is seldom so severe that life is endangered. Nevertheless a considerable number of deaths from severe hemorrhage have been reported.

ENCEPHALOTRIGEMINAL ANGIOMATOSIS

(Sturge-Weber Disease)

Encephalotrigeminal angiomatosis is a rather uncommon congenital condition characterized by the combination of a venous angioma of the leptomeninges over the cerebral cortex with ipsilateral angiomatous lesions of the face and,

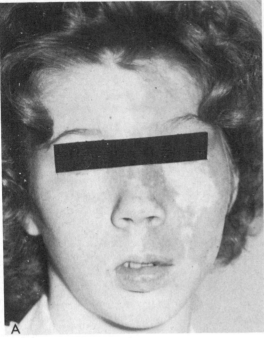

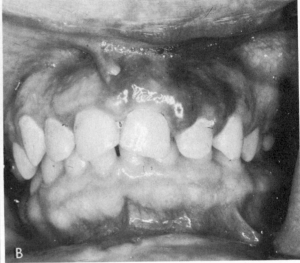

Figure 2–54. *Encephalotrigeminal angiomatosis.*
(Courtesy of Dr. George Mumford.)

sometimes, of the skull, jaws and oral soft tissues. Thus this disorder may be classified as a variant of the hemangioma. Peterman and his associates have reviewed the literature pertaining to the disease and studied 35 additional cases of their own.

Clinical Features. The typical dermal capillary-venous angiomas (or portwine nevi) are generally but not invariably present. These nevi are present at birth and are confined almost exclusively to the skin area supplied by the trigeminal nerve (Fig. 2–54, A). A second common feature is the presence of typical intracranial convolutional calcifications discernible in cranial roentgenograms. Ocular involvement occurs in some patients, consisting generally of glaucoma, exophthalmus, angioma of the choroid or other abnormalities.

Neurologic manifestations are among the most characteristic features of the disease and consist of convulsive disorders and spastic hemiplegia with or without mental retardation. These manifestations are directly related to the leptomeningeal angioma and calcifications, the latter being also related to the vascular disturbance.

Oral Manifestations. Occasionally, angiomatous lesions also involve the gingiva and buccal mucosa (Fig. 2–54, B). There is generally no difficulty in diagnosis because of the presence of the facial lesions.

Treatment. The treatment of the disease is essentially a neurosurgical problem, although the convulsions can sometimes be controlled by anticonvulsant drugs.

NASOPHARYNGEAL ANGIOFIBROMA
(Juvenile Nasopharyngeal Fibroma)

The nasopharyngeal angiofibroma is a relatively uncommon neoplasm occurring almost exclusively in the nasopharynx of adolescent males. Occasional cases have extended to involve the oral cavity, however, and for this reason the entity deserves consideration here.

Clinical Features. This benign tumor is a nonencapsulated, expansile and infiltrating lesion arising from the soft tissue of the nasopharynx. Few cases have ever been reported in females. Although the average age of occurrence, according to the series of 26 cases reported by Hubbard, is 16 years, occasional cases are seen in older patients. The same age of onset has been reported by Hicks and Nelson from a series of 58 cases in their excellent review of the clinical and pathologic nature of the nasopharyngeal fibroma. The frequent occurrence in young males has suggested an endocrine basis for the lesion, but the explanation for this relationship remains obscure.

The lesion is generally manifested by nasal obstruction, epistaxis and sinusitis. Care must be taken to differentiate this lesion from ordinary nasal polyps, which it may superficially resemble. As the tumor mass enlarges, inferior depression of the palate and facial deformity may occur.

Oral Manifestations. The oral manifestations of the nasopharyngeal angiofibroma are generally those of a palatal or tonsillar mass, often with nasal obstruction. Occasionally, however, lesions of the posterior portion of the maxilla and even of the mandible have been seen which are microscopically identical with the nasopharyngeal lesions, and they may be considered similar in nature.

Histologic Features. The tumor consists essentially of two basic and characteristic components: a vascular network and a connective tissue stroma. The vessels comprising the vascular network are of varying caliber, irregular in shape and generally consisting of a simple endothelial lining. The vascular element is generally most pronounced at the periphery of the lesion where active growth is occurring. Thrombosis and occlusion are frequently seen, usually in association with vasculitis.

The connective tissue stroma consists of both fine and coarse collagen fibrils, usually with an irregular, unoriented pattern, interspersed with plump, stellate cells arranged in a haphazard fashion. Hyalinized foci are sometimes present, as well as areas resembling myxomatous degeneration. When the stromal cells are abundant, the resemblance to the sclerosing hemangioma may be pronounced. Multinucleated stromal cells are sometimes present and, with the occasional atypical nuclear and cellular changes that may be found, the lesion may be mistaken for a sarcoma.

Treatment and Prognosis. The treatment for the nasopharyngeal angiofibroma has generally been surgery, sometimes accompanied by x-ray radiation, particularly if intracranial extension has occurred. This has been discussed by Sessions and his associates. Multiple recurrences are common, but malignant transformation probably does not occur.

Occasional cases have been reported to regress upon attaining sexual maturity. However, this is not a uniform occurrence and the waiting for such an event may only result in a larger tumor with greater damage to surrounding structures.

LYMPHANGIOMA

The lymphangioma, a benign tumor of lymphatic vessels, is the far less common counterpart of the hemangioma, and there have arisen arguments about the true nature of this lesion (neoplasm vs. hamartoma) similar to those about the hemangioma. A classification of the lymphangiomas has been suggested by Watson and McCarthy based upon their study of 41 cases. In this classification the following divisions are proposed: (1) simple lymphangioma, (2) cavernous lymphangioma, (3) cellular or hypertrophic lymphangioma, (4) diffuse systemic lymphangioma, and (5) cystic lymphangioma or hygroma.

Clinical Features. The majority of cases of lymphangioma are present at birth, according to Watson and McCarthy, in whose series 95 per cent of the tumors had arisen before the age of 10 years. The age at onset was under 15 years in only 71 per cent of 42 cases reported by Nix, while in the series of 132 patients reported by Hill and Briggs, 88 per cent of the lesions had developed by the end of the second year of life. In contrast to that of the hemangioma, the sex distribution of the lymphangioma is nearly evenly divided. The head and neck area in the series of Watson and McCarthy was the site of the tumor in 52 per cent of the cases.

Oral Manifestations. The intraoral lymphangioma most commonly occurs on the tongue, but is seen also on the palate, buccal mucosa, gingiva and lips (Fig. 2–55). The superficial lesions are manifested as papillary lesions which may be of the same color as the surrounding mucosa or of a slightly redder hue. The deeper lesions appear as diffuse nodules or masses without any significant change in surface texture or color. In some cases relatively large areas of tissue may be involved. If the tongue is affected, considerable enlargement may occur, and to this clinical feature the term "macroglossia" may be applied. A series of 46 cases of

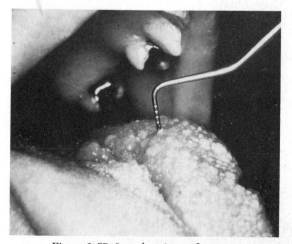

Figure 2–55. *Lymphangioma of tongue.*
(Courtesy of Dr. Max L. Schaeffer.)

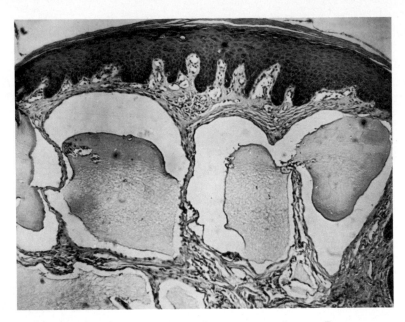

Figure 2–56. *Lymphangioma of buccal mucosa.*

lymphangioma of the tongue has been reviewed by Litzow and Lash. They pointed out that the anterior dorsal part of the tongue was most frequently affected. The irregular nodularity of the surface of the tongue with gray and pink projections is the commonest sign of the disease and, when associated with macroglossia, is pathognomonic of lymphangioma.

Lip involvement and its attendant deformity are referred to as macrocheilia. The cystic hygroma is a common and distinct entity that is not manifested in the oral cavity but occurs in the neck as a large, deep, diffuse swelling. This has been discussed in particular by Bill and Sumner and by Paletta.

An unusual form of lymphangioma termed *lymphangioma of the alveolar ridge in neonates* has been reported by Levin and his associates. They found small blue-domed fluid-filled lesions on the alveolar ridges in 55 (3.7 per cent) of 1470 normal black newborns; none were found in whites. Histologically, those biopsied were lymphangiomas. The natural history of this lesion is unknown, although spontaneous regression was noted in several cases.

Occasional cases of central lymphangioma of bone are also known to occur such as that in the tibia reported by Bullough and Goodfellow, as well as in the jaw.

Histologic Features. The lymphangioma, of which the cavernous type is the most common, consists of numerous dilated lymphatics, lined by endothelial cells and containing lymph (Fig. 2–56). Occasional channels may be filled with blood, a mixed hemangiolymphangioma.

Treatment and Prognosis. The treatment of the lymphangioma is considerably different from that of the hemangioma. Surgical excision is probably the treatment of choice, since the lymphangioma is more radioresistant and insensitive to sclerosing agents, such as sodium morrhuate, than the hemangioma. Spontaneous regression, according to most studies such as that of Saijo and his co-workers, is rare.

These lesions show a tendency to recur after removal, as evidenced by the series of Watson and McCarthy in which 41 per cent of the cases recurred. This tendency appears to increase with increasing age of the patient.

MYXOMA

The myxoma of the soft tissues is a tumor which has been described by Stout as a true neoplasm made up of tissue resembling primitive mesenchyme. Thus it is composed of stellate cells arranged in a loose mucoid stroma which also contains delicate reticulin fibers. The lesion is benign and does not metastasize, although it frequently infiltrates adjacent tissues.

Clinical Features. Most soft-tissue myxomas are deeply situated lesions, occurring in the skin or the subcutaneous tissues, the genitourinary tract, the gastrointestinal tract or in organs such as the liver, the spleen, or even the parotid gland.

This tumor may make its appearance at any age, approximately equal numbers of cases having been reported in every decade of life. There is no definite sex predilection of this neoplasm. A detailed study of 58 patients with 64 tumors has been reported by Ireland and his associates.

Oral Manifestations. The intraoral soft-tissue myxoma is an extremely rare lesion. The majority of oral cases undoubtedly represent only myxomatous degeneration in a fibrous tumor, and these cannot be considered true myxomas, although Elzay has presented 15 intraoral cases which he accepted as bona fide examples.

Other cases occurring centrally within the bone of the jaws have been classified, particularly in the dental literature, as odontogenic myxomas, i.e., as tumors derived from odontogenic tissue. Even though such tumors are sometimes associated with missing or displaced teeth, their dental origin is difficult, if not impossible, to establish. Nevertheless, for the sake of convenience, the central myxoma of bone is discussed under the odontogenic myxoma in the odontogenic tumor section (q.v.).

The *nerve sheath myxoma* is a benign tumor thought to arise from perineural cells of peripheral nerves and is characterized by the occurrence of stellate cells in a prominent mucoid matrix. A few cases have been reported in the oral cavity on the tongue, buccal mucosa and retromolar area and these have been reviewed by Sist and Greene. Their ultrastructural studies, along with those of Webb, supported the perineural origin of these lesions. They are treated by local excision and do not recur.

Oral focal mucinosis, the oral counterpart of a dermal lesion known as cutaneous focal mucinosis and/or cutaneous myxoid cyst, is the lesion most commonly misdiagnosed as an intraoral soft tissue myxoma, according to the study of Tomich. In fact, he has stated that most, if not all, cases diagnosed as oral soft tissue myxomas are in reality lesions of this entity. He reported eight cases of oral focal mucinosis, including the histologic and histochemical findings, postulating that the lesion develops because of a fibroblastic overproduction of hyaluronic acid due to an unknown stimulus.

Histologic Features. The soft-tissue myxoma is characteristically a loose-textured tissue containing moderate numbers of delicate reticulin fibers and mucoid material, probably hyaluronic acid. Oral focal mucinosis lacks this reticulin network. Interspersed throughout are varying numbers of stellate cells which occasionally assume a spindle shape. The tumor is not encapsulated and may invade surrounding tissue. This invasiveness is not characteristic of oral focal mucinosis.

Tomich has listed the "myxoid"-appearing lesions to be considered in the differential diagnosis as including: soft tissue myxoma, odontogenic myxoma, myxomatous degeneration in a fibrous lesion, oral focal mucinosis, nerve sheath myxoma, myxoid neurofibroma, mucous retention phenomenon and localized myxedema.

Treatment and Prognosis. The treatment of the myxoma is essentially surgical, since x-ray radiation is of little benefit. Recurrence is common, but this is not of grave concern, since the tumor does not metastasize. The attempt to avoid recurrence may necessitate the sacrifice of an appreciable amount of apparently uninvolved surrounding tissue, although this is generally not true of the intraoral lesion. In contrast, oral focal mucinosis has no tendency to recur.

CHONDROMA

The chondroma, a benign central tumor composed of mature cartilage, is a well-recognized entity in certain areas of the bony skeleton, but is uncommon in the bones of the maxilla or mandible. Reported cases were reviewed by MacGregor in 1952. A later review by Chaudhry and his co-workers contained only 18 cases from the English scientific literature between 1912 and 1959. The lesion is of considerable clinical importance because of the propensity of the tumor to undergo malignant degeneration in some instances, even after remaining quiescent for long periods of time.

The chondroma seldom develops in membrane bones, particularly if no vestigial cartilaginous rests are present, but since both the maxilla and mandible may contain such remnants, the tumor certainly may occur in these bones. Miles pointed out that areas of "secondary cartilage," cartilage not related to recognized parts of the chondrocranium, occur in the mandible in the mental region, coronoid process and condyle. At least in the embryo, cartilage is found in the maxilla on the lateral aspects near the malar process close to the molar teeth, as well as in the premaxillary area.

Clinical Features. This neoplasm may develop at any age and shows no apparent sex predilection. The chondroma usually arises as a painless, slowly progressive swelling of the jaw which, like many other neoplasms, may cause loosening of the teeth. The overlying mucosa is seldom ulcerated. The anterior portion of the maxilla is the most frequent site of involvement by this tumor because it is here that vestigial cartilage rests are found, particularly in the midline lingual to or between the central incisors. In the mandible the most common site of occurrence is posterior to the cuspid tooth, involving the body of the mandible, or the coronoid or condylar processes. It is also documented in the nasal septum and nasal spine and has been discussed here by Tomich and Hutton.

Occasional peripheral cases, outside bone, have been reported, such as that on the soft palate described by Gardner and Paterson or the relatively common chondroma or osteochondroma of the tongue. However, these may represent only islands of chondroid metaplasia or even a choristoma rather than a true neoplasm. Thus, they would be analogous to *osteoma mucosae* (q.v.). The relationship of these intraoral peripheral chondromas, especially those of the tongue, to the well-recognized *chondroma of soft parts*, reviewed by Chung and Enzinger, is not clearly established.

Roentgenographic Features. The roentgenogram shows an irregular radiolucent or mottled area in the bone. The chondroma is a destructive lesion and, in addition, has been shown to cause root resorption of teeth adjacent to it.

Histologic Features. The distinction between chondroma and chondrosarcoma is a narrow one and may offer a serious problem to the pathologist confronted with only a small biopsy specimen. The chondroma is made up of a mass of hyaline cartilage which may exhibit areas of calcification or of necrosis. The cartilage cells appear small, contain only single nuclei and do not exhibit great variation in size, shape or staining reaction. Cartilaginous tumors vary considerably in appearance from area to area, so that some malignant lesions present regions of apparent benignity. For this reason, care must be exercised in the unequivocal diagnosis of such a tumor from a small biopsy specimen.

Treatment and Prognosis. The treatment of the chondroma is surgical, since the tumor is resistant to x-ray radiation. The fact that sarcomatous change is not an unlikely occurrence suggests that somewhat more than a conservative enucleation should be carried out, although radical resection cannot be justified unless the tumor is of unusual size. Because of the dearth of reported cases, the prognosis of this disease in the jaws is not known, but to judge from cases in other parts of the body, it is probably good.

BENIGN CHONDROBLASTOMA

(Epiphyseal Chondromatous Giant Cell Tumor; Codman's Tumor)

The benign chondroblastoma of bone, named by Jaffe and Lichtenstein in 1942 but described earlier by Ewing in 1928 and Codman in 1931, is a distinct entity usually involving long bones but sometimes occurring in the cranial bones. Of 13 such cranial tumors reviewed by Al-Dewachi and his co-workers, 9 occurred in the temporal bone, 1 in the parietal, 2 in the mandible and 1 in the maxilla.

Clinical Features. This benign, primary central bone tumor occurs predominantly in young persons, nearly 90 per cent of a series of 69 cases reported by Schajowicz and Gallardo ranging between the ages of 5 and 25 years. Identical findings were reported in a series of 125 cases by Dahlin and Ivins. Males are involved more than females, usually in a ratio of about 2 to 1. The vast majority of cases involve the long bone of the upper and lower limbs. However, cases involving the mandibular condyle have been reported by Goodsell and Hubinger and by Dahlin and Ivins, while a case involving the anterior maxilla of a 13-year-old girl has been reported by Al-Dewachi and his associates. In addition, an extraskeletal chondroblastoma of the ear has been reported by Kingsley and Markel.

Histologic Features. The tumor is composed of relatively uniform, closely packed, polyhedral cells with occasional foci of chondroid matrix. A scattering of multinucleated giant cells may be found, usually associated with areas of hemorrhage, necrosis or calcification of the chondroid material. Formation of bone and osteoid also occurs and, as pointed out by Gravanis and Giansanti, is probably more common than is generally accepted. In addition, occasional cases have histologic features overlapping those of the chondromyxoid fibroma of bone.

Treatment. Conservative surgical excision is the usually accepted treatment, although recurrence is not uncommon. In a series of 25 cases reported by Huvos and his associates, an aneurysmal bone cyst was found engrafted on the primary bone lesion in 6 to 24 per cent of the cases, and the recurrence rate was higher in this group than in the group without the associated aneurysmal cysts.

CHONDROMYXOID FIBROMA

The chondromyxoid fibroma is an uncommon benign tumor of cartilage derivation first described as an entity in 1946 by Jaffé and Lichtenstein.

Clinical Features. This central bone tumor has a predilection for occurrence in young persons, approximately 75 per cent of patients being under the age of 25 years. There is no definite sex predilection. The majority of cases occur in long bones but it is also found in the small bones of the hands and feet, in the pelvic girdle and elsewhere sporadically. A case in the anterior mandible extending on either side of the symphysis of a 10-year-old girl has been reported by Schutt and Frost. It is extremely rare here, however, considering the relatively large series of cases of chondromyxoid fibroma in other bones reported, such as the 189 cases by Feldman and his associates, the 32 cases by Schajowicz and Gallardo, and the 76 cases by Rahimi and his associates. The possible cases in the jaws have been reviewed by Grotepass and his associates, adding an additional case, as have Davis and Tideman as well as Browne and Rivas.

Pain is the outstanding clinical characteristic of the lesion. Evident swelling is uncommon but does occur.

Histologic Features. This tumor characteristically exhibits lobulated myxomatous areas, fibrous areas and areas having a chondroid appearance, i.e., cells resembling chondroblasts and chondrocytes in lacunae in a chondroid matrix. In addition, foci of calcification are sometimes found. Care must be taken not to make a mistaken diagnosis of chondrosarcoma or mesenchymal chondrosarcoma.

Treatment. Conservative surgical excision is the preferred treatment for this benign tumor. However, recurrence of this tumor in other bones is not uncommon, particularly in young patients in whom the lesions appear to act somewhat more aggressively. Too few cases in the jaws have been reported to draw valid conclusions regarding biologic behavior here.

OSTEOMA

The osteoma is a benign neoplasm characterized by proliferation of either compact or cancellous bone usually in an endosteal or periosteal location. In many parts of the body it is not difficult to establish an incontrovertible diagnosis of osteoma. In the jaws, however, where infection is common, it is not always possible to differentiate a bony mass induced by irritation or inflammation from one of a true neoplastic nature. In addition, the so-called exo-

stoses and enostoses further complicate the picture, since they may produce a similar clinical, roentgenographic and histologic picture. Although their nature is unknown, they might more properly be considered developmental lesions.

Clinical Features. The osteoma is not a common oral lesion. Although it may arise at any age, it seems to be somewhat more common in the young adult. The lesion of periosteal origin manifests itself as a circumscribed swelling on the jaw producing obvious asymmetry, but it must not be confused with Garre's nonsuppurative sclerosing osteomyelitis or proliferative periostitis. The osteoma is a slow-growing tumor, and so the patient does not usually become alarmed. The osteoma of endosteal origin is slower to present clinical manifestations, since considerable growth must occur before there is expansion of the cortical plates (Fig. 2–57, *A, B*). There is seldom any pain associated with this tumor. Multiple osteomas of the jaws, as well as of long bones and skull, are a characteristic manifestation of Gardner's syndrome (q.v.).

The *soft-tissue osteoma* of the oral cavity is a relatively uncommon lesion, a total of 25 cases from the literature being reviewed and reported by Krolls and his co-workers. The lesion is also known as "osteoma mucosae," analogous to the well-recognized dermal lesion "osteoma cutis," and as "osseous choristoma" after Krolls. These lesions occur almost exclusively in the tongue, although occasional cases are found in the buccal mucosa. They occur at any age and present as a firm nodule ranging up to 2 cm. in diameter. Of the 25 reported cases, 18 occurred in females and only 7 in males but the significance of this is not known. The bone itself is normal, well-circumscribed lamellar bone, usually compact but sometimes showing fatty marrow (Fig. 2–58, *A, B*).

Roentgenographic Features. The central lesion usually appears within the jaw as a well-circumscribed radiopaque mass which is indistinguishable from scar bone (Fig. 2–57, *B*). Sometimes this osteoma is diffuse, but it must be differentiated from chronic sclerosing osteomyelitis. The periosteal form of the disease also is manifested as a sclerotic mass.

Histologic Features. The osteoma is composed either of extremely dense, compact bone or of coarse cancellous bone. In any given area the bone formed appears normal (Fig. 2–57, *C*). The lesion is most often well circumscribed, but not encapsulated. In some tumors foci of cartilage may be found, in which case the term "osteochondroma" is often used. Myxomatous

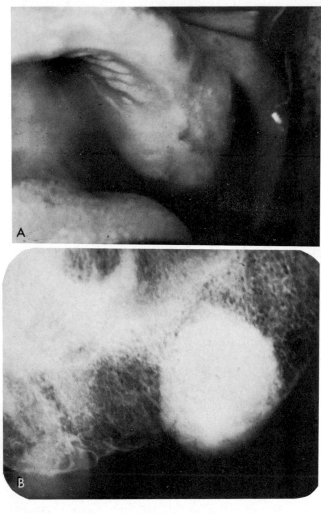

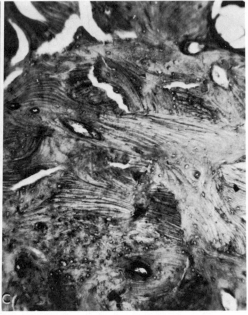

Figure 2–57. *Osteoma.*
The clinical expansion of the alveolar ridge (*A*) is seen on the roentgenogram (*B*) to be due to a well-circumscribed radiopaque mass. Microscopically, this was composed entirely of dense, compact bone (*C*).

tissue also may be intermingled on rare occasions.

Treatment and Prognosis. Treatment consists in surgical removal if the lesion is causing difficulty or if a prosthetic appliance is to be constructed, particularly when the tumor lies close to the surface of the alveolar bone. The osteoma does not recur after surgical removal.

Osteoid Osteoma

The osteoid osteoma is a benign tumor of bone which has seldom been described in the jaws. The true nature of this lesion is unknown. Jaffe and Lichtenstein have suggested that the lesion is a true neoplasm of osteoblastic derivation, but other workers have reported that the lesion occurs as a result of trauma or inflammation. In some instances it has been confused with chronic sclerosing osteomyelitis, and the

osteoid osteoma may actually represent a form of this osteomyelitis. A review of the literature with an additional report of 80 cases by Freiberger and his associates has supported the neoplastic theory.

Clinical Features. The osteoid osteoma usually occurs in young persons, seldom developing after the age of 30 years. Young children under the age of 10 years or even 5 years are frequently affected. In most series, males predominate over females by a ratio of at least 2 to 1. It has been reported most frequently in the femur or in the tibia, although other bones throughout the body have occasionally been involved. One of the chief symptoms of the condition is severe pain out of all proportion to the small size of the lesion. Localized swelling of the soft tissue over the involved area of bone may occur and may be tender.

Oral Manifestations. Greene and his associates have reviewed the literature and added

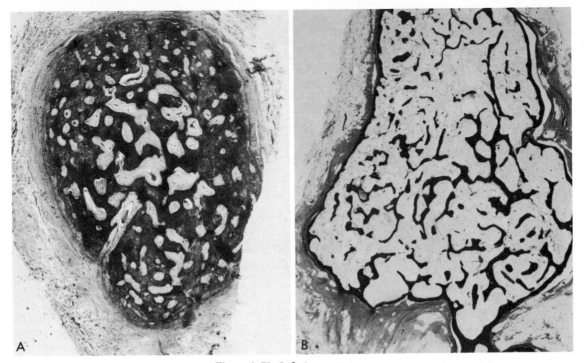

Figure 2–58. *Soft-tissue osteoma.*
The osteoma mucosae may be composed of quite dense bone (*A*) or very loose trabecular bone (*B*).

one more case, bringing the total number of cases of osteoid osteoma of the jaws to seven. Of these, four have occurred in the mandible and three in the maxilla. Of the mandibular lesions, three were in the body and one in the condyle, while one maxillary lesion involved the antrum.

Roentgenographic Features. Roentgenographically, the osteoid osteoma presents a pathognomonic picture characterized by a small ovoid or round radiolucent area surrounded by a rim of sclerotic bone. The central radiolucency may exhibit some calcification. The lesion seldom is larger than 1 cm. in diameter, but the overlying cortex does become thickened by subperiosteal new bone formation.

Histologic Features. The microscopic appearance of the osteoid osteoma is characteristic and consists of a central nidus composed of compact osteoid tissue, varying in degree of calcification, interspersed by a vascular connective tissue. Formation of definite trabeculae occurs, particularly in older lesions, outlined by active osteoblasts. Osteoclasts and foci of bone resorption are also usually evident. The overlying periosteum exhibits new bone formation, and in this interstitial tissue collections of lymphocytes may be noted.

Ultrastructural investigation of five cases of osteoid osteoma by Steiner has revealed the morphology of the osteoblasts to be similar to that of normal osteoblasts although atypical mitochondria could be seen. For comparison, the osteoblasts of a benign osteoblastoma were studied and were found to be essentially identical, including the atypical mitochondria. The author concluded that his observations supported the idea that the osteoid osteoma and the osteoblastoma are closely related lesions.

Treatment. The treatment of the osteoid osteoma consists of surgical removal of the lesion. If the lesion is completely excised, recurrence is not to be expected. There is fairly good circumstantial evidence that spontaneous regression may occur in at least some untreated cases.

BENIGN OSTEOBLASTOMA

(Giant Osteoid Osteoma)

The benign osteoblastoma was first described under the name "giant osteoid osteoma" by Dahlin and Johnson in 1954 and under the presently more accepted name by Jaffe and by Lichtenstein in 1956 in separate reports. The

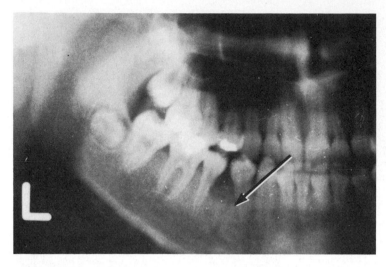

Figure 2–59. *Benign osteoblastoma.* (Courtesy of Dr. Ronald Vincent.)

lesion is not common but is nevertheless very important inasmuch as it is frequently mistaken for a malignant bone tumor even though it is actually entirely benign.

Clinical Features. This central bone tumor occurs most frequently in young persons, approximately 75 per cent of the patients being under 20 years of age and 90 per cent under 30 years of age. However, it does occur even in elderly adults. In most reported series, there is a definite predilection for occurrence in males. The lesion is characterized clinically by pain and swelling at the tumor site, the duration being just a few weeks to a year or more.

The most common site of occurrence is the vertebral column. Other frequently affected sites include the sacrum, long tubular bones and calvarium. The first case in the jaws was reported by Borello and Sedano in 1967, but it is now recognized that the benign osteoblastoma occurs in both the maxilla and mandible with some frequency, and a number of cases have been reported. These have been reviewed by Greer and Berman and, more recently, by Miller and his co-workers, who tabulated 26 cases: 14 mandible, 11 maxilla, and 1 unstated.

Roentgenographic Features. The lesion is not distinctive but, on the roentgenogram, appears rather well circumscribed. In some instances, there is purely bone destruction, while in other cases there is sufficient bone formation to produce a mottled, mixed radiolucent-radiopaque appearance (Fig. 2–59). A periosteal counterpart has been described by Goldman and such a case in the mandible is reported by Farman and his associates. The spectrum of the osteoblastoma is discussed by McLeod and his associates.

Histologic Features. There may be considerable variation in the microscopic appearance of the benign osteoblastoma. Nevertheless, the hallmark of the benign osteoblastoma consists of: (1) the vascularity of the lesion with many dilated capillaries scattered throughout the tissue, (2) the moderate numbers of multinucleated giant cells scattered throughout the tissue, and (3) the actively proliferating osteoblasts which pave the irregular trabeculae of new bone (Fig. 2–60). These osteoblasts often appear so active and are present in such numbers that, in the past, mistaken diagnoses of osteosarcoma have often been rendered. In addition, some cases bear remarkable resemblance to an aneurysmal bone cyst.

The osteoblastoma has been studied ultrastructurally by Steiner who noted that, with a few exceptions, the tumor osteoblasts resembled normal osteoblasts. Comparative differences of osteosarcoma cells from osteoblastoma cells also did not appear pathognomonic, so he concluded that the final diagnosis of osteoblastic tumors rested at the light microscope level.

A *malignant osteoblastoma* has been described by Schajowicz and Lemos on the basis of a histologically more bizarre pattern of cells: more abundant and often plump hyperchromatic nuclei, greater nuclear atypia, and numerous giant cells. While locally more aggressive than the benign osteoblastoma, it has a better prognosis than a conventional osteosarcoma.

Finally, malignant transformation of a previously benign osteoblastoma into an osteosarcoma has also been reported, such as the case discussed by Merryweather and his co-workers.

Treatment. Conservative surgical excision is

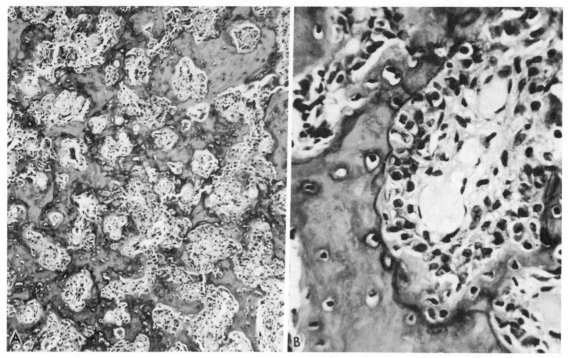

Figure 2–60. *Benign osteoblastoma.*

the preferred treatment for this tumor. Recurrence is rare.

TORUS PALATINUS

The torus palatinus is a slowly growing, flat-based bony protuberance or excrescence which occurs in the midline of the hard palate. Numerous theories have been suggested, but a plausible and thoroughly convincing explanation for this common oral lesion is still lacking. A study by Suzuki and Sakai offered evidence that both the torus palatinus and torus mandibularis are hereditary conditions, thought to follow a mendelian dominant pattern.

Clinical Features. The incidence of torus palatinus reported in the United States varies between 20 and 25 per cent. Women are affected more frequently than men, the approximate ratio found by Kolas and his associates being 2 to 1. Although the palatine torus may occur at any age, including the first decade, it appears to reach its peak incidence shortly before the age of 30 years. Certain races, such as the American Indian and the Eskimo, are reported to exhibit a much higher incidence of torus palatinus than the general population in this country, including blacks.

The torus palatinus presents itself as an out-growth in the midline of the palate and may assume a variety of shapes (Fig. 2–61; see also Plate III). It has been classified clinically on this basis as flat, spindle-shaped, nodular or lobular. The mucosa overlying the torus is intact, but occasionally appears blanched. It may become ulcerated if traumatized. The torus itself may be composed either of dense compact bone or of a shell of compact bone with a center of cancellous bone, and thus it is often visible on an intraoral palatal roentgenogram.

Treatment and Prognosis. There is little clinical significance attached to this lesion, since it is benign and never becomes malignant. The torus is usually not treated, although occasionally it may be of such size and shape that it is impossible or impractical to construct a full or partial denture over the structure because of undercuts, the probability of trauma to the overlying mucosa or inability to seat the denture, owing to rocking. In such cases the situation must be appraised and the torus removed surgically before the construction of the prosthetic appliance.

TORUS MANDIBULARIS

The torus mandibularis is an exostosis or outgrowth of bone found on the lingual surface

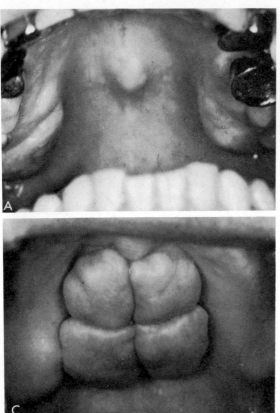

Figure 2–61. *Torus palatinus.*
This lesion may be a small outgrowth in the midline of the palate (A), a larger lobed mass (B), or may nearly completely fill the palatal vault (C).

of the mandible. Just as in the case of the palatine torus, numerous causes have been suggested, but the etiology of the torus mandibularis is actually still unknown.

A genetic or ethnic background is suggested, for example, by the high frequency of occurrence in Mongoloid groups and a low frequency in Caucasoid groups, as pointed out by Sellevold. Supporting this idea through familial investigations, Suzuki and Sakai have commented on its apparent hereditary nature. Essentially, their studies showed that when one or both parents had either type of torus, the frequency of occurrence of a torus in the children ranged between 40 and 64 per cent. When neither parent had a torus, the incidence of a torus in the children was only 5 to 8 per cent. In contrast, some studies seem to favor an environmental background as the more important factor. For example, it has been found that groups of the same population living in different environments have different frequencies of occurrence of this torus, while different racial groups living in approximately the same environment have similar frequencies of occurrence. It has been an idea held for many years

that a torus mandibularis will develop as a reinforcement of bone in this bicuspid area in response to the torsional stress created by heavy mastication.

Clinical Features. This growth on the lingual surface of the mandible occurs above the mylohyoid line, usually opposite the bicuspid teeth. Like the palatine torus, it may vary considerably in size and shape. Although the mandibular tori are usually bilateral, they are seen as a unilateral condition in about 20 per cent of the cases. Both unilateral and bilateral protuberances may be single or multiple, and they are frequently visible on dental periapical roentgenograms (Fig. 2–62). There is no correlation in the frequency of simultaneous occurrence of torus palatinus and torus mandibularis, according to the studies of Kolas and co-workers, suggesting that the two conditions are not related. Suzuki and Sakai reported a highly significant correlation in the frequency of simultaneous occurrence of the two tori, however.

The reported incidence in the United States varies between 6 and 8 per cent, with no differences between the sexes noted. Some

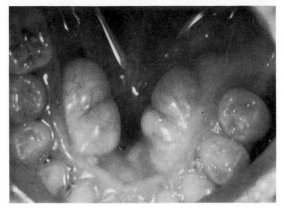

Figure 2–62. *Torus mandibularis.*
The bilateral bony growths on the lingual of the mandible may be lobed or multiple.

races, such as the Alaskan Eskimos and Aleuts, are reported to have a much higher incidence of mandibular tori. Among the general population in this country the torus mandibularis is infrequently seen in the first decade of life, but it usually has its onset by the age of 30 years.

Treatment and Prognosis. Surgical removal of the torus mandibularis may be necessary because of difficulties encountered in attempting to construct a denture over the outgrowth. The lesion is comparable to the torus palatinus in its benignity.

MULTIPLE EXOSTOSES

Multiple exostoses of the jaws are somewhat less common than the maxillary and mandibular tori and are usually found on the buccal surface of the maxilla below the mucobuccal fold in the

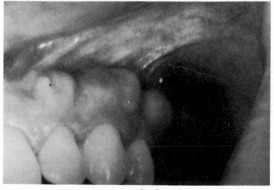

Figure 2–63. *Multiple exostoses.*
There are numerous small excrescences of bone on the buccal surface of the maxilla above the teeth and below the mucobuccal fold.

molar region. Clinically, these exostoses appear as small nodular protuberances over which the mucosa may appear blanched (Fig. 2–63).

Their etiology is unknown, and no figures are available as to their incidence or disposition. They are of no clinical significance except that, if large, they may interfere with the preparation or insertion of a prosthetic appliance.

MALIGNANT TUMORS OF CONNECTIVE TISSUE ORIGIN

FIBROSARCOMA

The fibrosarcoma was once considered to be one of the most common of the malignant soft-tissue neoplasms. However, the gradual separation of other tumors from this group as our knowledge of fibrous lesions increased has in effect reduced the apparent frequency of the disease, so that today fibrosarcoma, particularly of the head and neck area, is a quite uncommon neoplasm.

The sarcomas as a group differ from malignant epithelial neoplasms by their typical occurrence in relatively young persons and their greater tendency to metastasize through the blood stream rather than the lymphatics, thereby producing more widespread foci of secondary tumor growth.

Clinical Features. The fibrosarcoma may occur in any part of the body where the parent tissue is found. It does have a predilection for certain locations, however, and these include the skin and deeper subcutaneous tissue, muscles, tendons and tendon sheaths, and periosteum. In a series of 144 cases of fibrosarcoma of the soft tissues reported by Stout, 18 per cent occurred in the head and neck region.

The intraoral or paraoral fibrosarcoma may arise in any location, but is most commonly associated with the cheek, maxillary sinus, pharynx, palate, lip and periosteum of the maxilla or mandible. O'Day and his associates have reviewed the literature on oral soft-tissue fibrosarcoma and added 6 additional cases from the files of the Mayo Clinic. Of 13 cases of periosteal fibrosarcoma reported by Stout, 3 involved the mandible.

Dahlin and Ivins have reported a series of 114 cases of fibrosarcoma originating centrally in bone. Of these, 13 cases occurred in the mandible. In at least 4 of these cases there was some evidence of an odontogenic origin. One case was a postradiation sarcoma in a mandible affected by fibrous dysplasia. The investigators pointed out that differentiation of the central fibrosarcoma from other fibroblastic tumors, particularly the fibroblastic osteosarcoma, may be very difficult, but the distinction should be drawn because of the better 5-year survival rate of patients with fibrosarcoma of bone.

This neoplasm may have its onset at any age, but is most common before 50 years, 45 per cent of a series of 200 cases reported by Stout occurring between the ages of 20 and 40 years. Stout has also reported a series of 23 cases of fibrosarcoma occurring in infants and children, 3 of which involved the oral cavity—the tongue, gingiva and pharynx.

There is no particularly characteristic or pathognomonic clinical picture of fibrosarcoma about the head and neck. The tumor, which may develop rapidly or very slowly, tends to invade locally and to produce a fleshy, bulky lesion. This particular sarcoma does not exhibit a high frequency of metastasis. Ulceration, hemorrhage and secondary infection are seen in some cases, but the most typical finding is the asymmetric swelling and distortion.

Histologic Features. The fibrosarcoma is characterized by the proliferation of fibroblasts and the formation of collagen and reticulin fibers. Great variation exists between cases; some tumors appear extremely well differentiated and closely resemble the normal parent tissue, while others are poorly differentiated, the cells exhibiting all the features of a bizarre, highly anaplastic growth. The cells, which are usually spindle-shaped with elongated nuclei, and their associated fibers are generally arranged in interlacing bands or fascicles (Fig. 2–64). Since these bands run in different directions, the fibers may be seen in a variety of planes in any given tissue section and often produce a spiralling appearance.

Mitotic figures are prominent in the small group of poorly differentiated tumors, but in well-differentiated lesions they are difficult to find. Bizarre tumor giant cells are similarly uncommon.

Considerable difficulty is often encountered in differentiating this tumor from other lesions such as the liposarcoma, rhabdomyosarcoma and neurogenic sarcoma.

Treatment and Prognosis. The most accepted form of therapy for the fibrosarcoma is radical surgical excision. X-ray radiation is generally without effect, but a few cases have manifested a definite response to this type of treatment.

The prognosis of the fibrosarcoma is surprisingly favorable as compared to that of some other sarcomas. In a series of 145 cases reported by Stout, 52 per cent of the patients exhibited recurrence after treatment, but only 7 per cent of these patients had metastases and only 17 per cent are known to have died of their disease. A number of different factors enter into any consideration of survival, and one of the most important of these is the differentiation of the tumor cells. In the same series of 145 cases reported by Stout, 28 per cent were poorly

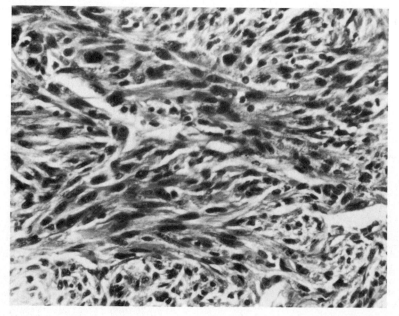

Figure 2–64. *Fibrosarcoma.*
The spindle cells show considerable nuclear variation with numerous mitotic figures.

differentiated, and of this group, 76 per cent recurred after treatment, 24 per cent metastasized, and 50 per cent of the patients died of tumor. The well differentiated lesions constituted 72 per cent of the group, and of these, 42 per cent recurred after treatment, none metastasized, and only 4 per cent of the patients died. The site of the tumor and its accessibility are also important factors in considering prognosis. In the series of fibrosarcoma of bone reported by Dahlin and Ivins, the 5-year survival rate was approximately 29 per cent, the prognosis being appreciably better in the histologically well-differentiated group. Although the majority of metastases occur through the blood stream, lymphatic involvement has been reported.

Miscellaneous Locally Aggressive Fibrous Lesions

There is a sizable group of locally aggressive but nonmetastasizing fibrous lesions which must always be differentiated from fibrosarcoma, particularly the well-differentiated type. In the past, many of these benign but locally aggressive lesions have been confused with sarcoma, and it is only in recent years that the pathologist has been able to separate these lesions with any assurance.

All of these lesions are quite uncommon in the oral cavity and, for this reason, no detailed description of them will be made here. This group consists chiefly of the following:

1. Nodular fasciitis (pseudosarcomatous fibromatosis)
2. Aggressive fibromatosis (extra-abdominal desmoid)
3. Proliferative myositis
4. Fibrous histiocytoma (fibroxanthoma)
5. Atypical fibroxanthoma (and malignant variant)
6. Desmoplastic fibroma of bone

Each of these lesions has been described in detail in the Atlas of Tumor Pathology Fascicle on Tumors of the Soft Tissues (AFIP) by Stout and Lattes and in the World Health Organization (WHO) publication on Histological Typing of Soft Tissue Tumors by Enzinger, Lattes and Torloni.

Definitions of each of the above lesions have been proposed in this WHO monograph and are reproduced as follows:

1. *Nodular fasciitis.* "A benign and probably reactive fibroblastic growth extending as a solitary nodule from the superficial fascia into the subcutaneous fat or, less frequently, into the subjacent muscle. Confusion with a sarcoma is possible because of its cellularity, its mitotic activity, its richly mucoid stroma, and its rapid growth. Other fibroblastic proliferations, such as proliferative myositis, are probably akin to this lesion. Nodular fasciitis is most common in the upper extremity, the trunk and the neck region of young adults."

Nodular fasciitis of the head and neck has been described in detail by Werning, who reported 41 cases in this area and reviewed the pertinent literature. In his series, lesions occurred in every age group but were most common in the third through the fifth decade of life. These lesions developed most often within subcutaneous tissues overlying the mandible and zygoma, although intraoral lesions of buccal mucosa, tongue and alveolar mucosa also occurred. Since so many of the cases occurred in areas which serve as sites of origin or insertion of muscles of mastication and which are particularly vulnerable to trauma, Werning has emphasized that this lends support to the theory that nodular fasciitis is a pseudoneoplastic exuberant fibroblastic or myofibroblastic reactive process. These were usually firm, painless masses but, on occasion, there was pain, tenderness and a history of rapid growth. The treatment for this lesion is surgical excision and recurrence is rare.

2. *Aggressive fibromatosis.* "A non-metastasizing tumour-like fibroblastic growth of unknown pathogenesis involving voluntary muscle as well as aponeurotic and fascial structures. Histologically, it is indistinguishable from an abdominal fibromatosis. The lesion has a strong tendency to local recurrence and aggressive, infiltrating growth. It is most common in the shoulder girdle, the thigh, and the buttock of young adults."

Aggressive fibromatosis of the oral or paraoral structures has been reported on occasion but it is quite uncommon in this location. Melrose and Abrams, reporting three cases involving the jaws of children, have discussed the protean nature of this group. For example, some are rapidly enlarging while others are of quite slow growth. Pain may or may not be present. When in apposition to bone, destruction of the bone occurs. The microscopic appearance of their lesions was quite uniform, however, consisting of cellular interlacing bundles of elongated fibroblasts showing no pleomorphism, little or no mitotic activity and no giant cells but typically with numerous slit-like vascular spaces not associated with inflammation. Treatment consists of complete surgical excision with generous margins of normal tissue. Recurrence is always a strong possibility and some workers recommend prolonged indefinite follow-up.

3. *Proliferative myositis.* "A rapidly growing, poorly circumscribed, probably reactive proliferation of fibroblasts and ganglion-cell-like giant cells involving chiefly the connective tissue framework of striated muscle tissue. In contrast to myositis ossificans, a history of preceding trauma is infrequent and the lesion occurs chiefly in patients older than 45 years. The lesion is benign and should not be mistaken for a rhabdomyosarcoma or some other malignant neoplasm. Proliferative myositis has been discussed in Chapter 17 on Diseases of Nerves and Muscles (q.v.).

4. *Fibrous histiocytoma.* "A benign, unencapsulated and often richly vascular growth made up of histiocytes and collagen-producing fibroblast-like cells, which are arranged in a whorled or cartwheel pattern. Frequently, the growth contains lipid-carrying macrophages. It may occur anywhere but is most common in the dermis."

The fibrous histiocytoma actually comprises a group of lesions with varying histologic features dependent upon the pathway of development or differentiation of the basic histiocyte inasmuch as it is now recognized that this cell may have a bimodal differentiation pattern: into a phagocytic histiocyte or into a collagen-forming fibroblast. Tumors, both benign and malignant, composed of these two forms of cells occur at many sites in the body. The benign tumor has borne many names, depending on histology and anatomic site, including xanthoma, fibroxanthoma, xanthogranuloma, sclerosing hemangioma, dermatofibroma, villonodular synovitis and giant cell tumor of tendon among others. While these are usually spoken of as tumors and even though there is a malignant counterpart, the malignant fibrous histiocytoma, there is not yet total agreement that this group of lesions represents true neoplasms and not reactive, proliferative hyperplasia of tissue.

Fibrous histiocytomas of the oral cavity are relatively uncommon. A total of five such cases have been reviewed and reported by Hoffman and Martinez. Children and young adults are most frequently affected and cases have occurred at a variety of sites such as lip, tongue and buccal mucosa. Treatment is surgical excision and there is no recurrence.

Malignant fibrous histiocytoma is now rec-

ognized as one of the more common sarcomas of the soft tissues of the body. It is often subclassified into four chief variants: fibrous, giant cell, inflammatory (interestingly, the most aggressive of the four) and myxoid. However, as an entity it is rare in the head and neck area and oral cavity. Van Hale and her associates have reviewed the reported cases, noting only nine in the mouth and only one of these originating in the soft tissues. The remainder occurred centrally in the maxilla or mandible. This lesion has been reported to metastasize in nearly one-fourth of all cases by Weiss and Enzinger and, therefore, must be treated very vigorously and promptly.

5. *Atypical fibroxanthoma.* "A probably benign growth, which is closely related to fibroxanthoma but shows a much greater degree of cellular pleomorphism with multinucleated giant cells and occasional giant cells of the Touton type as well as numerous mitotic figures, including atypical forms. The relatively small size of the lesion (generally less than 3 cm.), its prevalence in the sun-damaged or irradiated skin of elderly individuals, and the fact that it is usually well-circumscribed, help in the difficult differential diagnosis from malignant fibroxanthoma. It probably does not occur in the oral cavity.

6. *Desmoplastic fibroma of bone.* This is a lesion of bone, including the jaws, which is histologically indistinguishable from aggressive fibromatosis or the extra-abdominal desmoid. Although there is a wide spread in the age of occurrence, the vast majority of cases have occurred in the second decade. The lesion does not metastasize but often shows local recurrence. Wide local excision is, therefore, the treatment of choice.

The desmoplastic fibroma of the jaws has been reviewed by Freedman and his associates, who have analyzed and discussed 26 cases described in the literature. They found also that nearly all cases in this location occurred in the first three decades of life with the vast majority involving the mandible, particularly the molar-ramus-angle area. Swelling of the jaw was the common presenting complaint, pain or tenderness rarely being present. In a high percentage of cases, the lesions appeared as well-delineated radiolucencies, either unilocular or multilocular. The broadening of the microscopic parameters of this lesion was also emphasized by Freedman, who summarized the concept of the desmoplastic fibroma of bone as being composed of cells that may be either small and uniform, plump and uniform, or both in the same lesion, set in a variably collagenized stroma. The cells lack anaplastic forms or significant numbers of mitotic figures. Treatment of this lesion appears to be surgical excision or thorough curettage. Recurrence of jaw lesions has been uncommon.

SYNOVIAL SARCOMA

Synovial sarcoma is a distinctive malignancy usually arising from articular or para-articular sites, bursae or tendon sheaths, especially of the extremities. However, it does occur in other somatic soft tissues and in the head and neck area with some frequency.

Clinical Features. The synovial sarcoma of the neck area is predominantly a disease of young people, the median age being 19 years in a series of 24 cases reported by Roth and his associates. The presenting complaint is usually a painless, deep-seated swelling which may produce difficulties in breathing or swallowing. The majority of the cases in this series originated in the hypopharyngeal, retropharyngeal or hyoid areas. However, intraoral cases may occur, according to the review of Mitcherling and his co-workers. These sites include the submandibular area, cheek, tongue, floor of mouth and soft palate.

Histologic Features. The tumor is characterized by a biphasic cellular pattern of cleft-like or slit-like spaces lined by cuboidal epithelial-like cells. The spaces may contain a PAS-positive mucoid material. The second pattern is comprised of a fibrosarcoma-like proliferation of cells with associated collagen and reticulin. A monophasic pattern without the slit-like spaces exists but is very uncommon.

Treatment. Early radical excision probably offers the best results for synovial sarcoma of the head and neck, although experience with cases in this area is quite limited. In other sites, the 5-year survival rate has varied between about 25 and 50 per cent. However, these tumors can metastasize and, significantly, in at least one series, no patient with metastasis was cured. Although these tumors are relatively resistant to x-ray radiation, some workers have shown good results with combined surgery and radiation.

LIPOSARCOMA

Liposarcoma is an extremely uncommon malignant mesenchymal neoplasm, especially of the head and neck area. According to Baden and Newman in an excellent review of the tumor in this region, only 4 per cent of all liposarcomas are found in this site. This is in contrast to the lipoma in which the head and neck is a common location.

Clinical Features. The liposarcoma of the head and neck region occurs most frequently in adults over the age of 40 years, although there is a wide range, from children to the very elderly. There is a significant predilection for occurrence in males in a ratio of about 2 to 1 over females.

It characteristically has a slow, silent growth, submucosal or deep in location, producing a firm, resilient lesion, sometimes lobulated, and often suggestive of a cyst.

Histologic Features. The lesion has been classified in a number of ways, one of the most useful by Enzinger as: (1) myxoid, (2) round cell, (3) adult, and (4) pleomorphic types. In general, these tumors consist of fat cells and lipoblasts in varying degrees of differentiation and anaplasia, with a variable stromal component, all of which is indicative of the basic type of liposarcoma involved. The microscopic diagnosis requires skill and experience and the characteristic features of each individual type are too variable to be discussed succinctly here.

However, it has been noted by Baden and Newman that the majority of liposarcomas of the head and neck area (71 per cent of 35 reported cases) were myxoid liposarcomas and that the majority of these were well-differentiated neoplasms with an excellent prognosis.

Treatment and Prognosis. Surgical excision with or without radiation therapy has been used to treat these lesions. Prognosis depends upon many factors, especially cell type of the tumor, although according to the review by Saunders and his associates, less than half of reported patients were living without evidence of disease.

HEMANGIOENDOTHELIOMA

The hemangioendothelioma is a neoplasm of mesenchymal origin which is angiomatous in nature and derived from the endothelial cells. It was first reported under this name in 1899 by Bormann, who also proposed a complete histogenetic classification of the blood vessel tumors. At one time, this tumor was divided into a benign and a malignant form. At present, however, the term *benign hemangioendothelioma* is used only to describe an unusual vascular tumor of the liver. In addition, the term was considered at one time to be synonymous with *juvenile hemangioendothelioma,* although this latter lesion is currently recognized as being simply a cellular hemangioma. Thus, the proper usage of the term for the neoplasm under discussion here is malignant hemangioendothelioma or hemangioendotheliosarcoma, there being no recognized benign hemangioendothelioma except for the hepatic lesion mentioned above.

Clinical Features. This neoplasm may occur anywhere in the body, but is most commonly found in the skin and subcutaneous tissues. Primary lesions of the oral cavity, though not common, have been reported in a variety of locations, including the lips, palate, gingiva, tongue and centrally within the maxilla and mandible. The literature pertaining to malignant hemangioendotheliomas of the oral cavity was reviewed by Wesley and his associates and Zachariades and his co-workers, who tabulated 46 reported oral cases.

The hemangioendothelioma arises at any age and has been found present even at birth. Females appear to be affected almost twice as often as males. Localized swelling may be the primary manifestation of the lesion, although pain is occasionally present as well.

The malignant hemangioendothelioma is similar to the hemangioma in appearance and is usually manifested clinically as a flat or slightly raised lesion of varying size, dark red or bluish red, sometimes ulcerated and showing a tendency to bleed after even slight trauma. Bone may be involved by the tumor, producing a destructive process.

Histologic Features. The typical malignant hemangioendothelioma is composed of masses of endothelial cells often arranged in columns. Capillary formation is poorly defined, although anastomosing vascular channels may be discerned. A silver reticulin stain best demonstrates this vascularity, and characteristically the tumor cells lie within the reticulin sheath enclosing each vessel. The individual cells are pleomorphic, large, polyhedral or slightly flattened, with a faint outline and a round nucleus with multiple minute nucleoli. Mitotic figures are seen in some lesions, although they are not a constant finding. The malignant hemangioendothelioma is an infiltrative lesion and is not encapsulated.

Treatment and Prognosis. Both surgery and x-ray radiation have been utilized in the management of the malignant hemangioendothelioma. Repeated surgical intervention without complete removal appears to invite metastases to regional lymph nodes or to distant organs by blood-stream dissemination.

Seven cases have been reported by Stout, and, of these, five patients had metastases and three died of their neoplasm. Of those oral cases with the follow-up information reviewed by Zachariades and his associates, the 5-year post-treatment survival rate of 24 cases was only 25 per cent and two-year survival was only 50 per cent.

HEMANGIOPERICYTOMA

The hemangiopericytoma is a vascular neoplasm characterized by the proliferation of capillaries surrounded by masses of round or spindle-shaped cells. It resembles the glomus tumor, but lacks its organoid pattern, encapsulation and clinical manifestation of pain. Stout and Murray in 1942 suggested the term "hemangiopericytoma" after Murray had shown by tissue culture of the glomus tumor that the characteristic cell was probably the "pericyte" of Zimmerman, a cell with contractile properties, but no myofibrils, although it has been assumed to be related to smooth muscle cells. Stout subsequently studied an undefined group of tumors, noted the resemblance of the neoplastic cells to those of the glomus tumor cells which had been identified as pericytes, and named this group of neoplasms the hemangiopericytoma.

It is generally accepted that both a benign and a malignant form of this tumor exist but that there are serious difficulties in formulating dependable criteria for distinguishing between the two. That prediction of the biologic behavior of the lesion based on morphologic grounds has been found to be unreliable was emphasized by Angervall and his co-workers in their study.

Clinical Features. The hemangiopericytoma is an uncommon tumor which has been found to have a wide anatomic distribution, including the oral cavity. It appears to have no sex predilection, and the age range of patients reported is birth to old age, the majority of cases occurring before 50 years. Backwinkel and Diddams have presented a comprehensive review of the literature, finding 247 reported cases.

The lesions are firm, apparently circumscribed and often nodular, and may or may not exhibit redness indicative of their vascular nature (Fig. 2–65). Although the tumor may appear encapsulated at operation, this is often not confirmed microscopically. The majority of tu-

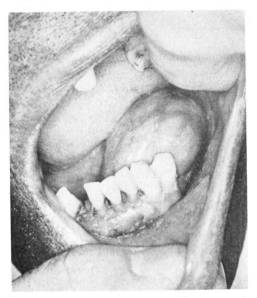

Figure 2–65. *Hemangiopericytoma of floor of mouth.*
(Courtesy of Dr. Irwin A. Small; from I. A. Small and
H. J. Bloom: J. Oral Surg., *17*:65, 1959.)

mors grow rapidly and are therefore of short
duration, although tumors with a history of
many years are known. Occasionally, central
hemangiopericytomas of bone occur, four such
cases being reported by Unni and his associates.

Only about 5 per cent of hemangiopericytomas in the series of Stout occurred in the oral
cavity and pharynx. An interesting case in the
floor of the mouth has been reported by Small
and Bloom.

Histologic Features.   The great histologic
variation between cases of hemangiopericytoma
often leads to considerable difficulty in their

diagnosis. The lesion is characterized by the
profuse proliferation of occult capillaries. Each
vessel in turn is surrounded by a connective
tissue sheath, outside of which are found masses
of tumor cells. This relation of tumor cells to
vessel sheaths may be demonstrated by a silver
stain and is important in differentiating this
tumor from the hemangioendothelioma. The
tumor cells of the hemangiopericytoma vary
considerably in size and shape, appearing large
or small, round to spindle-shaped. These cells
often show a characteristic tendency for concentric layering about the capillaries (Fig. 2–66).

Treatment and Prognosis.   The treatment of
most reported cases of hemangiopericytoma has
been surgical excision. Some patients have been
cured by this means, while others (13 per cent
in the series of Stout) have suffered metastases
not only in lymph nodes, but also in distant
organs. Stout has pointed out that no congenital
hemangiopericytoma is known to have been
malignant. However, according to the findings
of Backwinkel and Diddams in 224 cases with
available information, the total local and distant
recurrence rate of the hemangiopericytoma was
52 per cent.

MULTIPLE IDIOPATHIC HEMORRHAGIC SARCOMA OF KAPOSI

(Kaposi's Sarcoma; Angioreticuloendothelioma)

Kaposi's sarcoma is an unusual and uncommon disease of blood vessels which occasionally
manifests in the oral cavity. Although rare in
the United States, the disease is extremely

Figure 2–66. *Hemangiopericytoma.*
(Courtesy of Dr. Irwin A. Small;
from I. A. Small and H. J. Bloom: J.
Oral Surg., *17*:65, 1959.)

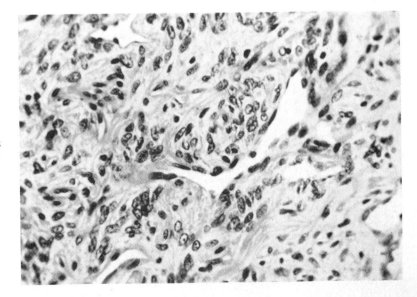

common in certain areas of Africa and is said to comprise over 10 per cent of all malignancies occurring in both children and adults there. Furthermore, the African form of the disease is very aggressive and has a rapidly ingravescent course in contrast to the usual indolent course of the disease in the United States.

The etiology of the disease is unknown, but the condition is considered by most workers to be neoplastic in nature. Other theories have proposed that Kaposi's sarcoma is an infectious granuloma or a reticuloendothelial hyperplasia. Within recent years increasing numbers of cases of Kaposi's sarcoma have been reported as developing simultaneously in patients with one of the malignant lymphomas or other forms of cancer. In fact, in a follow-up study of 63 patients with Kaposi's sarcoma by O'Brien and Brasfield, 31 per cent were found to have died of a second primary cancer, including lymphoma and myeloma as well as melanoma and carcinoma of the colon, breast, prostate, tongue, tonsil and pancreas. This is considered by most investigators to be more than a chance occurrence. Tedeschi has presented an extensive discussion of the nature of Kaposi's sarcoma with a thorough review of the literature.

Clinical Features. Kaposi's sarcoma may occur at any age, but is most common in the fifth, sixth and seventh decades, except in Africa where childhood involvement is common as well. Between 85 and 90 per cent of all reported cases have occurred in males, suggesting at least some endocrine basis. Choisser and Ramsey, in an excellent review of this subject, found that of the many reported cases in men, these were most frequent in laborers and out-of-door workers. Cox and Helwig have reviewed 50 additional cases of this disease and concluded, as have most other current investigators, that this is a neoplastic disease of the vascular system with multiple foci of origin.

The multiple skin lesions usually originate on the extremities, but subsequently involve the face and sometimes the oral cavity, as well as many visceral organs and lymph nodes. They appear as reddish or brownish-red nodules which may vary in size from a few millimeters to a centimeter or more in diameter and are usually tender or painful. The lesions of the oral mucosa are identical in appearance with the cutaneous nodules, and at least one case has been reported in which an oral lesion appeared before the skin manifestations (Fig. 2–67). Cervical lymph node and salivary gland involvement commonly precedes cutaneous and

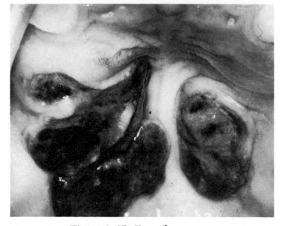

Figure 2–67. *Kaposi's sarcoma.*
Lesions of the palate are present in a patient with diffuse cutaneous involvement. (Courtesy of Dr. Stephen F. Dachi.)

visceral involvement in the disease in African children.

Histologic Features. The microscopic pattern of Kaposi's sarcoma is extremely variable. The lesion may consist of numerous, small capillary-type blood vessels which may or may not be blood-containing. When this feature predominates, the lesion may be confused with a hemangioma. Elsewhere, lesions in this disease may be extremely cellular, consisting of proliferating masses of embryonic-appearing spindle cells of varying size, shape and appearance showing occasional mitoses, with hyperemic vascular slits. Inflammatory cell infiltration is common, and Coburn and Morgan emphasized changes in the blood vessel walls similar to those seen in polyarteritis nodosa. They suggest that the development of the disease takes place in three stages: inflammation, granuloma and neoplasia, the initial lesion being primarily a polyvasculitis.

Treatment and Prognosis. Surgical eradication of the disease is difficult because of the multiplicity of lesions. Various forms of x-ray radiation have been used with considerable success, comparable to that in treatment of other vascular lesions. Chemotherapeutic agents have also been used beneficially.

The prognosis is good because of the chronic, slowly progressive nature of the condition. Many lesions will actually regress over a period of time. Cases have been reported which persisted for as long as 25 years only to terminate fatally. The mean survival time of a group of patients dying of the disease has been reported by O'Brien and Brasfield as being 9 years with a range of 1 to 22 years, while McCarthy and Pack estimated the mean duration between diagnosis and death to be 8 years.

Relation to Acquired Cellular Immune Deficiency Syndrome. A very unusual syndrome of diseases has been recognized within the past few years which appears related to a breakdown in the immune system of the body. The patients may first develop an unexplained fever, weight loss and lymphadenopathy. Medical examination may then reveal: (1) oral candidosis, (2) pneumocystis pneumonia, (3) cytomegalovirus viruria, (4) depressed T-lymphocytes and (5) Kaposi's sarcoma of a fulminating type similar to that seen in Africa, rather than the indolent form common in the United States. Each patient does not necessarily manifest all syndromic characteristics listed, however. The vast majority of patients discovered to date have been homosexual males, although a few heterosexual males and females have been afflicted as well. The disease has been most prevalent in California and New York, but numerous cases have occurred elsewhere. The death rate among these persons is exceptionally high, although the actual cause of death may be any one or more of the variable factors of the syndrome.

The cause of the disease is unknown. It appears to represent an acquired immune deficiency whose triggering mechanism is being sought intensely.

EWING'S SARCOMA

(Endothelial Myeloma; "Round Cell" Sarcoma)

Ewing's sarcoma is an uncommon malignant neoplasm which occurs as a primary destructive lesion of bone. The origin of the cells has been questioned ever since the original description of the tumor by James Ewing, who believed that they were derived from marrow endothelium. Some authorities think that the tumor arises from undifferentiated cells of the reticuloendothelial system. Yet even in the review of Ewing's sarcoma by Dahlin and his group and presentation of their series of 165 cases, it was concluded that the nature of the parent cell is still in dispute, so that use of the eponym must still be continued to distinguish this entity.

Clinical Features. This neoplastic disease occurs predominantly in children and young adults between the ages of 5 and 25 years, but is seen on occasion in older patients. In the series of 107 cases reported by Bhansali and Desai, 6 patients were over the age of 40 years,

the oldest being an 83-year-old woman. Thus it arises in the same general age group in which osteogenic sarcoma is most prevalent. It was reported to be approximately twice as common in males as in females in a series of cases of Geschickter and Copeland and also in the series of Dahlin and his associates and that of Pomeroy and Johnson. It is noteworthy that an episode of trauma often precedes the development of the tumor, although it must not be inferred that this is in any manner important in the etiology of the neoplasm.

Pain, usually of an intermittent nature, and swelling of the involved bone are often the earliest clinical signs and symptoms of Ewing's sarcoma. The bones most commonly affected are the long bones of the extremities, although the skull, clavicle, ribs and shoulder and pelvic girdles may be involved, as well as the maxilla and mandible. The jaws were involved in 13 per cent of a series of 126 cases reported by Geschickter and Copeland. Nine additional cases, eight in the mandible and one in the maxilla, have been reported by Potdar.

Facial neuralgia and lip paresthesia have been reported in cases of jaw involvement. The appearance of the jaw swelling is often a relatively rapid one, and the intraoral mass may become ulcerated. The patient may have a low-grade fever and an elevated white blood cell count, and these findings have often given rise to an erroneous tentative diagnosis of an infection.

An extraskeletal form of this tumor has been described by Angervall and Enzinger and termed *Ewing's sarcoma of soft tissues*. The ultrastructural characteristics of the cells constituting this tumor, studied by Gillespie and his associates, among others, are identical to those of the typical Ewing's cells.

Roentgenographic Features. The roentgenographic appearance of Ewing's sarcoma has been described as being suggestive but not pathognomonic of the disease. The lesion is a destructive one and produces an irregular, diffuse radiolucency, although lesions of the jaw resembling sclerosing osteomyelitis have been described.

A common characteristic roentgenographic feature is the formation of layers of new subperiosteal bone producing the so-called "onion-skin" appearance on the film. This thickened cortex is usually infiltrated by tumor. Osteophyte formation may also be visible on the roentgenogram and, in such cases, may be similar to the "sun-ray" appearance of osteosarcoma.

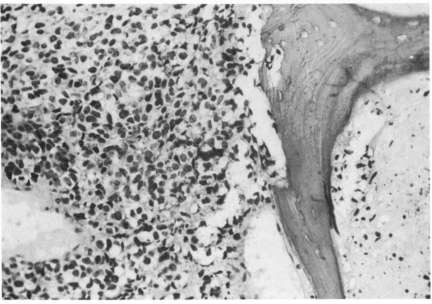

Figure 2–68. *Ewing's sarcoma.*
Encroachment of tumor cells on a bone trabecula causing its ragged resorption is apparent. Necrosis is also present on the opposite side of the fragment of bone.

Histologic Features. Ewing's sarcoma is an extremely cellular neoplasm composed of solid sheets or masses of small round cells with very little stroma, although a few connective tissue septa may be present (Fig. 2–68). The cells themselves are small and round, with little cytoplasm and relatively large round or ovoid nuclei. Mitotic figures are common. Many tiny vascular channels may also be present. There is a noteworthy absence of multinucleated giant cells. Necrosis is a common microscopic feature. However, as Telles and his associates pointed out in an autopsy study of 26 cases of Ewing's sarcoma, increased cellular pleomorphism and increased numbers of bizarre giant cells may be found in the lesions in patients treated with radiation and adjuvant chemotherapy.

The cells of Ewing's sarcoma can generally be differentiated from reticulum cell sarcoma with little difficulty. In some cases of Ewing's sarcoma, however, the cells are larger and may simulate the malignant lymphoma. Schajowicz has reported that tumor cells of Ewing's sarcoma contain histochemically demonstrable glycogen, which is absent in cells of the reticulum cell sarcoma, thus providing an easy method of differentiation. The importance of intracytoplasmic glycogen in the diagnosis of Ewing's sarcoma has been reaffirmed by Telles and his co-workers, who also emphasized that therapy did not alter the presence of this glycogen.

Treatment and Prognosis. This neoplasm is radiosensitive, but unfortunately, in the past, has seldom been cured by x-ray radiation. Radical surgical excision has been done, alone and coupled with x-ray radiation, but it has been common for metastatic foci to appear in other bones and organs, such as lungs and lymph nodes, within a matter of a few weeks or months. In a review of 646 cases by Bhansali and Desai, only 8.7 per cent of patients survived for 5 years.

Recently, a more aggressive therapeutic approach has been used involving a combination of surgery, radiation and chemotherapy. In a series of such patients, Rosen and his associates reported an 85 per cent survival free of disease for periods of up to 26 months.

CHONDROSARCOMA

The chondrosarcoma is the malignant counterpart of the chondroma and, like the benign lesion, may occur in either the maxilla or the mandible, as well as in many other bones in the body. It has been discussed in detail by Barnes and Catto. Until recent years this malignant neoplasm was indiscriminantly classed with osteosarcoma, but careful review of clinical data has indicated the need for their definite separation, since the cartilaginous tumor has a better prognosis. The chondrosarcoma is sometimes classified as primary or secondary in type. The secondary type is one which develops in a pre-existing benign cartilaginous tumor, whereas the primary type develops *de novo*. It is of considerable interest that malignant cartilaginous tumors of the jaws are far more common than benign cartilaginous tumors.

Clinical Features. There are no pathognomonic signs or symptoms presented by the chondrosarcoma, nor may it be differentiated from the chondroma purely on the basis of the clinical findings. The tumor can occur at any age between 10 and 80 years. However, in the series of 288 cases reported by Henderson and Dahlin, the peak incidence was between 30 and 60 years, while in the series of 151 cases of McKenna and his associates, it was between 30 and 50 years. The secondary chondrosarcoma occurs at an earlier age than the primary chondrosarcoma, by an average of about 10 years. In general, chondrosarcomas occur more often in males, in a ratio of about 2 to 1.

Mesenchymal chondrosarcoma is a characteristic and distinctive type of chondrosarcoma in which the majority of cases occur between the ages of 10 and 30 years, and in which there is an approximately equal sex distribution. In addition, the most common sites of origin are the jaws and ribs, according to Salvador and his associates.

Clear cell chondrosarcoma is a recognized variant of the usual chondrosarcoma from which it should be separated because of its slow growth pattern and its favorable clinical course with low metastatic potential and high probability of cure. Without radical excision, however, death can result. It may occur in the jaws, and such a case has been reported by Slootweg.

Oral Manifestations. Chaudhry and his associates have reviewed all cartilaginous tumors of the jaws reported in the English literature between 1912 and 1959. Both primary and secondary jaw chondrosarcomas appear as an expanding lesion which is frequently painless (Fig. 2–69, *A*). The mucosa is often intact. The tumor may occur in the mandible or the maxilla with primary involvement of the alveolar ridge, or sometimes in the maxilla near the antrum. Resorption and exfoliation of teeth sometimes occur. In general, these lesions are invasive and destructive and metastasize readily.

Roentgenographic Features. Roentgenographic findings do not differ remarkably from those seen in the benign chondroma unless the lesion is of relatively long standing and has produced considerable destruction of bone. Occasional tumors will appear as radiopaque lesions because of calcification of the neoplastic cartilage (Fig. 2–69, *B*, *C*).

Histologic Features. The microscopic examination of cartilage tumors commonly leads to an improper diagnosis if insufficient tissue is available for study, since different areas of the chondrosarcoma may show considerable variation. The neoplasm is composed of hyaline cartilage, and in this respect resembles the chondroma. It may also show ossification and thus resemble the osteogenic sarcoma. The important feature lies in the appearance of the cartilage cells. In the malignant form of this disease there is considerable variation in size of the cells, and binucleated cells are common (Fig. 2–69, *D*). The absence of mitotic figures is of little significance, however. The cytologic abnormalities merit greatest consideration, but in certain areas of these tumors anaplasticity is not a prominent feature. The cartilage may appear typical, but calcification or ossification is usually abnormal.

The *mesenchymal chondrosarcoma* consists of sheets of small, round or ovoid, undifferentiated cells interspersed by small islands of well-differentiated cartilage which often show calcification and metaplastic bone formation. Ultrastructural studies by Steiner and his associates have confirmed the presence of two cell types: a poorly differentiated mesenchymal cell and a cell with cartilaginous differentiation in an early stage of maturation.

The *clear cell chondrosarcoma* consists of single or clustered benign giant cells and tumor cells with clear cytoplasm. Conventional low-grade chondrosarcoma may sometimes be found in areas.

Treatment and Prognosis. The only beneficial treatment of the chondrosarcoma is surgery. The malignant nature of this tumor demands wide excision to ensure the greatest possibility for cure. X-ray radiation is of little value, since this type of neoplasm is resistant to such therapy. Neither does chemotherapy appear to be of significant benefit.

The data gathered from known cases of chondrosarcoma of the jaws indicate that the tumor in this location is exceedingly dangerous and often results in death, either from local invasion or from metastasis to distant sites. Although the lesion tends to grow slowly, surgical intervention often stimulates the growth rate and increases the tendency for metastasis.

The *mesenchymal chondrosarcoma* is even more variable in its clinical course, since metastasis may occur many years after the original surgical procedure and death is markedly delayed. Expression of "5-year survival" is of little significance in the case of this tumor.

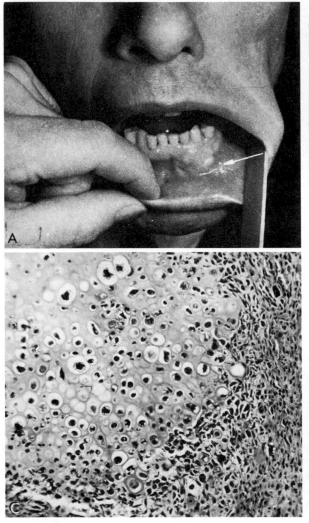

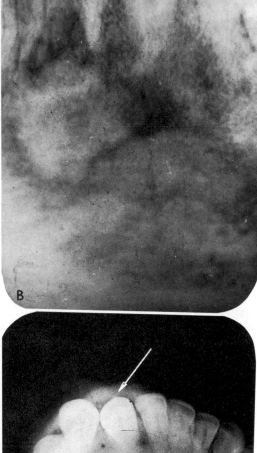

Figure 2–69. *Chondrosarcoma.*
The clinical expansion of the mandible (*A*) manifests obvious changes in the dental roentgenograms (*B*, *C*). The photomicrograph (*D*) illustrates malignant cartilage cells comprising the neoplasm. (Courtesy of Dr. Charles A. Waldron.)

OSTEOSARCOMA

(Osteogenic Sarcoma)

The osteosarcoma consists of a group of comparatively rare primary malignant neoplasms of bone which exhibit considerable variation not only in the clinical and histologic appearance, but also in the course and prognosis of the disease. The tumor as defined by most investi-gators is composed of cells and tissues in different stages of bone development, and for this reason one might expect a wide range of types. The Registry of Bone Sarcoma of the American College of Surgeons recognizes a classification of this disease based partially upon location (e.g., periosteal, medullary) and partially upon histologic pattern (e.g., telangiectatic type when vascularity is prominent). Such a classification is cumbersome and unnecessary here. For purposes of simplification, the osteosarcoma has often been divided into two forms: an osteoblastic or sclerosing type and an osteolytic type. The latter lesion is far less differentiated, since, as the name indicates, it does not reach the stage of bone formation. Coventry and Dahlin, in a critical review of 430 cases of osteosarcoma, classified the lesion histologically as either osteoblastic, chondroblastic or fibroblastic, but they point out that this division is arbitrary in some cases. Nevertheless, this classification is in wide use today.

Clinical Features. Osteosarcoma occurs chiefly in young persons, the majority between 10 and 25 years of age, with a decreasing incidence as age increases. Males are affected more frequently than females. The predominant site of this tumor is the long bones, chiefly the femur and tibia, although it may arise anywhere.

Pain and swelling of the involved bone are early features of this neoplasm, with a definite history of trauma preceding the development or at least the discovery of the tumor in approximately half of the reported cases. There is no evidence of a cause-and-effect relation, but it is not difficult to imagine that malignant transformation could take place in the rapidly proliferating bone cells in the callus after fracture or even in repairing tissues without fracture. However, pathologic fracture at the tumor site is uncommon.

Oral Manifestations. Several large series of cases of osteosarcoma of the jaws have been published in recent years, contributing greatly to our knowledge of this tumor. The largest series was that of Garrington and his associates who analyzed 56 cases and found that the most common presenting symptoms of the patients were swelling of the involved area, often producing facial deformity, and pain, followed by loose teeth, paresthesia, toothache, bleeding, nasal obstruction and a variety of other manifestations (Fig. 2–70).

The median age of the patients at the time of appearance of the first related symptom was about 27 years, nearly a decade older than patients with osteosarcoma of other bones of the skeleton. Of 44 cases of osteosarcoma of the jaws and facial bones reported by Kragh and his associates, the mean age of occurrence was 33 years. In all series, mandibular tumors are more common than those in the maxilla, and there is usually a predilection for occurrence in males.

As indicated previously, it has been reported

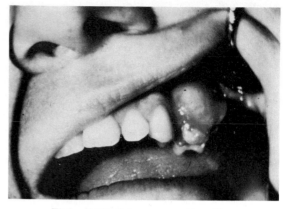

Figure 2–70. *Osteosarcoma of maxilla.*
(Courtesy of Dr. Wilbur C. Moorman.)

on numerous occasions that trauma to other sites in the skeleton has preceded the development of osteosarcoma at that site. Furthermore, it is recognized that osteosarcoma develops with considerable frequency in bone affected by osteitis deformans, or Paget's disease, as in the 80 cases studied by Price and Goldie. Finally, bone that has been subjected to therapeutic x-ray radiation may undergo malignant transformation, as in the 50 cases studied by Arlen and his associates. Surprisingly, in nearly all cases of osteosarcoma of the jaws, there is no preceding history of trauma or of Paget's disease. However, cases of osteosarcoma developing after x-ray radiation for benign jaw lesions such as fibrous dysplasia and giant cell granuloma are adequately documented: 43 such cases were discussed by De Lathouwer and Brocheriou in their review of the literature.

Parosteal (juxtacortical) osteosarcoma is a very uncommon form of osteosarcoma which occurs in many bones throughout the skeleton and is characterized by its slow growth and good prognosis because of its lower tendency for metastasis. It is exceedingly rare in the jaws, although 2 cases have been reported in a series of 20 osteosarcomas of the maxilla and mandible by Roca and his co-workers. A total of 7 cases in the jaws have now been reported, according to a recent review by Bras and his co-workers.

Periosteal osteosarcoma appears to be an aggressive variant of the parosteal osteosarcoma and has been separated out as an entity by Unni and his associates because of its more active biologic behavior. Nevertheless, it still has a much better prognosis than the conventional intramedullary osteosarcoma.

Extraosseous osteosarcoma involving extraskeletal osteosarcoma of soft tissue in the absence of a primary skeletal tumor occasionally occurs but is rare. Osteosarcoma occurring in certain organs, such as the breast, liver and kidney, may only represent malignant teratoma but, excluding these, a true soft-tissue osteosarcoma does exist. It is a highly malignant tumor and has been discussed by Miller and his associates.

Roentgenographic Features. The osteosarcoma may be primarily a sclerosing, bone-forming lesion or an osteolytic one with minimal calcified bone formation; however, there is commonly a combination of these features. The sclerosing form of osteosarcoma exhibits roentgenographic evidence of excessive production of bone, as the name implies. In some cases irregular spicules or trabeculae of new bone may be seen radiating outward on the periphery of the lesion, producing the so-called "sun-ray" appearance of osteosarcoma which is characteristic (Fig. 2–71). This pattern was present in about 25 per cent of the cases reported by Garrington and his associates. In the jaws the sclerosis may appear confined by the cortical plates in the early stage of the disease. There are commonly intermingled areas of radiolucency due to foci of bone destruction. As the tumor progresses, the cortical plates become involved by tumor, expanded and perforated.

The osteolytic form of osteosarcoma presents fewer characteristic features on the roentgenogram, and this imparts considerable difficulty to the diagnosis. The lesion is essentially a destructive one, producing an irregular radiolucency and demonstrating both expansion of the cortical plates and destruction.

A very important early manifestation of osteosarcoma of the jaws described by Garrington and his co-workers was the finding of a symmetrically widened periodontal ligament space about one or more teeth on the dental periapical roentgenogram. This appears before there is any other prominent roentgenographic evidence of the presence of the neoplasm, and this is of great diagnostic significance since it is not seen in any other disease except scleroderma or acrosclerosis. Cases of osteosarcoma of the jaws illustrating this widening of the periodontal ligament have also been reported by Gardner and Mills.

Histologic Features. Osteosarcoma is characterized by the proliferation of both atypical osteoblasts and their less differentiated precursors. These obviously atypical, neoplastic osteoblasts exhibit considerable variation in size and shape, show large, deeply staining nuclei and are arranged in a disorderly fashion about trabeculae of bone. In addition, there is a great deal of new tumor osteoid and bone formation, mostly in an irregular pattern and sometimes in solid sheets rather than in trabeculae (Fig. 2–72). This constitutes the osteoblastic type of osteosarcoma which comprised nearly 60 per cent of the jaw lesions of Garrington's group. Varying degrees of proliferation of anaplastic fibroblasts are also found and, in the absence of significant amounts of tumor osteoid or bone, when these cells predominate, the lesion is designated as a fibroblastic type of osteosarcoma. This type comprised about 34 per cent of the above group of jaw tumors. Some tumors show occasional areas of neoplastic myxomatous tissue and cartilage. Most authorities currently believe that even though a lesion is composed chiefly of malignant cartilage, it should be diagnosed as osteosarcoma if significant malignant osteoblasts and tumor osteoid or bone can be

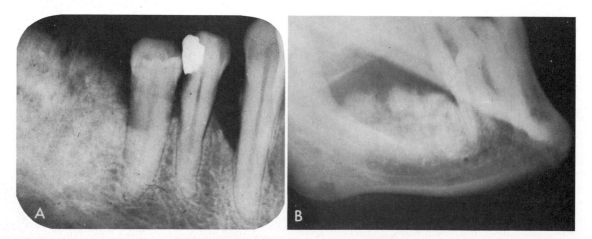

Figure 2–71. *Osteogenic sarcoma of mandible.*
A, Intraoral roentgenogram; B, lateral jaw roentgenogram.

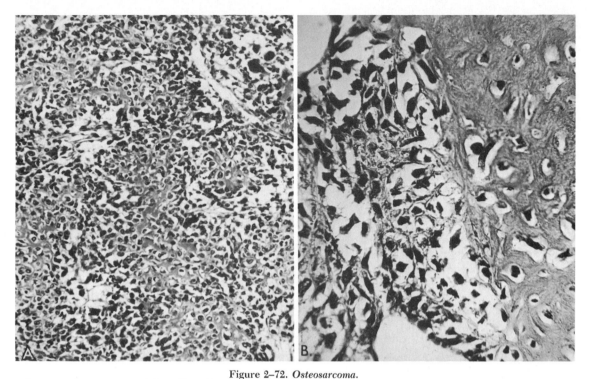

Figure 2–72. *Osteosarcoma.*
The atypical appearance of the cells and production of "tumor bone" are illustrated in the photomicrographs. *A* is low power, *B* high power.

identified, since the course of the lesion will probably be that of an osteosarcoma rather than of a chondrosarcoma. However, when only limited chondroid is present, it is termed chondroblastic type and this form accounts for less than 10 per cent of jaw osteosarcomas.

Vascular channels are often a common feature in the osteosarcoma, and when they are exceptionally prominent, the term "telangiectatic" is sometimes applied to the tumor. Finally, this tumor may contain small numbers of multinucleated giant cells, and care must be taken not to let their presence confuse the diagnosis.

Treatment and Prognosis. The treatment of osteosarcoma must be radical if there is to be hope of curing the patient. In the case of long bone involvement, amputation is a prime requisite. Primary x-ray radiation is of no avail. Neoplasms in other sites must be treated by radical resection, but, especially in the jaws, it is difficult to perform adequate and complete excision. More recently, adjuvant chemotherapy in combination with surgery, including resection of pulmonary metastases, has appeared to offer promise of increased survival from this disease.

The prognosis depends considerably upon the condition of the patient and the duration of the lesion when treatment is instituted. Under favorable conditions, when skeletal osteosarcoma was treated by proper radical means, the 5-year cure rate of a series of 183 cases of sclerosing osteosarcoma reported by Geschickter and Copeland was 21 per cent, while the 5-year cure rate for their series of 149 cases of osteolytic osteosarcoma was 16 per cent.

Of 45 cases of osteosarcoma of the jaws available for follow-up in the Garrington series, 50 per cent developed clinical evidence of metastasis, most commonly to the lung. The over-all 5-year survival rate for maxillary osteosarcoma was 25 per cent and for mandibular osteosarcoma, 41 per cent. There was no correlation between histologic characteristics of the tumor and prognosis.

MALIGNANT LYMPHOMA

The malignant lymphomas constitute a group of neoplasms of varying degrees of malignancy which are derived from the basic cells of lymphoid tissue, the lymphocytes and histiocytes in any of their developmental stages. For this reason these diseases are intimately related to each other, and a concise distinction cannot always be drawn even on histologic grounds. Lukes has rendered the following excellent definition of this disease process: "Malignant lymphoma is a neoplastic proliferative process of the lymphopoietic portion of the reticuloendothelial system that involves cells of either the lymphocytic or histiocytic series in varying degrees of differentiation and occurs in an essentially homogeneous population of a single cell type. The character of histologic involvement is either diffuse (uniform) or nodular and the distribution of involvement may be regional or systemic (generalized); however, the process is basically multicentric in character. Lymphomas and leukemias of lymphocytes and histiocytes are identical, and the variation in the frequency of cells appearing in the peripheral blood appears to be related to differences in distribution and is dependent usually upon the occurrence of bone marrow involvement."

The malignant lymphomas, with the exception of Hodgkin's disease which is well established nosologically, are currently in a state of change relative to a universally accepted classification. The non-Hodgkin's lymphomas, as they are known today, were called lymphosarcomas for many years. In the late 1930s and early 1940s, Gall and Mallory and Jackson and Parker developed classifications for the malignant lymphomas including Hodgkin's disease. These classifications were generally accepted, but in 1956, Rappaport and his colleagues presented a new classification of the malignant lymphomas. Rappaport revised this classification in 1966 and currently it is used by many pathologists because of its clinicopathologic relevance. However, many authorities claim that the modified Rappaport classification is scientifically inaccurate. In 1974, Lukes and Collins developed an immunologic classification of the non-Hodgkin's lymphomas which was scientifically accurate but difficult to use in a clinical situation. During the ensuing years, a number of classifications of non-Hodgkin's lymphomas have evolved. These too have not been based upon extensive clinicopathologic correlation and in addition have required modifications as new entities or variants of lymphomas were recognized.

At the present time, there are six well-described classifications of the non-Hodgkin's lymphomas. Each has its proponents, advantages and disadvantages. As a result, the National Cancer Institute sponsored an international study of nearly 1200 cases of non-Hodgkin's lymphoma. The panel consisted of six "expert" proponents of the respective classifications as well as six other pathologists with experience and expertise in lymph node pathology. The study was designed "to assess the clinical applicability and reproducibility of six major histopathologic systems of classification for the non-Hodgkin's lymphomas and to evaluate whether any classification was superior to others in these regards". Based upon morphologic criteria only, without the use of immunologic methods, a working classification of ten major types of non-Hodgkin's lymphoma was devised. This working classification has provided a means for translating a lymphoma into the various classifications but most importantly has reaffirmed the prognostic significance of a follicular architecture in the non-Hodgkin's lymphomas. Unfortunately, there is no unanimity of opinion as to whether this system is superior to the others or to the revised Rappaport classification insofar as clinical significance, scientific accuracy and reproducibility is concerned. Because these current classifications of the non-Hodgkin's lymphomas are as yet not finalized and universally accepted, only a division of the non-Hodgkin's lymphomas and Hodgkin's disease will be used here until there is unification of the lymphoma concept.

Non-Hodgkin's Lymphoma

The American Cancer Society predicted that approximately 23,000 cases of non-Hodgkin's lymphomas would occur in the United States in 1982. This accounts for approximately 70 per cent of all new cases of malignant lymphoma. The non-Hodgkin's lymphomas involve both lymph nodes and lymphoid organs as well as extranodal organs and tissues. The lymph nodes of the head and neck are commonly involved as well as the extranodal tissues of this area. Wong and his associates have discussed extranodal non-Hodgkin's lymphoma of the head and neck, including the oral cavity, and presented data on 128 cases from the files of the M. D. Anderson Hospital and Tumor Institute.

Clinical Features. The non-Hodgkin's lymphomas affect persons of all ages, from infants to the elderly, and occur in both sexes. The onset of symptoms may be acute or insidious and include lymphadenopathy, abdominal and mediastinal enlargement and, at times, constitutional symptoms such as fever, night sweats and weight loss.

Extranodal involvement of a wide variety of organs is known to occur. Thus, non-Hodgkin's lymphoma may present in the central nervous

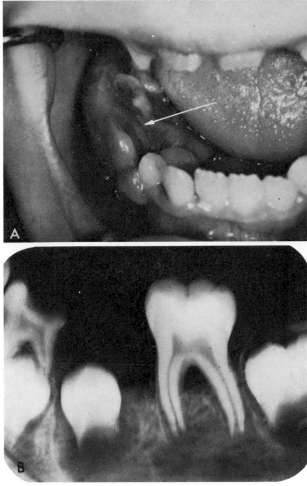

Figure 2–73. Non-Hodgkin's lymphoma.
A, The child had a fungating tissue mass after extraction of the second deciduous molar because of sudden looseness. *B*, The intraoral roentgenogram demonstrates loss of supporting bone around the first permanent molar, an unusual and serious finding in a child. *C*, The photomicrograph shows dense diffuse infiltration of the tissues by abnormal lymphocytes.

system, the gastrointestinal tract, the kidney, the testes, bone and skin. Nodal and extranodal involvement may occur concomitantly. A form of cutaneous T-cell lymphoma is known as *mycosis fungoides* and this may manifest as lesions of the oral mucosa and facial skin.

Extranodal involvement of the head and neck tissues is reported to occur primarily in persons over the age of 60 years. In the M. D. Anderson series, the male to female ratio was 3 to 2. Waldeyer's ring was the most common site of involvement but the paranasal sinuses, oral cavity and parotid gland were involved. Associated lymphadenopathy was found in 71 per cent of the cases.

Oral Manifestations. Numerous cases of non-Hodgkin's lymphoma of the oral cavity have been reported. In many instances, the oral involvement is simply a manifestation of disseminated disease. On the other hand, many lesions are the sole expression of the disease or the initial manifestation of generalized disease.

The oral lesions are characterized by swellings which may grow rapidly and then ulcerate. In some cases, these become large, fungating, necrotic, foul-smelling masses (Fig. 2–73). Pain is a variable feature. When underlying bone is involved, tooth mobility and pain may develop. A number of cases have been reported in which paresthesia of the mental nerve developed.

Tomich and Shafer reported 21 cases of malignant lymphomas in the hard palate. Reported as *lymphoproliferative disease of the hard palate,* all proved to be non-Hodgkin's lymphomas. These lesions occurred primarily in elderly men and women with an average age of 70 years. They presented as soft, fluctuant swellings which were occasionally bilateral. The swellings were ulcerated or discolored in some cases (Fig. 2–74). Eight of the 21 patients died of their disease. Blok and his co-workers confirmed the existence of this clinicopathologic entity by reporting eight additional cases. Their findings were similar to those reported by Tomich and

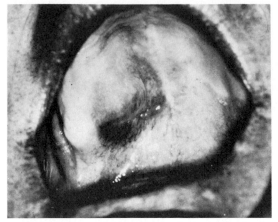

Figure 2–74. *Lymphoproliferative disease of the hard palate.*

Shafer. Although lymphoid lesions in the hard palate are very likely to be lymphomas, follicular lymphoid hyperplasia can present in this anatomic location and therefore careful histologic examination is of paramount importance. Harsany and his associates described such a condition and discussed the histologic differentiation between lymphoid hyperplasia, non-Hodgkin's lymphoma and benign lymphoepithelial lesion (q.v.).

Histologic Features. The non-Hodgkin's lymphomas present a histologic pattern which is described as either nodular or diffuse. In the nodular pattern, the neoplastic cells tend to aggregate in such a way that large clusters of cells are seen (Fig. 2–75, *A*). In contrast, the diffuse pattern is characterized by a monotonous distribution of cells with no evidence of nodu-

larity or germinal center formation. The diffuse lymphomas produce an entire effacement of normal lymph node architecture (Fig. 2–75, *B*). The histologic pattern of involvement is very important, since there is clinicopathologic and prognostic correlation between the two types. The nodular pattern is seen in lymphomas in adults more often than in children and is associated with a more favorable prognosis than the diffuse type. The histologic pattern of involvement, therefore, has been a basis for the classification of non-Hodgkin's lymphoma. A diagnosis of nodular or diffuse lymphoma is highly reproducible among pathologists and it has definite clinical significance.

The actual cell type involved in the non-Hodgkin's lymphoma has proven to be an enigma for histopathologists. Immunologic cell surface marking studies have shown that the nodular lymphomas are of B-cell origin. Many of the diffuse lymphomas are likewise of B-cell origin but some diffuse lymphomas prove to be of T-cell origin. From a purely morphologic observation, without the use of immunologic markers, the determination of the cell of origin is difficult. This has resulted in cells being interpreted as lymphocytes, reticulum cells and histiocytes in various degrees of differentiation. Currently, cells formerly interpreted as "reticulum cells" or "histiocytes" are known to represent large lymphocytes. However, it is thought that a histiocytic lymphoma does exist, albeit uncommon. The problem of cell identification on a morphologic, nonimmunologic basis is one of the major obstacles in arriving at a universally acceptable classification of the non-Hodgkin's lymphomas.

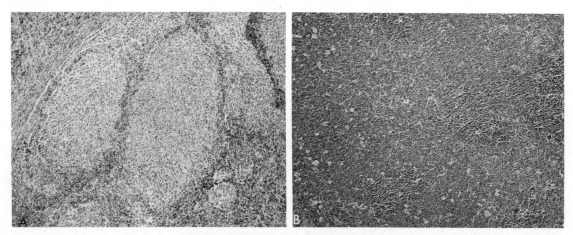

Figure 2–75. *Non-Hodgkin's lymphoma.*
The nodular pattern is characterized by large clusters of cells (*A*) while the diffuse pattern shows no such clustering but rather a monotonous population of cells (*B*).

Treatment and Prognosis. The non-Hodgkin's lymphomas are best treated by radiation or chemotherapy or both. Long-term remissions and cures are fairly common in some cases of lymphoma, particularly those with nodular histologic patterns. In a retrospective clinicopathologic study of 293 cases of non-Hodgkin's lymphoma, Patchefsky and his co-workers found that lymphomas with a nodular pattern, particularly a well-developed nodular pattern, was associated with a significantly better prognosis than lymphomas with a diffuse pattern.

Other factors which have a bearing on prognosis are the clinical stage of the disease (localized vs. regional vs. generalized) and the cell type. In regard to the latter, the well-differentiated lymphocytic lymphomas have a better prognosis than the poorly differentiated lymphocytic lymphomas. The "histiocytic" or large-cell lymphomas are known to have a poor long-term prognosis, regardless of the histologic pattern of involvement.

Although significant advances in lymphoma treatment have been made, the disease is still a serious one, and the prognosis for any particular patient should be a guarded, carefully considered one.

PRIMARY LYMPHOMA OF BONE

(Primary Reticulum Cell Sarcoma of Bone)

Primary lymphoma (reticulum cell sarcoma, as it was originally known) of bone was first described as a separate entity in a report by Parker and Jackson in 1939. They noted that the lesion had frequently been confused with Ewing's sarcoma, Hodgkin's disease, osteogenic sarcoma and even inflammation. Since their report, many cases have been recorded in the literature.

Clinical Features. This lymphoma of bone occurs in a wide age range. In the series of Parker and Jackson, over 75 per cent of the patients were under 40 years of age and 35 per cent were under 20 years. In a series of 150 primary cases reported by Dahlin, the disease occurred in all age groups but the very young.

Clinical signs and symptoms of the neoplasm are frequently absent except for the presence of localized swelling of the involved bone, usually an extremity, with or without attendant pain. Regional lymphadenopathy may be present, but the patient is nearly always in a remarkably good state of general health.

Oral Manifestations. Primary lymphoma of bone is not a common disease of the jaws, but it appears to be somewhat more frequent in the mandible than in the maxilla. Of the 150 primary cases of Dahlin, 22 or 15 per cent occurred in the mandible. There were no cases in the maxilla. It occurs in the jaws with a predilection for the male sex.

Gerry and Williams collected all the reported cases of primary lymphoma of the mandible and noted that the principal presenting symptom of the disease was pain, usually present for a period of several months to a year or more before the patient sought advice and treatment. Demonstrable swelling or enlargement of the bone was often noted.

The oral mucosa in this disease seldom is ulcerated over the involved bone, although there may be minor change in the texture or hue, sometimes appearing diffusely inflamed (Fig. 2–76). The teeth often become exceedingly loose, owing to destruction of bone. When the neoplasm involves the maxilla, there may be evidence of expansion of the bone as well as symptoms of nasal obstruction due to superior growth of the tumor into the floor of the nasal cavity. Aside from this local discomfort, the patient seldom exhibits systemic signs or symptoms of the disease.

Roentgenographic Features. The typical roentgenographic appearance of lymphoma of bone is one of an osteolytic invasive, malignant neoplasm. There is frequently a diffuse radiolucency involving the alveolar bone which may present destruction of the supporting bone of the teeth (Fig. 2–76, *B*). Seldom is there a significant periosteal reaction.

Although the features are suggestive of a malignant neoplasm, there is nothing roentgenographically pathognomonic of the disease.

Histologic Features. The primary cell of this osseous lesion is identical with that of the soft-tissue tumor, and diagnosis depends upon adequate biopsy with microscopic examination of the tissue by a competent and qualified pathologist (Fig. 2–76, *C*, *D*). Since the oral tissues frequently exhibit considerable inflammatory cell infiltration, confusion of this tumor with an inflammatory lesion sometimes occurs.

The diagnosis of this osseous lymphoma is often more difficult that that of the same tumor involving the soft tissues, since there are a number of lesions in bone which it closely resembles. Thus care must be taken by the pathologist not to confuse primary lymphoma with Ewing's tumor, osteolytic osteosarcoma,

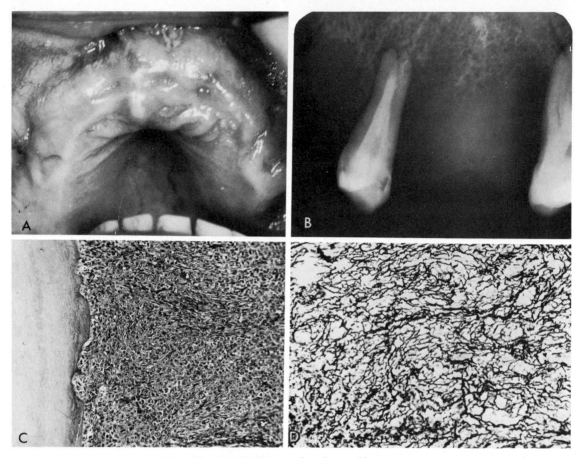

Figure 2–76. *Primary lymphoma of bone.*
A, The maxilla is diffusely involved by the neoplasm, but presents no remarkable changes in the oral mucosa. *B*, The intraoral roentgenogram, taken just before extraction of the few remaining teeth, shows bone destruction causing loosening of the teeth. *C*, The photomicrograph illustrates the cellular nature of the neoplasm in an area of tissue attached to one tooth. *D*, A special silver stain shows the profusion of reticulin fibers produced by the lesion.

plasma cell myeloma, and certain reticuloendothelial diseases.

Treatment and Prognosis. Primary lymphoma of bone has been treated by various means, chiefly radical surgical excision or x-ray radiation. The tumor appears to be radiosensitive, more so than most bone sarcomas. Since the response to radiation is usually good, radical surgery such as amputation or wide resection does not appear justified.

The data of Coley and his associates indicate a remarkably high 5-year survival rate of 73 per cent of patients and a 10-year survival rate of 56 per cent, when patients treated palliatively only were excluded. The fallacy of accepting a 5-year survival rate as indicative of a cure rate was stressed by these workers on the basis that recurrences frequently happened up to 10 years after treatment of the primary lesion. In a series of primary lymphoma reported by Boston and

his colleagues, 98 patients with long-term follow-up had a 5-year survival rate of 44 per cent.

It appears that primary lymphoma of bone is a far less serious form of lymphoma than the analogous lesion of soft tissue. Nevertheless the lesion is an exceedingly dangerous one, and the prognosis for any given patient should be a guarded one.

AFRICAN JAW LYMPHOMA

(Burkitt's Lymphoma)

In 1958–1959, Burkitt reported on a type of malignant lymphoma seen with undue frequency, particularly involving the jaws, in native children of Kampala, Uganda, in Central East Africa. Once recognized, it was found to constitute about 50 per cent of all malignant tumors seen in African children. At one time the tumor was thought to be confined to certain areas of Africa. However, it has now been found in many countries, including the United States. A series of 421 Americans were studied by the American Burkitt's Lymphoma Registry and the data reported by Levine and his associates. This large study has provided an excellent comparison between the endemic African cases and the nonendemic non-African cases.

Burkitt's lymphoma, a non-Hodgkin's lymphoma, has been shown to be a B-cell neoplasm by immunologic cell surface-marking studies. The climatic and geographic distribution of the endemic African cases originally suggested a mosquito-borne virus but none were identified. In 1964, Epstein and his co-workers identified a herpes-like virus in cultured Burkitt lymphoma cells studied by electron microscopy. This virus is now known as the Epstein-Barr virus (EBV). Further studies have shown that endemic African cases have significantly elevated antibody titers to EBV-determined antigens. Thus there is considerable but not totally conclusive evidence that the Epstein-Barr virus is causally related to Burkitt's lymphoma.

Clinical Features. The endemic African form of the disease is confined almost exclusively to children between 2 and 14 years of age. In contrast to most non-Hodgkin's lymphomas, it primarily involves extranodal tissues. It begins generally as a rapidly growing tumor mass of the jaws, destroying the bone and causing loosening of the teeth with extension commonly to involve the maxillary, ethmoid and sphenoid sinuses as well as the orbit. Visceral organ involvement also occurs frequently but seldom without jaw involvement.

The nonendemic non-African form of the disease tends to occur in a slightly older age group, although children and young adults are involved primarily. There is a peak age incidence of 10 to 12 years in American males, whereas the incidence of American females is relatively uniform throughout the first two decades of life. The disease occurs more commonly in American males until 13 years of age with an equal sex distribution thereafter. In contrast to the endemic African form, this form tends to involve lymph nodes and lymphoid tissues, particularly bone marrow, more often. Visceral involvement is more common and jaw involvement relatively uncommon. Thus, nonendemic Burkitt's lymphoma appears to be clinically heterogeneous.

Immunologic studies have shown that antibody titers to EBV-antigens are less commonly observed in the nonendemic disease although they are significantly higher than in nonaffected controls. Of interest is data from the American Burkitt's Lymphoma Registry that nonendemic cases with high antibody titers to EBV-antigen had a more favorable prognosis.

Histologic Features. The tumor consists of a monotonous overgrowth of undifferentiated monomorphic lymphoreticular cells, usually showing abundant mitotic activity. Macrophages with an abundant clear cytoplasm, often containing cellular debris, are usually found scattered uniformly throughout the tumor, producing the very characteristic "starry sky" effect.

Detailed study of the jaws and teeth in this lymphoma has been reported by Lehner. From his histologic studies, he has concluded that invasion of the jaw occurs from outside and that the dental tissues probably play no role in the pathogenesis of the tumor.

Treatment and Prognosis. The disease was rapidly and uniformly fatal at one time. However, it is now being treated by cytotoxic drugs with surprisingly good long-term survival and apparent cure in some cases.

HODGKIN'S DISEASE

Hodgkin's disease is considered as one of the two main types of malignant lymphoma. As with the non-Hodgkin's lymphomas, the etiology is unknown. The American Cancer Society predicted that approximately 7000 cases of Hodgkin's disease would occur in the United States in 1982. This accounts for approximately 23 per cent of all new cases of malignant lymphoma. Hodgkin's disease is primarily one of lymph nodes and lymphoid organs. The lymph nodes of the head and neck, particularly the cervical nodes, are often the initial site of involvement.

In contrast to the non-Hodgkin's lymphomas, the classification of Hodgkin's disease is well established and has been since 1966. The classification was originally devised by Lukes and Butler and it was then modified by a panel of experts who met in Rye, New York. The current (Rye) classification and its comparison with the Lukes and Butler classification and the traditional Jackson and Parker classification are shown in Table 2–8.

Clinical Features. Hodgkin's disease is characterized by a bimodal age incidence peak, one in young adults and the second in the fifth

Table 2–8.   Comparison of Classifications of Hodgkin's Disease

JACKSON AND PARKER	LUKES AND BUTLER	RYE (N.Y.)

Paragranuloma	Lymphocytic and/or histiocytic
	  a. Nodular
	  b. Diffuse
		Lymphocytic predominance

Granuloma	Nodular sclerosis Mixed cellularity Diffuse fibrosis	Nodular sclerosis Mixed cellularity Lymphocytic depletion
Sarcoma	Reticular	

From J. J. Butler: Relationship of histological findings to survival in Hodgkin's disease. Cancer Res., *31*:1770, 1971.

decade. The disease occurs in the younger age group with an equal distribution between the sexes, whereas in the older age group it occurs more commonly in males.

The clinical signs and symptoms of Hodgkin's disease are extremely protean. The first manifestation in the majority of cases is painless enlargement of one or more cervical lymph nodes, not an uncommon finding in other lymphomas or in cases of simple upper respiratory tract or oral infection (Fig. 2–77). Many cases of Hodgkin's disease have been manifested by persistence of lymphadenopathy after an upper respiratory tract infection. The nodes are usually firm and rubbery in consistency, and the overlying skin is normal.

Pain may develop in the abdomen and back, owing to splenic enlargement and pressure of enlarged nodes or involvement of the vertebrae. Generalized weakness is sometimes an early feature of the disease, as are loss of weight, cough and dyspnea, anorexia and sometimes a generalized itching of the skin. The patient may also complain of edema of the legs, dysphagia and hemoptysis or melena. Actually, nearly any organ in the body may be involved by Hodgkin's disease, although the diagnosis is usually made by lymph node biopsy.

Oral Manifestations.   Hodgkin's disease is primarily a disease of lymph nodes and, for this reason, seldom occurs as a disease primarily in the oral cavity. It is conceivable that the oral cavity could be involved secondarily, but this appears to be an exceedingly rare happening. A case of Hodgkin's disease secondarily involving the mandible and overlying alveolar mucosa has been reported by Forman and Wesson.

Histologic Features.   The essential histologic features of Hodgkin's disease consist of the multinucleated Reed-Sternberg cell in an appropriate cellular background. Although the Reed-Sternberg cell is generally considered to be the "malignant cell" of Hodgkin's disease, its precise nature is still obscure. Some investigators consider it to be derived from B-lymphocytes, while others advocate a monocyte-macrophage derivation. Ultrastructural studies generally have supported a lymphocyte origin, whereas immunologic and cell culture studies support a monocyte-macrophage origin.

There are four recognized histologic types of Hodgkin's disease which form the basis for its classification. *Lymphocyte predominant* Hodgkin's disease is characterized by abundant lymphocytes and few plasma cells with only occasional Reed-Sternberg cells. *Mixed cellularity* Hodgkin's disease is characterized by lymphocytes, plasma cells, eosinophils and easily identified Reed-Sternberg cells. The *lymphocyte depletion* type is characterized by sparse lymphocytes and stromal cells, fibrosis, and numerous but bizarre Reed-Sternberg cells. The

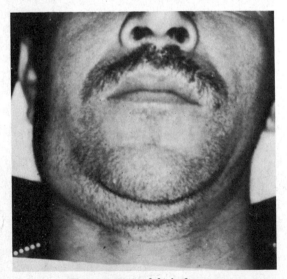

Figure 2–77. *Hodgkin's disease.*
There is cervical lymphadenopathy which is more pronounced on one side. (Courtesy of Dr. Cesar Lopez.)

nodular sclerosis type is characterized by lymphocytes, plasma cells, eosinophils and Reed-Sternberg cells surrounded by dense bands of collagen. The Reed-Sternberg cells in the nodular sclerosis type are histologic variants known as "lacunar" cells.

The histologic distinction between the types of Hodgkin's disease has clinical and prognostic significance. For example, the nodular sclerosis type has a remarkable female sex predilection whereas the mixed cellularity type occurs more often in males. The lymphocyte predominant and nodular sclerosis types generally have localized involvement on one side of the diaphragm, whereas the mixed cellularity and lymphocyte depletion types are more likely to be widespread.

Treatment and Prognosis. It is now recognized that proper treatment of Hodgkin's disease can lead to long-term remission and even cure. Radiation therapy and combination chemotherapy have been clearly shown to be effective in the management of Hodgkin's disease. The most important prognostic determinants are the histologic type and the clinical stage of the disease. The lymphocyte predominant type has the most favorable prognosis, followed by nodular sclerosis, mixed cellularity and lymphocyte depletion, the least favorable. Localized (Stage I) disease has a much better prognosis than disseminated (Stage IV) disease. Patchefsky and his associates have reported that male sex, older age and systemic symptoms also are associated with poor prognosis.

THE LEUKEMIAS

Both monocytic and lymphocytic leukemia are considered by most investigators to be related to the malignant lymphoma group because of the frequent transition from one of the lymphomas to a leukemia. Despite this close relationship, the leukemias are more fittingly described in the section on diseases of the blood (q.v.), and the clinical and histologic similarities are pointed out there.

MULTIPLE MYELOMA

(Plasma Cell Myeloma; Plasmacytoma)

Multiple myeloma is a neoplasm of bone that originates from cells of the bone marrow which bear a remarkable resemblance to plasma cells, common constituents of an inflammatory infiltrate. Some investigators believe that this lesion is closely related to the lymphoma group of malignant neoplasms, although at present it is not usually included within this category. Since numerous bones are involved by this disease, two ideas have arisen about its true nature. The neoplasm is thought by some authorities to be of multicentric origin, lesions arising in numerous areas at approximately the same time, but each independent of the other lesions and rarely producing metastases. Other workers have suggested that the disease begins as a single lesion which metastasizes widely.

According to Dahlin, the relative incidence of myeloma appears to be increasing. Nearly 53 per cent of all patients with malignant bone tumors seen at the Mayo Clinic between 1964 and 1975 had histologically verified myeloma. In 1976, the American Cancer Society predicted 8000 new cases of myeloma compared with 9600 for 1982. However, the relative incidence was virtually unchanged during this six-year period, although the actual incidence increased by 20 per cent. Kyle has presented an in-depth review of 869 cases of multiple myeloma seen and treated at the Mayo Clinic.

Clinical Features. Multiple myeloma occurs most frequently between the ages of 40 and 70 years, although it may occur in much younger persons. Men are affected more frequently than women.

Afflicted patients usually present pain as an early feature of the disease, and, because of the destruction of bone, pathologic fracture is fairly common. Occasionally, swelling over the areas of bone involvement may be detectable.

Oral Manifestations. Involvement of the jaws in cases of multiple myeloma has been reported on many occasions. Bruce and Royer studied a series of patients with this disease and concluded that the mandible is far more frequently involved than the maxilla, since nearly 95 per cent of their cases evidenced mandibular lesions. Furthermore, the ramus, angle and molar region of the mandible were the most frequent sites of the lesions. These correspond to the most active hematopoietic areas. Conversely, in the Mayo series 20 of the 28 cases with jaw lesions had maxillary involvement. Interestingly, two of the patients were only in the third decade of life. Cataldo and Meyer have confirmed the high frequency of jaw involvement in a series of 44 cases of multiple myeloma in which 70 per cent of the patients who had jaw roentgenograms taken had maxillary or mandibular lesions.

Other signs and symptoms of jaw involvement include pain, swelling, expansion of the jaw, numbness and mobility of teeth. In addition, extraosseous lesions occur which may resemble gingival enlargements or epulides. Extension of the disease to other sites outside the skeleton such as to lymph nodes, skin and viscera also occurs.

It is impossible to compute the over-all incidence of jaw involvement in patients with multiple myeloma, since most patients suffering from this disease do not receive a thorough oral examination with roentgenograms. Nevertheless studies indicate that the incidence may be somewhat higher than formerly believed because many such lesions may be asymptomatic.

Roentgenographic Features. Roentgenographic examination will usually reveal numerous sharply punched-out areas in a variety of bones, which may include the vertebrae, ribs, skull, jaws and ends of long bones (Fig. 2–78). Note that these are all sites of active hematopoiesis. These lesions may vary in size from a few millimeters to a centimeter or more in diameter, but there is usually no peripheral bone reaction. Diffuse destructive lesions of bone may also occur.

Laboratory Features. Certain laboratory findings are of considerable importance in establishing the diagnosis of multiple myeloma. Many patients, but not all, exhibit a hyperglobulinemia resulting in a reversal of the serum albumin-globulin ratio and an increase in total serum protein to a level of 8 to 16 gm. per cent. In addition, the presence of Bence-Jones protein in the urine is noted in 60 to 85 per cent of myeloma patients. This is an unusual protein which coagulates when the urine is heated to 40° to 60° C. and then disappears when the urine is boiled. It reappears as urine is cooled. Occasionally, Bence-Jones protein is found in the urine of patients with diseases other than multiple myeloma, such as leukemia and polycythemia. Furthermore, its absence does not rule out the presence of multiple myeloma. Anemia is also a common finding in multiple myeloma. Kyle has thoroughly discussed the laboratory findings in the Mayo Clinic cases.

Histologic Features. The usual lesion is composed of sheets of closely packed cells resembling plasma cells. These are round or ovoid cells with eccentrically placed nuclei exhibiting chromatin clumping in a "cartwheel" or "check-

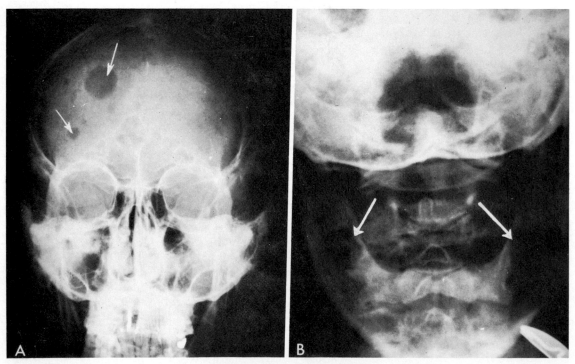

Figure 2–78. *Multiple myeloma.*

A, Numerous sharply punched-out areas are found in the skull film. *B,* The anteroposterior roentgenogram of another patient shows multiple bilateral radiolucent jaw lesions. (*B,* Courtesy of Dr. Clifford Brown.)

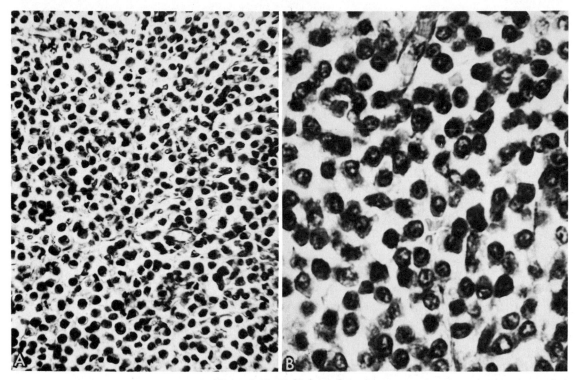

Figure 2–79. *Multiple myeloma.*
A, The uniform distribution of cells with very little stroma is characteristic of myeloma. *B,* Under high magnification, the resemblance of myeloma cells to inflammatory plasma cells is obvious.

erboard" pattern (Fig. 2–79). Two nuclei within a single cell membrane are seen occasionally, but mitotic activity is not great. A perinuclear halo may be present. Russell bodies are common as in chronic inflammatory lesions with numerous typical plasma cells, although it was once thought that their absence in myeloma was noteworthy.

Chen has studied the ultrastructure of a mandibular plasma cell myeloma. He noted numerous mitochondria in a perinuclear distribution as well as prominent Golgi complexes. The latter are most likely responsible for the perinuclear halo which is observed by light microscopy. Wright and his co-workers have discussed the diagnostic value of the immunoperoxidase technique in distinguishing between inflammatory and neoplastic lesions of the jaws which are composed of plasma cells. Inflammatory plasma cell lesions are characterized by polyclonal staining, whereas monoclonal staining is indicative of neoplasia.

Treatment and Prognosis. Chemotherapy is presently the treatment of choice for multiple myeloma and this has been discussed by Kyle and Elveback. Chemotherapy is associated with a variety of side effects, most notably bone marrow depression. Radiation therapy is also used, often in combination with chemotherapy. Unfortunately, the prognosis is poor, with the median survival time being two to three years. Infection, anemia and kidney failure are the most common immediate causes of death.

SOLITARY PLASMA CELL MYELOMA

(Plasmacytoma)

Solitary plasma cell myeloma is an unusual disease which some authorities believe to be unrelated to multiple myeloma even though the two are microscopically indistinguishable. As the name indicates, solitary myeloma involves only a single bone and has an excellent prognosis.

The criteria for establishing a diagnosis of solitary plasma cell myeloma have been recently enumerated by Bataille and Sany. These criteria are as follows: (1) presence of a solitary bone tumor; (2) a biopsy showing plasma cell histology; (3) absence of myeloma cells in bone marrow examination; (4) absence of anemia, hypercalcemia or renal involvement; (5) absence of or a low monoclonal component on serum electrophoresis; and (6) normal levels of immunoglobulins after treatment. Although these criteria seem precise, it is well known that many of the "solitary" lesions in time prove to be the forerunners of disseminated disease. Some authorities therefore are of the opinion that all "solitary" myelomas will eventuate into multiple myeloma if given sufficient time.

Clinical Features. There appears to be a greater range in the age incidence of solitary myeloma than of multiple myeloma. In the review of 114 cases by Bataille and Sany, 22 per cent of the patients were less than 40 years of age, although the mean age was 51 years. Males were affected more frequently than females, as in multiple myeloma.

The presenting symptoms of patients with solitary myeloma are similar to those with multiple myeloma. Thus pain, swelling and pathologic fracture are the most common findings.

Oral Manifestations. Occasional cases of solitary plasma cell myeloma of bone have been reported in the jaws, both maxilla and mandible. Caution must be exercised, however, in diagnosing a lesion of the jaws as solitary myeloma, since the finding of large numbers of plasma cells in granulomas associated with dental infection is common. It is in such cases that immunoperoxidase techniques may be of diagnostic value.

The *extramedullary solitary plasmacytoma* is a primary soft-tissue plasma cell tumor of the nasal, pharyngeal and oral mucous membranes occurring without apparent primary bone involvement. Stout and Kenney reviewed a series of 104 such cases, and a review by Dolin and Dewar summarized the findings in 126 cases. This extramedullary plasmacytoma may be situated on the gingiva, palate, floor of the mouth, tongue, tonsils and pillar as well as the nasal cavity, nasopharynx and paranasal sinuses. Visceral organs are the site of these lesions in occasional cases. The lesions are described as sessile or polypoid reddish masses in the mucous membranes, which become lobulated as they enlarge, but do not tend to ulcerate.

The nature of the extramedullary plasmacytoma is as obscure as that of the other forms of plasma cell lesions. It is undoubtedly different from the common plasma cell-containing granulomas and polyps which are commonly found in the upper air passages and oral cavity. Yet, though the majority of the reported cases of plasma cell tumors in this location remain localized lesions in the soft tissue, metastases have occurred to lymph nodes, bones and other sites. In a discussion of this disease by Kotner and Wang, it was pointed out that only 10 to 20 per cent of patients develop regional lymph node metastases.

Corwin and Lindberg studied 12 patients with extramedullary plasmacytoma. Two of the 12 developed multiple myeloma. Thus these tumors should be regarded as serious and potentially fatal, although they have a much more favorable prognosis than multiple myeloma.

Roentgenographic Features. Roentgenographic examination of the bones in solitary plasma cell myeloma reveals one of two types of lesions. One type is a purely destructive intramedullary lesion suggestive of metastatic carcinoma. The other type of lesion is an expansile one suggestive of a giant cell tumor. There is nothing pathognomonic or even characteristic of the roentgenographic picture of solitary myeloma.

Laboratory Features. Laboratory findings are interesting because few of the patients exhibit Bence-Jones protein in the urine. Furthermore, the characteristic hyperglobulinemia and anemia, so characteristic of multiple myeloma, are absent in solitary myeloma and extramedullary plasmacytoma.

Histologic Features. It has been stated previously that the histologic features of the solitary and multiple myeloma are similar. In the well-differentiated lesions of multiple myeloma it is impossible to distinguish between the two. The extramedullary plasmacytoma is also microscopically identical with the solitary myeloma. Nevertheless some cases of multiple myeloma present a variegated histologic picture which is not seen in solitary myeloma or the extramedullary plasmacytoma.

Treatment and Prognosis. The treatment of the solitary myeloma should be a relatively conservative procedure to eradicate the single lesion. This may be accomplished by surgery, by x-ray radiation or by a combination of the two. The prognosis of true solitary myeloma is excellent, although the difficulty in distinguishing this from multiple myeloma must be borne in mind.

BENIGN TUMORS OF MUSCLE TISSUE ORIGIN

LEIOMYOMA

The leiomyoma is a benign tumor derived from smooth muscle and is found in a variety of anatomic sites, including the skin, subcutaneous tissues and oral cavity. It is uncommon in the oral cavity, probably because of the general absence of smooth muscle there except in blood vessel walls and occasionally in the circumvallate papillae of the tongue. A review of the literature by Farman and Kay showed 51 cases of oral leiomyoma reported through 1975, with occasional cases described since then.

Clinical Features. The majority of cases of leiomyoma have occurred on the posterior portion of the tongue, although others have been found on the palate, cheeks, gingiva, lips and salivary glands. Of the reported cases, the majority of oral leiomyomas occur in adults in the middle decades of life, over 65 per cent being found in patients older than 30 years of age, although cases are described in young children in the first decade.

The oral leiomyoma is a slow-growing, painless lesion which is superficial and often pedunculated. The presenting symptoms of some of the patients in the reported cases have been "sore throat" or "tumor in the throat." The tumor does not ulcerate and resembles the normal mucosa in color and texture.

A *central leiomyoma* of the jaw is also known to occur but is exceedingly rare. A case in the mandible, with ultrastructural confirmation, has been reported by Goldblatt and Edesess, who have also reviewed the literature on the central lesions of bone.

Histologic Features. The leiomyoma is composed of interlacing bundles of smooth muscle fibers interspersed by varying amounts of fibrous connective tissue. The muscle nuclei are typically spindle-shaped with blunt ends and quite vesicular. The bundles of fibers appear to form whorls because of their fascicular arrangement in varying planes. Intracytoplasmic myofibrils are present and can be demonstrated by phosphotungstic acid-hematoxylin special stain. Masson's trichrome stain is also commonly used to differentiate between collagen and smooth muscle.

Treatment and Prognosis. This smooth muscle neoplasm is best treated by conservative surgical excision, since it does not tend to recur or become malignant.

ANGIOMYOMA

(Vascular Leiomyoma; Angioleiomyoma)

Leiomyomas and angiomyomas have commonly been treated as two forms of the same basic lesion in the past and reported together as an entity. Thus, some lesions are quite vascular, being composed of large numbers of blood vessels of an atypical nature with disoriented smooth muscle layers (the angiomyoma), while others are relatively avascular. The suggestion has even been made that there may be a progression of lesions: hemangioma, angioma with much nonstriated muscle, vascular leiomyoma, leiomyoma with many vessels and solid leiomyoma. Thus, it has been proposed that the vascular leiomyoma may be only a stage in the continuous process of smooth muscle proliferation.

Most investigators today believe that the angiomyoma probably represents a hamartomatous malformation, while the solid leiomyoma represents a true neoplasm and that, therefore, these two entities should be clearly separated. This has been discussed in detail by Damm and Neville. Since the two lesions have been combined in the literature, separation of their clinical characteristics at this time is not possible, although Reichart and Reznik-Schüler have reported the ultrastructure of an oral angiomyoma and discussed some of the cases classified under this term.

RHABDOMYOMA

The rhabdomyoma, or benign tumor of striated muscle origin, is an exceedingly rare lesion. The term "rhabdomyoma" has been used to refer to a lesion of the myocardium that is often associated with a hamartoma complex, including sebaceous adenomas, tuberous sclerosis, and hamartomas of the kidney and other organs. However, some investigators view the rhabdomyoma in that location as a developmental anomaly rather than a neoplasm. In other sites, the rhabdomyoma is exceedingly rare, the most common locations being the tongue and floor of the mouth. Additional sites of occurrence include the axilla, thoracic wall, neck, larynx, and pharynx, stomach, uterus, vulva and vagina according to the reviews of Moran and Enterline and Corio and Lewis. As pointed out by the latter authors, the cardiac and extracardiac rhabdomyomas have morphologic similarities but there appear to be clinical, light microscope, histochemical, enzymatic and ultrastructural differences between the two lesions.

Clinical Features. The intraoral rhabdomyoma usually presents as a well-circumscribed tumor mass which may have a known duration of months or even several years. According to the 16 cases reviewed by Corio and Lewis and the 13 additional ones which they reported, over 75 per cent of the cases occur in the fifth decade of life or later, with a male to female ratio of 2 to 1. The most common sites of occurrence are the floor of the mouth, tongue, soft palate, buccal mucosa and lower lip.

A fetal rhabdomyoma is a very rare form of this tumor, reported by Dehner and his associates, which usually occurs in children but may be found in adults. Intraoral cases are recognized.

Histologic Features. The tumor is composed of large, round cells that have a granular, eosinophilic cytoplasm and show irregular cross striations. This cytoplasm is rich in glycogen and glycoprotein. According to Corio and Lewis, lipid material is also present in the cytoplasm of some of the cells.

Kay has investigated a rhabdomyoma in the floor of the mouth and reported that these cells contain enlarged and abundant mitochondria, which would indicate that the cell is enzymatically and perhaps physiologically active. However, the haphazard arrangement of cross-striations would probably preclude its usual function of proper contraction.

Treatment. The rhabdomyoma is excised conservatively, usually enucleating with ease. However, recurrences were documented in 4 of the 13 cases reported by Corio and Lewis.

GRANULAR CELL MYOBLASTOMA

(Myoblastic Myoma; Granular Cell Tumor; Granular Cell Schwannoma)

The granular cell myoblastoma is an uncommon tumor which is of controversial origin. Since it has carried the name "myoblastoma" for many years, thus denoting an origin from muscle tissue, it will be discussed with lesions of this primary tissue. The granular cell myoblastoma occurs in many parts of the body, but by far the most common site of occurrence is the tongue. Bangle reported a study of 43 cases of myoblastoma, 21 of which were found in the tongue, the remainder being located in the skin, the lips, breast, subcutaneous tissue, vocal cord and floor of the mouth. Similar lesions have also been reported in the gastrointestinal tract and the neurohypophysis. In a more recent study, Strong and his associates have reported 110 lesions occurring in 95 patients, multiple lesions being present in 8 patients, and found that 39 of the lesions, or 35 per cent, occurred

in the tongue. Moscovic and Azar have reviewed over 500 myoblastomas from the literature.

Numerous theories on the histogenesis of the granular cell myoblastoma exist, all having arisen since the recognition by Abrikossoff in 1926 of the myoblastoma as a distinct and separate entity. Some investigators believe that the myoblastoma is derived from striated muscle, and it is interesting to note that the histologic appearance of the cells in some ways is reminiscent of those features seen in degenerating or regenerating skeletal muscle fibers. It should be pointed out that these tumors may be found in areas where striated muscle is normally absent, such as the breast and skin, and therefore it is difficult to explain such a lesion arising from this tissue. It is conceivable that the tumor might arise from embryonal rests of aberrant muscle, in which case one should find cells resembling myoblasts, but such cells are not found. Tissue culture studies in vitro of the myoblastoma by Murray have shown considerable resemblance between the growth pattern of this tumor and that of various forms of striated muscle.

Histiocytes have also been suggested as the cell of origin of the myoblastoma. Thus it is reasoned that the granules of the cells represent phagocytized or stored material.

The neural theory of origin proposed by Fust and Custer explains the origin of the myoblastoma from connective tissue of nerves, and these workers suggested the term "granular cell neural fibroma." Electron microscope studies of the myoblastoma, such as that of Fisher and Wechsler, have supported the derivation from Schwann cells. In addition, in a study reported by Stefansson and Wollmann, it was shown that all tumor cells in 10 different granular cell myoblastomas stained intensely with antiserum to S-100 protein. This protein is found outside the central nervous system only in Schwann cells and satellite cells of ganglia and, in addition, has been demonstrated also in schwannomas and neurofibromas, but is absent from soft-tissue tumors of non-neural origin. Thus, the results of this study support the concept of origin of the myoblastoma from Schwann cells.

As still another hypothesis, Aparacio and Lumsden have proposed that the granular cell lesion originates from a stem cell with a leiomyofibrillogenic capacity which may be some type of specialized smooth muscle cell peculiar to certain tissues that are found in characteristic sites for the tumor.

Finally, electron microscope studies of the myoblastoma by Sobel and his co-workers have suggested to them that the progenitor cell is an undifferentiated mesenchymal cell and that this cell was the source of another unusual cell found in the myoblastoma termed the angulate body cell, a cell intermediate between the undifferentiated mesenchymal cell and the mature granular cell.

In reviewing a series of granular cell tumors of the head and neck, including their own ultrastructural observations on the myoblastoma, Regezi and his associates have concluded that the evidence supports two hypotheses: (1) that the granular cells represent an unusual nonspecific degenerative process, and (2) that the histogenesis is from undifferentiated mes-

enchymal cells that subsequently undergo cytoplasmic autophagocytosis. They have recommended, as have other investigators, that until the cell of origin is firmly established, the granular cell myoblastoma would be better termed "granular cell tumor."

Clinical Features. The appearance of this lesion depends considerably upon the site. Those lesions found in the tongue are usually single nodules within the substance of the tongue itself, although there may be an elevation of the tissue evident (Fig. 2–80, A, B). Multiple lesions sometimes occur. The lesion is not ulcerated, and it may have a normal covering or may exhibit some clinical leukoplakia. The tumor appears to occur at any age with no definite predilection for any one decade. There

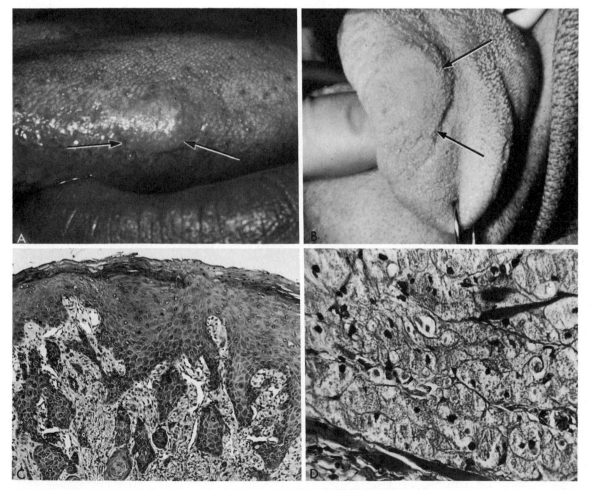

Figure 2–80. *Granular cell myoblastoma.*
A, The lesion appears as a small nodular growth on the lateral border of the tongue. B, The tumor may become quite large. C, The low-power photomicrograph illustrates the remarkable overlying pseudoepitheliomatous hyperplasia, which may be mistaken for epidermoid carcinoma. D, Under higher magnification the granular nature of the cells comprising the lesion can be seen. (B, Courtesy of Dr. Ronald Vincent.)

appears to be no difference in the incidence of occurrence between males and females, although a few studies have shown a predilection for females.

Histologic Features. The benign granular cell myoblastoma is made up of strands and fascicles of cells which are large, 20 to 40 microns in diameter, and show an extremely granular eosinophilic cytoplasm (Fig. 2–80, *C*, *D*). These granules may be fine or, in some instances, very coarse. Mitotic figures are not usually seen. The tumor cells themselves are sometimes intimately related to striated muscle fibers as well as to peripheral myelinated nerves. In some instances the tumor cells have been found arranged in concentric whorls around these myelinated nerve fibers. It is particularly common for the surface of the lesion to be covered by a layer of stratified squamous epithelium exhibiting remarkable pseudoepitheliomatous hyperplasia which has been confused with epidermoid carcinoma (Fig. 2–80, *C*).

Treatment and Prognosis. The treatment of the granular cell myoblastoma is surgical excision. Recurrence is not to be expected.

Congenital Epulis of the Newborn

The congenital epulis of the newborn bears an unusual resemblance to the granular cell myoblastoma and is considered by some persons to be the same lesion. Nevertheless there are certain features of the congenital epulis which are distinctly different from the granular cell myoblastoma and, as has been suggested by Custer and Fust, it is most likely a separate pathologic entity.

The congenital epulis is present at birth, as the name implies, and in this regard is distinctly different from the granular cell myoblastoma. It has been suggested that a protuberant mass of the maxilla, the typical site of the congenital epulis, would be more obvious than a lesion in the substance of the tongue, the usual site of the granular cell myoblastoma, and thus would be apt to be discovered at a far earlier age than the tongue lesion. On this basis it is conceivable that the two tumors are similar in nature, although actually the maxilla has been found to be a most unusual site for the occurrence of a myoblastoma.

A number of workers have suggested that these congenital epulides are malformations of the dental blastema and should be regarded as a type of embryonal hamartoma and not a true neoplasm. The basis for such a belief is the presence of numerous epithelial rests in some sections of these tumors. Remember, however, that such epithelial inclusions are remnants of the dental lamina and may be found normally in most jaws of infants. Their occurrence in the congenital epulis is more likely to be coincidental than associated with the development of the lesion. Other theories of origin include the fibroblastic, histiocytic, myogenic and neurogenic. These have been discussed in a centennial review of the congenital epulis by Fuhr and Krogh.

Clinical Features. This tumor is present at birth and is located on the maxillary or mandibular gingiva, although it is somewhat more common on the maxilla than the mandible, by a ratio of approximately 2 to 1. It is usually a pedunculated lesion found in the incisor region, apparently arising on the crest of the alveolar ridge or process (Fig. 2–81, *A*). It may vary considerably in size from just a few millimeters in diameter to several centimeters. Of 40 cases reported in the literature and reviewed by Custer and Fust, only three occurred in males. Of the 113 cases reported since the original description of a congenital epulis by Neumann in 1871, 80.5 per cent were females, 10.6 per cent were males and 8.9 per cent were of unstated sex, according to the review of Fuhr and Krogh.

Histologic Features. The congenital epulis is histologically similar to the granular cell myoblastoma, although pseudoepitheliomatous hyperplasia does not occur in the former lesion. Thus sheets of large, closely packed cells showing fine, granular, eosinophilic cytoplasm comprise the tumor mass (Fig. 2–81, *B*). Neither mitoses nor cross striations are visible, but capillaries are numerous. In fact, the vascular component is much more prominent than in the myoblastoma. Study by means of special staining techniques has not been highly informative.

An electron microscope study of a congenital epulis by Kay and his associates revealed junctional complexes between some of the granular cells which suggested that they might be of epithelial origin, although the studies were not entirely conclusive. However, Lack and his associates reported that their ultrastructural findings strongly supported a mesenchymal histogenesis. In addition, their tissue assay for estrogen receptors was negative, but considering the marked predilection of the lesion for females, a hormonal factor could not be ruled out in its development.

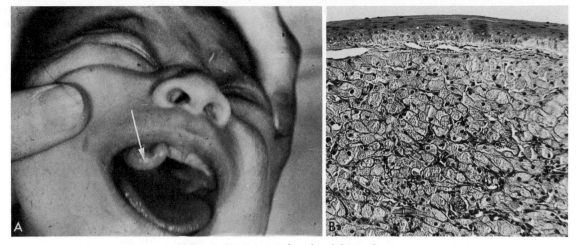

Figure 2–81. *Congenital epulis of the newborn.*
The nodular lesion of the maxilla (*A*), present at birth, was composed of large, closely packed cells with an eosinophilic, granular cytoplasm (*B*).

Treatment. The treatment for the congenital epulis is surgical excision with little possibility of recurrence. However, Welbury has suggested, on the basis of a few scattered reports, that the natural history of this lesion is one of spontaneous regression and that no treatment is required unless dictated by feeding or respiratory problems.

MALIGNANT TUMORS OF MUSCLE TISSUE ORIGIN

LEIOMYOSARCOMA

The leiomyosarcoma is a malignant tumor of smooth muscle origin. It is very rare in the oral cavity and whether it develops through malignant transformation of a leiomyoma or *de novo* is not known.

Clinical Features. Twelve cases of leiomyosarcoma of the mouth have been reported according to the review of Farman and Kay. Four of these have been in older adults, one case occurred in the tongue of an 11-month-old infant and four other patients were under the age of 12 years. The cheek and floor of mouth were the most common sites. At least one case developed central in the mandible. No sex predilection was apparent in these cases.

The lesions appear as a painful swelling but other clinical characteristics are not known.

Histologic Features. The leiomyosarcoma sometimes bears considerable resemblance to the leiomyoma, the number of mitoses present often being the most important criterion in distinguishing between the two. At other times, more obvious features of malignancy are present, such as nuclear pleomorphism, hyperchromatism and bizarre cell forms.

Treatment. Too few oral cases are recorded to be certain of proper treatment or prognosis. However, of the 12 reported cases, 4 patients had died in less than three years.

RHABDOMYOSARCOMA

The rhabdomyosarcoma, the malignant tumor of striated muscle, is a relatively uncommon tumor in the oral cavity. There are four separate types of rhabdomyosarcoma based on histologic appearance, and many of the clinical features are quite characteristic of certain of these. The four forms of rhabdomyosarcoma are: (1) pleomorphic, (2) alveolar, (3) embryonal, and (4) botryoid. The embryonal form of rhabdomyosarcoma is recognized as having a marked predilection for occurrence in the head and neck area.

Clinical Features. *Pleomorphic rhabdomyosarcoma* is a form of the tumor which, according to Patton and Horn, occurs more frequently in the extremities than in other sites and is generally seen in older individuals. In a series of 19 cases reported by these authors, the average age was 53 years.

Alveolar rhabdomyosarcoma, in an analysis of 110 cases by Enzinger and Shiraki, is reported to occur much earlier in life, generally between 10 and 20 years of age with a median of 15 years. However, the range in this group was 5 months to 58 years. While the majority of cases of this type also occurred in the extremities, approximately 18 per cent were found in the head and neck region.

Embryonal rhabdomyosarcoma occurs more commonly in the head and neck area than any of the other forms. Stobbe and Dargeon have pointed out that this neoplasm arises chiefly from the orbital, facial, and cervical musculature. Of 15 cases reported by Stobbe and Dargeon, the sites of occurrence included the orbit and inner canthus, the tonsil, soft palate, mastoid, internal ear and parotid, zygoma, and temporal and cervical regions. The average age of this group of patients was 6 years, ranging from 16 months to 16 years, with no sex predilection. In another review of 37 cases of this tumor by Moore and Grossi, the cheek, mandible and gingiva were found to be additional sites of occurrence. The youngest patient in this series was 7 weeks, although there is one case on record of an infant born with an embryonal rhabdomyosarcoma of the floor of the mouth. In a series of 48 patients with embryonal rhabdomyosarcoma reported by Lawrence and his associates, the ages at diagnosis ranged from 16 days to 14 years, with a mean of 5 years. Finally, a series of 11 cases of embryonal rhabdomyosarcoma of the oral soft tissues have been re-

ported by O'Day and his associates. The age of these patients ranged between 2 and 41 years of age, with a mean of 16 years. Of these oral tumors, four were in the soft palate, three in the cheek and one each in the upper and lower labial folds, lower buccal fold and lateral aspect of the tongue (Fig. 2–82).

Botryoid rhabdomyosarcoma (sarcoma botryoides) has been long recognized as a malignant tumor of the vagina, prostate, and base of the bladder in young children. Today, it is generally accepted as a variant of embryonal rhabdomyosarcoma and has been reported also involving the maxillary sinus, nasopharynx, common bile duct and middle ear. It was formerly separated out as an entity because of its unusual clinical growth pattern.

The chief presenting complaint of the patient with rhabdomyosarcoma, generally irrespective of the histologic type, is usually swelling, but pain may be present if there is nerve involvement. Depending upon the site of the lesion, the following phenomena may be recognized: divergence of an eye, abnormal phonation, dysphagia, cough, aural discharge or deviation of the jaw. The lesions are occasionally ulcerated and may invade underlying bone and develop distant metastases.

Histologic Features. *Pleomorphic rhabdo-*

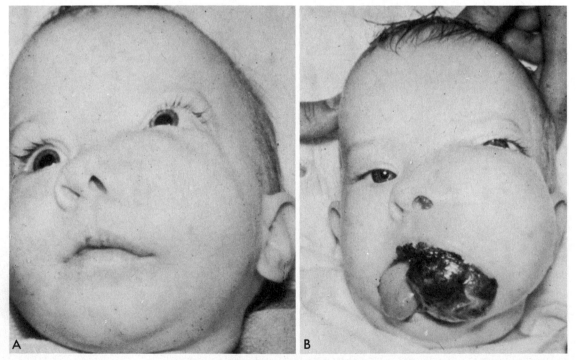

Figure 2–82. *Embryonal rhabdomyosarcoma.*
The rapidity of growth of this type of neoplasm can be judged by the fact that the two illustrations of this lesion, originating in the buccal mucosa, were taken only 14 days apart.

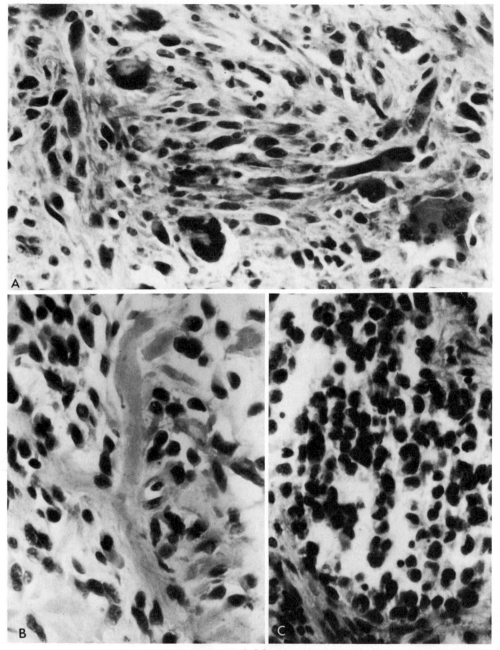

Figure 2–83. Rhabdomyosarcoma.
A, Pleomorphic type; B, embryonal type; C, alveolar type.

myosarcoma is composed chiefly of spindle cells in a haphazard arrangement. These cells are generally large and show considerable variation in appearance. The nuclei are ovoid or elongated with packed chromatin. A characteristic feature of this form of tumor is the large bizarre cells, the nuclei situated often in an expanded end of the cell, the "racquet" cell. "Strap" and "ribbon" cells typically show processes of long streaming cytoplasm. Mitoses, particularly atypical, are common. The cytoplasm is eosinophilic, and intracytoplasmic longitudinal fibrils as well as transverse cross-striations may be seen. Cytoplasmic vacuoles are also present as a result of large amounts of glycogen in the cell (Fig. 2–83, A).

Alveolar rhabdomyosarcoma is characterized by spaces lined by epithelium-like cells which appear to be "dropping off" from collagen trabeculae. The cells are often small, monomorphic, round or ovoid with dark-staining nuclei. Cells "floating" in the alveolar spaces are common (Fig. 2–83, *B*).

Embryonal rhabdomyosarcoma has been described by O'Day and his co-workers as exhibiting a mixture of four cell types: (1) eosinophilic spindle cells, usually arranged in interlacing fascicles; (2) round eosinophilic cells, large and intermediate in size, with a small nucleus and a granular eosinophilic cytoplasm, generally interspersed among other cell types; (3) broad elongated eosinophilic cells, occasionally with cross-striations; and (4) small round and spindle cells with dark-staining nuclei and little cytoplasm (Fig. 2–83, *C*).

Treatment. The recommended form of therapy for the various forms of rhabdomyosarcoma has been wide, radical surgical excision followed by supportive x-ray radiation. The prognosis of the pleomorphic and alveolar forms of rhabdomyosarcoma is generally poor. For example, in the series of 110 cases of alveolar rhabdomyosarcoma reported by Enzinger and Shiraki, 94, or 92 per cent, had died from widespread metastases within the first 4 years after diagnosis had been made. However, embryonal rhabdomyosarcoma in particular, and head and neck rhabdomyosarcoma of children in general, has received a great deal of attention in recent years, since it has been found possible to dramatically improve the survival rate through a multimodal therapeutic program. For example, prior to the establishment of this type of program, no large series of oral embryonal rhabdomyosarcoma with long-term follow-up are reported. However, of the 11 patients reported by O'Day, only 4 were alive and free of tumor between 3 to 18 years after treatment. Seven patients had died of their tumors. According to a preliminary report in 1977 of the Intergroup Rhabdomyosarcoma Study presented by Maurer and associates, in a group of 423 children with this tumor diagnosed since 1972 and treated by combined surgery, radiation and multichemotherapeutic agents, dramatic survival rates have been achieved. In some groups, depending on the extent of tumor and numerous other factors, over 80 per cent of patients have been alive and apparently controlled for significant periods of time. Similar findings are reported by Donaldson and his group with a 74 per cent 2-year survival rate and Fernandez and his group with a 68 per cent 3-year survival rate. Thus, while rhabdomyosarcoma is still a very serious neoplasm, the afflicted patient is not without hope today.

ALVEOLAR SOFT-PART SARCOMA
(Malignant Granular Cell Myoblastoma)

The alveolar soft-part sarcoma is a tumor of uncertain histogenesis originally described under this name by Christopherson and his co-workers in 1952. It is a rare tumor, thought by some investigators to be of striated muscle origin, although it differs in some respects from the alveolar type of rhabdomyosarcoma. Other workers believe that it may be of neural origin and related to the benign granular cell myoblastoma, or that it may arise in nonchromaffin paraganglionic tissue.

Clinical Features. The initial report of Christopherson indicated that this is predominantly a tumor of females, occurring usually in the teens or early twenties. A study of 53 cases by Lieberman and his associates has confirmed these findings. Of the 53 patients, 34 were female and 19 were male. The average age of their male patients was 30 years but that of their female patients, only 20 years. Occasional cases in older adults are reported.

The lesion occurs with greatest predilection in the muscles of the extremities, although lesions in the tongue and floor of the mouth have been reported by Caldwell and his associates. Only one of the 53 cases reported by Lieberman and his associates was intraoral and this occurred in the tongue. Font and his associates have reported 17 cases involving the orbit. The lesions are usually slow-growing, well-circumscribed masses with no distinguishing gross features.

Histologic Features. This tumor is composed of large cells with a finely granular cytoplasm that is not as eosinophilic as the cell of the rhabdomyosarcoma. These cells have a uniform pseudoalveolar or organoid pattern, arranged in relation to numerous delicate endothelial-lined vascular channels and septa (Fig. 2–84). The pattern is reminiscent of that seen in the nonchromaffin paraganglioma.

Marshall and Horn reported that the alveolar soft-part sarcoma consistently showed a strongly positive periodic acid–Schiff (PAS) reaction before and after treatment with diastase, similar to the benign granular cell myoblastoma, but in contrast to the alveolar rhabdomyosarcoma in which the PAS-positive material is removed by digestion with diastase. This PAS-positive

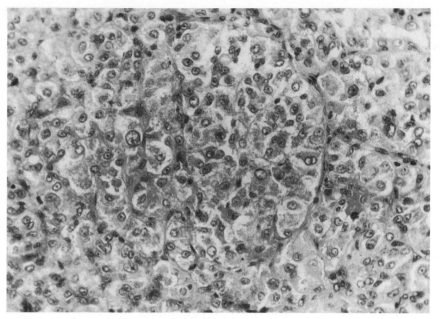

Figure 2–84. *Alveolar soft-part sarcoma.*

material in the cytoplasm of the alveolar soft-part sarcoma, described by Font and his co-workers as a highly characteristic and virtually pathognomonic finding of this lesion, represents crystalline structures composed of a protein-carbohydrate complex. They appear to form by coalescence of peculiar membrane-bound granules that exhibit acid-phosphatase activity.

Treatment and Prognosis. Radical surgical excision is the accepted treatment for this lesion because of the high frequency of recurrence, metastases and death of patients. Marshall and Horn reported the recurrence or metastatic rate as 70 per cent, 5-year survival being uncommon. Lieberman and his co-workers stated that they knew of no life-time cures.

BENIGN TUMORS OF NERVE TISSUE ORIGIN

Traumatic Neuroma

(Amputation Neuroma)

The traumatic (post-traumatic) or amputation neuroma is not a true neoplasm, but rather an exuberant attempt at repair of a damaged nerve trunk, i.e., a hyperplasia of nerve fibers and their supporting tissues. It most frequently follows accidental or purposeful sectioning of a nerve and may be incidental to difficult extraction. Cases also have occurred after an accident in which the lip or tongue was deeply lacerated by the teeth and nerve fibers were inadvertently severed.

Degeneration of the distal portion of the nerve after severance of the nerve fibers begins with swelling, fragmentation and disintegration of the axis cylinders and myelin sheaths. Macrophages serve to remove this tissue debris. The neurilemmal sheaths or tubes shrink until the distal degenerated fibers consist only of strands of connective tissue and the neurilemma. The nerve does not disappear completely.

Repair of a damaged nerve begins with proliferation of the axis cylinders, the cells of the neurilemmal sheaths and the endoneurium. Regeneration is facilitated by the persistence of the neurilemmal tubes, since new fibers proliferate through them and Schwann cells multiply around them.

Reinnervation usually occurs unless the proliferating proximal end meets some obstruction, such as scar tissue or a malaligned bone, in which case the nerve continues to proliferate into an unorganized bulbous or nodular mass of nerve fibers and Schwann cells in varying proportions. This constitutes a traumatic neuroma. The pathogenesis of this lesion has been reviewed by Swanson.

Clinical Features. The oral traumatic neuroma usually appears as a small nodule or swelling of the mucosa, typically near the men-

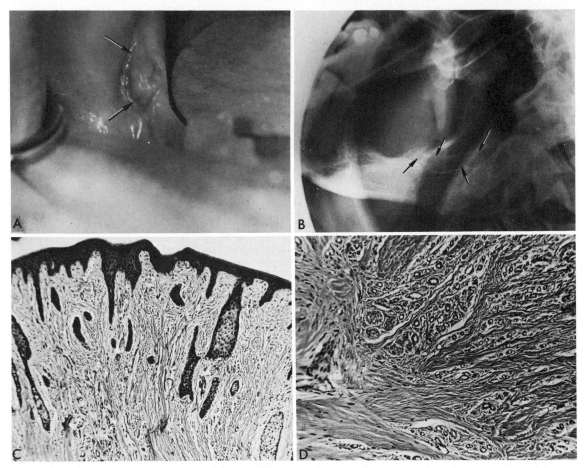

Figure 2–85. *Traumatic neuroma.*
The nodular growth in the retromolar area (*A*) represents the proliferating end of the mandibular nerve. The patient had sustained a fracture of the mandible many years previously that had resulted in the abnormal course of the mandibular nerve seen in the lateral jaw roentgenogram (*B*). This nerve was subsequently sectioned for "relief of pain." The photomicrographs (*C, D*) reveal the hyperplasia of nerve fibers in a fibrous stroma.

tal foramen, on the alveolar ridge in edentulous areas or on the lips or tongue (Fig. 2–85; see also Plate III). A central lesion within the substance of the bone associated with a nerve trunk may also occur. This is a slowly growing lesion and seldom reaches a size greater than a centimeter in diameter.

Digital pressure may cause considerable pain locally, and in some instances along the course of the nerve involved. Reflex neuralgia with distant pain associated with the face, eyes and head has been recorded. The traumatic neuroma has been discussed in detail by Robinson and Slavkin and by Sist and Greene, who also reported 31 cases.

The *palisaded, encapsulated neuroma* is not a form of traumatic neuroma but may represent a primary hyperplasia of nerve fibers, the axons and their sheath cells. An alternative theory is

that it represents a benign neoplasm. The lesion was first described by Reed and his co-workers as a clinically distinctive, solitary, benign cutaneous tumor occurring with equal frequency in both sexes and limited in its anatomic distribution (with rare exceptions) to areas bordering mucocutaneous junctions predominantly on the face. A case on the lower lip has been reported by Tomich and Moll.

Histologic Features. The histologic appearance of the neuroma is characteristic and shows a mass of irregular and often interlacing neurofibrils and Schwann cells situated in a connective tissue stroma of either scanty or plentiful proportions. Much of this connective tissue is probably derived from the perineurium. The proliferating nerve fibers themselves may occur either in small discrete bundles or spread diffusely throughout the tissue (Fig. 2–85, *C, D*).

Care must be taken to differentiate this lesion from both the neurofibroma and neurilemmoma. The histologic, histochemical and ultrastructural aspects of wallerian degeneration of nerves have been described by Fisher and Turano and by Sist and Greene.

Treatment and Prognosis. Because of the progressive nature of this neuroma and the attendant pain, it is best treated by surgical excision of the nodule along with a small proximal portion of the involved nerve. Recurrence is not common even though the sectioning of the nerve during treatment is similar to the injury that preceded the development of the tumor.

MULTIPLE ENDOCRINE NEOPLASIA SYNDROMES

(MEN Syndromes)

This is a group of syndromes characterized by tumors of various endocrine organs occurring in association with a variety of other pathologic features which are so manifold that the full range probably still remains to be delineated. Steiner and his associates proposed a classification dividing these syndromes into the multiple endocrine neoplasia syndrome, type I (MEN I) and type II (MEN II). A type III (MEN III) has been described by Khairi and his co-workers although other workers have subdivided type II into IIa (synonymous with the original Type II) and IIb (synonymous with Type III of Khairi et al.).

The multiple endocrine neoplasia syndromes each appear to be inherited as an autosomal dominant characteristic. Sporadic cases have been reported but this may reflect poor family screening.

Clinical Features. *MEN I* consists of tumors or hyperplasias of the pituitary, parathyroids, adrenal cortex and the pancreatic islets occurring in association with peptic ulcers and gastric hypersecretion.

MEN II (Sipple's syndrome, IIa) is characterized by parathyroid hyperplasia or adenoma but no tumors of the pancreas. However, in addition, these patients have pheochromocytomas of the adrenal medulla and medullary carcinoma of the thyroid gland. There is no peptic ulcer.

MEN III (IIb) is characterized by mucocutaneous neuromas, pheochromocytomas of the adrenal medulla, medullary carcinoma of the thyroid and frequently a marfanoid habitus. Other associated abnormalities frequently seen are hypertrophied corneal nerves, other skeletal defects and gastrointestinal difficulties such as intestinal ganglioneuromatosis, diarrhea, diverticulosis and megacolon.

The thyroid carcinoma occurs early in life, at a mean age of 20 years in the series of Khairi and his associates. In over 75 per cent of their patients the tumor had already metastasized at the time of initial diagnosis. About 40 per cent of the patients eventually died of widespread metastasis.

The adrenal pheochromocytomas are commonly bilateral in this syndrome, 63 per cent of the cases in the series of 41 patients reported by Khairi and co-workers. This tumor may cause sustained or paroxysmal hypertension.

The marfanoid habitus refers to a slender body build, with long, thin extremities, muscular hypotonicity and increased laxity of the joints. The face also appears long and thin.

Oral Manifestations. The most constant component of MEN III is the presence of neuromas, particularly the oral ones. These are most common on the lips, tongue and buccal mucosa. On the lips, they produce what are often described as "bumpy" lips since these neuromas, which may be multiple, are often present at birth or develop shortly thereafter and appear as small, elevated sessile nodules on the vermilion. Sometimes the lips are puffy and diffusely enlarged. On the tongue, they are commonly present on the anterior third. Similar neuromas may be found on the eyelids producing small sessile protruding growths or thickened lids.

Histologic Features. The oral neuromas appear as tortuous masses of nerve fibers surrounded by a thickened perineurium and these bear remarkable resemblance to traumatic neuromas. It has been suggested that these may represent hamartomatous growths rather than true tumors. Ultrastructural studies by Miller and his associates have also suggested that these lesions represent hypertrophy of axons similar to that noted in the amputation neuroma.

Treatment and Prognosis. The most important aspect of this syndrome is the medullary carcinoma of the thyroid because of its ability to metastasize and cause death. Therefore, the detection of the mucosal neuromas, a prodromal manifestation of more serious consequences to follow, may alert the clinician for early diagnosis and prompt treatment of the thyroid and adrenal lesions.

NEUROFIBROMA

(Neurofibromatosis; von Recklinghausen's Disease of Skin; Fibroma Molluscum)

The neurofibroma is a tumor of nerve tissue origin, although the specific cell involved is still a matter of controversy. The most widely accepted view, according to Holt, based on electron microscope and autoradiographic studies is that it arises from Schwann cells, fibroblasts and occasional perineurial cells with intermingled neurites or axons. Other investigators believe that the neurofibroma originates from perineural cells and does not involve Schwann cells. An in-depth review of our current knowledge of the neurofibroma and other tumors of the peripheral nervous system has been presented by Abell and his associates and more recently by Russell and Rubinstein. It most frequently involves the skin or oral mucosa and does not differ from the disseminated or multiple form of the disease, known as neurofibromatosis or von Recklinghausen's disease of skin, except that systemic or hereditary factors are usually not present. Since neurofibromatosis is the somewhat more common and interesting disease, the discussion will be limited to the consideration of this entity. Nevertheless all remarks pertinent to the clinical appearance of its individual lesions, their histologic features, treatment and prognosis may be considered applicable to the solitary neurofibroma.

Clinical Features. Neurofibromatosis, though not an exceedingly common disease, is by no means a clinical rarity. It has been reported in all races and does not exhibit a significant consistent sex predilection for occurrence. The hereditary nature of the disease has been recognized for many years and it is now known that it is inherited as a simple autosomal dominant trait with variable penetrance and a 50 per cent mutation rate. It occurs with a frequency of one case in approximately 3000 births in the general population.

The individual lesions are of two general types. In one form, numerous sessile or pedunculated, elevated smooth-surfaced nodules of variable size are scattered over the skin surface, chiefly the trunk, face and extremities (Fig. 2–86); in the other form there are deeper, more diffuse lesions which are often of greater proportions than the superficial nodules and are sometimes referred to as "elephantiasis neuromatosa" (Fig. 2–87). In addition, the majority of patients exhibit asymmetric areas of cutaneous melanin pigmentation, often described as "café-au-lait" spots. Axillary freckling is also

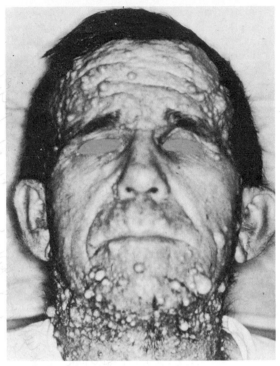

Figure 2–86. *Neurofibromatosis.*
(Courtesy of Dr. James H. Dirlam.)

common. The pigmentation and hirsutism which occur in some cases have suggested an endocrine disturbance to many investigators. In some instances loose overgrowths of thickened, pigmented skin may hang in folds. Many patients exhibit the cutaneous lesions in infancy or while still in childhood, although this is not invariably true.

The great clinical significance of neurofibromatosis, aside from the cosmetic problem, lies in the fact that in some patients malignant transformation subsequently occurs in one or more of their lesions. The incidence of sarcomatous transformation in neurofibromatosis has been placed at approximately 15 per cent of all cases by Hosoi and by Preston and his coworkers. The type of sarcoma has been variously described as fibrosarcoma, spindle cell sarcoma and neurogenic sarcoma. However, solitary neurofibromas seldom undergo malignant transformation. Preston and his co-investigators have reported other associated pathologic lesions, including osseous changes, mental disorders, congenital defects and ocular disease occurring in approximately 20 per cent of their patients.

Oral Manifestations. Oral lesions occur in patients with von Recklinghausen's disease of skin, but the percentage of patients presenting such manifestations is not definitely known. In

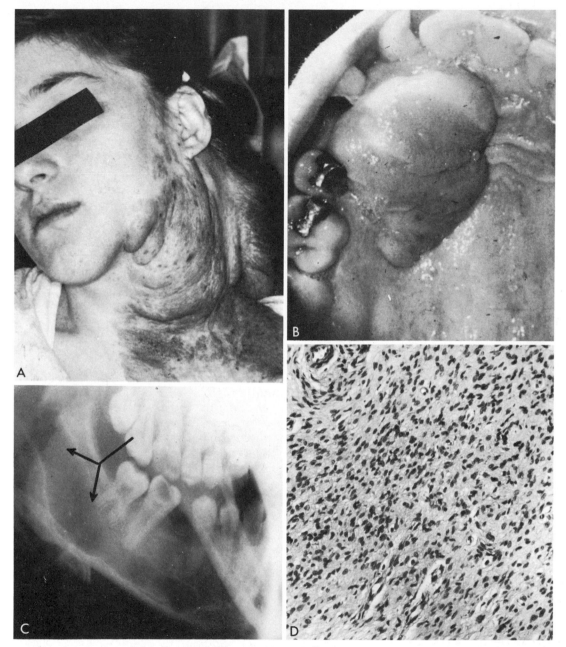

Figure 2–87. Neurofibroma.
A, The patient presented several pendulous, pigmented tumor masses of the skin. *B,* Neurofibroma of the palate in a patient without apparent neurofibromatosis. *C,* Central neurofibroma of the mandible in a patient with no apparent neurofibromatosis. *D,* The microscopic appearance of neurofibroma is similar in most cases. (Courtesy of Drs. Stephen F. Dachi, Robert Ewbank and George A. Gleason.)

the series reported by Preston and his associates, intraoral neurofibromas were present in 7 per cent of the patients. In contrast, Cherrick and Eversole reported that 20 per cent of a series of 19 cases of intraoral neurofibroma occurred in association with von Recklinghausen's disease.

Discrete, nonulcerated nodules, which tend to be of the same color as the normal mucosa, may be noted, usually occurring on the buccal mucosa, palate, alveolar ridge, vestibule and tongue (Fig. 2–87, *B*). Other cases exhibit diffuse masses of tissue which may involve the palate, buccal tissues and alveolar ridges and are composed of the same type of tissue as that seen in the isolated lesions. In addition, macroglossia due to diffuse involvement of the tongue is well recognized and has been reviewed by Ayres and his associates. Typical cases have been reported by Stillman to demonstrate these various intraoral manifestations of the disease. Chen and Miller have also reported a series of 55 cases of benign nerve tumors of the oral cavity and noted the preponderance of neurofibroma over the neurilemmoma.

Occasional cases of neurofibroma located centrally within the jaw are seen, and 16 such cases have been reviewed by Prescott and White. These are generally in the mandible, associated with the mandibular nerve, and roentgenographically show a fusiform enlargement of the mandibular canal (Fig. 2–87, C). Discomfort, pain or paresthesia are common clinical manifestations of the neurofibroma in this location. Ellis and his associates have also discussed central nerve sheath tumors of the jaws and found that very few of these reported were associated with multiple neurofibromatosis.

Histologic Features. The neurofibroma exhibits considerable variation in histologic structure but is generally composed of a proliferation of delicate spindle cells with thin, wavy nuclei intermingled with neurites in an irregular pattern as well as delicate, intertwining connective tissue fibrils. Cellular and myxoid patterns predominate; organoid features are not present. Melanocytes may sometimes be found in the tumor and mast cells are common (Fig. 2–87, D). The lesions may or may not be well circumscribed.

Treatment and Prognosis. There is no satisfactory treatment for neurofibromatosis. The lesions may be surgically excised, but their usual great number precludes any surgical attempts other than those carried out for cosmetic reasons on exposed surfaces. X-ray radiation is of no value. Solitary lesions may be excised conservatively and seldom recur.

Lesions which have undergone sarcomatous transformation have a poor prognosis, although occasional survivals are recorded following surgical removal of the tumor. Unfortunately these malignant lesions metastasize, and such cases are nearly always hopeless.

NEUROLEMMOMA

(Neurilemoma; Perineural Fibroblastoma;
Schwannoma; Neurinoma; Lemmoma)

The neurolemmoma is a rather common tumor accepted by most investigators today to be derived from Schwann cells. Neurites are not a component of the tumor as in the neurofibroma but may be found on the surface of the tumor. Tissue culture studies by Murray and Stout, who cultivated this tumor in vitro, lend credence to the idea of the Schwann cells as the site of origin.

Clinical Features. Available clinical evidence indicates that the neurolemmoma is a slowly growing lesion and is usually of long duration at the time of presentation by the patient. An occasional tumor does exhibit a relatively rapid course, however. The lesion does occur with some frequency in patients with neurofibromatosis. It may arise at any age, cases having been reported even during the first year of life as well as in elderly patients. There is no sex predilection.

Despite the fact that these tumors originate from nerve tissue, they are usually painless unless they are causing pressure on adjacent nerves rather than on the nerve of origin. The presenting symptom of the majority of patients is only the presence of a tumor mass.

Oral Manifestations. The head and neck are rather common regions for the development of this neoplasm, as shown by the report of Ehrlich and Martin, and a variety of oral and paraoral locations have been the site of development of the neurolemmoma. Furthermore, in a series of 303 patients with benign solitary neurolemmomas reported by Das Gupta and his associates, 136 occurred in the head and neck. Reported cases of intraoral soft-tissue neurolemmomas have been reviewed by Hatziotis and Asprides with the following frequency of occurrence: tongue, 59 cases; palate, 11 cases; floor of mouth, 10 cases; buccal mucosa, 9 cases; gingiva, 6 cases; lip, 6 cases; and vestibule, 5 cases. Other cases have involved the maxillary sinus and salivary glands, as well as the retropharyngeal, nasopharyngeal and retrotonsillar areas.

In addition, the neurolemmoma has been reported as a central lesion within bone, chiefly the mandible, apparently arising from the mandibular nerve. Eighteen such cases have been reviewed by Eversole, while Ellis and his coworkers have added additional cases.

The soft-tissue lesion is usually a single, circumscribed nodule of varying size that presents no pathognomonic features (Fig. 2–88, A, B). It may resemble any of a number of benign oral soft-tissue lesions. The central lesions in bone may produce considerable destruction of bone with expansion of the cortical plates and thus resemble a more serious lesion (Fig. 2–88, C).

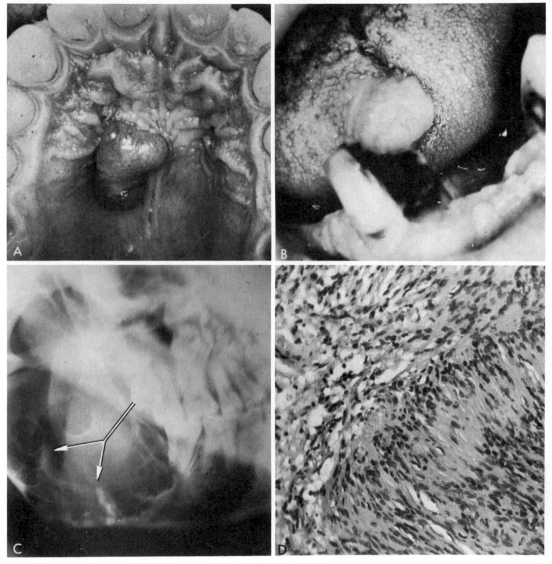

Figure 2–88. *Neurolemmoma.*
A, Palate; *B*, tongue; *C*, central in bone, probably originating from mandibular nerve; *D*, the microscopic features are characteristic. (*A*, Courtesy of Dr. Charles A. Waldron, and *B*, of Dr. Robert Ewbank.)

Pain and paresthesia may accompany these central lesions of bone.

Histologic Features. The microscopic picture of the neurolemmoma is characteristic and can seldom be confused with that of other lesions. The tumor is classically described as being composed of two types of tissue, Antoni type A and Antoni type B. Antoni type A tissue is made up of cells with elongated or spindle-shaped nuclei which are aligned to form a characteristic palisading pattern, while the intercellular fibers are arranged in parallel fashion between rows of nuclei. These fibers in some planes will give the impression of occurring in whorls or swirls. Antoni type B tissue does not

exhibit this characteristic palisading, but rather a disorderly arrangement of cells and fibers with areas of what appears to be edema fluid, and with the formation of microcysts. Verocay bodies, small hyaline structures, are also characteristically present in this tumor (Fig. 2–88, *D*). Of great importance is the fact that in nearly all instances the tumor is encapsulated.

Treatment and Prognosis. The treatment of the neurolemmoma is surgical excision. Like other nerve tumors, this lesion is not responsive to x-ray radiation. Since it is an encapsulated tumor, little difficulty is usually encountered in its complete removal, but it has been suggested that in instances in which complete removal cannot be accomplished a portion of tumor may be left without danger of recurrence. Such a procedure is poor clinical practice, however, except possibly in cases in which complete removal of the tumor would necessitate extensive sacrifice of structures and result in deformity. Recurrence is uncommon.

The neurolemmoma does not undergo malignant transformation, as may the neurofibroma after numerous episodes of surgical tampering.

MELANOTIC NEUROECTODERMAL TUMOR OF INFANCY

(Pigmented Ameloblastoma; Melanoameloblastoma; Melanotic Ameloblastoma; Retinal Anlage Tumor; Melanotic Progonoma)

The melanotic neuroectodermal tumor of infancy is a lesion which has had a long and controversial history concerning the nature of the tumor. This is underscored by the first case of this lesion reported by Krompecher in 1918 under the term "congenital melanocarcinoma," the second case reported by Mummery and Pitts in 1926 under the term "melanotic epithelial odontome," and a still later case reported by Halpert and Patzer in 1947 under the name "retinal anlage tumor." Thus, the three chief theories have suggested that it is derived from pigmented anlage of the retina of the eye; that it is of odontogenic origin; or that the tumor represents an atavism of sensory neuroectodermal development, and hence the term "melanotic progonoma." All available evidence now indicates that the tumor is of neural crest origin and the term "melanotic neuroectodermal tumor of infancy," suggested by Borello and Gorlin in their discussion of this lesion, is most widely accepted. The high urinary excretion of vanillylmandelic acid in the case reported by these authors strongly supports the neural crest origin since this is a recognized property of the neuroblastoma, the ganglioneuroblastoma and the pheochromocytoma, all neural crest tumors. Histochemical studies of Koudstaal and his associates also support this origin. Dooling and her associates also have drawn attention to the similarity in microscopic appearance between this tumor and the developing pineal gland and have suggested that the fetal pineal, a neural crest derivative itself, may be the precursor of the tumor.

Clinical Features. Nearly all cases of this lesion have occurred in infants under the age of six months with an approximately equal sex distribution in the 77 cases reported by Stowens

and Lin. Though most of the tumors have occurred in the jaws, chiefly the maxilla, there have been a few tumors reported in the mandible and skull as well as cases in the shoulder region, palate, mediastinum, brain, skin, epididymis and uterus.

The majority of reported cases have been rapidly growing, nonulcerated, darkly pigmented lesions which have given a roentgenographic appearance of an invasive malignant neoplasm (Fig. 2–89, *A,B*). There have been few reported recurrences of this lesion, however, even after very conservative surgical excision.

Histologic Features. The microscopic appearance of this tumor is characteristic. It is usually a nonencapsulated, infiltrating tumor mass of cells arranged in a pattern of alveolus-like spaces lined by cuboidal cells, many of which contain melanin pigment. The central portions of the alveolar spaces contain many small round neuroblast-like cells which show little cytoplasm and exhibit a round, deeply staining nucleus (Fig. 2–89, *C,D*).

Treatment and Prognosis. The treatment of this tumor appears to be conservative surgical excision, since the likelihood of recurrence is extremely low. One case, reported by Dehner and his co-workers, began in the maxilla of a 4-month-old boy, recurred locally after initial excision, metastasized to a cervical lymph node and finally, after widespread dissemination, caused his death at 38 months of age. Such an occurrence is exceedingly rare, however.

MALIGNANT TUMORS OF NERVE TISSUE ORIGIN

MALIGNANT SCHWANNOMA

(Neurogenic Sarcoma; Neurofibrosarcoma)

Malignant neoplasms arising from nerve tissue, specifically from nerve sheath cells, are extremely rare lesions in and about the oral cavity. Occasional cases do occur, however, and a thorough review and discussion of malignant peripheral nerve tumors of the oral cavity has been presented by DeVore and Waldron and more recently by Eversole and his associates. These latter authors have reviewed the literature and found six cases of peripheral malignant schwannomas, seven of central, and six of both central and peripheral. Some cases of malignant schwannoma originate in previously benign lesions of neurofibromatosis or von Recklinghau-

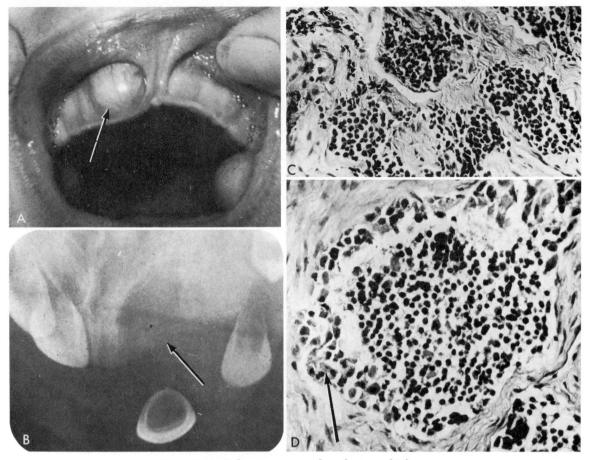

Figure 2–89. *Melanotic neuroectodermal tumor of infancy.*
There is a rapidly growing mass present on the anterior maxilla (*A*). The roentgenogram shows diffuse destruction of bone, suggestive of a malignant neoplasm (*B*). The photomicrographs demonstrate typical alveolus-like structures lined by an irregular layer of cuboidal cells containing melanin pigment (*C* and *D*). (*A*, Courtesy of Dr. Jan L. Silagi.)

sen's disease of skin, while others appear to occur *de novo* in solitary neurofibromas. In a series of 165 cases of malignant schwannoma, Sordillo and his associates found that 40 per cent of these occurred in patients with neurofibromatosis. Various studies indicate that 4 to 29 per cent of patients with neurofibromatosis may have malignant schwannoma at some time in their lives. Such sarcomatous transformation in neurofibromatosis is more apt to occur in the deep-seated lesions rather than in the superficial ones and is generally seen in adolescents and young adults. The *de novo* sarcomas are more apt to occur later in life than those originating in neurofibromatosis. Most authorities believe that malignant transformation in the neurolemmoma does not occur. Malignant schwannomas are reported occurring also in areas previously treated with radiation.

Clinical Features. The majority of reported cases of oral malignant schwannoma have occurred in the third to sixth decades, with no sex predilection. In the soft-tissue malignant schwannomas, the lip, gingiva, palate and buccal mucosa have been sites of involvement. In the central tumors, the mandible or mandibular nerve is more frequently affected than the maxilla. In some instances there is no complaint other than the presence of a mass, although in other cases pain and/or paresthesia are present.

Roentgenographic Features. The roentgenogram may reveal a diffuse radiolucency characteristic of a malignant infiltrating neoplasm (Fig. 2–90, *A*). On the other hand, the appearance may be that of only a smooth radiolucency, such as dilatation of the mandibular canal when the tumor is originating from this nerve. When this appearance prevails, the lesion may be mistaken on the roentgenogram for a benign one.

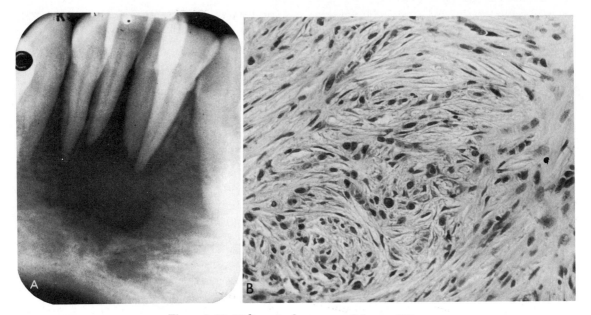

Figure 2–90. *Malignant schwannoma of the mandible.*
(Courtesy of Drs. Charles H. Redish and Norman S. Klein.)

Histologic Features. The malignant schwannoma in many cases is nearly identical in its microscopic appearance with the fibrosarcoma. If a palisading arrangement is present, it aids in diagnosis of the lesion, as do plump spindle-shaped cells arranged in streams and cords with tandem nuclei. Many pathologists contend that unless the neoplasm can actually be demonstrated microscopically arising from nerve bundles, a neurogenic origin cannot be definitively established. As with the fibrosarcoma, the malignant schwannoma exhibits all variations in degree of morphologic malignancy, ranging from tumors that are relatively acellular and show little cellular pleomorphism to tumors that are highly cellular with pleomorphism and bizarre mitotic activity (Fig. 2–90, *B*). Sordillo and his associates reported that the sarcomas of neurofibromatosis tend to be more collagenous and better differentiated than those of solitary neurofibromas, which tend to be highly cellular and undifferentiated—a paradox in view of the more aggressive behavior of the former lesion. Finally, foci of cartilaginous and osseous modulation are found in some malignant schwannomas.

Treatment and Prognosis. The malignant schwannoma has been treated by surgery and by radiation. It has a marked tendency for local recurrence, however, and the degree of malignancy frequently increases with each recurrence. This high recurrence rate is partly due to the tendency for the tumor to grow along the involved nerve, making total excision difficult. Lymphatic spread is rare. Pulmonary metastases have been reported in between 40 and 50 per cent of cases of the series reported by Sordillo. The use of adjuvant therapy after surgery may be of some benefit. The over-all prognosis will vary greatly, depending upon the location of the tumor, its degree of differentiation, its duration before discovery and the method of treatment.

OLFACTORY NEUROBLASTOMA

(Esthesioneuroblastoma; Esthesioneuroepithelioma)

The olfactory neuroblastoma is a rare tumor apparently originating from the olfactory apparatus and, therefore, found most frequently in the nasal cavity and nasopharynx. Occasional cases have been reported either originating in or invading the maxillary sinus. Such examples have been described by Church and Uhler and by Mashberg and his associates.

Clinical Features. The lesion generally appears as a painful swelling in the area of the nasal fossa. It is an invasive, destructive tumor, but only rarely metastasizes, chiefly to cervical lymph nodes and lungs. In contrast to other types of neuroblastoma, this lesion usually occurs in adults rather than children.

Histologic Features. The appearance of the tumor characteristically is one of densely packed masses of small darkly staining cells each with a poorly defined eosinophilic cytoplasm and a regular round vesicular nucleus, sometimes with stippled chromatin. Rosette formation is common. This is a pseudoglandular structure lined by a single layer of nonciliated columnar cells with a basal nucleus and a cuticular border at the apex of the cell. These resemble the sustentacular and olfactory cells of the olfactory mucosa. Eosinophilic neurofibrils extend into the lumen from the cell borders. Pseudorosettes also occur. Mitotic figures are often present, but not in large numbers. The stroma has a fibrillar neuroid pattern. The difficulty in microscopic diagnosis, however, has been emphasized by Oberman and Rice.

Treatment. The treatment is generally surgery, radiation or the two in combination. Although recurrence of the lesion is rather common, its prognosis is generally fair. In a series of nearly 100 cases reviewed by Skolnik and his co-workers, the 5-year survival rate was 52 per cent.

METASTATIC TUMORS OF THE JAWS

Malignant neoplasms of the jaws metastatic from primary sites elsewhere in the body do not constitute a numerically large group of lesions. These tumors are of great clinical significance, however, since their appearance may be the first indication of an undiscovered malignancy at a distant site. Furthermore, a tumor of the jaws may be the first evidence of dissemination of a known tumor from its primary site.

It has been suggested that metastatic lesions of the jaws are rare, since they have seldom been reported in critical analytical studies dealing with the distribution of such lesions throughout the body. It should be pointed out, however, that the usual method of determining the distribution of metastatic tumors is by means of a roentgenographic skeletal survey of a given patient. This consists of roentgenograms of the limbs, pelvis, chest, vertebral column and skull. Seldom does such a survey include separate films of the mandible and maxilla, and the presence of a lesion of these two bones is impossible to establish by most routine skull films.

Thus there is good reason to believe, and the ever-increasing number of reports in the literature dealing with metastatic tumors of the jaws bears this out, that such lesions are far more common than was formerly believed.

Clinical Features. The metastatic lesions of the jaw may be completely asymptomatic. Usually, however, the patient is aware of slight discomfort or pain, followed in many cases by paresthesia or anesthesia of the lip or chin due to involvement of the mandibular nerve. The importance of this clinical finding has been emphasized by Moorman and Shafer. The teeth in the affected area may become loose and extruded. Unfortunately, these teeth may be extracted simply because they are loose without an attempt by the dentist to learn the cause of this phenomenon. In some cases, pain described as a toothache has been the chief complaint of the patient. A definite swelling or expansion of the jaw is also an almost constant finding, according to Cash and his associates.

The mandible is affected far more frequently than the maxilla by metastatic tumor. For example, in a series of 97 cases of metastatic jaw tumors reviewed by Clausen and Poulsen, 82 per cent were in the mandible, while 85 per cent were in the mandible in a series of 20 cases reported by Meyer and Shklar. The molar area is predominantly involved, apparently because this region contains a rich deposit of hematopoietic tissue, and, since the mode of spread is usually hematogenous, tumor cells tend to be deposited in this vascular medullary tissue. This mechanism of metastasis has been discussed by Stockdale, who cited the extreme importance of the plexus of vertebral veins, or Batson's plexus, as a dissemination pathway. The physiologic significance of this plexus has been discussed in detail by Eckenhoff.

Roentgenographic Features. Metastatic lesions produce no pathognomonic roentgenographic appearance. Although most of such metastases produce osteolytic lesions and thus appear as a radiolucency on the roentgenogram, certain tumors produce osteoplastic lesions or lesions characterized by the production of bone (Fig. 2–91). Such lesions are manifested as radiopaque or sclerotic areas and are most often associated with carcinoma of the prostate and, occasionally, of the breast and lung. The metastases in the roentgenogram may be relatively well demarcated and confined or they may exhibit diffuse, poorly outlined involvement of a considerable portion of bone. Because of the destruction of bone which may occur, pathologic fracture is occasionally seen.

Certain neoplasms exhibit a greater propensity for metastasis to bone than do others. Castigliano and Rominger reviewed the literature dealing with metastatic tumors of the jaws and found 176 cases reported between 1902 and 1953. Since that time, many additional cases

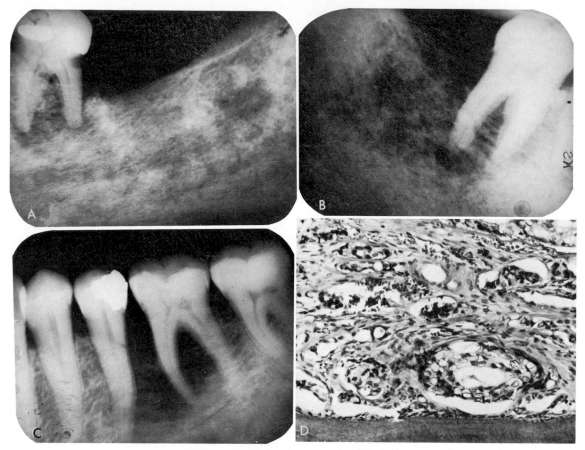

Figure 2–91. *Metastatic carcinoma of the jaw.*

A, Carcinoma metastatic from the breast, an osteoplastic lesion. *B*, Carcinoma metastatic from the breast, an osteolytic lesion. *C*, Carcinoma metastatic from the lung. *D*, Photomicrograph of metastatic carcinoma in periodontal membrane area adjacent to tooth. (*A*, Courtesy of Dr. George A. Gleason; *B*, of Dr. Arnold E. Felten; and *C*, of Dr. John E. Davidson.)

have been reported, according to the excellent review and discussion of metastatic jaw tumors by Cash and his co-workers in 1961.

There is a wide variety of primary tumors which metastasize to the jaws. For example, Clausen and Paulsen, in their 97 cases of metastatic carcinoma of the jaws, found the following distribution of primary tumors:

Breast	31%	Melanocarcinoma	5%
Lung	18	Testis	3
Kidney	15	Bladder	1
Thyroid	6	Liver	1
Prostate	6	Uterine cervix	1
Colon	6	Ovary	1
Stomach	5		

In addition, the malignant lymphomas and multiple myeloma are often found in the jaws, although it is debatable whether these should be considered true examples of metastatic lesions. In the series reported by Castigliano and Rominger, carcinoma of the thyroid was the

most common metastatic tumor of the jaws. But the remarkable increase in carcinoma of the lung in the past few decades, with subsequent jaw metastases in many cases, has accounted for a relative decrease in the incidence of metastatic thyroid cancer in the recent experience of most investigators. Other tumors also may evidence metastases to the jaws more frequently than previously suspected, such as the neuroblastoma of the adrenal, which was metastatic to the osseous structures of the oral cavity in 25 per cent of a series of 83 cases reported by Stern and his associates.

The importance of obtaining a thorough past medical history of all patients in whom the possibility of a metastatic tumor is entertained cannot be overemphasized. In addition, a thorough oral clinical and roentgenographic examination should be carried out in such cases, and if a suspicious lesion is discovered, a final diagnosis must be established by biopsy. Such a diagnosis can often be made because of the similarity in histologic appearance between the primary and metastatic lesions. Some tumors, however, are not sufficiently characteristic to suggest the primary site.

Finally, the pathologist must exercise great caution not to mistake a normal microscopic structure for cancer, particularly metastatic carcinoma. An excellent example of a problem of this nature is the correct recognition of the *juxtaoral organ of Chievitz*. This is a cluster of nests of squamous epithelial cells, sometimes with a ductlike appearance, found microscopically in tissue taken from the approximate site used by the dentist for injection of the inferior alveolar nerve, i.e., just medial to the mandibular internal oblique ridge and the pterygomandibular raphe, and from where a biopsy, for one reason or another, might be taken. These epithelial islands are usually intimately associated with myelinated nerves and the suggestion has been made, but not universally accepted, that they might represent neuroepithelial structures with a neuroendocrine receptor function. An excellent discussion of this problem has been published by Danforth and Baughman, while Wysocki and Wright have elaborated on the further presence of epithelial islands at other sites within nerves, representing odontogenic rests, and in the anterior maxilla, representing remnants of the nasopalatine duct. The development of the juxtaoral organ of Chievitz, its morphology and clinical aspects as well as its comparative anatomy, have been described in detail in the monograph by Zenker.

Treatment and Prognosis. It should be recognized that the demonstration of metastatic bone lesions involves a grave prognosis, since they are nearly always a late sign of the neoplastic disease. Considerable relief of symptoms and prolonged palliation have been accomplished by a variety of measures, including, singly or in combination, x-ray radiation, administration of sex hormones, adrenalectomy, administration of a wide variety of chemotherapeutic agents and even hypophysectomy. In general, however, the disease is fatal.

REFERENCES

Abell, M. R., Hart, W. R., and Olson, J. R.: Tumors of the peripheral nervous system. Hum. Pathol., *1*:503, 1970.

Abbey, L. M., Page, D. G., and Sawyer, D. R.: The clinical and histopathologic features of a series of 464 oral squamous cell papillomas. Oral Surg., *49*:419, 1980.

Abels, J. C., Reckers, P. E., Martin, H., and Rhoads, C. P.: The relationship between dietary deficiency and the occurrence of papillary atrophy of the tongue and oral leukoplakia. Cancer Res. 2:381, 1942.

Abrams, B., and Shear, M.: A histological comparison of the giant cells in the central giant cell granuloma of the jaws and the giant cell tumour of long bone. J. Oral Path., 3:217, 1974.

Abrikossoff, A. J.: Uber Myome, ausgehend von der quergestriebenen willkurlichen Muskulatur. Virchows Arch. [Pathol. Anat.], 260:215, 1926.

Ackerman, L. V.: Verrucous carcinoma of the oral cavity. Surgery, 23:670, 1948.

Ackerman, L. V., and del Regato, J. A.: Cancer: Diagnosis, Treatment and Prognosis. 4th ed. St. Louis, C. V. Mosby Company, 1970.

Ackerman, L. V., and Johnson, R.: Present day concepts of intraoral histopathology. Proceedings of the Second National Cancer Conference; American Cancer Society, Inc., 1954.

Ahuja, S. C., Villacin, A. B., Smith, J., Bullough, P. G., Huvos, A. G. and Marcove, R. C.: Juxtacortical (parosteal) osteogenic sarcoma. Histological grading and prognosis. J. Bone Joint Surg., 59A:632, 1977.

Ainsworth, A. M., Folberg, R., Reed, R. J., and Clark, W. H., Jr.: Melanocytic nevi, melanocytomas, melanocytic dysplasias, and uncommon forms of melanoma; in W. H. Clark Jr., L. I. Goldman and M. J. Mastrangelo: (eds.) Human Malignant Melanoma. New York, Grune & Stratton, 1979.

Al-Dewachi, H. S., Al-Naib, N., and Sangal, B. C.: Benign chondroblastoma of the maxilla: a case report and review of chondroblastomas in cranial bones. Br. J. Oral Surg., 18:150, 1980.

Allan, C. J., and Soule, E. H.: Osteogenic sarcoma of the somatic soft tissues. Cancer, 27:1121, 1971.

Allen, A. C.: A reorientation on the histogenesis and clinical significance of cutaneous nevi and melanomas. Cancer, 2:28, 1949.

Idem: Juvenile melanomas of children and adults and melanocarcinomas of children. Arch. Dermatol., 82:325, 1960.

Allen, A. C., and Spitz, S.: Malignant melanoma: a clinicopathological analysis of the criteria for diagnosis and prognosis. Cancer, 6:1, 1953.

Andersen, L., Fejerskov, O., and Philipsen, H. P.: Oral giant cell granulomas. A clinical and histological study of 129 new cases. Acta Pathol. Microbiol. Scand., [A] 81:606, 1973.

Anderson, W. A. D. and Kissane, J. M.: Pathology. 7th ed. St. Louis, C. V. Mosby Company, 1977.

Angervall, L., and Enzinger, F. M.: Extraskeletal neoplasm resembling Ewing's sarcoma. Cancer, 36:240, 1975.

Angervall, L., Kindblom, L.-G., Nielsen, J. M., Stener, B., and Svendsen, P.: Hemangiopericytoma. A clinicopathologic, angiographic and microangiographic study. Cancer, 42:2412, 1978.

Aparacio, S. R., and Lumsden, C. E.: Light- and electron-microscope studies on the granular cell myoblastoma of the tongue. J. Pathol., 97:339, 1969.

Apostol, J. V., and Frazell, E. L.: Juvenile nasopharyngeal angiofibroma. A clinical study. Cancer, 18:869, 1965.

Archard, H. O., Carlson, K. P., and Stanley, H. R.: Leukoedema of the human oral mucosa. Oral Surg., 25:717, 1968.

Arlen, M., Higinbotham, N. L., Huvos, A. G., Marcove, R. C., Miller, T., and Shah, I. C.: Radiation-induced sarcoma of bone. Cancer, 28:1087, 1971.

Ash, C. L., and Millar, O. B.: Radiotherapy of cancer of

the tongue and floor of the mouth. Am. J. Roentgenol. Radium Ther. Nucl. Med., 73:611, 1955.

Austin, L. T., Jr., Dahlin, D. C., and Royer, R. Q.: Giant-cell reparative granuloma and related conditions affecting the jawbones. Oral Surg., 12:1285, 1959.

Axéll, T., and Henricsson, V.: Leukoedema—an epidemiologic study with special reference to the influence of tobacco habits. Oral Epidemiol., 9:142, 1981.

Ayres, W. W., Delaney, A. J., and Backer, M. H.: Congenital neurofibromatous macroglossia associated in some cases with von Recklinghausen's disease. Cancer, 5:721, 1952.

Backwinkel, K. D., and Diddams, J. A.: Hemangiopericytoma. Report of a case and comprehensive review of the literature. Cancer, 25:896, 1970.

Baden, E., and Newman, R.: Liposarcoma of the oropharyngeal region. Review of the literature and report of two cases. Oral Surg., 44:889, 1977.

Baden, E., Pierce, H. E., and Jackson, W. F.: Multiple neurofibromatosis with oral lesions. Oral Surg., 8:263, 1955.

Ballard, B. R., Suess, G. R., Pickren, J. W., Greene, G. W., Jr., and Shedd, D. P.: Squamous-cell carcinoma of the floor of the mouth. Oral Surg., 45:568, 1978.

Bang, G.: Metastatic carcinoma of the mandible. Acta Odontol. Scand., 23:103, 1965.

Bangle, R., Jr.: A morphological and histochemical study of the granular-cell myoblastoma. Cancer, 5:950, 1952.

Bánóczy, J.: Follow-up studies in oral leukoplakia. J. Maxillofac. Surg., 5:69, 1977.

Bánóczy, J., and Sugár, L.: Progressive and regressive changes in Hungarian oral leukoplakias in the course of longitudinal studies. Community Dent. Oral Epidemiol., 3:194, 1975.

Barber, C. Z.: Reactive bone formation in Ewing's sarcoma. Cancer, 4:839, 1951.

Barcos, M., Herrmann, R., Pickren, J. W., Naeher, C., Han, T., Stutzman, L., and Henderson, E. S.: The influence of histologic type on survival in non-Hodgkin's lymphoma. Cancer, 47:2894, 1981.

Barnes, R., and Catto, M.: Chondrosarcoma of bone. J. Bone Joint Surg. [Br.], 48:729, 1966.

Barnett, M. L., Bosshardt, L. L., and Morgan, A. F.: Double lip and double lip with blepharachalosis (Ascher's syndrome). Oral Surg., 34:727, 1972.

Barr, R. J., and Plank, C. J.: Verruciform xanthoma of the skin. J. Cutan. Pathol., 7:422, 1980.

Barrock, J. J.: Hereditary hemorrhagic telangiectasia. Wis. Med. J., 43:805, 1944.

Bataille, R., and Sany, J.: Solitary myeloma: clinical and prognostic features of a review of 114 cases. Cancer, 48:845, 1981.

Batsakis, J. G.: Tumors of the Head and Neck: Clinical and Pathological Considerations. 2nd ed. The Williams & Wilkins Company, Baltimore, 1979.

Batsakis, J. G., Fries, G. T., Goldman, R. T., and Karlsberg, R. C.: Upper respiratory tract plasmacytoma. Arch. Otolaryngol., 79:613, 1964.

Batsakis, J. G., Regezi, J. A., Solomon, A. R., and Rice, D. H.: The pathology of head and neck tumors: mucosal melanomas, part 13. Head Neck Surg., 4:404, 1982.

Batson, O. V.: The function of the vertebral veins and their role in the spread of metastasis. Ann. Surg., 112:138, 1940.

Bauer, W. H., and Bauer, J. D.: The so-called "congenital epulis." Oral Surg., 6:1065, 1953.

Berard, C., O'Conor, G. T., Thomas, L. B., and Torloni,

H.: Histopathological definition of Burkitt's tumour. Bull. W.H.O., 40:601, 1969.

Bernick, S.: Growths of the gingiva and palate. I. Chronic inflammatory lesions. II. Connective tissue tumors. III. Epithelial growths. Oral Surg., 1:1029, 1098, 1948; 2:217, 1949.

Bernier, J. L., and Bhaskar, S. N.: Aneurysmal bone cysts of the mandible. Oral Surg., 11:1018, 1958.

Berry, H. H., and Landwerlen, J. R.: Cigarette smoker's lip lesion in psychiatric patients. J. Am. Dent. Assoc., 86:657, 1973.

Bhansali, S. K., and Desai, P. B.: Ewing's sarcoma. Observations on 107 cases. J. Bone Joint Surg. [Am.], 45:541, 1963.

Bhaskar, S. N., and Akamine, R.: Congenital epulis (congenital granular cell fibroblastoma). Oral Surg., 8:517, 1955.

Bhaskar, S. N., and Cutright, D. E.: Multiple enostosis: report of 16 cases. J. Oral Surg., 26:321, 1968.

Bhaskar, S. N., and Jacoway, J. R.: Peripheral fibroma and peripheral fibroma with calcification: report of 376 cases. J. Am. Dent. Assoc., 73:1312, 1966.

Bhawan, J.: Melanocytic nevi. A review. J. Cutan. Pathol., 6:153, 1979.

Biesecker, L. J., Marcove, R. C., Huvos, A. G., and Miké, V.: Aneurysmal bone cysts: a clinicopathologic study of 66 cases. Cancer, 26:615, 1970.

Bill, A. H., Jr., and Sumner, D. S.: A unified concept of lymphangioma and cystic hygroma. Surg. Gynecol. Obstet., 120:79, 1965.

Bizzozero, O. J., Jr., Johnson, K. G., and Ciocco, A.: Radiation-related leukemia in Hiroshima and Nagasaki, 1946–1964. I. Distribution, incidence, and appearance time. N. Engl. J. Med., 274:1095, 1966.

Blok, P., van Delden, L., and van der Waal, I.: Non-Hodgkin's lymphoma of the hard palate. Oral Surg., 47:445, 1979.

Bloom, S. M.: Cancer of the nasopharynx: with special reference to the significance of histopathology. Laryngoscope, 71:1207, 1961.

Boies, L. R., Peterson, R. G., Waldron, C. W., and Stenstrom, K. W.: Osteogenic sarcoma of the maxilla: report of a case. J. Oral Surg., 4:56, 1946.

Borello, E. D., and Gorlin, R. J.: Melanotic neuroectodermal tumor of infancy: a neoplasm of neural crest origin. Cancer, 19:196, 1966.

Borello, E. D., and Sedano, H. O.: Giant osteoid osteoma of the maxilla. Report of a case. Oral Surg., 23:563, 1967.

Boston, H. C., Jr., Dahlin, D. C., Ivins, J. C., and Cupps, R. E.: Malignant lymphoma (so-called reticulum cell sarcoma) of bone. Cancer, 34:1131, 1974.

Bras, J. M., Donner, R., van der Kwast, W. A. M., Snow, G. B., and van der Waal, I.: Juxtacortical osteogenic sarcoma of the jaws. Oral Surg., 50:535, 1980.

Breslow, A.: Thickness, cross sectional areas and depth of invasion in the prognosis of cutaneous melanoma. Ann. Surg., 172:902, 1970.

Broders, A. C.: The grading of carcinoma. Minn. Med., 8:726, 1925.

Brown, R. L., Suh, J. M., Scarborough, J. E., Wilkins, S. A., and Smith, R. R.: Snuff dippers' intraoral cancer: clinical characteristics and response to therapy. Cancer, 18:2, 1965.

Browne, R. M., and Rivas, P. H.: Chondromyxoid fibroma of the mandible: a case report. Br. J. Oral Surg., 15:19, 1977.

Brownstein, M. H., Wolf, M., and Bikowski, J. B.: Cowden's disease. A cutaneous marker of breast cancer. Cancer, 41:2393, 1978.

Bruce, K. W.: Solitary neurofibroma (neurilemmoma, schwannoma) of the oral cavity. Oral Surg., 7:1150, 1954.

Bruce, K. W., and Royer, R. Q.: Lipoma of the oral cavity. Oral Surg., 7:930, 1954.

Idem: Multiple myeloma occurring in the jaws. Oral Surg., 6:729, 1953.

Buchner, A., and Hansen, L. S.: Pigmented nevi of the oral mucosa: a clinicopathologic study of 32 new cases and review of 75 cases from the literature. Part I. A clinicopathologic study of 32 new cases. Oral Surg., 48:131, 1979.

Buchner, A., and Hansen, L. S.: Pigmented nevi of the oral mucosa: a clinicopathologic study of 32 new cases and review of 75 cases from the literature. Part II. Analysis of 107 cases. Oral Surg., 49:55, 1980.

Bullough, P. G., and Goodfellow, J. W.: Solitary lymphangioma of bone. A case report. J. Bone Joint Surg., 58A:418, 1976.

Bundens, W. D., Jr., and Brighton, C. T.: Malignant hemangioendothelioma of bone: report of two cases and review of the literature. J. Bone Joint Surg. [Am], 47:762, 1965.

Bunting, H., Strauss, M. J., and Banfield, W. G.: Cytology of skin papillomas that yield virus-like particles. Am. J. Pathol., 28:985, 1952.

Burch, R. J.: Metastasis of neuroblastoma to the mandible: report of case. J. Oral Surg., 10:160, 1952.

Burford, W. N., Ackerman, L. V., and Robinson, H. B. G.: Leiomyoma of the tongue. Am. J. Orthod. Oral Surg., 30:395, 1944.

Burket, L. W.: Oral Medicine: Diagnosis and Treatment. 6th ed. Philadelphia, J. B. Lippincott Company, 1971.

Burkitt, D.: A sarcoma involving the jaws in African children. Br. J. Surg., 46:218, 1958.

Burkitt, D., and O'Conor, G. T.: Malignant lymphoma in African children. I. A clinical syndrome. Cancer, 14:258, 1961.

Burkitt, D. P., and Wright, D. H.: Burkitt's Lymphoma. Edinburgh and London, E and S Livingstone, 1970.

Burrows, M. T.: The mechanism of cancer metastasis. Arch. Intern. Med., 37:453, 1926.

Butler, J. J.: Relationship of histological findings to survival in Hodgkin's disease. Cancer Res., 31:1770, 1971.

Byers, R. M.: Squamous cell carcinoma of the oral tongue in patients less than thirty years of age. Am. J. Surg., 130:475, 1975.

Cadotte, M.: Malignant granular-cell myoblastoma. Cancer, 33:1417, 1974.

Caldwell, J. B., Hughes, K. W., and Fadell, E. J.: Alveolar soft-part sarcoma of the tongue. J. Oral Surg., 14:342, 1956.

Carney, J. A., Sizemore, G. W., and Lovestedt, S. A.: Mucosal ganglioneuromatosis, medullary thyroid carcinoma, and pheochromocytoma: Multiple endocrine neoplasia, type 2b. Oral Surg., 41:739, 1976.

Carr, M. W.: Congenital bilateral hemangioendothelioma: clinicopathologic report. J. Oral Surg., 6:341, 1948.

Cash, C. D., Royer, R. Q., and Dahlin, D. C.: Metastatic tumors of the jaws. Oral Surg., 14:897, 1961.

Casino, A. J., Sciubba, J. J., Ohri, G. L., Rosner, F., Winston, J., Yunis, M., and Wolk, D.: Oral-facial manifestations of the multiple endocrine neoplasia syndrome. Oral Surg., 51:516, 1981.

Castigliano, S. G., and Rominger, C. J.: Metastatic malignancy of the jaws. Am. J. Surg., 87:496, 1954.

Castro, L., de la Pava, S., and Webster, J. H.: Esthesioneuroblastomas: a report of 7 cases. Am. J. Roentgenol. Radium Ther. Nucl. Med., 105:7, 1969.

Cataldo, E., and Meyer, I.: Solitary and multiple plasmacell tumors of the jaws and oral cavity. Oral Surg., 22:628, 1966.

Cataldo, E., Shklar, G., and Meyer, I.: Osteoma of the tongue. Arch. Otolaryngol., 85:202, 1967.

Catlin, D.: Mucosal melanomas of the head and neck. Am. J. Roentgenol. Radium Ther. Nucl. Med., 99:809, 1967.

Cawson, R. A.: Chronic oral candidiasis and leukoplakia. Oral Surg., 22:582, 1966.

Cawson, R. A., and Lehner, T.: Chronic hyperplastic candidiasis—candidal leukoplakia. Br. J. Dermatol., 80:9, 1968.

Chaudhry, A. P., Gorlin, R. J., and Mosser, D. G.: Carcinoma of the antrum. Oral Surg., 13:269, 1960.

Chaudhry, A. P., Hampel, A., and Gorlin, R. J.: Primary malignant melanoma of the oral cavity. Cancer, 11:923, 1958.

Chaudhry, A. P., Robinovitch, M. R., and Mitchell, D. F.: Chondrogenic tumors of the jaws. Am. J. Surg., 102:403, 1961.

Chen, S.–Y.: Ultrastructure of a plasma-cell myeloma in the mandible. Oral Surg., 48:57, 1979.

Chen, S.–Y., and Harwick, R. D.: Ultrastructure of oral squamous-cell carcinoma. Oral Surg., 44:744, 1977.

Chen, S.–Y., and Miller, A. S.: Neurofibroma and schwannoma of the oral cavity. Oral Surg., 47:522, 1979.

Cherrick, H. M., and Eversole, L. R.: Benign neural sheath neoplasm of the oral cavity. Report of thirty-seven cases. Oral Surg., 32:900, 1971.

Cherrick, H. M., Dunlap, C. L., and King, O. H., Jr.: Leiomyomas of the oral cavity. Oral Surg., 35:54, 1973.

Choisser, R. M., and Ramsey, E. M.: Angioreticuloendothelioma (Kaposi's disease) of the heart. Am. J. Pathol., 15:155, 1939.

Christensen, R. W.: Lymphangioma of the tongue: report of case. Oral Surg., 6:593, 1953.

Christopherson, W. M., Foote, F. W., Jr., and Stewart, F. W.: Alveolar soft-part sarcomas. Cancer, 5:100, 1952.

Chung, E. B., and Enzinger, F. M.: Benign lipoblastomatosis. An analysis of 35 cases. Cancer, 32:482, 1973.

Chung, E. B., and Enzinger, F. M.: Chondroma of soft parts. Cancer, 41:1414, 1978.

Church, L. E., and Uhler, I. V.: Olfactory neuroblastoma. Oral Surg., 12:1040, 1959.

Clark, W. H., Jr., and Mihm, M. C., Jr.: Lentigo maligna and lentigo-maligna melanoma. Am. J. Pathol., 55:39, 1969.

Clark, W. H., Jr., From, L., Bernardino, E. A., and Mihm, M. C.: The histogenesis and biologic behavior of primary human malignant melanomas of the skin. Cancer Res., 29:705, 1969.

Clark, W. H., Jr., Ainsworth, A. M., Bernardino, E. A., Yang, C.–H., Mihm, M. C., Jr., and Reed, R. J.: The developmental biology of primary human malignant melanomas. Semin. Oncol., 2:83, 1975.

Clark, W. H., Jr., Goldman, L. I., and Mastrangelo, M. J.: Human Malignant Melanoma. New York, Grune & Stratton, 1979.

Clark, W. H., Jr., Reimer, R. R., Greene, M., Ainsworth, A. M., and Mastrangelo, M. J.: Origin of familial malignant melanomas from heritable melanocytic lesions. Arch. Dermatol., 114:732, 1978.

Clarke, C. A., Howel-Evans, A. W., and McConnell, R.

B.: Carcinoma of esophagus associated with tylosis. Br. Med. J., *1*:945, 1957.

Clausen, F., and Poulsen, H.: Metastatic carcinoma to the jaws. Acta Pathol. Microbiol. Scand., 57:361, 1963.

Clinical staging system for carcinoma of the oral cavity. C. A., *18*:163, 1968.

Cobb, C. M., Holt, R., and Denys, F. R.: Ultrastructural features of the verruciform xanthoma. J. Oral Pathol., 5:42, 1976.

Coburn, J. G., and Morgan, J. K.: Multiple idiopathic hemorrhagic sarcoma of Kaposi. Arch. Dermatol. Syph., *71*:618, 1955.

Cohan, W. G., Woddard, H. Q., Higinbotham, N. L., Stewart, F. W., and Coley, B. L.: Sarcoma arising in irradiated bone. Cancer, *1*:3, 1948.

Colberg, J. E.: Granular cell myoblastoma. Surg. Gynecol. Obstet., *115*:205, 1962.

Cole, L. J., and Nowell, P. C.: Radiation carcinogenesis: the sequence of events. Science, *150*:1782, 1965.

Coleman, W. P., III, Loria, P. R., Reed, R. J., and Krementz, E. T.: Acral lentiginous melanoma. Arch. Dermatol., *116*:773, 1980.

Coley, B. L., Higinbotham, N. L., and Groesbeck, H. P.: Primary reticulum cell sarcoma of bone. Radiology, 55:641, 1950.

Conley, J., and Pack, G. T.: Melanoma of the mucous membranes of the head and neck. Arch. Otolaryngol., 99:315, 1974.

Cook, T. J., and Zbar, M. J.: Arteriovenous aneurysm of the mandible. Oral Surg., *15*:442, 1962.

Cooke, B. E. C.: Leukoplakia buccalis and oral epithelial naevi. A clinical and histological study. Br. J. Dermatol., 68:151, 1956.

Corio, R. L., and Lewis, D. M.: Intraoral rhabdomyomas. Oral Surg., *48*:525, 1979.

Correa, J. N., Bosch, A. and Marcial, V. A.: Carcinoma of the floor of the mouth: review of clinical factors and results of treatment. Am. J. Roentgenol. Radium Ther. Nucl. Med., 99:302, 1967.

Corwin, J., and Lindberg, R. D.: Solitary plasmacytoma of bone vs. extramedullary plasmacytoma and their relationship to multiple myeloma. Cancer, *43*:1007, 1979.

Costanza, M. E., Dayal, Y., Binder, S., and Nathanson, L.: Metastatic basal cell carcinoma: review, report of a case, and chemotherapy. Cancer, *34*:230, 1974.

Cotran, R. S.: Metastasizing basal cell carcinomas. Cancer, *14*:1036, 1961.

Coventry, M. B., and Dahlin, D. C.: Osteogenic sarcomas. J. Bone Joint Surg. [Am], 39:741, 1957.

Cox, F. H., and Helwig, E. B.: Kaposi's sarcoma. Cancer, *12*:289, 1959.

Cramer, L. M.: Gardner's syndrome. J. Plast. Reconstr. Surg., 29:402, 1962.

Cross, J. E., Guralnick, E., and Daland, E. M.: Carcinoma of the lip. Surg. Gynecol. Obstet., 87:153, 1948.

Crowley, R. E.: Neurofibroma. N.Y. Dent. J., *17*:457, 1951.

Cundiff, E. J.: Peripheral ossifying fibroma: a review of 365 cases. M.S.D. Thesis, Indiana University, 1972.

Curkovic, M.: Osteoma of the maxillary sinuses; report of case. Arch. Otolaryngol., *54*:53, 1951.

Custer, R. P.: The interrelationship of Hodgkin's disease and other lymphatic tumors. Am. J. Med. Sci., *216*:625, 1948.

Custer, R. P., and Fust, J. A.: Congenital epulis. Am. J. Clin. Pathol., 22:1044, 1952.

Cutler, S. J., and Young, J. L., Jr. (eds.): Third national cancer survey: incidence data. Natl. Cancer Inst. Monogr., *41*, 1975.

Dabelsteen, E., Roed-Petersen, B., Smith, C. J., and Pindborg, J. J.: The limitations of exfoliative cytology for the detection of epithelial atypia in oral leukoplakias. Br. J. Cancer, 25:21, 1971.

Dabska, M., and Buraczewski, J.: Aneurysmal bone cyst: pathology, clinical course and radiologic appearances. Cancer, 23:371, 1969.

D'Agostino, A. N., Soule, E. H., and Miller, R. H.: Primary malignant neoplasms of nerves (malignant neurilemmomas) in patients without manifestations of multiple neurofibromatosis (Von Recklinghausen's disease). Cancer, *16*:1003, 1963.

Idem: Sarcomas of the peripheral nerves and somatic soft tissues associated with multiple neurofibromatosis (Von Recklinghausen's disease). Cancer, *16*:1015, 1963.

Dahlin, D. C.: Bone Tumors. General Aspects and Data on 6,221 Cases. 3rd ed. Charles C Thomas, Springfield, Ill., 1978.

Dahlin, D. C., and Ivins, J. C.: Benign chondroblastoma. A study of 125 cases. Cancer, *30*:401, 1972.

Idem: Fibrosarcoma of bone. A study of 144 cases. Cancer, 23:35, 1969.

Dahlin, D. C., and Johnson, E. W., Jr.: Giant osteoid osteoma. J. Bone Joint Surg. [Am.], 36:559, 1954.

Dahlin, D. C., Cupps, R. E., and Johnson, E. W., Jr.: Giant-cell tumor: a study of 195 cases. Cancer, 25:1061, 1970.

Dahlin, D. C., Coventry, M. B., and Scanlon, P. W.: Ewing's sarcoma. J. Bone Joint Surg. [Am.], *43*:185, 1961.

Damm, D. D., and Neville, B. W.: Oral leiomyomas. Oral Surg., 47:343, 1979.

Danforth, R. A., and Baughman, R. A.: Chievitz's organ: a potential pitfall in oral cancer diagnosis. Oral Surg., *48*:231, 1979.

Das Gupta, T. K., Brasfield, R. D., Strong, E. W., and Hajdu, S. I.: Benign solitary Schwannomas (neurilemmomas). Cancer, 24:355, 1969.

Davis, G. B., and Tideman, H.: Chondromyxoid fibroma of the mandible. Case report. Int. J. Oral Surg., 7:23, 1978.

Dehner, L. P., Enzinger, F. M., and Font, R. L.: Fetal rhabdomyoma. An analysis of nine cases. Cancer, *30*:160, 1972.

Dehner, L. P., Sibley, R. K., Sauk, J. J., Jr., Vickers, R. A., Nesbit, M. E., Leonard, A. S., Waite, D. E., Neeley, J. E., and Ophoven, J.: Malignant melanotic neuroectodermal tumor of infancy. A clinical, pathologic, ultrastructural and tissue culture study. Cancer, *43*:1389, 1979.

De Lathouwer, C., and Brocheriou, C.: Sarcoma arising in irradiated jawbones. Possible relationship with previous non-malignant bone lesions. Report of 6 cases and review of the literature. J. Maxillofac. Surg., *4*:8, 1976.

Desforges, J. F., Rutherford, C. J., and Piro, A.: Hodgkin's Disease. N. Engl. J. Med. *301*:1212, 1979.

DeVore, D. T., and Waldron, C. A.: Malignant peripheral nerve tumors of the oral cavity. Review of the literature and report of a case. Oral Surg., *14*:56, 1961.

Dolin, S., and Dewar, J. P.: Extramedullary plasmacytoma. Am. J. Pathol., *32*:83, 1956.

Donaldson, D., and Myall, R. W. T.: Hereditary hemorrhagic telangiectasia, Raynaud's disease, and the C.R.S.T. syndrome. Oral Surg., *36*:512, 1973.

Donaldson, S. S., Castro, J. R., Wilbur, J. R., and Jesse, R. H., Jr.: Rhabdomyosarcoma of head and neck in children. Combination treatment by surgery, irradiation, and chemotherapy. Cancer, 31:26, 1973.

Dooling, E. C., Chi, J. G., and Gilles, F. H.: Melanotic neuroectodermal tumor of infancy. Its histological similarities to fetal pineal gland. Cancer, 39:1535, 1977.

Dorfman, H. D., Steiner, G. C., and Jaffe, H. L.: Vascular tumors of bone. Hum. Pathol., 2:349, 1971.

Echevarria, R., and Ackerman, L. V.: Spindle and epithelioid cell nevi in the adult: clinicopathologic report of 26 cases. Cancer, 20:175, 1967.

Eckenhoff, J. E.: The physiologic significance of the vertebral venus plexus. Surg. Gynecol. Obstet., 131:72, 1970.

Ehrlich, H. E., and Martin, H.: Schwannomas (neurilemmomas) in the head and neck. Surg. Gynecol. Obstet., 76:577, 1943.

Einhorn, J., and Wersäll, J.: Incidence of oral carcinoma in patients with leukoplakia of the oral mucosa. Cancer, 20:2189, 1967.

Ellis, G. L., Abrams, A. M., and Melrose, R. J.: Intraosseous benign neural sheath neoplasms of the jaws. Oral Surg., 44:731, 1977.

Ellis, G. L., and Corio, R. L.: Spindle cell carcinoma of the oral cavity. Oral Surg., 50:523, 1980.

Elwood, J. M., and Lee, J. A. H.: Recent data on epidemiology of malignant melanoma. Semin. Oncol., 2:149, 1975.

Elzay, R. P., and Dutz, W.: Myxomas of the paraoral-oral soft tissue. Oral Surg., 45:246, 1978.

Enzinger, F. M., and Shiraki, M.: Alveolar rhabdomyosarcoma: an analysis of 110 cases. Cancer, 24:18, 1969.

Enzinger, F. M., Lattes, R., and Torloni, H.: Histological Typing of Soft Tissue Tumours. International Histological Classification of Tumours Monograph No. 3, World Health Organization, 1969.

Epstein, M. A., Achong, B. G., and Barr, Y. M.: Virus particles in cultured lymphoblasts from Burkitt's lymphoma. Lancet, 2:702, 1964.

Evans, H. L., Ayala, A. G., and Romsdahl, M. M.: Prognostic factors in chondrosarcoma of bone. A clinicopathologic analysis with emphasis on histologic grading. Cancer, 40:818, 1977.

Eversole, L. R.: Central benign and malignant neural neoplasms of the jaws: a review. J. Oral Surg., 27:716, 1969.

Eversole, L. R., and Rovin, S.: Reactive lesions of the gingiva. J. Oral Pathol., 1:30, 1972.

Eversole, L. R., Schwartz, W. D., and Sabes, W. R.: Central and peripheral fibrogenic and neurogenic sarcoma of the oral regions. Oral Surg., 36:49, 1973.

Ewing, J.: Lymphoepithelioma. Am. J. Pathol., 5:99, 1929.

Farman, A. G., and Kay, S.: Oral leiomyosarcoma. Report of a case and review of the literature pertaining to smooth-muscle tumors of the oral cavity. Oral Surg., 43:402, 1977.

Farman, A. G., Jortjé, C. J., and Grotepass, F.: Periosteal benign osteoblastoma of the mandible. Report of a case and review of the literature pertaining to benign osteoblastic neoplasms of the jaws. Br. J. Oral Surg., 14:12, 1976.

Fawcett, K. J., and Dahlin, D. C.: Neurilemmoma of bone. Am. J. Clin. Pathol., 47:759, 1967.

Feldman, F., Hecht, H. L., and Johnston, A. D.: Chondromyxoid fibroma of bone. Radiology, 94:249, 1970.

Ferlito, A., and Recher, G.: Ackerman's tumor (verrucous carcinoma) of the larynx. A clinicopathologic study of 77 cases. Cancer, 46:1617, 1980.

Fernandez, C. H., Sutow, W. W., Merino, O. R., and George, S. L.: Childhood rhabdomyosarcoma. Analysis of coordinated therapy and results. Am. J. Roentgenol., 123:588, 1975.

Fisher, E. R., and Turano, A.: Schwann cells in Wallerian degeneration. Arch. Pathol., 75:517, 1963.

Fisher, E. R., and Vuzevski, V. D.: Cytogenesis of Schwannoma (neurilemoma), neurofibroma, dermatofibroma, and dermatofibrosarcoma as revealed by electron microscopy. Am. J. Clin. Pathol., 49:141, 1968.

Fisher, E. R., and Wechsler, H.: Granular cell myoblastoma—a misnomer: electron microscopic and histochemical evidence concerning its Schwann cell derivation and nature (granular cell Schwannoma). Cancer, 15:936, 1962.

Fitzpatrick, T. B., Miyamoto, M., and Ishikawa, K.: The evolution of concepts of melanin biology. Arch. Dermatol., 96:305, 1967.

Flamant, R., Hayem, M., Lazar, P., and Denoix, P.: Cancer of the tongue: a study of 904 cases. Cancer, 17:377, 1964.

Font, R. L., Jurco, S., and Zimmerman, L. E.: Alveolar soft-part sarcoma of the orbit: a clinicopathologic analysis of seventeen cases and a review of the literature. Hum. Pathol., 13:569, 1982.

Forman, G.: Chondrosarcoma of the tongue. Br. J. Oral Surg., 4:218, 1967.

Forman, G. H., and Wesson, C. M.: Hodgkin's disease of the mandible. Br. J. Oral Surg., 7:146, 1970.

Franklin, C. D., Craig, G. T., and Smith, C. J.: Quantitative analysis of histological parameters in giant cell lesions of the jaws and long bones. Histopathology, 3:511, 1979.

Frazell, E. L., and Lucas, J. C., Jr.: Cancer of the tongue. Report of the management of 1,554 patients. Cancer, 15:1085, 1962.

Freedman, P. D., Cardo, V. A., Kerpel, S. M., and Lumerman, H.: Desmoplastic fibroma (fibromatosis) of the jawbones. Report of a case and review of the literature. Oral Surg., 46:386, 1978.

Freedman, P. D., Kerpel, S. M., Begel, H., and Lumerman, H.: Solitary intraoral keratoacanthoma. Oral Surg., 47:74, 1979.

Freiberger, R. H., Loitman, B. S., Helpern, M., and Thompson, T. C.: Osteoid osteoma: a report on 80 cases. Am. J. Roentgenol. Radium Ther. Nucl. Med., 82:194, 1959.

Fuhr, A. H., and Krogh, P. H.: Congenital epulis of the newborn: centennial review of the literature and a report of case. J. Oral Surg., 30:30, 1972.

Fust, J. A., and Custer, R. P.: On the neurogenesis of so-called granular-cell myoblastoma. Am. J. Clin. Pathol., 19:522, 1949.

Gall, E. A., and Mallory, T. B.: Malignant lymphoma. A clinicopathological survey of 618 cases. Am. J. Path., 18:381, 1942.

Gambardella, R. J.: Kaposi's sarcoma and its oral manifestations. Oral Surg., 38:591, 1974.

Gamez-Araujo, J. J., Toth, B. B., and Luna, M. A.: Central hemangioma of the mandible and maxilla: Review of a vascular lesion. Oral Surg., 37:230, 1974.

Garancis, J. C., Komorowski, R. A., and Kuzma, J. F.: Granular cell myoblastoma. Cancer, 25:542, 1970.

Gardner, D. G.: The peripheral odontogenic fibroma: an attempt at clarification. Oral Surg., 54:40, 1982.

Gardner, D. G., and Mills, D. M.: The widened periodontal ligament of osteosarcoma of the jaws. Oral Surg., 41:652, 1976.

Gardner, D. G., and Paterson, J. C.: Chondroma or metaplastic chondrosis of soft palate. Oral Surg., 26:601, 1968.

Garland, H. G., and Anning, S. T.: Hereditary hemorrhagic telangiectasia. Br. J. Dermatol. Syph., 62:289, 1950.

Garrington, G. E., Scofield, H. H., Cornyn, J., and Hooker, S. P.: Osteosarcoma of the jaws: analysis of 56 cases. Cancer, 20:377, 1967.

Gerard-Marchant, R., and Micheau, C.: Microscopical diagnosis of olfactory esthesioneuromas: general review and report of five cases. J. Natl. Cancer Inst., 35:75, 1965.

Gerry, R. G., and Williams, S. F.: Primary reticulum-cell sarcoma of the mandible. Oral Surg., 8:568, 1955.

Geschickter, C. F., and Copeland, M.: Tumors of Bone. 3rd ed. Philadelphia, J. B. Lippincott Company, 1949.

Gettinger, R.: Papilloma of the palate, tongue, retromolar area and cheek. Arch. Clin. Oral Pathol., 3:45, 51, 56, 63, 1939.

Ghadially, F. N., Barton, B. W., and Kerridge, D. F.: The etiology of keratoacanthoma. Cancer, 16:603, 1963.

Giansanti, J. S., and Waldron, C. A.: Peripheral giant cell granuloma: review of 720 cases. J. Oral Surg., 27:787, 1969.

Gibbel, M. I., Cross, J. H., and Ariel, I. M.: Cancer of the tongue: review of 330 cases. Cancer, 2:411, 1949.

Gillespie, J. J., Roth, L. M., Wills, E. R., Einhorn, L. H., and Willman, J.: Extraskeletal Ewing's sarcoma. Histologic and ultrastructural observations in three cases. Am. J. Surg. Pathol., 3:99, 1979.

Gius, J. A., Boyle, D. E., Castle, D. D., and Congdon, R. H.: Vascular formations of the lip and peptic ulcer. J.A.M.A., 183:725, 1963.

Goette, D. K., and Carson, T. E.: Erythroplasia of Queyrat. Treatment with topical 5-fluorouracil. Cancer, 38:1498, 1976.

Goldblatt, L. I., and Edesess, R. B.: Central leiomyoma of the mandible. Report of a case with ultrastructural confirmation. Oral Surg., 43:591, 1977.

Goldenberg, R. R., Campbell, C. J., and Bonfiglio, M.: Giant-cell tumor of bone: an analysis of two hundred and eighteen cases. J. Bone Joint Surg. [Am], 52:619, 1970.

Goldman, R. L.: The periosteal counterpart of benign osteoblastoma. Am. J. Clin. Pathol., 56:73, 1971.

Goldman, R. L., Klein, H. Z., and Sung, M.: Adenoid squamous cell carcinoma of the oral cavity. Report of the first case arising in the tongue. Arch Otolaryngol., 103:496, 1977.

Goldstein, B. H., and Laskin, D. M.: Giant cell tumor of the maxilla complicating Paget's disease of bone. J. Oral Surg., 32:209, 1974.

Gomes, M. M. R., and Bernatz, P. E.: Arteriovenous fistulas: a review and ten-year experience at the Mayo Clinic. Mayo Clin. Proc., 45:81, 1970.

Goodsell, J. O., and Hubinger, H. L.: Benign chondroblastoma of mandibular condyle: report of a case. J. Oral Surg., 22:355, 1964.

Gordon, R. S. (ed.): "From the NIH." Human wart virus found in many papillomas. J.A.M.A., 244:2041, 1980.

Gorlin, R. J.: Bowen's disease of the mucous membrane of the mouth. Oral Surg., 3:35, 1950.

Gorlin, R. J., Sedano, H. O., Vickers, R. A., and Cervenka, J.: Multiple mucosal neuromas, pheochromocytoma and medullary carcinoma of the thyroid: a syndrome. Cancer, 22:293, 1968.

Gorlin, R. J., Vickers, R. A., Kelln, E., and Williamson, J. J.: The multiple basal-cell nevi syndrome: an analysis of a syndrome consisting of multiple nevoid-basal-cell carcinoma, jaw cysts, skeletal anomalies, medulloblastoma, and hyporesponsiveness to parathormone. Cancer, 18:89, 1965.

Gowen, G. F., and de Suto-Nagy, G.: The incidence and sites of distant metastases in head and neck carcinoma. Surg. Gynecol. Obstet., 116:603, 1963.

Graham, S., Dayal, H., Rohrer, T., Swanson, M., Sultz, H., Shedd, D., and Fischman, S.: Dentition, diet, tobacco, and alcohol in the epidemiology of oral cancer. J. Natl. Cancer Inst., 59:1611, 1977.

Granstein, R. D., and Sober, A. J.: Current concepts in ultraviolet carcinogenesis. Proc. Soc. Exp. Biol. Med., 170:115, 1982.

Gravanis, M. B., and Giansanti, J. S.: Benign chondroblastoma: report of four cases with a discussion of the presence of ossification. Am. J. Clin. Pathol., 55:624, 1971.

Greene, G. W., Jr., Natiella, J. R., and Spring, P. N., Jr.: Osteoid osteoma of the jaws. Report of a case. Oral Surg., 26:342, 1968.

Greer, R. O., and Berman, D. N.: Osteoblastoma of the jaws: current concepts and differential diagnosis. J. Oral Surg., 36:304, 1978.

Greer, R. O., and Goldman, H. M.: Oral papillomas. Clinicopathologic evaluation and retrospective examination for dyskeratosis in 110 lesions. Oral Surg., 38:435, 1974.

Greer, R. O., and Richardson, J. F.: The nature of lipomas and their significance in the oral cavity. A review and report of cases. Oral Surg., 36:551, 1973.

Griffith, J. G., and Irby, W. B.: Desmoplastic fibroma. Report of a rare tumor of the oral structures. Oral Surg., 20:269, 1965.

Grossman, H., Winchester, P. H., Bragg, D. G., Tan, C., and Murphy, M. L.: Roentgenographic changes in childhood Hodgkin's disease. Am. J. Roentgenol. Radium Ther. Nucl. Med., 108:354, 1970.

Grotepass, F. W., Farman, A. G., and Nortje, C. J.: Chondromyxoid fibroma of the mandible. J. Oral Surg., 34:988, 1976.

Hagy, D. M., Halperin, V., and Wood, C., III: Leiomyoma of the oral cavity. Review of the literature and report of a case. Oral Surg., 17:748, 1964.

Hall, A. F.: Relationships of sunlight, complexion and heredity to skin carcinogenesis. Arch. Dermatol. Syph., 61:589, 1950.

Hamner, J. E., III, and Fullmer, H. M.: Oxytalan fibers in benign fibro-osseous jaw lesions. Arch. Pathol., 82:35, 1966.

Hamperl, H.: Benign and malignant oncocytoma. Cancer, 15:1019, 1962.

Hansen, L. S.: Diagnosis of oral keratotic lesions. J. Oral Surg. Anesth. Hosp. Dent. Serv., 17:60, 1959.

Hansen, L. S., and Buchner, A.: Changing concepts of the junctional nevus and melanoma: review of the literature and report of case. J. Oral Surg., 39:961, 1981.

Hardman, F. G.: Keratoacanthoma on the lips. Br. J. Oral Surg., 9:46, 1971.

Harsany, D. L., Ross, J., and Fee, W. E., Jr.: Follicular lymphoid hyperplasia of the hard palate simulating lymphoma. Otolaryngol. Head Neck Surg., 88:349, 1980.

Hashimoto, K., and Pritzker, M. S.: Heredity hemorrhagic telangiectasia. Oral Surg., 34:751, 1972.

Hatziotis, J. C., and Asprides, H.: Neurilemoma (schwannoma) of the oral cavity. Oral Surg., 24:510, 1967.

Hazel, O. G., Charles, G. W., and Diamond, L. E.: Leukoplakia buccalis. Arch. Dermatol. Syph., 61:781, 1950.

Hazen, H. H., and Eichenlaub, F. J.: Leukoplakia buccalis. J.A.M.A., 79:1487, 1922.

Henderson, E. D., and Dahlin, D. C.: Chondrosarcoma of bone: a study of two hundred and eighty-eight cases. J. Bone Joint Surg. [Am], 45:1450, 1963.

Henle, W.: Evidence for viruses in acute leukemia and Burkitt's tumor. Cancer, 21:580, 1968.

Hickey, M. J., and Feinman, J.: Chondrosarcoma of mandible. N.Y. Dent. J., 15:577, 1949.

Hicks, J. I.., and Nelson, J. F.: Juvenile nasopharyngeal angiofibroma. Oral Surg., 35:807, 1973.

Hill, J. T., and Briggs, J. D.: Lymphangioma. West. J. Surg. Obstet. Gynecol., 69:78, 1961.

Hillerup, S., and Hjørting-Hansen, E.: Aneurysmal bone cyst—simple bone cyst, two aspects of the same pathologic entity? Int. J. Oral Surg., 7:16, 1978.

Hirschl, S., and Katz, A.: Giant cell reparative granuloma outside the jaw bone. Diagnostic criteria and review of the literature with the first case described in the temporal bone. Hum. Pathol., 5:171, 1974.

Hobaek, A.: Leukoplakia oris. Acta Odontol. Scand., 7:61, 1946.

Hoffman, S., and Martinez, M. G., Jr.: Fibrous histiocytomas of the oral mucosa. Oral Surg., 52:277, 1981.

Holland, D. J.: Metastatic carcinoma to the mandible. Oral Surg., 6:567, 1953.

Holman, C. B., and Miller, W. E.: Juvenile nasopharyngeal fibroma: roentgenologic characteristics. Am. J. Roentgenol. Radium Ther. Nucl. Med., 94:292, 1965.

Holt, J. F.: Neurofibromatosis in children. Am. J. Roentgenol., 130:615, 1978.

Horn, R. C., Jr., and Enterline, H. T.: Rhabdomyosarcoma: a clinicopathological study and classification of 39 cases. Cancer, 11:181, 1958.

Hosoi, K.: Multiple neurofibromatosis (von Recklinghausen's disease): with special reference to malignant transformation. Arch. Surg., 22:258, 1931.

Houston, G. D.: The giant cell fibroma. A review of 464 cases. Oral Surg., 53:582, 1982.

Howell, J. B., Anderson, D. E., and McClendon, J. L.: Multiple cutaneous cancers in children: the nevoid basal cell carcinoma syndrome. J. Pediatr., 69:97, 1966.

Hubbard, E. M.: Nasopharyngeal angiofibromas. Arch. Pathol., 65:192, 1958.

Hutter, R. V. P., Stewart, F. W., and Foote, F. W., Jr.: Fasciitis. A report of 70 cases with follow-up proving the benignity of the lesion. Cancer, 15:992, 1962.

Hutter, R. V. P., Worcester, J. N., Jr., Francis, K. C., Foote, F. W., Jr., and Stewart, F. W.: Benign and malignant giant cell tumors of bone. A clinicopathological analysis of the natural history of the disease. Cancer, 15:653, 1962.

Huvos, A. G., Marcove, R. C., Erlandson, R. A., and Miké, V.: Chondroblastoma of bone. A clinicopathologic and electron microscopic study. Cancer, 29:760, 1972.

Ingram, R. C., and Coker, J. L., Jr.: Palatal aneurysm. Oral Surg., 11:1158, 1958.

Ireland, D. C. R., Soule, E. H., and Ivins, J. C.: Myxoma of somatic soft tissues. A report of 58 patients, 3 with multiple tumors and fibrous dysplasia of bone. Mayo Clin. Proc., 48:401, 1973.

Ivey, D. M., Delfino, J. J., Sclaroff, A., and Pritchard, L. J.: Intramuscular hemangioma. Oral Surg., 50:295, 1980.

Jackson, H., Jr., and Parker, F., Jr.: Hodgkin's Disease and Allied Disorders. New York, Oxford University Press, 1947.

Jacoway, J. R., Nelson, J. F., and Boyers, R. C.: Adenoid squamous-cell carcinoma (adenoacanthoma) of the oral labial mucosa. A clinicopathologic study of fifteen cases. Oral Surg., 32:444, 1971.

Jaffe, H. L.: Benign osteoblastoma. Bull. Hosp. Joint Dis., 17:141, 1956.

Idem: Giant-cell reparative granuloma, traumatic bone cyst, and fibrous (fibro-osseous) dysplasia of the jawbones. Oral Surg., 6:159, 1953.

Idem: Osteoid-osteoma. Arch. Surg., 31:709, 1935.

James, J. N.: Cavernous haemangioma of the mandible. Proc. R. Soc. Med., 47:797, 1964.

Järvi, O. H., Saxén, A. E., Hopsu-Havu, V. K., Wartiovaara, J. J., and Vaissalo, V. T.: Elastofibroma: a degenerative pseudotumor. Cancer, 23:42, 1969.

Jenson, A. B., Lancaster, W. D., Hartman, D-P., and Shaffer, E. L. Jr.: Frequency and distribution of papillomavirus structural antigens in verrucae, multiple papillomas, and condylomata of the oral cavity. Am. J. Pathol., 107:212, 1982.

Johnson, W. C., and Helwig, E. B.: Adenoid squamous cell carcinoma (adenoacanthoma). Cancer, 19:1639, 1966.

Jones, R. E., Jr., Cash, M. E., and Ackerman, A. B.: Malignant melanomas mistaken histologically for junctional nevi; in A. B. Ackerman (ed): Pathology of Malignant Melanoma. New York, Masson Publishing USA, Inc., 1981.

Ju, D. M. C.: On the etiology of cancer of the lower lip. Plast. Reconstr. Surg., 52:151, 1973.

Kaplan, E. N.: The risk of malignancy in large congenital nevi. Plast. Reconstr. Surg., 53:421, 1974.

Kay, S.: Subcutaneous pseudosarcomatous fibromatosis: report of 4 cases. Am. J. Clin. Pathol., 33:433, 1960.

Kay, S., Elzay, R. P., and Wilson, M. A.: Ultrastructural observations on a gingival granular cell tumor (congenital epulis). Cancer, 27:674, 1971.

Kay, S., Gerszten, E., and Dennison, S. M.: Light and electron microscopic study of a rhabdomyoma arising in the floor of the mouth. Cancer, 23:708, 1969.

Kauffman, S. L., and Stout, A. P.: Histiocytic tumors (fibrous xanthoma and histiocytoma) in children. Cancer, 14:469, 1961.

Keller, A. R., Kaplan, H. S., Lukes, R. J., and Rappaport, H.: Correlation of histopathology with other prognostic indicators in Hodgkin's disease. Cancer, 22:487, 1968.

Keller, A. Z.: Cirrhosis of the liver, alcoholism and heavy smoking associated with cancer of the mouth and pharynx. Cancer, 20:1015, 1967.

Kempson, R. L., and McGavran, M. H.: Atypical fibroxanthomas of the skin. Cancer, 17:1463, 1964.

Kerr, D. A.: Nicotine stomatitis. J. Mich. Dent. Soc., 30:90, 1948.

Idem: Myoblastic myoma. Oral Surg., 2:41, 1949.

Kerr, D. A., and Pullon, P. A.: A study of the pigmented tumors of the jaws of infants (melanotic ameloblastoma, retinal anlage tumor, progonoma). Oral Surg., 18:759, 1964.

Khairi, M. R. A., Dexter, R. N., Burzynski, N. J., and Johnston, C. C., Jr.: Mucosal neuroma, pheochromocytoma and medullary thyroid carcinoma: multiple endocrine neoplasia type 3. Medicine, 54:89, 1975.

Kingsley, T. C., and Markel, S. F.: Extraskeletal chondroblastoma: a report of the first recorded case. Cancer, 27:203, 1971.

Kjaerheim, A., and Stokke, T.: Juvenile xanthogranuloma of the oral cavity. Oral Surg., 38:414, 1974.

Klug, H., and Gunther, W.: Ultrastructural differences in human malignant melanomata. Br. J. Dermatol., 86:395, 1972.

Kohn, M. W., and Eversole, L. R.: Keratoacanthoma of the lower lip: report of cases. J. Oral Surg., 30:522, 1972.

Kolas, S., Halperin, V., Jefferis, K., Huddleston, S. D., and Robinson, H. B. G.: The occurrence of torus palatinus and torus mandibularis in 2,478 dental patients. Oral Surg., 6:1134, 1953.

Kollar, J. A., Jr., Finley, C. W., Nabers, J. M., Ritchey, B., and Orban, B. J.: Leukoplakia. J. Am. Dent. Assoc., 49:538, 1954.

Kolmeier, K. H., and Bayrd, E. D.: Familial leukemia: report of instance and review of the literature. Mayo Clin. Proc., 38:523, 1963.

Kostrubala, J. G., Thurston, E. W., and Chapin, M. E.: Metastatic dysgerminoma of the mandible. Oral Surg., 3:1184, 1950.

Kotner, L. M., and Wang, C. C.: Plasmacytoma of the upper air and food passages. Cancer, 30:414, 1972.

Koudstaal, J., Oldhoff, J., Panders, A. K., and Hardonk, M. J.: Melanotic neuroectodermal tumor of infancy. Cancer, 22:151, 1968.

Kraemer, B. B., Schmidt, W. A., Foucar, E., and Rosen, T.: Verruciform xanthoma of the penis. Arch. Dermatol., 117:516, 1981.

Kragh, L. V., Dahlin, D. C., and Erich, J. B.: Cartilaginous tumors of the jaws and facial regions. Am. J. Surg., 99:852, 1960.

Idem: Osteogenic sarcoma of the jaws and facial bones. Am. J. Surg., 96:496, 1958.

Kramer, I. R. H.: Carcinoma-in-situ of the oral mucosa. Int. Dent. J., 23:94, 1973.

Kramer, I. R. H., El-Labban, N., and Lee, K. W.: The clinical features and risk of malignant transformation in sublingual keratosis. Br. Dent. J., 144:171, 1978.

Kreshover, S. J., and Salley, J. J.: Predisposing factors in oral cancer. J. Am. Dent. Assoc., 54:509, 1957.

Krolls, S. O., and Hoffman, S.: Squamous cell carcinoma of the oral soft tissues: a statistical analysis of 14,253 cases by age, sex and race of patients. J. Am. Dent. Assoc., 92:571, 1976.

Krolls, S. O., Jacoway, J. R., and Alexander, W. N.: Osseous choristomas (osteomas) of intraoral soft tissues. Oral Surg., 32:588, 1971.

Krugman, M. E., Rosin, H. D., and Toker, C.: Synovial sarcoma of the head and neck. Arch. Otolaryngol., 98:53, 1973.

Kwapis, B. W., and Keubel, J. O.: Bronchogenic carcinoma with probable metastasis to the gingiva: report of case. J. Oral Surg., 10:255, 1952.

Kyle, R. A.: Multiple myeloma. Review of 869 cases. Mayo Clin. Proc., 50:29, 1975.

Kyle, R. A., and Elveback, L. R.: Management and prognosis of multiple myeloma. Mayo Clin. Proc., 51:751, 1976.

Lack, E. E., Perez-Atayde, A. R., McGill, T. J., and Vawter, G. F.: Gingival granular cell tumor of the newborn (congenital "epulis"): ultrastructural observations relating to histogenesis. Hum. Pathol., 13:686, 1982.

Lain, E. S.: Lesions of the oral cavity caused by physical and by physiochemical factors. Arch. Dermatol. Syph., 41:295, 1941.

Langdon, J. D., Rapidis, A. D., and Patel, M. F.: Ossifying fibroma—one disease or six? An analysis of 39 fibro-osseous lesions of the jaws. Br. J. Oral Surg., 14:1, 1976.

Lapertico, P., and Ibanez, M. L.: Nasal glioma (encephalochoristoma nasofrontalis): report of a case. Arch. Otolaryngol., 79:628, 1964.

Lapins, N. A., and Helwig, E. B.: Perineural invasion by keratoacanthoma. Arch. Dermatol., 116:791, 1980.

Lawrence, W., Jr., Jegge, G., and Foote, F. W., Jr.: Embryonal rhabdomyosarcoma: a clinicopathological study. Cancer, 17:361, 1964.

Lehner, T.: The jaws and teeth in Burkitt's tumour (African lymphoma). J. Path. Bacteriol., 88:581, 1964.

Leifer, C., Miller, A. S., Butong, P. B., and Min, B. H.: Spindle-cell carcinoma of the oral mucosa. A light and electron microscopic study of apparent sarcomatous metastasis to cervical lymph nodes. Cancer, 34:597, 1974.

Lever, W. F., and Schaumberg-Lever, G.: Histopathology of the Skin. 5th ed. Philadelphia, J. B. Lippincott Company, 1975.

Levin, L. S., Jorgenson, R. J., and Jarvey, B. A.: Lymphangiomas of the alveolar ridges in neonates. Pediatrics, 58:881, 1976.

Levine, G. D.: Hibernoma. An electron microscopic study. Hum. Pathol., 3:351, 1972.

Levine, P. H., Kamaraju, L. S., Connelly, R. R., Berard, C. W., Dorfman, R. F., Magrath, I., and Easton, J. M.: The American Burkitt's Lymphoma Registry: eight years' experience. Cancer, 49:1016, 1982.

Levy, W. M., Miller, A. S., Bonakdarpour, A., and Aegerter, E.: Aneurysmal bone cyst secondary to other osseous lesions. Report of 57 cases. Am. J. Clin. Pathol., 63:1, 1975.

Lichtenstein, L.: Aneurysmal bone cyst. Observations on fifty cases. J. Bone Joint Surg. [Am], 39:873, 1957.

Idem: Benign osteoblastoma; a category of osteoid and bone forming tumors other than classical osteoid osteoma which may be mistaken for giant cell tumor or osteogenic sarcoma. Cancer, 9:1044, 1956.

Idem: Bone Tumors. 4th ed. St. Louis, C. V. Mosby Company, 1972.

Idem: Classification of primary tumors of bone. Cancer, 4:335, 1951.

Lichtiger, B., Mackay, B., and Tessmer, C. F.: Spindle-cell variant of squamous carcinoma: a light and electron microscopic study of 13 cases. Cancer, 26:1311, 1970.

Lieberman, P. H., Foote, F. W., Jr., Stewart, F. W., and Berg, J. W.: Alveolar soft-part sarcoma. J. A. M. A., 198:1047, 1966.

Lighterman, I.: Hemangioendothelioma of the tongue: report of case. J. Oral Surg., 10:163, 1952.

Link, J. F.: Chondrosarcoma of the maxilla. Oral Surg., 7:140, 1954.

Litzow, T. J., and Lash, H.: Lymphangiomas of the tongue. Mayo Clin. Proc., 36:229, 1961.

Lowe, R. S., Robinson, D. W., Ketchum, L. D., and Masters, F. W.: Nasal gliomata. Plast. Reconstr. Surg., 47:1, 1971.

Lukes, R. J.: Criteria for involvement of lymph node, bone marrow, spleen, and liver in Hodgkin's disease. Cancer Res., 31:1755, 1971.

Idem: The American concept of malignant lymphoma. Saishin Igaku, 19:1630, 1964.

Idem: Updated Hodgkin's disease: prognosis and relationship of histologic features to clinical stage. J.A.M.A., 222:1294, 1972.

Lukes, R. J., and Collins, R. D.: Immunological characterization of human malignant lymphomas. Cancer, 34:1488, 1974.

Lund, B. A., and Dahlin, D. C.: Hemangiomas of the mandible and maxilla. J. Oral Surg., 22:234, 1964.

Lund, H. Z.: Tumors of the Skin. (Atlas of Tumor Pathology, Section I, Fascicle 2.) Washington, D.C., Armed Forces Institute of Pathology, 1957.

Lund, H. Z., and Kraus, J. M. K.: Melanotic Tumors of the Skin. (Atlas of Tumor Pathology, Section I, Fascicle 3.) Washington, D.C., Armed Forces Institute of Pathology, 1962.

MacGregor, A. B.: Chondroma of the maxilla. Br. Dent. J., 94:39, 1952.

Mackenzie, I. C., Dabelsteen, E., and Squier, C. A. (eds.): Oral premalignancy. Iowa City, University of Iowa Press, 1980.

Mann, R. B., Jaffe, E. S., and Berard, C. W.: Malignant lymphomas—a conceptual understanding of morphologic diversity. A review. Am. J. Pathol., 94:105, 1979.

Marcove, R. C., Miké, V., Hajek, J. V., Levin, A. G., and Hutter, R. V. P.: Osteogenic sarcoma under the age of twenty-one. J. Bone Joint Surg. [Am], 52:411, 1970.

Marshall, R. B., and Horn, R. C., Jr.: Nonchromaffin paraganglioma. Cancer, 14:779, 1961.

Martin, H. E.: Cancer of the gums (gingivae). Am. J. Surg., 54:765, 1941.

Idem: Cancer of the head and neck. J.A.M.A., 137:1306, 1366, 1948.

Idem: Five year end-results in the treatment of cancer of the tongue, lip and cheek. Surg. Gynecol. Obstet., 65:793, 1937.

Idem: Mouth cancer and the dentist. J. Am. Dent. Assoc., 33:845, 1946.

Martin, H. E., and Sugarbaker, E. D.: Cancer of the floor of the mouth. Surg. Gynecol. Obstet., 71:347, 1940.

Martin, H. E., Munster, H., and Sugarbaker, E. D.: Cancer of the tongue. Arch. Surg., 41:888, 1940.

Mashberg, A., and Meyers, H.: Anatomical site and size of 222 early asymptomatic oral squamous cell carcinomas. A continuing prospective study of oral cancer, II. Cancer, 37:2149, 1976.

Mashberg, A., Morrissey, J. B., and Garfinkel, L.: A study of the appearance of early asymptomatic oral squamous cell carcinoma. Cancer, 32:1436, 1973.

Mashberg, A., Thoma, K. H., and Wasilewski, E. J.: Olfactory neuroblastoma (esthesioneuroepithelioma) of the maxillary sinus. Oral Surg., 13:908, 1960.

Massarelli, G., Tanda, F., and Salis, B.: Synovial sarcoma of the soft palate: report of a case. Hum. Pathol., 9:341, 1978.

Masson, P.: My conception of cellular nevi. Cancer, 4:9, 1951.

Mathis, H., and Herrmann, D.: Erythroplasie de Queyrat an der Mundschleimhaut. Z. Stomatol., 60:170, 1963.

Maurer, H. M., Moon, T., Donaldson, M., Fernandez, C., Gehan, E. A., Hammond, D., Hays, D. M., Lawrence, W., Jr., Newton, W., Ragab, A., Raney, B., Soule, E. H., Sutow, W. W., and Tefft, M.: The intergroup rhabdomyosarcoma study. A preliminary report. Cancer, 40:2015, 1977.

McCaffrey, T. V., Neel, H. B., III, and Gaffey, T. A.: Malignant melanoma of the oral cavity: review of 10 cases. Laryngoscope, 90:1329, 1980.

McCarthy, F. P.: Etiology, pathology and treatment of leukoplakia buccalis, with report of 316 cases. Arch. Dermatol. Syph, 34:612, 1936.

McCarthy, F. P., and McCarthy, P. L.: Diseases of mouth. N. Engl. J. Med., 250:493, 1954.

McCarthy, W. P., and Pack, G. T.: Malignant blood vessel tumors. Surg. Gynecol. Obstet., 91:465, 1950.

McClatchey, K. D., Batsakis, J. G., and Young, S. K.: Intravascular angiomatosis. Oral Surg., 46:70, 1978.

McComb, R. J., and Trott, J. R.: Spontaneous oral haemorrhage: arteriovenous aneurysm. An unusual case. Br. Dent. J., 128:239, 1970.

McCormack, L. J., and Gallivan, W. F.: Hemangiopericytoma. Cancer, 7:595, 1954.

McCoy, J. M., and Waldron, C. A.: Verrucous carcinoma of the oral cavity. A review of forty-nine cases. Oral Surg., 52:623, 1981.

McCrea, M. W., Miller, A. S., and Rosenthal, S. L.: Intraoral blue nevi. Oral Surg., 25:590, 1968.

McGovern, V. J.: The nature of melanoma. A critical review. J. Cutan. Pathol., 9:61, 1982.

McGowan, D. A., and Jones, J. H.: Angioma (vascular leiomyoma) of the oral cavity. Oral Surg., 27:649, 1969.

McGrath, P. J.: Giant-cell tumour of bone. An analysis of fifty-two cases. J. Bone Joint Surg. [Br], 54:216, 1972.

McKenna, R. J., Schwinn, C. P., Soong, K. Y., and Higinbotham, N. L.: Osteogenic sarcoma arising in Paget's disease. Cancer, 17:42, 1964.

Idem: Sarcomata of the osteogenic series (osteosarcoma, fibrosarcoma, chondrosarcoma, parosteal osteogenic sarcoma, and sarcomata arising in abnormal bone). J. Bone Joint Surg. [Am], 48:1, 1966.

McLeod, R. A., Dahlin, D. C., and Beabout, J. W.: The spectrum of osteoblastoma. Am. J. Roentgenol., 126:321, 1976.

Mehregan, A. H., and Pinkus, H.: Intraepidermal epithelioma: a critical study. Cancer, 17:609, 1964.

Melrose, R. J., and Abrams, A. M.: Juvenile fibromatosis affecting the jaws. Report of three cases. Oral Surg., 49:317, 1980.

Merryweather, R., Middlemiss, J. H., and Sanerkin, N. G.: Malignant transformation of osteoblastoma. J. Bone Joint Surg., 62:381, 1980.

Meyer, I., and Abbey, L. M.: The relationship of syphilis to primary carcinoma of the tongue. Oral Surg., 30:678, 1970.

Meyer, I., and Shklar, G.: Malignant tumors metastatic to mouth and jaws. Oral Surg., 20:350, 1965.

Idem: Multiple malignant tumors involving the oral mucosa and the gastrointestinal tract. Oral Surg., 13:295, 1960.

Miles, A. E. W.: Chondrosarcoma of the maxilla. Br. Dent. J., 88:257, 1950.

Miller, A. P., and Owens, J. B., Jr.: Teratoma of the tongue. Cancer, 19:1583, 1966.

Miller, A. S., Leifer, C., Chen, S.–Y., and Harwick, D.: Oral granular-cell tumors. Report of twenty-five cases with electron microscopy. Oral Surg., 44:227, 1977.

Miller, A. S., Rambo, H. M., Bowser, M. W., and Gross, M.: Benign osteoblastoma of the jaws: report of three cases. J. Oral Surg., 38:694, 1980.

Miller, R. L., Burzynski, N. J., and Giammara, B. L.: The ultrastructure of oral neuromas in multiple mucosal neuromas, pheochromocytoma, medullary thyroid carcinoma syndrome. J. Oral Pathol., 6:253, 1977.

Miller, W. B., Jr., Wirman, J. A., and McKinney, P.: Extraosseous osteogenic sarcoma of forearm. Arch. Pathol., 97:246, 1974.

Mincer, H. H., and Spears, K. D.: Nerve sheath myxoma in the tongue. Oral Surg., 37:428, 1974.

Mintz, G. A., Abrams, A. M., Carlsen, G. D., Melrose, R. J., and Fister, H. W.: Primary malignant giant cell tumor of the mandible. Report of a case and review of the literature. Oral Surg., 51:164, 1981.

Mitcherling, J. J., Collins, E. M., Tomich, C. E., Bianco, R. P., and Cooper, W. K.: Synovial sarcoma of the neck: report of case. J. Oral Surg., 34:64, 1976.

Mnaymneh, W. A., Dudley, H. R., and Mnaymneh, L.

G.: Giant cell tumor of bone: an analysis and follow-up study of the forty-one cases observed at the Massachusetts General Hospital between 1925 and 1961. J. Bone Joint Surg. [Am], 46:63, 1964.

Modlin, J., and Johnson, R. E.: The surgical treatment of cancer of the buccal mucosa and lower gingivae. Am. J. Roentgenol., 73:620, 1955.

Moertel, C. G., and Foss, E. L.: Multicentric carcinomas of the oral cavity. Surg. Gynecol. Obstet., 106:652, 1958.

Monkman, G. R., Orwoll, G., and Ivins, J. C.: Trauma and oncogenesis. Mayo Clin. Proc., 49:157, 1974.

Montgomery, H.: Precancerous dermatoses and epithelioma in situ. Arch. Dermatol. Syph., 39:387, 1939.

Moore, C.: Smoking and cancer of the mouth, pharynx, and larynx. J.A.M.A., 191:283, 1965.

Moore, O., and Grossi, C.: Embryonal rhabdomyosarcoma of the head and neck. Cancer, 12:69, 1959.

Moorman, W. C., and Shafer, W. G.: Metastatic carcinoma of the mandible. J. Oral Surg., 12:205, 1954.

Moran, J. J., and Enterline, H. T.: Benign rhabdomyoma of the pharynx: a case report, review of the literature, and comparison with cardiac rhabdomyoma. Am. J. Clin. Pathol., 42:174, 1964.

Morrison, R., and Deeley, T. J.: Intra-alveolar carcinoma of the jaw: treatment by supervoltage radiotherapy. Br. J. Radiol., 35:321, 1962.

Moscovic, E. A., and Azar, H. A.: Multiple granular cell tumors ("myoblastoma"); case report with electron microscopic observations and review of the literature. Cancer, 20:2032, 1967.

Mulay, D. N., and Urbach, F.: Local therapy of oral leukoplakia with vitamin A. Arch. Dermatol. Syph., 78:637, 1958.

Mummery, J. H., and Pitts, A. T.: A melanotic epithelial odontome in a child. Br. Dent. J., 47:121, 1926.

Murray, M.: Cultural characteristics of three granular-cell myoblastomas. Cancer, 4:857, 1951.

Murray, M., and Stout, A. P.: Characteristics of human Schwann cells in vitro. Anat. Rec., 84:275, 1942.

Mustard, R. A., and Rosen, I. B.: Cervical lymph node involvement in oral cancer. Am. J. Roentgenol. Radium Ther. Nucl. Med., 90:978, 1963.

Nathanson, I. T., and Weisberger, D. B.: The treatment of leukoplakia buccalis and related lesions with estrogenic hormones. N. Engl. J. Med., 221:556, 1939.

Nathwani, B. N.: A critical analysis of the classifications of non-Hodgkin's lymphomas. Cancer, 44:347, 1979.

Neumann-Jensen, B., and Praetorius, F.: Et usaedvanligt tilfaelde of aneurysmal knoglecyste. Tandlaegebladet, 81:230, 1977.

Neville, B. W., and Weathers, D. R.: Verruciform xanthoma. Oral Surg., 49:429, 1980.

New, G. B., and Hallberg, O. E.: The end-results of the treatment of malignant tumors of the palate. Surg. Gynecol. Obstet., 73:520, 1941.

Nieburgs, H. E., Herman, B. E., and Reisman, H.: Buccal cell changes in patients with malignant tumors. Lab. Invest., 11:80, 1962.

Nix, J. T.: Lymphangioma. Am. Surg., 20:556, 1954.

Oberman, H. A., and Rice, D. H.: Olfactory neuroblastomas. A clinicopathologic study. Cancer, 38:2494, 1976.

Oberman, H. A., Holtz, F., Sheffer, L. A., and Magielski, J. E.: Chemodectomas (nonchromaffin paragangliomas) of the head and neck: a clinicopathologic study. Cancer, 21:838, 1968.

O'Brien, J. E., and Stout, A. P.: Malignant fibrous xanthomas. Cancer, 17:1445, 1964.

O'Brien, P. H., and Brasfield, R. D.: Hemangiopericytoma. Cancer, 18:249, 1965.

Idem: Kaposi's sarcoma. Cancer, 19:1497, 1966.

O'Conor, G. T.: Malignant lymphoma in African children. II. A pathological entity. Cancer, 14:270, 1961.

O'Connor, G. T., Rappaport, H., and Smith, E. B.: Childhood lymphoma resembling "Burkitt Tumor" in the United States. Cancer, 18:411, 1965.

O'Day, R. A., Soule, E. H., and Gores, R. J.: Embryonal rhabdomyosarcoma of the oral soft tissues. Oral Surg., 20:85, 1965.

Idem: Soft tissue sarcomas of the oral cavity. Mayo Clin. Proc., 39:169, 1964.

Oliver, W. M.: Hereditary hemorrhagic telangiectasia. Oral Surg., 16:658, 1963.

Orbach, S.: Congenital arteriovenous malformations of the face. Report of a case. Oral Surg., 42:2, 1976.

Oringer, M. J.: Neuroma of the mandible. Oral Surg., 1:1135, 1948.

Paissat, D. K.: Oral submucous fibrosis. Int. J. Oral Surg., 10:307, 1981.

Paletta, F. X.: Lymphangioma. Plast. Reconstr. Surg., 237:269, 1966.

Parker, F., Jr., and Jackson, H., Jr.: Primary reticulum cell sarcoma of bone. Surg. Gynecol. Obstet., 68:45, 1939.

Patchefsky, A. S., Brodovsky, H., Southard, M., Menduke, H., Gray, S., and Hoch, W. S.: Hodgkin's Disease. A clinical and pathologic study of 235 cases. Cancer, 32:150, 1973.

Patchefsky, A. S., Brodovsky, H. S., Menduke, H., Southard, M., Brooks, J., Nicklas, D., and Hoch, W. S.: Non-Hodgkin's Lymphomas: A clinicopathologic study of 293 cases. Cancer, 34:1173, 1974.

Patterson, C. N.: Juvenile nasopharyngeal angiofibroma. Arch. Otolaryngol, 81:270, 1965.

Patton, R. B., and Horn, R. C., Jr.: Rhabdomyosarcoma: clinical and pathological features and comparison with human fetal and embryonal skeletal muscle. Surgery, 52:572, 1962.

Peacock, E. E., Jr., Greenberg, B. G., and Brawley, B. W.: The effect of snuff and tobacco on the production of oral carcinoma: an experimental and epidemiological study. Ann. Surg., 151:542, 1960.

Pearse, A. G.: The histogenesis of granular-cell myoblastoma (granular-cell perineural fibroblastoma). J. Pathol. Bacteriol., 62:351, 1950.

Peterman, A. F., Hayles, A. B., Dockerty, M. B., and Love, J. G.: Encephalotrigeminal angiomatosis (Sturge-Weber disease). Clinical study of thirty-five cases. J.A.M.A., 167:2169, 1958.

Petit, V. D., Chamness, J. T., and Ackerman, L. V.: Fibromatosis and fibrosarcoma following irradiation therapy. Cancer, 7:149, 1954.

Pimpinella, R. J.: The nasopharyngeal angiofibroma in the adolescent male. J. Pediatr., 64:260, 1964.

Pindborg, J. J.: Fibrous dysplasia or fibro-osteoma. Acta Radiol., 36:196, 1951.

Idem: Oral leukoplakia. Aust. Dent. J., 16:83, 1971.

Idem: Is submucous fibrosis a precancerous condition in the oral cavity? Int. Dent. J., 22:474, 1972.

Pindborg, J. J., and Sirsat, S. M.: Oral submucous fibrosis. Oral Surg., 22:764, 1966.

Pindborg, J. J., and Zachariah, J.: Frequency of oral submucous fibrosis among 100 south Indians with oral cancer. Bull. W.H.O., 32:750, 1965.

Pindborg, J. J., Kramer, I. R. M., and Torloni, H.: Histological typing of odontogenic tumours, jaw cysts and allied lesions, international histological classification of tumours No. 5, Geneva, World Health Organization, 1971.

Pindborg, J. J., Mehta, F. S., and Daftary, D. K.: Incidence of oral cancer among 30,000 villagers in India in a 7-year follow-up study of oral precancerous lesions. Community Dent. Oral Epidemiol., 3:86, 1975.

Pindborg, J. J., Chawla, T. N., Srivastava, A. N., and Gupta, D.: Epithelial changes in oral submucous fibrosis. Acta Odontol. Scand., 23:277, 1965.

Pindborg, J. J., Chawla, T. N., Srivastava, A. N., Gupta, D., and Mehrotra, M. L.: Clinical aspects of oral submucous fibrosis. Acta Odontol. Scand., 22:679, 1964.

Pindborg, J. J., Jølst, O., Renstrup, G., and Roed-Petersen, B.: Studies in oral leukoplakia: a report on the period prevalence of malignant transformation in leukoplakia based on a follow-up study of 248 patients. J. Am. Dent. Assoc., 76:767, 1968.

Pindborg, J. J., Mehta, F. S., Gupta, P. C., and Daftary, D. K.: Prevalence of oral submucous fibrosis among 50,915 Indian villagers. Br. J. Cancer, 22:646, 1968.

Pindborg, J. J., Reibel, J., Roed-Petersen, B., and Mehta, F. S.: Tobacco-induced changes in oral leukoplakic epithelium. Cancer, 45:2330, 1980.

Pindborg, J. J., Renstrup, G., Poulsen, H. E., and Silverman, S., Jr.: Studies in oral leukoplakias. Acta Odontol. Scand., 21:407, 1963.

Pinkus, G. S., and Said, J. W.: Characterization of non-Hodgkin's lymphomas using multiple cell markers. Immunologic, morphologic, and cytochemical studies of 72 cases. Am. J. Pathol., 94:349, 1979.

Pinkus, H.: Keratosis senilis: a biologic concept of its pathogenesis and diagnosis based on the study of normal epidermis and 1730 seborrheic and senile keratoses. Am. J. Clin. Pathol., 29:193, 1958.

Platkajs, M. A.: A clinicopathologic study of oral leukoplakia with emphasis on the keratinization pattern. J. Can. Dent. Assoc., 3:107, 1979.

Pliskin, M. E.: Malignant melanoma of the oral cavity; in W. H. Clark, Jr., L. I. Goldman, and M. J. Mastrangelo: Human Malignant Melanoma. New York, Grune & Stratton, 1979.

Pomeroy, T. C., and Johnson, R. E.: Prognostic factors for survival in Ewing's sarcoma. Am. J. Roentgenol., 123:598, 1975.

Potdar, G. G.: Ewing's tumors of the jaws. Oral Surg., 29:505, 1970.

Praetorius-Clausen, F.: Historadiographic study of oral leukoplakias. Scand. J. Dent. Res., 78:479, 1970.

Prescott, G. H., and White, R. E.: Solitary, central neurofibroma of the mandible: report of case and review of the literature. J. Oral Surg., 28:305, 1970.

Preston, F. W., Walsh, W. S., and Clarke, T. H.: Cutaneous neurofibromatosis (von Recklinghausen's disease): clinical manifestations and incidence of sarcoma in sixty-one male patients. Arch. Surg., 64:813, 1952.

Price, C. H. G., and Goldie, W.: Paget's sarcoma of bone. A study of eighty cases from the Bristol and the Leeds bone tumour registries. J. Bone Joint Surg. [Br], 51:205, 1969.

Quick, D., and Cutler, M.: Transitional cell epidermoid carcinoma: a radiosensitive type of intraoral tumor. Surg. Gynecol. Obstet., 45:320, 1927.

Quigley, L. F., Jr., Cobb, C. M., Schoenfeld, S., Hunt, E. E., Sr., and Williams, P.: Reverse smoking and its oral consequences in Caribbean and South American peoples. J. Am. Dent. Assoc., 69:427, 1964.

Rahausen, A., and Sayago, C.: Treatment of carcinoma of the tongue. Am. J. Roentgenol. Radium Ther. Nucl. Med., 71:243, 1954.

Rahimi, A., Beabout, J. W., Ivins, J. C., and Dahlin, D. C.: Chondromyxoid fibroma: a clinicopathologic study of 76 cases. Cancer, 30:726, 1972.

Rappaport, H.: Tumors of the Hematopoietic System. (Atlas of Tumor Pathology, Section III, Fascicle 8.) Washington, D.C., Armed Forces Institute of Pathology, 1966.

Rappaport, H. M.: Neurofibromatosis of the oral cavity: report of case. Oral Surg., 6:599, 1953.

Reed, R. J.: New Concepts in Surgical Pathology of the Skin. New York, John Wiley & Sons, 1976.

Reed, R. J., Fine, R. M., and Meltzer, H. D.: Palisaded, encapsulated neuromas of the skin. Arch. Derm., 106:865, 1972.

Regezi, J. A., Batsakis, J. G., and Courtney, R. M.: Granular cell tumors of the head and neck. J. Oral Surg., 37:402, 1979.

Regezi, J. A., Hayward, J. R., and Pickens, T. N.: Superficial melanomas of oral mucous membranes. Oral Surg., 45:703, 1978.

Reichart, P., and Reznik-Schüller, H.: The ultrastructure of an oral angiomyoma. J. Oral Pathol., 6:25, 1977.

Renstrup, G.: Leukoplakia of the oral cavity. Acta Odontol. Scand., 16:99, 1958.

Idem: Occurrence of candida in oral leukoplakias. Acta Pathol. Microbiol. Scand., 78:421, 1970.

Richards, G. E.: Radiation therapy of carcinoma of the buccal mucosa (cheek); in G. T. Pack and E. M. Livingston (eds.): Treatment of Cancer and Allied Diseases. New York, Paul B. Hoeber, Inc., 1940.

Robbins, S. L., and Cotran, R. S.: Pathologic Basis of Disease. 2nd ed. W. B. Saunders Company, Philadelphia, 1979.

Robinson, L., and Hukill, P. B.: Hutchinson's melanotic freckle in oral mucous membrane. Cancer, 26:297, 1970.

Robinson, M., and Slavkin, H. C.: Dental amputation neuromas. J. Am. Dent. Assoc., 70:662, 1965.

Roca, A. N., Smith, J. L., and Jing, B-S.: Osteosarcoma and parosteal osteogenic sarcoma of the maxilla and mandible: study of 20 cases. Am. J. Clin. Pathol., 54:625, 1970.

Rodriguez, H. A., and Ackerman, L. V.: Cellular blue nevus. Clinicopathologic study of forty-five cases. Cancer, 21:393, 1968.

Roed-Petersen, B.: Cancer development in oral leukoplakia: follow-up of 331 patients. J. Dent. Res., 50:711, 1971.

Roed-Petersen, B., and Pindborg, J. J.: A study of Danish snuff-induced oral leukoplakias. J. Oral Pathol., 2:301, 1973.

Roed-Petersen, B., Renstrup, G., and Pindborg, J. J.: Candida in oral leukoplakias: a histologic and exfoliative study. Scand. J. Dent. Res., 78:323, 1970.

Roffo, A. H.: Leucoplasie expérimentale produite par le tobac. Rev. Stomatol., 32:699, 1930.

Rosen, G., Caparros, B., Mosende, C., McCormick, B., Huvos, A. G., and Marcove, R. C.: Curability of Ewing's sarcoma and considerations for future therapeutic trials. Cancer, 41:888, 1978.

Rosenberg Gertzman, G. B., Clark, M., and Gaston, G.: Multiple hamartoma and neoplasia syndrome (Cowden's syndrome). Oral Surg., 49:314, 1980.

Rosenberg, S. A.: National Cancer Institute Sponsored Study of Classifications of Non-Hodgkin's Lymphomas. Summary and description of a working formulation for clinical usage. Cancer, 49:2112, 1982.

Roth, J. A., Enzinger, F. M., and Tannenbaum, M.: Synovial sarcoma of the neck: a follow-up study of 24 cases. Cancer, 35:1243, 1975.

Roth, S. I., Stowell, R. E., and Helwig, E. B.: Cutaneous ossification: report of 120 cases and review of the literature. Arch. Pathol., 76:44, 1963.

Roy, J. J., Klein, H. Z., and Tipton, D. L.: Osteochondroma of the tongue. Arch. Pathol., 89:565, 1970.

Royster, H. P., Moyers E. D., Jr., Williams, R. B., and Horn, R. C., Jr.: A study of cervical lymph node metastasis in squamous cell carcinoma of the oral cavity. Am. J. Roentgenol. Radium Ther. Nucl. Med., 69:792, 1953.

Ruschak, P. J., Kauh, Y. C., and Luscombe, H. A.: Cowden's disease associated with immunodeficiency. Arch. Dermatol., 117:573, 1981.

Russell, D. S., and Rubinstein, L. J.: Pathology of Tumors of the Nervous System. 4th ed. London, Arnold Ltd. 1977.

Sachs, W., and Sachs, P. M.: Erythroplasia of Queyrat: report of 10 cases. Arch. Dermatol. Syph., 58:184, 1948.

Saijo, M., Munro, I. R., and Mancer, K.: Lymphangioma. A long-term follow-up study. Plast. Reconstr. Surg., 56:642, 1975.

Salvador, A. H., Beabout, J. W., and Dahlin, D. C.: Mesenchymal chondrosarcoma: observations on 30 new cases. Cancer, 28:605, 1971.

Samter, T. G., Vellios, F., and Shafer, W. G.: Neurilemmoma of bone. Report of 3 cases with a review of the literature. Radiology, 75:215, 1960.

Sandler, H. C.: Morphological characteristics of malignant cells from mouth lesions. Acta Cytol., 9:282, 1965.

Sandstead, H. R., and Lowe, J. W.: Leukoedema and keratosis in relation to leukoplakia of buccal mucosa in man. J. Natl. Cancer Inst., 14:423, 1953.

Santa Cruz, D. J., and Martin, S. A.: Verruciform xanthoma of the vulva: report of two cases. Am. J. Clin. Pathol., 71:224, 1979.

Sapp, J. P.: Ultrastructure and histogenesis of peripheral giant cell reparative granuloma of the jaws. Cancer, 30:1119, 1972.

Saunders, J. R., Jaques, D. A., Casterline, P. F., Percarpio, B., and Goodloe, S., Jr.: Liposarcomas of the head and neck. A review of the literature and addition of four cases. Cancer, 43:162, 1979.

Saunders, W. H.: Nicotine stomatitis of the palate. Ann. Otol. Rhinol. Laryngol., 67:618, 1958.

Schajowicz, F.: Ewing's sarcoma and reticulum-cell sarcoma of bone. With special reference to the histochemical demonstration of glycogen as an aid to differential diagnosis. J. Bone Joint Surg. [Am], 41:394, 1959.

Idem: Giant-cell tumors of bone (osteoclastoma). A pathological and histochemical study. J. Bone Joint Surg. [Am], 43:1, 1961.

Schajowicz, F., and Gallardo, H.: Chondromyxoid fibroma (fibromyxoid chondroma) of bone. J. Bone Joint Surg. [Br], 53:198, 1971.

Idem: Epiphysial chondroblastoma of bone. A clinicopathological study of sixty-nine cases. J. Bone Joint Surg. [Br], 52:205, 1970.

Schajowicz, F., and Lemos, C.: Malignant osteoblastoma. J. Bone Joint Surg., 58:202, 1976.

Schreiber, M. M., Bozzo, P. D., and Moon, T. E.: Malignant melanoma in southern Arizona. Arch. Dermatol., 117:6, 1981.

Schreiner, B. F., and Christy, C..J.: Results of irradiation treatment of the cancer of the lip: analysis of 636 cases from 1926–1936. Radiology, 39:293, 1942.

Schuller, D. E., Lawrence, T. L., and Newton, W. A., Jr.: Childhood rhabdomyosarcomas of the head and neck. Arch. Otolaryngol., 105:689, 1979.

Schutt, P. G., and Frost, H. M.: Chondromyxoid fibroma. Clin. Orthop., 78:323, 1971.

Schwartz, J.: Atrophia Idiopathia (Tropica) Mucosae Oris. Demonstrated at the Eleventh International Dental Congress, London, 1952.

Schwarz, E.: Ossifying fibroma of the face and skull. Am. J. Roentgenol. Radium Ther. Nucl. Med., 91:1012, 1964.

Scofield, H. H.: Epidermoid carcinoma of the nasal and pharyngeal regions: a statistical and morphological analysis of two hundred and fourteen cases. M. S. Thesis, Georgetown University, 1952.

Idem: The blue (Jadassohn-Tieche) nevus: a previously unreported intraoral lesion. J. Oral Surg., 17:4, 1959.

Scopp, I. W., and Quart, A.: Hereditary hemorrhagic telangiectasia involving the oral cavity. Oral Surg., 11:1138, 1958.

Seelig, C. A.: Carcinoma of the antrum. Ann. Otol. Rhinol. Laryngol., 58:168, 1949.

Seldin, H. M., Seldin, S. D., Rakower, W., and Jarrett, W. J.: Lipomas of the oral cavity: report of 26 cases. J. Oral Surg., 25:270, 1967.

Sellevold, B. J.: Mandibular torus morphology. Am. J. Phys. Anthropol., 53:569, 1980.

Sessions, R. B., Zarin, D. P., and Bryan, R. N.: Juvenile nasopharyngeal angiofibroma. Am. J. Dis. Child., 135:535, 1981.

Shafer, W. G.: Oral carcinoma in situ. Oral Surg., 39:227, 1975.

Idem: Verruciform xanthoma. Oral Surg., 31:784, 1971.

Idem: Verrucous carcinoma. Int. Dent. J., 22:451, 1972.

Idem: Basic clinical features of oral premalignant lesions; in I. C. Mackenzie, E. Dabelsteen, and C. A. Squier (eds.): Oral Premalignancy. University of Iowa Press, Iowa City, 1980.

Shafer, W. G., and Moorman, W. C.: Traumatic (amputation) neuroma. J. Oral Surg., 15:253, 1957.

Shafer, W. G., and Waldron, C. A.: A clinical and histopathological study of oral leukoplakia. Surg. Gynecol. Obstet., 112:411, 1961.

Idem: Erythroplakia of the oral cavity. Cancer, 36:1021, 1975.

Idem: Fibro-osseous Lesions of the Jaws. American Academy of Oral Pathology. Continuing Education Course. 1982.

Shapiro, M. J., and Mix, B. S.: Heterotopic brain tissue of the palate: a report of two cases. Arch. Otolaryngol., 87:96, 1968.

Sharp, G. S.: Cancer of the oral cavity. Oral Surg., 1:614, 1948.

Shear, M.: Erythroplakia of the mouth. Int. Dent. J., 22:460, 1972.

Idem: Lipoblastomatosis of the cheek. Br. J. Oral Surg., 5:173, 1967.

Shear, M., and Pindborg, J. J.: Verrucous hyperplasia of the oral mucosa. Cancer, 46:1855, 1980.

Shillitoe, E. J., and Silverman, S., Jr.: Oral cancer and herpes simplex virus—a review. Oral Surg., 48:216, 1979.

Shillitoe, E. J., Greenspan, D., Greenspan, J. S., Hansen, L. S., and Silverman, S., Jr.: Neutralizing antibody to herpes simplex virus type I in patients with oral cancer. Cancer, 49:2315, 1982.

Shira, R. B.: Diagnosis of common lesions of the oral cavity. J. Oral Surg., 15:95, 1957.

Shklar, G., and Cataldo, E.: The gingival giant cell granuloma. Histochemical observations. Periodont., 5:303, 1967.

Shklar, G., and Meyer, I.: Giant cell tumors of the mandible and maxilla. Oral Surg., 14:809, 1961.

Silverberg, E.: Cancer statistics, 1982. CA, 32:15, 1982.

Silverman, S., Jr., and Griffith, M.: Smoking characteristics of patients with oral carcinoma and the risk for second oral primary carcinoma. J. Am. Dent. Assoc., 85:637, 1972.

Silverman, S., Jr., Renstrup, G., and Pindborg, J. J.: Studies in oral leukoplakias. Acta Odontol. Scand., 21:271, 1963.

Sist, T. C., Jr., and Greene, G. W.: Traumatic neuroma of the oral cavity. Report of thirty-one new cases and review of the literature. Oral Surg., 51:394, 1981.

Idem: Benign nerve sheath myxoma: light and electron microscopic features of two cases. Oral Surg., 47:441, 1979.

Skolnik, E. M., Massari, F. S., and Tenta, L. T.: Olfactory neuroepithelioma. Arch. Otolaryngol., 84:84, 1966.

Slaughter, D. P., Southwick, H. W., and Smejkal, W.: "Field cancerization" in oral stratified squamous epithelium: clinical implications of multicentric origin. Cancer, 6:693, 1953.

Slootweg, P. J.: Clear-cell chondrosarcoma of the maxilla. Report of a case. Oral Surg., 50:233, 1980.

Small, I. A., and Bloom, H. J.: Hemangiopericytoma of the sublingual fossa: report of a case. J. Oral Surg. Anesth. Hosp. Dent. Serv., 17:65, 1959.

Smith, C.: Carcinoma in situ. Hum. Pathol., 9:373, 1978.

Smith, C., and Pindborg, J. J.: Histological Grading of Oral Epithelial Atypia by the Use of Photographic Standards. World Health Organization's International Reference Centre for Oral Precancerous Conditions, Copenhagen, 1969.

Smith, J. B.: Cancer of the floor of the mouth. J. Oral Surg., 6:106, 1948.

Sobel, H. J., and Churg, J.: Granular cells and granular cell lesions. Arch. Pathol., 77:132, 1964.

Sobel, H. J., Schwartz, R., and Marguet, E.: Light- and electron-microscope study of the origin of granular-cell myoblastoma. J. Path., 109:101, 1973.

Sober, A. J., and Fitzpatrick, T. B.: Melanoma fact sheet. CA, 29:276, 1979.

Solomon, M. P., and Sutton, A. L.: Malignant fibrous histiocytoma of the soft tissues of the mandible. Oral Surg., 35:653, 1973.

Sordillo, P. P., Helson, L., Hajdu, S. I., Magill, G. B., Kosloff, C., Golbey, R. B., and Beattie, E. J.: Malignant schwannoma—clinical characteristics, survival, and response to therapy. Cancer, 47:2503, 1981.

Sovadina, M.: Ad leukoplacia oris. Czas. Stomatol., 55:116, 1955.

Spouge, J. D.: Odontogenic tumors. A unitarian concept. Oral Surg., 24:392, 1967.

Stefansson, K., and Wollmann, R. L.: S–100 protein in granular cell tumors (granular cell myoblastomas). Cancer, 49:1834, 1982.

Stein, J. J., James, A. G., and King, E. R.: The management of the teeth, bone, and soft tissues in patients receiving treatment for oral cancer. Am. J. Roentgenol. Radium Ther. Nucl. Med., 108:257, 1970.

Steiner, A. L., Goodman, A. D., and Powers, S. R.: Study of a kindred with pheochromocytoma, medullary thyroid carcinoma, hyperparathyroidism and Cushing's disease: multiple endocrine neoplasia, type 2. Medicine, 47:371, 1968.

Steiner, G. C.: Ultrastructure of osteoblastoma. Cancer, 39:2127, 1977.

Idem: Ultrastructure of osteoid osteoma. Hum. Pathol., 7:309, 1976.

Steiner, G. C., Mirra, J. M., and Bullough, P. G.: Mesenchymal chondrosarcoma. A study of the ultrastructure. Cancer, 32:926, 1973.

Stern, M. H., Turner, J. E., and Coburn, T. P.: Oral involvement in neuroblastoma. J. Am. Dent. Assoc., 88:346, 1974.

Stewart, R. E., and Prescott, G. H.: Oral Facial Genetics. St. Louis, C. V. Mosby Company, 1976.

Stillman, F. S.: Neurofibromatosis. J. Oral Surg., 10:112, 1952.

Stobbe, G. D., and Dargeon, H. W.: Embryonal rhabdomyosarcoma of the head and neck in children and adolescents. Cancer, 3:826, 1950.

Stock, M. F.: Hereditary hemorrhagic telangiectasia (Osler's disease). Arch. Otolaryngol., 40:108, 1944.

Stockdale, C. R.: Metastatic carcinoma of the jaws secondary to primary carcinoma of the breast. Oral Surg., 12:1095, 1959.

Stoddart, T. G.: Conference on cancer of the lip (based on a series of 3166 cases). Can. Med. Assoc. J., 90:666, 1964.

Stout, A. P.: Fibrosarcoma in infants and children. Cancer, 15:1028, 1962.

Idem: Fibrosarcoma: malignant tumor of fibroblasts. Cancer, 1:30, 1948.

Idem: Hemangiopericytoma: a study of twenty-five new cases. Cancer, 3:1027, 1949.

Idem: Leiomyoma of the oral cavity. Am. J. Cancer, 34:31, 1938.

Idem: Malignant manifestations of Bowen's disease. N.Y. J. Med., 39:801, 1939.

Idem: Myxoma, the tumor of primitive mesenchyme. Ann. Surg., 127:706, 1948.

Stout, A. P., and Kenney, F. R.: Primary plasma-cell tumors of the upper air passages and oral cavity. Cancer, 2:261, 1949.

Stout, A. P., and Lattes, R.: Tumors of the Soft Tissues. (Atlas of Tumor Pathology, Section II, Fascicle 1.) Washington, D.C., Armed Forces Institute of Pathology, 1967.

Stowens, D., and Lin, T.–H.: Melanotic progonoma of the brain. Hum. Pathol., 5:105, 1974.

Strong, E. W., McDivitt, R. W., and Brasfield, R. D.: Granular cell myoblastoma. Cancer, 25:415, 1970.

Sturgis, S. H., and Lund, C. C.: Leukoplakia buccalis and keratosis labialis. N. Engl. J. Med., 210:996, 1934.

Suzuki, M., and Sakai, T.: A familial study of torus palatinus and torus mandibularis. Am. J. Phys. Anthropol., 18:263, 1960.

Svirsky, J. A., Freedman, P. D., and Lumerman, H.: Solitary intraoral keratoacanthoma. Oral Surg., 43:116, 1977.

Swanson, H. H.: Traumatic neuromas. Oral Surg., 14:317, 1961.

Symmers, D.: Lymphoid diseases. Arch. Pathol., 45:73, 1948.

Syrop, H. M., and Krantz, S.: Kaposi's disease. Oral Surg., 4:337, 1951.

Takagi, M., Ishikawa, G., and Mori, W.: Primary malignant melanoma of the oral cavity in Japan, with special reference to mucosal melanosis. Cancer, 34:358, 1974.

Takagi, M., Sakota, Y., Takayama, S., and Ishikawa, G.: Adenoid squamous cell carcinoma of the oral mucosa. Report of two autopsy cases. Cancer, 40:2250, 1977.

Taylor, H. B., and Helwig, E. B.: Dermatofibrosarcoma protuberans: a study of 115 cases. Cancer, 15:717, 1962.

Tedeschi, C. G.: Some considerations concerning the nature of the so-called sarcoma of Kaposi. Arch. Pathol., 66:656, 1958.

Telles, N. C., Rabson, A. S., and Pomeroy, T. C.: Ewing's sarcoma: an autopsy study. Cancer, 41:2321, 1978.

Tepperman, B. S., and Fitzpatrick, P. J.: Second respiratory and upper digestive tract cancers after oral cancer. Lancet, ii:547, 1981.

Thoma, K. H.: Rhabdomyoma of the tongue. Am. J. Orthod. Oral Surg., 27:235, 1941.

Idem: Stomatitis nicotina and its effect on the palate. Am. J. Orthod. Oral Surg., 27:38, 1941.

Idem: Sturge-Kalischer-Weber syndrome with pregnancy tumors. Oral Surg., 5:1124, 1952.

Idem: Torus palatinus. Int. J. Orthod. Oral Surg., 23:194, 1937.

Thomas, G.: Solitary plasmacytoma of the upper air passages. J. Laryngol. Otolaryngol., 79:498, 1965.

Tiecke, R. W., and Bernier, J. L.: Statistical and morphological analysis of four hundred and one cases of intraoral squamous cell carcinoma. J. Am. Dent. Assoc., 49:684, 1954.

Tillman, B. P., Dahlin, D. C., Lipscomb, P. R., and Stewart, J. R.: Aneurysmal bone cyst: an analysis of 95 cases. Mayo Clin. Proc., 43:478, 1968.

Tomich, C. E.: Oral focal mucinosis. Oral Surg., 38:714, 1974.

Tomich, C. E., and Hutton, C. E.: Adenoid squamous cell carcinoma of the lip: report of cases. J. Oral Surg., 30:592, 1972.

Idem: Chondroma of the anterior nasal spine. J. Oral Surg., 34:911, 1976.

Tomich, C. E., and Moll, M. C.: Palisaded, encapsulated neuroma of the lip. J. Oral Surg., 34:265, 1976.

Tomich, C. E., and Shafer, W. G.: Lymphoproliferative disease of the hard palate: A clinicopathologic entity. Oral Surg., 39:754, 1975.

Idem: Squamous acanthoma of the oral mucosa. Oral Surg., 38:755, 1974.

Toto, P. D.: Mucopolysaccharide keratin dystrophy of the oral epithelium. Oral Surg., 22:47, 1966.

Trieger, N., Ship, I. I., Taylor, G. W., and Weisberger, D.: Cirrhosis and other predisposing factors in carcinoma of the tongue. Cancer, 11:357, 1958.

Trieger, N., Taylor, G. W., and Weisberger, D.: The significance of liver dysfunction in mouth cancer. Surg. Gynecol. Obstet., 108:230, 1959.

Trodahl, J. N., and Sprague, W. G.: Benign and malignant melanocytic lesions of the oral mucosa: an analysis of 135 cases. Cancer, 25:812, 1970.

Tsukada, Y., de la Pava, S., and Pickren, J. W.: Granular-cell ameloblastoma with metastasis to the lungs: report of a case and review of the literature. Cancer, 18:916, 1965.

Tyldesley, W. R., and Kempson, S. A.: Ultrastructure of the oral epithelium in leukoplakia associated with tylosis and esophageal carcinoma. J. Oral. Pathol., 4:49, 1975.

Tyldesley, W. R., and Osborne Hughes, R.: Tylosis, leukoplakia and esophageal carcinoma. Br. Med. J., 4:427, 1973.

Unni, K. K., Dahlin, D. C., and Beabout, J. W.: Periosteal osteogenic sarcoma. Cancer, 37:2476, 1976.

Unni, K. K., Dahlin, D. C., Beabout, J. W., and Ivins, J. C.: Parosteal osteogenic sarcoma. Cancer, 37:2466, 1976.

Unni, K. K., Ivins, J. C., Beabout, J. W., and Dahlin, D. C.: Hemangioma, hemangiopericytoma, and heman-gioendothelioma (angiosarcoma) of bone. Cancer, 27:1403, 1971.

Van Hale, H. M., Handlers, J. P., Abrams, A. M., and Strahs, G.: Malignant fibrous histiocytoma, myxoid variant metastatic to the oral cavity. Report of a case and review of the literature. Oral Surg., 51:156, 1981.

Van Wyck, C. W.: The oral lesion caused by snuff: a clinicopathological study. Med. Proc., 11:531, 1965.

Vellios, F., Baez, J., and Shumacker, H. B.: Lipoblastomatosis: a tumor of fetal fat different from hibernoma. Report of a case with observations on the embryogenesis of human adipose tissue. Am. J. Pathol., 34:1149, 1958.

Waldron, C. A.: Giant cell tumors of the jawbones. Oral Surg., 6:1055, 1953.

Idem: Metastatic carcinoma of the mandible; adenocarcinoma of the lung with metastatic lesion of mandible as first clinical sign. Oral Surg., 5:185, 1952.

Idem: Ossifying fibroma of the mandible. Oral Surg., 6:464, 1953.

Waldron, C. A., and Shafer, W. G.: Current concepts of leukoplakia. Int. Dent. J., 10:350, 1960.

Idem: The central giant cell reparative granuloma of the jaws: an analysis of 38 cases. Am. J. Clin. Pathol., 45:437, 1966.

Idem: Leukoplakia revisited. A clinicopathologic study of 3256 oral leukoplakias. Cancer, 36:1386, 1975.

Walsh, T. S., Jr., and Tompkins, V. N.: Some observations on the strawberry nevus of infancy. Cancer, 9:869, 1956.

Wang, C. C., and James, A. E., Jr.: Chordoma: brief review of the literature and report of a case with widespread metastases. Cancer, 22:162, 1968.

Watanabe, S.: The metastasizability of tumor cells. Cancer, 7:215, 1954.

Watson, W. L., and McCarthy, W. D.: Blood and lymph vessel tumors: a report of 1,056 cases. Surg. Gynecol. Obstet., 71:569, 1940.

Wayte, D. M., and Helwig, E. B.: Melanotic freckle of Hutchinson. Cancer, 21:893, 1968.

Weary, P. E., Gorlin, R. J., Gentry, W. C., Jr., Comer, J. E., and Greer, K. E.: Multiple hamartoma syndrome (Cowden's disease). Arch. Dermatol., 106:682, 1972.

Weathers, D. R.: Benign nevi of the oral mucosa: a report of six cases. Arch. Dermatol., 99:688, 1969.

Weathers, D. R., and Callihan, M. D.: Giant-cell fibroma. Oral Surg., 37:374, 1974.

Weathers, D. R., and Campbell, W. G.: Ultrastructure of the giant-cell fibroma of the oral mucosa. Oral Surg., 38:550, 1974.

Webb, H. E., Harrison, E. G., Masson, J. K., and ReMine, W. H.: Solitary extramedullary myeloma (plasmacytoma) of the upper part of the respiratory tract and oropharynx. Cancer, 15:1142, 1962.

Webb, J. N.: The histogenesis of nerve sheath myxoma: report of a case with electron microscopy. J. Path., 127:35, 1979.

Weedon, D., and Little, J. H.: Spindle and epithelioid cell nevi in children and adults. A review of 211 cases of the Spitz nevus. Cancer, 40:217, 1977.

Weiss, S. W., and Enzinger, F. M.: Myxoid variant of malignant fibrous histiocytoma. Cancer, 39:1672, 1977.

Weitzner, S.: Clear-cell acanthoma of vermilion mucosa of lower lip. Oral Surg., 37:911, 1974.

Weitzner, S., Lockey, M. W., and Lockard, V. G.: Adult rhabdomyoma of soft palate. Oral Surg., 47:70, 1979.

Welbury, R. R.: Congenital epulis of the newborn. Br. J. Oral Surg., 18:238, 1980.

Werning, J. T.: Nodular fasciitis of the orofacial region. Oral Surg., 48:441, 1979.

Wesley, R. K., Mintz, S. M., and Wertheimer, F. W.: Primary malignant hemangioendothelioma of the gingiva. Oral Surg., 39:103, 1975.

White, D. K., Miller, A. S., and Gomez, L.: Occurrence of oral squamous cell carcinoma in persons under 50 years of age. Phila. Med., 74:442, 1978.

Whitten, J. B.: The fine structure of an intraoral granular-cell myoblastoma. Oral Surg., 26:202, 1968.

WHO Collaborating Centre for Oral Precancerous Lesions: Definition of leukoplakia and related lesions: an aid to studies on oral precancer. Oral Surg., 46:518, 1978.

Widmann, B. P.: Cancer of the lip. Am. J. Roentgenol. Radium Ther. Nucl. Med., 63:13, 1950.

Williamson, J. J.: Erythroplasia of Queyrat of the buccal mucous membrane. Oral Surg., 17:308, 1964.

Wolbach, S. B.: Pathologic changes resulting from vitamin deficiency. J.A.M.A., 108:7, 1937.

Wolfe, J. J., and Platt, W. R.: Postirradiation osteogenic sarcoma of the nasal bone: a report of two cases. Cancer, 2:438, 1949.

Wong, D. S., Fuller, L. M., Butler J. J., and Shullenberger, C. C.: Extranodal non-Hodgkin's lymphomas of the head and neck. Am. J. Roentgenol. Radium Ther. Nucl. Med., 123:471, 1975.

Wood, J. S., Jr., Holyoke, E. D., Clason, W. P., Sommers, S. C., and Warren, S.: An experimental study of the relationship between tumor size and number of lung metastases. Cancer, 7:437, 1954.

Woodbridge, H.: Carcinoma in situ. Oral Surg., 3:1447, 1950.

Wright, B. A., Wysocki, G. P., and Bannerjee, D.: Diagnostic use of immunoperoxidase techniques for plasma cell lesions of the jaws.Oral Surg., 52:615, 1981.

Wynder, E. L., Bross, I. J., and Feldman, R. M.: A study of the etiological factors in cancer of the mouth. Cancer, 10:1300, 1957.

Wysocki, G. P., and Hardie, J.: Ultrastructural studies of intraoral verruca vulgaris. Oral Surg., 47:58, 1979.

Wysocki, G. P., and Wright, B. A.: Intraneural and perineural epithelial structures. Head Neck Surg., 4:69, 1981.

Zachariades, N., Papadakou, A., Koundouris, J., Constantinidis, J., and Angelopoulos, A. P.: Primary hemangioendotheliosarcoma of the mandible: review of the literature and report of a case. J. Oral Surg., 38:288, 1980.

Zegarelli, E. V., Kutscher, A. H., and Silvers, H. F.: Keratotic lesions of the oral mucous membranes treated with high dosage topical systemic vitamin A. N.Y. State Dent. J., 25:244, 1959.

Zegarelli, D. J., Zegarelli-Schmidt, E. C., and Zegarelli, E. V.: Verruciform xanthoma. Oral Surg., 38:725, 1974.

Idem: Verruciform xanthoma. Oral Surg., 40:246, 1975.

Zenker, W.: Juxtaoral Organ (Chievitz' Organ): Morphology and Clinical Aspects. Baltimore, Urban & Schwarzenberg, 1982.

Ziegler, J. L.: Burkitt's Lymphoma. N. Engl. J. Med., 305:735, 1981.

Ziskin, D. E.: Effects of certain hormones on gingival and oral mucous membranes. J. Am. Dent. Assoc., 25:422, 1938.

Idem: Effects of male sex hormones on gingivae and oral mucous membranes. J. Dent. Res., 20:419, 1941.

Ziskin, D. E., Blackberg, S. N., and Slanetz, C. A.: Effects of subcutaneous injections of estrogenic and gonadotrophic hormones on gums and oral mucous membranes of normal and castrated rhesus monkeys. J. Dent. Res., 15:407, 1935–36.

CHAPTER 3

Tumors of the Salivary Glands

Tumors of the salivary glands constitute a heterogeneous group of lesions of great morphologic variation and, for this reason, present many difficulties in classification. Until recent years there were few concerted efforts made to study large numbers of either major or accessory intraoral salivary gland tumors with the view of obtaining a better understanding of their natural history. Since these tumors are relatively uncommon, investigators were handicapped by insufficient material for study. With the publication of several large series of cases, accompanied by serious discussions of the nature of tumors of the salivary glands based upon a cumulative clinical experience of many years, considerable progress has been made in broadening our knowledge of these lesions. Among these studies have been those of Evans and Cruickshank, Thackray and Lucas, and the World Health Organization.

Foote and Frazell were among the first investigators to provide a usable classification of salivary gland tumors. More recently, Spiro and his associates, Thackray and Sobin, and Batsakis have proposed classifications for practical use that are based on clinical behavior or specific histologic criteria. However, Eversole has proposed a histogenetic classification of salivary gland tumors, implicating two cell types as possible progenitors: the intercalated duct cell and the excretory duct reserve cell. The various types of salivary gland tumors are best distinguished by their histologic patterns. The clinical behavior of these various lesions may be based, as in most tumors, on the type of tumor as well as on the method of treatment utilized.

It is important to recognize that neoplasms may arise not only from the major salivary glands, although tumors of the sublingual gland are extremely rare, but also from any of the numerous, diffuse, intraoral accessory salivary glands. Thus one may expect to see tumors originating from the glands in the lip, palate, tongue, buccal mucosa, floor of the mouth and retromolar area. Salivary gland tumors are much more common on the hard palate than on the soft, probably because there are a greater number of gland aggregates on the hard palate than on the soft palate. With only occasional exceptions, any type of tumor which occurs in a major salivary gland may also arise in an intraoral accessory gland. Thus in the following discussion the general features described under each tumor will hold true for both major and minor salivary gland lesions. There appear to be no truly specific, recognized tumors native only to the intraoral glands. Eneroth has presented data on over 2300 tumors of the major salivary glands (Table 3–1), while a complete review of the intraoral minor salivary gland tumors has been published by Chaudhry and his co-workers, with much valuable information obtained from the analysis of over 1300 cases (Table 3–2).

BENIGN TUMORS OF THE SALIVARY GLANDS

PLEOMORPHIC ADENOMA

("Mixed" Tumor)

The benign "mixed" tumor of salivary glands has masqueraded under a great variety of names throughout the years (e.g., enclavoma, branchioma, endothelioma, enchondroma), but the term "pleomorphic adenoma" suggested by Willis characterizes closely the unusual histologic pattern of the lesion. It is almost universally agreed that this tumor is not a "mixed" tumor in the true sense of being teratomatous

230

Table 3–1. Occurrence of Major Salivary Gland Tumors

	PAROTID	SUBMAXILLARY	TOTAL (No.)	TOTAL (%)
Benign tumors:				
Pleomorphic adenoma...............	1658	102	1760	75.6
Papillary cystadenoma				
lymphomatosum...................	101	4	105	4.5
Oxyphilic cell adenoma..............	21	1	22	0.9
Malignant tumors:				
Carcinoma in pleomorphic adenoma...	32	3	35	1.5
Mucoepidermoid carcinoma..........	88	6	94	4.0
Adenoid cystic carcinoma............	49	26	75	3.2
Acinic cell carcinoma...............	66	1	67	2.9
Mucus-producing adenopapillary	52	—	52	2.2
carcinoma......................				
Solid undifferentiated carcinoma......	84	15	99	4.3
Epidermoid carcinoma	7	12	19	0.8
Total.............................	2158	170	2328	100.0

Data from C.-M. Eneroth: Salivary gland tumors in the parotid gland, submandibular gland and the palate region. Cancer, 27:1415, 1971.

or derived from more than one primary tissue. Its morphologic complexity is the result of the differentiation of the tumor cells, and the fibrous, hyalinized, myxoid, chondroid and even osseous areas are the result of metaplasia or are actually products of the tumor cells per se. It is the most common of all salivary gland tumors, constituting over 50 per cent of all cases of tumors of both major and minor salivary gland origin and approximately 90 per cent of all benign salivary gland tumors.

Histogenesis. Numerous theories have been advanced to explain the histogenesis of this bizarre tumor. Currently, these center around the myoepithelial cell and a reserve cell in the intercalated duct. Ultrastructural studies have confirmed the presence of both ductal and myoepithelial cells in pleomorphic adenomas. It follows that possibly either or both may play active roles in the histogenesis of the tumor. Hübner and his associates have postulated that the myoepithelial cell is responsible for the morphologic diversity of the tumor, including the production of the fibrous, mucinous, chondroid and osseous areas. Regezi and Batsakis postulated that the intercalated duct reserve cell can differentiate into ductal and myoepithelial cells and the latter, in turn, can undergo mesenchymal metaplasia, since they inherently have smooth muscle-like properties. Further differentiation into other mesenchymal cells then can occur. More recently, Batsakis has

Table 3–2. Occurrence of Intraoral Accessory Salivary Gland Tumors

	PALATE	LIP UPPER	LIP LOWER	LIP NS	CHEEK	TONGUE	RETROMOLAR	OTHERS	TOTAL (NO.)	TOTAL (%)
Benign tumors:										
Pleomorphic adenoma	476	105	13	15	38	18	40	28	733	55.7
Simple adenoma	18	2	0	0	0	4	0	0	24	1.8
Myoepithelioma	12	1	0	0	4	0	0	0	17	1.3
Cystadenoma (incl. papillary)....	12	1	0	0	4	1	1	1	20	1.5
Canalicular adenoma	1	0	0	2	1	0	0	0	4	0.3
Oxyphilic adenoma	0	0	0	0	0	1	1	0	2	0.2
Malignant tumors:										
Malignant pleomorphic adenoma .	13	1	0	0	5	0	5	2	26	2.0
Adenocarcinoma:										
Adenoid cystic carcinoma	104	6	1	5	17	62	12	8	215	16.3
Acinar cell adenocarcinoma	2	1	0	0	0	0	2	2	7	0.5
Miscellaneous forms	80	3	0	12	17	26	6	18	162	12.3
Mucoepidermoid carcinoma	43	0	0	2	15	23	22	2	107	8.0
Epidermoid carcinoma	1	0	0	0	2	0	0	0	3	0.2
Total	762	120	14	36	103	135	89	61	1320	100.
	(57.7%)	(9.1%)	(1.0%)	(2.7%)	(7.7%)	(10.2%)	(6.7%)	(4.6%)		

Data from A. P. Chaudhry, R. A. Vickers, and R. J. Gorlin: Intraoral minor salivary gland tumors. Oral Surg., *14:* 1194, 1961.

discussed salivary gland tumorigenesis and, while still implicating the intercalated duct reserve cell as the histogenetic precursor of the pleomorphic adenoma, stated that the role of the myoepithelial cell is still uncertain and that it may be either an active or passive participant histogenetically. Finally, Dardick and his associates recently have questioned the role of both ductal reserve and myoepithelial cells. They state that a neoplastically altered epithelial cell with the potential for multidirectional differentiation may be histogenetically responsible for the pleomorphic adenoma.

Clinical Features. Of the major salivary glands, the parotid gland is the most common site of the pleomorphic adenoma, 90 per cent of a group of nearly 1900 such tumors reported by Eneroth occurring there. It may occur, however, in any of the major glands or in the widely distributed intraoral accessory salivary glands. It is somewhat more frequent in women than in men, the ratio approximating 6:4, although not all series record this slight difference. The majority of the lesions are found in patients in the fourth to sixth decades, but they are also relatively common in young adults and have been known to occur in children. Interesting analyses of salivary gland tumors in children have been made by Castro and associates and by Krolls and associates.

The history presented by the patient is usually that of a small, painless, quiescent nodule which slowly begins to increase in size, sometimes showing intermittent growth (Fig. 3–1). The pleomorphic adenoma, particularly of the parotid gland, is typically a lesion that does not show fixation either to the deeper tissues or to the overlying skin (Fig. 3–2, A). It is usually an irregular nodular lesion which is firm in consistency, although areas of cystic degeneration may sometimes be palpated if they are superficial. The skin seldom ulcerates even though these tumors may reach a fantastic size, lesions having been recorded which weighed several pounds (Fig. 3–2, B). Pain is not a common symptom of the pleomorphic adenoma, but local discomfort is frequently present. Facial nerve involvement manifested by facial paralysis is rare.

The pleomorphic adenoma of intraoral accessory glands seldom is allowed to attain a size greater than 1 to 2 cm. in diameter. Because this tumor causes the patient difficulties in mastication, talking and breathing, it is detected and treated earlier than tumors of the major glands. The palatal glands are frequently the site of origin of tumors of this type (Fig. 3–3), as are the glands of the lip (Fig. 3–4) and occasionally other sites. Except for size, the intraoral tumor does not differ remarkably from its counterpart in a major gland. The palatal pleomorphic adenoma may appear fixed to the underlying bone, but is not invasive. In other sites the tumor is usually freely movable and easily palpated.

Histologic Features. Greater variation exists in this group of lesions than in most other types of salivary gland tumors. The diverse histologic pattern of this neoplasm is in fact one of its most characteristic features (Fig. 3–5). Seldom do individual cases resemble each other.

Some areas present cuboidal cells arranged in tubes or ductlike structures which bear striking resemblance to normal ductal epithelium. These ductlike spaces not uncommonly contain an eosinophilic coagulum. There is often proliferation of epithelium in strands or sheets about these tubular structures. In other areas the tumor cells assume a stellate, polyhedral or spindle form and may be relatively few in number. Lomax-Smith and Azzopardi described a "hyaline cell" with a plasmacytoid morphology in 70 and 10 per cent respectively of minor and major gland pleomorphic adenomas studied. Buchner and his colleagues recently found such cells in all 124 pleomorphic adenomas studied and, based on ultrastructural analysis, suggested that "hyaline cells" are modified myoepithelial cells. Squamous epithelial cells are relatively common and exhibit typical intercellular bridges and sometimes actual keratin pearls. Loose myxoid material is frequently a predominant feature of the lesion, while foci of

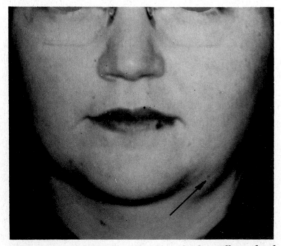

Figure 3–1. *Pleomorphic adenoma of submaxillary gland.*

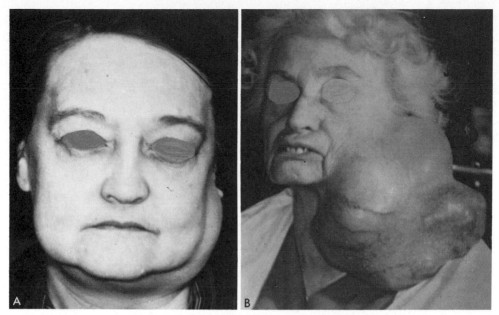

Figure 3–2. *Pleomorphic adenoma of parotid gland.*
A, Typical appearance of pleomorphic adenoma of parotid gland. *B*, The lesion here is used not to illustrate the usual clinical appearance of a pleomorphic adenoma of the parotid gland, but to demonstrate the size which these tumors may attain. This lesion was present for eighteen years.

hyalinized connective tissue, or cartilage-like material and even bone, are common. Finally, a mucoid material, originating from the tumor cells, may be collected in areas. The tumor is always encapsulated (Fig. 3–6), although tumor cells are often present in the connective tissue capsule. When the pleomorphic pattern of the stroma is absent, and the tumor is highly cellular, it is often referred to as a "cellular adenoma." When myoepithelial proliferation predominates, the diagnosis of "myoepithelioma" (q.v.) is generally made.

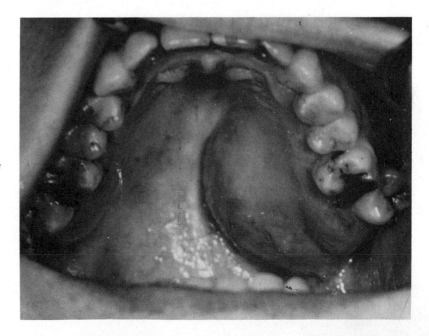

Figure 3–3. *Pleomorphic adenoma of palate.*

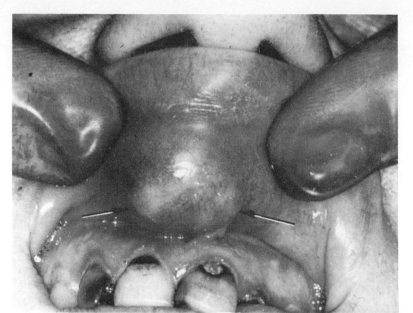

Figure 3–4. *Pleomorphic adenoma of lip.*

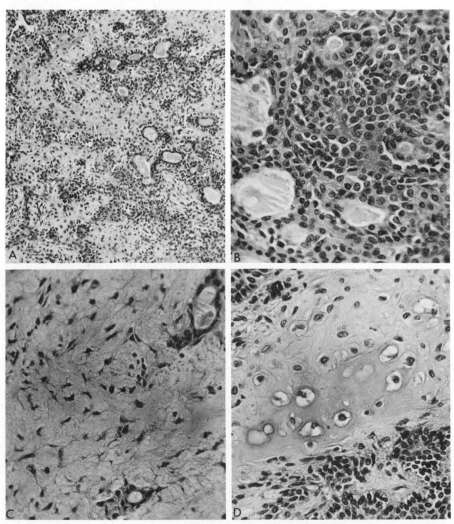

Figure 3–5. *Pleomorphic adenoma.*

Photomicrographs taken through different areas of a typical pleomorphic adenoma to show (A) the pleomorphic nature of the tumor, (B) sheets of epithelial cells, some of which have formed ducts, (C) myxomatous tissue, and (D) chondroid tissue.

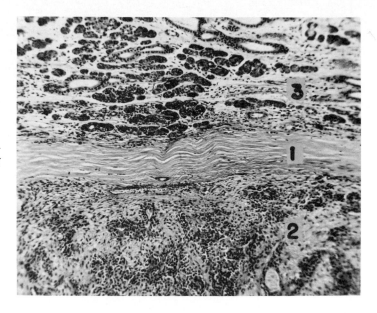

Figure 3–6. *Pleomorphic adenoma.* Photomicrograph illustrating the connective tissue capsule (*1*) separating the tumor (*2*) from the normal gland (*3*).

Treatment and Prognosis. The accepted treatment for this tumor is surgical excision. In the parotid gland, treatment must conform to established principles of parotid surgery, and thus the tumor and the involved lobe of the gland must be removed. Submaxillary gland tumors are treated by removal of the gland and tumor in continuity. The intraoral lesions can be treated somewhat more conservatively by extracapsular excision. In general, lesions of the hard palate should be excised with the overlying mucosa, while those in lining mucosa, such as the lips, soft palate and buccal mucosa often can be treated successfully by enucleation or extracapsular excision. Since these tumors are radioresistant, the use of radiation therapy is of little benefit and is therefore contraindicated.

In the past, recurrence of the pleomorphic adenoma in all locations was a common clinical problem, either because of inadequate treatment, because of tumor cells within the capsule or because of irregularities in the capsular surface. In a study of the growth patterns and recurrence of pleomorphic adenomas, Naeim and associates found incomplete resection, hypocellularity and incomplete encapsulation to be features associated with recurrence. In a long-term follow-up study of 89 patients with such tumors, Krolls and Boyers found a recurrence rate of 44 per cent. The high rate of recurrence was due to an initial inadequate surgical procedure.

It is now well-recognized that benign pleomorphic adenomas may undergo malignant transformation. The malignant component may be a carcinoma, an adenocarcinoma or "cylin-

dromatous." This transformation may take place in a long-standing untreated tumor or in a recurrent one, or the malignant element may be present at the time of initial surgery. The rate of malignant transformation is uncertain but has been estimated by various workers to be 3 to 15 percent. LiVolsi and Perzin have studied 47 such cases in both major and minor glands.

MONOMORPHIC ADENOMA

It has long been recognized that not all benign salivary gland tumors possess a "mixed" or "pleomorphic" appearance, although it was not until 1967 that Kleinsasser and Klein separated a group of tumors with a monomorphic pattern from those with a pleomorphic pattern. The term "monomorphic adenoma" was first proposed by Thackray and Sobin in the World Health Organization's monograph on salivary gland tumors.

The World Health Organization classification subdivides the monomorphic adenomas into three groups: (1) adenolymphoma (Warthin's tumor); (2) oxyphilic adenoma; and (3) others. The latter includes tubular, alveolar or trabecular, basal cell and clear cell adenomas. Although the oxyphilic adenoma is monomorphous, it is a separate well-recognized entity, as is the Warthin's tumor, and thus neither are included here in the discussion of monomorphic adenomas.

A number of other classifications of monomorphic adenomas have been proposed and, as

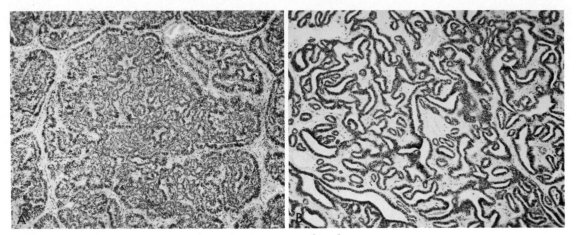

Figure 3–7. *Monomorphic adenoma.*
A, Basal cell adenoma. *B,* Canalicular adenoma.

yet, there is no unanimity of opinion. However, two main histologic patterns have evolved, the *basal cell adenoma* and the *canalicular adenoma*. While some authorities consider the canalicular adenoma to be a variant of basal cell adenoma, sufficient differences exist in clinical presentation and histologic features to separate them, at least presently, into separate tumors.

Batsakis and associates have discussed monomorphic adenomas of the major salivary glands and reported 96 new cases. Mintz and his colleagues recently reviewed the world literature on monomorphic adenomas of the major and minor salivary glands and added 21 new cases, 15 of which were in minor glands and 6 in major glands.

Basal Cell Adenoma

The basal cell adenoma was first reported as a distinct entity by Kleinsasser and Klein in 1967. Batsakis is credited with reporting the first case in the American literature in 1972, and suggested that the intercalated duct or reserve cell is the histogenetic source of the basal cell adenoma.

Clinical Features. Basal cell adenomas tend to occur primarily in the major salivary glands, particularly the parotid gland. In the series reported by Batsakis and associates, 48 of 50 tumors were in the parotid gland and 2 were in the submaxillary gland. The tumors are usually painless and are characterized by slow growth. There is a 5:1 male predilection and the majority of patients are over 60 years of age. The tumor can occur in younger persons, however; Canalis and his co-workers reported a basal cell

adenoma in the submaxillary gland of a newborn male. Basal cell adenomas of minor salivary glands have been reported by Fantasia and Neville. These tend to occur primarily in the upper lip of elderly persons.

Histologic Features. Basal cell adenomas have a fairly well-defined connective tissue capsule. The cells are isomorphic and basaloid in appearance with basophilic round to oval nuclei. Cytoplasm is scanty and ill-defined. The tumor cells are arranged in solid nests with the peripheral cells often showing a palisaded arrangement (Fig. 3–7 *A*). In other tumors, the cells may be arranged in ribbons and cords. Only scanty stroma is found between the nests of tumor cells.

Electron microscopic studies suggest that the tumor cells bear similarity to secretory cells of the intercalated duct. Most ultrastructural studies have failed to demonstrate the presence of myoepithelial cells, although Jao and co-workers found occasional myoepithelial cells at the periphery of the tumor cell masses.

Treatment and Prognosis. The tumor is treated by excision and recurrences are seldom seen.

Canalicular Adenoma

The canalicular adenoma is a distinctive variant of the monomorphic adenoma. Nelson and Jacoway have reported 29 cases, and Mader and Nelson recently reported a case and reviewed the literature.

Clinical Features. This lesion originates primarily in the intraoral accessory salivary glands, and in the vast majority of cases, it occurs in the upper lip. However, cases are known in which the lesion occurred in the palate, buccal mucosa and lower lip. Only one was noted in the parotid gland in the series reported by Nelson and Jacoway. The tumor occurs far more commonly in patients over 60 years of age, but there is no particular sex predilection.

The tumor generally presents as a slowly growing, well-circumscribed, firm nodule which, particularly in the lip, is not fixed and may be moved through the tissue for some distance. Occasionally, two separate and distinct tumors may occur in the upper lip of an individual.

Histologic Features. The canalicular adenoma has a strikingly characteristic picture: it is composed of long strands or cords of epithelial cells, almost invariably arranged in a double row and usually showing a "party wall." In some instances, cystic spaces of varying sizes are enclosed by these cords. The cystic spaces are usually filled with an eosinophilic coagulum. The supporting stroma is loose and fibrillar with delicate vascularity (Fig. 3–7 *B*). The tumor has, at times, been mistaken for an adenoid cystic carcinoma and care should be taken to prevent this error. As Mader and Nelson have pointed out, the adenoid cystic carcinoma rarely occurs in the upper lip and is seldom freely movable.

Chen and Miller recently have studied the ultrastructure of a canalicular adenoma of the upper lip. The component tall columnar and small basal cells most closely resembled those of salivary gland excretory ducts. The tumor did not show any multilayered basal lamina as is observed in the adenoid cystic carcinoma.

Treatment and Prognosis. The tumor can be treated by enucleation or simple surgical excision; recurrence is rare.

Papillary Cystadenoma Lymphomatosum

(Warthin's Tumor; Adenolymphoma)

This unusual type of salivary gland tumor occurs almost exclusively in the parotid gland, although occasional cases have been reported in the submaxillary gland. The intraoral accessory salivary glands are rarely affected; two cases involving the palate were reported by Fantasia and Miller. Baden and his associates also reported two cases and reviewed the literature on the intraoral tumor.

Histogenesis. Numerous theories have been advanced to account for the peculiar nature of this tumor and these have been reviewed in detail by Little. The currently accepted theory is that the tumor arises in salivary gland tissue entrapped within paraparotid or intraparotid lymph nodes during embryogenesis. However, Allegra has suggested that the Warthin's tumor is most likely a delayed hypersensitivity disease, the lymphocytes being an immune reaction to the salivary ducts which undergo oncocytic change. Hsu and co-workers recently studied the tumor immunohistochemically and have suggested that the lymphoid component of the tumor is an exaggerated secretory immune response.

Chaudhry and Gorlin carried out an extensive review of 357 cases of papillary cystadenoma lymphomatosum, while Bernier and Bhaskar reviewed 186 cases of lymphoepithelial lesions of the salivary glands, including papillary cystadenoma lymphomatosum.

Clinical Features. The papillary cystadenoma lymphomatosum exhibits a definite predilection for men. The study of Chaudhry and Gorlin recorded 257 cases occurring in men, but only 49 in women, a ratio of 5:1. In this same study the average age of the patients at the time of discovery of the lesion was 56 years, 82 per cent of the patients being between 41 and 70 years of age, with an average duration of symptoms of 3 years. In approximately 7 per cent of 210 cases reviewed by Chaudhry and Gorlin in which the site was stated, the tumors were bilateral.

The tumor is generally superficial, lying just beneath the parotid capsule or protruding through it. Seldom does the lesion attain a size exceeding 3 to 4 cm. in diameter. It is not painful, is firm to palpation and is clinically indistinguishable from other benign lesions of the parotid gland.

Histologic Features. This tumor is made up of two histologic components: epithelial and lymphoid tissue. As the name would indicate, the lesion is essentially an adenoma exhibiting cyst formation, with papillary projections into the cystic spaces and a lymphoid matrix showing germinal centers (Fig. 3–8). The epithelial cells covering the papillary projections are columnar or cuboidal cells usually arranged in two rows, although the inner layer may be several cells thick. These cells are eosinophilic, containing hyperchromatic or pyknotic nuclei and vast numbers of mitochondria, as demonstrated by Tandler under the electron microscope. There is frequently an eosinophilic coagulum present within the cystic spaces, which appears as a chocolate-colored fluid in the gross specimen.

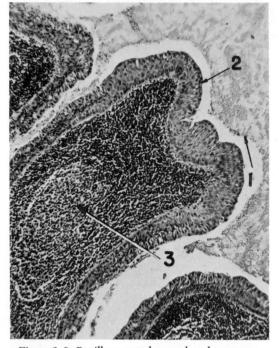

Figure 3–8. *Papillary cystadenoma lymphomatosum.*
Photomicrograph illustrating cystic cavity (*1*), epithelium
(*2*), and lymphocytes and lymphoid follicle (*3*). (Courtesy of
Dr. Frank Vellios.)

The abundant lymphoid component may represent the normal lymphoid tissue of the lymph node within which the tumor developed or it may actually represent a reactive cellular infiltrate which involves both humoral and cell-mediated mechanisms.

Treatment and Prognosis. The accepted treatment of the papillary cystadenoma lymphomatosum is surgical excision. This can almost invariably be accomplished without injury to the facial nerve, particularly since the lesion is usually small and superficial. These tumors are well encapsulated and seldom recur after removal.

Malignant transformation is exceedingly rare in either the epithelial or lymphoid component. Assor reported a carcinoma arising in a Warthin's tumor.

OXYPHILIC ADENOMA

(Oncocytoma; Acidophilic Adenoma)

This rare salivary gland tumor is a small benign lesion which usually occurs in the parotid gland. Except that it does not generally attain any great size, it does not differ in its clinical characteristics from other benign salivary gland tumors. For this reason a clinical diagnosis is difficult if not impossible to establish.

The name "oncocytoma" is derived from the resemblance of these tumor cells to apparently normal cells which have been termed "oncocytes" and which are found in a great number of locations, including the salivary glands, respiratory tract, breast, thyroid, pancreas, parathyroid, pituitary, testicle, fallopian tube, liver and stomach. These cells are predominantly seen in duct linings of glands in elderly persons, but little is actually known of their mode of development or significance (Fig. 3–9). Electron microscope studies have shown that the cytoplasm of the oncocyte is choked with mitochondria.

Clinical Features. The oxyphilic adenoma is somewhat more common in women than in men and occurs almost exclusively in elderly persons. Chaudhry and Gorlin, who reviewed the literature, found 29 cases of oxyphilic adenoma and added four new cases to those reported. Only occasionally does this tumor arise before the age of 60 years, 80 per cent of cases occurring between the ages of 51 and 80 years. The tumor usually measures 3 to 5 cm. in diameter and appears as a discrete, encapsulated mass which is sometimes nodular. Pain is generally absent.

An interesting condition called diffuse multinodular oncocytoma or "oncocytosis" of the parotid gland has been described by Schwartz and Feldman. This condition is characterized by nodules of oncocytes which involve the entire gland or large portions of it.

Histologic Features. The oxyphilic adenoma is characterized microscopically by large cells which have an eosinophilic cytoplasm and distinct cell membrane and which tend to be arranged in narrow rows or cords (Fig. 3–9). Sometimes the cells occur in sheets and may demonstrate an alveolar or lobular pattern. These cells, exhibiting few mitotic figures, are closely packed, and there is little supportive stroma. Lymphoid tissue is frequently present, but does not appear to be an integral part of the lesion. Ultrastructural studies of parotid oncocytomas by Tandler and associates and Kay and Still have shown that the cells are engorged with enlarged and morphologically altered mitochondria.

A variant of the oxyphilic adenoma is sometimes seen in intraoral salivary glands, particularly in the buccal mucosa and upper lip. This

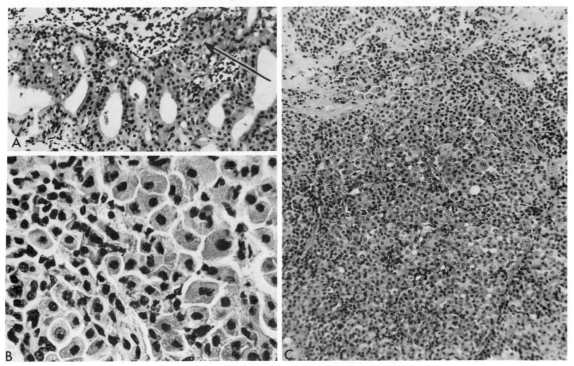

Figure 3–9. *Oxyphilic adenoma.*
A, Normal oncocytes in accessory salivary gland ducts of elderly patient. *B*, High-power photomicrograph, and *C*, low-power photomicrograph of oncocytoma.

has been termed an oncocytic cystadenoma since it is a tumor-like nodule composed chiefly of numerous dilated ductlike or cystlike structures lined with oncocytes.

Treatment and Prognosis. The treatment of choice is surgical excision, and the tumor does not tend to recur. Malignant transformation is uncommon, but malignant oncocytoma is now a well-established entity. Johns and associates reviewed the literature on malignant oncocytomas and reported three additional cases. Other well-documented cases have been those of Lee and Roth, and Gray and his co-workers.

MYOEPITHELIOMA

The myoepithelioma is an uncommon salivary gland tumor which accounts for less than one per cent of all major and minor salivary tumors. Nonetheless, it is important in that the component cell constitutes such a prominent place in salivary gland neoplasia. Many authorities, including Batsakis, consider the myoepithelioma to be a "one-sided" variant at the opposite end of the spectrum from the pleomorphic adenoma.

Sciubba and Brannon recently reported 23 myoepitheliomas of major and minor salivary glands. Chaudhry and his co-workers and Luna and associates studied the ultrastructure of myoepitheliomas in the parotid and palate respectively.

Clinical Features. There are no clinical features which can serve to separate the myoepithelioma from the more common pleomorphic adenoma. It occurs in adults with an equal sex distribution. The parotid gland is most commonly involved and the palate is the most frequent intraoral site of occurrence. Sciubba and Brannon reported lesions in the retromolar glands and the upper lip.

Histologic Features. The tumor is composed of spindle-shaped or plasmacytoid cells or a combination of the two cell types. The cells may be set in a myxomatous background which varies from scanty to copious. The tumor is often difficult to diagnose definitively at the light microscopic level. Of the 23 cases studied by Sciubba and Brannon, only one case was interpreted as a myoepithelioma by the original contributing pathologist, the remainder being interpreted as a variety of benign and malignant neoplasms.

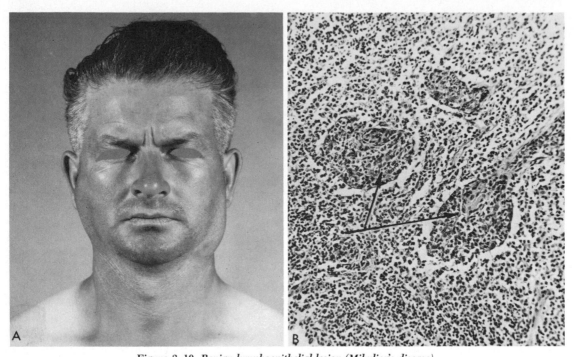

Figure 3–10. *Benign lymphoepithelial lesion (Mikulicz's disease).*
A, There is enlargement of the parotid, submaxillary and lacrimal glands. *B*, The photomicrograph illustrates the diffuse lymphocytic infiltrate and the typical epimyoepithelial islands. (Courtesy of Dr. Frank Vellios.)

Definitive diagnosis lies in the ultrastructural identification of myoepithelial cells. The myoepithelial cell exhibits a basal lamina and fine intracytoplasmic myofilaments. Desmosomes are encountered between adjacent cells.

Treatment and Prognosis. The tumor is treated by surgical excision. The same surgical principles apply as in treating pleomorphic adenomas. Only one recurrence was noted in 16 cases in which follow-up was available.

DUCTAL PAPILLOMAS

Papillomas arising from the excretory ducts of the major and especially minor salivary glands are known to occur. These present in three forms: (1) simple ductal papilloma, (2) inverted ductal papilloma, and (3) sialadenoma papilliferum.

The *simple ductal papilloma* presents as an exophytic lesion with a papillary surface and a pedunculated base. It is usually reddish in color and presents on the buccal mucosa or palate. It consists of nonkeratinized epithelium, often columnar, supported by cores of vascular fibrous connective tissue. It is treated by excision, including the base, and it does not recur if completely removed.

The *inverted ductal papilloma* has been recently reported by White and co-workers. The lesion presents as a nodule of the oral mucosa of adults and has no distinctive clinical features. This papilloma histologically resembles the inverted papilloma of the sino-nasal tract. It consists of squamous, cuboidal or columnar epithelium which proliferates into a salivary gland duct to form broad bulbous masses. Mucous cells and small microcysts with mucus may be seen. The lesion is treated by excision.

The *sialadenoma papilliferum* is the salivary gland analogue of the syringadenoma papilliferum of skin. It was originally described by Abrams and Fink. Drummond and associates and Freedman and Lumerman recently have reported cases. The lesion occurs in adults, generally as an exophytic papillary lesion of the hard palate. It consists of a luminal layer of columnar cells resting on a cuboidal basal layer. The connective tissue papillae typically contain plasma cells. The lesion is treated by simple surgical excision.

BENIGN LYMPHOEPITHELIAL LESION
(Mikulicz's Disease)

This particular lesion of salivary glands is a rather uncommon one, but is very interesting in that it exhibits both inflammatory and neoplastic characteristics. There is increasing evidence that the disease is closely related to Sjögren's syndrome (q.v.) and that both are actually autoimmune diseases in which the patient's own salivary gland tissue becomes antigenic. Since more work on this aspect of the etiology has been carried out on patients with Sjögren's syndrome than on patients with the benign lymphoepithelial lesion, a more detailed discussion will be found under that condition.

Clinical Features. The benign lymphoepithelial lesion is manifested essentially as a unilateral or bilateral enlargement of the parotid and/ or submaxillary glands, associated in some cases with mild local discomfort, occasional pain and xerostomia (Fig. 3–10, *A*). The onset of the lesion is sometimes associated with fever, upper respiratory tract infection, oral infection, tooth extraction or some other local inflammatory disorder. There is often a diffuse, poorly outlined enlargement of the salivary gland rather than formation of a discrete tumor nodule. The enlargements vary in size, but are generally just a few centimeters in diameter. There is sometimes a history of an alternating increase and decrease in the size of the mass from time to time. The duration of the tumor mass may be only a few months or many years. Sometimes the lacrimal glands are enlarged also.

Studies of the benign lymphoepithelial lesion by Godwin and by Swinton and Warren have indicated that it occurs far more frequently in women, particularly those in middle or later life. In some series 85 per cent of the affected patients are female. In the series of 55 cases reported by Bernier and Bhaskar, however, there was an approximately equal distribution between men and women.

Histologic Features. The disease is characterized by an orderly lymphocytic infiltration of the salivary gland tissue, destroying or replacing the acini, with the persistence of islands of epithelial cells which probably represent residua of gland ducts (Fig. 3–10, *B*). Although the lymphoid element is usually diffuse, actual germinal centers are occasionally present. The epithelium may consist of ducts showing cellular proliferation and loss of polarity or, as the disease persists, solid nests or clumps of poorly defined epithelial cells which Morgan and Castleman termed "epimyoepithelial islands." These sometimes seem to form a syncytium. It has been suggested that such islands arise as a result of proliferation of both ductal cells and peripheral myoepithelial cells. A characteristic change also found in advanced lesions is the deposition of eosinophilic, hyaline material in the epithelial islands.

Great care must be taken in differentiating between the benign lymphoepithelial tumor and a malignant lymphoma involving the salivary glands. In the latter disease, epimyoepithelial islands are not present, the lymphoid element is atypical, and there is infiltration of the interlobular septa by lymphoid tissue. The epithelial islands, on the other hand, may be mistaken for metastatic carcinoma. Other histologically similar lesions which must be considered in the differential diagnosis are chronic sialadenitis, papillary cystadenoma lymphomatosum and uveoparotitis.

Treatment and Prognosis. The benign lymphoepithelial lesion has been treated by both surgical excision and radiation. In mild cases, no treatment is indicated once the diagnosis is made. In some cases, the swelling even regresses spontaneously. Persistent disease may be treated by surgical excision. Most authorities currently are opposed to the routine use of radiation therapy in view of the possibility of radiation-induced malignancy.

In general, the prognosis of benign lymphoepithelial lesion is good. However, malignancy associated with the condition is well documented. Hyman and Wolff have reported four cases of malignant lymphoma which developed in patients with benign lymphoepithelial lesion. An interesting case of a 63-year-old woman with benign lymphoepithelial lesion which transformed to a malignant lymphoma while on phenytoin (Dilantin) therapy was reported by Lapes and his associates. A remarkable number of cases of anaplastic carcinomas arising in Alaskan natives (Eskimo, Indian and Aleut) with benign lymphoepithelial lesion have been reported by Arthaud. Altogether, 17 such cases have been reported. There is no explanation for this epidemiologic oddity.

Relation to Mikulicz's Disease. The disease originally described by Mikulicz in 1888 was a condition characterized by a symmetric or bilateral, chronic, painless enlargement of the lacrimal and salivary glands. Subsequently, numerous cases were recorded which had similar clinical findings, but which often ran a rapidly fatal course. These latter cases in many instances proved to be examples of malignant lymphoma, leukemia or even tuberculosis. Since Mikulicz's patient manifested a benign course without involvement of the lymphatic system, it is now believed in the light of present knowledge that the disease described by Mikulicz and the benign lymphoepithelial lesion are identical in nature.

The term "Mikulicz's syndrome" has also found its way into the literature and has been used to describe the condition of salivary gland enlargement, usually accompanied by lymph node enlargement, due to some generalized specific disease such as one of the lymphomas or tuberculosis. The application of this term in such cases cannot be justified, since it does nothing to indicate the true nature of the disease.

SJÖGREN'S SYNDROME

(Sicca Syndrome; Gougerat-Sjögren Syndrome)

Sjögren's syndrome is a condition originally described as a triad consisting of keratoconjunctivitis sicca, xerostomia and rheumatoid arthritis. Subsequently, it has been found that some patients present only with dry eyes and dry mouth (sicca complex or primary Sjögren's syndrome), while others also develop systemic lupus erythematosus, polyarteritis nodosa, polymyositis or scleroderma, as well as rheumatoid arthritis (secondary Sjögren's syndrome). As Sjögren pointed out, cases of xerostomia and arthritis without keratoconjunctivitis sicca have been observed. A comprehensive review of the pathogenetic, clinical and laboratory features of Sjögren's syndrome has been published by Moutsopoulos and co-workers.

Etiology. Various causes of this disease have been suggested: genetic, hormonal, infectious and immunologic, among others. It may well be that a combination of factors, both extrinsic and intrinsic, play a role in the etiology of this condition. Most authorities consider an altered immunologic response to be the main intrinsic factor which is responsible for the disease. Laboratory findings support the autoimmune etiologic role (q.v.). Bertram has reported that 75 per cent of a series of 35 patients with Sjögren's syndrome had in their sera antisalivary duct antibody. Similar antibody was found in the sera of 24 per cent of a group of 29 patients with systemic lupus erythematosus, a documented autoimmune disease. In addition,

the sicca complex and Sjögren's syndrome have been found to be associated with the HLA system, specifically HLA–DR3 and DR4.

Kessler has described an animal model for Sjögren's syndrome, the New Zealand Black (NZB) and White (NZW) mice. These animals spontaneously develop lymphoid infiltrates of the salivary glands which are similar to those in Sjögren's syndrome. They also develop lupus erythematosus and lymphoid neoplasms. They have been shown to have abnormalities of the cellular and humoral immune systems.

Clinical Features. This disease occurs predominantly in women over 40 years of age, although children or young adults may be affected. The female:male ratio is approximately 10:1.

The typical features of the disease are dryness of the mouth and eyes as a result of hypofunction of the salivary and lacrimal glands. This often results in painful, burning sensations of the oral mucosa. In addition, various secretory glands of the nose, larynx, pharynx and tracheobronchial tree (buccopharyngolaryngitis sicca), as well as of the vagina, are involved with this dryness. Schall and his associates have evaluated the degree of xerostomia by means of sequential salivary scintigraphy. Chisholm and Mason have quantified saliva production in patients with the sicca complex and Sjögren's syndrome. Reduced salivary flow was noted in both groups. Sialochemistry studies by Ben-Aryeh and co-workers have demonstrated significantly elevated levels of IgA, potassium and sodium in the saliva of patients with the sicca complex.

Moutsopoulos has reported that 80 per cent of patients with primary Sjögren's syndrome have parotid enlargement in contrast to only 14 per cent with secondary Sjögren's syndrome. Lymphadenopathy is more than twice as common in the primary form of the disease.

Rheumatoid arthritis, as mentioned, is an integral part of secondary Sjögren's syndrome. It has been shown that patients with Sjögren's syndrome with rheumatoid arthritis have certain different clinical manifestations than patients with sicca complex, despite similar histologic findings and some laboratory findings. In this regard, patients without rheumatoid arthritis, that is, sicca complex or primary Sjögren's syndrome, more frequently manifest parotid gland enlargement, lymphadenopathy, purpura, Raynaud's phenomenon, kidney involvement and myositis.

Histologic Features. Three types of histologic alterations in the major salivary glands have been described. In one case, there may be intense lymphocytic infiltration of the gland replacing all acinar structures although the lobular architecture is preserved. In another, there may be proliferation of ductal epithelium and myoepithelium to form "epimyoepithelial islands." Both of these histologic changes are identical with those occurring in the benign lymphoepithelial lesion in Mikulicz's disease. The third alteration may be simply an atrophy of the glands sequential to the lymphocytic infiltration.

Interestingly, Bertram and Hjørting-Hansen have reported that 85 per cent of a group of patients with Sjögren's syndrome exhibited alterations in the accessory salivary glands of the lip characteristically similar to those in the major glands; they also have suggested biopsy of the labial mucosa as an aid in establishing the diagnosis of the disease. Similar findings in accessory glands, as well as the demonstration of antisalivary duct antibody by an immunofluorescent technique, have been reported by Tarpley, Anderson and White.

Laboratory Findings. Over 75 per cent of patients with primary Sjögren's syndrome have a polyclonal hyperglobulinemia and many develop cryoglobulins. Multiple organ- or tissue-specific antibodies are found, including antisalivary duct antibodies, rheumatoid factor and antinuclear antibodies. An increased sedimentation rate is present in 80 per cent of these patients. Interestingly, the presence of antisalivary duct antibody is three times more common in those with secondary Sjögren's syndrome as compared to those with the sicca complex.

Roentgenographic Features. Sialography may be of diagnostic value in Sjögren's syndrome. Sialographs demonstrate the formation of punctate, cavitary defects which are filled with radiopaque contrast media. These filling defects have been said to produce a "cherry blossom" or "branchless fruit-laden tree" effect radiographically. Som and his associates have suggested that the contrast material actually extravasates through the weakened salivary gland ducts to produce the sialographic features. Poor elimination of contrast media is noted, as might be expected, with retention of the material for over a month.

Treatment and Prognosis. There is no satisfactory treatment for Sjögren's syndrome. Most patients are treated symptomatically. Keratoconjunctivitis is treated by instillation of ocular lubricants such as artificial tears containing methylcellulose, and xerostomia is treated by saliva substitutes such as those used in the treatment of persons with xerostomia secondary to radiation therapy. Extensive dental caries is a complication which is quite common, and scrupulous oral hygiene and frequent fluoride application is indicated to reduce this problem. There is no specific treatment for enlargement of the salivary glands. Surgery has been employed but is generally recommended only in patients with discomfort. Although radiation therapy has been recommended in the past, its use is not advocated currently.

A major complicating factor in patients with Sjögren's syndrome is the development of pseudolymphoma and malignant lymphoma. In an extensive National Institutes of Health (NIH) study, 136 patients with Sjögren's syndrome were followed for an average period of over eight years. Nonlymphoma malignancies were no more common than would be expected, whereas lymphomas were observed in nearly 44 times the expected incidence rate. The risk of lymphoma in Sjögren's patients is 6.4 cases per 100 cases per year. Most lymphomas are non-Hodgkin's types and are B-cell in origin. Macroglobulinemia of Waldenström also has been noted to develop in these patients.

Thus, the relation between the benign lymphoepithelial lesion, Mikulicz's disease and Sjögren's syndrome is possibly a very close one. Mikulicz's disease, but not Mikulicz's syndrome, is probably identical with the lymphoepithelial lesion. This entity shares several features in common with Sjögren's syndrome. Both diseases are manifested, often but not invariably, by a swelling of the major salivary glands and lacrimal glands, singly or in pairs. In both diseases the patient has xerostomia, which probably is related to the displacement and destruction of acinar tissue. Finally, both diseases occur chiefly in middle-aged or elderly women.

It is likely that the benign lymphoepithelial lesion is a mild form of Sjögren's syndrome, but it should not be inferred that lymphoepithelial lesions will eventually terminate in Sjögren's disease. More aptly, the two diseases may be considered two forms of the same disease with a probably common etiology.

MALIGNANT TUMORS OF THE SALIVARY GLANDS

MALIGNANT PLEOMORPHIC ADENOMA

*(Malignant "Mixed" Tumor; Carcinoma
Ex Pleomorphic Adenoma)*

Occasionally salivary gland tumors occur that appear histologically benign, and yet have proved metastases resembling the primary lesion, or resemble the benign pleomorphic adenoma, but exhibit cytologically malignant areas. Such lesions are rare, but must be classified as malignant pleomorphic adenomas.

It is uncertain whether these tumors represent previously benign lesions which have undergone transformation into malignant tumors, or lesions which were malignant from the onset. Foote and Frazell favor the former view, since they found that the average age of patients with a malignant pleomorphic adenoma is about ten years older than that of patients with the benign form of the neoplasm. This differential would allow time for the malignant transformation. Furthermore, they indicated that patients with the malignant lesion usually give a history of a mass which had been present for a number of years, but only recently had shown a remarkably increased growth rate.

However, in the series of cases reported by Gerughty and his co-workers, there was no age differential between the benign and malignant lesions; the majority of their cases presented initially as malignant tumors without a history of sudden rapid growth in a long-standing tumor. Therefore, their data suggest that these tumors were malignant from the onset.

Clinical Features. There are no obvious clinical differences between the benign and the malignant pleomorphic adenoma in many instances. Foote and Frazell pointed out that the malignant tumors are usually larger than the benign ones, but this fact is of no significance in the differential clinical diagnosis, since both forms vary greatly in size. There is often fixation of the malignant tumor to underlying structures as well as to the overlying skin or mucosa, as is true in general for malignant salivary gland lesions, and surface ulceration is also variably present. Pain is more frequently a feature in the malignant than in the benign pleomorphic adenoma. LiVolsi and Perzin have reported a clinicopathologic study of 47 cases of carcinomas arising in benign mixed tumors. Seventeen of these arose in intraoral accessory glands, primarily in the palate.

Histologic Features. In some malignant pleomorphic adenomas the malignant component appears to overgrow the benign element, so that histologically benign areas are difficult to demonstrate. In other cases the bulk of the lesion may appear benign, and the malignant foci may be found only after diligent search. For this reason there is need for careful study of all supposedly benign salivary gland tumors, and the pathologist should take particular care to examine sections from numerous blocks of tissue cut from many areas throughout the tumor.

The specific criteria for recognizing a malignant "mixed" tumor are not completely established. Nevertheless, they appear to include those nuclear changes usually held as indicative of malignancy (nuclear hyperchromatism and pleomorphism, increased or abnormal mitoses and increased nuclear/cytoplasmic ratio); invasion of blood vessels, lymphatics or nerves; focal necrosis; and obvious peripheral infiltration and destruction of normal tissue. Nagao and co-workers have studied the histologic features of 48 cases of carcinomas arising in parotid gland pleomorphic adenomas and have elaborated upon the important criteria for the diagnosis.

The malignant cell pattern of transformation appears to be into epidermoid carcinoma or into adenocarcinoma, and some malignant tumors show both types of cells. Spindle cell and giant cell transformation also occur.

Treatment and Prognosis. The treatment of the malignant pleomorphic adenoma is essentially surgical, although lesions which have shown a tendency for local recurrence are sometimes treated by combined surgery and radiation therapy.

These malignant neoplasms exhibit a high recurrence rate after surgical removal, as well as a high incidence of regional lymph node involvement. Distant metastases to lungs, bones, viscera and brain frequently develop.

ADENOID CYSTIC CARCINOMA

(Cylindroma; Adenocystic Carcinoma; Adenocystic Basal Cell Carcinoma; Pseudoadenomatous Basal Cell Carcinoma; Basaloid Mixed Tumor)

The adenoid cystic carcinoma is a form of adenocarcinoma which is sufficiently distinctive to warrant separation in the classification of malignant glandular tumors. Histologically similar lesions occur in the intraoral accessory salivary glands as well as in the lacrimal glands and the glands of the paranasal sinuses, pharynx, trachea and bronchi, skin and breast. Tarpley and Giansanti have studied 50 cases of oral adenoid cystic carcinomas. The palatal mucosa was the most frequent site of occurrence.

Clinical Features. The salivary glands most commonly involved by this tumor are the parotid, the submaxillary and the accessory glands in the palate and tongue (Fig. 3–11, *A*). The

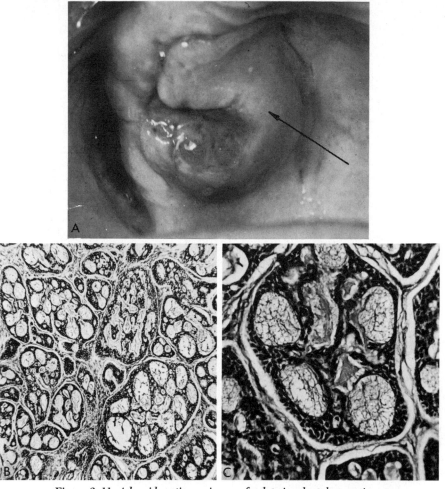

Figure 3–11. *Adenoid cystic carcinoma of palate in edentulous patient.*
A, Clinical picture; *B*, low-power photomicrograph showing pattern of tumor; *C*, high-power photomicrograph showing greater detail.

adenoid cystic carcinoma occurs most commonly during the fifth and sixth decades of life, but it is by no means rare even in the third decade. Many of the patients exhibit clinical manifestations of a typical malignant salivary gland tumor: early local pain, facial nerve paralysis in the case of parotid tumors, fixation to deeper structures and local invasion. Some of the lesions, particularly the intraoral ones, exhibit surface ulceration. There may be clinical resemblance in some cases to the pleomorphic adenoma.

Histologic Features. The adenoid cystic carcinoma is composed of small, deeply staining uniform cells resembling basal cells that are commonly arranged in anastomosing cords or a ductlike pattern, the central portion of which may contain a mucoid material (Fig. 3–11, *B*, *C*), producing the typical cribriform, "honey-comb" or "Swiss cheese" pattern. Characteristically, the stromal connective tissue becomes hyalinized and surrounds the tumor cells, forming a structural pattern of cylinders from which the lesion originally derived the name "cylindroma." Growth of cells in a solid form sometimes occurs, and there may be little typical cystic glandular pattern. In other instances only thin, delicate anastomosing cords of neoplastic cells are dispersed throughout an abundant stroma. A pseudoameloblastoma form of the tumor also occurs on rare occasions. Spread of the tumor cells along the perineural spaces or perineural sheaths is a common feature of this neoplasm (Fig. 3–12). It is of interest that, despite the malignant nature of the lesion, mitotic figures are extremely rare. Great variation in the histologic pattern is seen in different cases. Care must be exercised not to confuse

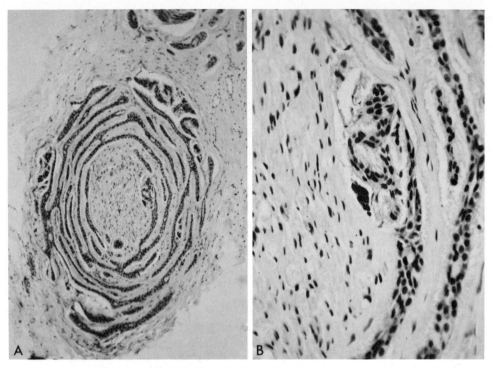

Figure 3–12. *Adenoid cystic carcinoma.*
The perineural invasion by tumor cells is evident. (Courtesy of Dr. James K. Jacoby.)

this lesion with a benign adenoma, because of the vastly different prognosis between the two.

Treatment and Prognosis. The treatment of the adenoid cystic carcinoma is chiefly surgical, although in some cases surgery has been successfully coupled with x-ray radiation. Radiation alone is not recommended. In general, this tumor is a slowly growing lesion which tends to metastasize only late in its course. Cervical node involvement eventually occurs in about 30 per cent of the cases, however, and distant metastases to lung, bones and brain occur in a high proportion of the patients. The cure rate for patients with this disease, though varying somewhat from series to series, is discouragingly low.

Factors influencing prognosis are the site of occurrence and the histologic pattern of the tumor. Conley and Dingman found that there is a marked difference in the clinical behavior of major and minor gland adenoid cystic carcinomas. Only 28 per cent of 78 patients with minor gland tumors were alive with no evidence of disease in a 4- to 14-year follow-up study. Sixty-four per cent of 54 patients with major gland tumors studied over a comparable period were alive and free of disease. A number of studies, including one by Perzin and his co-

workers, have shown that tumors with a solid histologic pattern have a poorer prognosis than those with a tubular or cribriform pattern.

ACINIC CELL CARCINOMA

(Acinar Cell or Serous Cell Adenoma and Adenocarcinoma)

Most salivary gland tumors arise from the epithelium of the duct apparatus, but occasionally lesions seem to show acinar cell differentiation. Batsakis and his colleagues have suggested origin of the tumor from cells of terminal salivary gland ducts. Some authors advocate the existence of both benign and malignant acinic cell neoplasms, whereas others are of the opinion that all acinic cell neoplasms are malignant. Unfortunately, the criteria for distinguishing between benign and malignant acinar cell tumors, if such a distinction exists, have not been clearly established. In an extensive study of acinic cell tumors of the major salivary glands by Abrams and his co-workers, it was concluded that most investigators believe that all tumors of this type have at least a low-grade malignant potential.

Clinical Features. The acinic cell carcinoma closely resembles the pleomorphic adenoma in gross appearance, tending to be encapsulated and lobulated. Although this tumor has been reported occurring chiefly in the parotid, it does occur occasionally in the other major glands and in the accessory intraoral glands. Abrams and Melrose, Chen and associates, and Gardner and his colleagues have reported series of acinic cell carcinomas of intraoral salivary glands. Approximately 80 well-documented cases are in the literature. The most common intraoral sites are the lips and buccal mucosa. The acinic cell carcinoma occurs predominantly in persons in middle age or somewhat older, but has been encountered before the age of 20 years. Of 77 cases reported by Abrams and his associates, approximately 35 per cent were in the third decade of life. In the series of 51 cases reported by Perzin and LiVolsi, 72 per cent of the patients were 40 years of age or older. The youngest patient was 13, while the oldest was 74 years. Patients with bilateral synchronous tumors have been reported.

Histologic Features. The acinic cell carcinoma, which is frequently surrounded by a thin capsule, may be composed of cells of varying degrees of differentiation. Well-differentiated cells bear remarkable resemblance to normal acinar cells, whereas less differentiated cells resemble embryonic ducts and immature acinar cells (Fig. 3–13 A, B). Abrams and his associates have described four growth patterns: (1) solid, (2) papillary-cystic, (3) follicular, and (4) microcystic. In general, one pattern predominates, although combinations can occur.

Lymphoid elements are commonly found in parotid acinic cell carcinomas, a feature which is helpful in the diagnosis. Such features are not found in the intraoral tumors. Apparently the acinic cell carcinoma can arise from embryologically entrapped salivary gland tissue in lymph nodes in or near the parotid compartment.

Although "clear cells," have been described in acinic cell carcinomas, they most likely represent cells altered by fixation or they may actually represent the component cells of a clear cell carcinoma (q.v.), a recently recognized entity.

Treatment and Prognosis. The treatment of the acinic cell carcinoma in most cases has been surgical. Perzin and LiVolsi recommend total excision of parotid gland tumors with preser-

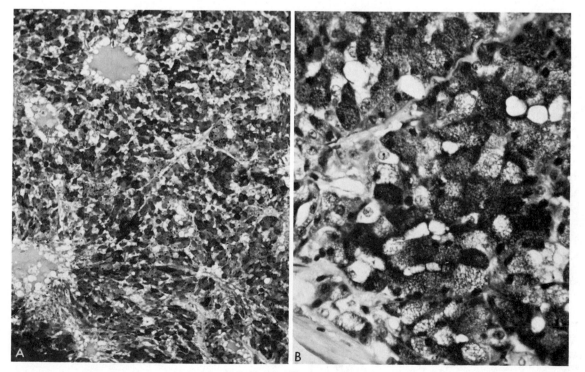

Figure 3–13. *Acinic cell adenocarcinoma.*
The granular nature of the cytoplasm of the tumor cells is prominent. (Courtesy of Dr. Gisle Bang.)

vation of the facial nerve unless it is involved. Lymph node dissection is indicated only in the presence of clinical involvement and not as a routine procedure. Radiation therapy has not been shown to be of therapeutic value. Intraoral tumors are treated by surgical excision.

The recurrence rate of acinic cell carcinoma varies from 8 to 59 per cent. High recurrence rates are seen in tumors treated by enucleation and limited excision. It is important to recognize that recurrences may occur many years after surgery. Metastasis takes place in approximately 20 per cent of patients, again, often occurring many years after the initial surgery. Hematogenous metastases to bone and lung are most common.

Although the five-year survival rate of patients with acinic cell carcinoma is quite good, long-term studies show that a significant number of individuals may die 15 to 20 years after the initial treatment. Thus, long-term follow-up is necessary.

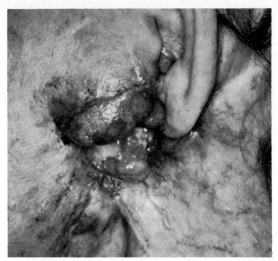

Figure 3–14. *Recurrent mucoepidermoid carcinoma of parotid gland.*

MUCOEPIDERMOID CARCINOMA

The mucoepidermoid carcinoma is an unusual type of salivary gland tumor first studied and described as a separate entity by Stewart, Foote and Becker in 1945. As the name implies, the tumor is composed of both mucus-secreting cells and epidermoid-type cells in varying proportions.

Clinical Features. The majority of mucoepidermoid carcinomas involving the major salivary glands occur in the parotid gland (Fig. 3–14), although the other major glands and especially the intraoral accessory glands may also be their site of origin (Fig. 3–15). Stewart and his co-workers attempted to classify the mucoepidermoid tumor into two varieties, a benign and a malignant form, based upon the clinical nature and histologic features of the lesions. It has subsequently become apparent that such a classification is probably not justified, and many authorities now consider the entire group to be malignant neoplasms presenting varying degrees or grades of malignancy.

Spiro and his associates reported an extensive study of 367 cases of mucoepidermoid carcinomas involving both the major and accessory salivary glands and pointed out that, on the basis of their data, all mucoepidermoid "tumors" were malignant. Healey, Perzin and Smith concurred with such a viewpoint. On the other hand, Melrose and his colleagues challenged the concept based upon their analysis of 54 cases involving intraoral minor salivary glands.

Mucoepidermoid carcinoma occurs with an equal distribution between men and women. It occurs primarily in the third to fifth decades of life but actually can occur in virtually all decades. It is the most common malignant salivary gland tumor of children. Castro and his colleagues reported 15 mucoepidermoid carcinomas in children, while Krolls, Trodahl and Boyers reviewed 20 such cases.

The tumor of low-grade malignancy usually appears as a slowly enlarging, painless mass which simulates the pleomorphic adenoma. Unlike the pleomorphic adenoma, however, the low-grade mucoepidermoid carcinoma seldom exceeds 5 cm. in diameter, is not completely encapsulated and often contains cysts which may be filled with a viscid, mucoid material. Intraoral tumors of this type frequently occur in such sites as the palate, buccal mucosa, tongue and retromolar area. Because of their tendency to develop cystic areas, these intraoral lesions may bear close clinical resemblance to the mucous retention phenomenon or mucocele, especially those in the retromolar area.

The tumor of high-grade malignancy grows rapidly and does produce pain as an early symptom. Facial nerve paralysis is frequent in parotid tumors. The mucoepidermoid carcinoma is not encapsulated, but tends to infiltrate the surrounding tissue and, in a high percentage of cases, to metastasize to regional lymph nodes. Distant metastases to lung, bone, brain and subcutaneous tissues are also common.

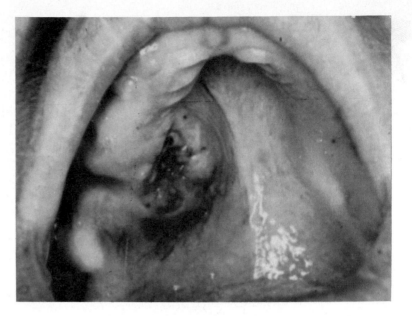

Figure 3–15. *Mucoepidermoid carcinoma of palate.*

In 1968, Gerughty and his co-workers described a malignant salivary gland tumor which had features of both adenocarcinoma and carcinoma. They designated the neoplasm *adenosquamous carcinoma.* The tumors arose in minor salivary glands of the oral and nasal cavities and larynx. They proved to be extremely aggressive, with a marked tendency for regional lymph node and distant metastasis. A number of authorities, including Batsakis and his associates, consider the adenosquamous carcinoma to be similar to, if not identical with, a high-grade mucoepidermoid carcinoma.

Histologic Features. The mucoepidermoid carcinoma is a pleomorphic tumor composed of mucus-secreting cells, epidermoid-type cells and intermediate cells (Fig. 3–16). In low-grade tumors all three types of cells are present, although the epidermoid and mucus-secreting cells predominate. The intermediate cell is seldom the dominant cell, although it appears that it may undergo transformation into either mucous or epidermoid cells. On occasion, clusters of clear cells, often in abundance, may be present. These clear cells are generally mucin- and glycogen-free. This tumor seems to arise from ductal epithelium, since ductal proliferation adjacent to the tumor is common.

Essentially, these tumors show sheets or nests of epidermoid cells and similar nests of mucous cells, usually arranged in a glandular pattern and sometimes showing microcyst formation (Fig. 3–17). These cysts may rupture, liberating mucus which may pool in the connective tissue and evoke an inflammatory reaction. Special stain is often necessary to demonstrate the mucous cells present. In the higher-grade tumors the mucous cell element is not prominent. It may be so inconspicuous and the epidermoid cell may be so outstanding that a mistaken diagnosis of epidermoid carcinoma may be made.

Treatment and Prognosis. The treatment of the mucoepidermoid carcinoma is chiefly surgical, although recent data have shown favorable responses to radiation therapy. Currently, surgery followed by radiation treatment is recommended for intermediate-grade and high-grade tumors; low-grade tumors can be managed by surgery alone. Elective lymph node dissection is not necessary in patients with low-grade and intermediate-grade tumors; however, such a procedure is recommended in high-grade tumors, since occult cervical metastases have been reported in two-thirds of these cases.

Spiro and his associates reported distant metastases in 15 per cent of their cases. When viewed with respect to the histologic grade of the tumor, the rates were 2, 16 and 35 per cent for low-, intermediate- and high-grade tumors respectively. Low-grade lesions had a five-year cure rate of 92 per cent, whereas the intermediate-grade and high-grade lesions had a 49 per cent five-year cure rate. All types showed additional deaths due to tumor at 10 and 15 years, thus showing the necessity for long-term follow-up of patients with malignant salivary gland tumors of this type.

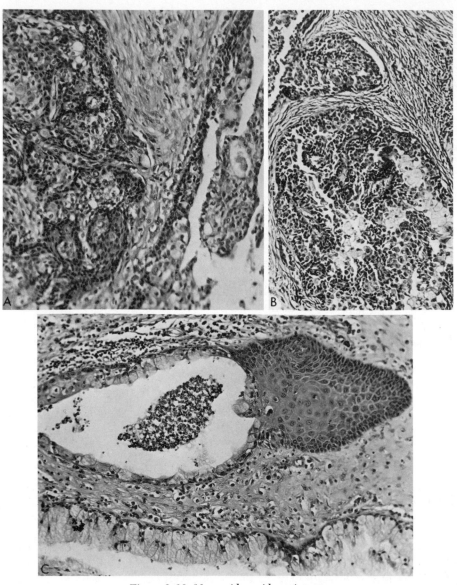

Figure 3–16. *Mucoepidermoid carcinoma.*
A, B, Photomicrographs illustrate the association of the pale-staining, mucus-containing cells associated with darker-staining epidermoid cells in a moderately high-grade mucoepidermoid carcinoma. *C,* In one ductlike structure the lining consists partially of squamous epithelium and partially of mucous cells. (From F. Vellios: Am. J. Clin. Pathol., 25:147, 1955.)

CENTRAL MUCOEPIDERMOID CARCINOMA OF THE JAW

Mucoepidermoid carcinoma central within the jaws is a recognized entity. Browand and Waldron reported 9 cases and reviewed the 41 previously reported cases. The majority of these lesions have occurred in the mandible, although a few have developed in the maxilla; in most cases, the lesions occurred in the premolar-molar area and did not extend anteriorly beyond the premolar region.

Several theories have been advanced to account for the occurrence of these lesions within the jaws. It has been suggested that they may originate from: (1) entrapment of retromolar mucous glands within the mandible, which subsequently undergo neoplastic transformation; (2) developmentally included embryonic remnants of the submaxillary gland within the man-

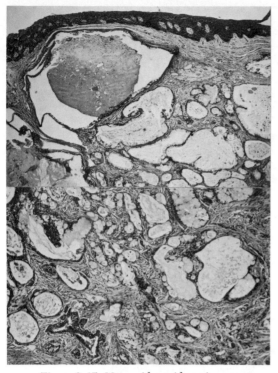

Figure 3–17. Mucoepidermoid carcinoma.
The photomicrograph illustrates a low-grade mucoepidermoid carcinoma characterized chiefly by proliferation of mucus-secreting cells, pools of mucus and minimal epidermoid cell proliferation.

dible; and (3) neoplastic transformation of the mucous-secreting cells commonly found in the epithelial lining of dentigerous cysts associated with impacted third molars. Inasmuch as a number of the cases of central mucoepidermoid carcinomas have appeared to resemble dentigerous cysts, clinically or radiographically, it appears likely that the source of many of these mucoepidermoid carcinomas is in the pluripotential epithelium of such a cyst. It is difficult to explain those lesions found in the posterior portion of the maxilla; a mucoepidermoid carcinoma originating from the lining of the maxillary sinus and invading the alveolar bone, in such cases, cannot be excluded.

There appears to be no significant difference in age or sex distribution between the central mucoepidermoid carcinomas and those occurring in the major and minor salivary glands. In addition, the same degree of histologic variation is found in those tumors central within the jaws, as that reported in the major and minor salivary gland mucoepidermoid carcinomas. However, in the reported cases of central tumors, metastases have been more regional than widespread.

Occasional salivary gland tumors other than mucoepidermoid carcinoma also have been reported to occur central in the jaws. Miller and Winnick have reviewed the literature on such lesions and have found that these included the benign mixed tumor, adenoid cystic carcinoma and malignant mixed tumor.

CLEAR CELL CARCINOMA

The clear cell carcinoma of salivary gland origin is a relatively recently recognized lesion. Corridan is credited with the first report of a clear cell tumor in 1956 and other isolated cases were reported by British and German authors. Reports of the tumor in the American literature have been found only in the last decade. Early investigators reported both benign (adenomas) and malignant (carcinomas) clear cell tumors. Currently, most authorities view all clear cell tumors as at least low-grade malignancies.

The origin of the clear cell is somewhat controversial. The semipluripotential intercalated duct cell has been implicated by some investigators. Others, including Saksela and associates, have implicated the myoepithelial cell as the progenitor of the clear cell. Donath and his colleagues have designated a group of clear cell neoplasms as *epithelial-myoepithelial carcinoma of intercalated duct origin* (also called the Donath-Seifert tumor). The bicellular histologic appearance of this tumor has been explained by the participation of both ductal and myoepithelial cells. Corio and his colleagues recently reported 16 cases of epithelial-myoepithelial carcinomas, 15 of which occurred in the major salivary glands and 1 in the buccal mucosa.

The clear cell carcinoma is found primarily in the major salivary glands, especially the parotid. It may, however, be found in intraoral sites. It occurs in elderly adults and, on the basis of cases reported thus far, tends to occur more often in females.

Clear cell carcinomas are composed of clusters of cells surrounded by thin septa of fibrous connective tissue. This often produces somewhat of an "organoid" appearance (Fig. 3–18A). Glycogen may be demonstrated in the cells in many cases by the periodic acid-Schiff (PAS) reaction. The epithelial-myoepithelial carcinoma consists of an inner layer of ductal cells surrounded by a layer of clear cells (Fig. 3–18B). Histologically, clear cell carcinomas of salivary gland origin bear close similarity to the

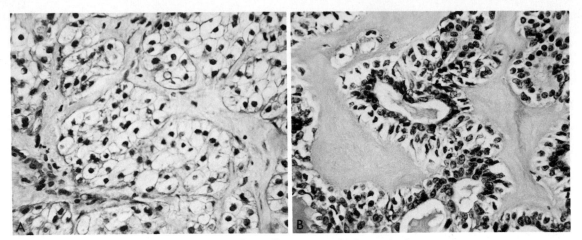

Figure 3–18. *Clear cell carcinoma of salivary gland.*
A, Clusters of clear cells in an organoid arrangement. B, Epithelial-myoepithelial carcinoma of intercalated duct origin.

clear cell carcinoma of the kidney (hypernephroma). Therefore, a metastatic renal malignancy should be considered in the histologic differential diagnosis of these lesions.

Clear cell carcinomas are treated by surgical excision. The tumor has a relatively favorable prognosis in that less than one-third recur and fewer metastasize. Nonetheless, the tumor can behave aggressively and there are no means by which such behavior can be predicted.

ADENOCARCINOMA OF MISCELLANEOUS FORMS

The lesions which may be classed in this nonspecific category are a histologically heterogeneous group. They vary from highly anaplastic adenocarcinomas to moderately well-differentiated lesions, such as the trabecular adenocarcinoma, papillary cystadenocarcinoma and adenocarcinoma with a pseudoadamantine pattern—i.e., made up of columnar cells suggesting ameloblasts and a developing tooth germ.

Despite the microscopic variation in pattern, these tumors as a group exhibit the usual features of malignant neoplasms, including local infiltrative growth, tendency for recurrence and frequency of metastasis. These lesions generally tend to grow rapidly and act aggressively (Fig. 3–19).

The treatment of these tumors as a class is surgical excision. A high recurrence rate is to be expected, and the survival rate of patients with such tumors is low.

EPIDERMOID CARCINOMA

(Squamous Cell Carcinoma)

This type of malignancy occurring in the salivary glands involves a grave prognosis, since the tumor exhibits infiltrative properties, metastasizes early and recurs readily. Fortunately it is not a common lesion. Although it appears to arise more frequently in the major salivary glands, particularly the parotid and submaxillary, it may arise in accessory salivary gland tissue.

The exact site from which epidermoid carcinomas of the salivary gland arise has not been

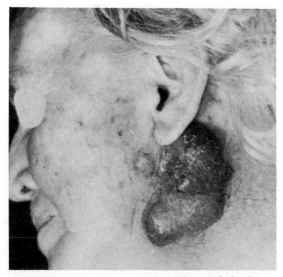

Figure 3–19. *Adenocarcinoma of parotid gland.*

definitely established. It appears most likely that they are of ductal origin, since the ducts may undergo squamous metaplasia with ease. Standish has shown that the ducts of experimental animal salivary glands may undergo squamous metaplasia within a matter of days after implantation of a carcinogenic hydrocarbon such as 7,12-dimethylbenz(α)-anthracene, and then subsequently develop epidermoid carcinoma.

Squamous metaplasia of the salivary gland ducts and acini following x-ray radiation of the mouth and oropharynx also has been reported by Friedman and Hall as an incidental finding, although these investigators did not think this represented a precancerous phenomenon. Ionizing radiation has been associated with the development of both benign and malignant salivary gland tumors. Rice, Batsakis and McClatchey reviewed 22 malignant salivary gland tumors associated with prior exposure to ionizing radiation and added an additional case of the tumor in the parotid gland of a person who received x-ray treatment for acne 20 years previously. Interestingly, Belsky and his associates reported a more than fivefold increase in the incidence of salivary gland tumors in Japanese survivors of the atomic bombs when compared with nonirradiated controls.

Treatment and Prognosis. The combined use of surgery and radiotherapy is more apt to be of benefit in this type of salivary gland tumor than in most of the others. Since regional lymph node metastasis is a common finding associated with this tumor, a radical neck dissection of the local lymphatic chain is often carried out, provided the primary lesion appears to be controlled.

NECROTIZING SIALOMETAPLASIA

Necrotizing sialometaplasia is a benign, inflammatory reaction of salivary gland tissue which both clinically and histologically mimics a salivary gland malignancy. Although the phenomenon had been recognized for a number of years previously, Abrams and his colleagues were the first to report the condition in the literature in 1973 as a distinctive clinicopathologic entity. Since the original report, a number of cases have appeared in both the dental and medical literature. Unfortunately, some have been cases in which the diagnosis was made retrospectively after mutilating surgery. Lynch and his associates have reviewed the literature and have added two cases of their own.

Etiology and Pathogenesis. The most likely cause of necrotizing sialometaplasia is local ischemia. The acinar necrosis is fairly typical of coagulation necrosis, and it is well-recognized that salivary gland ducts exhibit squamous metaplasia when the blood supply is compromised. Standish and Shafer have shown that acinar necrosis and ductal squamous metaplasia occur in the salivary glands of rats which have had ligation of the arterial blood supply. The precise cause of the ischemic process is unknown. Many patients with the condition use tobacco or alcohol or both; however, there is no proof that either plays an etiologic role. Surprisingly, the occurrence of necrotizing sialometaplasia in persons with peripheral vascular disorders is unusual, although Rye, Calhoun and Redman reported a case in a patient with documented thromboangiitis obliterans (Buerger's disease) complicated by Raynaud's phenomenon.

Clinical Features. Necrotizing sialometaplasia occurs somewhat more commonly in men than in women. Most patients are in the fourth and fifth decades, but the lesion is reported in all ages except children. Most cases occur in the palate, but other intraoral sites such as buccal mucosa, lip and retromolar area have been affected. Occasionally, extraoral sites such as the nasopharynx may be involved. Cases have been reported in the parotid gland as a postsurgical sequela.

The lesion generally presents as an ulcer (Fig. 3–20). Swelling and feeling of "fullness" may precede some lesions. Pain is not a common complaint despite the often large areas of ulceration.

Histologic Features. Necrotizing sialometaplasia is characterized histologically by ulcerated

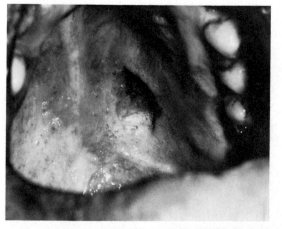

Figure 3–20. *Necrotizing sialometaplasia of palate.*
(Courtesy of Dr. Jack E. Schaaf.)

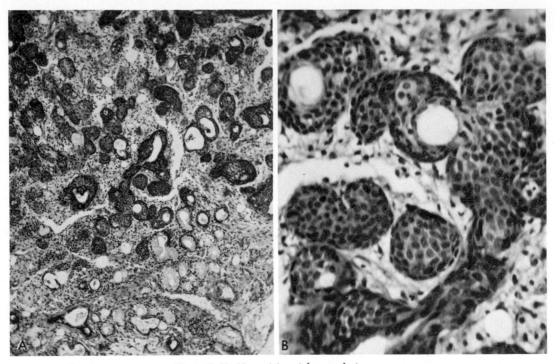

Figure 3–21. *Necrotizing sialometaplasia.*

mucosa, pseudoepitheliomatous hyperplasia of the mucosal epithelium, acinar necrosis and squamous metaplasia of salivary ducts. Importantly, there is preservation of the lobular architecture despite the necrosis (Fig. 3–21). Inflammatory cells may be found in and around the lobular areas of necrosis. Granulation tissue or fibrosis in variable amounts is present. The pseudoepitheliomatous hyperplasia, necrosis and ductal squamous metaplasia are the features which have led to erroneous diagnoses of carcinoma or mucoepidermoid carcinoma.

Treatment and Prognosis. The lesion is essentially self-limiting and heals by secondary intention. Debridement and saline rinses may aid the healing process. Recurrence is not usually encountered.

STROMAL SALIVARY GLAND TUMORS

The previous discussion deals with tumors which arise from the glandular or ductal epithelial elements of the salivary glands. Such tumors make up most of the neoplasms occurring in the salivary glands. A limited group of tumors do occur, however, which are derived from the stromal tissue rather than the parenchyma. Benign stromal salivary gland tumors include the

hemangioma or juvenile hemangioendothelioma, various forms of nerve tumors and the lipoma. Malignant lesions in the group include the lymphomas, rhabdomyosarcoma, melanoma and fibrosarcoma, as well as metastatic tumors from many sites.

REFERENCES

Abrams, A. M., and Finck, F. M.: Sialadenoma papilliferum. A previously unreported salivary gland tumor. Cancer, 24:1057, 1969.

Abrams, A. M., and Melrose, R. J.: Acinic cell tumors of minor salivary gland origin. Oral Surg., 46:220, 1978.

Abrams, A. M., Melrose, R. J., and Howell, F. V.: Necrotizing sialometaplasia. A disease simulating malignancy. Cancer, 32:130, 1973.

Abrams, A. M., Cornyn, J., Scofield, H. H., and Hansen, L. S.: Acinic cell adenocarcinoma of the major salivary glands. Cancer, 18:1145, 1965.

Allegra, S. R.: Warthin's tumor: a hypersensitivity disease? Ultrastructural, light and immunofluorescent study. Hum. Pathol., 2:403, 1971.

Arthaud, J. B.: Anaplastic parotid carcinoma ("malignant lymphoepithelial lesion") in seven Alaskan natives. Am. J. Clin. Pathol., 57:275, 1972.

Assor, D.: Bilateral carcinoma of the parotid, one cancer arising in a Warthin's tumor. Am. J. Clin. Pathol., 61:270, 1974.

Baden, E., Pierce, M., Selman, A. J., Roberts, T. W., and Doyle, J. L.: Intraoral papillary cystadenoma lymphomatosum. J. Oral Surg., 34:533, 1976.

Batsakis, J. G.: Basal cell adenoma of the parotid gland. Cancer, 29:226, 1972.

Idem: Tumors of the Head and Neck. Clinical and Pathological Considerations. 2nd ed. Baltimore, Williams & Wilkins Company, 1979.

Idem: Salivary gland neoplasia: an outcome of modified morphogenesis and cytodifferentiation. Oral Surg., 49:229, 1980.

Batsakis, J. G., and Regezi, J. A.: Selected controversial lesions of salivary tissues. Otolaryngol. Clin. North Am., 10:309, 1977.

Batsakis, J. G., Brannon, R. B., and Sciubba, J. J.: Monomorphic adenomas of major salivary glands: a histologic study of 96 tumours. Clin. Otolaryngol., 6:129, 1981.

Batsakis, J. G., Wozniak, K. J., and Regezi, J. A.: Acinous cell carcinoma: a histogenetic hypothesis. J. Oral Surg., 35:904, 1977.

Belsky, J. L., Tachikawa, K., Cihak, R. W., and Yamamoto, T.: Salivary gland tumors in atomic bomb survivors, Hiroshima-Nagasaki, 1957 to 1970. J.A.M.A., 219:864, 1972.

Ben-Aryeh, H., Scharf, J., Gutman, D., Szargel, R., and Zonis, S.: Sialochemistry of KCS patients. Int. J. Oral Surg., 7:172, 1978.

Bernier, J. L., and Bhaskar, S. N.: Lymphoepithelial lesions of salivary glands. Histogenesis and classification based on 186 cases. Cancer, 11:1156, 1958.

Bertram, U.: Xerostomia. Acta Odontol. Scand., 25:Suppl. 49, 1967.

Bertram, U., and Hjørting-Hansen, E.: Punch-biopsy of minor salivary glands in the diagnosis of Sjögren's syndrome. Scand. J. Dent. Res., 78:295, 1970.

Bertram, U., Pindborg, J. J., Seedorff, H. H., and Videbaek, A. A.: Sjögren's syndrome. Ugeskr. Laeger, 123:1085, 1961.

Bhaskar, S. N.: Acinic-cell carcinoma of salivary glands. Report of twenty-one cases. Oral Surg., 17:62, 1964.

Bhaskar, S. N., and Bernier, J. L.: Mucoepidermoid tumors of major and minor salivary glands. Cancer, 15:801, 1962.

Browand, B. C., and Waldron, C. A.: Central mucoepidermoid tumors of the jaws. Oral Surg., 40:631, 1975.

Buchner, A., David, R., and Hansen, L. S.: "Hyaline cells" in pleomorphic adenoma of salivary gland origin. Oral Surg., 52:506, 1981.

Canalis, R. F., Mok, M. W., Fishman, S. M., and Hemenway, W. G.: Congenital basal cell adenoma of the submandibular gland. Arch. Otolaryngol., 106:284, 1980.

Castro, E. B., Huvos, A. G., Strong, E. W., and Foote, F. W., Jr.: Tumors of the major salivary glands in children. Cancer, 29:312, 1972.

Chaudhry, A. P., and Gorlin, R. J.: Papillary cystadenoma lymphomatosum (adenolymphoma). A review of the literature. Am. J. Surg., 95:923, 1958.

Idem: Oxyphilic granular cell adenoma (oncocytoma). Oral Surg., 11:897, 1958.

Chaudhry, A. P., Vickers, R. A., and Gorlin, R. J.: Intraoral minor salivary gland tumors. Oral Surg., 14:1194, 1961.

Chaudhry, A. P., Satchidanand, S., Peer, R., and Cutler, L. S.: Myoepithelial cell adenoma of the parotid gland: a light and ultrastructural study. Cancer, 49:288, 1982.

Chen, S.-Y., and Miller, A. S.: Canalicular adenoma of the upper lip. An electron microscopic study. Cancer, 46:552, 1980.

Chen, S.-Y., Brannon, R. B., Miller, A. S., White, D. K., and Hooker, S. P.: Acinic cell adenocarcinoma of minor salivary glands. Cancer, 42:678, 1978.

Chisholm, D. M., and Mason, D. K.: Salivary gland function in Sjögren's syndrome. A review. Br. Dent. J., 135:393, 1973.

Chisholm, D. M., Waterhouse, J. P., Kraucunas, E., and Sciubba, J. J.: A quantitative ultrastructural study of the pleomorphic adenoma (mixed tumor) of human minor salivary glands. Cancer, 34:1631, 1974.

Conley, J., and Dingman, D. L.: Adenoid cystic carcinoma in the head and neck (cylindroma). Arch. Otolaryngol., 100:81, 1974.

Corio, R. L., Sciubba, J. J., Brannon, R. B., and Batsakis, J. G.: Epithelial-myoepithelial carcinoma of intercalated duct origin. A clinicopathologic and ultrastructural assessment of sixteen cases. Oral Surg., 53:280, 1982.

Cossman, J., Deegan, M. J., and Batsakis, J. G.: Warthin tumor. B-lymphocytes within the lymphoid infiltrates. Arch. Pathol. Lab. Med., 101:354, 1977.

Cummings, N. A. (mod.): Sjögren's syndrome: newer aspects of research, diagnosis and therapy. Ann. Intern. Med., 75:937, 1971.

Dardick, I., van Nostrand, P., and Phillips, M. J.: Histogenesis of salivary gland pleomorphic adenoma (mixed tumor) with an evaluation of the role of the myoepithelial cell. Hum. Pathol., 13:62, 1982.

Drummond, J. F., Giansanti, J. S., Sabes, W. R., and Smith, C. R.: Sialadenoma papilliferum of the oral cavity. Oral Surg., 45:72, 1978.

Dunlap, C. L., and Barker, B. F.: Necrotizing sialometaplasia. Oral Surg., 37:722, 1974.

Echevarria, R. A.: Ultrastructure of the acinic cell carcinoma and clear cell carcinoma of the parotid gland. Cancer, 20:563, 1967.

Evans, R. W., and Cruickshank, A. H.: Epithelial Tumors of the Salivary Glands. Philadelphia, W. B. Saunders Company, 1970.

Eversole, L. R.: Histogenic classification of salivary tumors. Arch. Pathol., 92:433, 1971.

Fantasia, J. E., and Miller, A. S.: Papillary cystadenoma lymphomatosum arising in minor salivary glands. Oral Surg., 52:411, 1981.

Fantasia, J. E., and Neville, B. W.: Basal cell adenomas of the minor salivary glands. A clinicopathologic study of seventeen new cases and a review of the literature. Oral Surg., 50:433, 1980.

Foote, F. W., Jr., and Frazell, E. L.: Tumors of the major salivary glands. Cancer, 6:1065, 1953.

Freedman, P. D., and Lumerman, H.: Sialadenoma papilliferum. Oral Surg., 45:88, 1978.

Friedman, M., and Hall, J. W.: Radiation-induced squamous metaplasia and hyperplasia of the normal mucous glands of the oral cavity. Radiology, 55:848, 1950.

Gardner, D. G., Bell, M. E. A., Wesley, R. K., and Wysocki, G. P.: Acinic cell tumors of minor salivary glands. Oral Surg., 50:545, 1980.

Gerughty, R. M., Hennigar, G. R., and Brown, F. M.: Adenosquamous carcinoma of the nasal, oral and laryngeal cavities. A clinicopathologic survey of ten cases. Cancer, 22:1140, 1968.

Gerughty, R. M., Scofield, H. H., Brown, F. M., and Hennigar, G. R.: Malignant mixed tumors of salivary gland origin. Cancer, 24:471, 1969.

Godwin, J. T.: Benign lymphoepithelial lesion of the parotid gland (adenolymphoma, chronic inflammation, lymphoepithelioma, lymphocytic tumor, Mikulicz disease): report of eleven cases. Cancer, 5:1089, 1952.

Godwin, J. T., Foote, F. W., Jr., and Frazell, E. L.: Acinic cell adenocarcinoma of the parotid gland: report of twenty-seven cases. Am. J. Pathol., 30:465, 1954.

Gray, S. R., Cornog, J. L., Jr., and Seo, I. S.: Oncocytic

neoplasms of salivary glands. A report of fifteen cases including two malignant oncocytomas. Cancer, 38:1306, 1976.

Greenspan, J. S., Daniels, T. E., Talal, N., and Sylvester, R. A.: The histopathology of Sjögren's syndrome in labial salivary gland biopsies. Oral Surg., 37:217, 1974.

Healey, W. V., Perzin, K. H., and Smith, L.: Mucoepidermoid carcinoma of salivary gland origin. Classification, clinical-pathologic correlation, and results of treatment. Cancer, 26:368, 1970.

Hsu, S.-M., Hsu, P.-L., and Nayak, R. N.: Warthin's tumor: an immunohistochemical study of its lymphoid stroma. Hum. Pathol., 12:251, 1981.

Hübner, G., Klein, H. J., and Schiefer, H. G.: Role of myoepithelial cells in the development of salivary gland tumors. Cancer, 27:1255, 1971.

Hyman, G. A., and Wolff, M.: Malignant lymphomas of the salivary glands. Review of the literature and report of 33 new cases, including four cases associated with the lymphoepithelial lesion. Am. J. Clin. Pathol., 65:421, 1976.

Jao, W., Keh, P. C., and Swerdlow, M. A.: Ultrastructure of the basal cell adenoma of parotid gland. Cancer, 37:1322, 1976.

Johns, M. E., Regezi, J. A., and Batsakis, J. G.: Oncocytic neoplasms of salivary glands: an ultrastructural study. Laryngoscope, 87:862, 1977.

Kay, S., and Still, W. J. S.: Electron microscopic observations on a parotid oncocytoma. Arch. Pathol., 96:186, 1973.

Kessler, H. S.: A laboratory model for Sjögren's syndrome. Am. J. Pathol., 52:671, 1968.

Krolls, S. O., and Boyers, R. C.: Mixed tumors of salivary glands. Long-term follow-up. Cancer, 30:276, 1972.

Krolls, S. O., and Hicks, J. L.: Mixed tumors of the lower lip. Oral Surg., 35:212, 1973.

Krolls, S. O., Trodahl, J. N., and Boyers, R. C.: Salivary gland lesions in children. A survey of 430 cases. Cancer, 30:459, 1972.

Lapes, M., Antoniades, K., Gartner, W., Jr., and Vivacqua, R.: Conversion of a benign lymphoepithelial salivary gland lesion to lymphocytic lymphoma during Dilantin therapy. Correlation with Dilantin-induced lymphocyte transformation in vitro. Cancer, 38:1318, 1976.

Lee, S. C., and Roth, L. M.: Malignant oncocytoma of the parotid gland. A light and electron microscopic study. Cancer, 37:1607, 1976.

Little, J. W.: The histogenesis of papillary cystadenoma lymphomatosum. Oral Surg., 22:72, 1966.

LiVolsi, V. A., and Perzin, K. H.: Malignant mixed tumors arising in salivary glands. I. Carcinomas arising in benign mixed tumors: a clinicopathologic study. Cancer, 39:2209, 1977.

Lomax-Smith, J. D., and Azzopardi, J. G.: The hyaline cell: a distinctive feature of "mixed" salivary tumours. Histopathology, 2:77, 1978.

Luna, M. A., Mackay, B., and Gamez-Araujo, J.: Myoepithelioma of the palate. Report of a case with histochemical and electron microscopic observations. Cancer, 32:1429, 1973.

Lynch, D. P., Crago, C. A., and Martinez, M. G., Jr.: Necrotizing sialometaplasia. A review of the literature and report of two additional cases. Oral Surg., 47:63, 1979.

Mader, C. L., and Nelson, J. F.: Monomorphic adenoma of the minor salivary glands. J. Am. Dent. Assoc., 102:657, 1981.

Martinez-Mora, J., Boix-Ochoa, J., and Tresserra, L.: Vascular tumors of the parotid region in children. Surg. Gynecol. Obstet., 133:973, 1971.

McGavran, M. H., Bauer, W. C., and Ackerman, L. V.: Sebaceous lymphadenoma of the parotid salivary gland. Cancer, 13:1185, 1960.

Melrose, R. J., Abrams, A. M., and Howell, F. V.: Mucoepidermoid tumors of the intraoral minor salivary glands: a clinicopathologic study of 54 cases. J. Oral Pathol., 2:314, 1973.

Miller, A. S., and McCrea, M. W.: Sebaceous gland adenoma of buccal mucosa. J. Oral Surg., 26:593, 1968.

Miller, A. S., and Winnick, M.: Salivary gland inclusion in the anterior mandible. Oral Surg., 31:790, 1971.

Mintz, G. A., Abrams, A. M., and Melrose, R. J.: Monomorphic adenomas of the major and minor salivary glands. Oral Surg., 53:375, 1982.

Morgan, W. S., and Castleman, B.: A clinicopathologic study of "Mikulicz's disease." Am. J. Path., 29:471, 1953.

Moutsopoulos, H. M. (mod.): Sjögren's syndrome (sicca syndrome): current issues. Ann. Intern. Med., 92:212, 1980.

Naeim, F., Forsberg, M. I., Jr., Waisman, J., and Coulson, W. F.: Mixed tumors of the salivary glands. Growth pattern and recurrence. Arch. Pathol. Lab. Med., 100:271, 1976.

Nagao, K., Matsuzaki, O., Saiga, H., Sugano, I., Shigematsu, H., Kaneko, T., Katoh, T., and Kitamura, T.: Histopathologic studies on carcinoma in pleomorphic adenoma of the parotid gland. Cancer, 48:113, 1981.

Nelson, J. F., and Jacoway, J. R.: Monomorphic adenoma (canalicular type). Report of 29 cases. Cancer, 31:1511, 1973.

Perzin, K. H., Gullane, P., and Clairmont, A. C.: Adenoid cystic carcinomas arising in salivary glands. A correlation of histologic features and clinical course. Cancer, 42:265, 1978.

Perzin, K. H., and LiVolsi, V.: Acinic cell carcinomas arising in salivary glands. A clinicopathologic study. Cancer, 44:1434, 1979.

Regezi, J. A., and Batsakis, J. G.: Histogenesis of salivary gland neoplasms. Otolaryngol. Clin. North Am., 10:297, 1977.

Rice, D. H., Batsakis, J. G., and McClatchey, K. D.: Postirradiation malignant salivary gland tumor. Arch. Otolaryngol., 102:699, 1976.

Rye, L. A., Calhoun, N. R., and Redman, R. S.: Necrotizing sialometaplasia in a patient with Buerger's disease and Raynaud's phenomenon. Oral Surg., 49:233, 1980.

Saksela, E., Tarkkanen, J., and Wartiovaara, J.: Parotid clear-cell adenoma of possible myoepithelial origin. Cancer, 30:742, 1972.

Schall, G. L., Anderson, L. G., Wolf, R. O., Herdt, J. R., Tarpley, T. M., Jr., Cummings, N. A., Zeiger, L. S., and Talal, N.: Xerostomia in Sjögren's syndrome. Evaluation by sequential salivary scintigraphy. J.A.M.A., 216:2109, 1971.

Schwartz, I. S., and Feldman, M.: Diffuse multinodular oncocytoma ("oncocytosis") of the parotid gland. Cancer, 23:636, 1969.

Sciubba, J. J., and Brannon, R. B.: Myoepithelioma of salivary glands: report of 23 cases. Cancer, 49:562, 1982.

Silverglade, L. B., Alvares, O. F., and Olech, E.: Central mucoepidermoid tumors of the jaws. Cancer, 22:650, 1968.

Sjögren, H.: Some problems concerning keratoconjunctivitis sicca and the sicca-syndrome. Acta Opthalmol., 29:33, 1951.

Smith, R. L., Dahlin, D. C., and Waite, D. E.: Mucoepidermoid carcinomas of the jawbones. J. Oral Surg., 26:387, 1968.

Som, P. M., Shugar, J. M. A., Train, J. S., and Biller, H. F.: Manifestations of parotid gland enlargement: radiographic, pathologic, and clinical correlations. Part I. The autoimmune pseudosialectasias. Radiology, 141:415, 1981.

Spiro, R. H., Huvos, A. G., and Strong, E. W.: Acinic cell carcinoma of salivary origin. A clinicopathologic study of 67 cases. Cancer, 41:924, 1978.

Spiro, R. H., Huvos, A. G., Berk, R., and Strong, E. W.: Mucoepidermoid carcinoma of salivary gland origin. A clinicopathologic study of 367 cases. Am. J. Surg., 136:461, 1978.

Spiro, R. H., Koss, L. G., Hajdu, S. I., and Strong, E. W.: Tumors of minor salivary origin. A clinicopathologic study of 492 cases. Cancer 31:117, 1973.

Standish, S. M.: Early histologic changes in induced tumors of the submaxillary salivary glands of the rat. Am. J. Pathol., 33:671, 1957.

Standish, S. M., and Shafer, W. G.: Serial histologic effects of rat submaxillary and sublingual salivary gland duct and blood vessel ligation. J. Dent. Res. 36:866, 1957.

Stewart, F. W., Foote, F. W., and Becker, W. F.: Mucoepidermoid tumors of salivary glands. Ann. Surg., 122:820, 1945.

Tandler, B.: Warthin's tumor. Arch. Otolaryngol., 84:68, 1966.

Tandler, B., Hutter, R. V. P., and Erlandson, R. A.: Ultrastructure of oncocytoma of the parotid gland. Lab. Invest., 23:567, 1970.

Tarpley, T. M., Jr., and Giansanti, J. S.: Adenoid cystic carcinoma. Oral Surg., 41:484, 1976.

Tarpley, T. M., Jr., Anderson, L. G., and White, C. L.: Minor salivary gland involvement in Sjögren's syndrome. Oral Surg., 37:64, 1974.

Thackray, A. C., and Lucas, R. B.: Tumors of the Major Salivary Glands. Fascicle 10, Second Series. Washington, D.C., Armed Forces Institute of Pathology, 1974.

Thackray, A. C., and Sobin, L. H.: Histological Typing of Salivary Gland Tumours. Geneva, World Health Organization, 1972.

Vellios, F., and Davidson, D.: The natural history of tumors peculiar to the salivary glands. Am. J. Clin. Pathol., 25:147, 1955.

Vellios, F., and Shafer, W. G.: Tumors of the intraoral accessory salivary glands. Surg., Gynecol. Obstet., 108:450, 1959.

Warthin, A. S.: Papillary cystadenoma lymphomatosum: a rare teratoid of the parotid region. J. Cancer Res., 13:116, 1929.

White, D. K., Miller, A. S., McDaniel, R. K., and Rothman, B. N.: Inverted ductal papilloma: a distinctive lesion of minor salivary gland. Cancer, 49:519, 1982.

CHAPTER 4

Cysts and Tumors of Odontogenic Origin

Tumors derived from the odontogenic tissues constitute an unusually diverse group of lesions. This multiformity reflects the complex development of the dental structures, since these tumors all originate through some aberration from the normal pattern of odontogenesis. An understanding of the pathogenesis of the odontogenic tumors is predicated upon an understanding of the histogenesis of the tooth.

Certain of the lesions discussed here represent only minor alterations in odontogenesis and not true neoplasms. The odontogenic cysts are included here because they too represent an aberration at some stage of odontogenesis and, in fact, may be intimately associated with the development of certain of the odontogenic tumors. All of the various lesions are grouped here because of their common origin from a uniquely specialized group of tissues, and their classification is based upon this origin from the various germ layers.

The World Health Organization (WHO) established an International Reference Center for the Histological Definition and Classification of Odontogenic Tumors, Jaw Cysts and Allied Lesions at Copenhagen in 1966. This was chiefly in recognition of the complexity of this group of tumors and in an attempt to achieve international cooperation in discussion and dissemination of knowledge and ideas. Some of the concepts and principles included in this chapter derive from or were crystallized by the meetings and deliberations of this group, whose work culminated in the monograph of the WHO International Histological Classification of Tumours Series dealing with these odontogenic tumors, cysts and related lesions, by Pindborg, Kramer and Torloni (1971).

ODONTOGENIC CYSTS

The odontogenic cysts are derived from epithelium associated with the development of the dental apparatus. Since several types of these cysts may occur, dependent chiefly upon the stage of odontogenesis during which they originate, various investigators have attempted to devise a classification and system of nomenclature of the lesions. Some of these classifications have not been entirely satisfactory because they generally failed to recognize the mode of origin and development of the cysts and did not unite the views of the oral surgeon, the radiologist and the pathologist. A simple yet practical classification follows:

1. Primordial cyst
2. Dentigerous cyst
   a. Eruption cyst
3. Periodontal cyst
   a. Apical
   b. Lateral
4. Gingival cyst
   a. Newborn (dental lamina cyst)
   b. Adult
5. Odontogenic keratocyst
   a. Basal cell nevus–bifid rib syndrome
6. Calcifying odontogenic cyst

A cyst is defined as a pathologic epithelium-lined cavity usually containing fluid or semisolid material. All odontogenic cysts satisfy these criteria, with the possible exception of the calcifying odontogenic cyst, and, in addition, are often but not always enclosed within bone. The epithelium associated with each of the odontogenic cysts is derived from one of the following sources: (1) a tooth germ, (2) the reduced enamel epithelium of a tooth crown, (3) the epithelial rests of Malassez, remnants of the sheath of Hertwig, (4) remnants of the dental lamina, or (5) possibly the basal layer of oral epithelium.

The diagnosis of any of the odontogenic cysts and their correct identification as to type depend upon microscopic examination of the tissue coupled with close study of the clinical and roentgenographic findings.

Primordial Cyst

The primordial cyst is one of the less common types of odontogenic cyst. It develops through cystic degeneration and liquefaction of the stellate reticulum in an enamel organ before any calcified enamel or dentin has been formed. Thus the primordial cyst is found *in place of* a tooth rather than directly associated with one. It may also originate from a supernumerary tooth organ so that a normal complement of teeth is present in some cases. In a patient who has had several teeth extracted previously, a cyst of the jaw may be found not closely associated with a tooth. This may resemble a primordial cyst and yet actually be a residual cyst of the periodontal type or even of the dentigerous type, and microscopic examination cannot distingush one from the other. These circumstances exemplify the difficulty sometimes involved in establishing the diagnosis of a primordial cyst.

Soskolne and Shear have reviewed a series of 50 primordial cysts from a group of 39 patients, 7 having multiple cysts, and stated that, in addition to the above sources, a primordial cyst may also originate directly from dental lamina. They found that all of their primordial cysts, according to their definition of the lesion, showed keratin or parakeratin formation by the lining epithelium and, therefore, were all odontogenic keratocysts (q.v.). However, in his classical clinicopathologic study of 312 cases of odontogenic keratocyst, Brannon found that only 44 per cent of primordial cysts, according to his definition of this cyst, were odontogenic keratocysts.

This disparity has been explained in part by Forssell and Sainio, who emphasized that the term "primordial cyst" has been used by some persons to indicate a cyst developing from degeneration of the enamel organ, and by others to indicate a cyst developing from an odontogenic primordium, the dental lamina. Because the latter cyst is almost invariably characterized by those histologic features that are pathognomonic of the odontogenic keratocyst, the terms primordial cyst (used in the latter sense) and odontogenic keratocyst have come to be used synonymously by some to the confusion of many. The term "primordial cyst" as used here refers to a cyst developing through degeneration of the enamel organ, thus occurring in place of a tooth, and has no histologic connotation regarding keratin formation. The odontogenic keratocyst will be discussed separately (q.v.)

Clinical Features. The primordial cyst varies widely in size but has the potential for expanding bone and displacing adjacent teeth by pressure. It is occasionally associated with a retained, erupted deciduous tooth, and roentgenographic examination will reveal a radiolucent area in place of the underlying normal permanent tooth. The lesion is not painful unless it becomes secondarily infected, and it seldom presents obvious clinical manifestations. This cyst undoubtedly forms early in life, but may not be discovered until much later.

Roentgenographic Features. The primordial cyst appears as a round or ovoid, well-demarcated radiolucent lesion which may show a sclerotic or reactive border and which may be unilocular or multilocular. It may be situated below the roots of teeth, between the roots of adjacent teeth or near the crest of the ridge in place of a congenitally missing tooth, particularly an upper or lower third molar (Fig. 4–1). The propensity for involvement of the third molar has not been satisfactorily explained.

Histologic Features. The microscopic appearance of the primordial cyst is similar to that of some of the other odontogenic cysts. The wall is composed of parallel bundles of collagen fibers, which vary in degree of compactness. It is lined on the inner surface facing the lumen by an intact or interrupted layer of stratified squamous epithelium. In some cases, this epithelium is nonkeratinized and exhibits a very prominent spinous layer with elongated and sometimes confluent rete pegs and a basal layer that is present but not prominent. In other instances, the epithelium may exhibit a surface layer of orthokeratin, while the spinous layer may be relatively thin or of moderate thickness. The basal cell layer is not prominent and is sometimes flattened. In still other cases, the epithelium is covered by a layer of parakeratin and exhibits a typical corrugated appearance, while the remainder of the epithelium is exceptionally uniform in thickness, usually 6 to 10 cells thick, with an extremely prominent basal layer, the cells arranged in a "picket fence" or

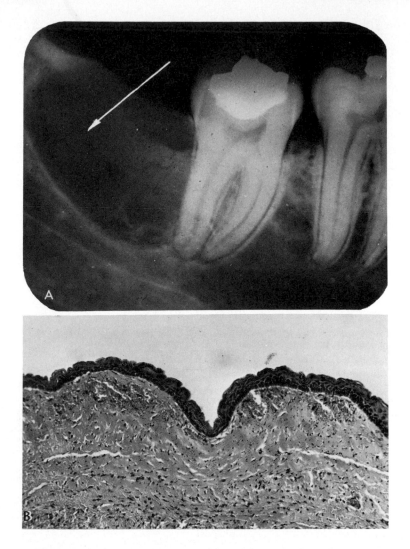

Figure 4–1. *Primordial cyst.*
The roentgenogram (*A*) shows a cystlike lesion in place of the mandibular third molar, which has failed to develop. The photomicrograph (*B*) is taken through the thin wall of the specimen and shows the connective tissue lined by a thin, regular layer of stratified squamous epithelium with the characteristic features of an odontogenic keratocyst, in this particular case.

"tombstone" pattern and showing no rete peg formation. This latter type of lining represents the characteristic odontogenic keratocyst (q.v.) which is apparent in some of these primordial cysts (Fig. 4–1). The presence of chronic inflammatory cells, chiefly lymphocytes and plasma cells, admixed with polymorphonuclear leukocytes in the adjacent subepithelial zone of the connective tissue is a variable finding.

Treatment. The treatment of the primordial cyst consists in its surgical removal with thorough curettage of the bone, particularly if any fragmentation of the lining occurs, to ensure complete removal of the epithelium. The recurrence rate is relatively high if the cyst represents an odontogenic keratocyst (q.v.). Otherwise, the recurrence rate is probably low, although data based on significant series are lacking.

Dentigerous Cyst

(Follicular Cyst)

The dentigerous cyst is a far more common type of odontogenic cyst than the primordial cyst. It originates *after* the crown of the tooth has been completely formed by accumulation of fluid between the reduced enamel epithelium and the tooth crown. If the cyst were to originate *before* tooth crown formation were completed, the result would be either a primordial cyst or a cyst involving a tooth exhibiting enamel hypoplasia, and such is not the case. An alternative or additional explanation for the pathogenesis of the dentigerous cyst has been that it may originate initially by proliferation and cystic transformation of islands of epithelium in the connective tissue wall of the dental follicle or even outside the follicle and this transformed epithelium then unites with the lining follicular epithelium, forming a solitary cystic cavity around the tooth crown. While conceivable, such an occurrence must be considered unlikely or at least uncommon.

The dentigerous cyst nearly always involves or is associated with the crown of a normal permanent tooth. Seldom is a deciduous tooth involved. The diagnosis is ordinarily easy to establish from the roentgenogram alone, although sometimes this may not be true.

Dachi and Howell have reported that 37 per cent of impacted mandibular third molars and 15 per cent of impacted maxillary third molars roentgenographically showed a circumcoronal radiolucency, and this was large enough to be considered a dentigerous cyst in about 10 per cent of these cases. Their study was based on examination of 3874 routine full-mouth roentgenograms of persons over 20 years of age and, of this series, approximately 17 per cent of the patients had at least one impacted tooth.

Clinical Features. This cyst is always associated initially with the crown of an impacted, embedded or unerupted tooth. A dentigerous cyst may also be found enclosing a complex compound odontoma or involving a supernumerary tooth. The most common sites of this cyst are the mandibular and maxillary third molar and maxillary cuspid areas, since these are the most commonly impacted teeth.

The dentigerous cyst is potentially capable of becoming an aggressive lesion. Expansion of bone with subsequent facial asymmetry, extreme displacement of teeth, severe root resorption of adjacent teeth and pain are all possible sequelae brought about by continued enlargement of the cyst. Cystic involvement of an unerupted mandibular third molar may result in a "hollowing-out" of the entire ramus extending up to the coronoid process and condyle as well as in expansion of the cortical plate due to the pressure exerted by the lesion. Associated with this reaction may be displacement of the third molar to such an extent that it sometimes comes to lie compressed against the inferior border of the mandible. In the case of a cyst associated with a maxillary cuspid, expansion of the anterior maxilla often occurs and may superficially resemble an acute sinusitis or cellulitis.

A specific type of cyst which must be classified as a form of dentigerous cyst is frequently associated with erupting deciduous or permanent teeth in children. This cyst has often been termed an *"eruption cyst"* or "eruption hema-

toma." It is essentially a dilatation of the normal follicular space about the crown of the erupting tooth caused by the accumulation of tissue fluid or blood. Seward has reported that this is a relatively common lesion, since she found such a cyst occurring in 11 per cent of infants during eruption of the incisors and in 30 per cent of infants during eruption of the canines and molars. Clinically, the lesion appears as a circumscribed, fluctuant, often translucent swelling of the alveolar ridge over the site of the erupting tooth (Fig. 4–2). When the circumcoronal cystic cavity contains blood, the swelling appears purple or deep blue; hence the term "eruption hematoma." The cause for the development of this form of dentigerous cyst is not known. The cyst often requires no treatment, since the tooth generally erupts into the oral cavity without any significant delay. However, a small portion of tissue overlying the tooth is sometimes removed to facilitate eruption.

Roentgenographic Features. Roentgenographic examination of the jaw involved by a dentigerous cyst will reveal a radiolucent area associated in some fashion with an unerupted tooth crown (Fig. 4–3, A). The impacted or otherwise unerupted tooth crown may be surrounded symmetrically by this radiolucency, although the distinction between a small dentigerous cyst and an enlarged dental follicle or follicular space is quite arbitrary, especially since the small cyst and the enlarged follicle would be histologically identical. Only when the size of the radiolucency is grossly pathologic can the distinction be made with assurance.

In other cases the radiolucent area may appear to project laterally from the tooth crown, particularly if the cyst is relatively large or if there has been displacement of the tooth. The term *lateral dentigerous cyst* is frequently applied to such a situation (Fig. 4–4, A). Still another type is the *circumferential dentigerous cyst*, described by Thoma, in which the cyst surrounds the entire crown of the tooth, without involving the occlusal surface, so that the tooth may erupt through the cyst as "through the hole of a doughnut." This cyst becomes located then around the roots of a normal tooth, similar to an apical periodontal cyst. The *paradental cyst* is a cyst of uncertain pathogenesis, described in detail by Craig, that is thought to be related to the dentigerous cyst, since its epithelial lining appears to originate from reduced enamel epithelium. It arises in relation to a partly erupted vital tooth involved by pericoronitis, usually adjacent to a mandibular third

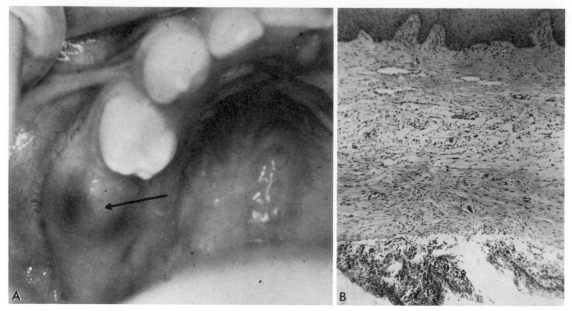

Figure 4–2. *Eruption cyst.*

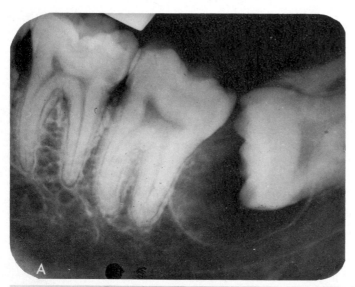

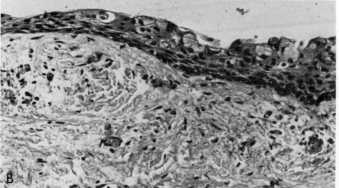

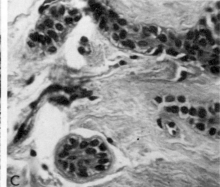

Figure 4–3. *Dentigerous cyst.*
The roentgenogram *(A)* demonstrates a large radiolucent area associated with the crown of the impacted mandibular third molar. The photomicrograph *(B)* shows this cyst to be lined by a thin layer of stratified squamous epithelium similar in appearance to the primordial cyst. Occasional mucus-containing cells are present in the epithelium. Small islands of odontogenic epithelium *(C)* are often present in the connective tissue wall.

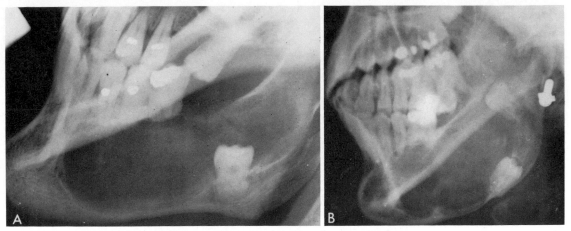

Figure 4–4. *Dentigerous cyst.*
The lesion in both cases had displaced the associated tooth and caused destruction of bone.

molar which has an anomalous enamel projection extending from the cemento-enamel junction into the buccal bifurcation.

The dentigerous cyst is usually a smooth, unilocular lesion, but occasionally one with a multilocular appearance may occur. In actuality, the various compartments are all united by the continuous cystic membrane. Sometimes the radiolucent area is surrounded by a thin sclerotic line representing bony reaction. In cases of apparently multiple dentigerous cysts, care should be taken to rule out the possible occurrence of the odontogenic keratocyst-basal cell nevus-bifid rib syndrome (q.v.)

Histologic Features. There are no characteristic microscopic features which can be used reliably to distinguish the dentigerous cyst from the other types of odontogenic cysts. It is usually composed of a thin connective tissue wall with a thin layer of stratified squamous epithelium lining the lumen (Fig. 4–3, *B*). Rete peg formation is generally absent except in cases that are secondarily infected. The connective tissue wall is frequently quite thickened and composed of a very loose fibrous connective tissue or of a sparsely collagenized myxomatous tissue, each of which has been sometimes mistakenly diagnosed as either an odontogenic fibroma or an odontogenic myxoma. A hyperplastic dental follicle is not necessarily associated with inflammation. An additional feature of the connective tissue walls of both normal dental follicles and dentigerous cysts is the presence of varying numbers of islands of odontogenic epithelium (Fig. 4–3, *C*). These are sometime very sparse and obviously inactive, while at other times they are present in sufficient numbers to be mistaken for an ameloblas-

toma. While this latter odontogenic tumor can originate in this situation, care must be taken to differentiate between it and simply odontogenic epithelial rests. Inflammatory cell infiltration of the connective tissue is common although the cause for this is not always apparent. An additional finding, especially in cysts which exhibit inflammation, is the presence of Rushton bodies within the lining epithelium. These are peculiar linear, often curved, hyaline bodies with variable stainability which are of uncertain origin, questionable nature and unknown significance. Even electron microscope studies, such as those of El-Labban, have only been of partial help in determining that the structures are probably of hematogenous origin, although it is not clear why they have such an intimate relationship to epithelium. The content of the cyst lumen is usually a thin, watery yellow fluid, occasionally blood tinged.

It was reported by Brannon in his excellent clinicopathologic study of 312 cases of odontogenic keratocysts that 8.5 per cent of a series of 1850 dentigerous cysts were odontogenic keratocysts (q.v.) with the characteristic histologic findings in the epithelium of a parakeratinized, corrugated surface, a remarkable uniformity of a 6- to 10-cell thickness without rete peg formation, and a polarized and palisaded basal layer of cells. This percentage of dentigerous cysts which are odontogenic keratocysts is in close agreement with the findings of Pindborg and his co-workers (7.1 per cent) and Payne (8.5 per cent).

The pluripotentialities of the epithelium in mandibular dentigerous cysts has been further emphasized by Gorlin, who described mucus-secreting cells in the lining stratified squamous

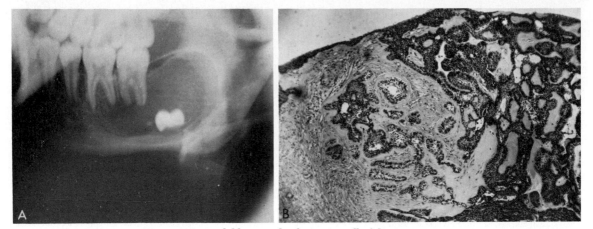

Figure 4–5. *Ameloblastoma developing in wall of dentigerous cyst.*

epithelium, respiratory epithelial lining, sebaceous cells in the connective tissue wall, and lymphoid follicles with germinal centers.

Treatment. The treatment of the dentigerous cyst is usually dictated by the size of the lesion. Smaller lesions can be surgically removed in their entirety with little difficulty. The larger cysts which involve serious loss of bone and thin the bone dangerously are often treated by insertion of a surgical drain or marsupialization. This procedure results in relief of pressure and the gradual shrinking of the cystic space by peripheral apposition of new bone. Such a procedure is often necessary because of the potential danger of fracturing the jaw if complete surgical removal were attempted.

Recurrence is relatively uncommon unless there has been fragmentation of the cyst lining with remnants allowed to remain. If the lesion is a keratocyst the possibility of recurrence is remarkably increased.

Potential Complications. Several relatively serious potential complications exist stemming from the dentigerous cyst, besides simply the possibility of recurrence following incomplete surgical removal. These include: (1) the development of an ameloblastoma either from the lining epithelium or from rests of odontogenic epithelium in the wall of the cyst; (2) the development of epidermoid carcinoma from the same two sources of epithelium; and (3) the development of a mucoepidermoid carcinoma, basically a malignant salivary gland tumor, from the lining epithelium of the dentigerous cyst which contains mucus-secreting cells, or at least cells with this potential, most commonly seen in dentigerous cysts associated with impacted mandibular third molars.

It is of great clinical significance that numerous cases of ameloblastoma have been reported developing in the wall of dentigerous cysts from the lining epithelium or associated epithelial rests (Fig. 4–5). Stanley and Diehl have reviewed a series of 641 cases of ameloblastoma and have found that at least 108 cases of this neoplasm, approximately 17 per cent, were definitely associated with an impacted tooth and/or a follicular or dentigerous cyst. The disposition for neoplastic epithelial proliferation in the form of an ameloblastoma is far more pronounced in the dentigerous cyst than in the other odontogenic cysts. The formation of such a tumor manifests itself as a nodular thickening in the cyst wall, the mural ameloblastoma, but this is seldom obvious clinically. Therefore, it is not only good clinical practice, but also an absolute requisite that all tissue from dentigerous cysts be submitted to a qualified oral pathologist for thorough gross and microscopic examination. In reviewing the histologic changes sought by the oral pathologist which occur in the dentigerous cyst as a premonitory manifestation of ameloblastoma, Vickers and Gorlin have stressed that hyperchromatism of basal cell nuclei, palisading with polarization of basal cells and cytoplasmic vacuolization with intercellular spacing of the lining epithelium, *when observed together*, are manifestations of impending neoplasia. These findings may occur *individually* in other rather harmless conditions. The presence of sprouting or budding and protruding of epithelial islands from lining epithelium has been claimed to be evidence of neoplastic transformation, but this in itself was not considered such an indication by Vickers and Gorlin.

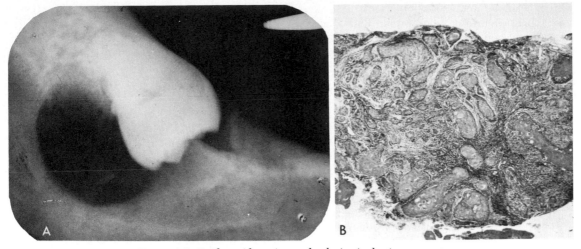

Figure 4–6. *Epidermoid carcinoma developing in dentigerous cyst.*

The development of epidermoid carcinoma from the lining epithelium of the dentigerous cyst also has been adequately documented in the literature reviewed by Gardner, who reported 8 acceptable cases among 25 cases of carcinoma developing in odontogenic cysts of all types combined. Browne and Gough have reported two additional cases of malignant transformation in dental cysts and suggested that keratin metaplasia in long-standing cyst lining appears to precede the development of the carcinomatous change, although there is little evidence that the odontogenic keratocyst is associated with malignant change more commonly than other types of odontogenic cysts. The predisposing factors and mechanism of development of this malignancy are unknown, but its occurrence appears unequivocal (Fig. 4–6, A, B).

Finally, the development of a mucoepidermoid carcinoma, a type of salivary gland tumor, is less well documented than the epidermoid carcinoma of this origin, but it also appears to be a potentiality. The inclusion of normal salivary gland tissue in the posterior portion of the body of the mandible has been reported and, undoubtedly, some central salivary gland tumors in this location originate from this source. However, cases of central mucoepidermoid carcinoma (q.v.) have been discovered in association with dentigerous cysts involving impacted mandibular third molars and, considering the frequency with which mucus-secreting cells are found in this lining epithelium indicative of the pluripotentiality of this epithelium, this very distinct possibility must always be considered.

Apical Periodontal Cyst

(Radicular Cyst; Periapical Cyst; Dental Root End Cyst; Etc.)

The apical periodontal cyst is the most common of the odontogenic cysts. In contrast to the other types of cysts, it involves the apex of an erupted tooth and is most frequently a result of infection via the pulp chamber and root canal through carious involvement of the tooth. The term "residual cyst" is frequently applied to a periodontal cyst which remains after or develops subsequent to extraction of a tooth, although this same term can be applied to any cyst of the jaw which remains following a surgical procedure.

The epithelial lining of the apical periodontal cyst is derived from the epithelial rests of Malassez in the periodontal ligament and does not seem to exhibit the tendency for ameloblastomatous transformation that occurs in the dentigerous cyst. Since the apical periodontal cyst is most commonly a sequela of a carious tooth, detailed discussion of this lesion will be deferred to the section on diseases of the periapical tissues. In addition to the apical periodontal cyst occurring at the apex of a tooth, a lateral periodontal cyst developing in the lateral periodontal ligament is recognized.

Lateral Periodontal Cyst

The lateral periodontal cyst is an uncommon but well-recognized type of developmental odontogenic cyst. The various theories concerning the etiology and pathogenesis of the lesion have been reviewed by Standish and Shafer. These cysts appear to arise in intimate association with the lateral root surface of an erupted tooth, with a predilection for the mandibular bicuspid area. The possibilities which have been offered to explain their origin and mode of development include: (1) origin initially as a dentigerous cyst developing along the lateral surface of the crown and, as the tooth erupts, the cyst assumes a position in approximation to the lateral surface of the root; (2) origin from proliferation of rests of Malassez in the periodontal ligament although the stimulus for this proliferation is unknown; (3) origin simply as a primordial cyst of a supernumerary tooth germ, since the predilection for occurrence of the lateral periodontal cyst in the mandibular bicuspid area corresponds well with the known high incidence of supernumerary teeth in this same region; and (4) origin from proliferation and cystic transformation of rests of dental lamina, which are in a post-functional state and therefore have only a limited growth potential that is in accordance with the usual small size of these cysts.

This latter theory, including the suggestion that the lateral periodontal cyst and the gingival cyst of the adult (q.v.) share this common histogenesis from post-functional dental lamina rests and that these two cysts represent basically the central or intraosseous and peripheral or extraosseous manifestations of the same lesion, has been discussed in detail by Wysocki and his colleagues. At present, it seems the most appropriate one. They have also pointed out the important fact that in many reports of the lateral periodontal cyst in the previous literature, the term has been used to designate any cyst that may be positioned against the lateral root surface of a tooth (e.g., lateral radicular cyst related to pulp infection, odontogenic keratocyst, etc.). This positional use of the term should be avoided and the designation applied only to that specific developmental lesion with characteristic features.

An unusual form of cyst was reported in 1973 by Weathers and Waldron under the term *botryoid odontogenic cyst*. They described two cases of cysts which had a multilocular pattern apparent roentgenographically, histologically and even clinically at the time of surgical removal. Additional experience with this cyst, as indicated by Wysocki and his associates, now strongly suggests that this is simply a polycystic variant of the lateral periodontal cyst developing through cystic transformation of multiple islands of dental lamina rests. The epithelial lining in the two cysts is identical, as are its clinical features, including age of predilection and sites of occurrence. In addition, a multilocular extraosseous form analogous to the gingival cyst of the adult also occurs.

Clinical Features. The lateral periodontal cyst occurs chiefly in adults, according to the series of 39 cases reported by Wysocki and his associates in which there was a mean age of 50 years and an age range of 22 to 85 years. In this series, there was a predilection for occurrence in males over females, 67:28 per cent with 5 per cent unknown. The location of the lesion was extremely limited in this study: 67 per cent of cases were in the mandibular bicuspid/cuspid/incisor area, while 33 per cent were in the maxillary lateral incisor area. Lesions were found at no other sites and this has also been the experience of most other investigators. No rational explanation has been offered for this localization.

The majority of cases have presented no clinical signs or symptoms and have been discovered during routine roentgenographic examination of the teeth. Occasionally, when the cyst is located on the labial surface of the root, there may be a slight mass obvious, although the overlying mucosa is normal. Unless otherwise affected, the associated tooth is vital. If the cyst becomes infected, it may resemble a lateral periodontal abscess and even seek to establish drainage.

Roentgenographic Features. The periapical roentgenogram discloses the lateral periodontal cyst as a radiolucent area in apposition to the lateral surface of a tooth root (Fig. 4–7, *A*, *B*, *C*, *D*). The lesion is usually small, seldom over 1 cm. in diameter, and may or may not be well circumscribed. In most cases the border is definitive and is even surrounded sometimes by a thin layer of sclerotic bone. The botryoid odontogenic cyst appears similar except that its polycystic nature is often evident through its multilocular pattern on the roentgenogram (Fig. 4–9).

Histologic Features. The cyst is comprised essentially of a hollow sac with a connective tissue wall lined on the inner surface by a layer of epithelium which may range from a single flat layer of cells to one that is several cells thick, a thin stratified squamous type. Cuboidal or even columnar cells may be found composing the lining. Many of the lining cells have a clear, vacuolated, glycogen-rich cytoplasm (Fig. 4–8).

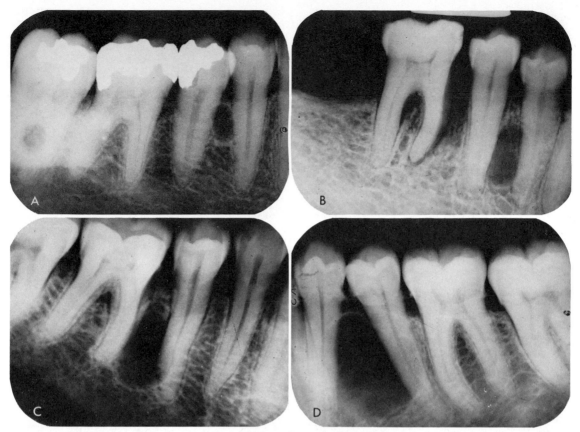

Figure 4–7. *Lateral periodontal cysts.*

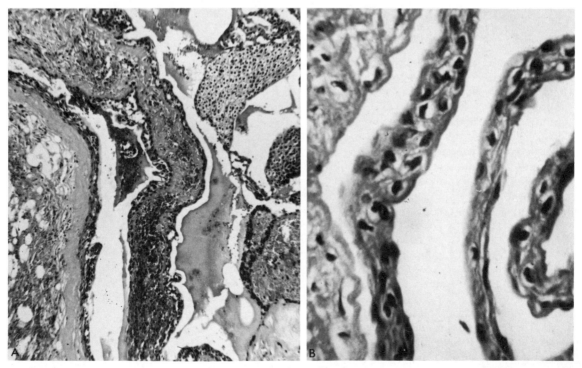

Figure 4–8. *Lateral periodontal cysts.*

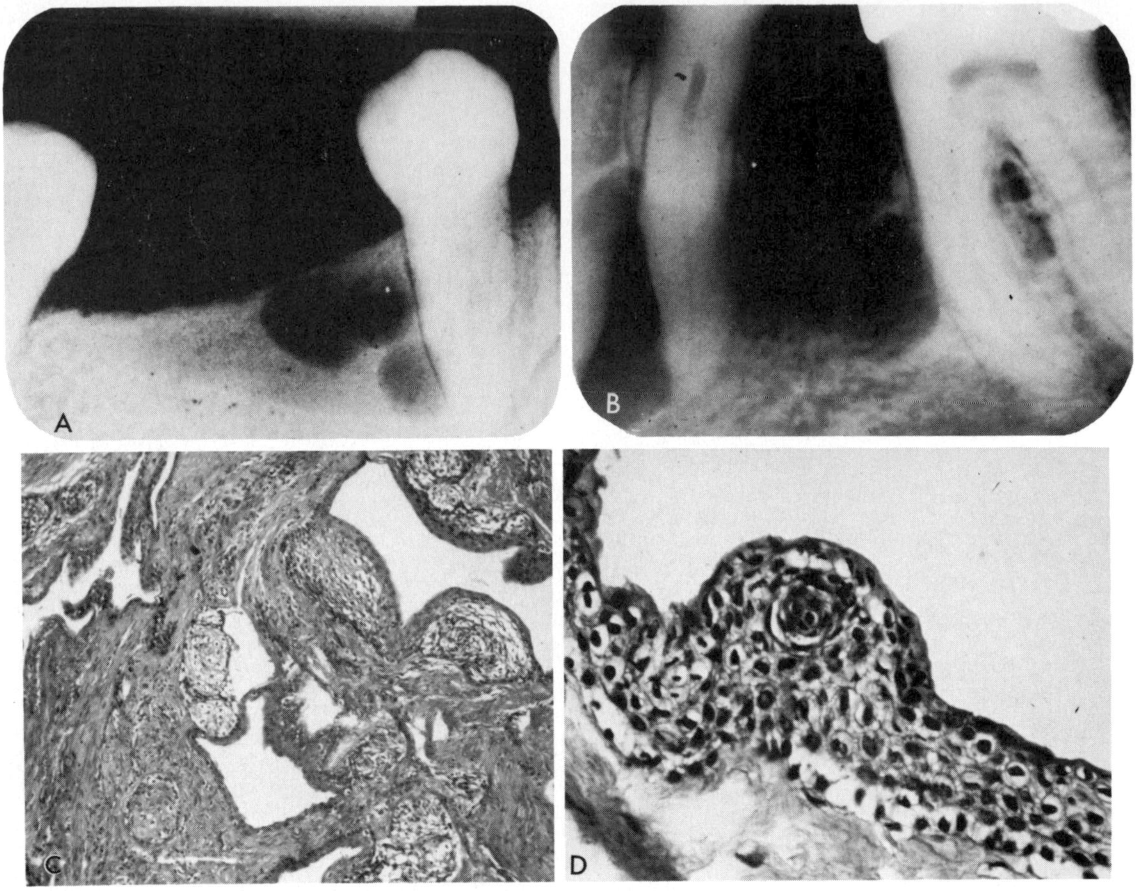

Figure 4–9. *Botryoid odontogenic cysts.*
The multilocular appearance *(A,B)* is indicative of their polycystic nature. The lining epithelium *(C,D)* of the numerous small cysts is thin and shows focal areas of thickening.

Focal thickened plaques of proliferating lining cells often project into the lumen in areas. These are especially prominent in the botryoid odontogenic cyst (Fig. 4–8). Rests of dental lamina are sometimes found in the connective tissue wall and these similarly are frequently composed of glycogen-rich clear cells. These also appear to be more common in the botryoid-type cyst. Papillary infoldings of the lateral periodontal cyst wall are sometimes seen and inflammatory cells may be present, but this is a secondary reaction. The histologic characteristics of these cysts have been detailed by Wysocki and his colleagues as well as by Shear and Pindborg.

Treatment and Prognosis. The lateral periodontal cyst must be surgically removed if at all possible without extracting the associated tooth. If this cannot be accomplished, the tooth must be sacrificed. It is especially important that the diagnosis be established because of the similarity in appearance between this cyst and other

more serious lesions such as an early ameloblastoma. There is no reported tendency for recurrence of this type of cyst following its surgical excision.

Dental Lamina Cyst of the Newborn

(Gingival Cyst of the Newborn; Epstein's Pearls; Bohn's Nodules)

Dental lamina cysts of the newborn are multiple, occasionally solitary, nodules on the alveolar ridge of newborn or very young infants which represent cysts originating from remnants of the dental lamina. The eponyms "Epstein's pearls" and "Bohn's nodules" have both been applied to this odontogenic cyst of dental lamina origin, but incorrectly so. As originally described, Epstein's pearls arc cystic, keratin-filled nodules found along the midpalatine raphe, probably derived from entrapped epithelial remnants along the line of fusion (q.v.).

Bohn's nodules are keratin-filled cysts scattered over the palate, most numerous along the junction of the hard and soft palate and apparently derived from palatal salivary gland structures (q.v.). Discussions of these various types of cysts in the newborn have been published by Fromm and by Cataldo and Berkman.

In studying sections of the maxillae and mandibles of 17 infants, Kreshover reported finding 65 examples of gingival cysts (38 multiple and 27 single). These cysts were localized in the corium below the surface epithelium. Those in the anterior portion of the jaws were usually displaced lingually with respect to the deciduous incisors and cuspids. Those in the posterior portion of the jaw were found occlusal to the crown of the molars. Kreshover stated that in all instances the cystic lesions were seen to arise from cells of the dental lamina. The etiology of these cysts has been thoroughly discussed by Maher and Swindle.

Clinical Features. Occasionally these dental lamina cysts in infants become sufficiently large to be clinically obvious as small discrete white swellings of the alveolar ridge, sometimes appearing blanched as though from internal pressure (Fig. 4–10, A). These probably correspond to those structures described in the older literature as the "predeciduous dentition." These lesions appear to be asymptomatic and do not seem to produce discomfort in the infants.

Histologic Features. These are true cysts with a thin epithelial lining, and show a lumen usually filled with desquamated keratin, occasionally containing inflammatory cells. (Fig. 4–10, B). Interestingly, dystrophic calcification and hyaline bodies of Rushton (q.v.), commonly found in dentigerous cysts, are also sometimes found in this lesion.

Treatment. No treatment is required inasmuch as these lesions almost invariably will disappear by opening onto the surface of the mucosa or through disruption by erupting teeth.

Gingival Cyst of the Adult

The gingival cyst of the adult is an uncommon cyst of gingival soft tissue, occurring in either the free or attached gingiva.

The etiology and pathogenesis of this lesion have been reviewed by Ritchey and Orban, who suggested possible sources of cystic formation as (1) heterotopic glandular tissue, (2) degenerative changes in a proliferating epithelial peg, (3) remnants of the dental lamina, enamel organ or epithelial islands of the periodontal membrane, and (4) traumatic implantation of epithelium. Of these possibilities, only the last two appear valid, and on this basis there do appear to be two recognizable forms of gingival cyst: (1) that arising from cystic transformation of dental lamina or the "glands" or rests of Serres, and (2) that arising from traumatic implantation of surface epithelium (and, therefore, not truly an odontogenic cyst).

The origin of the gingival cyst of the adult has been evaluated by Wysocki and his colleagues, who concluded that it does arise from post-functional rests of dental lamina and thus represents the extraosseous counterpart of the lateral periodontal cyst, with which it shares a common histogenesis. Buchner and Hansen have reported essentially the same conclusions.

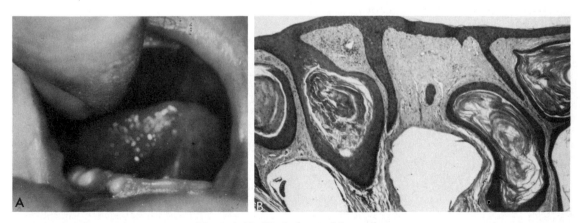

Figure 4–10. *Gingival cyst of the newborn.*
(Courtesy of Drs. Ralph E. McDonald and Alfred Fromm.)

The similarities between the lateral periodontal cyst and the gingival cyst of the adult in clinical behavior, morphologic appearance, anatomic site of occurrence and age predilection are too striking to be coincidental.

The vast majority of these gingival cysts appear to originate in the fashion described from dental lamina, including a soft tissue counterpart of the multilocular botryoid odontogenic cyst. However, an implantation type of cyst can occur lined by a more mature keratinizing stratified squamous epithelium lining derived from surface mucosal epithelium. Finally, as suggested by Buchner and Hansen, there is some evidence that a dental lamina cyst of the newborn may persist into adulthood, as judged by the finding of cysts packed with orthokeratin that appear identical to those in the newborn.

Clinical Features. The gingival cyst may occur at any age but is most common in adults. In the review of the literature by Reeve and Levy, the majority of patients were over 40 years of age. The mean age in the 33 cases reported by Buchner and Hansen was 48 years and that of the 10 cases reported by Wysocki and his associates was 51 years. The location of the lesion closely follows that of the lateral periodontal cyst. Thus, all except one cyst in the series of Wysocki and his coworkers were in the mandibular bicuspid-cuspid incisor area, the one exception being in the maxillary lateral incisor area. The locations in the series of Buchner and Hansen were virtually identical except that they had several cases also in the maxillary arch from cuspid to first molar.

This lesion presents generally as a small, well-circumscribed, painless swelling of the gingiva, sometimes closely resembling a superficial mucocele (Fig. 4–11). The lesion is of the same color as the adjacent normal mucosa and seldom measures over 1 cm. in diameter, generally much less. Although this cyst may occur in either the free or attached gingiva, some gingival cysts occur in the gingival papilla itself.

Roentgenographic Features. The gingival cyst is a soft tissue lesion and does not generally manifest itself on the dental roentgenogram. If it enlarges to sufficient size, it may cause superficial erosion of the cortical plate of bone, but this is still generally not visible on the roentgenogram. If a circumscribed, radiolucent cystic lesion of alveolar bone with some swelling of the soft tissue is present, the cyst probably represents a lateral periodontal cyst rather than a gingival cyst.

Histologic Features. The gingival cyst of the adult is a true cyst, since it is a pathologic epithelium-lined cavity which usually contains fluid (Fig. 4–11, *B*). The lining epithelium is generally identical to that found in the lateral periodontal cyst, with the occasional exceptions noted above. The epithelium ranges in thickness from simply one flattened cell to several cells, a thin stratified squamous epithelium. Glycogen-rich clear cells may be present, especially in the focal thickenings or plaques of the lining. Dental lamina rests may also be found in the connective tissue wall and these are commonly composed of the same type of glycogen-rich clear cells. As noted earlier, these lesions may be unicystic or polycystic. Since the cyst lies free in the connective tissue of the gingiva, it may or may not exhibit an associated inflammatory reaction.

In cases of the traumatic or implantation type of gingival cyst, calcification or even ectopic ossification on rare occasions may be associated with the cystic lesion, reminiscent of the ossification occurring after experimental implantation of bladder epithelium into subcutaneous tissues.

Treatment. Local surgical excision of the lesion in adults is usually recommended, and the lesions do not tend to recur. A neoplastic potential has never been reported.

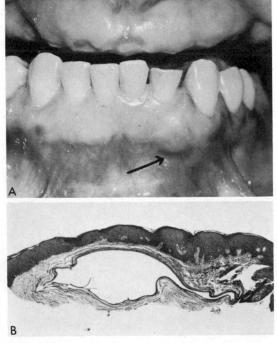

Figure 4–11. *Gingival cyst of the adult.*

Odontogenic Keratocyst

The term "odontogenic keratocyst" was first used by Philipsen in 1956, while Pindborg and Hansen in 1963 described the essential features of this type of cyst. There is general agreement at present that it is a cyst with very well-defined histologic criteria and one which possesses one clinical feature warranting its recognition and separation as a distinctive entity: the exceedingly high recurrence rate.

The term "primordial cyst" has been widely used in the literature synonymously with the term "odontogenic keratocyst." Unfortunately, this has led to much confusion, since not all primordial cysts are odontogenic keratocysts in the original context of a primordial cyst being one developing in place of a tooth through degeneration of an enamel organ. Certainly not all odontogenic keratocysts are primordial cysts in the similar context. This has been discussed at greater length under the section on primordial cysts. As Browne has wisely pointed out, to avoid confusion, usage of the term "primordial cyst" should be restricted to its original sense, and cysts of the nature to be described in this section should be termed "odontogenic keratocysts."

Many different types of cysts may exhibit keratinization of the lining epithelium including nonodontogenic cysts such as the fissural cysts and dermoid-epidermoid cysts. In addition, certain odontogenic cysts may exhibit keratinization, such as the primordial cyst, the dentigerous cyst and, on rare occasions, the apical periodontal cyst. The keratin formed by the lining epithelium may be parakeratin (persisting nuclei) or orthokeratin (absence of nuclei). A stratum granulosum is usually present with orthokeratin but not parakeratin. The spinous layer of cells may be thin or thick and may be of uniform width or variable width with or without rete pegs. The basal layer of cells may have their usual nondistinctive cuboidal shape, be quite flattened or be tall, columnar, and palisading.

Those cysts which are characterized by (1) a parakeratinized surface which is typically corrugated, (2) a remarkable uniformity of thickness of the epithelium, usually ranging from 6 to 10 cells thick, and (3) a prominent palisaded, polarized basal layer of cells often described as having a "picket fence" or "tombstone" appearance are known as odontogenic keratocysts.

The origin of this cyst has not been definitively established, although it is generally accepted by most investigators today to originate from dental lamina which still possess marked growth potential or, alternatively, from proliferation of basal cells as "basal cell hamartias," a residue or remnant of oral epithelium as discussed by Stoelinga and Peters, albeit the stimulus for the cellular proliferation is unknown. The epithelium of the odontogenic keratocyst has been shown to be far more active than that in most other odontogenic cysts as judged by greater mitotic activity, according to both Main and Browne, and by increased thymidine uptake by cyst lining explants indicative of increased DNA synthesis, reported by Toller.

Clinical Features. The largest and most detailed series of cases of odontogenic keratocyst has been published by Brannon, and his data are probably most representative of this lesion. The cyst may occur at any age, from the very young to the very elderly, although Brannon found it to be exceedingly rare under the age of 10 years, there being only 2 such patients in his series of 283 persons. The peak incidence is in the second and third decades of life, with a gradual decline thereafter. The data of Browne (104 patients) and of Forssell (119 patients) are virtually identical. In all series, there is a predilection for occurrence in males, ranging from 1.44:1 (Brannon) and 1.46:1 (Browne) to 1.79:1 (Forssell).

The mandible is invariably affected more frequently than the maxilla: in the series of Brannon, 65 per cent versus 35 per cent, in the series of Browne, 79 per cent versus 21 per cent, and in that of Forssell, 78 per cent versus 22 per cent. In the mandible, the majority of the cysts occur in the ramus–third molar area, followed by the first and second molar area and then the anterior mandible. In the maxilla, the most common site is the third molar area followed by the cuspid region.

Multiple odontogenic keratocysts occur with some frequency. In some instances, these are associated with the jaw cyst-basal cell nevus-bifid rib syndrome (q.v.), which will be discussed subsequently. However, at other times, these multiple cysts are independent of the syndrome. A rather remarkable parallelism between the odontogenic keratocyst and the ameloblastoma with respect to mean age of occurrence, predilection for site of occurrence, roentgenographic findings and recurrence rate has also been pointed out by Browne.

There are no characteristic clinical manifestations of the keratocyst, although about 50 per cent of the patients in Brannon's series were symptomatic prior to seeking treatment. Among the more common features are pain, soft-tissue

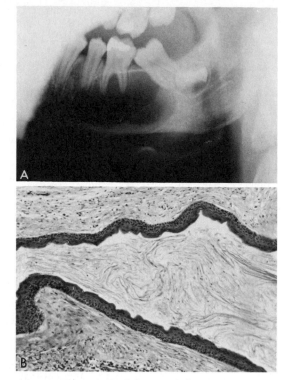

Figure 4–12. *Odontogenic keratocyst.*

swelling and expansion of bone, drainage and various neurologic manifestations such as paresthesia of the lip or teeth.

Roentgenographic Features. The lesion may appear as either a unilocular or multilocular radiolucency, frequently with a thin sclerotic border representing reactive bone (Fig. 4–12). This border may be smooth or scalloped, but is generally sharply demarcated. In the series of Browne, approximately 40 per cent of the cysts appeared to be dentigerous since they were associated with impacted or unerupted teeth. However, in the majority of these cases, the cysts were found at the time of surgery to be separated from the tooth by a layer of fibrous tissue. It is of interest also that in the study of Brannon, approximately 24.4 per cent of cysts originally diagnosed as lateral periodontal cysts and 9.0 per cent of those originally diagnosed as globulomaxillary cysts, each chiefly because of location and roentgenographic appearance, were found histologically to be odontogenic keratocysts. Proximity to the roots of adjacent normal teeth sometimes causes resorption of these roots, although displacement is more common. Sometimes these cysts displace the neurovascular bundle. The roentgenographic

findings in these cysts have been discussed in detail by Smith and Shear and by Forssell.

Histologic Features. The odontogenic keratocyst wall is usually rather thin unless there has been superimposed inflammation. The lining epithelium is highly characteristic, as described previously, and is composed of: (1) a parakeratin surface which is usually corrugated, rippled or wrinkled, (2) a uniformity of thickness of the epithelium, generally between 6 and 10 cells in depth without rete peg formation, and (3) a polarized, palisaded basal layer of cells (Fig. 4–12). Occasionally, orthokeratin is found but, if present, parakeratin is also usually evident. In such cases, a granular layer is not found.

The connective tissue wall often shows small islands of epithelium similar to the lining epithelium; some of these islands may be small cysts. In at least some cases, the apparent islands of epithelium and small satellite or "daughter" cysts actually represent the ends of folds of the lining epithelium of the main cystic cavity which have been cut in cross-section; the linings of these cysts are very commonly folded. Forssell and his associates have studied this problem using serial sections of cysts and found microcysts in the wall in 20 per cent and epithelial islands in 50 per cent of their cases. In 35 per cent of the cases apparent microcysts were found to be part of the main cyst by the serial sections, while pseudoislands of epithelium were found in 75 per cent of the cases.

The lumen of the keratocyst may be filled with a thin straw-colored fluid or with a thicker creamy material. Sometimes the lumen contains a great deal of keratin, while at other times it has little. Cholesterol, as well as hyaline bodies at the sites of inflammation, may also be present. The electrophoretic measurement of fluid from these cysts has been reported by Toller to show that it contains a very low content of soluble protein compared with the patient's own serum.

Dysplastic and neoplastic transformation of the lining epithelium in the odontogenic keratocyst is an uncommon occurrence but has been reported. Of the 312 keratocysts studied by Brannon, only two exhibited cellular atypia. Occasional other cases have also been described in the literature. Areen and his associates have recently reported a case of epidermoid carcinoma developing in an odontogenic keratocyst and, in reviewing the literature, have emphasized the necessity for careful microscopic examination of all such cysts.

Finally, the highly characteristic nature of

the parakeratinized lining epithelium and its relationship to the high recurrence rate have been emphasized by a report dealing with orthokeratinized odontogenic cysts and their recurrence rate. Wright investigated 59 cases of orthokeratinized odontogenic cysts and found they showed a predilection for occurrence in males, most commonly in the second to fifth decade. These cysts were located predominantly in the posterior mandible, where they most typically appeared as dentigerous cysts. The thin, uniform lining epithelium was covered with orthokeratin and showed a prominent granular layer and a cuboidal to flattened basal layer. Follow-up of 24 of these patients revealed only one case of recurrence. This difference in biologic behavior would further underscore the necessity for very strict application of the definition of the term odontogenic keratocyst in diagnosis of the lesion.

Treatment and Prognosis. The odontogenic keratocyst should be surgically excised. However, clinical experience has shown that complete eradication of the cyst may be difficult because the wall of the cyst is very thin and friable and may easily fragment. In addition, perforation of cortical bone, particularly in lesions involving the ramus, is common and this complicates total removal.

The most important feature of the odontogenic keratocyst is its extraordinary recurrence rate. This has been reported as being between 13 and 60 per cent. A review of 763 cases of odontogenic keratocysts in 13 different reported series of cases has shown the average recurrence rate to be 26 per cent, with the majority occurring within five years of the surgical procedure. Browne found no significant differences in recurrence rate following three basic methods of treating the lesions: (1) marsupialization, (2) enucleation and primary closure, and (3) enucleation and packing open. Furthermore, recurrence does not appear related to the presence of satellite cysts. On this basis, Browne concluded that recurrence of the keratocyst is due to the nature of the lesion itself, i.e., the presence of additional remnants of dental lamina from which a cyst may develop, and is not related to its method of treatment. Since recurrence may be long delayed in this lesion, follow-up of any case of odontogenic keratocyst with annual roentgenograms is essential for at least five years after surgery. It is also essential that patients with an odontogenic keratocyst, especially if multiple, be evaluated medically to rule out the possibility of the jaw cyst-basal cell nevus-bifid rib syndrome (q.v.).

Jaw Cyst-Basal Cell Nevus-Bifid Rib Syndrome

(Basal Cell Nevus Syndrome; Hereditary Cutaneomandibular Polyoncosis; Gorlin and Goltz Syndrome)

This syndrome, first described by Binkley and Johnson in 1951, has been thoroughly reviewed by Gorlin and his co-workers. A hereditary condition, it is transmitted as an autosomal dominant trait, with high penetrance and variable expressivity.

Clinical Features. The syndrome is very complex and includes a great variety of possible abnormalities. These may be briefly summarized as follows: (1) *cutaneous anomalies,* including basal cell carcinoma, other benign dermal cysts and tumors, palmar pitting, palmar and plantar keratosis and dermal calcinosis; (2) *dental and osseous anomalies,* including odontogenic keratocysts (often multiple), mild mandibular prognathism, rib anomalies (often bifid), vertebral anomalies and brachymetacarpalism; (3) *ophthalmologic abnormalities,* including hypertelorism with wide nasal bridge, dystopia canthorum, congenital blindness and internal strabismus; (4) *neurologic anomalies,* including mental retardation, dural calcification, agenesis of corpus callosum, congenital hydrocephalus and occurrence of medulloblastomas with greater than normal frequency; and (5) *sexual abnormalities,* including hypogonadism in males and ovarian tumors.

Some of these patients have shown a lack of response to parathormone as judged by the lack of phosphate diuresis which, coupled with shortened fourth metacarpals in some patients, has suggested that there may be some relationship to pseudohypoparathyroidism.

Oral Manifestations. The odontogenic keratocysts are indistinguishable from those previously described by that term which are not associated with this syndrome (Fig. 4–13). Because they often develop early in life, deformity and displacement of developing teeth may occur. However, they may not develop until middle age even though the basal cell skin tumors have occurred early in life.

Treatment and Prognosis. The recurrence rate of the keratocysts associated with this syndrome appears to be as high as that of the unassociated keratocyst. In addition, several cases of ameloblastoma have developed in cysts of this syndrome, thus emphasizing the importance of surgical removal of the cysts and their histologic examination. Whenever a diagnosis of odontogenic keratocyst is received by the

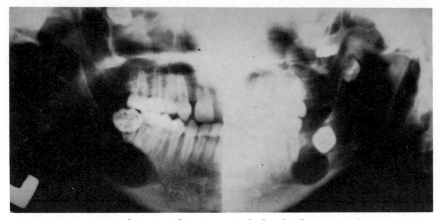

Figure 4–13. Odontogenic keratocysts in the basal cell nevus syndrome.

dentist, he must be certain to rule out the presence of this syndrome because of the many associated problems which these patients ultimately will face.

Calcifying Odontogenic Cyst

(Keratinizing and/or Calcifying Epithelial Odontogenic Cyst; Gorlin Cyst; Cystic Keratinizing Tumor)

A unique odontogenic lesion was first described in 1962 by Gorlin and his co-workers under the term "calcifying epithelial odontogenic cyst." The lesion is unusual in that it has some features of a cyst but also has many characteristics of a solid neoplasm. Prior to the separation of this lesion as an entity, it had often been misdiagnosed as some form of an ameloblastoma.

There has been a complete re-evaluation of the calcifying odontogenic cyst recently by Praetorius, Hjørting-Hansen, Gorlin and Vickers because of the many apparent discrepancies and variations which were reported under the title of this condition subsequent to that first description. This recent study, based on 16 cases of the calcifying odontogenic cyst, was directed chiefly toward clarification of its range, variations and neoplastic potential. The findings, representing the consensus of opinions of this group, which has dealt with the condition as thoroughly as any other group of investigators, will form the basis for the following discussion. While many of the concepts and ideas put forth by this group and summarized here vary considerably from previous reports in the literature, they do appear fundamentally sound,

definitely reconcile many conflicting ideas and findings of earlier investigators and no doubt will be confirmed as further studies provide additional information.

One major conclusion of Praetorius and his colleagues was that this condition as it has been described actually contains two entities, a cyst and a neoplasm. The cystic form occurred as three chief variants, whereas the neoplasm appeared too unusual to be included any longer in the category of calcifying odontogenic cyst, and its separation as an entity was recommended.

Clinical and Histologic Features. The three cystic variants of this lesion were described by Praetorius and his co-workers as: Type 1A, the *simple unicystic type*; type 1B, the *odontome producing type*; and type 1C, the *ameloblastomatous proliferating type* (Fig. 4–14).

Type 1A appears to occur at any age in life and may be either an intraosseous or extraosseous lesion. The epithelium of the cyst lining is chiefly low cuboidal or squamous, two to three cells thick. Focal areas of stellate reticulum and "ghost" cells may be present as well as sparse amounts of dentinoid. No other hard tissue is found.

These "ghost" cells were identified by Gorlin in his original report as being characteristically present in this lesion and, at that time, suggested to him that this cyst may represent the oral counterpart of the dermal calcifying epithelioma of Malherbe. "Ghost" cells are pale, eosinophilic, swollen epithelial cells that have lost the nucleus but show a faint outline of the cellular and nuclear membrane. They contain many tonofibrils. However, their presence is not confined to the calcifying odontogenic cyst;

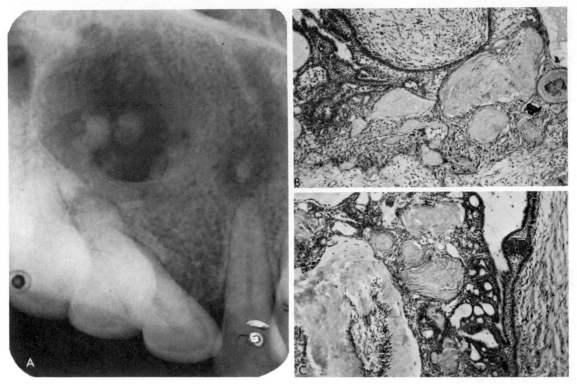

Figure 4–14. *Calcifying odontogenic cyst.*
(Courtesy of Dr. Robert Johnson.)

they are also found in ameloblastic fibro-odon-tomas, complex and compound odontomas (q.v.), and craniopharyngiomas, and have been observed by Praetorius and his associates in ameloblastomas and carcinomas.

Type 1B has a predilection for occurrence between the ages of 10 and 29 years. It also may be either intraosseous or extraosseous in location. This is histologically a unilocular cyst with a similar type of lining to type 1A, but in addition, it exhibits formation of calcified tissues in the cyst wall similar to those found in compound and complex odontomas. Furthermore, proliferation of tissue similar to an ameloblastic fibroma may be seen in the cyst wall and this may invade surrounding bone.

Type 1C only was represented by one example, an intraosseous lesion. The cystic lesion histologically presents ameloblastoma-like proliferations in the connective tissue of the fibrous capsule as well as in the lumen of the cyst.

The *type II* neoplasm-like lesion exhibits an entirely different structure, consisting of ameloblastoma-like strands and islands of odontogenic epithelium infiltrating into mature connective tissue. "Ghost" cells in varying numbers are present, as well as varying amounts of dentinoid in contact with the odontogenic epithelium. This lesion appears to occur predominantly in later life, may be either intraosseous or extraosseous and may recur after cystectomy. Praetorius and his colleagues suggested separation and designation of this lesion by the term *dentinogenic ghost cell tumor*.

Roentgenographic Features. The central intrabony lesions appear as a radiolucency, usually rather well circumscribed, although this is not invariably the case. Variable amounts of calcified radiopaque material are usually scattered throughout the radiolucency, ranging from tiny flecks to large masses, depending upon the particular type of calcifying odontogenic cyst (Fig. 4–14). They may become very large lesions, many centimeters in diameter, and may involve much of the jaw, although small lesions are the more common finding.

Treatment and Prognosis. Because of the propensity of the lesion for continued growth, it should be surgically excised when found. Lack of recurrence is dependent upon completeness of excision. Carcinomatous transformation has been recorded.

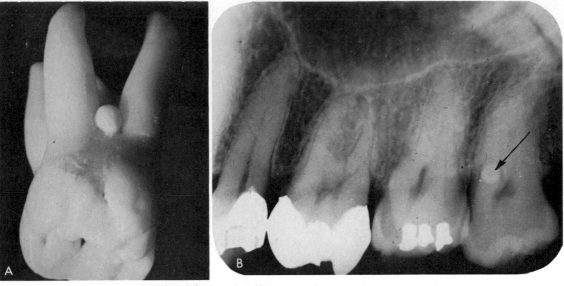

Figure 4–15. *Enameloma.*
A, A nodular mass of enamel is shown in the interradicular area of the extracted maxillary molar. *B*, The roentgenogram demonstrates the appearance of the condition in situ.

ECTODERMAL TUMORS OF ODONTOGENIC ORIGIN

ENAMELOMA

(Enamel Drop; Enamel Pearl)

The enameloma is not a true neoplasm and may be classified as a tumor only by virtue of the fact that it constitutes a small, focal excessive mass of enamel on the surface of a tooth. The enamel pearl is most frequently found near or in the bifurcation or trifurcation of the roots of teeth or on the root surface near the cementoenamel junction. It appears as a tiny globule of enamel, firmly adherent to the tooth, which arises from a small group of misplaced ameloblasts (Fig. 4–15, A), This enamel sometimes contains a small core of dentin and rarely a small strand of pulp tissue extending from the pulp chamber or root canal of the tooth. Cavanha has described the histomorphology of enamel pearls in detail.

Turner reported observing 23 enamel pearls in 1000 maxillary molars, but only 3 in 1000 mandibular molars. In addition, he found no pearls on teeth anterior to the molars. Thus the enamel drop is not a common finding and is of no clinical significance except that, clinically and roentgenographically, it may occasionally be mistaken for calculus (Fig. 4–15, *B*).

AMELOBLASTOMA

(Adamantinoma; Adamantoblastoma; Multilocular Cyst)

The ameloblastoma is a true neoplasm of enamel organ–type tissue which does not undergo differentiation to the point of enamel formation. It has been described very aptly by Robinson as being a tumor that is "usually unicentric, nonfunctional, intermittent in growth, anatomically benign and clinically persistent."

The term "ameloblastoma" as applied to this particular tumor was suggested by Churchill in 1934 to replace the term "adamantinoma," coined by Malassez in 1885, since the latter term implies the formation of hard tissue, and no such material is present in this lesion. The first neoplasm of this nature reported in the scientific literature is credited to Broca in 1868, although Guzack reported a tumor of the jaw in 1826 which may be the first recorded instance of an ameloblastoma. In any event, the first thorough description of an ameloblastoma is that of Falkson in 1879.

Pathogenesis. The earlier workers noted the resemblance between the odontogenic apparatus and the ameloblastoma and suggested that the neoplasm was derived from a portion of this apparatus or from cells potentially capable of forming dental tissue. Malassez described small collections of epithelial cells adjacent to the roots of teeth in the periodontal ligament and suggested that the "adamantine epithelioma" was produced by proliferation of these cell rests.

At present most authorities consider the ameloblastoma to be of varied origin, although the stimulus initiating the process is unknown. Thus the tumor conceivably may be derived from (1) cell rests of the enamel organ, either remnants of the dental lamina or remnants of Hertwig's sheath, the epithelial rests of Malassez; (2) epithelium of odontogenic cysts, particularly the dentigerous cyst, and odontomas; (3) disturbances of the developing enamel organ; (4) basal cells of the surface epithelium of the jaws; or (5) heterotopic epithelium in other parts of the body, especially the pituitary gland.

Cahn in 1933 reported a case of ameloblastoma originating in the wall of a dentigerous cyst, and numerous cases have subsequently been recognized as developing in this fashion. It should be reiterated that Stanley and Diehl, in reviewing 641 cases of ameloblastoma, found that 108 of these tumors, approximately 17 per cent, were definitely associated with an impacted tooth and/or a follicular (dentigerous) cyst. They also noted a marked reduction in the prevalence of such cases after the age of 30, presumably because of the loss of the ameloblastomatous potential of the odontogenic epithelium in impacted tooth follicles and follicular cysts as patients age. Such a significant finding emphasizes the dangerous potential of the dentigerous cyst and the need for careful microscopic examination of every such lesion. This is discussed in greater detail in the section on the dentigerous cyst (q.v.). Since a dentigerous cyst may develop in association with an odontoma, as well as with an impacted tooth, it is suggested that these too be examined by the pathologist. There is apparently little tendency for the development of the ameloblastoma in the ordinary apical periodontal or radicular cyst.

Peripheral (Extraosseous) Ameloblastoma. This is a tumor which histologically resembles the typical central or intraosseous ameloblastoma but which occurs in the soft tissue outside and overlying the alveolar bone. In addition, a number of cases of lesions in a similar location and with similar histologic features have been reported under the term "basal cell carcinoma of the gingiva." Many investigators consider these the same basic lesion, including Gardner, who has reviewed the literature, adding 7 additional unpublished cases for a total of 21 examples of peripheral ameloblastoma. Occasional other cases have since been reported, such as those of Greer and Hammond and of Gould and his colleagues.

This tumor appears to originate from either surface epithelium or remnants of dental lamina. In some instances, the tumor exhibits one or more areas of continuity with the surface epithelium, while in other cases, even with serial sectioning, no evidence of continuity between the two can be found.

The ages of the patients in the 21 cases reviewed by Gardner ranged between 23 and 82 years, with 10 patients between 30 and 50 years of age. There was a slight predilection for occurrence in males, 13 cases to 8 cases in females. There was an approximately 2:1 ratio of occurrence in the mandible over the maxilla. The lesions, all of which appeared as nodules on the gingiva, varied in size from 3 mm. to 2 cm. in diameter. In only two cases was roentgenographically evident superficial erosion of bone present.

The peripheral ameloblastoma histologically may exhibit the same patterns seen in the intraosseous ameloblastoma. However, while some lesions appeared to be of the follicular type, the vast majority were acanthomatous, at least in areas. Greer and Hammond have studied the ultrastructural characteristics of their case and found the electron microscopic appearance to be similar to that of the intraosseous ameloblastoma and the cutaneous basal cell carcinoma. In a similar ultrastructural study, Gould and his associates found that the features of their tumor was characteristic of origin from either surface epithelium or odontogenic remnants, thereby precluding definitive conclusions regarding site of origin. In terms of differential diagnosis, one must always consider the possibility of the peripheral odontogenic fibroma, which is also a peripheral lesion of the gingiva with variable amounts of odontogenic epithelium. The distinction on the basis of the connective tissue parenchyma of the odontogenic fibroma is usually not difficult, although cases with features of both lesions may occur, such as that reported by Sciubba and Zola.

One of the most important aspects of the peripheral ameloblastoma, emphasizing the need for its careful identification as a peripheral lesion and separation from the intraosseous counterpart, is the difference in clinical behavior. The peripheral lesion is relatively innocuous, lacks the persistent invasiveness of the intraosseous lesion and has very limited tend-

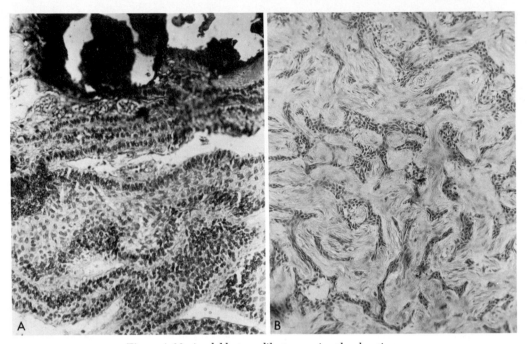

Figure 4–16. *Ameloblastoma-like tumors in other locations.*
A, Craniopharyngioma showing typical ameloblastoma-like formation with calcification. B, Adamantinoma of tibia. (Courtesy of Drs. William G. Sprague and David C. Dahlin.)

ency for recurrence. For this reason, it may be excised locally, although follow-up examination is always good practice.

Pituitary Ameloblastoma (Craniopharyngioma, Rathke's Pouch Tumor). This is a neoplasm involving the central nervous system which grows as a pseudoencapsulated mass, usually in the suprasellar area but occasionally in the intrasellar area, and often destroys the pituitary gland. The peak incidence is reported to be between 13 and 23 years of age. According to Zulch, the pituitary ameloblastoma is the most common tumor of childhood and adolescence. In his series of 6000 CNS tumors, it constituted 2.5 per cent of the total in all patients regardless of age.

It is generally thought to originate from the unobliterated portions of the fetal craniopharyngeal duct, which itself is derived from Rathke's pouch. This pouch is a recess arising as a result of invagination of a portion of the stomadeal ectoderm, and the pituitary gland forms by fusion of this pouch with a process of the forebrain. Epithelial remnants of this craniopharyngeal duct are extremely common in the adult. These cell rests have a certain pluripotential and on occasion may give rise to tumors histologically similar to the ameloblastoma of the jaw.

Microscopic features of the craniopharyngioma not generally found in the ameloblastoma include the almost universal occurrence of irregular calcified masses as well as occasional foci of metaplastic bone or cartilage (Fig. 4–16, A). In addition, many investigators have noted the similarity between the craniopharyngioma and the calcifying odontogenic cyst because of the presence in the pituitary lesion of islands and nests of "ghost" cells, as well as the calcifications and the fact that cyst formation is common. Several cases of craniopharyngioma with tooth formation have also been reported, such as that of Seemayer and his associates.

There is great variability in the rate of growth of the pituitary ameloblastoma. Depending upon its exact location, there may be a gamut of clinical features eventually manifested, such as evidence of endocrine disturbance, drowsiness or even toxic symptoms. The treatment of this neoplasm is a neurosurgical problem.

Adamantinoma of Long Bones. This tumor has been discussed by Baker, Dockerty and Coventry, who reviewed the literature and concluded that the true nature of the lesion is still unknown. The tumor, which bears a superficial microscopic resemblance to the ameloblastoma of the jaws, has occurred in the tibia in approximately 90 per cent of the slightly over 100 reported cases, but also has been recorded in the ulna, femur and fibula (Fig. 4–16, *B*). Changus and his co-workers suggested that the lesion is actually a malignant angioblastoma, and this view is supported by Huvos and Marcove in their investigation of 14 cases. In contrast, Unni and his co-workers studied 29 cases, with ultrastructural microscopy of 3 of the tumors, and concluded that this provided evidence that the islands of tumor cells were epithelial in origin. Thus, although the histogenetic origin of this tumor is unknown, most authorities agree that it is not related to the ameloblastoma of the jaws, even though they support retention of the term "adamantinoma" because of its acceptance through usage and for lack of a better name.

Clinical Features. The survey of the literature of 379 cases of ameloblastoma of the jaw by Robinson in 1937 has been of inestimable aid in adding to our knowledge of this tumor. A later survey by Small and Waldron, including 984 published cases and 62 unpublished ones, has shown results very similar to those of Robinson in the clinical features of the ameloblastoma. The few more recent series, such as the 126 cases reported by Mehlisch and his coworkers, the 92 cases reported by Sehdev and his associates and the 78 cases reported by Regezi and his colleagues, have all exhibited data essentially identical with those of the previously reported series. Since the study of Small and Waldron consisted of over 1000 cases, including the 379 of Robinson, it will be used as the basis for the discussion of the clinical features of this neoplasm (Table 4–1).

The occurrence of the ameloblastoma is approximately evenly divided between the sexes, the slight difference noted being an insignificant one. A predominance for a specific race is difficult to evaluate. Kegel reported that blacks are more commonly affected than whites, but this is uncertain. The average age of the patient at the time of discovery of the lesion is approximately 33 years, while the average duration of the tumor after discovery is approximately six years. Nevertheless *the ameloblastoma may occur at any age*, even though nearly half of the tumors do occur between the ages of 20 and 40 years.

The ameloblastoma originates in the mandible in 80 per cent of the cases, and nearly three-fourths of these occur in the molar-ramus area. The less common lesions in the maxilla are found most frequently in the molar area, antrum and floor of the nose.

Table 4–1. Ameloblastomas of the Jaws: Statistical Analysis of the Literature

	NO.	%
Total cases	1036	
Sex (987 cases):		
Male	514	52
Female	473	48
Race (594 cases):		
Caucasian	371	
Negro	121	
Chinese	71	
Egyptian	15	
Indian	15	
Filipino	1	
Average age at time of report	38.9 years	
Average duration of tumor	5.8 years	
Average age at time of discovery	32.7 years	
Site of growth (925 cases):		
Mandible	752	81
Maxilla	173	19
Structural characteristics (465 cases):		
Cystic (includes those called cystic and solid)	365	78
Solid	100	22
Location:		
Mandible:		
Molar-ramus area	170	70
Premolar area	49	20
Symphysis area	27	10
Maxilla:		
Molar area	21	47
Antrum and floor of nose	15	33
Premolar area	4	9
Canine area	4	9
Palate	1	2

From I. A. Small and C. A. Waldron: Ameloblastomas of the jaws. Oral Surg., 8:281, 1955.

The typical ameloblastoma begins insidiously as a central lesion of bone which is slowly destructive, but tends to expand the bone rather than perforate it. The tumor is seldom painful unless secondarily infected, and it does not often produce signs or symptoms of nerve involvement. Occasionally patients allow an ameloblastoma to persist for many years without treatment, and in such cases, though the expansion may be extremely disfiguring, the fungating, ulcerative type of growth characteristic of carcinoma does not occur. Seldom is there breakdown of the oral mucosa.

It is noteworthy that trauma has often been associated with development of the ameloblastoma. Some investigators claim that this neoplasm is frequently preceded by the extraction of teeth, cystectomy or some other traumatic episode. As in the case of other types of tumors, the extraction of teeth is frequently the effect of a tumor (i.e., the tumor caused loosening of the teeth) rather than its cause. Furthermore, since the infliction of trauma to the jaws is a common occurrence, its relation to the ameloblastoma is nearly impossible to assess. The resorption of roots of teeth is an extremely common finding in association with ameloblastomas. For example, Struthers and Shear found root resorption of associated teeth in 81 per cent of a series of 32 cases of ameloblastoma in contrast to resorption in only 55 per cent of 20 cases of dentigerous cyst and 18 per cent of 33 cases of apical periodontal cyst.

Malignant ameloblastoma has been reported occasionally in the literature. Small and Waldron listed 33 such cases, but point out that 12 of these are unacceptable and a number of the remainder are doubtful. Carr and Halperin have reviewed the literature on malignant ameloblastoma, subsequent to the period covered by Small and Waldron. They regarded 5 cases as proven malignant, 12 cases as possibly malignant, and 5 of the reported cases as doubtful malignant. Thus the incidence of malignant ameloblastoma has been placed at approximately 2 per cent, but even this figure is probably too high. The diagnosis of malignancy must depend upon the demonstration of metastatic lesions. Too frequently the histologic examination of the "metastases" has not been carried out. Nevertheless in some cases microscopic study has shown evidence of ameloblastoma in lymph nodes and lung. The literature dealing with metastatic ameloblastoma has been reviewed by Lee and his co-workers. The argument is often raised that demonstrable lung lesions are a result of aspiration implantation, and such a possibility cannot be denied, particularly since some such lesions are found in sites where aspirated foreign bodies are frequently found. The statement of Robinson that the ameloblastoma is a persistent, not malignant, tumor appears well founded.

A distinction is usually made between the terms "malignant ameloblastoma" and "ameloblastic carcinoma." As used by most investigators, the term "malignant ameloblastoma" has been defined as that particular ameloblastoma which has given evidence of truly malignant behavior, judged chiefly by the occurrence of metastasis, but in which the metastatic lesions have shown no significant histologic differences from the primary tumor. In other words, the metastatic tumor still resembles the primary ameloblastoma with no histologic transformation. On the other hand, the term "ameloblastic carcinoma" has been defined as that type of ameloblastoma in which there has been obvious histologically malignant transformation of the epithelial component (Fig. 4–17) and in which the tumor has behaved in a malignant fashion so that the metastatic lesions do not bear resemblance to the primary odontogenic tumor but, rather, to a less well differentiated carcinoma, usually an epidermoid carcinoma.

These malignant forms of ameloblastoma should be separated from the lesion described by Shear as a *primary intra-alveolar epidermoid carcinoma* (q.v.) and retitled by the World Health Organization (WHO) group the *primary intraosseous carcinoma*. This subject of the

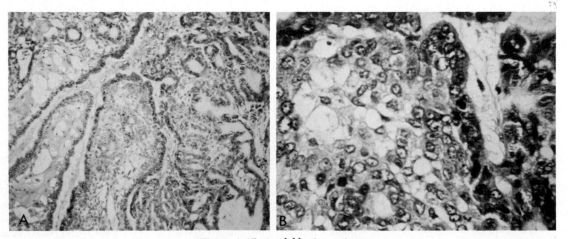

Figure 4–17. *Ameloblastic carcinoma.*
The pattern of the original ameloblastoma is still evident (*A*), but there has been cytologically malignant transformation of the tumor (*B*) which corresponded to its sudden extremely aggressive clinical behavior. (Courtesy of Dr. Charles L. Dunlap.)

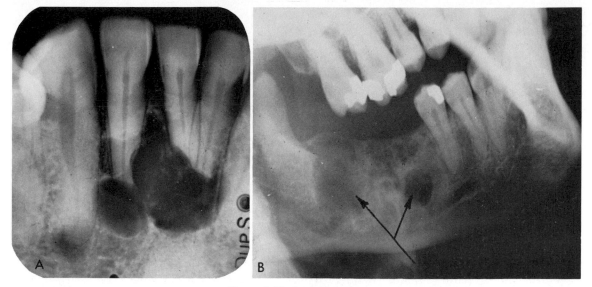

Figure 4–18. *Ameloblastoma.*
A, The typical loculations which often occur are clearly seen. B, This lateral jaw roentgenogram reveals an early lesion with no loculations, but with several focal areas of bone destruction.

classification of malignant primary intrabony tumors of the jaws has been discussed both by Shear and Altini and by Elzay.

Shear and Altini have pointed out that the WHO publication (Pindborg et al, 1971) considers all such malignant lesions under the broad title of odontogenic carcinomas with three categories: (1) malignant ameloblastoma, (2) primary intraosseous carcinoma, and (3) other carcinomas arising from odontogenic epithelium, including those arising from odontogenic cysts.

Elzay has liberalized his proposed classification under the broad title of primary intraosseous carcinoma with three types: (1) those arising from odontogenic cysts; (2) those arising from an ameloblastoma, either well differentiated (malignant ameloblastoma) or poorly differentiated (ameloblastic carcinoma); and (3) those arising de novo from odontogenic epithelial residues, either keratinizing or nonkeratinizing.

These classifications do not differ in their basic substantive nature, only in their terminology, and this serves to emphasize the importance of understanding the fundamental potentials of the odontogenic tissues regardless of the nomenclature.

Roentgenographic Features. The ameloblastoma has been described classically as a multilocular cystlike lesion of the jaw. This is especially true in advanced cases of ameloblastoma. Here, the tumor exhibits a compartmented appearance with septa of bone extending into the radiolucent tumor mass (Fig. 4–18, A). In many cases, however, the lesion is a unilocular one and presents no characteristic or pathognomonic features (Figs. 4–18, B, and 4–19). The periphery of the lesion on the roentgenogram is usually smooth, although this regularity may not be borne out at the time of operation. In the advanced lesion producing jaw expansion, thinning of the cortical plate may be seen on the roentgenogram (Fig. 4–20).

The term "cystic ameloblastoma" is frequently used in referring to certain of these neoplasms. It is important to note that there is no correlation between the term thus used clinically and the appearance of the tumor on the roentgenogram. The roentgenographic film does nothing more than indicate the relative presence or absence of calcified tissue, and a variety of lesions may manifest themselves in a manner similar to that of the ameloblastoma.

Histologic Features. The ameloblastoma closely resembles the enamel organ, although different cases may be distinguished by their similarity to different stages of odontogenesis. Since the histologic pattern of the ameloblastoma varies greatly, a number of different types are commonly described (Fig. 4–21).

The *follicular* (simple) ameloblastoma is composed of many small discrete islands of tumor composed of a peripheral layer of cuboidal or columnar cells whose nuclei are generally well polarized. These cells strongly resemble ameloblasts or preameloblasts and these enclose a

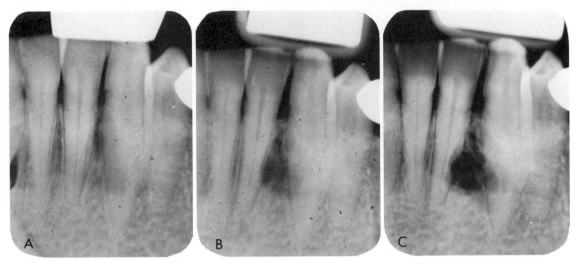

Figure 4–19. *Developing ameloblastoma.*
Each roentgenogram was taken at intervals of two years. The slow growth of the ameloblastoma over the four-year period is typical. (Courtesy of Drs. Harry R. Kerr Jr. and G. Thaddeus Gregory.)

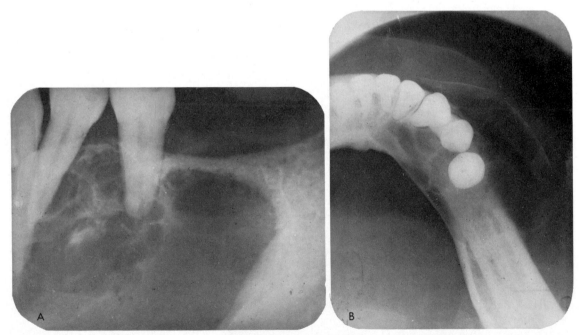

Figure 4–20. *Ameloblastoma.*
The periapical *(A)* and occlusal *(B)* roentgenograms show the destruction and expansion of bone which frequently occur.

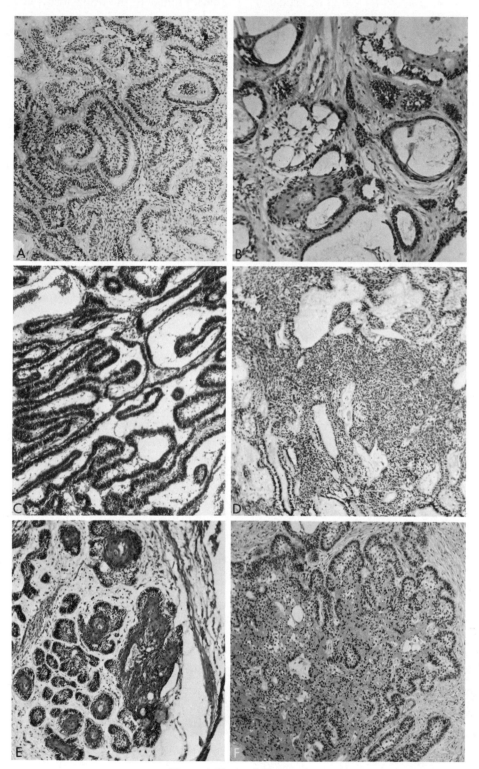

Figure 4–21. *Ameloblastoma.*
A, Follicular type; *B*, follicular type showing cystic degeneration and squamous metaplasia; *C*, plexiform type; *D*, basal cell type; *E*, acanthomatous type; *F*, granular cell type.

central mass of polyhedral, loosely arranged cells resembling the stellate reticulum. The terms "solid" and "cystic" have often been applied to the ameloblastoma and have variously referred to the clinical or histologic appearance of the tumor. Clinically, some cases exhibit tiny cysts that are grossly evident when the lesion is excised and examined carefully. In such instances, the stellate reticulum-like tissue has undergone complete breakdown or cystic degeneration and, in such cases, there is often flattening of the peripheral columnar cells so that they resemble low cuboidal or even squamous cells. Cyst formation is relatively common in this follicular type of ameloblastoma.

In the *plexiform* ameloblastoma, the ameloblast-like tumor cells are arranged in irregular masses or, more frequently, as a network of interconnecting strands of cells. Each of these masses or strands is bounded by a layer of columnar cells, and between these layers may be found stellate reticulum-like cells. Sometimes double rows of columnar cells are lined up back to back. However, the stellate reticulum-like tissue is much less prominent in the plexiform type than in the follicular type of ameloblastoma. Areas of cystic degeneration of stroma are also common.

In the *acanthomatous* ameloblastoma, the cells occupying the position of the stellate reticulum undergo squamous metaplasia, sometimes with keratin formation in the central portion of the tumor islands. This usually occurs in the follicular type of ameloblastoma. On occasion, epithelial or keratin pearls may even be observed.

In the *granular cell* ameloblastoma, there is marked transformation of the cytoplasm, usually of the stellate reticulum-like cells, so that it takes on a very coarse, granular, eosinophilic appearance. This often extends to include the peripheral columnar or cuboidal cells as well. Ultrastructural studies, such as that of Tandler and Rossi, have shown that these cytoplasmic granules represent lysosomal aggregates with no recognizable cellular components. Hartman has reported a series of 20 cases of granular cell ameloblastoma and emphasized that this granular cell type appears to be an aggressive lesion with a marked proclivity for recurrence unless appropriate surgical measures are instituted at the first operation. In addition, several cases of this type have been reported as metastasizing. However, all other clinical features of the lesion appear similar to the other forms of ameloblastoma.

The *basal cell* type of ameloblastoma bears considerable resemblance to the basal cell carcinoma of the skin. Thus, the epithelial tumor cells are more primitive and less columnar, and are generally arranged in sheets, more so than in the other tumor types. This is the least common of the different types of ameloblastoma.

The connective tissue stroma, associated with all of these types of ameloblastoma, may vary somewhat but generally is made up of bundles of collagen fibers which may be either relatively loose or dense.

Unicystic ameloblastoma is a lesion that has been documented most recently by Robinson and Martinez, who reported 20 cases. This is a unilocular, cystic lesion whose clinical features are those of a non-neoplastic cyst and which mimics a dentigerous cyst in most instances, although they were unable to determine whether the ameloblastoma began in an antecedent non-neoplastic cyst. The lesion tends to occur in younger patients than the ordinary ameloblastoma, more commonly in the mandible and often in association with an unerupted third molar. The unicystic ameloblastoma is characterized by one or more of the following features: (1) lining epithelium exhibiting alterations virtually identical with those described by Vickers and Gorlin as representing early ameloblastomatous changes in the dentigerous cyst (q.v.), (2) nodules of tumor projecting intraluminally, (3) ameloblastomatous lining epithelium proliferating into the connective tissue wall, and (4) islands of ameloblastoma occurring isolated in the connective tissue wall. The recurrence rate of this lesion is distinctly lower than that for the characteristic ameloblastoma, thus indicating a less aggressive type of lesion.

Plexiform unicystic ameloblastoma is a term introduced by Gardner to designate a plexiform type of epithelial proliferation occurring in the dentigerous cyst which does not exhibit the usual histologic characteristics for ameloblastoma developing in such cyst lining but yet which he considers to represent a form of ameloblastoma. The use of this term is unfortunate because of its similarity to the term "plexiform ameloblastoma," with which it has no relationship other than the fact that the epithelium in each case proliferates in a retiform or network pattern. Gardner has reported that this form of epithelial prolferation frequently but not invariably occurs in association with a histologically characteristic ameloblastoma elsewhere in the lesion. Furthermore, while these lesions were unicystic, they did not exhibit epithelium typical of that described by Vickers and Gorlin as indicative of ameloblastomatous transformation or of that described by Robinson and Martinez in the unicystic ameloblastoma. Of the 19 cases reported in this series, the majority occurred in the second and third decades of life, similar to the unicystic ameloblastoma. Follow-up information was only available in 3 of the 19 cases and there was recurrence in 1 of the 3. Such a fact could be consistent with either a benign neoplasm of a low degree of aggressiveness or simply a cyst. Whether the designation of the cases occurring without an associated ameloblastoma should be that of a neoplasm or not must await substantially more experience with this lesion than is now available.

Treatment and Prognosis. There is some difference of opinion about the preferable method of treatment of the ameloblastoma. The only unanimity centers around the fact that complete removal of the neoplasm, regardless of how it is accomplished, will result in a cure of the patient.

The types of treatment that have been used include both radical and conservative surgical excision, curettage, chemical and electrocautery, radiation therapy or a combination of surgery and radiation. The majority of workers today prefer some form of surgical excision. Curettage is least desirable, since it is associated with the highest incidence of recurrence. The basic principles of treatment have been discussed in detail by Gardner and by Mehlisch and his colleagues.

Frissell reviewed the reported cases in which radiation therapy was utilized and found that there was considerable variance of opinion as to its benefit. The report of Kimm, supported by study of serial biopsy, on the treatment of the ameloblastoma by radiation indicated that this neoplasm is generally highly radioresistant and that the use of this form of therapy is not warranted. Wide clinical experience has shown the truth of this finding. Regardless of the form of treatment, long-term follow-up of the patient is an absolute necessity.

The prognosis for patients afflicted with this form of neoplastic disease is favorable. Since it

is essentially a local problem, metastases seldom occurring, it may cause disfigurement, but seldom causes death unless vital structures are involved by local invasion.

PRIMARY INTRA-ALVEOLAR EPIDERMOID CARCINOMA
(Primary Intraosseous Carcinoma)

The primary intra-alveolar epidermoid carcinoma of the jaw has been described as a definite entity, although it is a very uncommon disease. Carcinomas may be found within the jaws in a variety of situations: invading from the overlying soft tissues, through malignant transformation of the epithelial lining of odontogenic or nonodontogenic cysts, through malignant transformation of ameloblastomas, by metastasis from different sites or, in the case of the maxilla, from primary tumors of the maxillary sinus. This lesion, however, represents a primary carcinoma developing within bone from either odontogenic epithelial remnants, such as rests of Malassez, or enclaved epithelium along fusion lines of embryonic processes. It appears that the vast majority of lesions are odontogenic in origin. The classification of lesions of this nature has been discussed under the preceding section on malignant ameloblastoma (q.v.).

Clinical Features. Shear has reviewed the literature concerning this lesion and has found that there is a rather wide age distribution of cases, although the majority of patients were in the sixth and seventh decades at the time of diagnosis. Of reported cases, the disease appears to occur about twice as frequently in men as in women. In addition, nearly 90 per cent of the cases occurred in the mandible; the maxilla seems rarely affected. The early symptoms of this form of carcinoma are swelling of the jaw, with pain and mobility of the teeth before ulceration has occurred.

McGowan has reviewed six additional cases reported since those of Shear, including two of his own, and has emphasized the difficulties encountered in diagnosing this rare but dangerous lesion, the chief being mistaking initial symptoms for a dental problem and not suspecting the serious nature of the disease for a considerable period of time.

Roentgenographic Features. The roentgenographic appearance of the lesion is not characteristic. It presents as simply a diffuse radiolucency similar to other central malignant neoplasms of the jaw.

Histologic Features. The intra-alveolar epidermoid carcinoma generally has an alveolar or plexiform pattern with the peripheral cells of the tumor masses showing palisading, thereby resembling odontogenic epithelium. The tumor, generally nonkeratinizing, is usually of the basal cell type, although on occasion spinous cells may be found. The tumor cells themselves generally exhibit nuclear pleomorphism and hyperchromatism; mitotic activity varies from case to case.

Treatment and Prognosis. Central carcinomas of bone of this type are generally treated by surgical resection rather than by radiotherapy, although the number of cases of this particular lesion are insufficient to compare results with different modalities of treatment. Metastasis of tumor to regional lymph nodes occurs frequently, as do distant metastases. The over-all 5-year-survival rate for reported cases is between 30 and 40 per cent. However, the presence of metastases at the time of treatment confers a much graver prognosis.

Calcifying Epithelial Odontogenic Tumor

(Pindborg Tumor)

The calcifying epithelial odontogenic tumor was first described as an entity by Pindborg in 1956. Although undoubtedly of odontogenic origin, it bears little microscopic similarity to the typical ameloblastoma, and the two lesions should be separated.

Clinical Features. A report by Franklin and Pindborg in 1976 shows that 113 cases of this intraosseous tumor have been described in the literature since Pindborg's original paper. As the number of reported cases continues to increase, we are rapidly improving our knowledge of this lesion.

This tumor occurs most frequently in middle-age. Of the reported cases, the mean age of occurrence at the time of diagnosis was 40 years of age in both men and women, with a range of 8 to 92 years. There is no significant difference in occurrence between the sexes, since 49 per cent of the cases were in men and 51 per cent in women.

There is a predilection for occurrence of the tumor in the mandible over the maxilla by a ratio of 2:1, and the prevalence in the molar region is three times that in the bicuspid region,

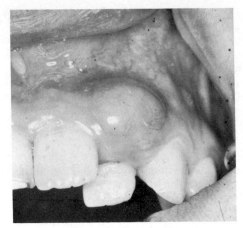

Figure 4–22. *Extraosseous calcifying epithelial odontogenic tumor.*
(Courtesy of Dr. Jens J. Pindborg: Acta Odontol. Scand., 24:419, 1966.)

whereas in other sites in the jaws there is a relatively even distribution. In these two respects, i.e., age and site, the Pindborg tumor is very similar to the ameloblastoma.

Most patients with this lesion are asymptomatic and are aware only of a painless swelling. It is significant, however, that 52 per cent of the reported cases have been definitely associated with an unerupted or impacted tooth.

An extraosseous calcifying epithelial odontogenic tumor is also known to occur but is quite rare, with only eight reported cases, according to the review by Wertheimer and his associates in 1977. This extraosseous lesion has had a mean age of occurrence of 35 years and an approximately equal sex distribution. With the exception of one equivocal lesion on the upper lip, all cases have occurred on the gingiva, five mandibular and two maxillary, and almost invariably in the anterior segment (Fig. 4–22). The extraosseous lesion is histologically identical with the intraosseous one.

Roentgenographic Features. The tumor may show considerable roentgenographic variation. In some cases the lesion appears as either a diffuse or a well-circumscribed unilocular radiolucent area, while in other cases there may appear to be a combined pattern of radiolucency and radiopacity with many small, irregular bony trabeculae traversing the radiolucent area in many directions, producing a multilocular or honeycomb pattern. Scattered flecks of calcification throughout the radiolucency have given rise to the descriptive term of a "driven snow" appearance. In some instances, the lesion is totally radiolucent and is in association with an

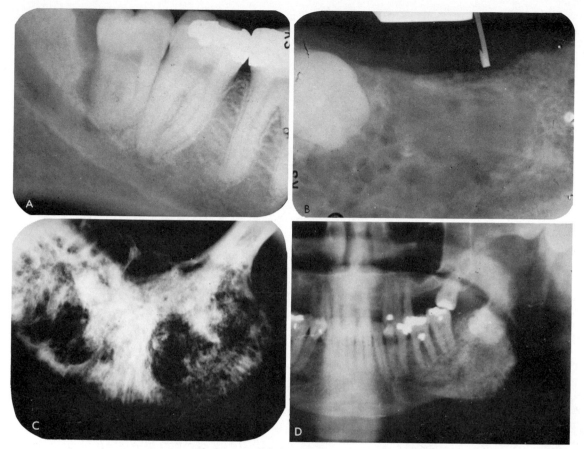

Figure 4–23. *Calcifying epithelial odontogenic tumor of Pindborg.*
(Courtesy of Drs. Charles Redish, Robert Bresick, Charles Hutton, and Ronald Vincent.)

impacted tooth, thus leading to a mistaken clinical diagnosis of dentigerous cyst (Fig. 4–23).

Histologic Features. The calcifying epithelial odontogenic tumor is composed of polyhedral epithelial cells, sometimes closely packed in large sheets but other times consisting chiefly of scattered small islands of cells in a bland fibrous connective tissue stroma (Fig. 4–24). Occasionally, the cells are arranged in cords or rows, mimicking adenocarcinoma. The tumor cells have a well-outlined cell border with a finely granular eosinophilic cytoplasm, and intercellular bridges are often prominent. The nuclei are frequently pleomorphic, with giant nuclei and multinucleation being quite common but mitotic figures rare. The tumor cells in some lesions are characterized by extreme morphologic variation with severe cellular abnormalities, mimicking those often seen in some highly malignant neoplasms, while other cases of the calcifying epithelial odontogenic tumor are composed of very monomorphic, innocuous-appearing tumor cells; yet, to the best of our knowledge, the biologic behavior does not differ between the two.

A well-recognized form of this neoplasm is the *clear-cell variant*. In this type, the tumor cells exhibit a clear vacuolated cytoplasm rather than an eosinophilic cytoplasm. The nucleus may remain round or oval in the center of the cells or be flattened against the cell membrane. According to Krolls and Pindborg, who have discussed these histomorphologic variations, most of the clear cells are mucicarmine-negative, although a few may show a faint tinge. In some tumors, the clear cells comprise the bulk of the tumor cells, while in others, they consist of only a few scattered foci. Inasmuch as a variety of other types of tumors, both primary (e.g., mucoepidermoid carcinoma) and metastatic (e.g., hypernephroma), may exhibit clear cells, great care must be utilized in their interpretation and diagnosis.

This tumor has been investigated under the electron microscope by many researchers in-

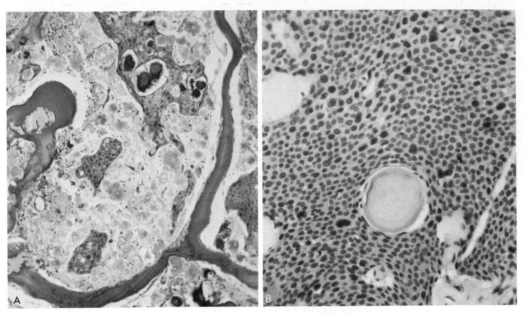

Figure 4–24. *Calcifying epithelial odontogenic tumor of Pindborg.*

cluding Anderson and his co-workers, who have demonstrated that the tumor cells exhibit the features commonly seen in epidermal cells such as intercellular bridges with desmosomes, intracytoplasmic tonofilaments and well-developed hemidesmosomes.

One of the characteristic microscopic features of this tumor is the presence of a homogeneous, eosinophilic substance which has been variously interpreted as amyloid, comparable glycoprotein, basal lamina, keratin or enamel matrix. In at least some instances, this appears to form intracellularly and then is extruded into the extracellular compartment as a result of cell secretion or degeneration. This homogeneous eosinophilic material may be present in large or very limited quantities. In most cases, it stains metachromatically with crystal violet, positively with Congo red, and fluoresces under ultraviolet light with thioflavin T, all in a fashion similar to amyloid. Ultrastructural studies have shown that this amyloid-like material is composed of at least three different types of fibrils, but that they have a smaller size than the fibers of "conventional" amyloid, although this term is a rapidly expanding one. Some forms of amyloid are now suggested to arise from light chain fragments of immunoglobulin molecules, called immunamyloid, while another form is thought to originate from cells of certain endocrine tumors (e.g., medullary carcinoma of the thyroid) which may be derived from the endo-

crine polypeptide cells of neural crest origin of the amine precursor uptake and decarboxylation (APUD) system, called apudamyloid. On the evidence available at present, the exact nature of the amyloid-like substance in the calcifying epithelial odontogenic tumor cannot be definitively assessed.

Another characteristic feature of the Pindborg tumor is the presence of calcification, sometimes in large amounts, and often in the form of Liesegang rings. This calcification actually appears to occur in some instances in globules of the amyloid-like material, many of which have coalesced and are transformed from being PAS (periodic acid-Schiff)-negative to PAS-positive during this calcification process. There does not appear to be necessarily a relationship between the amount of amyloid material formed in a given lesion and the amount of calcification occurring.

The source of the epithelial cells comprising this tumor was originally suggested by Pindborg to be the reduced enamel epithelium of the associated unerupted tooth. Today, most investigators believe that the cells originate from the stratum intermedium because of the morphologic similarity of the tumor cells to the normal cells of this layer of the odontogenic apparatus. Unfortunately, this does not explain those cases of tumor apparently occurring without an associated unerupted tooth or those extraosseous cases outside the jaw.

Treatment and Prognosis. There has been some attempt to equate the treatment and prognosis of the calcifying epithelial odontogenic tumor with the ameloblastoma because of certain features that these two lesions share in common. However, since far fewer data are available for the present lesion because of its more recent recognition as an entity, such parallel evaluation does not appear justified.

It is generally agreed that this tumor is of slow growth and is locally invasive, although Krolls and Pindborg have stated that it does not seem to extend into intertrabecular spaces as readily as the ameloblastoma. Unfortunately, the methods of treatment in the past have been extremely variable, ranging from simple enucleation to radical resection, so that end results have been difficult to evaluate. Furthermore, follow-up information on reported cases is quite limited and long-term follow-up is rare (16 cases were reported followed for 10 years or more). Nevertheless, the known recurrence rate is only 14 per cent, a relatively low figure although recurrence of this lesion may not be manifested for many years. The recurrence data and the known biologic behavior of this tumor would suggest that a radical surgical treatment is not warranted.

Adenomatoid Odontogenic Tumor

(Adenoameloblastoma; Ameloblastic Adenomatoid Tumor)

The adenomatoid odontogenic tumor is an uncommon histologic type of odontogenic tumor which is characterized by the formation of ductlike structures by the epithelial component of the lesion. Whether it represents a true neoplasm is not known, since it is of uncertain histogenesis. While it has been considered a benign neoplasm by some investigators, others have categorized it as a hamartomatous malformation or as an odontogenic cyst.

Clinical Features. There have been slightly over 100 cases of the adenomatoid odontogenic tumor reported in the literature up to 1970, according to the review of Giansanti and associates, and slightly over 150 by 1975, according to Courtney and Kerr. The mean age of these patients was approximately 18 years, with a range of 5 to 53 years. However, 73 per cent of the patients were under 20 years of age. There is a marked predilection for occurrence of the tumor in females—64 per cent contrasted to 36 per cent developing in males.

The site of occurrence is greater in the maxilla (65 per cent) than in the mandible (35 per cent). In contrast to the ameloblastoma, this tumor occurs more frequently in the anterior part of the jaws with 76 per cent developing anterior to the cuspid in the maxilla and mandible. Only very rarely does the lesion occur distal to the premolar area. It is of some interest that in at least 74 per cent of the cases, the tumors were associated with an unerupted tooth, and in over two-thirds of the cases, this tooth was the maxillary or mandibular cuspid.

The vast majority of the lesions measured between 1.5 and 3.0 cm., although large lesions, exceeding 7.0 cm., have been reported. A large proportion of these tumors produced an obvious clinical swelling although they were generally asymptomatic. Five tumors reported in the literature have been extraosseous in their occurrence, according to Swinson.

Giansanti and his co-workers have pointed out that the high percentage of these lesions being associated with unerupted teeth and present as dentigerous cysts would strongly suggest that they are related to some late disturbance in odontogenesis. Since none of the associated teeth were described as morphologically defective, the disturbance must occur after odontogenesis is complete.

Roentgenographic Features. The dental roentgenogram reveals a destructive lesion of the jaw which may or may not be well circumscribed but, in the majority of reported cases, has resembled a dentigerous cyst. In such cases, however, it extends apically further than the cementoenamel junction. The lesions are almost invariably unilocular radiolucencies but may contain faint to dense radiopaque foci. Separation of roots or displacement of adjacent teeth occurs frequently; root resorption is rare (Fig. 4–25, A, B).

Histologic Features. The adenomatoid odontogenic tumor is made up of epithelial cells, usually with only a scanty stroma of connective tissue. These epithelial cells, often polyhedral or even spindle-shaped, vary in their pattern from nests, sworls or cords to cells of a definite columnar or cuboidal variety arranged in ductlike or adenomatoid fashion (Fig. 4–25, C). Mitotic activity is uncommon. The lumina of these ductlike structures sometimes contain an eosinophilic coagulum. Droplets of unusual amorphous eosinophilic material are frequently found between epithelial cells arranged in solid nests, in the ductlike structures and sometimes in the midst of cells arranged in a rosette

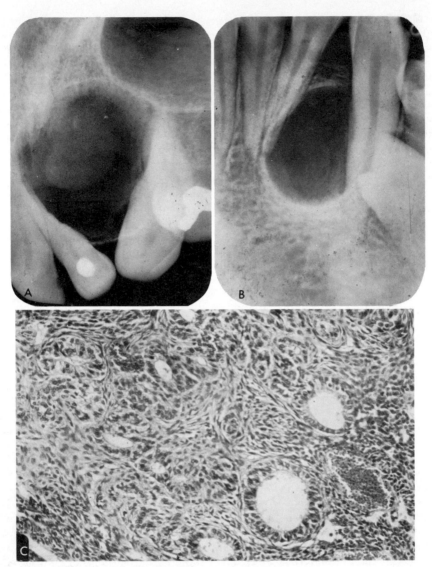

Figure 4–25. *Adenomatoid odontogenic tumor.*
The tumor in *A* roentgenographically resembled a globulo-maxillary cyst. The tumor in *B* was associated with an impacted tooth and superficially resembled a dentigerous cyst. The photomicrograph (*C*) shows the typical ductlike structures. (Courtesy of Drs. Charles Redish and Charles A. Waldron.)

pattern. Some of this material is PAS-positive, exhibits positive birefringence after alkaline Congo red staining, is metachromatic with crystal violet and shows a characteristic fluorescence with thioflavin T, all in a fashion similar to known liver amyloid. Thus, in the studies reported by Moro and his associates, the amyloid-like material was limited chiefly to the solid nests of cells. However, in other studies such as those of Smith and his co-workers, amyloid-like material was demonstrated in association with the columnar or cuboidal cells or the ductlike structures. Still other studies, such as

that of Buchner and David, have even denied the presence of amyloid. Thus, there is considerable controversy regarding this product. Foci of calcification are often seen scattered throughout the tumor and these have been interpreted by some investigators as attempted enamel formation, but by others as dentin or even cementum. Finally, the lesion is almost invariably encapsulated, thereby precluding any local invasion.

A variety of ultrastructural studies attempting to clarify the origin of this tumor have been carried out. Nearly all investigations have agreed upon the similarity of structures of the lesion to the normal enamel organ. Schlosnagle and Sameren have stated that the cells lining the ductlike structures under the electron microscopic resemble the cells of the inner enamel epithelium as they develop through the pre-ameloblast stage. They also concluded that the spindle-shaped cells of the tumor, constituting the other significant component, ultrastructurally resembled the cells of the stellate reticulum and the stratum intermedium. These findings agree with those of other workers, such as Smith and his colleagues. In addition, Hatakeyama and Suzuki have described cells present in the tumor similar to cells of the outer enamel epithelium, while Khan and his co-workers have described cells resembling odontoblasts. The identification of these two cell types awaits further confirmation.

Treatment and Prognosis. The majority of tumors of this variety have been treated by conservative surgical excision and recurrence, if it ever occurs, is exceedingly rare.

SQUAMOUS ODONTOGENIC TUMOR

(Benign Epithelial Odontogenic Tumor)

The squamous odontogenic tumor is a lesion which had been recognized as an apparent entity for a number of years but had not been named or reported until 1975, when Pullon and a small group of other oral pathologists combined their material and published six cases. Several additional cases have been reported since the original study, including five further cases by Goldblatt and his colleagues, who also reviewed the literature and commented further on this lesion.

The most important aspect of this lesion is its mistaken histologic identification as an acanthomatous ameloblastoma or as a well-differentiated epidermoid carcinoma. Most investigators believe that it represents a benign odontogenic neoplasm, probably arising from rests of Malassez, although a hamartomatous epithelial proliferation has also been considered.

Clinical Features. The age at discovery of the 16 cases evaluated by Goldblatt and his co-workers ranged from 11 to 67 years with 10 cases being between 19 and 31 years of age. There were 6 males and 10 females in the series.

The lesions occurred with approximately equal frequency of involvement of the maxilla and mandible. In the maxilla, lesions centered around the incisor-cuspid area, whereas in the mandible, lesions had a predilection for the bicuspid-molar area. However, several cases exhibited multiple site involvement, including both maxillary and mandibular involvement in the same patient.

The lesions were often asymptomatic but presenting manifestations included mobility of involved teeth, pain, tenderness to percussion and occasionally abnormal sensations.

Roentgenographic Features. There are no roentgenographic features sufficiently characteristic to suggest the diagnosis of this condition. It presents as a semicircular or roughly triangular radiolucent area, with or without a sclerotic border, usually in association with the cervical portion of the tooth root (Fig. 4–26, A,B).

Histologic Features. The squamous odontogenic tumor is composed entirely of islands of mature squamous epithelium without a peripheral palisaded or polarized columnar layer (Fig. 4–26, C,D). This peripheral layer is usually quite flattened or at least cuboidal. The squamous cells are very uniform and exhibit no pleomorphism, nuclear hyperchromatism or mitotic activity. Occasionally, individual cell keratinization is present but no epithelial pearls. Intercellular bridges are usually seen with no difficulty. Three other variable findings are microcyst formation involving only small portions of the epithelial islands, laminar calcifications in the epithelium and globular, hyalin, eosinophilic structures within the islands, which are not amyloid. The fibrous stroma of the tumor is simply mature bundles of collagen fibers and is devoid of any peri-insular inductive effect.

Squamous odontogenic tumor-like proliferations have been reported by Wright in the walls of odontogenic cysts, such as dentigerous or apical periodontal cysts. These proliferations may appear histologically nearly identical with those in the squamous odontogenic tumor, but they do not appear to cause any alteration in the usual biologic behavior of the cyst and do not appear to develop into the tumor. Care must be used, however, in differentiating between these proliferations and the tumor itself.

Treatment. Most reported cases of squamous odontogenic tumor have been treated by conservative excision with no recurrence. Maxillary lesions occasionally are more diffuse and require wider excision. Since occasional lesions also are multicentric, rigid treatment recommendations cannot be established, especially in view of the limited number of cases reported and the short history of the tumor as an entity.

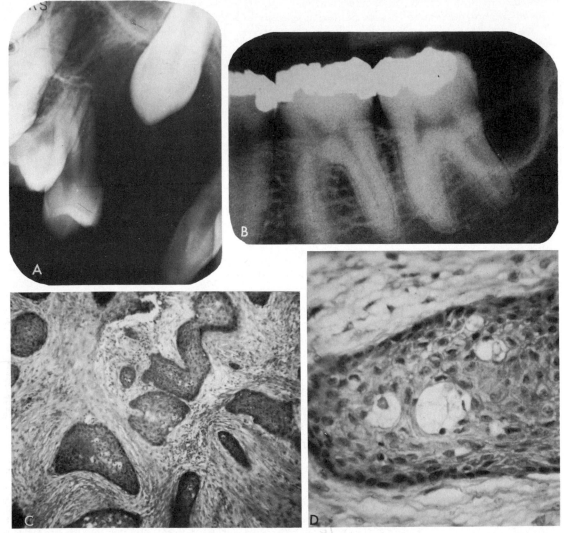

Figure 4–26. *Squamous odontogenic tumor.*

The roentgenographic appearance of the lesion (*A,B*) is nonspecific. However, the innocuous-appearing islands of squamous epithelium are quite characteristic (*C,D*). (*B*, courtesy of Drs. Richard P. Elzay and Bennet Malbon.)

MESODERMAL TUMORS OF ODONTOGENIC ORIGIN

PERIPHERAL ODONTOGENIC FIBROMA

(Peripheral Ossifying Fibroma; Odontogenic Gingival Epithelial Hamartoma; Peripheral Ameloblastic Fibrodentinoma; Peripheral Hamartoma of Dental Lamina Rests; Calcifying Fibrous Epulis)

There are a variety of different types of focal proliferative lesions which may occur on the gingiva, some neoplastic but others inflammatory, including such entities as the peripheral giant cell granuloma, pyogenic granuloma, giant cell fibroma, the simple fibroma, and the peripheral ossifying fibroma (q.v.). At one time, the terms "peripheral ossifying fibroma" and "peripheral odontogenic fibroma" were used quite interchangeably for one of these lesions. However, the World Health Organization (WHO), in its classification of odontogenic tumors, has used the term "peripheral odontogenic fibroma" for a specific entity, quite separate from the peripheral ossifying fibroma, and designated specifically in the past also as an "odontogenic gingival epithelial hamartoma" by Baden and his co-workers and as a "peripheral ameloblastic fibrodentinoma" by numerous oral pathologists such as McKelvy and Cherrick.

The peripheral ossifying fibroma has been separated here from the peripheral odontogenic fibroma and is discussed in Chapter 2 in the Benign Connective Tissue Tumors section. The peripheral odontogenic fibroma, sometimes characterized as the "WHO type," is considered here as an odontogenic tumor. An attempt at clarifying the distinction between these two conditions has been published recently by Gardner.

Clinical Features. The peripheral odontogenic fibroma, in distinct contrast to the peripheral ossifying fibroma, is a rare lesion. The largest series of cases reported has been that of Farman, who found only 5 cases in an extensive review of the English-language literature and added 10 new cases. There was no sex predilection in the 15 reported cases, while the ages of the patients ranged from 5 to 65 years, spaced throughout the various decades. There did seem to be a predilection for occurrence in the mandible, which was the site of 11 cases compared with only 4 cases in the maxilla.

The lesions appear to be slow growing, often present for a number of years. They are generally described as a solid, firmly attached gingival mass, sometimes arising between teeth and sometimes displacing teeth (Fig. 4–27, A). Some lesions are found to contain a calcified stalk at the time of surgery and this, or other islands of calcified material, may be seen as radiopaque flecks on the roentgenogram.

Histologic Features. The peripheral odontogenic fibroma consists of a markedly cellular fibrous connective tissue parenchyma, not the usual bland, acellular collagenous stroma of many tumors, with non-neoplastic islands, strands and cords of columnar or cuboidal, sometimes vacuolated odontogenic epithelium ranging from scanty to numerous. When nu-

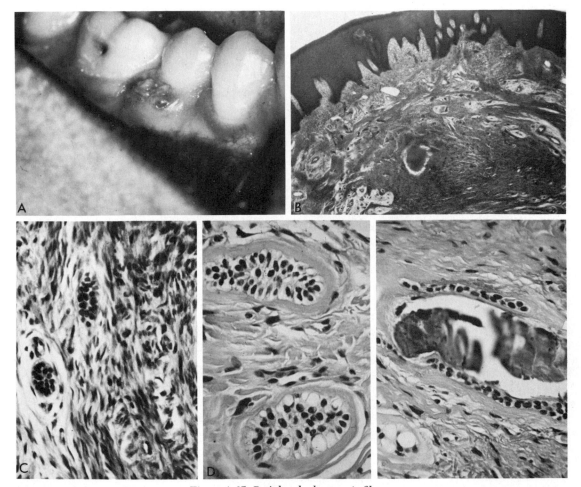

Figure 4–27. *Peripheral odontogenic fibroma.*
The mass on the gingiva (A) is characterized histologically by a cellular connective tissue containing islands of odontogenic epithelial cells, some of which show a clear vacuolated cytoplasm, and few foci of calcifications (B,C,D,E). (A, courtesy of Dr. Richard Henry; D and E, courtesy of Dr. Howard Goldstein.)

merous, the peripheral odontogenic fibroma has been occasionally mistaken for an epithelial neoplasm such as a peripheral ameloblastoma (Fig. 4–27, *B, C, D, E*). This epithelium is usually deep in the lesion, away from the surface epithelium and is sometimes found "cuffing" calcifications. Calcified tissue may or may not be present in the peripheral odontogenic fibroma. If found, it may resemble trabeculae of bone or osteoid, dentin or osteodentin (sometimes described as dysplastic dentin), or cementum-like material. Mature fibrous connective tissue stroma is present and is sometimes highly vascularized, particularly in the less cellular areas. Myxomatous changes may also be found in the stroma, and the presence of inflammation is variable.

Treatment. The lesion is treated by surgical excision. In the series reported by Farman, no lesion was known to recur.

Central Odontogenic Fibroma

The odontogenic fibroma is a central tumor of the jaws which is seen so infrequently that little is known about this neoplasm. Of all the odontogenic tumors, this lesion has the most poorly defined parameters. The major explanation for the uncertainty regarding this tumor, as discussed by Gardner in his attempt at unification of the concept of the central odontogenic fibroma, is the lack of unanimity of definition of the lesion.

Three basic concepts have existed concerning this tumor: (1) it is a lesion around the crown of an unerupted tooth resembling a small dentigerous cyst, although most investigators regard this as simply a hyperplastic dental follicle and not an odontogenic tumor; (2) it is a lesion of fibrous connective tissue, with scattered islands of odontogenic epithelium, bearing some resemblance to the dental follicle but because of the size which it may attain appearing to constitute a neoplasm; and (3) it is a lesion which has been described by the World Health Organization (WHO) as a fibroblastic neoplasm containing varying amounts of odontogenic epithelium and, in some cases, calcified material resembling dysplastic dentin or cementum-like material; thus, except for location, it is histologically identical to the peripheral odontogenic fibroma as described by the WHO group.

Since the occurrence of the latter two lesions in the jaws is undeniable even though their histogenesis is uncertain, Gardner has suggested referring to the tumor made up of connective tissue and odontogenic islands resembling dental follicle as the *simple central odontogenic fibroma* and to the tumor described by the WHO as the *WHO-type central odontogenic fibroma*. Until more cases of each are reported to clarify their histogenesis and their relationship, if any, this approach appears reasonable.

The simple central odontogenic fibroma has been discussed by Wesley and his associates, who reviewed eight cases, including one of their own, which they believed met the histologic criteria for this form of the lesion, while Dahl and her associates have added two more cases. Farman has reviewed eight cases of the WHO type of central odontogenic fibroma from the literature in his paper dealing basically with the peripheral form of this neoplasm. Thus, it may be seen that too few examples of either type of central odontogenic fibroma have been reported from which one may draw any significant conclusions regarding specific clinical features, treatment or prognosis.

Clinical Features. The odontogenic fibroma appears to occur more frequently in children and young adults, although a few cases have been reported in older persons, and has a predilection for occurrence in the mandible. It is generally asymptomatic except for swelling of the jaw.

Roentgenographic Features. This tumor sometimes produces an expansile, multilocular radiolucency similar to that of the ameloblastoma (Fig. 4–28, *A*).

Histologic Features. The odontogenic fibroma of both types has been described above. The *simple type* is characterized by a tumor mass made up of mature collagen fibers interspersed usually by many plump interspersed fibroblasts that are very uniform in their placement and tend to be equidistant from each other. Small nests or islands of odontogenic epithelium that appear entirely inactive are present in variable but usually quite minimal amounts (Fig. 4–28, *B*).

The *WHO type* also consists of relatively mature but quite cellular fibrous connective tissue with few to many islands of odontogenic epithelium. Osteoid, dysplastic dentin or cementum-like material is also variably present.

Care must be exercised not to misdiagnose other fibrous lesions of the jaws as an odontogenic fibroma. Lesions to be considered in the differential diagnosis include neurofibroma and desmoplastic fibroma.

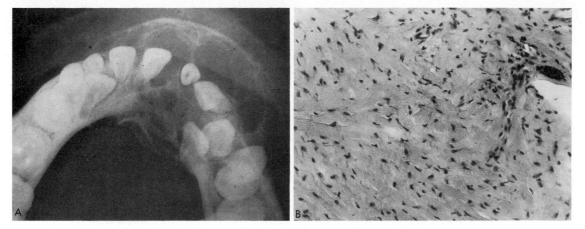

Figure 4–28. *Central odontogenic fibroma.*
The roentgenogram *(A)* exhibits expansion of the mandible with thinning of the cortical plates. The roentgenographic appearance is suggestive of ameloblastoma. The photomicrograph *(B)* shows the bundles of collagen fibers and an epithelial rest. (Courtesy of Dr. Charles A. Waldron.)

Treatment and Prognosis. The treatment of this neoplasm is surgical excision. Little is known about recurrence.

ODONTOGENIC FIBROSARCOMA

The odontogenic fibrosarcoma is the malignant counterpart of the odontogenic fibroma, but is a rare tumor. It originates from the same mesenchymal tissues as the central fibroma, but acts much more aggressively. It is a destructive lesion which produces a fleshy, bulky growth. Pain may be a feature of this neoplasm.

Histologic Features. The designation of odontogenic fibrosarcoma actually may be theoretical since the histologic appearance of this tumor is identical with that of the fibrosarcoma of non-odontogenic origin. The cellular element may or may not be more prominent than the fibrillar component. The cells often exhibit considerable mitotic activity. They resemble immature fibroblasts and appear as elongated cells containing ovoid nuclei with varying degrees of pleomorphism, situated in a fibrous meshwork which may or may not exhibit foci of odontogenic epithelium.

Treatment and Prognosis. The treatment of the odontogenic fibrosarcoma is radical surgical removal with resection of the jaw. The prognosis is poor.

ODONTOGENIC MYXOMA

(Odontogenic Fibromyxoma or Myxofibroma)

The odontogenic myxoma is a tumor of the jaws which apparently arises from the mesenchymal portion of the tooth germ, either the dental papilla, the follicle or the periodontal ligament. Previous reports of this tumor have been discussed by many investigators, most recently White and his colleagues, who summarized pertinent data on over 90 individual and series of cases of odontogenic myxoma of the jaws, including their own group of 9 cases. Absolute proof of origin from the odontogenic apparatus is lacking for this lesion, but it appears most likely because of the frequent occurrence of this lesion in the jaws and almost universal absence in any other bone of the skeleton. For example, in a study by McClure and Dahlin of 6000 cases of bone tumors at the Mayo Clinic up to 1976, no cases involving bones other than the jaws were found.

Clinical Features. The odontogenic myxoma occurs most frequently in the second or third decade of life, the average age in the various reported series ranging from 23 to 30 years. It rarely occurs before the age of 10 years or after the age of 50. There is no particular sex predilection in the occurrence of this tumor, and there is a slight predilection for occurrence in the mandible. Occasional cases occur outside the tooth-bearing areas, several cases having been reported in the condyle or neck of the condyle. In the series reported by Thoma and Goldman nearly every case was associated with missing or embedded teeth. However, in many instances this is not the case.

The odontogenic myxoma is a central lesion of the jaws which expands the bone and may cause destruction of the cortex. It is not a rapidly growing lesion, and pain may or may not be a feature.

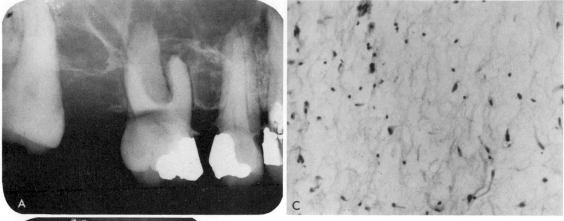

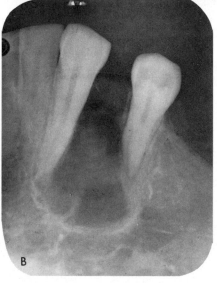

Figure 4–29. *Odontogenic myxoma.*
(Courtesy of Drs. Paul and Emmett Jurgens.)

Roentgenographic Features. The roentgenogram may present a mottled or honeycombed appearance of bone in some cases, while others may appear as a destructive, expanding radiolucency which sometimes has a multilocular pattern (Fig. 4–29, *A, B*). Displacement of teeth by the tumor mass is a relatively common finding, but root resorption is less frequent. The tumor is often extensive before being discovered. Invasion of the antrum occurs frequently in lesions of the maxilla.

Histologic Features. The myxoma is made up of loosely arranged, spindle-shaped and stellate cells, many of which have long fibrillar processes that tend to intermesh (Fig. 4–29, *C*). The loose tissue is not highly cellular, and those cells present do not show evidence of significant activity (pleomorphism, prominent nucleoli or mitotic figures). The intercellular substance is mucoid. The tumor is usually interspersed with a variable number of tiny capillaries and occasionally strands of collagen. Nests of odontogenic epithelium may be found infrequently.

Hodson and Prout have reported the presence of two acid mucopolysaccharides in the odontogenic myxoma: relatively large quantities of hyaluronic acid and lesser amounts of chondroitin sulfate. They have suggested that this high hyaluronic acid component may be a significant factor in the neoplastic behavior of the tumor.

Histochemical studies by Mori and his associates have shown that the tumor cells with long anastomosing processes in the odontogenic myxoma exhibited high alkaline phosphatase and lactate dehydrogenase activity, while there was low acid phosphatase, glucose-6-phosphate dehydrogenase and isocitrate dehydrogenase activity. These enzymatic reactions differed from those present in osteogenic sarcomas or even benign proliferating fibrous lesions such as osteogenic fibroma or a fracture callus. This suggested to the investigators that the tumor cells of the myxoma are not as biologically active as other tumors of the jaws.

Ultrastructural studies have also been reported by several investigators. White and his associates described "pale" cells which probably represented active secretory cells, the "secretion" actually representing transportation of synthesized material thought to be nonsulfated mucopolysaccharide, the myxoid material, into the intercellular compartment. The other cell type, the "dark" cell, contained collagen fibrils, and this suggested a disturbance in the secretory process of collagen molecules so that they became crystallized into fibrils intracellularly.

The ultrastructural studies of Goldblatt have also led him to conclude that the myxoma cell is not a typical fibroblast, that there is an attempt at collagen fibrillogenesis with little ultimate success and that prominent secretory activity within tumor cells appears to result in excess production of acid mucopolysaccharide matrix. He also pointed out that, according to other investigators, there may be actual phagocytosis by tumor cells of the small amount of collagen present. Finally he concluded that, while the myxoma cells showed many characteristics of fibroblasts of the odontogenic apparatus, tumor origin from nonodontogenic mesenchyme cannot be ruled out by existing ultrastructural studies.

Care must be used in distinguishing the odontogenic myxoma histologically from a variety of other myxoid lesions, including myxoid neurofibroma, myxoid liposarcoma, and myxoid chondrosarcoma.

Treatment and Prognosis. The treatment of odontogenic myxomas is surgical excision, followed by cautery. Extensive lesions may require resection to eradicate the tumor. Although this is a benign neoplasm, it frequently exhibits insidious local invasion, making its complete removal difficult, a problem augmented by the loose, gelatinous nature of the tissue itself. The prognosis is good despite unpredictable recurrence. The tumor is not sensitive to x-ray radiation.

A frankly malignant form of this tumor—an odontogenic myxosarcoma—is known but is exceedingly rare.

PERIAPICAL CEMENTAL DYSPLASIA

(Cementoma; Periapical Osteofibroma or Osteofibrosis; Cementifying Fibroma; Localized Fibro-osteoma; Cementoblastoma; Periapical Fibrous Dysplasia)

Periapical cemental dysplasia as classically described is a lesion of rather common occurrence, but it is still a puzzling one to investigators who have attempted to explain its nature. Some adhere strongly to a theory of its origin from odontogenic tissue, the cementum, while others believe that it represents only an unusual reaction of the periapical bone. It is not considered a neoplasm in the usual sense of the term.

Etiology. The etiology of the condition is unknown, although it has been suggested to occur as a result of mild chronic trauma, perhaps traumatogenic occlusion.

The study of Zegarelli and Ziskin considered carefully both the medical and the dental history of the patients involved, but could reach

Table 4–2. Clinical Nature of Periapical Cemental Dysplasia

	NO. OF CASES	SEX M (%)	SEX F (%)	AVERAGE AGE (YRS.)	RACE CAUCASIAN (%)	NEGRO (%)	TYPE OF LESION SINGLE (%)	TYPE OF LESION MULTIPLE (%)	LOCATION MAX. (%)	LOCATION MAND. (%)
Stafne (1934)	65	29	71	43	—	—	(130 teeth involved in the 65 cases)		5	95
Zegarelli and Ziskin (1943)	50	0	100	40	34	66	36	64	13	87
Bernier and Thompson (1946)	15	46	54	37	67	33	87	13	4	96
Chaudhry, Spink and Gorlin (1958)	30	13	87	37	90	10	(51 teeth involved in the 30 cases)		6	94
Zegarelli and co-workers (1964)	230	15	85	—	29	71	30	70	6	94

no conclusions about the etiology. The lesion could not be related to obvious trauma or infection of the tooth, a past history of syphilis or a hormonal disturbance.

The true nature of the condition, despite the fact that it is relatively common, is as obscure today as it was nearly 50 years ago following one of the earliest large surveys of the lesion by Stafne.

Clinical Features. Several series of cases have been reported in the literature, and these provide considerable information about the clinical features of the lesion. These data have been summarized in Table 4–2. In most series the patients with periapical cemental dysplasia are nearly always over 20 years of age, and women appear to be affected far more often than men. In some series, the lesions have occurred predominantly, even almost exclusively, in blacks.

The lesion occurs in and near the periodontal ligament around the apex of a tooth, usually a mandibular incisor. Most cases actually present multiple lesions, the cementomas involving the apices of several mandibular anterior teeth or bicuspids. The maxilla is only rarely the site of a cementoma. Seldom are there any clinical manifestations of the lesion.

Stafne, in an attempt to determine the incidence of the lesion, found 24 cases involving a total of 52 teeth in 10,000 consecutive adult patients, while Chaudhry and his co-workers found 30 cases involving 51 teeth in a review of 10,500 roentgenograms.

Roentgenographic Features. In most instances, it is discovered accidentally during routine intraoral roentgenographic examination of the patient, since the lesion is almost invariably asymptomatic. Occasional lesions localized near the mental foramen appear to impinge on the mental nerve and produce pain, paresthesia or even anesthesia. Whether this is actually cause and effect is questionable. Periapical cemental dysplasia has a definite pattern in its natural history, and for this reason it may present a varied roentgenographic picture depending upon its stage at discovery.

The earliest stage in its development is the formation of a circumscribed area of periapical fibrosis accompanied by localized destruction of the bone. This initial step has been called the *osteolytic stage*. Since there is loss of bony substance and replacement by connective tissue, the lesion appears radiolucent on the roentgenogram (*1* in Fig. 4–30, *A*). Thus it bears close resemblance to periapical lesions such as the granuloma or cyst arising as a result of death

of the pulp through infection or trauma. There can be no doubt that many teeth have been extracted needlessly because of failure of the dentist to recognize the noninfectious nature of the condition. Unless they are coincidentally involved by caries or trauma, teeth exhibiting periapical cemental dysplasia are vital.

The second stage in the development of the lesion is the beginning of calcification in the radiolucent area of fibrosis (Fig. 4–30, *B*, and *2* in Fig. 4–30, *A*). This has been described as increased cementoblastic activity with the deposition of spicules of cementum or cementicles and has been referred to as the *cementoblastic stage*. The stimulus for the formation of this calcified material has not been determined.

The third stage in the natural history of this lesion is the so-called *mature stage*, in which an excessive amount of calcified material is deposited in the focal area and appears on the roentgenogram as a well defined radiopacity that is usually bordered by a thin radiolucent line or band (Fig. 4–30, *C*). Thus there may be considerable roentgenographic similarity between the mature stage of periapical cemental dysplasia and the so-called condensing osteitis or chronic focal sclerosing osteomyelitis, a periapical reaction of bone usually in response to infection (q.v.).

Treatment and Prognosis. The treatment of this lesion consists simply in recognition of the condition and periodic observation, since it is harmless. Under no circumstances should one extract the tooth, institute endodontic procedures or otherwise disturb the tooth unless for reasons not related to the condition. Since difficulty may occasionally be encountered in distinguishing roentgenographically between this and a periapical granuloma, the necessity of testing the pulp for vitality must be strongly emphasized.

CENTRAL CEMENTIFYING FIBROMA

The central cementifying fibroma is a neoplasm of bone which has caused considerable controversy because of confusion of terminology and criteria of diagnosis. It now appears that this represents a definite entity which should be separated from fibrous dysplasia of bone and certain other fibro-osseous lesions which do not represent true neoplasms. This concept has been discussed by Pindborg, by Waldron and many others.

It has been suggested by Shafer and Waldron

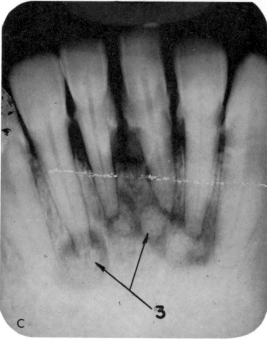

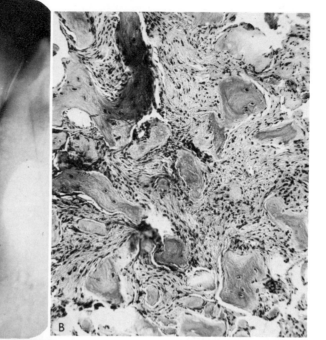

Figure 4–30. *Periapical cemental dysplasia.*
A, The roentgenogram shows a cementoma in the early or "osteolytic" stage *(1)* and a later or "cementoblastic" stage *(2)*. *B,* The photomicrograph is a section of a cementoma in the "cementoblastic" stage. The similarity of the calcified tissue to bone is obvious. *C,* The roentgenogram demonstrates a typical mature case of cementoma *(3)*.

that a close histogenetic relationship exists between the central cementifying fibroma and the central ossifying fibroma (q.v.). They have stated that, based on the marked similarity between the two regarding predilection for age of occurrence, sex, race, location, roentgenographic appearance and clinical behavior, these two lesions represent the same basic neoplastic process, the only difference being in the cell involved with its end product: cementum in one case, bone in the other. Furthermore, many tumors in this general category are characterized by the presence of both types of cells, but probably the same progenitor cell, thus giving rise to the well-recognized hybrid form of the tumor: the cemento-ossifying fibroma.

Clinical Features. The central cementifying fibroma may occur at any age, but is more common in young and middle-aged adults, with a mean age of occurrence of 35 years. Furthermore, there is a marked predilection for occurrence in females by a ratio of about 2:1. Either jaw may be involved, but there appears to be a marked predilection for the mandible, as confirmed by the series reported by Hamner and his associates. Of the 43 cases in the series of Shafer and Waldron, approximately 80 per cent occurred in the mandible.

The lesion is generally asymptomatic until the growth produces a noticeable swelling and mild deformity; displacement of teeth may be an early clinical feature. It is a relatively slow-growing tumor and may be present for some years before discovery. Because of this slow growth, the cortical plates of bone and overlying mucosa or skin are almost invariably intact.

Roentgenographic Features. The neoplasm presents an extremely variable roentgeno-

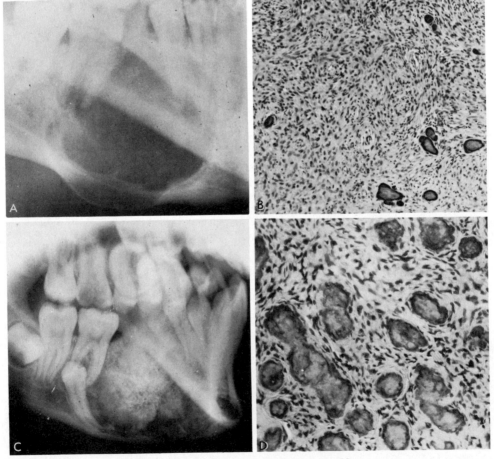

Figure 4–31. *Central cementifying fibroma of bone.*
A, The well-circumscribed radiolucency represents an early stage of the disease as characterized in *B* by the cellular, fibrillar stroma with few cementum-like structures. *C*, A more mature form of cementifying fibroma showing a similar well-circumscribed lesion. It is radiopaque, owing to the great number of cemental structures in *D*. (Courtesy of Drs. C. E. Hopkins and Wilbur C. Moorman.)

graphic appearance depending upon its stage of development. Yet despite the stage of development, the lesion is always well circumscribed and demarcated from surrounding bone, in contrast to true fibrous dysplasia.

In its early stages, or at least in one form of the disease, the cementifying fibroma appears as a radiolucent lesion with no evidence of internal radiopacities (Fig. 4–31, A). As the tumor apparently matures, there is increasing calcification, so that the radiolucent area becomes flecked with opacities until, ultimately, the lesion appears as an extremely radiopaque mass (Fig. 4–31,C). This may actually represent another form of the disease rather than maturation of a given case. Displacement of adjacent teeth is common, as well as impingement upon other adjacent structures.

One additional important diagnostic feature of this lesion is its effect upon the inferior border of the mandible when the lesion reaches such a size as to encroach upon it. The central cementifying fibroma and its related lesions, the central ossifying fibroma and central cemento-ossifying fibroma, have a centrifugal growth pattern rather than a linear one. Therefore, the lesions grow by expansion equally in all directions and present as a round tumor mass. When the mass reaches the inferior border of the mandible, it produces an expansion whose outline is in continuity with the outline of the tumor mass above. These three related lesions are the only three central tumors of the mandible which produce this characteristic phenomenon. Other lesions (e.g., fibrous dysplasia of bone) expand cortex linearly and the outline of the expanded mandible is not in continuity with the remainder of the outline of the lesion.

Histologic Features. The lesion is composed basically of many delicate interlacing collagen fibers, seldom arranged in discrete bundles, interspersed by large numbers of active, proliferating fibroblasts or cementoblasts. Although mitotic figures may be present in small numbers, there is seldom any remarkable cellular pleomorphism. This connective tissue characteristically presents many small foci of basophilic masses of cementum-like tissue (Fig. 4–31, B). These islands are generally irregularly round, ovoid or slightly elongated, often lobulated, and do not present the bizarre Chinese-character shape of the bony trabeculae in fibrous dysplasia of bone (q.v.).

As the lesion matures, the islands of cementum increase in number, enlarge and ultimately coalesce (Fig. 4–31, D). This, with the probable increase in degree of calcification, accounts for increasing radiopaqueness of the lesion on the roentgenogram. The microscopic features of this lesion are characteristic, and it should be carefully separated from other fibro-osseous lesions.

In some cases, instead of the lesion being composed entirely of globules of cementum-like tissue, there will be varying amounts of trabeculae of bone scattered throughout. To recognize the mixed nature of the tumor, the term "cemento-ossifying fibroma" has been applied to such cases.

Treatment and Prognosis. The lesion, which is almost invariably sharply circumscribed and demarcated from bone, should be excised conservatively. Recurrence is rare.

BENIGN CEMENTOBLASTOMA

(True Cementoma)

The benign cementoblastoma is probably a true neoplasm of functional cementoblasts which form a large mass of cementum or cementum-like tissue on the tooth root. It is quite distinctive but relatively uncommon, although 55 cases have been reported up to 1979, according to Farman and his associates.

Clinical Features. The benign cementoblastoma occurs most frequently under the age of 25 years, with no significant sex predilection. More than half of the tumors have occurred in persons under 20 years of age, although the range has been 10 to 72 years. When the site has been specified, the mandible is affected three times more frequently than the maxilla. The mandibular first permanent molar is the most frequently affected tooth. In fact, only one case is reported involving the deciduous dentition. Involvement of this mandibular first molar has accounted for approximately 50 per cent of all reported cases. However, other teeth involved have included mandibular second and third molars, mandibular bicuspids, maxillary bicuspids and first, second and third molars. The associated tooth is vital unless coincidentally involved. The lesion is slow-growing and may cause expansion of cortical plates of bone, but is usually otherwise asymptomatic. Pain has been reported, but this may have been related to associated caries rather than to the lesion.

Roentgenographic Features. The tumor mass is attached to the tooth root and appears as a well-circumscribed dense radiopaque mass often surrounded by a thin, uniform radiolucent line (Fig. 4–32, A, B). The outline of the affected root is generally obliterated because of

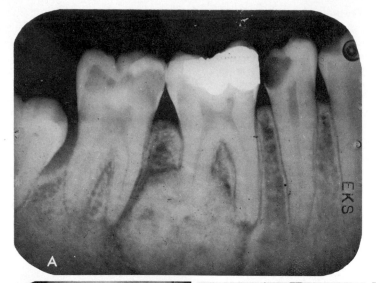

Figure 4–32. *Benign cementoblastoma.*
The large calcified mass present associated with the distal root of the mandibular first molar in the periapical roentgenogram *(A)* is producing bulging of the lingual plate of the mandible *(B)*. The photomicrograph *(C)* shows the mass to be continuous and identical with the cementum, while the extreme cellular activity bordering the trabeculae of matrix is evident *(D)*.

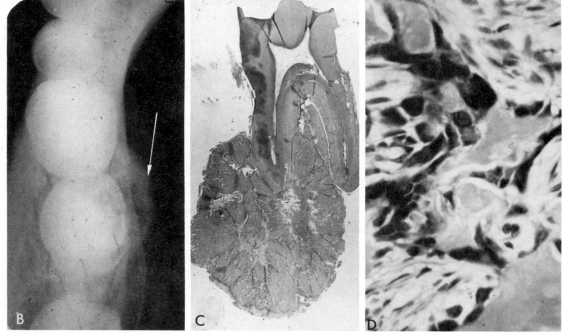

resorption of the root and fusion of the mass to the tooth.

Histologic Features. The main bulk of the tumor mass is composed of sheets of cementum-like tissue, sometimes resembling secondary cellular cementum but other times being deposited in a globular pattern resembling giant cementicles (Fig. 4–32, *C*). Reversal lines scattered throughout this calcified tissue are often quite prevalent. There is a variable soft-tissue component consisting of fibrillar, vascular and cellular elements. Many of the cemental trabeculae in areas of activity are bordered by layers of cementoblasts (Fig. 4–32, *D*). Away from these trabecular surfaces, cementoclasts may be evident. In such active areas, the lesion is frequently microscopically indistinguishable from the benign osteoblastoma or giant osteoid osteoma, and this relationship has been discussed by Larsson and his associates. In fact, some areas are so cellularly active that they bear strong resemblance to osteosarcoma.

This calcified mass will be found united to the tooth root through obliteration of the periodontal ligament, resorption of portion of the root and replacement by the tumor tissue. The periphery of the tumor generally shows a soft tissue cellular layer resembling a capsule. At this periphery, the cemental trabeculae are almost invariably arranged at right angles.

Treatment and Prognosis. Because of the tendency for expansion of the jaw, it is believed that extraction of the tooth is justified despite the fact that the pulp is vital. Care must be taken to distinguish this lesion from severe hypercementosis or chronic focal sclerosing osteomyelitis (i.e., condensing osteitis), both of which it may superficially resemble. The lesion does not appear to recur.

GIGANTIFORM CEMENTOMA

(Familial Multiple Cementoma)

The gigantiform cementoma is a very rare condition which may or may not prove to be a distinct entity. In several cases reported by Agazzi and Belloni, the lesions had their onset at a young age, developed slowly and involved all four jaw quadrants. The lesions occurred in families and appeared to be inherited as an autosomal dominant characteristic, although other reported cases are nonfamilial and do not support this claim.

Other cases have been reported to be most common in adult black females. Most present as diffuse radiopaque masses scattered throughout the jaws, sometimes expanding the jaw. These have been described as consisting of dense, highly calcified, almost totally acellular cementum which is poorly vascularized and frequently becomes infected with ensuing suppuration and sequestration.

The scanty literature dealing with the gigantiform cementoma has been reviewed by Punniamoorthy, who has noted that the origin of the lesion is still a mystery, although it has been suggested by Pindborg and his colleagues in the World Health Organization (WHO) Odontogenic Group to be some form of dysplasia or even a hamartomatous condition. Punniamoorthy has also pointed out that numerous cases of lesions of the jaws have been reported in the literature which are very similar to the gigantiform cementoma in clinical, roentgenographic and histologic features but yet have been described under different terms such as chronic sclerosing osteomyelitis, sclerotic cemental masses, chronic productive osteitis, osseous dysplasia and multiple enostosis, among others. It has also been emphasized that similar masses occur in some cases of osteitis deformans or Paget's disease of bone.

There must be further clarification of this disease entity if, in fact, it actually proves to be such, in order to separate it from other diseases with certain similar features.

DENTINOMA

The dentinoma is an extremely rare tumor of odontogenic origin composed of immature connective tissue, odontogenic epithelium and irregular or dysplastic dentin, according to the WHO Odontogenic Group. Pindborg reviewed the literature and found only nine published cases, some of which are controversial. In fact, the entire concept of this tumor is controversial and some authorities do not accept the lesion as an entity.

Clinical Features. The dentinoma seems to occur predominantly central in the mandible, especially in the molar area, and frequently is associated with an impacted tooth. The patients are usually young, the average age in the cases reviewed by Pindborg being 26 years; there is no apparent sex predilection. The majority of patients noted swelling present for a variable period of time; pain, perforation of mucosa and subsequent infection also have been presenting complaints.

Roentgenographic Features. The roentgenographic findings are not specific, but usually there is a radiolucent area in the bone containing either a large, solitary, opaque mass or numerous smaller, irregular, radiopaque masses of calcified material which vary considerably in size. Such findings are similar to those noted in the simple odontoma as well as in the ameloblastic fibro-odontoma.

In some cases, the dentin is present in relatively small quantities or is only poorly calcified so that there are no opacities in the radiolucency.

Histologic Features. The dentinoma is composed of masses of irregular dentin which has been termed "dentinoid" or "osteodentin." The connective tissue often resembles the dental papilla but the degree of cellularity varies. It is difficult to justify the diagnosis of dentinoma unless recognizable dentinal tubules are present. The occurrence of enamel or enamel matrix precludes the diagnosis of dentinoma, since, by definition, an irregular mass of enamel and dentin should be designated as a complex composite odontoma.

The presence of undifferentiated odontogenic epithelium has been found to be quite characteristic. This is not surprising, since it is well established that odontogenic epithelium is necessary for the differentiation of odontoblasts. The unusual feature is the lack of enamel formation, since it is equally well established that enamel formation is induced by dentin deposition and takes place after dentin deposition has begun. The general pattern of the primitive odontogenic epithelium and connective tissue is similar to that of the ameloblastic fibroma. On occasion, the epithelial component has been found to be proliferating in a neoplastic fashion, along with the connective tissue portion of the lesion, with dysplastic dentin being formed; and in these cases, the term "ameloblastic fibrodentinoma" has been applied. Its relationship, if any, to the WHO type of central odontogenic fibroma remains unsettled.

Treatment and Prognosis. The treatment of the dentinoma is surgical excision with thorough curettage of the area. Some lesions are reported to have a connective tissue capsule which, if remnants are left at the time of operation, may be the basis for recurrence of the dentinoma.

The lesion is benign in that it never metastasizes, but there may be considerable local destruction of bone by the tumor.

MIXED TISSUE TUMORS OF ODONTOGENIC ORIGIN

AMELOBLASTIC FIBROMA

(Soft Mixed Odontogenic Tumor; Soft Mixed Odontoma; Fibroadamantoblastoma)

The ameloblastic fibroma is a relatively uncommon neoplasm of odontogenic origin which is characterized by the simultaneous proliferation of both epithelial and mesenchymal tissue without the formation of enamel or dentin. Thus this may be viewed as an example of a true mixed tumor.

Some investigators have suggested, however, that the ameloblastic fibroma represents an immature complex odontoma and that, if the tumor is left undisturbed, it will ultimately differentiate or mature further into a lesion known as an ameloblastic fibro-odontoma (q.v.) and then continue maturation into a completely differentiated odontoma. In contrast, Eversole and his co-workers, in a discussion of the histogenesis of odontogenic tumors, have proposed that the mixed odontogenic tumors are solely and totally dependent upon the presence of differentiation factors which are or are not elab-

orated by a particular tumor. Thus, they have concluded that there is little probability of sequential differentiating events resulting in the progression of an immature entity such as the ameloblastic fibroma into a highly differentiated entity such as the complex odontoma. As Eversole and his associates discussed and as Slootweg has emphasized, if these three lesions— the ameloblastic fibroma, the ameloblastic fibro-odontoma and the odontoma—were simply stages in a continuum, clinical data on each of the lesions should support this. For example, the ameloblastic fibroma should occur in younger patients, the odontoma in somewhat older patients and the ameloblastic fibro-odontoma in an intermediate age group. In addition, the sex predilection and the distribution of all lesions should be the same. Slootweg has investigated this problem utilizing data from 55 reported cases of ameloblastic fibroma, 50 cases of ameloblastic fibro-odontoma, 77 cases of complex odontoma and 48 cases of compound odontoma. While correction had to be made for the fact that the odontogenic apparatus is active in various parts of the jaws at various ages, Slootweg concluded that the ameloblastic fibroma represents a separate specific neoplastic entity that does not develop into a more differentiated odontogenic lesion. He also concluded from his data that the ameloblastic fibro-odontoma does represent an immature complex odontoma, a hamartomatous rather than neoplastic odontogenic lesion.

Clinical Features. The ameloblastic fibroma, arising most commonly in the molar region of the mandible, is similar in location to the simple ameloblastoma. Nearly 75 per cent of the 55 cases reviewed by Slootweg occurred in this location. There is a considerable difference, however, in the age group of patients most commonly affected. Whereas the simple ameloblastoma occurs typically in middle-aged persons, the average age of the patient at the time of discovery being approximately 33 years according to Small and Waldron, the ameloblastic fibroma occurs in much younger persons. In the review of 55 cases, Slootweg found that the average age of patients with the ameloblastic fibroma was 14.6 years, with 40 per cent of the patients under the age of 10 years. He also reported that there was a very slight predilection for occurrence in males.

This tumor exhibits somewhat slower clinical growth than the simple ameloblastoma and does not tend to infiltrate between trabeculae of bone. Instead it enlarges by gradual expansion

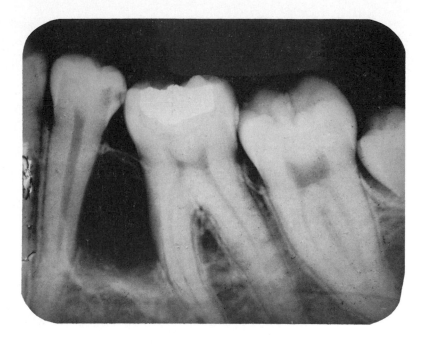

Figure 4–33. *Ameloblastic fibroma.*
The neoplasm was asymptomatic and was discovered during routine roentgenographic examination.

so that the periphery of the lesion often remains smooth. It will frequently cause no complaint on the part of the patient and has been discovered accidentally during roentgenographic examination. Pain, tenderness or mild swelling of the jaw may induce the patient to seek aid from the dentist, however.

Roentgenographic Features. No constant significant differences between the appearance of the simple ameloblastoma and that of the ameloblastic fibroma are found. The latter is manifested as a unilocular or multilocular, radiolucent lesion which has a rather smooth outline, often with a sclerotic border, and which may or may not produce evident bulging of bone (Fig. 4–33) In the study of 24 cases by Trodahl, most of the lesions were associated with unerupted teeth. In addition, he found considerable variation roentgenographically in the size of lesions, there being a range of 1 to 8.5 cm. in diameter.

Histologic Features. The microscopic appearance of this odontogenic neoplasm is characteristic. The ectodermal portion consists of scattered islands of epithelial cells in a variety of patterns, including rosettes, long finger-like strands, nest and cords. These epithelial cells are usually of a cuboidal or columnar type and bear close resemblance to primitive odontogenic epithelium. Mitotic activity is not common. Because the pattern of these cells is one of strands and cords, tissue resembling stellate reticulum is often not seen. However, occa-

sional cases occur in which some of these tumor islands are found "opening," with the formation of stellate reticulum. The resemblance to the dental lamina is far more striking in this lesion than in the simple ameloblastoma (Fig. 4–34, A, B).

The mesenchymal component is made up of a primitive connective tissue that in some cases shows closely intertwining fibrils interspersed by large connective tissue cells closely resembling those of the dental papilla. There may be a paucity of blood vessels, and juxtaepithelial hyalinization of areas of the connective tissue occurs. On occasion, this may even resemble dysplastic dentin. Electron microscope studies have suggested that this apparent hyalinization may, instead, actually represent exuberant basal lamina.

Treatment and Prognosis. The treatment of the ameloblastic fibroma has been somewhat more conservative than that of the simple ameloblastoma, since it does not appear to infiltrate bone as actively or as widely as the ameloblastoma. It also tends to separate from the bone more readily.

At one time the ameloblastic fibroma was regarded as exhibiting little tendency for recurrence, even following the most conservative surgical removal. This was based in part on the review by Gorlin and his associates of 35 documented cases with only 2 instances of recurrence (approximately 6 per cent). In contrast,

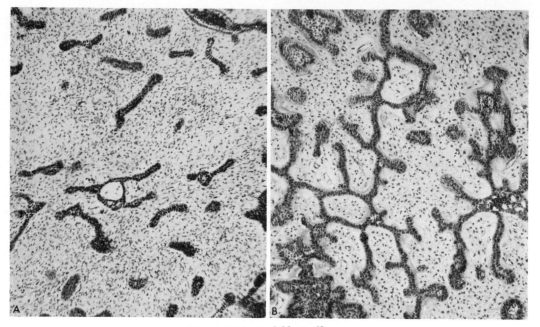

Figure 4–34. *Ameloblastic fibroma.*

Trodahl subsequently reported 10 recurrences in his series of 24 cases (approximately 44 per cent). Since these two series, numerous other instances of recurrent lesions have been reported, and these have been reviewed and discussed by Zallen and his colleagues, who noted a total cumulative recurrence rate of 18.3 per cent for this lesion. In addition, there have been a surprising number of cases reported of ameloblastic fibrosarcoma originating, at least in some instances, in a recurrent ameloblastic fibroma, as in the cases of Leider and his associates. Thus, it would seem that a somewhat more aggressive surgical removal, rather than simple curettage, should be considered for this lesion.

AMELOBLASTIC FIBROSARCOMA

(Ameloblastic Sarcoma)

The ameloblastic fibrosarcoma is the malignant counterpart of the ameloblastic fibroma in which the mesenchymal element has become malignant. The tumor is exceedingly rare, although 17 cases had been reported according to the review of Lieder and his associates, while 5 additional cases were reviewed by Howell and Burkes, who added 2 new cases originating from ameloblastic fibro-odontomas. However, one of these latter cases contained dysplastic dentin, but no enamel, with the malignant mesenchymal component and therefore corresponds to the lesion described by Altini and Shear as an *ameloblastic dentinosarcoma*. This appears to represent a form of that exceedingly rare tumor termed an *ameloblastic odontosarcoma*, which has been defined by the WHO group as a tumor similar to the ameloblastic fibrosarcoma but one in which limited amounts of dysplastic dentin and enamel have formed.

Clinical Features. The ameloblastic fibrosarcoma occurs most frequently in young adults, as does its benign counterpart, although the latter is seen at an even earlier age. Of the cases reported in the literature, the average age was 30 years, with no sex predilection. The lesion occurs more frequently in the mandible than in the maxilla.

The tumor is almost uniformly painful, generally grows rapidly and causes destruction of bone with loosening of the teeth. In addition, ulceration and bleeding of the overlying mucosa have been reported.

Roentgenographic Features. The roentgenographic appearance of this neoplasm is generally one of severe bone destruction, with irregular and poorly defined margins. There may also be gross expansion and thinning of cortical bone. In maxillary lesions, involvement of the antrum may occur. Thus, the picture is not specific and resembles only that of any malignant destructive neoplasm.

Histologic Features. The majority of reported cases appear to arise through malignant transformation of a benign pre-existing ameloblastic fibroma. There is no apparent remarkable change in the odontogenic epithelium in the malignant tumor and it maintains its benign appearance. In some lesions, it is diminished in quantity, apparently as a result of overgrowth of the malignant mesenchymal portion of the lesion. This mesenchymal tissue exhibits a remarkable increase in cellularity, the malignant fibroblasts being bizarre and pleomorphic, with hyperchromatic nuclei and numerous atypical mitotic figures.

Treatment and Prognosis. The treatment for the ameloblastic fibrosarcoma is radical resection. As with most sarcomas, recurrence may be expected and the prognosis is relatively poor. Of the 24 reported cases, about one-half of the patients had one or more recurrences, although a number were lost to follow-up. Six patients were known to have died of their disease.

AMELOBLASTIC FIBRO-ODONTOMA

The ameloblastic fibro-odontoma has been confused in the earlier literature with a lesion of similar nomenclature, the ameloblastic odontoma (q.v.), although a clear distinction between the two was finally drawn by Hooker in 1967 at the annual meeting of the American Academy of Oral Pathology. It has been emphasized that some investigators, furthermore,

have believed that the ameloblastic fibroma (q.v.) represents an early, undifferentiated complex odontoma and that the ameloblastic fibro-odontoma is simply a further differentiated maturing odontoma. After investigating this problem, Slootweg concluded that the ameloblastic fibroma is a true neoplasm and does not differentiate into an ameloblastic fibro-odontoma. This evidence has been discussed in the section on ameloblastic fibroma. He also concluded that the ameloblastic fibro-odontoma to be discussed here did in fact represent an immature complex odontoma and, therefore, represented a hamartomatous rather than a neoplastic odontogenic lesion.

Clinical Features. The original report by Hooker consisted of 26 cases of ameloblastic fibro-odontoma. Of these 26 cases, there were 20 male and 6 female for a ratio of 3.3:1 in favor of the males. However, of the 50 cases reviewed by Slootweg, which did not include the 26 cases of Hooker, there were 28 males and 22 females. The age range of the cases in the series of Hooker was 0.5 to 39 years with the mean being 11.5 years of age. Nineteen of the 26 cases occurred under the age of 15, only 2 cases over the age of 20. In the Slootweg series, the mean age was 8.1 years, with 62 per cent of the patients under the age of 10 years. Hooker's cases were evenly divided between the maxilla and mandible with 13 each. Nine of the 13 cases in the maxilla, and 10 of the 13 in the mandible occurred in the molar area. All cases were associated with an impacted tooth and 3 cases involved the maxillary sinus. Of Slootweg's cases, 38 per cent were in the maxilla

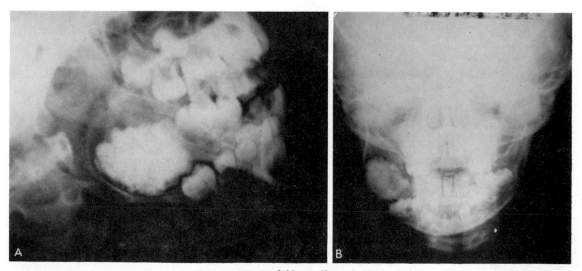

Figure 4–35. *Ameloblastic fibro-odontoma.*

and 62 per cent in the mandible, with 54 per cent occurring in the posterior mandible.

Clinical manifestations of the lesion are often absent. The two most common presenting complaints are swelling and failure of tooth eruption.

Roentgenographic Features. The ameloblastic fibro-odontoma is almost invariably a well-circumscribed lesion, presenting as an expansile radiolucency generally containing either a solitary radiopaque mass or multiple small opacities representing the odontoma portion of the lesion (Fig. 4–35). Some of the lesions are relatively small when first detected, measuring not over 1 to 2 cm. in diameter, while others may be exceedingly large, involving a considerable portion of the body of the mandible and even extending into the ramus. Occasionally, these lesions will become huge. A case was illustrated by Miller and his associates in their series that showed the calcified mass alone to measure 6 cm. by 7 cm. and that had produced a terrible facial deformity.

Histologic Features. The lesion consists of the same apparent type of tissue as seen in the ameloblastic fibroma. Thus, there is found cords, fingers, strands and rosettes of primitive odontogenic columnar or cuboidal epithelial cells, often resembling dental lamina. The mesenchymal component is an embryonic fibrous connective tissue with delicate fibrils interspersed by large primitive fibroblasts, all resembling dental papilla. In addition, typical composite odontoma is found.

Treatment and Prognosis. The ameloblastic fibro-odontoma is treated by curettage, since it does not appear to locally invade bone. There appears to be little tendency for recurrence of the ameloblastic fibro-odontoma. Tsagaris reviewed a total of 77 cases, including Hooker's 26 cases from the Armed Forces Institute of Pathology, and, of 29 cases which he was able to follow up, found only one recurrence.

ODONTOMA

The term "odontoma," by definition alone, refers to any tumor of odontogenic origin. Through usage, however, it has come to mean a growth in which both the epithelial and the mesenchymal cells exhibit complete differentiation, with the result that functional ameloblasts and odontoblasts form enamel and dentin. This enamel and dentin are usually laid down in an abnormal pattern because the organization of the odontogenic cells fails to reach a normal state of morpho-differentiation. Most authorities accept the view today that the odontoma represents a hamartomatous malformation rather than a neoplasm. This lesion is composed of more than one type of tissue and, for this reason, has been called a composite odontoma. In some composite odontomas the enamel and dentin are laid down in such a fashion that the structures bear considerable anatomic resemblance to normal teeth, except that they are often smaller than typical teeth. They have been termed *compound composite odontomas* when there is at least superficial anatomic similarity to normal teeth. On the other hand, when the calcified dental tissues are simply an irregular mass bearing no morphologic similarity even to rudimentary teeth, the term *complex composite odontoma* is used. The complex form of odontoma is less common than the compound type.

Etiology. The etiology of the odontoma is unknown. It has been suggested that local trauma or infection may lead to the production of such a lesion. This is entirely possible, but it would appear more likely that in such an event hypoplasia would be the end-result, depending upon the stage of odontogenesis. There is no seeming predilection for occurrence of the odontoma in particular sites of the oral cavity; it does not appear to be associated especially with supernumerary teeth, as might be suggested were it to occur with great frequency between the maxillary central incisors or distal to the maxillary third molar.

It has been suggested by Hitchin that odontomas are either inherited or are due to a mutant gene or interference, possibly postnatal, with the genetic control of tooth development. On the other hand, Levy has reported the experimental production of this lesion in the rat by traumatic injury.

Clinical Features. The odontoma may be discovered at any age in any location of the dental arch, maxillary or mandibular. Budnick has compiled an analysis of 149 cases of odontoma (76 complex and 73 compound) from the literature (65 cases) and from the files of Emory University (84 cases). While it may be discovered·at any age, from the very young to the very elderly, he found the mean age of detection to be 14.8 years, with the most prevalent age for diagnosis and treatment being the second decade of life. He also found a slight predilection for occurrence in males (59 per cent) compared with females (41 per cent).

Of all odontomas combined, 67 per cent

occurred in the maxilla and 33 per cent in the mandible. The compound odontoma had predilection in this study for the anterior maxilla (61 per cent), whereas only 34 per cent of complex odontomas occurred here. In general, complex odontomas had a predilection for the posterior jaws (59 per cent) and lastly the premolar area (7 per cent). Interestingly, both types of odontomas occurred more frequently on the right side of the jaw than on the left (compound, 62 per cent; complex, 68 per cent). The odontoma usually remains small, the diameter of the mass only occasionally greatly exceeding that of a tooth. Occasionally it does become large and may produce expansion of

bone with consequent facial asymmetry. This is particularly true if a dentigerous cyst develops around the odontoma.

Most odontomas are asymptomatic, although occasionally signs and symptoms relating to their presence do occur. These generally consist of unerupted or impacted teeth, retained deciduous teeth, swelling and evidence of infection.

Roentgenographic Features. The roentgenographic appearance of the odontoma is characteristic. Since most odontomas are clinically asymptomatic and are discovered by routine roentgenographic examination, the dentist should be familiar with their appearance. They are often situated between the roots of teeth

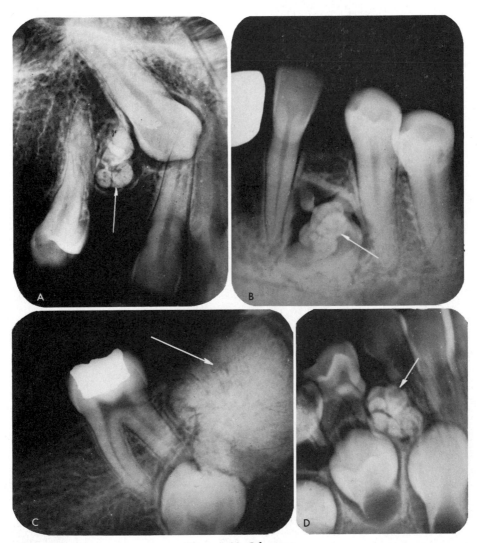

Figure 4–36. *Odontoma.*

Roentgenograms *A* and *B* illustrate two examples of compound composite odontoma, and *C* shows an example of a complex composite odontoma. The odontoma may also occur in young children, as seen in roentgenogram *D*. (Illustration *C* courtesy of Dr. Wilbur C. Moorman.)

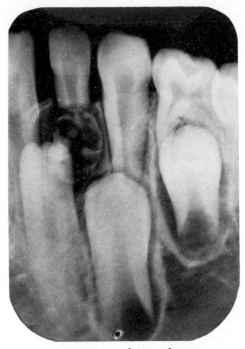

Figure 4–37. *Developing odontoma.*

contain several dozen (Fig. 4–36). Both forms of odontoma are frequently associated with unerupted teeth. It is of interest that the majority of odontomas in the anterior segments of the jaws are compound composite in type, while the majority in the posterior areas are complex composite. This latter odontoma may appear also as a calcified mass overlying the crown of an unerupted or impacted tooth. A developing odontoma may be discovered on the routine roentgenogram and present difficulty in diagnosis because of the lack of calcification (Fig. 4–37).

Histologic Features. The histologic appearance of the odontoma is not spectacular. One finds normal-appearing enamel or enamel matrix, dentin, pulp tissue and cementum which may or may not exhibit a normal relation to one another (Fig. 4–38). If the morphologic resemblance to teeth does exist, the structures are usually single-rooted. The connective tissue capsule around the odontoma is similar in all respects to the follicle surrounding a normal tooth.

One additional interesting feature is the presence of "ghost" cells in odontomas. These are the same cells described in the calcifying odontogenic cyst (q.v.) and have been reported by Levy to be present in nearly 20 per cent of a series of 43 odontomas which he investigated. This has been substantiated by Sedano and Pindborg, although they could find no significance attached to the presence of these cells

and appear either as an irregular mass of calcified material surrounded by a narrow radiolucent band with a smooth outer periphery (Fig. 4–36), or as a variable number of toothlike structures with the same peripheral outline. This latter type of odontoma may contain only a few structures resembling teeth, or it may

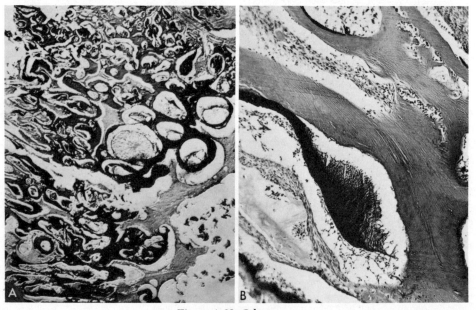

Figure 4–38. *Odontoma.*
The admixture of dental tissues is illustrated in the photomicrographs.

regarding prognosis or treatment of the odontoma.

Treatment and Prognosis. The treatment of the odontoma is surgical removal, and there is no expectancy of recurrence. Since both the ameloblastic odontoma and the ameloblastic fibro-odontoma bear great resemblance to the common odontoma, particularly on the roentgenogram, it is suggested that all odontomas be sent to a qualified oral pathologist for microscopic examination.

AMELOBLASTIC ODONTOMA

(Odontoameloblastoma; Adamanto-odontoma; Soft and Calcified Odontoma)

The ameloblastic odontoma is an odontogenic neoplasm characterized by the simultaneous occurrence of an ameloblastoma and a composite odontoma. As judged by the reported cases reviewed by Frissell and Shafer, it is a rare clinical entity. It should not be inferred that this tumor represents two separate neoplasms growing in unison; there exists, rather, a peculiar proliferation of tissue of the odontogenic apparatus in an unrestrained pattern, including complete morphodifferentiation, as well as apposition and even calcification. The lesion is unusual in that a relatively undifferentiated neoplastic tissue is associated with a highly differentiated tissue, both of which may show recurrence after inadequate removal.

Clinical Features. So few cases of this tumor have been reported that any statistical information may not be valid. However, the ameloblastic odontoma appears to occur at any age, but more frequently in children, and is somewhat more common in the mandible than in the maxilla. It is a slowly expanding lesion of bone which produces considerable facial deformity or asymmetry if left untreated. Since it is a central lesion, considerable destruction of bone occurs. Mild pain may be a presenting complaint, as well as delayed eruption of teeth.

Roentgenographic Features. Central destruction of bone with expansion of the cortical plates is prominent. The characteristic feature is the presence within the lesion proper of numerous small radiopaque masses which may or may not bear resemblance to formed, albeit miniature, teeth (Fig. 4–39, A). In other instances there is only a single, irregular radiopaque mass of calcified tissue present. Thus the roentgenographic appearance of the ameloblastic odontoma is identical with that of the composite odontoma of one form or another.

Histologic Features. The microscopic appearance of this tumor is both unusual and characteristic. It consists of a great variety of cells and

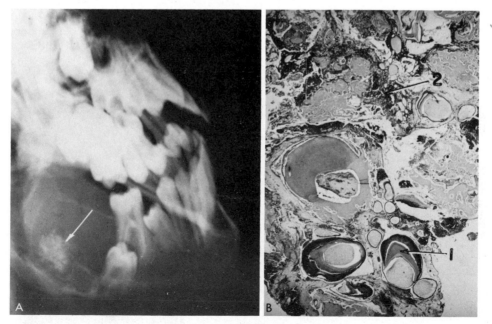

Figure 4–39. *Ameloblastic odontoma.*
The roentgenogram *(A)* shows the destructive lesion of the mandible containing numerous small, irregular calcified masses. The photomicrograph *(B)* reveals that these are dental tissue, enamel and dentin *(1)*, in association with an ameloblastoma *(2)*.

tissues in a complex distribution, including columnar, squamous and undifferentiated epithelial cells, as well as ameloblasts, enamel and enamel matrix, dentin, osteodentin, dentinoid and osteoid material, stellate reticulum-like tissue, dental papilla, bone and cementum as well as stromal connective tissue (Fig. 4–39, *B*). Many structures resembling normal or atypical tooth germs may be found, with or without the presence of calcified dental tissues. In addition, an outstanding characteristic is the presence of sheets of typical ameloblastoma of one or another of the recognized types—usually basal cell, follicular or plexiform. Few mitotic figures are present even though the proliferative tendencies of the epithelial cells are obvious.

Treatment and Prognosis. The treatment of the ameloblastic odontoma is controversial, probably because there are few published cases. Some investigators believe that recurrence, associated with continued destruction of tissue, is common after conservative curettage or enucleation and that a more radical approach is necessary. Resection of the jaw, if possible preserving the inferior border of the mandible when this area is uninvolved, will certainly result in a permanent cure. The general behavior of this lesion is the same as that of the ameloblastoma component and therefore the same philosophy of management would also apply here as for the ameloblastoma.

TERATOMA

(Teratoblastoma; Teratoid Tumor)

The teratoma is a true neoplasm made up of a number of different types of tissue which are not native to the area in which the tumor occurs. The teratoma should be differentiated from non-neoplastic lesions which represent simply heterotopic collections of various forms of tissue and which are common. It is *not* odontogenic in origin, but is discussed here under the odontogenic tumors only because of the interesting common occurrence of teeth in the lesion.

Clinical Features. The teratoma occurs in a variety of locations, including the ovaries, testes, anterior mediastinum, retroperitoneal area, presacral and coccygeal regions, pineal region, head, neck and abdominal viscera. Except for the teratomas occurring in the ovaries, testes or mediastinum, the neoplasms are usually known to be present at birth or are discovered shortly thereafter. The ovarian, testicular and mediastinal teratomas are usually discovered in early adult life, at the average age of 30 years. The ovarian and mediastinal teratomas are usually benign lesions and grow relatively slowly. The testicular teratomas, however, are frequently malignant.

Gross Features. The benign teratomas are usually cystic lesions with solid thickenings in the wall of the lesion. They often contain recognizable hair, sebaceous material and teeth. Although the usual teratoma contains only a few teeth, cases have been recorded in which the tumor enclosed dozens or even several hundred small teeth (Fig. 4–40). Teeth are uncommon in the malignant form of teratoma.

Histologic Features. The benign teratoma is made up of a vast variety of different tissues, including epithelium and various epithelial appendages such as hair, sweat glands, sebaceous

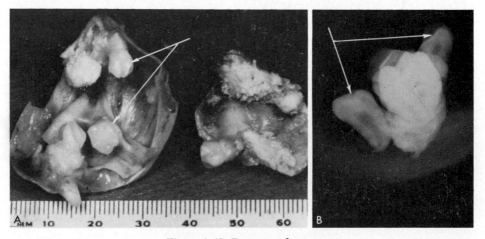

Figure 4–40. *Teratoma of ovary.*
Several teeth are seen in the gross specimen (*A*), and these seem to have reasonably normal roentgenographic appearance (*B*). (Courtesy of Dr. Frank Vellios.)

glands, salivary glands and teeth, as well as discrete epithelial organs such as thyroid gland and pancreas. It is not unusual to find respiratory epithelium as well as intestinal epithelium present in various areas in the teratoma in well-differentiated form. In addition, nervous tissue is seen in some tumors, as are cartilage and bone. The tissue seen in malignant teratomas is usually not as well differentiated as in the benign form.

The teeth present are frequently normal teeth and resemble bicuspids; they seldom are multirooted. They are sometimes situated in an alveolar socket and exhibit a typical periodontal membrane, all supporting and adjacent structures often appearing normal. Inflammatory cell infiltration of the gingiva, resembling "gingivitis," is commonly observed.

REFERENCES

Abrams, A. M., and Howell, F. V.: Calcifying epithelial odontogenic tumors: report of four cases. J. Am. Dent. Assoc., 74:1231, 1967.

Idem: The calcifying odontogenic cyst. Oral Surg., 25:594, 1968.

Abrams, A. M., Melrose, R. J., and Howell, F. V.: Adeno-ameloblastoma: a clinical pathologic study of ten new cases. Cancer, 22:175, 1968.

Abrams, A. M., Kirby, J. W., and Melrose, R. J.: Cementoblastoma. Oral Surg., 38:394, 1974.

Agazzi, C., and Belloni, L.: Gli odontomi duri dei mascellari. Arch. Ital. Otol., LXIV (Suppl. XVI): 1953.

Aisenberg, M. S.: Adamantinohemangioma. Oral Surg., 3:798, 1950.

Idem: Histopathology of ameloblastoma. Oral Surg., 6:1111, 1953.

Altini, M., and Smith, I.: Ameloblastic dentinosarcoma (a case report). Int. J. Oral Surg. 5:142, 1976.

Anderson, H. C., Byunghoon, K., and Minkowitz, S.: Calcifying epithelial odontogenic tumor of Pindborg: an electron microscopic study. Cancer, 24:585, 1969.

Areen, R. G., McClatchey, K. D., and Baker, H. L.: Squamous cell carcinoma developing in an odontogenic keratocyst. Arch. Otolaryngol., 107:568, 1981.

Baden, E.: Terminology of the ameloblastoma: history and current usage. J. Oral Surg., 23:40, 1965.

Baden, E., Moskow, B. S., and Moskow, R.: Odontogenic gingival epithelial hamartoma. J. Oral Surg., 26:702, 1968.

Baker, P. L., Dockerty, M. B., and Coventry, M. B.: Adamantinoma (so-called) of the long bones. J. Bone Joint Surg., 36A:704, 1954.

Baker, R. D., D'Onofrio, E. D., Corio, R. L., Crawford, B. E., and Terry, B. C.: Squamous-cell carcinoma arising in a lateral periodontal cyst. Oral Surg., 47:495, 1979.

Barros, R. E., Dominguez, F. V., and Cabrini, R. L.: Myxoma of the jaws. Oral Surg., 27:225, 1969.

Becker, M. H., Lopf, A. W., and Lande, A.: Basal cell nevus syndrome: its roentgenologic significance. Am. J. Roentgenol., Radium Ther. Nucl. Med., 99:817, 1967.

Bernier, J. L.: Ameloblastoma: report of 34 cases. J. Dent. Res., 21:529, 1942.

Bernier, J. L., and Thompson, H. C.: The histogenesis of the cementoma. Am. J. Orthod. Oral Surg., 32:543, 1946.

Bhaskar, S. N.: Adenoameloblastoma: its histogenesis and report of 15 new cases. J. Oral Surg., Anesth. Hosp. Dent. Serv., 22:218, 1964.

Bhaskar, S. N., and Jacoway, J. R.: Peripheral fibroma and peripheral fibroma with calcification: report of 376 cases. J. Am. Dent. Assoc., 73:1312, 1966.

Bhaskar, S. N., and Laskin, D. M.: Gingival cysts. Oral Surg., 8:803, 1955.

Blake, H., and Blake, F. S.: Ameloblastic odontoma, report of case. J. Oral Surg., 9:240, 1951.

Bohn, H.: Die Mundkrankheiten der Kinder. Leipzig, W. Engelmann, 1866.

Bradley, J. L.: Multiple cementoma. J. Oral Surg., 2:278, 1944.

Brandon, S. A.: Adamantinoma of the left maxillary area: report of case. J. Oral Surg., 7:252, 1949.

Brannon, R. B.: The odontogenic keratocyst. A clinicopathologic study of 312 cases. Part I: Clinical features. Oral Surg., 42:54, 1976. Part II: Histologic features. Oral Surg., 43:233, 1977.

Browne, R. M.: The odontogenic keratocyst: clinical aspects. Br. Dent. J., 128:255, 1970.

Idem: The odontogenic keratocyst: histological features and their correlation with clinical behavior. Br. Dent. J., 131:249, 1971.

Idem: The origin of cholesterol in odontogenic cysts in man. Arch. Oral Biol., 16:107, 1971.

Idem: The pathogenesis of odontogenic cysts: a review. J. Oral Path., 4:31, 1975.

Browne, R. M., and Gough, N. G.: Malignant change in the epithelium lining odontogenic cysts. Cancer, 29:1199, 1972.

Buchner, A., and Hansen, L. S.: The histomorphologic spectrum of the gingival cyst in the adult. Oral Surg., 48:532, 1979.

Budnick, S. D.: Compound and complex odontomas. Oral Surg., 42:501, 1976.

Cahn, L. R.: The dentigerous cyst as a potential adamantinoma. Dent. Cosmos, 75:889, 1933.

Carr, R. F., and Halperin, V.: Malignant ameloblastomas from 1953 to 1966. Review of the literature and report of a case. Oral Surg., 26:514, 1968.

Cataldo, E., and Berkman, M. D.: Cysts of the oral mucosa in newborns. Am. J. Dis. Child., 116:44, 1968.

Cavanha, A. O.: Enamel pearls. Oral Surg., 19:373, 1965.

Changus, G. W., Speed, J. S., and Stewart, F. W.: Malignant angioblastoma of bone; reappraisal of adamantinoma of long bone. Cancer, 10:540, 1957.

Chaudhry, A. P., Spink, J. H., and Gorlin, R. J.: Periapical fibrous dysplasia (cementoma). J. Oral Surg., 16:483, 1958.

Chen, S.-Y., Fantasia, J. E., and Miller, A. S.: Hyaline bodies in the connective tissue wall of odontogenic cysts. J. Oral Pathol., 10:147, 1981.

Cherrick, H. M., King, O. H., Jr., Lucatorto, F. M., and Suggs, D. M.: Benign cementoblastoma. Oral Surg., 37:54, 1974.

Churchill, H. R.: Histological differentiation between certain dentigerous cysts and ameloblastomata. Dent. Cosmos, 76:1173, 1934.

Corio, R. L., Crawford, B. E., and Schaberg, S. J.: Benign cementoblastoma. Oral Surg. 41:524, 1976.

Couch, R. D., Morris, E. E., and Vellios, F.: Granular cell ameloblastic fibroma: report of two cases in adults, with observations on its similarity to congenital epulis. Am. J. Clin. Pathol., *37*:398, 1962.

Courtney, R. M., and Kerr, D. A.: The odontogenic adenomatoid tumor. Oral Surg., *39*:424, 1975.

Craig, G. T.: The paradental cyst. A specific inflammatory odontogenic cyst. Br. Dent. J., *141*:9, 1976.

Critchley, M., and Ironside, R. N.: The pituitary adamantinomata. Brain, *49*:473, 1926.

Cundiff, E. J.: Peripheral ossifying fibroma. A review of 365 cases. M.S.D. Thesis, Indiana University, 1972.

Dachi, S. F., and Howell, F. V.: A survey of 3,875 routine full-mouth radiographs. II. A study of impacted teeth. Oral Surg., *14*:1165, 1961.

Dahl, E. C., Wolfson, S. H., and Haugen, J. C.: Central odontogenic fibroma: review of literature and report of cases. J. Oral Surg., *39*:120, 1981.

Darlington, C. G., Ehrlich, H. E., and Seldin, H. M.: Malignant transformation of odontogenic cyst: report of case. J. Oral Surg., *11*:64, 1953.

El-Labban, N.: Electron microscopic investigation of hyaline bodies in odontogenic cysts. J. Oral Pathol., *8*:81, 1979.

Elzay, R. P.: Primary intraosseous carcinoma of the jaws. Review and update of odontogenic carcinomas. Oral Surg., *54*:299, 1982.

Epstein, A.: Ueber Epithelperlen in der Mundhöhle Neurgeborener Kinder. Ztsch. für Heilkunde, *1*:59, 1880.

Eversole, L. R., Tomich, C. E., and Cherrick, H. M.: Histogenesis of odontogenic tumors. Oral Surg., *32*:569, 1971.

Fantasia, J. E.: Lateral periodontal cyst. Oral Surg., *48*:237, 1979.

Farman, A. G.: The peripheral odontogenic fibroma. Oral Surg., *40*:82, 1975.

Farman, A. G., Köhler, W. W., Nortjé, C. J., and Van Wyk, C. W.: Cementoblastoma: report of a case. J. Oral Surg., *37*:198, 1979.

Field, H. J., and Ackerman, A. A.: Calcifying fibro-adamantoblastoma. Am. J. Orthod. Oral Surg., *28*:543, 1942.

Forssell, K.: The primordial cyst. A clinical and radiographic study. Academic dissertation, Turku, Finland, 1980.

Forssell, K., and Sainio, P.: Clinicopathological study of keratinized cysts of the jaws. Proc. Finn. Dent. Soc., *75*:36, 1979.

Forssell, K., Kallioniemi, H., and Sainio, P.: Microcysts and epithelial islands in primordial cysts. Proc. Finn. Dent. Soc., *75*:99, 1979.

Forssell, K., Sorvari, T. E., and Oksala, E.: An analysis of the recurrence of odontogenic keratocysts. Proc. Finn. Dent. Soc., *70*:135, 1974.

Franklin, C. D., and Pindborg, J. J.: The calcifying epithelial odontogenic tumor. Oral Surg., *42*:753, 1976.

Freedman, P. D., Lumerman, H., and Gee, J. K.: Calcifying odontogenic cyst. Oral Surg., *40*:93, 1975.

Frissell, C. T.: Ameloblastoma: a statistical study of two hundred sixty-one cases, including fifteen previously unreported from the Indiana University Medical Center, M.S. Thesis, Indiana University, 1952.

Frissell, C. T., and Shafer, W. G.: Ameloblastic odontoma; report of case. Oral Surg., *6*:1129, 1953.

Fromm, A.: Epstein's pearls, Bohn's nodules and inclusion-cysts of the oral cavity. J. Dent. Child., *34*:275, 1967.

Gardner, A. F.: Proliferation of dental lamina in the wall of a primordial cyst. Oral Surg., *8*:510, 1955.

Idem: The odontogenic cyst as a potential carcinoma: a clinico-pathologic appraisal. J. Am. Dent. Assoc., *78*:746, 1969.

Gardner, D. G.: Peripheral ameloblastoma. A study of 21 cases, including 5 reported as basal cell carcinoma of the gingiva. Cancer, *39*:1625, 1977.

Idem: The concept of hamartomas: its relevance to the pathogenesis of odontogenic lesions. Oral Surg., *45*:884, 1978.

Idem: The central odontogenic fibroma: an attempt at clarification. Oral Surg., *50*:425, 1980.

Idem: Plexiform unicystic ameloblastoma: a diagnostic problem in dentigerous cysts. Cancer, *47*:1358, 1981.

Idem: The peripheral odontogenic fibroma: an attempt at clarification. Oral Surg., *54*:40, 1982.

Gardner, D. G., Michaels, L., and Liepa, E.: Calcifying epithelial odontogenic tumor: an amyloid-producing neoplasm. Oral Surg., *26*:812, 1968.

Gardner, D. G., and Pecak, A. M. J.: The treatment of ameloblastoma based on pathologic and anatomic principles. Cancer, *46*:2514, 1980.

Gardner, D. G., Smith, F. A., and Weinberg, S.: Ameloblastic fibroma: a benign tumour treatable by curettage. J. Can. Dent. Assoc., *35*:306, 1976.

Ghatak, N. R., Hirano, A., and Zimmerman, H. M.: Ultrastructure of a craniopharyngioma. Cancer, *27*:1465, 1971.

Giansanti, J. S., Someren, A., and Waldron, C. A.: Odontogenic adenomatoid tumor (adenoameloblastoma). Oral Surg., Oral Med. & Oral Pathol., *30*:69, 1970.

Glickman, I., and Robinson, L.: Destruction of calcified dental tissue in an ovarian dermoid cyst. Oral Surg., *2*:902, 1949.

Goldblatt, L. I.: Ultrastructural study of an odontogenic myxoma. Oral Surg., *42*:206, 1976.

Goldblatt, L. I., Brannon, R. B., and Ellis, G. L.: Squamous odontogenic tumor. Report of five cases and review of the literature. Oral Surg., *54*:187, 1982.

Gorlin, R. J.: Potentialities of oral epithelium manifest by mandibular dentigerous cysts. Oral Surg., *10*:271, 1957.

Gorlin, R. J., and Chaudhry, A. P.: The ameloblastoma and the craniopharyngioma: their similarities and differences. Oral Surg., *12*:199, 1959.

Gorlin, R. J., Chaudhry, A. P., and Pindborg, J. J.: Odontogenic tumors. Classification, histopathology, and clinical behavior in man and domesticated animals. Cancer, *14*:73, 1961.

Gorlin, R. J., and Goltz, R. W.: Multiple nevoid basal-cell epithelioma, jaw cysts and bifid rib. N. Engl. J. Med., *262*:908, 1960.

Gorlin, R. J., Meskin, L. H., and Brodey, R.: Odontogenic tumors in man and animals: pathologic classification and clinical behavior—a review. Ann. N.Y. Acad. Sci., *108*:722, 1963.

Gorlin, R. J., Pindborg, J. J., Clausen, F. P., and Vickers, R. A.: The calcifying odontogenic cyst: a possible analogue of the cutaneous calcifying epithelioma of Malherbe. Oral Surg., *15*:1235, 1962.

Gorlin, R. J., Pindborg, J. J., Redman, R. S., Williamson, J. J., and Hansen, L. S.: The calcifying odontogenic cyst: a new entity and possible analogue of the cutaneous calcifying epithelioma of Malherbe. Cancer, *17*:723, 1964.

Gorlin, R. J., Vickers, R. A., Kelln, E., and Williamson, J. J.: The multiple basal-cell nevi syndrome. An analysis of a syndrome consisting of multiple nevoid basal-cell carcinoma, jaw cysts, skeletal anomalies, medulloblastoma, and hyporesponsiveness to parathormone. Cancer, *18*:89, 1965.

Gould, A. R., Farman, A. G., DeJean, E. K., and Van Arsdall, L. R.: Peripheral ameloblastoma: an ultrastructural analysis. J. Oral Pathol., *11*:90, 1982.

Greer, R. O., Jr., and Hammond, W. S.: Extraosseous

ameloblastoma: light microscopic and ultrastructural observations. J. Oral Surg., 36:553, 1978.

Grimes, O. F., and Stephen, H. B.: Adamantinoma of the maxilla metastatic to the lung. Ann. Surg., 128:999, 1948.

Hamner, J. E., III, and Pizer, M. E.: Ameloblastic odontoma: report of two cases. Am. J. Dis. Child., 115:332, 1968.

Hamner, J. E., III, Scofield, H. H., and Cornyn, J.: Benign fibro-osseous jaw lesions of periodontal membrane origin: an analysis of 249 cases. Cancer, 22:861, 1968.

Hartman, K. S.: Granular-cell ameloblastoma. Oral Surg., 38:241, 1974.

Hatakeyama, S., and Suzuki, A.: Ultrastructural study of adenomatoid odontogenic tumor. J. Oral Pathol., 7:295, 1978.

Hietanen, J., Calonius, P. E. B., Collan, Y., and Poikkeus, P.: Histology and ultrastructure of an ameloblastic fibroma. A case report. Proc. Finn. Dent. Soc., 69:129, 1973.

Hitchin, A. D.: The etiology of the calcified composite odontomes. Br. Dent. J., 130:475, 1971.

Hjørting-Hansen, E., Andreasen, J. O., and Robinson, L. H.: A study of odontogenic cysts with special reference to location of keratocysts: Part 1. Br. J. Oral Surg., 7:15, 1969.

Hodson, J. J., and Prout, R. E. S.: Chemical and histochemical characterization of mucopolysaccharides in a jaw myxoma. J. Clin. Pathol., 21:582, 1968.

Hoke, H. F., Jr., and Harrelson, A. B.: Granular cell ameloblastoma with metastasis to the cervicular vertebrae: observations on the origin of the granular cells. Cancer, 20:991, 1967.

Hooker, S. P.: Ameloblastic odontoma: an analysis of twenty-six cases. Oral Surg., 24:375, 1967 (Abst.).

Howell, R. M., and Burkes, E. J., Jr.: Malignant transformation of ameloblastic fibro-odontoma to ameloblastic fibrosarcoma. Oral Surg., 43:391, 1977.

Huvos, A. G., and Marcove, R. C.: Adamantinoma of long bones. A clinicopathological study of fourteen cases with vascular origin suggested. J. Bone Joint Surg., 57:148, 1975.

Ingham, G. G.: Dentinoma. Oral Surg., 5:353, 1952.

Kemper, J. W., and Root, R. W.: Adamanto-odontoma: report of case. Am. J. Orthod. Oral Surg., 30:709, 1944.

Khan, M. Y., Kwee, H., Schneider, L. C., and Saber, I.: Adenomatoid odontogenic tumor resembling a globulomaxillary cyst: Light and electron microscopic studies. J. Oral Surg., 35:739, 1977.

Kimm, H. T.: The radiosensitivity of adamantinoma. Chin. Med. J., 59:497, 1941.

Kreshover, S. J.: The incidence and pathogenesis of gingival cysts. Presented at 35th General Meeting, International Association for Dental Research, March, 1957.

Krikos, G. A.: Histochemical studies of mucins of odontogenic cysts exhibiting mucous metaplasia. Arch. Oral Biol., 11:633, 1966.

Krolls, S. O., and Pindborg, J. J.: Calcifying epithelial odontogenic tumor. A survey of 23 cases and discussion of histomorphologic variations. Arch. Pathol., 98:206, 1974.

Larsson, A., Forsberg, O., and Sjögren, S.: Benign cementoblastoma—cementum analogue of benign osteoblastoma? J. Oral Surg., 36:299, 1978.

Lee, K. W.: A light and electron microscopic study of the adenomatoid odontogenic tumors. Int. J. Oral Surg., 3:183, 1974.

Lee, R. E., White, W. L., and Totten, R. S.: Ameloblastoma with distant metastases. Arch. Pathol., 68:23, 1959.

Leider, A. S., Nelson, J. F., and Trodahl, J. N.: Ameloblastic fibrosarcoma of the jaws. Oral Surg., 33:559, 1972.

Levy, B. A.: Effects of experimental trauma on developing first molar teeth in rats. J. Dent. Res., 47:323, 1968.

Idem: Ghost cells and odontomas. Oral Surg., 36:851, 1973.

Lucas, R. B.: Neoplasia in odontogenic cysts. Oral Surg., 7:1227, 1954.

Lurie, H. I.: Congenital melanocarcinoma, melanotic adamantinoma, retinal anlage tumor, progonoma, and pigmented epulis of infancy. Cancer, 14:1090, 1961.

Maher, W. P., and Swindle, P. F.: Etiology and vascularization of dental lamina cysts. Oral Surg., 29:590, 1970.

Main, D. M. G.: The enlargement of epithelial jaw cysts. Odontol. Revy, 21:29, 1970.

Idem: Epithelial jaw cysts: a clinicopathological reappraisal. Br. J. Oral Surg., 8:114, 1970.

McClure, D. K., and Dahlin, D. C.: Myxoma of bone. Report of three cases. Mayo Clin. Proc., 52:249, 1977.

McGowan, R. H.: Primary intra-alveolar carcinoma. A difficult diagnosis. Br. J. Oral Surg., 18:259, 1980.

McKelvy, B. D., and Cherrick, H. M.: Peripheral ameloblastic fibrodentinoma. J. Oral Surg., 34:826, 1976.

Mehlisch, D. R., Dahlin, D. C., and Masson, J. K.: Ameloblastoma: a clinicopathologic report. J. Oral Surg., 30:9, 1972.

Miller, A. S., López, C. F., Pullon, P. A., and Elzay, R. P.: Ameloblastic fibro-odontoma. Oral Surg., 41:354, 1976.

Mori, M., Murakami, M., Hirose, I., and Shimozato, T.: Histochemical studies of myxoma of the jaws. J. Oral Surg., 33:529, 1975.

Moro, I., Okamura, N., Okuda, S., Komiyama, K., and Umemura, S.: The eosinophilic and amyloid-like materials in adenomatoid odontogenic tumor. J. Oral Pathol., 11:138, 1982.

Moskow, B. S., Siegel, K., Zegarelli, E. V., Kutscher, A. H., and Rothenberg, F.: Gingival and lateral periodontal cysts. J. Periodontol., 41:9, 1970.

Nichamin, S. J., and Kaufman, M.: Gingival microcysts in infancy. Pediatrics, 31:412, 1963.

Payne, T. P.: An analysis of the clinical and histopathologic parameters of the odontogenic keratocyst. Oral Surg., 53:538, 1972.

Peterson, W. C., and Gorlin, R. J.: Possible analogous cutaneous and odontogenic tumors. Arch. Dermatol., 90:255, 1964.

Philipsen, H. P.: Om keratocyster (kolesteatomer) i kaeberne. Tandlaegebladet, 60:693, 1956.

Philipsen, H. P., and Birn, H.: The adenomatoid odontogenic tumour: ameloblastic, adenomatoid tumour or adeno-ameloblastoma. Acta Pathol. Microbiol. Scand. (A), 75:375, 1969.

Pincock, L. D., and Bruce, K. W.: Odontogenic fibroma. Oral Surg., 7:307, 1954.

Pindborg, J. J.: A calcifying epithelial odontogenic tumor. Cancer, 11:838, 1958.

Idem: Ameloblastic sarcoma in the maxilla. Report of a case. Cancer, 13:917, 1960.

Idem: Calcifying epithelial odontogenic tumors. Acta Pathol. Microbiol. Scand., 111 (Suppl.):71, 1956.

Idem: On dentinomas. Acta. Pathol. Microbiol. Scand., 105(Suppl.):135, 1955.

Idem: The calcifying epithelial odontogenic tumor: review of literature and report of an extra-osseous case. Acta Odontol. Scand., 24:419, 1966.

Pindborg, J. J., and Clausen, F.: Classification of odontogenic tumors. Acta Odontol. Scand., 16:293, 1958.

Pindborg, J. J., and Hansen, J.: Studies on odontogenic cyst epithelium. 2. Clinical and roentgenologic aspects of odontogenic keratocysts. Acta Pathol. Microbiol. Scand. (A), 58:283, 1963.

Pindborg, J. J., and Hjørting-Hansen, E.: Atlas of Diseases of the Jaws. Philadelphia, W. B. Saunders Company, 1974.

Pindborg, J. J., Kramer, I. R. H., and Torloni, H.: Histological Typing of Odontogenic Tumours, Jaw Cysts, and Allied Lesions. International Histological Classification of Tumours, No. 5. Geneva, World Health Organization, 1971.

Pindborg, J. J., Philipsen, H. P., and Henriksen, J.: Studies on odontogenic cyst epithelium; in: Fundamentals of Keratinization. Publication No. 70. Washington, D.C., American Association for the Advancement of Science. 1962, pp. 151–160.

Praetorius, F., Hjørting-Hansen, E., Gorlin, R. J., and Vickers, R. A.: Calcifying odontogenic cyst. Range, variations and neoplastic potential. Acta. Odontol. Scand., 39:227, 1981.

Pullon, P. A., Shafer, W. G., Elzay, R. P., Kerr, D. A., and Corio, R. L.: Squamous odontogenic tumor. Oral Surg., 40:616, 1975.

Punniamoorthy, A.: Gigantiform cementoma: a review of the literature and a case report. Br. J. Oral Surg., 18:221, 1980.

Ranløv, P., and Pindborg, J. J.: The amyloid nature of the homogeneous substance in the calcifying epithelial odontogenic tumor. Acta Pathol. Microbiol. Scand. (A), 68:169, 1966.

Rater, C. J., Selke, A. C., and Van Epps, E. F.: Basal cell nevus syndrome. Am. J. Roentgenol. Radium Ther. Nucl. Med., 103:589, 1968.

Reeve, C. M., and Levy, B. P.: Gingival cysts: a review of the literature and a report of four cases. Period. 6:115, 1968.

Regezi, J. A., Kerr, D. A., and Courtney, R. M.: Odontogenic tumors: analysis of 706 cases. J. Oral Surg., 36:771, 1978.

Richardson, J. F., Balogh, K., Merk, F., and Booth, D.: Pigmented odontogenic tumor of jawbone. A previously undescribed expression of neoplastic potential. Cancer, 34:1244, 1974.

Ritchey, B., and Orban, B.: Cysts of the gingiva. Oral Surg., 6:765, 1953.

Robinson, H. B. G.: Ameloblastoma: a survey of 379 cases from the literature. Arch. Pathol., 23:831, 1937.

Idem: Classification of cysts of the jaws. Am. J. Orthod. Oral Surg., 31:370, 1945.

Idem: Histologic study of ameloblastoma. Arch. Pathol., 23:664, 1937.

Robinson, H. B. G., and Koch, W. E., Jr.: Diagnosis of cysts of the jaw. J. Mo. Dent. Assoc., 21:187, 1941.

Robinson, H. B. G., Koch, W. E., Jr., and Kolas, S.: Radiographic interpretation of oral cysts. Dent. Radiogr. Photogr., 29:61, 1956.

Robinson, L., and Martinez, M. G.: Unicystic ameloblastoma. A prognostically distinct entity. Cancer, 40:227, 1977.

Rosai, J.: Adamantinoma of the tibia: electron microscopic evidence of its epithelial origin. Am. J. Clin. Pathol., 51:786, 1969.

Rud, J., and Pindborg, J. J.: Odontogenic keratocysts: a follow-up study of 21 cases. J. Oral Surg., 27:323, 1969.

Scannell, J. M., Jr.: Cementoma. Oral Surg., 2:1169, 1949.

Schlosnagle, D. C., and Someren, A.: The ultrastructure of the adenomatoid odontogenic tumor. Oral Surg., 52:154, 1981.

Schweitzer, F. C., and Barnfield, W. F.: Ameloblastoma of the mandible with metastasis to the lungs; report of a case. J. Oral Surg., 1:287, 1943.

Sciubba, J. J., and Zola, M. B.: Odontogenic epithelial hamartoma. Oral Surg., 45:261, 1978.

Sedano, H. O., and Pindborg, J. J.: Ghost cell epithelium in odontomas. J. Oral Pathol., 4:27, 1975.

Seeman, G. F.: Sacrococcygeal cystic teratoma with traumatic hemorrhage. Oral Surg., 1:308, 1948.

Seemayer, T. A., Blundell, J. S., and Wiglesworth, F. W.: Pituitary craniopharyngioma with tooth formation. Cancer, 29:423, 1972.

Sehdev, M. K., Huvos, A. G., Strong, E. W., Gerold, F. P., and Willis, G. W.: Ameloblastoma of maxilla and mandible. Cancer, 33:324, 1974.

Seward, M. H.: Eruption cyst: an analysis of its clinical features. J. Oral Surg., 31:31, 1973.

Shafer, W. G.: Ameloblastic fibroma. J. Oral Surg., 13:317, 1955.

Shafer, W. G., and Frissell, C. T.: The melano-ameloblastoma and retinal anlage tumors. Cancer, 6:360, 1953.

Shafer, W. G., and Waldron, C. A.: Fibro-osseous Lesions of the Jaws. American Academy of Oral Pathology Continuing Education Course, Reno, Nevada, May 1982.

Shear, M.: Primary intra-alveolar epidermoid carcinoma of the jaw. J. Pathol., 97:645, 1969.

Idem: Induction of bone by the dental lamina. J. Dent. Assoc. S. Afr., 21:1, 1966.

Idem: The histogenesis of the dental cyst. Dent. Pract., 13:238, 1963.

Idem: The histogenesis of the "tumour of enamel organ epithelium." Br. Dent. J., 112:494, 1962.

Shear, M., and Altini, M.: Malignant odontogenic tumours. J. Dent. Assoc. S. Afr., 37:547, 1982.

Shear, M., and Pindborg, J. J.: Microscopic features of the lateral periodontal cyst. Scand. J. Dent. Res., 83:103, 1975.

Sherman, R. S., and Caumartin, H.: The roentgen appearance of adamantinoma of the mandible. Radiology, 65:361, 1955.

Slootweg, P. J.: An analysis of the interrelationship of the mixed odontogenic tumors—ameloblastic fibroma, ameloblastic fibro-odontoma, and the odontomas. Oral Surg., 51:266, 1981.

Small, I. A., and Waldron, C. A.: Ameloblastomas of the jaws. Oral Surg., 8:281, 1955.

Smith, I., and Shear, M.: Radiological features of mandibular primordial cysts (keratocysts). J. Max.-Fac. Surg., 6:147, 1978.

Smith, R. R. L., Olson, J. L., Hutchins, G. M., Crawley, W. A., and Levin, L. S.: Adenomatoid odontogenic tumor. Ultrastructural demonstration of two cell types and amyloid. Cancer, 43:505, 1979.

Soskolne, W. A., and Shear, M.: Observations on the pathogenesis of primordial cysts. Br. Dent. J., 123:321, 1967.

Spouge, J. D.: Odontogenic tumors. Oral Surg., 24:392, 1967.

Stafne, E. C.: Periapical osteofibrosis with formation of cementoma. J. Am. Dent. Assoc., 21:1822, 1934.

Standish, S. M., and Shafer, W. G.: The lateral periodontal cyst. J. Periodontol., 29:27, 1958.

Stanley, H. R., and Diehl, D. L.: Ameloblastoma potential of follicular cysts. Oral Surg., 20:260, 1965.

Stasinopoulos, M.: Mixed calcified odontogenic tumours. Br. J. Oral Surg., 8:93, 1970.

Stoelinga, P. J. W., and Peters, J. H.: A note on the origin of keratocysts of the jaws. Int. J. Oral Surg., 2:37, 1973.

Struthers, P., and Shear, M.: Root resorption by ameloblastomas and cysts of the jaws. Int. J. Oral Surg., 5:128, 1976.

Swinson, T. W.: An extraosseous adenomatoid odontogenic tumor. Br. J. Oral Surg., 15:32, 1977.

Tandler, B., and Rossi, E. P.: Granular cell ameloblastoma: electron microscopic observations. J. Oral Pathol., 6:401, 1977.

Thoma, K. H.: Cementoblastoma. Int. J. Orthod., 23:1127, 1937.

Idem: Diagnosis and treatment of odontogenic and fissural cysts. Oral Surg., 3:961, 1950.

Idem: Pathogenesis of the odontogenic tumors. Oral Surg., 4:1262, 1951.

Idem: Adenoameloblastoma. Oral Surg., 8:441, 1955.

Idem: The circumferential dentigerous cyst. Oral Surg., 18:368, 1964.

Thoma, K. H., and Goldman, H. M.: Odontogenic tumors: a classification based on observations of the epithelial, mesenchymal and mixed varieties. Am. J. Pathol., 22:433, 1946.

Idem: Odontogenic tumors: survey of 75 cases. Am. J. Orthod. Oral Surg., 32:763, 1946.

Idem: Central myxoma of the jaw. Am. J. Orthod. Oral Surg., 33:532, 1947.

Tiecke, R. W., and Bernier, J. L.: Melanotic ameloblastoma. Oral Surg., 9:1197, 1956.

Toller, P.: Origin and growth of cysts of the jaws. Ann. R. Coll. Surg., Engl., 40:306, 1967.

Idem: Permeability of cyst walls in vivo: investigations with radioactive tracers. Proc. R. Soc. Med., 59:724, 1966.

Toller, P. A.: Protein substances in odontogenic cyst fluids. Br. Dent. J., 128:317, 1970.

Idem: Autoradiography of explants from odontogenic cysts. Br. Dent. J., 131:57, 1971.

Tratman, E. K.: Classification of odontomas. Br. Dent. J., 91:167, 1951.

Trodahl, J. N.: Ameloblastic fibroma. A survey of cases from the Armed Forces Institute of Pathology. Oral Surg., 33:547, 1972.

Tsagaris, G. T.: A review of the ameloblastic fibro-odontoma. M.S. Thesis, George Washington University, Washington, D.C., 1972.

Tsukada, Y., de la Pava, S., and Pickren, J. W.: Granular-cell ameloblastoma with metastasis to the lungs. Report of a case and review of the literature. Cancer, 18:916, 1965.

Turner, J. G.: A note on enamel nodules. Br. Dent. J., 78:39, 1945.

Unni, K. K., Dahlin, D. C., Beabout, J. W., and Ivins, J. C.: Adamantinomas of long bones. Cancer, 34:1796, 1974.

Valderhaug, J., and Zander, H. A.: Relationship of "epithelial rests of Malassez" to other periodontal structures. J. Am. Soc. Periodontol., 5:254, 1967.

Van der Waal, I., and Van der Kwast, W. A. M.: A case of gigantiform cementoma. Int. J. Oral Surg., 3:440, 1974.

Vap, D. R., Dahlin, D. C., and Turlington, E. G.: Pindborg tumor: the so-called calcifying epithelial odontogenic tumor. Cancer, 25:629, 1970.

Vickers, R. A., Dahlin, D. C., and Gorlin, R. J.: Amyloid-containing odontogenic tumors. Oral Surg., 20:476, 1965.

Vickers, R. A., and Gorlin, R. J.: Ameloblastoma: delineation of early histopathologic features of neoplasia. Cancer, 26:699, 1970.

Villa, V. G.: Ameloblastic sarcoma in the mandible: report of case. Oral Surg., 8:123, 1955.

Vindenes, H., Nilsen, R., and Gilhuus-Moe, O.: Benign cementoblastoma. Int. J. Oral Surg., 8:318, 1979.

Waldron, C. A., Giansanti, J. S., and Browand, B. C.: Sclerotic cemental masses of the jaws (so-called chronic sclerosing osteomyelitis, sclerosing osteitis, multiple enostosis, and gigantiform cementoma). Oral Surg., 39:590, 1975.

Weathers, D. R., and Waldron, C. A.: Unusual multilocular cysts of the jaws (botryoid odontogenic cysts). Oral Surg., 36:235, 1973.

Wertheimer, F. W., Fullmer, H. M., and Hansen, L. S.: A histochemical study of hyaline bodies in odontogenic cysts and a comparison to the human secondary dental cuticle. Oral Surg., 15:1466, 1962.

Wertheimer, F. W., Zielinski, R. J., and Wesley, R. K.: Extraosseous calcifying epithelial odontogenic tumor (Pindborg tumor). Int. J. Oral Surg., 6:266, 1977.

Wesley, R. K., Wysocki, G. P., and Mintz, S. M.: The central odontogenic fibroma. Clinical and morphologic studies. Oral Surg., 40:235, 1975.

White, D. K., Chen, S.-Y., Mohnac, S. M., and Miller, A. S.: Odontogenic myxoma. Oral Surg., 39:901, 1975.

Willis, R. A.: Teratomas. Atlas of Tumor Pathology, Section III, Fascicle 9. Washington, D.C., Armed Forces Institute of Pathology, 1951.

Winer, H. J., Goepp, R. A., and Olsen, R. E.: Gigantiform cementoma resembling Paget's disease. Report of a case. J. Oral Surg., 30:517, 1972.

Wright, B. A., and Jennings, E. H.: Oxytalan fibers in peripheral odontogenic fibromas. A histochemical study of eighteen cases. Oral Surg., 48:451, 1979.

Wright, J. M., Jr.: Squamous odontogenic tumorlike proliferations in odontogenic cysts. Oral Surg., 47:354, 1979.

Idem: The odontogenic keratocyst: orthokeratinized variant. Oral Surg., 51:609, 1981.

Wysocki, G. P., Brannon, R. B., Gardner, D. G., and Sapp, P.: Histogenesis of the lateral periodontal cyst and the gingival cyst of the adult. Oral Surg., 50:327, 1980.

Wysocki, G. P., and Sapp, J. P.: Scanning and transmission electron microscopy of odontogenic keratocysts. Oral Surg., 40:494, 1975.

Zallen, R. D., Preskar, M. H., and McClary, S. A.: Ameloblastic fibroma. J. Oral Maxillofac. Surg., 40:513, 1982.

Zegarelli, E. V., and Ziskin, D. E.: Cementomas: a report of 50 cases. Am. J. Orthod. Oral Surg., 29:285, 1943.

Zegarelli, E. V., Napoli, N., and Hoffman, P.: The cementoma. A study of 230 patients with 435 cementomas. Oral Surg., 17:219, 1964.

CHAPTER 5

Regressive Alterations of the Teeth

Regressive changes in the dental tissues include a variety of alterations that are not necessarily related either etiologically or pathogenetically. Some of the changes to be considered here are associated with the general aging process of the individual. Others arise as a result of injury to the tissues. Still other regressive changes of teeth occur with such frequency that there is some doubt whether they should actually be considered pathologic. None of the lesions discussed here can be regarded as developmental abnormalities or as inflammatory lesions. They are brought together in this section because they do represent what must be considered lesions of a retrograde nature.

ATTRITION, ABRASION, AND EROSION

Attrition, abrasion, and erosion are three separate and distinct processes, each of which results in loss of tooth substance. The terms are frequently used interchangeably, but such careless terminology serves only to confuse the recognition of the etiology and to delay institution of proper treatment.

ATTRITION

Attrition may be defined as the physiologic wearing away of a tooth as a result of tooth-to-tooth contact, as in mastication. This occurs only on the occlusal, incisal, and proximal surfaces of teeth, not on other surfaces unless a very unusual occlusal relation or malocclusion exists. *This phenomenon is physiologic rather than pathologic*, and it is associated with the aging process. The older a person becomes, the more attrition is exhibited.

Attrition commences at the time contact or occlusion occurs between adjacent or opposing teeth. It may be seen in the deciduous dentition as well as in the permanent, but severe attrition is seldom seen in primary teeth because they are not retained normally for any great period of time. Occasionally, however, children may suffer from either dentinogenesis imperfecta or amelogenesis imperfecta, and in both diseases pronounced attrition may result from ordinary masticatory stresses.

The first clinical manifestation of attrition may be the appearance of a small polished facet on a cusp tip or ridge or a slight flattening of an incisal edge. Because of the slight mobility of the teeth in their sockets, a manifestation of the resiliency of the periodontal ligament, similar facets occur at the contact points on the proximal surfaces of the teeth. As the person becomes older and the wear continues, there is gradual reduction in cusp height and consequent flattening of the occlusal inclined planes. According to Robinson and his associates, there is also shortening of the length of the dental arch due to reduction in the mesiodistal diameters of the teeth through proximal attrition.

Only minor variation in the hardness of tooth enamel exists between individuals; nevertheless considerable variation in the degree of attrition is observed clinically. Men usually exhibit more severe attrition than women of comparable age, probably as a result of the greater masticatory force of men. Variation also may be a result of differences in the coarseness of the diet or of habits such as chewing tobacco or bruxism, either of which would predispose to more rapid attrition. Certain occupations, in which the worker is exposed to an atmosphere of abrasive dust and cannot avoid getting the material into his mouth, also are important in the etiology of severe attrition.

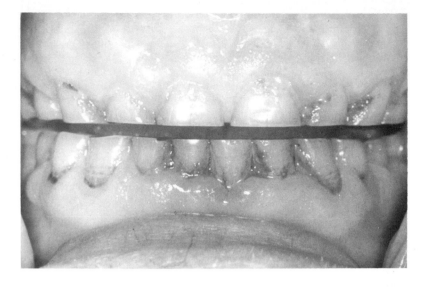

Figure 5–1. *Advanced attrition.* There is severe flattening of the incisal plane.

Advanced attrition, in which the enamel has been completely worn away in one or more areas, sometimes results in an extrinsic yellow or brown staining of the exposed dentin from food or tobacco (Figs. 5–1, 5–2). Provided there is no premature loss of the teeth, attrition may progress to the point of complete loss of cuspal interdigitation. In some cases the teeth may be

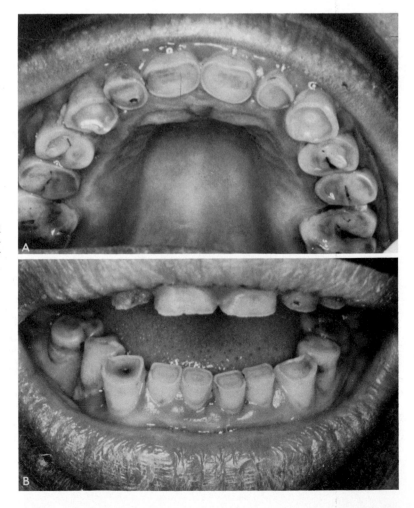

Figure 5–2. *Advanced attrition.* There is flattening of the incisal and occlusal surfaces and replacement of pulp chambers by secondary dentin. (Courtesy of Dr. Stephen F. Dachi.)

worn down nearly to the gingiva, but this extreme is unusual even in elderly persons.

The exposure of dentinal tubules and the subsequent irritation of odontoblastic processes result in formation of secondary dentin (q.v.) pulpal to the primary dentin, and this serves as an aid to protect the pulp from further injury. The rate of secondary dentin deposition is usually sufficient to preclude the possibility of pulp exposure through attrition alone. Sometimes, as the teeth wear down by attrition, little tendrils of pulp horn remain and are exposed to the oral cavity. These can be seen only when the tooth is examined carefully under a magnifying lens.

ABRASION

Abrasion is the pathologic wearing away of tooth substance through some abnormal mechanical process. Abrasion usually occurs on the exposed root surfaces of teeth, but under certain circumstances it may be seen elsewhere, such as on incisal or proximal surfaces.

Robinson stated that the most common cause of abrasion of root surfaces is the use of an abrasive dentifrice. Although modern dentifrices are not sufficiently abrasive to damage intact enamel severely, they can cause remarkable wear of cementum and dentin if the toothbrush carrying the dentifrice is injudiciously used, particularly in a horizontal rather than vertical direction. In such cases abrasion caused by a dentifrice manifests itself usually as a V-shaped or wedge-shaped ditch on the root side of the cementoenamel junction in teeth with some gingival recession (Fig. 5–3). The angle formed in the depth of the lesion, as well as that at the enamel edge, is a rather sharp one, and the exposed dentin appears highly polished. It has been shown by Kitchin and by Ervin and Bucher that some degree of tooth root exposure is a common clinical finding, and a 66 per cent incidence of abrasion among 1252 patients examined was reported by Ervin and Bucher. The fact that abrasion was more common on the left side of the mouth in right-handed people, and vice versa, suggested that improper toothbrushing caused abrasion. The results of a study by the American Dental Association on the comparative abrasiveness of a number of popular dentifrices are shown in Table 5–1 and indicate the wide variation among the commercial products.

Other less common forms of abrasion may be related to habit or to the occupation of the patient. The habitual opening of bobby pins with the teeth may result in a notching of the incisal edge of one maxillary central incisor (Fig. 5–4). Similar notching may be noted in carpenters, shoemakers, or tailors who hold nails, tacks, or pins between their teeth. Habitual pipe smokers may develop notching of the teeth that conforms to the shape of the pipe stem (Fig. 5–5). The improper use of dental floss and toothpicks may produce lesions on the proximal exposed root surface, which also should be considered a form of abrasion.

It is apparent that though the etiology of

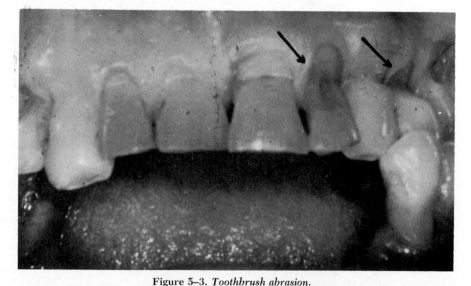

Figure 5–3. *Toothbrush abrasion.*
Severe gingival notching of the teeth as a result of improper toothbrushing habits is clearly seen.

Table 5–1. Abrasiveness of Dentifrices

PRODUCT	MANUFACTURER	ABRASIVITY INDEX
T-Lak	Laboratories Cazé	20 (20–21)† (Lowest)
Thermodent	Chas. Pfizer & Co.	24 (23–24)
Listerine	Warner-Lambert Pharm. Co.	26 (22–30)
Pepsodent*	Lever Brothers Co.	26 (23–29)
Amm-i-dent	Block Drug Co.	33 (31–34)
Colgate with MFP	Colgate-Palmolive Co.	51 (46–56)
Ultra-Brite	Colgate-Palmolive Co.	64 (52–82)
Macleans*, spearmint	Beecham Inc.	66 (66)
Macleans*, regular	Beecham Inc.	70 (68–72)
Pearl Drops	Cameo Chemicals	72 (65–83)
Crest, mint*	Procter & Gamble Co.	81 (71–90)
Close-up	Lever Brothers Co.	87 (70–101)
Macleans, spearmint	Beecham Inc.	93 (85–99)
Macleans, regular	Beecham Inc.	93 (74–103)
Crest, regular*	Procter & Gamble Co.	95 (77–110)
Gleem	Procter & Gamble Co.	106 (88–136)
Phillips	Sterling Drug Inc.	114 (111–116)
Vote	Bristol-Myers Co.	134 (112–162)
Sensodyne	Block Drug Co., Inc.	157 (151–168)
Iodent No. 2	Iodent Co.	174 (172–176)
Smokers Tooth Paste	Walgreen Lab., Inc.	202 (198–205) (Highest)

Modified from American Dental Association Report of the Council on Dental Therapeutics: Abrasivity of current dentifrices. J. Am. Dent. Assoc., *81*:1177, 1970. Copyright by the American Dental Association. Reprinted by permission.
*New formulation.
†Average and range.

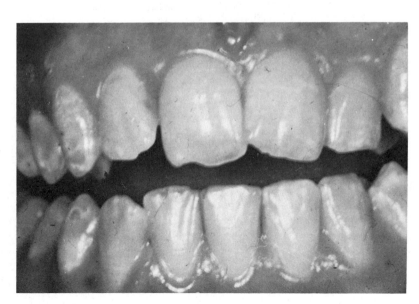

Figure 5–4. *Abrasion of maxillary central incisor caused by habitual opening of bobby pins with tooth.*

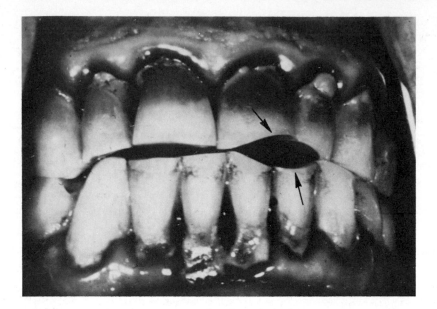

Figure 5–5. *Abrasion of teeth caused by pipestem.*

abrasion can be varied, the pathogenesis under these different conditions is essentially identical. The loss of tooth substance that occurs by one means or another is certainly pathologic but should present no problem in diagnosis.

The exposure of dentinal tubules and the consequent irritation of the odontoblastic processes stimulate the formation of secondary dentin similar to that seen in cases of attrition. Unless the form of abrasion is an extremely severe and rapidly progressive one, the rate of secondary dentin formation is usually sufficient to protect the tooth against pulp exposure.

EROSION

Erosion is defined as a loss of tooth substance by a chemical process that does not involve known bacterial action. The smooth lesions, which exhibit no chalkiness, occur most frequently on the labial and buccal surfaces of the teeth. They also may occur on proximal surfaces. The loss of tooth substance is usually manifested by a shallow, broad, smooth, highly polished, scooped-out depression on the enamel surface adjacent to the cementoenamel junction. Although generally confined to the gingival third of the labial surfaces of anterior teeth, erosion may affect the labial surfaces of any teeth. The lesions, which may exhibit considerable variation in size and shape, usually involve several teeth.

Some cases of erosion may progress to involve the dentin and thereby provoke a secondary

dentin response similar to that seen in cases of attrition and abrasion.

The etiology of this disease is unknown in the majority of cases. The work of McClure and Ruzicka and of Zipkin and McClure suggested that erosion may be related to the citrate content of saliva. Shulman and Robinson, however, were unable to correlate this citrate content of the saliva with the occurrence of erosion in the human being. It has also been suggested that the decalcification may be due to local acidosis in the periodontal tissues resulting from damage due to traumatogenic occlusion. Since traumatogenic occlusion is so common and erosion so rare, however, nearly all authorities agree that there is no relation between the two conditions.

Erosion may occur also as a result of obvious decalcification of teeth. In cases of chronic vomiting, the lingual surfaces of the teeth, particularly of the anterior teeth, may exhibit complete loss of enamel through dissolution by gastric hydrochloric acid. Similarly, the labial surfaces of the teeth of persons who drink large quantities of highly acidic carbonated beverages or lemon juice or who habitually suck lemons or other acid citrus fruits may be affected. Mannerberg has reported that excessive consumption of acid fruit juices is the initial causative factor in many cases of erosion.

This erosion or gastric acid decalcification of teeth is a common finding in patients with *anorexia nervosa*. This is a psychosomatic disease mainly affecting young women, which appears to be increasing in frequency in very recent years. The disease is characterized by induced chronic vomiting, often after bouts of uncontrolled eating that are interspersed between periods of starvation because of an inner rejection of food. The oral manifestations of this disease have been discussed by Hellström and more recently by Brady, who stressed the occurrence of the acid erosion of the teeth from chronic vomiting and also from excessive intake of fruits and juices by many of these patients in an attempt to relieve their thirst after vomiting. It was noted that severe dental caries is also a feature of this disease because of excessive carbohydrate intake.

Dental erosion is also a well-recognized hazard in many industries involving the use of acids. It has been reported by ten Bruggen Cate that in a survey of 555 acid workers, 176 (about 32 per cent) exhibited dental erosion. The various industries involved where acids were utilized included plating, galvanizing, acid pickling, battery manufacture, sanitary cleanser manufacture, munitions manufacture, soft-drinks manufacture, process engraving, crystal glassworks, dyestuffs-container cleaning, and enamel manufacture.

DENTINAL SCLEROSIS

(Transparent Dentin)

Sclerosis of primary dentin is a regressive alteration in tooth substance that is character-ized by calcification of the dentinal tubules. It occurs not only as a result of injury to the dentin by caries or abrasion but also as a manifestation of the normal aging process. For many years it has been known that if a ground section of a tooth with a very shallow carious lesion of the dentin is examined by transmitted light, a translucent zone can be seen in the dentin underlying the cavity (Fig. 5–6, A). This was readily recognized as being due to a difference between the refractive indices of the sclerotic or calcified dentinal tubules and the adjacent normal tubules. Both Beust and Fish showed that dyes do not penetrate those dentinal tubules that are sclerotic as a result either of age or of a slowly progressive type of dental caries.

The exact mechanism of dentinal sclerosis or the deposition of calcium salts in the tubules is not understood, although the most likely source of the calcium salts is the fluid or "dental lymph" within the tubules. The increased mineralization of the tooth decreases the conductivity of the odontoblastic processes. In addition, the sclerosis slows an advancing carious process.

Sclerotic dentin under a carious lesion was shown by Hodge and McKay to be actually harder than adjacent normal dentin. Subsequently Van Huysen, Hodge, and Warren confirmed the fact that sclerotic dentin is more highly calcified than normal dentin by employing a unique adaptation of the x-ray absorption technique in which ground slabs of teeth were

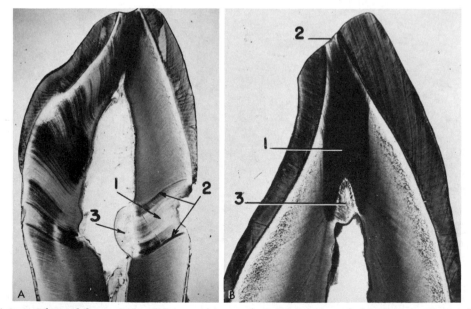

Figure 5–6. A, Sclerosed dentin (1) beneath a cervical cavity bounded on either side by "dead tracts" (2) and below by secondary dentin (3); B, "dead tract" (1) beneath an area of incisal attrition (2). Secondary dentin (3).

photographed by x-rays and the degree of radiopacity in areas of normal and sclerotic dentin
was measured.

"DEAD TRACTS"

"Dead tracts" in dentin are seen in ground
sections of teeth and are manifested as a black
zone by transmitted light but as a white zone
by reflected light (Fig. 5–6, A, B). This optical
phenomenon is due to differences in the refractive indices of the affected tubules and normal
tubules. The nature of the change in the affected tubules is not known, although these
tubules are not calcified and are permeable to
the penetration of dyes.

SECONDARY DENTIN

(Irregular Dentin)

Secondary dentin, which is formed after deposition of the primary dentin has been completed, is characterized by its irregular morphologic pattern. Physiologically, it occurs as a part
of the response of the tooth to stimuli associated
with the normal aging process. Pathologically,
it results from stimulation of exposed dentinal
tubules and odontoblastic processes in a variety
of circumstances, including dental caries, abrasion, attrition, erosion, tooth fracture, and cavity preparation. This dentin, formed as a response to abnormal irritation, has sometimes
been called "adventitious" dentin.

In recent years, a distinction has been drawn
between secondary and tertiary dentin. According to Kuttler, tertiary dentin develops when
pulp irritants are more intense—e.g., abrasion;
mechanical, chemical and thermal insults; erosion; caries; cavity and crown preparations; and
so forth. Tertiary dentin differs from secondary
dentin in that it is localized exclusively adjacent
to the irritated zone, its tubules being very
irregular, tortuous, and reduced in number or
even absent. In contrast, Kuttler has considered
secondary dentin as that which forms in response to the slight aggressive effects of normal
biologic function. Taintor and his associates
have also discussed this terminology, pointing
out that the terms "irregular dentin," "reparative dentin," and "irritation dentin" have been
used as synonyms for "tertiary dentin." However, the term "secondary dentin" is so firmly
ingrained in the vocabulary of most practicing
dentists to designate any dentin that is not

primary dentin that no attempt will be made
here to alter the terminology accepted for many
years, since such a change might result in undue
confusion.

Clinical Features. There are no significant
clinical features that may be used to determine
when teeth have formed secondary dentin, although there is an evident decrease in tooth
sensitivity when secondary dentin formation is
extensive, as it is in elderly persons. This type
of dentin forms an additional insulating layer of
calcified tissue between the pulp and the particular pathologic process that initiated the dentinal response. Thus the eventual pulp involvement is usually delayed. Although secondary
dentin occurs in all teeth, including those of
the deciduous dentition, a study by Bevelander
and Benzer indicated that the anterior teeth
exhibit a higher incidence of secondary dentin
formation than the molar teeth.

Roentgenographic Features. Secondary dentin often may be visualized on the dental roentgenogram if it occurs in an area that is not
overshadowed by other calcified tissue, either
bone or tooth substance. Such secondary dentin
formation may be noted particularly in the pulp
horn areas as well as on the proximal walls of
teeth with proximal caries.

The decrease in size of the pulp chamber and
root canals that occurs with advancing age as a
result of secondary dentin formation is obvious
roentgenographically.

Histologic Features. Physiologic secondary
dentin is usually similar in appearance to primary dentin, but in decalcified stained sections
it often exhibits a different tinctorial reaction
and may be rather well demarcated from the
primary dentin by a deeply staining "resting
line." This type of secondary dentin exhibits
somewhat fewer tubules, although their course
is not especially irregular.

Adventitious secondary dentin arising in response to irritation is usually irregular in nature,
being composed of few tubules that may be
tortuous in appearance (Figs. 5–6, 5–7). In
some instances tubules are inconspicuous if not
completely absent. Occasionally, this secondary
dentin is formed at a rapid rate and odontoblasts
may become entrapped, producing a superficial
resemblance to bone. Such calcified tissue has
been termed "osteodentin."

Stanley and his associates have studied the
rate of reparative dentin formation in human
teeth following cavity preparation under a variety of clinical conditions. They found that
reparative dentin formation was insignificant in
the first postoperative month. Between one and

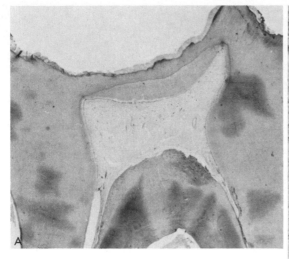

Figure 5–7. *Secondary dentin.*
Secondary dentin beneath carious lesion *(A)*. Normal dentin *(1)*, resting line *(2)*, secondary dentin *(3)*, and pulp *(4)* are shown in higher magnification *(B)*.

one-and-a-half months, new dentin formation reached a maximum rate of approximately 3.5 microns per day. After this period, new dentin formation rapidly decreased.

RETICULAR ATROPHY OF THE PULP

Reticular atrophy of the pulp and more discrete vacuolization of the pulpal tissue and cells have often been described as degenerative or regressive changes of pulp, particularly when they occur as an age change in elderly persons. It has been stated that teeth so affected are clinically symptomless and respond normally to vitality tests. Histologically, reticular atrophy has been described as being characterized by the presence of large vacuolated spaces in the pulp, with a reduction in the number of cellular elements. Accompanying these changes are degeneration and disappearance of the odontoblasts.

It is most interesting and significant that alterations in the pulp tissue identical with those described above can be produced by improper fixation of the tooth and pulp after extraction preparatory to histologic sectioning. Most investigators now believe that this condition is purely an artefact brought about by autolysis of the pulp tissue and does not occur in vivo.

PULP CALCIFICATION

Various forms of calcification within the pulps of teeth are found with such frequency that it may be questioned whether their presence represents a pathologic state or merely an occurrence within the range of normal biologic variation. These calcifications may be located in any portion of the pulp tissue, although certain types are more common in the pulp chamber and others in the root canal.

A number of studies have been carried out to determine the actual incidence of pulp calcification, and the results of these investigations are in essential agreement. For example, Willman reported that of a series of 164 teeth picked at random and examined histologically, 143 (or 87 per cent) exhibited calcification in the pulp. Interestingly, only 15 per cent of the areas of calcification were large enough to be seen on the dental roentgenogram. These findings confirm the investigations of Hill, who reported calcifications in 66 per cent of all teeth examined in young persons between the ages of 10 and 20 years and in 90 per cent of all teeth examined in persons between the ages of 50 and 70 years. There is no apparent difference in the frequency of occurrence either between the sexes or among the various teeth in the dental arch.

The two chief morphologic forms of pulp calcifications are discrete pulp stones (denticles,

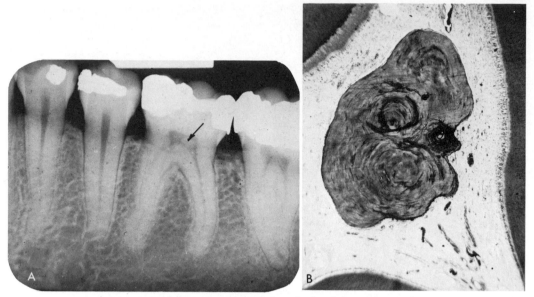

Figure 5–8. *Denticle in pulp chamber.*
Roentgenogram *(A)* and histologic section *(B)*.

pulp nodules) and diffuse calcification. Pulp stones have been classified as either true or false stones, depending upon their microscopic structure.

True denticles are made up of localized masses of calcified tissue that resemble dentin because of their tubular structure. Actually, these nodules bear greater resemblance to secondary dentin than to primary dentin, since the tubules are irregular and few in number. They are considerably more common in the pulp chamber than in the root canal.

True denticles may be subdivided further according to whether or not they are attached to the wall of the pulp chamber. Denticles lying entirely within the pulp tissue and not attached to the dentinal walls are called "free denticles," while those that are continuous with dentinal walls are referred to as "attached denticles." The latter type of calcification is somewhat more common than the former. It should be remembered that though a denticle may appear free in the one plane of section in which it is visualized, it may be attached in another plane. Thus, without serial section of an entire tooth pulp, one cannot state with any degree of assurance that a given denticle is free and not attached.

False denticles are composed of localized masses of calcified material and, unlike true denticles, do not exhibit dentinal tubules. Instead, the nodule appears to be made up of concentric layers or lamellae deposited around a central nidus (Fig. 5–8). The exact nature of this nidus is unknown, although Johnson and Bevelander believe that it is composed of cells, as yet unidentified, around which is laid down a layer of reticular fibers that subsequently calcify.

The false denticle also may be classified as free or attached. As the concentric deposition of calcified material continues, it approximates and finally is in apposition with the dentinal wall. Here it eventually may become surrounded by secondary dentin, and it is then referred to as an "interstitial denticle." False denticles, which occur more commonly in the pulp chamber than in the root canal, are generally somewhat larger than true denticles. They may fill nearly the entire pulp chamber, while true denticles are seldom larger than a fraction of a millimeter in diameter.

Johnson and Bevelander concluded from their studies that a differentiation between "true" and "false" denticles should not be drawn, since all denticles originally show no tubules even though they subsequently may become surrounded by tissue containing dentinal tubules.

Diffuse calcification is most commonly seen in the root canals of teeth and resembles the calcification seen in other tissues of the body following degeneration. This type of calcification is frequently termed "calcific degeneration." Its usual pattern is in amorphous, unorganized linear strands or columns paralleling

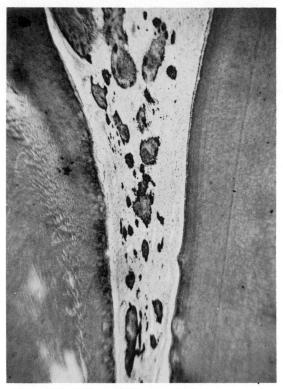

Figure 5-9. *Diffuse calcification of pulp in root canals.*

the blood vessels and nerves of the pulp (Fig. 5-9).

Etiology. The etiology of the various types of pulp calcification is unknown. Although the incidence appears to increase with the age of the persons, there is no definite association with pulpal irritation or inflammation such as that arising from caries or trauma. Since pulp calcifications have been described in unerupted teeth, it is doubtful whether pulpal disease such as inflammation is of any significance. Stafne

and Szabo attempted to correlate pulp nodules with various local or systemic diseases including cholelithiasis, renal lithiasis, arteriosclerosis, gout, acromegaly, osteitis deformans, hypercementosis, and torus palatinus or mandibularis. Their data indicate that no clear-cut relation exists between any of these conditions and pulp calcification.

Kretschmer and Seybold reported that an extremely high percentage of pulp stones yield a pure growth of streptococci upon culture. On this basis it has been suggested that microorganisms are the cause of pulp calcifications. Since the pulps of the affected teeth were reportedly normal, aside from the calcification, and since it is well recognized that bacteria may be forced into the pulp tissue at the time of tooth extraction, it is most unlikely that bacteria are of any significance in the development of these pulp nodules.

More recently, Sundell and his associates have attempted to determine whether the degree of pulp response elicited by cutting procedures and restorative materials was capable of increasing the incidence of pulp stone nidi and pulp stones. They found no significant correlation between pulp stones or nidi and the age or sex of the patient, the thickness of remaining dentin beneath the cavity preparation, the preparation time, or the traumatic potential of the operative procedure. In addition, these workers have proposed the following schematic diagram incorporating several hypotheses from the literature and, concomitantly, including the mechanism of thrombosis or vascular wall injury or both, leading to pulp-stone formation (see below).

Clinical Significance. The clinical significance of pulp calcification is not completely understood. It has been reported upon numer-

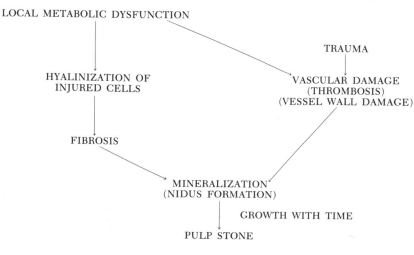

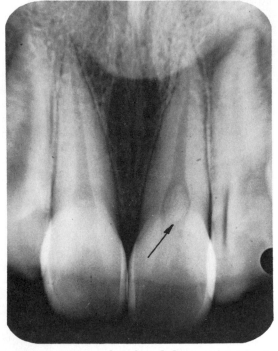

Figure 5–10. *Large denticle occluding entrance to root canal.*

ous occasions that pulp stones are a cause of pain, varying from mild pulpal neuralgia to severe, excruciating pain resembling that of tic douloureux. The consensus is that though denticles may seem to impinge on nerves of the pulp, they probably do not. Most investigators now believe that seldom, if ever, are pulp stones the cause of dental pain. Therefore, the extraction of teeth with roentgenographically demonstrable pulp stones in the hope of relieving dental pain or vague facial neuralgia cannot be defended. Neither can the view that the presence of pulp stones indicates pulpal infection be condoned. In the light of our present knowledge, pulp calcification is a purely coincidental finding without clinical significance. Difficulty may be encountered in extirpating the pulp during root canal therapy if calcifications are present (Fig. 5–10).

RESORPTION OF TEETH

Resorption of teeth occurs in many circumstances other than the normal process associated with the shedding of deciduous teeth. The roots of permanent teeth may undergo resorption in response to a variety of stimuli; moreover, it is recognized that root resorption in permanent

teeth occurs to a slight degree even under apparently normal conditions. Since resorption of a tooth may begin either on the external surface (arising as a result of a tissue reaction in the periodontal or pericoronal tissue) or inside the tooth (from a pulpal tissue reaction), the general terms "external resorption" and "internal resorption" are used to distinguish between the two types. The chief causes or situations in which resorption may occur are as follows:

1. External resorption
    a. Periapical inflammation
    b. Reimplantation of teeth
    c. Tumors and cysts
    d. Excessive mechanical or occlusal forces
    e. Impaction of teeth
    f. Idiopathic
2. Internal resorption
    a. Idiopathic

EXTERNAL RESORPTION

RESORPTION ASSOCIATED WITH PERIAPICAL INFLAMMATION. Resorption of calcified dental tissues occurs in the same fashion as that of bone and, in most instances, the presence of osteoclasts is an outstanding feature in areas of active resorption. It should be pointed out, however, that there is considerable evidence indicating that osteoclasts may not be essential for the resorption of calcified tissues.

A periapical granuloma (q.v.) arising as a result of pulpal infection or trauma occasionally causes subsequent resorption of the root apex if the inflammatory lesion persists for a sufficient period of time (Fig. 5–11). Most teeth involved by a periapical granuloma, however, do not exhibit any significant degree of resorption. The reason for the occasional occurrence is not known. It is generally agreed that bone resorption occurs more readily in highly vascular areas than in relatively avascular areas and, since the periapical granuloma is quite vascular, it is surprising that resorption of the root is not more frequently seen. That bone is more readily resorbed than dental tissue is borne out by the fact that bone is always destroyed when a periapical granuloma develops, whereas resorption of the tooth root without loss of bone seldom occurs except at a microscopic level.

In those cases of periapical granuloma in which root resorption does occur, it is usually obvious on the dental roentgenogram. It appears as a slight raggedness or blunting of the

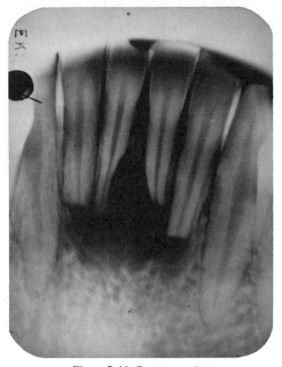

Figure 5–11. *Root resorption.*
Diffuse periapical granuloma resulting from death of pulp caused by traumatic injury has resulted in resorption of roots.

teeth, however, exhibit complete resorption of the root and are exfoliated.

TUMORS AND CYSTS. The resorption of roots brought about by tumors is similar to that seen in teeth involved by cysts (Fig. 5–12). In many instances resorption by tumors or cysts appears to be essentially a pressure phenomenon. This is to be expected, since the phenomenon of resorption of bone under pressure is well recognized and actually forms the basis of orthodontic practice.

Both benign and malignant tumors may cause root resorption, although benign lesions are more likely to produce displacement than actual destruction of the tooth. In most cases connective tissue is present between the tumor and the tooth, and it is from this tissue that cells develop, chiefly osteoclasts, which appear responsible for the root resorption. This is particularly true of epithelial tumors that invade the jaws. Occasionally tumors are seen in which, histologically, the neoplastic cells are found adjacent to and within the ragged resorption lacunae on the root surface.

Cysts cause root resorption in a manner similar to resorption caused by benign tumors, that is, chiefly by pressure, although displacement of the tooth is more common than resorption. An apical periodontal cyst arising as a result of pulp infection may exert such pressure on the

root apex in the early stages, proceeding to a severe loss of tooth substance. In a tooth that has had the root canal treated and filled, but around which periapical inflammation persists, resorption of the root may occur and ultimately leave only the root canal filling projecting out of the shortened root. The roentgenographic picture of this phenomenon presents an unusual appearance and superficially resembles overfilling of the root canal.

REIMPLANTED TEETH. The reimplantation, or transplantation, of teeth (q.v.) almost invariably results in severe resorption of the root. The tooth substance, regardless of whether the root canal has been filled or not, must be considered nonvital tissue, except in the case of transplanted developing teeth when the vascular supply to the tooth may be reestablished and its vitality maintained. Thus the implanted tooth is analogous to a bone graft which acts only as a temporary scaffold and is ultimately resorbed and replaced. The tooth root is resorbed and replaced by bone, producing an ankylosis. If the tooth root does not become completely resorbed, the ensuing ankylosis may result in a functional tooth. Many reimplanted

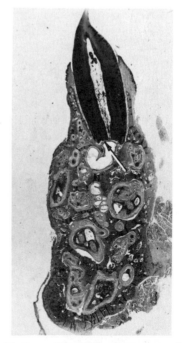

Figure 5–12. *Resorption of the root apex associated with an ameloblastoma.*

apex of the involved or adjacent tooth that the intervening connective tissue is stimulated, osteoclasts form, and resorption begins. This reaction may occur with any type of cyst that progressively expands, but it is more common with the periodontal cyst than with the dentigerous, primordial, or fissural cysts.

EXCESSIVE MECHANICAL OR OCCLUSAL FORCES. The usual form of excessive mechanical force with which root resorption may be associated is that applied during orthodontic treatment. It has been recognized for many years, at least since the work of Ketcham, that patients who have undergone orthodontic treatment frequently exhibit multiple areas of root resorption irrespective of the manner of treatment, i.e., the type of appliance or the duration and degree of force exerted. In some patients this resorption is mild and involves only a few teeth; in others there may be loss of over 50 per cent of the root length of most of the teeth.

The cause for this extreme variation under apparently similar clinical conditions is unknown. Becks reported that systemic disturbances, the chief among these being hypothyroidism, may predispose to root resorption, particularly in the patient who is receiving orthodontic treatment. The influence of the systemic factor remains to be confirmed, however.

It is fortunate that bone undergoes resorption far more readily than cementum when force is exerted upon the tooth by orthodontic appliances or by occlusal trauma. This pressure upon the supporting bone invariably results in destruction, primarily of bone. Small lacunae often appear on the surface of the cementum and ultimately extend into the dentin, indicating early tooth resorption. Probably most cases of this minor type of resorption are soon repaired by the deposition of bone or cementum in these ragged lacunae, particularly if the occlusal force or orthodontic pressure is relieved.

Some investigators have questioned the clinical significance of root resorption secondary to mechanical or occlusal forces since, regardless

of the severity or degree of the resorption, seldom is a tooth ever exfoliated. There may be destruction of the apical two thirds of the root of a tooth with no evidence of looseness or other signs of impending difficulties.

IMPACTED TEETH. Teeth that are completely impacted or embedded in bone occasionally will undergo resorption of the crown or of both crown and root. Stafne and Austin pointed out that although this resorption most commonly begins on the crown of the tooth, destruction of all the enamel epithelium is not a prerequisite for the onset of resorption. In some cases only a limited amount of epithelium appears to be destroyed, allowing the connective tissue to come in contact with the crown and thus initiating the resorptive process. Stafne and Austin reported that teeth that are completely embedded are those most apt to undergo resorption. In a study of 226 embedded teeth in which resorption occurred, they found that 78 per cent of the teeth were in the maxillary arch and that 60 per cent of these maxillary teeth were cuspids (Table 5–2). This finding is unusual and significant because, although maxillary and mandibular third molars far outnumber maxillary cuspids in incidence of impaction, the cuspids undergo resorption more frequently than the third molars. The reason for this is unknown. Impacted supernumerary teeth, particularly mesiodens, also are prone to undergo resorption.

The roentgenographic picture presented by these teeth is an unusual one, particularly when the resorption occurs on the tooth crown. The irregular destruction frequently has suggested that the impacted or embedded tooth is involved by caries, an obvious impossibility (Fig. 5–13).

Impacted teeth also may cause resorption of the roots of adjacent teeth without being resorbed themselves. This is particularly common in the case of a horizontally or mesioangularly impacted mandibular third molar impinging on the roots of the second molar. There is always connective tissue interposed between the sec-

Table 5–2. Distribution of Embedded Teeth Exhibiting Roentgenographic Evidence of Resorption

	CENTRAL INCISOR	LATERAL INCISOR	CUSPID	2ND BICUSPID	3RD MOLAR	TOTAL NO.	%
Maxilla	4	1	106	2	64	177	78
Mandible	1	0	17	7	24	49	22

From E. C. Stafne and L. T. Austin: Resorption of embedded teeth. J. Am. Dent. Assoc., 32:1003, 1945.

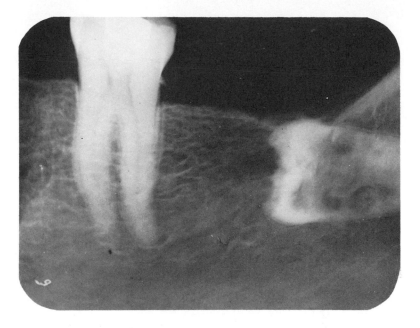

Figure 5–13. *Resorption of impacted tooth.* (Courtesy of Drs. Paul and Emmett Jurgens.)

ond and third molars, and the pressure of the third molar appears to activate the resorptive cells, thus setting the stage for tooth destruction.

IDIOPATHIC RESORPTION. Many investigators have reported that the roots of permanent teeth may undergo a certain amount of resorption in apparently normal adults without any obvious cause (Fig. 5–14). The term "idiopathic root resorption" has been applied to this phenomenon. The actual incidence of this form of resorption was not appreciated until the study of Massler and Perreault, in which it was found that of 301 young (18 to 25 years old) male and female patients, *all* exhibited some degree of

root resorption in four or more teeth, as judged by roentgenographic examination alone. Furthermore, it was reported that 82 per cent of the teeth in the men and 91 per cent of the teeth in the women showed some evidence of resorption. In less than three per cent of the cases was there any indication as to the cause of this condition. The teeth most commonly involved by root resorption were the maxillary bicuspids, while the mandibular incisors and molars exhibited the least resorption. Massler and Perreault pointed out, however, that this finding is in contradistinction to nearly all other reported studies, including those of Becks and of Stafne and Slocumb (Table 5–3), in which

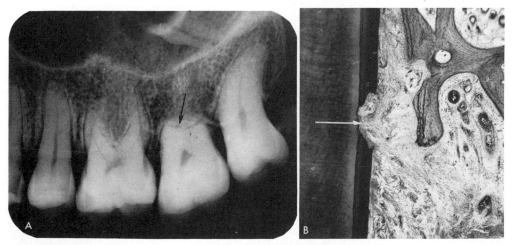

Figure 5–14. *Root resorption.*
A, Severe idiopathic root resorption of maxillary second molar. B, Mild root resorption, visible only microscopically.

Table 5–3. Teeth Involved in Idiopathic Resorption

TEETH INVOLVED*	MAXILLA		MANDIBLE	
	NO.	%	NO.	%
Central incisor	45	22.5	44	22.0
Lateral incisor	15	7.5	11	5.0
Cuspid	18	9.0	14	7.0
Premolar	10	5.0	25	12.5
Molar	0	0	18	9.0
Total	88	44.0	112	56.0

From E. C. Stafne and C. H. Slocumb: Idiopathic resorption of teeth. Am. J. Orthod. Oral Surg., *30*:41, 1944.

*No attempt was made to differentiate between external and internal resorption in this study, since such a distinction could not be drawn in many instances.

the maxillary and mandibular central incisors were shown to be most frequently involved.

It appears that root resorption is far more common than was formerly believed. The majority of cases of idiopathic resorption are mild (Fig. 5–14, *B*). According to the data of Massler and Perreault, over 75 per cent of the teeth exhibiting resorption showed loss of less than 4 mm. of the root apex. Although the etiology remains unknown, several possibilities present themselves. The resorption may be related to one or more systemic disorders, the most obvious being some form of endocrine disturbance. A genetic characteristic governing the resorption potential of bone and tooth substance has been demonstrated in animals and is conceivable in human beings. Finally, the possibility that root resorption, with subsequent repair, is no more pathologic than an analogous resorption and repair of bone must be considered.

A rare form of multiple idiopathic root resorption may occur that involves all or nearly all of the teeth. The resorption may begin at the cementoenamel junction or nearer to the root apex. This disease has been discussed by Kerr and his associates, who pointed out that these patients are medically normal and have no past history such as orthodontic treatment or radiation that might explain the phenomenon.

INTERNAL RESORPTION

(Chronic Perforating Hyperplasia of the Pulp; Internal Granuloma; Odontoclastoma; Pink Tooth of Mummery)

Internal resorption is an unusual form of tooth resorption that begins centrally within the tooth, apparently initiated in most cases by a peculiar inflammatory hyperplasia of the pulp. The cause of the pulpal inflammation and subsequent resorption of tooth substance is unknown, although an obvious carious exposure and accompanying pulp infection are sometimes present. It is even possible that true internal resorption does not exist but rather is a result of resorption of the tooth and invasion of the pulp by granulation tissue arising in the periodontium. An excellent discussion of the problem of idiopathic tooth resorption, both external and internal, has been published by Sullivan and Jolly, while Sweet has presented a historic review of the internal resorption of teeth, beginning with the first description of the problem by Bell in 1830.

Clinical Features. Most cases of internal resorption present no early clinical symptoms. The first evidence of the lesion may be the appearance of a pink-hued area on the crown of the tooth, which represents the hyperplastic, vascular pulp tissue filling the resorbed area and showing through the remaining overlying tooth substance (Fig. 5–15). In the event that the resorption begins in the root, there are no significant clinical findings.

It is unusual for more than one tooth in any given patient to be affected by internal resorption, although cases of multiple tooth involvement have been recorded. There appears to be no specific predilection for occurrence in one jaw rather than the other, although no large enough series of cases has been reported to justify drawing any significant conclusions. The individual tooth involved may be any tooth, and examples of internal resorption in incisors, cuspids, bicuspids and molars have all been reported at one time or another.

Roentgenographic Features. Roentgenographic examination may provide the first revelation of pulpal disease when the patient appears for a routine checkup. The involved tooth exhibits a round or ovoid radiolucent area in the central portion of the tooth, associated with the pulp but not with the external surface of the tooth unless the condition is of such duration that perforation has occurred (Fig. 5–16). Complete perforation is not an uncommon finding if the tooth is left untreated.

Histologic Features. Microscopic examination of a tooth with internal resorption shows a variable degree of resorption of the inner or pulpal surface of the dentin and proliferation of the pulp tissue filling the defect. The resorption is of an irregular lacunar variety showing occasional osteoclasts or "odontoclasts," hence the

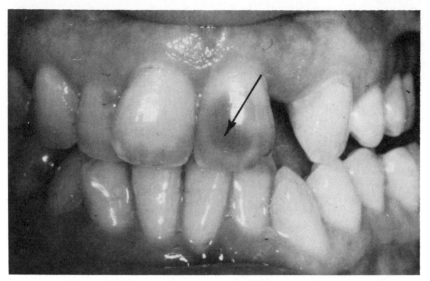

Figure 5–15. *Internal resorption of maxillary central incisor.*
The dark shadow represents pulp tissue visible through the tooth substance.

term "odontoclastoma." The pulp tissue usually exhibits a chronic inflammatory reaction but little else to explain the cause for this unusual condition (Fig. 5–17).

Sometimes the tooth exhibits alternating periods of resorption and repair, as manifested by irregular lacuna-like areas in the dentin that are partially or completely filled in with irregular.

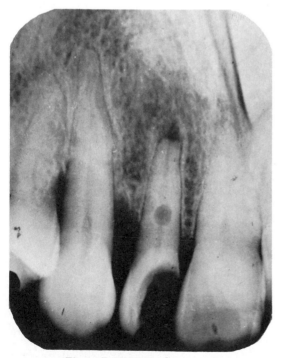

Figure 5–16. *Internal resorption.*

dentin or osteodentin, which itself is undergoing resorption. As the resorptive process advances, the dentin may be completely resorbed in a narrow segment. The enamel is also resorbed if the lesion is situated in the coronal portion of the tooth. If the lesion is in the root of the tooth, perforation of the dentin and cementum may occur, which, if left untreated, may eventually result in complete separation of the apical portion from the remainder of the tooth. When the root surface is perforated, it is impossible to determine whether the lesion began "externally" or "internally."

Treatment and Prognosis. If the condition is discovered before perforation of the crown or root has occurred, root canal therapy may be carried out with the expectation of a fairly high degree of success. Once perforation has occurred, the tooth must usually be extracted.

There are a few cases known in which spontaneous regression of the internal resorption occurred, with the lesion either remaining but showing no further progress or with actual repair by deposition of calcified tissue. The cause of the abrupt cessation of tissue destruction is as obscure as the cause of its initiation.

HYPERCEMENTOSIS

(Cementum Hyperplasia)

Hypercementosis may be regarded as a regressive change of teeth characterized by the deposition of excessive amounts of secondary cementum on root surfaces. This most com-

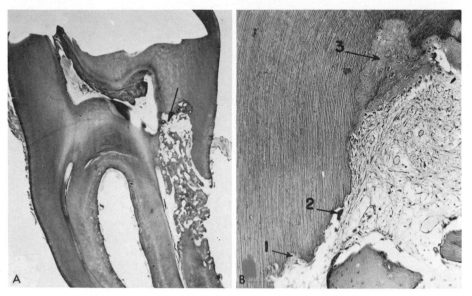

Figure 5–17. *Internal resorption.*
Low-power photomicrograph *(A)* and high-power photomicrograph *(B)* showing resorption lacuna *(1)*, osteoclasts *(2)*, and area of repair *(3)*.

monly involves nearly the entire root area, although in some instances the cementum formation is focal, usually occurring only at the apex of a tooth.

Etiology. A variety of circumstances may favor the deposition of excessive amounts of cementum. These include: (1) accelerated elongation of a tooth, (2) inflammation about a tooth, (3) tooth repair, and (4) osteitis deformans, or Paget's disease of bone. In addition, hypercementosis of unknown etiology may occur either in a generalized form, involving all the teeth, or in a localized form, involving one tooth. Tooth function does not appear to favor the increased deposition of cementum on root surfaces. Actually, studies have indicated that the thickness of cementum is increased in nonfunctioning teeth, including embedded or impacted teeth. The stimulus in these instances is unknown.

Acceleration in the elongation of a tooth owing to loss of an antagonist is accompanied by hyperplasia of the cementum, apparently as a result of the inherent tendency for maintenance of the normal width of the periodontal ligament. This hypercementosis is most prominent at the apex of the root, although deposition of secondary cementum usually involves the entire root, tapering off in thickness toward the cervical portion of the tooth.

Inflammation at the apex of a tooth root, usually occurring as a result of pulpal infection, sometimes stimulates excessive deposition of cementum. This does not occur at the apex of the root directly adjacent to the area of inflammation, since the cementoblasts and their direct precursors in this area have been lost as a result of the inflammatory process. Instead, the cementum is laid down on the root surface at some distance above the apex, apparently being induced by the inflammatory reaction that, at some distance from its center, acts as a stimulus to cementoblasts. At the apex of the involved root itself it is not uncommon for actual resorption of cementum and dentin to occur. Thoma and Goldman pointed out that the periapical inflammation tends to cause some increase in eruption of the tooth, and this also favors the deposition of cementum in attempting to maintain the width of the periodontal ligament.

Tooth repair does not occasion the deposition of remarkable amounts of secondary cementum. Nevertheless, the cementum that is formed is often laid down with such rapidity that a mild form of hypercementosis is simulated. On occasion, occlusal trauma results in mild root resorption. Such resorption is repaired by secondary cementum. Root fracture is also repaired on occasion by deposition of cementum between the root fragments as well as on their periphery. Finally, cemental tears, detachment of strips of cementum from the root due to trauma, are repaired by cementum growing into and filling the defects and eventually uniting with the torn cementum.

Osteitis deformans, or Paget's disease of bone

(q.v.), is a generalized skeletal disease characterized by deposition of excessive amounts of secondary cementum on the roots of the teeth and by the apparent disappearance of the lamina dura of the teeth, as well as by other features related to the bone itself. Although the bone changes are the most prominent features of the disease, generalized hypercementosis should always suggest the possibility of the presence of osteitis deformans.

Spike formation of cementum is an uncommon condition characterized by the occurrence of small spikes or outgrowths of cementum on the root surface. These cemental spikes appear in some cases of excessive occlusal trauma, probably as a result of deposition of irregular cementum in focal groups of fibers of the periodontal ligament. The exact mechanism of spike formation is unknown, and its significance is obscure.

Clinical Features. Hypercementosis produces no significant clinical signs or symptoms indicative of its presence. There is no increase or decrease in tooth sensitivity, no sensitivity to percussion unless periapical inflammation is present, and no visible changes in gross appearance in situ. When the tooth with hypercementosis is extracted, the root or roots appear larger in diameter than normal and present rounded apices.

Roentgenographic Features. On the periapical roentgenogram most cases of hypercementosis, at least of any significant degree, are distinguished by the thickening and apparent blunting of the roots. The roots lose their typical "sharpened" or "spiked" appearance and exhibit rounding of the apex (Fig. 5–18). It is generally impossible to differentiate the root dentin from the primary or secondary cementum roentgenographically; therefore the diagnosis of hypercementosis is established by the shape or outline of the root rather than by any differences in radiodensity of the tooth structure.

Histologic Features. The microscopic appearance of hypercementosis is a characteristic one in which an excessive amount of secondary or cellular cementum is found deposited directly over the typically thin layer of primary acellular cementum (Fig. 5–19). The area involved may be the entire root or only a portion, typically the apical region. The secondary cementum has been termed "osteocementum" because of its cellular nature and its resemblance to bone. This cementum typically is arranged in concentric layers around the root and frequently shows numerous resting lines, indicated by deeply staining hematoxyphilic lines parallel to the root surface.

Treatment and Prognosis. No treatment is indicated for teeth exhibiting hypercementosis, since the condition in itself is innocuous. In those cases in which the overproduction of cementum is due to inflammation of pulpal origin, treatment of the primary condition is obviously necessary. The extraction of teeth because of hypercementosis is contraindicated, since the prognosis of such teeth is excellent in the absence of concomitant infection.

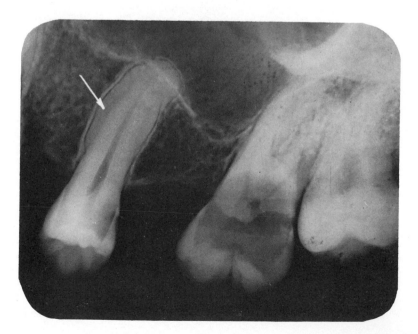

Figure 5–18. *Hypercementosis.*

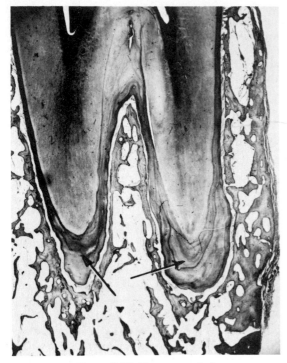

Figure 5–19. *Hypercementosis.*

CEMENTICLES

Cementicles are small foci of calcified tissue, not necessarily true cementum, which lie free in the periodontal ligament of the lateral and apical root areas. The exact cause for their formation is unknown, but it is generally agreed that in most instances they represent areas of dystrophic calcification and thus are an example of a regressive or degenerative change.

It is recognized that actually a variety of calcified bodies may occur in the periodontal ligament, not all of which have the morphologic characteristics of cementum. Nevertheless, they have all been commonly known as cementicles. These various types of calcifications have been reviewed by Moskow.

The most common manner in which cementicles develop is by calcification of nests of epithelial cells, i.e., epithelial rests, in the periodontal ligament as a result of degenerative change. These bodies enlarge by further deposition of calcium salts in the adjacent surrounding connective tissue (Fig. 5–20, A). The continued peripheral calcification of the connective tissue may result in the eventual union of the cementicle with, and even inclusion in, root cementum or alveolar bone. The pattern of calcification often gives the appearance of a circular lamellated structure. When only partially embedded in the root cementum, the cementicle may impart a roughened globular outline to the root surface (Fig. 5–20, B).

Cementicles may arise from focal calcification of connective tissue between Sharpey's bundles with no apparent central nidus. This calcification occurs as small round or ovoid globules of calcium salts.

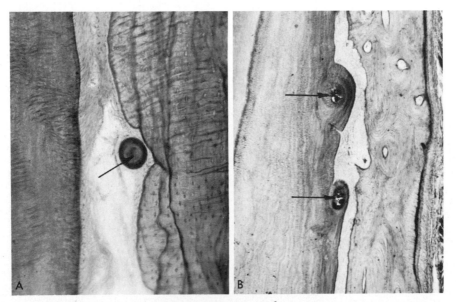

Figure 5–20. *Cementicles.*
A, Free cementicle. B, Attached cementicle.

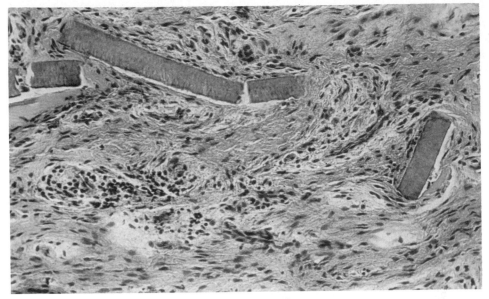

Figure 5–21. *Cemental tears.*
Small strips of primary cementum lying free in the periodontal membrane after traumatic injury.

Small spicules of cementum torn from the root surface—i.e., cemental tears—or fragments of bone detached from the alveolar plate, if lying free in the periodontal ligament may resemble cementicles, particularly after they have undergone some remodeling through resorption and subsequent repair (Fig. 5–21).

Finally, cementicles appear to arise through calcification of thrombosed capillaries in the periodontal ligament and, as Mikola and Bauer pointed out in their excellent discussion of the formation of cementicles, are analogous to phleboliths that can occur elsewhere in the body. Although all cementicles are composed of calcified material, they are too small to be seen on the intraoral roentgenogram, seldom being larger than 0.2 to 0.3 mm. in diameter. Clusters of cementicles may form, and at the apices of teeth these have sometimes been regarded as a cementoma (q.v.), particularly as the clusters unite through interstitial deposition of bone or cementum.

Cementicles are of no clinical significance and, as far as can be determined, are not detrimental to tooth function.

REFERENCES

Applebaum, E.: Internal resorption of teeth. Dent. Cosmos, 76:847, 1934.

Becks, H.: Root resorptions and their relation to pathologic bone formation. Int. J. Orthod. Oral Surg., 22:445, 1936.

Becks, H., and Cowden, R. C.: Root resorptions and their relation to pathologic bone formation. Am. J. Orthod. Oral Surg., 28:513, 1942.

Beust, T. B.: Physiologic changes in the dentin. J. Dent. Res., 11:267, 1931.

Bevelander, G., and Benzer, S.: Morphology and incidence of secondary dentin in human teeth. J. Am. Dent. Assoc., 30:1075, 1943.

Brady, W. F.: The anorexia nervosa syndrome. Oral Surg., 50:509, 1980.

Browne, W. G.: Idiopathic tooth resorption in association with metaplasia. Oral Surg., 7:1298, 1954.

Cahn, L. R.: Calcifications of the dental pulp. Dent. Items Interest, 48:808, 1926.

Coolidge, E. D.: The reaction of cementum in the presence of injury and infection. J. Am. Dent. Assoc., 18:499, 1931.

Ervin, J. C., and Bucher, E. M.: Prevalence of tooth root exposure and abrasion among dental patients. Dent. Items Interest, 66:760, 1944.

Fish, E. W.: Lesions of the dentine and their significance in the production of dental caries. J. Am. Dent. Assoc., 17:992, 1930.

Gardner, B. S., and Goldstein, H.: The significance of hypercementosis. Dent. Cosmos, 73:1065, 1931.

Gottlieb, B.: Biology of the cementum. J. Periodontol., 13:13, 1942.

Held, A. J.: Cementogenesis and the normal and pathologic structure of cementum. Oral Surg., 4:53, 1951.

Hellström, I.: Oral complications in anorexia nervosa. Scand. J. Dent. Res., 85:71, 1977.

Henry, J. L., and Weinmann, J. P.: The pattern of resorption and repair of human cementum. J. Am. Dent. Assoc., 42:270, 1951.

Hill, T. J.: Pathology of the dental pulp. J. Am. Dent. Assoc., 21:820, 1934.

Hodge, H. C., and McKay, H.: The micro-hardness of teeth. J. Am. Dent. Assoc., 20:227, 1933.

Johnson, P. L., and Bevelander, G.: Histogenesis and histochemistry of pulpal calcification. J. Dent. Res., 35:714, 1956.

Kerr, D. A., Courtney, R. M., and Burkes, E. J.: Multiple idiopathic root resorption. Oral Surg., 29:552, 1970.

Ketcham, A. H.: A progress report of an investigation of apical root resorption of vital permanent teeth. Int. J. Orthod. Oral Surg., 15:310, 1929.

Kitchin, P. C., and Robinson, H. B. G.: The abrasiveness of dentifrices as measured on the cervical areas of extracted teeth. J. Dent. Res., 27:195, 1948.

Kretschmer, O. S., and Seybold, J. W.: The bacteriology of dental pulp stones. Dent. Cosmos, 78:292, 1936.

Kronfeld, R.: The biology of the cementum. J. Am. Dent. Assoc. and Dent. Cosmos, 25:1451, 1938.

Kuttler, Y.: Classification of dentin into primary, secondary and tertiary. Oral Surg., 12:996, 1959.

Manly, R. S.: The abrasion of cementum and dentin by modern dentifrices. J. Dent. Res., 20:583, 1941.

Mannerberg, F.: Salivary factors in cases of erosion. Odontol. Revy, 14:156, 1963.

Massler, M., and Perreault, J. G.: Root resorption in the permanent teeth of young adults. J. Dent. Child., 21:158, 1954.

McClure, F. J., and Ruzicka, S. J.: The destructive effect of citrate vs. lactate ions on rats' molar tooth surfaces, in vivo. J. Dent. Res., 25:1, 1946.

Mikola, O. J., and Bauer, W. H.: "Cementicles" and fragments of cementum in the periodontal membrane. Oral Surg., 2:1063, 1949.

Moskow, B. S.: Origin, histogenesis and fate of calcified bodies in the periodontal ligament. J. Periodontol., 42:131, 1971.

Mummery, J. H.: The pathology of "pink spots" on teeth. Br. Dent. J., 41:300, 1920.

Pindborg, J. J.: Pathology of the Dental Hard Tissues. Philadelphia, W. B. Saunders Company, 1970.

Rabinovitch, B. Z.: Internal resorption. Oral Surg., 10:193, 1957.

Robinson, H. B. G.: Abrasion, attrition and erosion of the teeth. Health Center J. Ohio State Univ., 3:21, 1949.

Robinson, H. B. G., Boling, L. R., and Lischer, B. E.; in E. V. Cowdry: Problems on Ageing. 2nd ed. Baltimore, Williams & Wilkins Company, 1941.

Rudolph, C. E.: A comparative study in root resorption in permanent teeth. J. Am. Dent. Assoc., 23:822, 1936.

Shulman, E., and Robinson, H. B. G.: Salivary citrate content and erosion of teeth. J. Dent. Res., 27:541, 1948.

Sicher, H.: The biology of attrition. Oral Surg., 6:406, 1953.

Stafne, E. C., and Austin, L. T.: Resorption of embedded teeth. J. Am. Dent. Assoc., 32:1003, 1945.

Stafne, E. C., and Lovestedt, S. A.: Dissolution of tooth substance by lemon juice, acid beverages and acids from some other sources. J. Am. Dent. Assoc., 34:586, 1947.

Stafne, E. C., and Szabo, S. E.: The significance of pulp nodules. Dent. Cosmos, 75:160, 1933.

Stanley, H. R., White, C. L., and McCray, L.: The rate of tertiary (reparative) dentine formation in the human tooth. Oral Surg., 21:180, 1966.

Sullivan, H. R., and Jolly, M.: Idiopathic resorption. Aust. Dent. J., 2:193, 1957.

Sundell, J. R., Stanley, H. R., and White, C. L.: The relationship of coronal pulp stone formation to experimental operative procedures. Oral Surg., 25:579, 1968.

Sweet, A. P. S.: Internal resorption, a chronology. Dent. Radiogr. Photogr., 38:75, 1965.

Taintor, J. F., Biesterfeld, R. C., and Langeland, K.: Irritational or reparative dentin. Oral Surg., 51:442, 1981.

ten Bruggen Cate, H. J.: Dental erosion in industry. Br. J. Indust. Med., 25:249, 1968.

Thoma, K. H., and Goldman, H. M.: The pathology of dental cementum. J. Am. Dent. Assoc., 26:1943, 1939.

Van Huysen, G., Hodge, H. C., and Warren, S. L.: A quantitative roentgen-densitometric study of the changes in teeth due to attrition. J. Dent. Res., 16:243, 1937.

Warner, G. R., Orban, B., Hine, M. K., and Ritchey, B. T.: Internal resorption of teeth: interpretation of histologic findings. J. Am. Dent. Assoc., 34:468, 1947.

Weinberger, A.: Attritioning of teeth. Oral Surg., 8:1048, 1955.

Idem: The clinical significance of hypercementosis. Oral Surg., 7:79, 1954.

Willman, W.: Calcifications in the pulp. Bur, 34:73, 1934.

Zipkin, I., and McClure, F. J.: Salivary citrate and dental erosion. J. Dent. Res., 28:613, 1949.

SECTION II

DISEASES OF MICROBIAL ORIGIN

CHAPTER 6

Bacterial, Viral and Mycotic Infections

Certain bacteria, viruses and fungi produce diseases which are manifested in or about the oral cavity. Some of these diseases or lesions are of a specific nature and are produced by a specific microorganism. Others are clinically specific, but may be caused by any of a broad group of microorganisms. This microbial specificity or nonspecificity is characteristic of infectious diseases wherever they may occur in the body, and is not necessarily confined to those of the oral cavity.

BACTERIAL INFECTIONS

SCARLET FEVER

(Scarlatina)

Scarlet fever, a disease that occurs predominantly in children during the winter months, is caused by infection with streptococcal organisms of the beta hemolytic type that elaborate an erythrogenic toxin. It is similar in many respects to acute tonsillitis and pharyngitis caused by streptococci, paralleling the occurrence of these conditions in its epidemiology, and is regarded as a separate entity only because of the nature of the toxin. A number of different strains of streptococci may produce the disease. A widespread immunity exists, particularly among adults, owing to repeated mild experiences with streptococci which may never have produced clinical evidence of disease, but an immunity against the exanthema toxin does not protect against streptococcal infection.

Clinical Features. After the entrance of the microorganisms into the body, which is believed to occur usually through the pharynx, there is an incubation period of three to five days, after which the patient exhibits severe pharyngitis and tonsillitis, headache, chills, fever and vomiting. Accompanying these symptoms may be enlargement and tenderness of the regional cervical lymph nodes. The diagnosis of scarlet fever is frequently not established until the characteristic diffuse, bright scarlet skin rash appears on the second or third day of the illness. This rash, which is particularly prominent in the areas of the skin folds, is a result of the toxic injury to the vascular endothelium which produces dilatation of the small blood vessels and consequent hyperemia.

Oral Manifestations. The chief oral manifestations of scarlet fever have been referred to as "stomatitis scarlatina." The mucosa, particularly of the palate, may appear congested, and the throat is often fiery red. The tonsils and faucial pillars are usually swollen and sometimes covered with a grayish exudate.

More important are the changes occurring in the tongue. Early in the course of the disease the tongue exhibits a white coating, and the fungiform papillae are edematous and hyperemic, projecting above the surface as small red knobs. This phenomenon has been described clinically as a "strawberry tongue." The coating of the tongue is soon lost, beginning at the tip and lateral margins, and this organ becomes deep red, glistening and smooth except for the swollen, hyperemic papillae. The tongue in this phase has been termed the "raspberry tongue." In severe cases of scarlet fever, ulceration of the buccal mucosa and palate has been reported, but this appears to be due to secondary infection.

Signaling the clinical termination of the disease is the desquamation of the skin, which usually occurs within a week or 10 days. Soon after, the tongue and the remainder of the mucosa assume a normal appearance.

Complications. Occasional complications may arise referable to local or generalized bacterial dissemination or to hypersensitivity reactions to the bacterial toxins. These may include peritonsillar abscess, rhinitis and sinusitis, otitis media and mastoiditis, meningitis, pneumonia, glomerulonephritis, rheumatic fever and arthritis.

Prevention and Treatment. There are no available methods for the prevention of scarlet fever, although the disease at present in the United States appears to be a relatively mild one. The administration of antibiotics not only will ameliorate the disease, but also will aid in controlling possible complications.

DIPHTHERIA

Diphtheria is an acute contagious disease caused by a gram-positive bacillus, *Corynebacterium diphtheriae*, or the Klebs-Loeffler bacillus. This infection occurs most frequently in children during the fall and winter months. The microorganism inhabits the upper respiratory tract of man and is transmitted only by him, usually through droplet infection or by direct contact. In some instances carriers of the disease, unaffected themselves, are responsible for dissemination of the microorganisms. Exposure to the diphtheria bacillus, particularly in the adult, may result in a subclinical infection which is usually sufficient to establish immunity through development of circulating antitoxins.

Clinical Features. The incubation period for diphtheria is only a few days. The disease is manifested initially by listlessness, malaise, headache, fever and occasional vomiting. Within a short time the patient may complain of a sore throat, although this is not inevitably present. Mild redness and edema of the pharynx can usually be observed, and cervical lymphadenopathy is frequently present.

Oral Manifestations. Characteristically, there is formation of a patchy "diphtheritic membrane" which often begins on the tonsils and enlarges, becoming confluent over the surface. This false membrane is a grayish, thick, fibrinous, gelatinous-appearing exudate which contains dead cells, leukocytes and bacteria overlying necrotic, ulcerated areas of the mucosa and covering the tonsils, pharynx and larynx. It tends to be adherent and leaves a bleeding

surface if stripped away. Occasionally the diphtheritic membrane forms on the uvula, soft palate and gingiva. It also has been observed at the site of erupting teeth and on the buccal mucosa, but this is uncommon.

The soft palate may become temporarily paralyzed, usually during the third to fifth weeks of the disease. These patients have a peculiar nasal twang, and may exhibit nasal regurgitation of liquids during drinking. The paralysis usually disappears in a few weeks, or a few months at the most.

If the infection spreads unchecked in the respiratory tract, the larynx may become edematous and covered by the pseudomembrane. This is especially serious because it produces a mechanical respiratory obstruction and the typical cough or diphtheritic croup. If the airway is not cleared, suffocation may result.

Complications. During or after this disease, complications frequently arise in the cardiovascular and nervous systems as a result of toxemia. Thus both myocarditis and polyneuritis may develop, but usually there is complete recovery. Kidney lesions, particularly acute interstitial nephritis, are also possible serious sequelae. The mortality rate is still of such proportions that diphtheria should be considered a serious disease.

Prevention. The disease may be prevented by prophylactic active immunization with diphtheria toxoid. Once the disease has developed, it is treated with antitoxin, usually in combination with antibiotics, as soon as the diagnosis is suspected.

TUBERCULOSIS

Tuberculosis is an infectious granulomatous disease caused by the acid-fast bacillus *Mycobacterium tuberculosis* or, rarely, *Mycobacterium bovis*, although it is now recognized that a variety of other species of mycobacteria are also potentially pathogenic for humans. The disease occurs in all parts of the world, but there is a distinctive variation in the death rate between persons in different geographic areas and between persons of different races. In the United States there has been a great reduction in the mortality rate from tuberculosis since the early part of the twentieth century, although studies have shown that there is a lesser reduction in the actual incidence of infection. This would imply that the present population in this country is more resistant to the disease, probably because of the increasingly better standard of living, improved health laws and greater attention to nutritional needs. There has been a drastic reduction in the number of tuberculin-positive schoolchildren in very recent years, so that the majority of cases of actual tuberculous infection today do not represent new infections but rather those in older persons who had been infected some years earlier.

Pulmonary tuberculosis is the chief form of the disease, although infection may also occur by way of the intestinal tract, tonsils and skin. The primary lung infection may occur at any age and may either extend locally, become disseminated or, more commonly, become completely walled off and healed by fibrosis and calcification. A reinfection or exacerbation of the primary lesion may occur at any time by yielding to host-dependent factors, but a reinfection is usually mild.

Clinical Features. The clinical signs and symptoms of tuberculosis are often remarkably inconspicuous. The patient may suffer episodic fever and chills, but easy fatigability and malaise are often the chief early features of the disease. There may be gradual loss of weight accompanied by a persistent cough with or without associated hemoptysis.

The microorganisms may become disseminated by either blood stream or lymphatic metastasis and, in the former case, give rise to widespread involvement of many organs such as the kidney or liver. This is *miliary tuberculosis*. Lymphatic spread of the tubercle bacilli is usually less extensive, and the microorganisms frequently localize in the lymph nodes.

Tuberculous infection of submaxillary and cervical lymph nodes, or *scrofula*, a tuberculous lymphadenitis, may progress to the formation of an actual abscess or remain as a typical granulomatous lesion. In either case, swelling of the nodes is obvious clinically. They are tender or painful, often show inflammation of the overlying skin and, when an actual abscess exists, typically perforate and discharge pus. It has been suggested that this specific form of tuberculosis probably arises as a result of lymphatic spread of organisms from a focus of infection in the oral cavity such as the tonsils. However, as Popowich and Heydt have stated, no published studies have confirmed the relationship between tuberculous cervical lymphadenitis and a primary source of infection elsewhere. For example, in the series of 22 cases reported by Ord and Matz, there was no history or clinical evidence of pulmonary tuberculosis

in any patient. These investigators also emphasized that this disease can be caused by atypical mycobacteria and also that organisms frequently cannot be cultured from the lesions.

Primary tuberculosis of the skin, or *lupus vulgaris*, may occur in either children or adults and is a notoriously persistent disease. It appears as papular nodules which frequently ulcerate. These are particularly common on the face, but may occur anywhere.

Oral Manifestations. Tuberculous lesions of the oral cavity do occur, but are relatively uncommon. Reported studies on incidence vary considerably. The studies of Farber and his associates indicated that less than 0.1 per cent of the tuberculous patients whom they examined exhibited oral lesions. Katz, on the other hand, found that approximately 20 per cent of a series of 141 patients examined at autopsy manifested such lesions, the majority of which occurred on the base of the tongue and were not discovered clinically. The obscure location of the tuberculous lesions found by Katz might account for the disparity in incidence of occurrence in these studies.

There is general agreement that lesions of the oral mucosa are seldom primary, but rather are secondary to a pulmonary disease. Although the mechanism of inoculation has not been definitely established, it appears most likely that the organisms are carried in the sputum and enter the mucosal tissue through a small break in the surface. It is possible that the organisms may be carried to the oral tissues by a hematogenous route, to be deposited in the submucosa and subsequently to proliferate and ulcerate the overlying mucosa.

The possibility that the dentist may contract an infection from his contact with living tubercle bacilli in the mouths of patients who have pulmonary or oral tuberculosis is a problem of great clinical significance. It has been shown on numerous occasions that the viable acid-fast microorganisms may be recovered from swabs or washings of the oral cavities of tuberculous patients. Abbott and his associates reported that tubercle bacilli were cultured from 45 per cent of 300 samples of water used to wash the teeth and gingiva of 111 tuberculous patients.

Lesions may occur at any site on the oral mucous membrane, but the tongue is most commonly affected, followed by the palate, lips, buccal mucosa, gingiva and frenula. The usual tuberculous lesion is an irregular, superficial or deep, painful ulcer which tends to increase slowly in size (Fig. 6–1, *A*, *B*, *C*). It is frequently

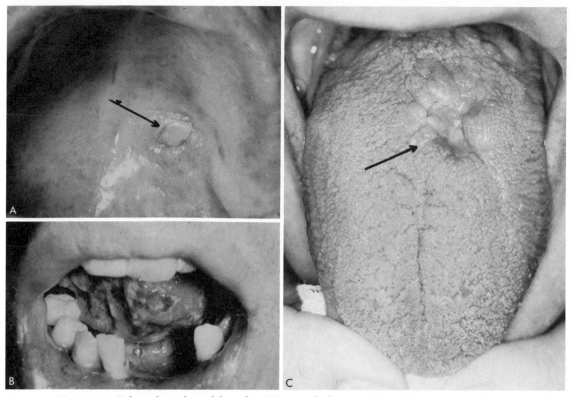

Figure 6–1. Tuberculous ulcer of the palate *(A)*, ventral of tongue *(B)*, and dorsum of tongue *(C)*.

found in areas of trauma and may be mistaken clinically for a simple traumatic ulcer or even carcinoma. Occasional mucosal lesions show swelling or fissuring, but no obvious clinical ulceration. Tuberculous gingivitis is an unusual form of tuberculosis which may appear as a diffuse, hyperemic, nodular or papillary proliferation of the gingival tissues (Fig. 6–2).

Tuberculosis may also involve the bone of the maxilla or mandible. One common mode of entry for the microorganisms is into an area of periapical inflammation by way of the blood

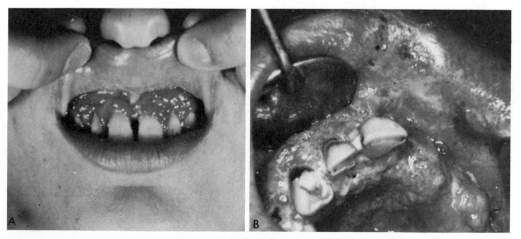

Figure 6–2. *Tuberculous gingivitis.*
The infection in *A* was restricted to the gingival tissues, but in *B* had extended to the palate and lip. (*B*, Courtesy of Dr. Cesar Lopez.)

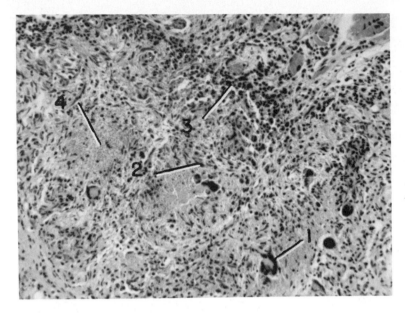

Figure 6–3. *Oral tuberculosis.* Photomicrograph of biopsy of tuberculous ulcer of tongue showing *(1)* giant cells, *(2)* epithelioid cells, *(3)* lymphocytes, and *(4)* areas of caseous necrosis.

stream, an anachoretic effect that has been noted in the oral cavity under other circumstances. It is conceivable also that these microorganisms may enter the periapical tissues by direct immigration through the pulp chamber and root canal of a tooth with an open cavity. The lesion produced is essentially a tuberculous periapical granuloma or tuberculoma. In a study of a group of tuberculous patients, Brodsky reported that periapical tuberculous granulomas were prevalent. These lesions were usually painful and sometimes involved a considerable amount of bone by relatively rapid extension.

Diffuse involvement of the maxilla or mandible may also occur, usually by hematogenous spread of infection, but sometimes by direct extension or even after tooth extraction. Tuberculous osteomyelitis frequently occurs in the later stages of the disease and has an unfavorable prognosis.

Histologic Features. Tuberculous lesions in the mouth do not differ microscopically from tuberculous lesions in other organs of the body. They exhibit foci of caseous necrosis surrounded by epithelioid cells, lymphocytes and occasional multinucleated giant cells (Fig. 6–3). Caseous necrosis is not inevitably present, however. The diagnosis of tuberculosis can be confirmed only by microscopic examination of the tissue with demonstration of the organisms in the lesion, coupled with culture and animal inoculation.

Treatment. The treatment of oral tuberculosis is secondary to treatment of the primary lesions.

SARCOIDOSIS

(Boeck's Sarcoid; Besnier-Boeck-Schaumann Disease)

This disease, of unknown etiology, has been regarded by many investigators in the past as an atypical tuberculosis because of certain points of similarity to that infection. This concept has now been discarded, although it is discussed in this section because of the similarities to tuberculosis.

Sarcoidosis may be best described as a multisystem granulomatous disease of unknown cause most commonly affecting young adults and presenting most frequently with hilar lymphadenopathy, pulmonary infiltration and skin and eye lesions. Thus, lesions of sarcoid are most common in the lungs, skin, lymph nodes, salivary glands, spleen and bones, but may be found to involve practically any site, including the mouth. The disease is characterized by a depression of delayed-type hypersensitivity suggesting an impaired cell-mediated immunity, and raised or abnormal serum immunoglobulins suggesting lymphoproliferation. There are numerous contributing background factors even though the precipitating cause of the disease is unknown. Prolonged antigenemia, circulating immune complexes and serum inhibitors all contribute to the granulomatous disorder, according to James and his colleagues.

Clinical Features. Sarcoidosis is so insidious a disease that the clinical signs and symptoms frequently are not severe enough to cause alarm. While it is most commonly seen in young and middle-aged adults, it may occur later in life and is considerably more prevalent in blacks. Mild malaise and cough may be the chief features, although involvement of a specific organ may occur and be evidenced by dysfunction of that organ.

Cutaneous lesions, which are present in approximately 25 to 35 per cent of all patients with sarcoidosis, may be the only distinct manifestation of the disease. These appear as multiple, raised red patches that occur in groups, grow slowly and do not tend to ulcerate or crust. Erythema nodosum occurs in about 15 per cent of the patients. Involvement of lymph nodes or salivary glands is manifested only by nodular enlargement, while hepatomegaly and splenomegaly may occur, owing to presence of the disease in the liver and spleen.

Oral Manifestations. Since there are no series of cases of sarcoidosis of the oral cavity and jaws reported in the literature, only scattered case reports, it is difficult to describe typical lesions. There are a number of reports in the literature of oral biopsies of clinically normal tissue in patients with proven sarcoidosis that revealed lesions which were microscopically consistent with the disease. For example, Cahn and his associates found sarcoid granulomas in 38 per cent of such a series of 23 patients known to have the disease; Nessan and Jacoway found similar granulomas in the labial glands of 58 per cent of a group of 75 patients with the disease. Lesions on the lips that have been reported were manifested clinically as small, papular nodules or plaques, or resembled herpetic lesions or "fever blisters." On the palate and buccal mucosa, the lesions have been described as bleblike, containing a clear yellowish fluid, or as solid nodules. It also appears that sarcoid may produce diffuse destruction of the bone. These oral manifestations have been discussed by Hillerup and by van Maarsseveen and his colleagues.

Histologic Features. Sarcoid lesions closely resemble proliferative noncaseating nodules of tuberculosis, and the differential diagnosis is frequently difficult to establish. However, no acid-fast organisms can be demonstrated in tissue sections of sarcoidosis. Nests of epithelioid cells, with multinucleated giant cells, are one of the chief microscopic features of the fibrous granulomatous nodules. These granulomas also contain T and B cells, as well as various immunoglobulins that can be identified by appropriate immunofluorescence. Caseation and ne-

crosis do not occur, although the granuloma ultimately transforms into a solid, amorphous, eosinophilic, hyaline mass as it ages.

In spite of the microscopic similarity of tuberculosis and sarcoidosis, it should be pointed out that the tuberculin reaction is positive in no higher a percentage of the patients with sarcoid than in the general population. Moreover, there is a low incidence of complement-fixing antibodies against tuberculosis in these patients and, when present at all, this antibody titer is usually low.

An intracutaneous test for the diagnosis of sarcoidosis, the Kveim-Siltzbach test, has been devised, utilizing a suspension of human known sarcoidal tissue as the test agent. A study by Siltzbach on 311 patients with sarcoidosis has indicated a high degree of specificity of the test with few false-positive reactions. Thus the Kveim-Siltzbach test may be an important aid in the early and accurate diagnosis of the disease.

UVEOPAROTID FEVER
(Uveoparotitis; Heerfordt's Syndrome)

Uveoparotid fever is considered by most investigators to be a form of sarcoidosis in which characteristically there is firm, painless, usually bilateral enlargement of the parotid glands, accompanied by inflammation of the uveal tracts of the eye and cranial nerve involvement. The submaxillary and sublingual glands may be similarly involved, and even the lacrimal glands may be swollen, all features suggestive of Mikulicz's disease or Sjögren's syndrome. A chronic, low-grade fever is often present, and the patient may complain of lassitude, malaise and vague gastrointestinal disturbances or even nausea and vomiting. Xerostomia is common. A patchy erythema of the skin has also been reported to be present early in the course of the disease. Enlargement of the cervical lymph nodes is seen in some cases.

The most common eye lesion in uveoparotitis, and often the earliest symptom, is uveitis, but conjunctivitis, keratitis and corneal herpes among others also have been reported. Although the uveitis may begin unilaterally, it eventually becomes bilateral and in most cases results in some permanent visual impairment. The most common nerve involvement is unilateral or bilateral seventh nerve paralysis, which is said to occur in from one-third to one-half of all cases.

The signs and symptoms of this syndrome usually disappear in time, although some swelling of the parotid glands and visual disturbance may persist.

Leprosy

(Hansen's Disease)

Leprosy is a chronic granulomatous infection caused by an acid-fast bacillus, *Mycobacterium leprae*. The disease is only slightly contagious. Although rare in the United States, it reaches endemic proportions in some parts of the world. A most thorough and concise review of this disease has been published by Binford and his colleagues.

Clinical Features. The most recent standardized classification of leprosy is that of Ridley and Jopling, who have divided the disease into two polarized categories, tuberculoid leprosy (TT) and lepromatous leprosy (LL) with three intermediate groups: borderline tuberculoid (BT), borderline leprosy (BB) and borderline lepromatous (BL).

The tuberculoid lesions are characterized by single or multiple macular, erythematous eruptions, with dermal nerve and peripheral nerve trunk involvement resulting in loss of sensation. The lepromatous lesions develop early erythematous macules or papules that subsequently lead to progressive thickening of the skin and the characteristic nodules. These may develop in considerable numbers on any skin area and produce severe disfigurement.

Facial paralysis occurs with some frequency due to nerve involvement, and this has been discussed recently by Reichart and his co-workers.

Although the disease is a crippling and disfiguring one, it runs a chronic course and seldom causes sudden death.

Oral Manifestations. The oral lesions that have been reported have generally consisted of small tumor-like masses called lepromas, which develop on the tongue, lips or hard palate. These nodules show a tendency to break down and ulcerate. Gingival hyperplasia with loosening of the teeth has also been described, but Reichart and his associates found that most of the gingival and periodontal changes occurring in a group of 30 leprosy patients were nonspecific.

Epker and Via have reviewed the oral and perioral findings in leprosy, adding an additional case, as have Southam and Venkataraman.

Histologic Features. The typical granulomatous nodule shows collections of epithelioid cells and lymphocytes in a fibrous stroma. Langhanstype giant cells are variably present. Vacuolated macrophages called lepra cells are scattered throughout the lesions and often contain the bacilli.

Treatment. Specific long-term chemotherapy is initiated upon diagnosis. However, drug regimen evaluation is very difficult in this disease.

Actinomycosis

Actinomycosis is a chronic granulomatous, suppurative, and fibrosing disease caused by anaerobic, gram-positive, nonacid-fast, branched, filamentous bacteria, the most commonly isolated organism being *Actinomyces israelii*, although *A. naeslundi*, *A. viscosus*, *A. odontolyticus* and *A. propionica* have been shown also to cause the human disease. These are all normal components of the oral flora, and none are known to be recoverable from the environment. *A. bovis* produces "lumpy jaw" in cattle but is seldom found to be a pathogen in humans.

Historically, these microorganisms were at one time believed to be fungi. However, as our knowledge of their biochemical and serologic aspects evolved, it became apparent that they were actually bacteria, the filaments frequently breaking up into bacillary and coccoid forms.

An aerobic microorganism known as Nocardia, with some physical characteristics similar to the actinomycetes, was at one time classified as an aerobic form of the latter organisms. Recently, however, it has been placed in a separate family of Nocardiaceae and 3 of the 31 known species are pathogens for humans: *N. asteroides*, *N. brasiliensis* and *N. caviae*. Two diseases produced in the human by these organisms are systemic nocardiosis and mycetoma. It is significant that none of the Nocardiae—all being normal inhabitants of the soil—are found as a part of the normal oral flora.

The usual pattern of this disease is one characterized chiefly by the formation of abscesses which tend to drain by the formation of sinus tracts. If the pus from the abscesses is carefully examined on a clean glass slide, it shows the typical "sulfur granules," or colonies of organisms which appear in the suppurative material as tiny yellow grains.

Actinomycosis is classified anatomically according to the location of the lesions, and thus we recognize (1) cervicofacial, (2) abdominal, and (3) pulmonary forms.

It is well established that the actinomycete is a common inhabitant of the oral cavity even in the complete absence of any clinical manifestations of mycotic infection. Thus the organisms may be cultured from carious teeth, tonsillar areas, calculus or a variety of the normal incubation zones which exist in the mouth.

The pathogenesis of actinomycosis is not entirely clear. It appears to be an endogenous infection and not communicable. Furthermore, it does not appear to be an opportunistic infection in a situation of depressed cell-mediated immunity. Trauma seems to play a role in some cases by initiating a portal of entry for the organisms, since they are not highly invasive. Thus the extraction of teeth or abrasion of the mucosa may precede the infection. It has been reported that the infecting agent does have the ability to enter the tissues through a carious tooth or a periodontal pocket. This is not unequivocal, however.

Clinical Features. *Cervicofacial actinomycosis* is the most common form of this disease and is of greatest interest to the dentist. It has been emphasized by Norman that two-thirds of all cases are of this type. A series of 39 cases of cervicofacial and intraoral actinomycosis have been reported by Stenhouse and his associates, who also emphasized the surprisingly high incidence of occurrence of actinomyces in routine pathologic and bacteriologic specimens. The organisms may enter the tissues through the oral mucous membranes and may either remain localized in the subjacent soft tissues or spread to involve the salivary glands, bone or even the skin of the face and neck, producing swelling and induration of the tissue. These soft tissue swellings eventually develop into one or more abscesses which tend to discharge upon a skin surface, rarely a mucosal surface, liberating pus containing the typical "sulfur granules" (Fig. 6–4). The skin overlying the abscess is purplish red and indurated or often fluctuant. It is common for the sinus through which the abscess has drained to heal, but because of the chronicity of the disease, new abscesses develop and perforate the skin surface. Thus the patient over a period of time may show a great deal of scarring and disfigurement of the skin. (See also Plate IV.)

The infection of the soft tissues may extend to involve the mandible or, less commonly, the maxilla. If the bone of the maxilla is invaded, the ensuing specific osteomyelitis may eventually involve the cranium, meninges or the brain itself. Once the infection reaches the bone, destruction of tissue may be extensive.

Such destructive lesions within bone may occur or localize at the apex of one or more teeth and simulate a pulp-related infection such as a periapical granuloma or cyst. Such a case has been reported by Wesley and his colleagues, who noted 12 other similar cases in the literature.

Abdominal actinomycosis is an extremely serious form of the disease and carries a high

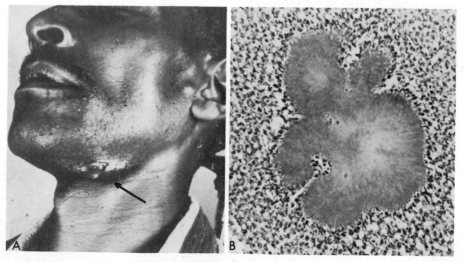

Figure 6–4. *Cervicofacial actinomycosis.*
Clinical photograph *(A)* and photomicrograph *B* of actinomycotic colony in a smear of the pus.

PLATE IV

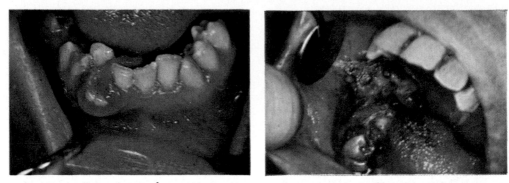

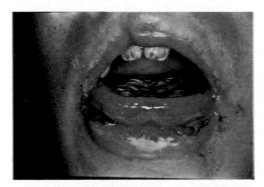

Pyogenic granuloma   Noma

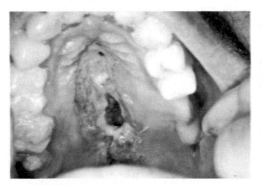

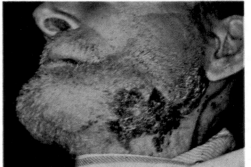

Midline lethal granuloma   Actinomycosis

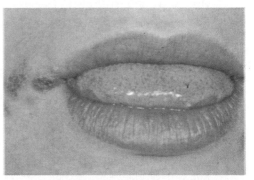

Primary herpetic gingivostomatitis   Recurrent herpes labialis

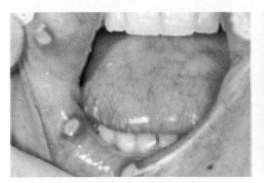

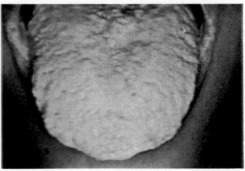

Recurrent aphthous stomatitis   Candidiasis

mortality rate. In addition to generalized signs and symptoms of fever, chills, nausea and vomiting, intestinal manifestations develop, followed by symptoms of involvement of other organs such as the liver and spleen.

Pulmonary actinomycosis produces similar findings of fever and chills accompanied by a productive cough and pleural pain. The organisms may spread beyond the lungs to involve adjacent structures.

Histologic Features. The typical lesion of actinomycosis, either in soft tissue or in bone, is essentially a granulomatous one showing central abscess formation within which may be seen the characteristic colonies of microorganisms. These colonies appear to be floating in a sea of polymorphonuclear leukocytes, often associated with multinucleated giant cells and macrophages particularly around the periphery of the lesion. The individual colony, which may appear round or lobulated, is made up of a meshwork of filaments that stains with hematoxylin, but shows eosinophilia of the peripheral club-shaped ends of the filaments (Fig. 6–4,*B*). This peculiar appearance of the colonies, with the peripheral radiating filaments, is the basis for the often-used term "ray fungus." The tissue surrounding the lesion may be fibrous.

The diagnosis of actinomycosis is dependent not only upon the clinical findings in the patient and the demonstration of the organisms in tissue section or smear, but also upon their culture. However, as Brown pointed out in his extensive review of 181 cases of actinomycosis, the organisms are difficult to culture. Of the 67 cases in which culture was attempted, the organism was isolated in only 16 instances. Use of a thin-needle aspiration biopsy technique for morphologic studies and collection of material for microbiologic isolation has been demonstrated by Pollock and his associates.

Treatment and Prognosis. The treatment of this disease is difficult and has not been uniformly successful. Penicillin and tetracyclines have been used most frequently, but the course of the disease is still often prolonged.

BOTRYOMYCOSIS

(Bacterial Actinophytosis; Actinobacillosis)

Botryomycosis is a granulomatous disease which was recognized over 100 years ago when it was first found to affect horses. Since that time, approximately 50 cases occurring in hu-

mans have been reported in the literature, and the first case involving the oral cavity was reported by Small and Kobernick.

There is some confusion as to the actual causative organism in this disease, although an Actinobacillus has been thought to be the one involved. Nevertheless, a variety of other types of organisms have been reported which may or may not represent secondary invaders. The Actinobacillus is often characterized as an "associate" organism with the actinomycetes, and some workers feel that the presence of actinobacilli is necessary for the disease process of actinomycosis. However, actinomycosis is known to occur from a "pure culture" of actinomycetes. Whether "pure cultures" of actinobacilli can produce botryomycosis is not known, but many workers believe that a number of common bacteria such as Staphylococcus, Streptococcus, Escherichia, Pseudomonas and probably many others may serve as etiologic agents of the disease.

Clinical Features. Human botryomycosis is usually a localized granulomatous infection of the skin or mucosa. It may disseminate, involving the liver, lungs, or kidneys, in which case the disease is usually fatal. The significance of this disease lies in the fact that the localized infection may closely mimic actinomycosis by producing a chronic granulomatous mass with multiple ulcers and sinuses. The oral case reported by Small and Kobernick involved the tongue and presented clinically as a firm, nodular infiltration of the body and base of the tongue. However, there were no sinuses present.

Histologic Features. The chronic granulomatous nodules are characterized by the presence of suppurative foci which contain grains or granules that are recognized as forming around microorganisms in certain cases as apparently a nonspecific reaction between agent and host, possibly related to hypersensitivity. In the ordinary H and E–stained section, these granules may be indistinguishable from those of actinomycosis. These grains or granules are eosinophilic and PAS-negative and negative to methenamine silver. The eosinophilic, peripheral club formations typical of actinomycetes are usually not identifiable in this disease.

Treatment. The suggestion has been made that botryomycosis may be caused by a variety of different microorganisms of low virulence and, therefore, the pathogenesis may be related more to a modified host resistance or tissue hypersensitivity than to a specific microorganism. Therefore, treatment is nonspecific.

TULAREMIA

(Rabbit Fever)

Tularemia is a disease caused by the gram-negative bacillus *Pasteurella tularensis*, and, in most cases in the United States, is contracted through contact with infected rabbits, muskrats, ground squirrels and other wild game, particularly of the rodent family. This exposure and subsequent infection may occur during skinning and dressing freshly killed infected animals, through eating only partially cooked contaminated meat from infected animals or through the bite of an infected deer fly or tick.

Clinical Features. Tularemia may be classified into several types, and these include the cutaneous, ophthalmic, pleuropulmonary, oral and abdominal forms. After a variable incubation period of up to seven days, the patient usually suffers a sudden headache, nausea, vomiting, chills and fever. A single cut or sore on the skin develops into a suppurative ulcer. The lymphatic vessels become swollen and painful and the lymph nodes remarkably enlarged. This general sequence of events is the most common course of the disease and is called ulceroglandular tularemia. The eyes also become involved, with conjunctivitis developing through localization of the disease in the conjunctival sac: oculoglandular tularemia. Tularemic pneumonia and pleuritis are also complications of the disease, which may eventuate in gangrene and lung abscesses.

The disease occurs most frequently in adults. However, as Hughes has reported, children are sometimes affected and, in such cases, the correct diagnosis may be easily overlooked.

Oral Manifestations. The oral lesions are manifested as necrotic ulcers of the oral mucosa or pharynx, usually accompanied by severe pain. In some cases it has been reported that a generalized stomatitis develops rather than isolated lesions; single nodular masses eventually developing into abscesses have also been described. Regional lymphadenitis may arise in the submaxillary and the cervical groups of nodes.

Treatment. The disease responds to antibiotic therapy. Before the availability of the newer antibiotics, the disease was considered a serious one, and even today in some persons it may run such a fulminating course that death occurs despite all forms of therapy.

MELIOIDOSIS

Melioidosis is a specific infection in man, caused by the bacillus *Pseudomonas pseudomallei*, which is endemic in certain areas of the Far East, including Burma, Ceylon, India, Indochina, Malaysia, Thailand and the Dutch East Indies. Military operations in that part of the world by United States Armed Forces have increased the significance of this disease, and cases have now been diagnosed in American servicemen who have returned from duty in Southeast Asia.

Clinical Features. There are two recognized forms of the disease: acute and chronic. In the acute form, the patients rapidly develop a high fever, evidence of acute pulmonary infection, diarrhea and hemoptysis. There is widespread visceral involvement as a result of hematogenous dissemination of microorganisms. Death as a result of fulminating septicemia may occur in a few days to weeks.

The chronic form of the disease usually develops in patients who have survived the acute form. It is characterized by multiple, small, nonspecific abscesses occurring subcutaneously or in the viscera, lymph nodes or bones, which often develop draining sinus tracts. These may involve the cervicofacial area and mimic fungal infection or tuberculosis.

The mode of transmission is not from one man to another man. The causative organism is abundant in soil and stagnant water where the disease occurs. It is believed that most human infections occur through contamination of skin abrasions by this soil or water.

Treatment. Incision and drainage, accompanied by massive antibiotic therapy, have proven moderately successful in treating the disease.

TETANUS

("Lock-jaw")

Tetanus is a disease of the nervous system characterized by intense activity of motor neurons and resulting in severe muscle spasms. It is caused by the exotoxin of the anaerobic gram-positive bacillus *Clostridium tetani*, which acts at the synapse of the interneurons of inhibitory pathways and motor neurons to produce blockade of spinal inhibition. The organisms can enter the body through even the most trivial injury.

Throughout the world, but mostly in underdeveloped countries, it is responsible for several hundred thousand deaths each year, chiefly in the form of neonatal tetanus. The mortality rate exceeds 60 per cent.

Clinical Features. There is a wide range in the incubation period, but clinical manifestations usually appear within 14 days. These consist of pain and stiffness in the jaws and neck muscles, with muscle rigidity producing trismus and dysphagia. Rigidity of facial muscles may also occur, producing the typical "risus sardonicus," and sometimes the entire body becomes affected, with characteristic opisthotonos. Reflex spasms frequently develop after stimuli.

"Cephalic tetanus" is tetanus which is either localized or generalized, occurring in association with cranial nerve palsy, most commonly the seventh cranial nerve.

This disease, which has been reviewed in depth by Smith and Myall, is of significance to the dentist because of the acute trismus which may develop in these patients and simulate acute oral infection, trauma, temporomandibular dysfunction and even hysteria.

Treatment. All patients with the disease should receive antimicrobial drugs, active and passive immunization, surgical wound care and anticonvulsants, if indicated.

SYPHILIS

(Lues)

Syphilis is a centuries-old infectious disease that has protean clinical features. In recent years, with the advent of antibiotic therapy and other epidemiologic control measures, its incidence was greatly reduced. However, within the past three decades there has been an astonishing upsurge in the incidence of the disease, much of it in teen-age individuals. It has been pointed out by Fiumara and Lessell that, in the 12-year period from 1958 to 1969, there was more than a 200 per cent increase in reported cases of primary and secondary syphilis in the United States and that, as a result, congenital syphilis in children under one year of age rose by 117 per cent during the 10-year period from 1960 to 1969. According to the Centers for Disease Control (CDC) in Atlanta, an annual increase in primary and secondary syphilis is still occurring. The total number of reported cases in the United States in 1979 was over 25,000; in 1980, it was over 27,000; and in 1981, over 31,000. Inasmuch as the number of unreported cases of primary and secondary syphilis is variously estimated to be between two and four times that of reported cases, it is obvious that the over-all incidence of this disease in this country is extremely serious. Fortunately, the incidence of congenital syphilis in those under one year of age has been decreasing since 1972 and now totals approximately 100 cases annually.

Syphilis is caused by infection with a spirochete, *Treponema pallidum.* This is a motile spirillar form which may be best demonstrated by the darkfield microscope, since it stains poorly except by silver impregnation.

Syphilis may be classified as either acquired or congenital, although this latter term is somewhat misleading, since the congenital form is "acquired" from an infected mother.

ACQUIRED SYPHILIS. The acquired form of syphilis is contracted primarily as a venereal disease, after sexual intercourse with an infected partner, although many cases have been innocently acquired by persons, such as dentists, working on infected patients in a contagious stage. The disease, if untreated, manifests three distinctive stages throughout its course, so that it is customary to speak of primary, secondary and tertiary lesions of acquired syphilis.

In the *primary stage* the lesion develops at the site of inoculation approximately three weeks after contact with the infection. This lesion, the chancre, most commonly occurs on the penis in the male and on the vulva or cervix in the female. About 95 per cent of the chancres occur on the genitalia, but they are found also in other areas. In recent years, there appears to have been an increase in occurrence of extragenital syphilis as a result of an increase in oral-genital activity and increased contact among infected male homosexuals. Of particular interest to the dentist are those lesions occurring on the lips, tongue, palate, gingiva and tonsils. The chancre has been reported as developing even at the site of a fresh extraction wound. The usual primary lesion is an elevated, ulcerated nodule showing local induration and producing regional lymphadenitis. Such a lesion on the lip may have a brownish, crusted appearance (Fig. 6–5).

The intraoral chancre is an ulcerated lesion covered by a grayish-white membrane which

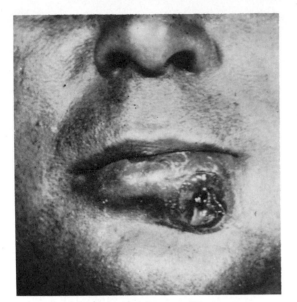

Figure 6–5. *Chancre of lip.*
(Courtesy of Dr. Boynton H. Booth.)

may be painful because of secondary infection. The chancre abounds with spirochetes, easily demonstrable by darkfield examination of a smear, and is highly infectious. The *Treponema microdentium*, which is found in many non-syphilitic people, may be confused with *T. pallidum* on darkfield examination. Therefore lesions contaminated by saliva should not be diagnosed by darkfield examination of the lesion, but by darkfield examination of an affected regional lymph node. An enlarged lymph node is almost always found along the lymphatics draining the area of the chancre.

The chancre appears microscopically as a superficial ulcer showing a rather intense in-

flammatory infiltrate. Plasma cells are particularly numerous. The microorganisms are present in the tissue and may be demonstrated by silver stain, although the diagnosis should not be established by this means but, rather, by any one of a variety of serologic tests. Of considerable importance is the fact that not every patient with a primary lesion exhibits a positive serologic reaction despite the presence of a spirochetemia. The chancre heals spontaneously in three weeks to two months.

The *secondary or metastatic stage*, usually commencing about six weeks after the primary lesion, is characterized by diffuse eruptions of the skin and mucous membranes. On the skin, the lesions may have a multiplicity of forms, but often appear as macules or papules. The oral lesions, called "mucous patches," are usually multiple, painless, grayish-white plaques overlying an ulcerated surface (Fig. 6–6). They occur most frequently on the tongue, gingiva or buccal mucosa. They are often ovoid or irregular in shape and are surrounded by an erythematous zone. Mucous patches are also highly infectious, since they contain vast numbers of microorganisms. In the secondary stage the serologic reaction is always positive. The lesions of the secondary stage undergo spontaneous remission within a few weeks, but exacerbations may continue to occur for months or several years.

Tertiary lesions, also called late syphilis, do not usually appear for several years and involve chiefly the cardiovascular system, the central nervous system and certain other tissues and organs. Late syphilis is noninfectious. The gumma is the chief localized tertiary lesion and occurs most frequently in the skin and mucous

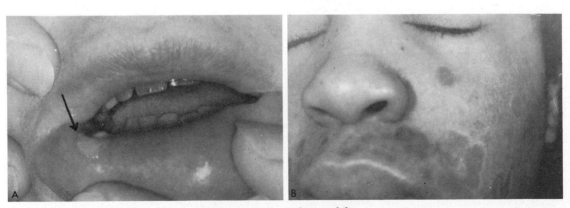

Figure 6–6. *Secondary syphilis.*
A, Mucous patch of lip in secondary syphilis. *B,* Annular, circinate lesions of skin in secondary syphilis. (Courtesy of Dr. Edward V. Zegarelli.)

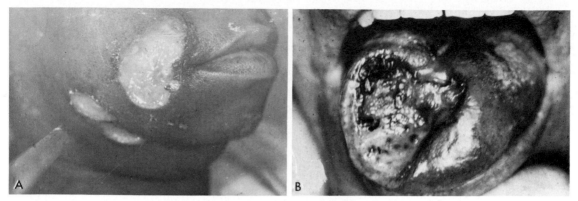

Figure 6–7. Tertiary syphilis.
A, Gumma of skin. B, Gumma of tongue. (Courtesy of Dr. Charles A. Waldron.)

membranes, liver, testes and bone. It consists of a focal, granulomatous inflammatory process with central necrosis. The lesion may vary in size from a millimeter or less to several centimeters in diameter.

The intraoral gumma most commonly involves the tongue and palate. In either situation the lesion appears as a firm nodular mass in the tissue which may subsequently ulcerate and, in the case of lesions of the palate, cause perforation by sloughing of the necrotic mass of tissue (Fig. 6–7). Such an occurrence frequently follows vigorous antibiotic therapy, a Herxheimer reaction.

Meyer and Shklar have reported the oral manifestations in 81 cases of acquired syphilis, and have stressed that tertiary lesions are far more common than lesions in either primary or secondary syphilis. This ratio is probably changing, however. They also emphasized that atrophic or interstitial glossitis is the most characteristic and important lesion of syphilis.

The predilection for luetic glossitis to undergo carcinomatous transformation has been recognized for many years. The incidence of such malignant transformation has ranged as high as 30 per cent in various reported series. However, in the series of Meyer and Shklar, the development of epidermoid carcinoma in luetic glossitis occurred in only 19 per cent of the cases. In a separate study, the same authors reported that only 7.5 per cent of the patients in a series of 210 cases of carcinoma of the tongue had a past history of syphilis. The prominent apparent decrease in the relationship between syphilis and lingual carcinoma was suggested to be related to the early and intensive treatment of the disease with antibiotics since 1940.

CONGENITAL (PRENATAL) SYPHILIS. Congenital syphilis is transmitted to the offspring only by an infected mother and is not inherited. Today it is a rare disease, for compulsory blood examination as a requirement for a marriage license in many states and routine serologic examination of pregnant women have done much to decrease the incidence of congenital syphilis and, consequently, the number of stillbirths due to syphilis. Nevertheless, Fiumara and Lessell have pointed out that there was a 168 per cent increase in the number of reported cases of congenital syphilis in the United States in children under 10 years of age between 1960 and 1969. However, the incidence has since decreased and plateaued. It is recognized that if treatment with antibiotics is begun in infected pregnant women before their fourth month of pregnancy, approximately 95 per cent of the offspring of these mothers will be free of the disease.

Persons with congenital syphilis manifest a great variety of lesions, including frontal bossae (found in 87 per cent of a series of 271 patients with congenital syphilis reported by Fiumara and Lessell), short maxilla (in 84 per cent), high palatal arch (in 76 per cent), saddle nose (in 73 per cent), mulberry molars (in 70 per cent), Higouménakis's sign or irregular thickening of the sternoclavicular portion of the clavicle (in 39 per cent), relative protuberance of mandible (in 26 per cent), rhagades (in 7 per cent), and saber shin (in 4 per cent) (Fig. 6–8). Reportedly pathognomonic of the disease is the occurrence of Hutchinson's triad: hypoplasia of the incisor and molar teeth, eighth nerve deafness and interstitial keratitis (q.v.).

In the above reported series, 75 per cent of the persons with congenital syphilis had one or

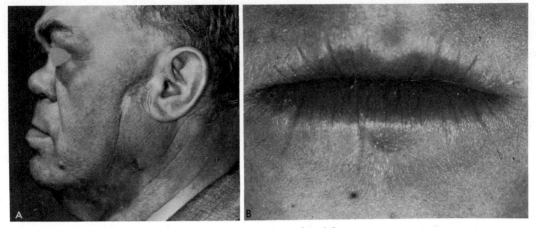

Figure 6–8. *Congenital syphilis.*
Saddle-nose *(A)* and rhagades or radiating fissures *(B)* of congenital syphilis. (Courtesy of Drs. Wilbur C. Moorman and Robert J. Gorlin.)

more of the components of Hutchinson's triad. It is unusual, however, for all features of this triad to occur simultaneously in the same person.

GONORRHEA

Gonorrhea is primarily a venereal disease affecting the male and female genitourinary tract and is transmitted by sexual intercourse. It is the most common reportable infectious disease in the United States today, with about one million cases being reported each year, although it is estimated that at least an additional one million cases occur but are not reported.

Oral Manifestations. Extragenital gonorrheal infection of the oral cavity is being seen with increasing frequency, especially among but not confined to homosexuals, and occurs as a result of oral-genital contact or inoculation through infected hands. Transmission by fomites is rare.

Schmidt and his co-workers have reviewed the literature on gonococcal stomatitis and have pointed out the clinical similarity between the oral lesions of this disease and the oral lesions of erythema multiforme, erosive or bullous lichen planus and herpetic stomatitis. Chue has also reviewed this disease, describing the various oral lesions in detail. The lips may develop acute painful ulceration, limiting motion; the gingiva may become erythematous, with or without necrosis; and the tongue may present red, dry ulcerations or become glazed and swollen with painful erosions, with similar lesions on the buccal mucosa and palate.

Gonococcal pharyngitis and tonsillitis are also well-recognized lesions. These appear as vesicles or ulcers with a gray or white pseudomembrane. Oral lesions are commonly accompanied by a fever and regional lymphadenopathy. Finally, gonococcal parotitis, presumably a result of an ascending infection from the duct to the gland, has been reported on numerous occasions.

Diagnosis. Diagnosis is established by bacteriologic examination of a smear, or cultures if indicated, of the oral lesions, coupled with a careful, detailed history of the sexual activity of the patient.

GRANULOMA INGUINALE
(Granuloma Venereum; Donovanosis)

Granuloma inguinale is a chronic, infectious, granulomatous disease caused by microorganisms, probably bacilli, formerly designated as *Donovania granulomatis* and popularly called Donovan bodies, but now carrying the name *Calymmatobacterium granulomatis*. Their taxonomic status is uncertain. It is considered to be a venereal disease, but is only mildly contagious. Care should be exercised not to confuse granuloma inguinale with lymphogranuloma venereum, a venereal disease that is caused by strains of *Chlamydia trachomatis*, once designated as viruses but now morphologically classified as bacteria. The oral cavity is not notably involved in this latter disease.

Clinical Features. The disease is most prevalent in the tropical zones, but is found in the southern portion of the United States. It chiefly affects adult blacks of either sex, but may occur in any race.

The primary lesions of granuloma inguinale appear on the external genitalia and in the inguinal region. They are manifested as papules or nodules which ulcerate to form clean, granular lesions with rolled margins and which show a tendency for peripheral enlargement. Satellite lesions often arise through lymphatic extension. Inguinal ulceration is commonly secondary to the genital lesions and arises initially as a fluctuant swelling known as a pseudobubo.

Extragenital lesions also may occur on the oral mucous membranes, usually through autoinoculation rather than as a primary infection, as well as in the pharynx, esophagus and larynx. Finally, metastatic spread to bones and soft subcutaneous tissues has been reported. Two separate investigators have reported an incidence of extragenital lesions of granuloma inguinale to be 6 per cent and 1.5 per cent, respectively.

Oral Manifestations. Oral lesions appear to be the most common extragenital form of granuloma inguinale. The reported cases have been reviewed by Ferro and Richter, who described additional cases. The lesions of the oral cavity are usually secondary to active genital lesions and appear in a variable period of time after the primary lesion, frequently months to several years later. The definitive diagnosis rests upon the demonstration of Donovan bodies in tissue from the lesions.

Lesions may occur in any oral location such as the lips, buccal mucosa or palate, or they may diffusely involve the mucosal surfaces. The varied clinical appearance of the lesions is the basis for their classification into one of three types: ulcerative, exuberant and cicatricial. Thus there may be painful ulcerated lesions, sometimes bleeding, suggestive but not pathognomonic of the disease. Or, in other instances, the lesions may appear as proliferative granular masses, with an intact epithelial covering. The mucous membrane generally may be inflamed and edematous. Cicatrization is one of the most characteristic of the oral manifestations of granuloma inguinale. Fibrous scar formation may become extensive and, if present in areas such as the cheek or lip, may so limit mouth opening as to necessitate surgical relief.

Histologic Features. The microscopic pattern of the various forms of granuloma inguinale is one of granulation tissue with infiltration of polymorphonuclear leukocytes and plasma cells. There is usually a marked overlying pseudoepitheliomatous hyperplasia. Pathognomonic of the disease is the presence of large mononuclear phagocytes, each containing tiny intracytoplasmic cysts within which are found the Donovan bodies. These bodies are tiny, elongated basophilic and argyrophilic rods and are present in profuse numbers within the macrophages.

It has been noted that, after treatment, improvement of the genital lesions is usually accompanied by improvement of the extragenital oral lesion; conversely, exacerbation of genital lesions usually results in worsening of the oral condition.

RHINOSCLEROMA

(Scleroma)

Rhinoscleroma is an unusual chronic infectious disease caused by the bacillus *Klebsiella rhinoscleromatis* (Klebsiellae type 3). This etiologic agent has been discussed in detail by Hoffman. The disease is most common in certain sections of Europe and Central and South America, although it is also reported in the United States. The mode of transmission of the disease is unknown.

The granulomatous, nodular lesions that occur in rhinoscleroma are found chiefly in the upper respiratory tract, often originating in the nose, but involvement of the lacrimal glands, orbit, skin, paranasal sinuses and intracranial invasion have also been described. The proliferative nasal masses may produce the configuration known as the "Hebra nose," which is typical of this disease.

Oral lesions appearing as proliferative granulomas are also known to occur. In addition, anesthesia of the soft palate and enlargement of the uvula are described. Three cases of rhinoscleroma seen in a maxillo-facial practice in Nigeria have been discussed by Edwards and his associates, who have included an extensive bibliography of the disease.

MIDLINE LETHAL GRANULOMA

(Malignant Granuloma; Lethal Granuloma; Midline Lethal Granulomatous Ulceration)

The lethal granuloma is a most unusual condition, resembling a serious infection, which has been best described as an idiopathic progressive destruction of the nose, paranasal sinuses, palate, face and pharynx. It was first extensively reviewed by Stewart in 1933. The person afflicted characteristically appears to exhibit complete lack of resistance to the insidious progress of the disease.

It is now recognized that many different specific diseases may have the same clinical manifestations as originally described for the midline lethal granuloma. These diseases have been listed by Tsokos and her colleagues, and are shown in Table 6–1. Some of these are infectious diseases, while others are neoplastic and, unquestionably, many of the early reports of midline lethal granuloma were in fact what is now recognized as polymorphic reticulosis or midline malignant reticulosis or even a conventional malignant lymphoma of the nose. Nevertheless, when all diseases in these first two categories are eliminated, there still remains a third group of lesions characterized by nonspecific acute and chronic inflammation without any evidence of the presence of causative microorganisms or malignancy. The two diseases in this category are Wegener's granulomatosis and the true midline lethal granuloma or "idi-

Table 6–1. Diseases Which May Appear Clinically as Midline Lethal Granuloma

I. Infectious Diseases
  A. Bacterial
    1. Brucellosis
    2. Rhinoscleroma
    3. Leprosy
    4. Actinomycosis
    5. Tuberculosis
    6. Syphilis
  B. Fungal
    1. Histoplasmosis
    2. Candidiasis
    3. Coccidioidomycosis
    4. Blastomycosis
    5. Rhinosporidiosis
    6. Phycomycosis
  C. Parasitic
    1. Leishmaniasis
    2. Myiasis

II. Neoplastic Diseases
  1. Squamous cell carcinoma
  2. Rhabdomyosarcoma
  3. Polymorphic reticulosis/lymphomatoid granulomatosis
  4. Conventional lymphoma

III. Inflammatory Diseases of Unknown Etiology
  1. Wegener's granulomatosis
  2. Idiopathic midline destructive disease

Modified from M. Tsokos, A. S. Fauci, and J. Costa: Idiopathic midline destructive disease (IMDD). Am. J. Clin. Pathol., 77:162, 1982.

opathic midline destructive disease," as termed by Tsokos and her co-workers. At one time, these two latter diseases were thought to be closely related. However, since Wegener's granulomatosis is a systemic disease and the lethal granuloma a purely localized one, they have been clearly separated and Wegener's disease will be discussed in another section. In a discussion of this subject in 1949, Williams presented the view that the lethal granuloma is due to a dysfunction of the immune mechanisms normally responsible for granuloma formation. In essence, a vascular "allergy" occurs, either the Arthus phenomenon or periarteritis nodosa, depending on whether capillaries or arterioles are affected, and the hyperimmune tissues become necrotic because of obstruction of the blood supply. Little additional information has been added to our knowledge of the etiology of this disease. Today, it is usually theorized that it represents a fulminant hypersensitivity response to an unidentified antigen. No etiologic association has been made with prior allergic rhinitis, chronic sinusitis or known infection.

Clinical Features. The peculiar granulomatous lesion may begin as a superficial ulceration of the palate or nasal septum, often preceded by a feeling of stuffiness in the nose. It may bear close clinical resemblance to carcinoma. This prodromal stage, described by Stewart and others, may persist for a month or two to several years. Eventually the ulceration spreads from the palate to the inside of the nose and thence to the outside. The palatal, nasal and malar bones may become involved, undergoing necrosis, and eventually sequestrate. Destruction becomes the prominent feature of the disease, and loss of the entire palate is not uncommon. The patient may exhibit purulent discharge from the eyes and nose; perforating sinus tracts may develop, and much of the soft tissue of the face finally may slough away, leaving a direct opening into the nasopharynx and oral cavity (see Plate IV). The patient ultimately dies of exhaustion or of hemorrhage if a large blood vessel becomes eroded. A patient studied at autopsy has been reported in detail by Hamilton and his co-workers.

Histologic Features. Microscopic examination of the affected tissue reveals extensive necrosis with infiltration of some inflammatory cells and the formation of occasional new capillaries.

Because of the clinical appearance of the lesion, extensive search and repeated biopsies are often carried out in an attempt to find neoplastic tissue. The innocuous appearance of the tissue belies its serious clinical nature. The diagnosis of the disease is typically one of exclusion.

Treatment. While the disease is usually fatal, corticosteroid therapy has proven of benefit in some cases, particularly when coupled with antibiotics for secondary infection. However, some authorities believe that the disease is best treated by high-dose radiation therapy.

WEGENER'S GRANULOMATOSIS

Wegener's granulomatosis is a disease of unknown etiology which basically involves the vascular, renal and respiratory systems. It does have certain features in common with the midline lethal granuloma but is now considered to represent a separate disease entity. Some investigators originally believed it to be a variant of polyarteritis nodosa. While the etiology is still unknown, it is generally thought to be an aberrant hypersensitivity reaction to an unknown antigen. The disease has been discussed in detail by Kornblut and his associates and by DeRemee and his co-workers, who proposed a unifying concept between midline lethal granuloma and Wegener's granulomatosis. The relationship between these two diseases has been discussed by Tsokos and her colleagues.

Clinical Features. Wegener's granulomatosis may occur at any age, from infants to the very elderly, although the majority of cases are in the fourth and fifth decades of life. There is a slight predilection for occurrence in males.

It is best described as a multisystem disease which is usually first characterized clinically by the development of rhinitis, sinusitis and otitis or ocular symptoms. The patient soon develops a cough and hemoptysis as well as fever and joint pains. Hemorrhagic or vesicular skin lesions are also commonly present. Granulomatous lesions of the lungs are found on the chest roentgenogram, while the glomerulonephritis which develops ultimately leads to uremia and terminal renal failure.

Oral Manifestations. Involvement of the oral cavity occurs with considerable frequency in Wegener's granulomatosis. However, only rarely are the oral lesions the first manifestation of the disease. In reported cases, involvement of the gingiva has been the most common manifestation. Brooke, in reviewing reported cases with oral lesions of this nature, has pointed out that the gingival lesions may be ulcerations, friable granular lesions or simply enlargements of the gingiva. Israelson and his associates have reported a case characterized by hyperplastic gingivitis in which this was the patient's main complaint. A similar case was reviewed by Eveson and Slaney as well as by Edwards and Buckerfield. However, as Cawson has pointed out, other lesions may occur such as ulceration of the palate by extension of the disease from the nose, where destruction of the nasal septum may develop; also occurring are small ulcerations resembling aphthae, diffuse ulcerative stomatitis, spontaneous exfoliation of teeth, and failure of tooth sockets to heal following extraction.

Laboratory Findings. Laboratory findings include an anemia, leukocytosis, elevated sedimentation rate and a hyperglobulinemia. Because of kidney involvement, hematuria is common as well as the finding of albumin, casts and leukocytes in the urine.

Circulating immune complexes have been demonstrated in some patients, but this is not a consistent finding.

Histologic Findings. The lesions in the upper respiratory tract and lungs consist of giant cell necrotizing granulomatous lesions showing vasculitis. The gingival and other lesions show a similar, nonspecific granulomatous process with scattered giant cells.

Treatment. The majority of cases of Wegener's granulomatosis formerly terminated fatally. However, cytotoxic agents, especially cyclophosphamide, have provided a good prognosis for these patients, with many known long-term remissions.

CHRONIC GRANULOMATOUS DISEASE

Chronic granulomatous disease, first described as a specific entity in 1957, is an uncommon hereditary disease with an X-linked mode of transmission, although there appears to be a variant transmitted as an autosomal recessive characteristic. Thus, the majority of patients are males, although affected females have been reported. The disease is generally found in infants and children but is also seen in young adults. One variant of this disease is known as familial lipochrome histiocytosis.

The condition is characterized by severe recurrent infections as a result of a defect of intracellular leukocyte enzymatic function with a decreased oxidative metabolism in which there is failure to destroy certain catalase-positive microorganisms, including staphylococci, enteric bacilli (Klebsiella, Aerobacter, *E. coli*, *S. marcescens*, Pseudomonas, Proteus and Salmonella) and certain fungi (Candida, Aspergillus and Nocardia). Other microorganisms such as streptococci and pneumococci are readily destroyed by the leukocytes. The chemotactic and phagocytic functions of the leukocytes are generally unimpaired.

Clinical Features. The disease is characterized by widespread infection from infancy, usually affecting lymph nodes, lung, liver, spleen, bone and skin, the latter commencing with eczematous lesions about the face leading to tissue necrosis and granuloma formation. Abscesses, septicemia, pneumonia, pericarditis, meningitis and osteomyelitis are but examples of the various forms which the disease may take.

Oral Manifestations. Oral lesions have been reported in a number of cases of chronic granulomatous disease and have been discussed by Wysocki and Brooke. The lesions have consisted chiefly of a diffuse stomatitis with or without solitary or multiple ulcerations. One patient with over a dozen oral ulcers of the buccal mucosa has been reported by Wolf and Ebel. In several patients, benign migratory glossitis has also been present but its relationship to the disease, if any, is not clear. In addition, Scully has reported enamel hypoplasia of permanent teeth in three cases, probably a result of the severe early infection.

Histologic Features. Microscopic examination of ulcerated lesions of the oral mucosa have been described as consisting of small granulomas with mononuclear histiocytes and multinucleated giant cells. Central necrosis with polymorphonuclear leukocytes may also be present.

Diagnosis. The diagnosis is established by neutrophil function tests—the impairment of in vitro microbicidal activity and failure of reduction of nitroblue tetrazolium (NBT test).

Treatment. Treatment is solely vigorous treatment of the infection.

NOMA

(Cancrum Oris; Gangrenous Stomatitis)

Noma is a rapidly spreading gangrene of the oral and facial tissues that occurs usually in debilitated or nutritionally deficient persons. It is seen chiefly in children, but is found also in adults under certain conditions, such as those existing among the malnourished internees of the Belsen concentration camp reported by

Dawson after World War II. Today, the disease is rare in North America and Western Europe. Most cases occur in Africa, Southeast Asia and South America. For example, one of the last reports of an extensive series was that of Enwonwu, who described 69 cases of noma in "miserably malnourished" Nigerian children between the ages of 2 and 7 years. He also documented the occurrence of necrotizing ulcerative gingivitis (NUG) in 27 per cent of Nigerian children hospitalized for treatment of protein-calorie malnutrition.

Predisposing factors play an important role in the development of the condition, since it occurs chiefly in persons who are undernourished or debilitated from infections such as diphtheria, dysentery, measles, pneumonia, scarlet fever, syphilis, tuberculosis and blood dyscrasias, including anemia. Thus noma may be considered a secondary complication of systemic disease rather than a primary disease.

Noma appears to originate as a specific infection by Vincent's organisms, an acute necrotizing gingivostomatitis, which is soon complicated by secondary invasion of many other microbial forms, including streptococci, staphylococci and diphtheria bacilli.

Selye reported the production of a noma-like condition in rats as a result of simultaneous administration of cortisone and clipping of the mandibular incisors, forcing the animals to chew with their gingiva and thus to cause excessive mechanical injury to the mucosa. The condition usually began around the gingiva and progressed to destruction of the floor of the mouth and the lower lip. The increase in susceptibility of the rat tissues to injury, induced by the cortisone, could be eliminated by the simultaneous administration of pituitary growth hormone (somatotropic hormone, or STH). On the basis of his experimental findings, Selye suggested that noma may not necessarily be due to a specific pathogenic agent, but may be due to a "pathogenic situation" resulting from faulty adaptation to a nonspecific injury or "stress."

Clinical Features. Noma usually begins as a small ulcer of the gingival mucosa which rapidly spreads and involves the surrounding tissues of the jaws, lips and cheeks by gangrenous necrosis (see Plate IV). The initial site is commonly an area of stagnation around a fixed bridge or crown. The overlying skin becomes inflamed, edematous and finally necrotic, with the result that a line of demarcation develops between healthy and dead tissue, and large masses of the tissue may slough out, leaving the jaw exposed. The commencement of gangrene is denoted by the appearance of blackening of the skin. It is reported that the subcutaneous fat pad and buccal fat pad undergo necrosis in advance of the other adjoining tissues. The odor arising from the gangrenous tissues is extremely foul. The palate and occasionally the tongue may become involved by this process, but this is not common. Patients have a high temperature during the course of the disease, suffer secondary infection and may die from toxemia or pneumonia.

Treatment and Prognosis. The mortality rate of noma approximated 75 per cent before the availability of antibiotics. Although the disease is still serious, the prognosis is considerably better if antibiotics are administered before the patient reaches the final stages. Immediate treatment of any existing malnutrition further improves the probability of saving the patient.

PYOGENIC GRANULOMA

(Granuloma Pyogenicum)

The pyogenic granuloma is a distinctive clinical entity originating as a response of the tissues to a nonspecific infection. It is of particular significance because of its common intraoral occurrence and because of its sometimes alarming clinical course.

Etiology. The pyogenic granuloma was originally believed to be a botryomycotic infection, an infection in horses thought to be transmissible to man. Subsequent work suggested that the lesion was due to infection by either staphylococci or streptococci, partially because it was shown that these microorganisms could produce colonies with fungus-like characteristics. It is now generally agreed, however, that the pyogenic granuloma arises as a result of some minor trauma to the tissues, which provides a pathway for the invasion of nonspecific types of microorganisms. The tissues respond in a characteristic manner to these organisms of low virulence by the overzealous proliferation of a vascular type of connective tissue. Some investigators think that penetration of microorganisms into the tissues does not occur or is negligible, since microorganisms can seldom be demonstrated deep in the lesion with appropriate bacterial staining techniques. The surface of the pyogenic granuloma, especially in areas of ulceration, abounds with typical colonies of saprophytic organisms.

This tissue response reiterates the well-known biologic principle that any irritant applied to living tissue may act either as a stimulus or as a destructive agent, or as both. In adult tissues the relative quiescence of the cells may be due either to an active restraint of growth or to a passive absence of stimulus for growth. Tissue culture studies of adult cells have shown that there is no active restraint of growth. It may then be assumed that tissues of embryos and young animals contain stimuli for the proliferation of cells. The sulfhydryl radical is probably one of the most essential stimulating agents. Burrows believed that all cells give off a stimulating substance. If many cells are present in a small volume of tissue and there is a relative reduction of blood flow through the area, as in inflammation, the concentration of this stimulating substance will be high and growth will be stimulated. As differentiation and maturation are attained, the cells become widely separated; the concentration of the substance falls, and little growth occurs. In the type of inflammation which results in the formation of pyogenic granuloma, the destruction of the fixed tissue cells is slight, but the stimulus to proliferation of the vascular endothelium persists and exerts its influence over a long period of time.

Clinical Features. The pyogenic granuloma of the oral cavity arises most frequently on the gingiva, but may also be found on the lips, tongue and buccal mucosa and occasionally on other areas. The lesion is usually an elevated, pedunculated or sessile mass with a smooth, lobulated or even a warty surface which commonly is ulcerated and shows a tendency for hemorrhage either spontaneously or upon slight trauma (Fig. 6–9). Sometimes there is exudation of purulent material, but this is not a characteristic feature despite the suggestive name of this lesion. It is deep red or reddish purple, depending upon its vascularity, painless, and rather soft in consistency. Some lesions have a brown cast if hemorrhage has occurred into the tissue. (See also Plate IV.)

The pyogenic granuloma may develop rapidly, reach full size and then remain static for an indefinite period. The lesions in different cases may vary considerably in size, ranging from a few millimeters to a centimeter or more in diameter. In an excellent study of the pyogenic granuloma, in which he reported 289 cases, Kerr stated that the age group incidence was not significant, cases having been seen in both very young infants and elderly persons with no apparent predilection for any one age

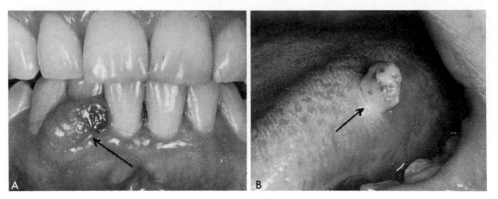

Figure 6–9. *Pyogenic granuloma.*
Gingiva *(A)* and tongue *(B).*

group. Nor were any significant differences in occurrence found between the sexes. However, in a series of 835 cases discussed by Angelopoulous, he noted that about 60 per cent of the lesions occurred in persons between 11 and 40 years of age, and that over 70 per cent involved females.

An *intravenous pyogenic granuloma* occurring on the neck and upper extremities has been reported by Cooper and his associates in a series of 18 patients between 15 and 66 years of age. These lesions, which appear to represent a different entity from that known as intravascular papillary endothelial hyperplasia (q.v.), have not been reported in the oral cavity.

Histologic Features. The histologic appearance of the pyogenic granuloma is similar to that of granulation tissue except that it is exuberant and is usually well localized (Fig. 6–10). The overlying epithelium, if present, is gener-

ally thin and atrophic, but may be hyperplastic. If the lesion is ulcerated, it shows a fibrinous exudate of varying thickness over the surface. The most startling features are the occurrence of vast numbers of endothelium-lined vascular spaces and the extreme proliferation of fibroblasts and budding endothelial cells. In addition, there is usually a moderately intense infiltration of polymorphonuclear leukocytes, lymphocytes and plasma cells, but this finding will vary, depending upon the presence or absence of ulceration. The connective tissue stroma is typically delicate, although frequently fasciculi of collagen fibers are noted coursing through the tissue mass. If the lesion is not surgically excised, there is gradual obliteration of the many capillaries, and it assumes a more fibrous appearance. This maturation of the connective tissue elements is construed as evidence of healing of the lesion. Both clinically and

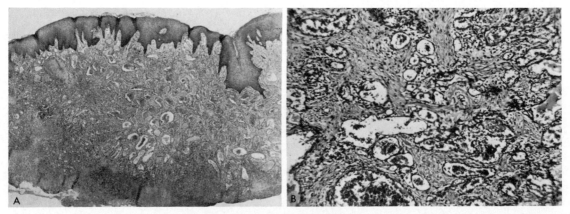

Figure 6–10. *Pyogenic granuloma.*
A, Low-power photomicrograph of pyogenic granuloma covered on one surface by epithelium and on the other by a fibrinous exudate; the vascularity of the lesion is obvious. *B,* High-power photomicrograph of *A* demonstrates the numerous endothelium-lined blood channels and fibroblasts.

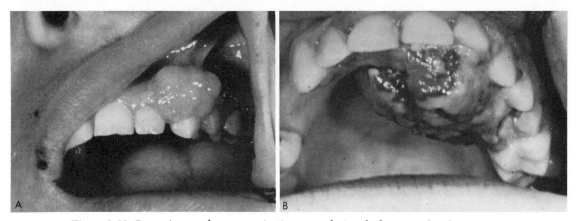

Figure 6–11. *Pyogenic granuloma occurring in women during the later months of pregnancy.*

microscopically, an old lesion may resemble a fibroepithelial polyp or even a typical fibroma, and it is likely that many so-called intraoral fibromas are healed pyogenic granulomas.

"PREGNANCY TUMOR." A lesion histologically identical to pyogenic granuloma of the gingiva frequently occurs during pregnancy and often has been called the "pregnancy tumor." This is a well-defined lesion which appears about the third month of pregnancy or sometimes later, gradually increases in size and, after delivery, may or may not regress (Fig. 6–11). If surgically removed during pregnancy, it frequently recurs. It is now believed by most workers that the "pregnancy tumor" is simply a pyogenic granuloma which occurs as a result of local minor trauma or irritation and in which the tissue reaction is probably intensified by the endocrine alteration occurring during pregnancy. There appears to be no justification for retaining the term "pregnancy tumor," since lesions of an identical clinical and histologic nature are seen in men as well as in nonpregnant women.

Treatment and Prognosis. The pyogenic granuloma is treated by surgical excision. The lesion occasionally recurs because it is not encapsulated, and the surgeon may have difficulty in determining its limits and excising it adequately. Some recurrent lesions may represent examples of a second episode of irritation with reinfection of tissue.

When excising a pyogenic granuloma of the gingiva, extreme care should always be taken to scale the adjacent tooth and make certain that it is free of calculus, since the calculus may act as the irritation leading to recurrence of the lesion. Careful microscopic examination of excised pyogenic granulomas will almost invaria-

bly reveal fragments of calculus on the inner surface of the lesion which was adjacent to the tooth.

PYOSTOMATITIS VEGETANS

Pyostomatitis vegetans is an uncommon inflammatory disease of the oral cavity originally described by McCarthy in 1949. The name was suggested because of the clinical similarity between the oral lesions of this disease and the skin lesions in a dermatologic disease known as "Pyodermatite végétante." The disease has been described in even greater detail by McCarthy and Shklar, who pointed out that the oral lesions are one part of a syndrome in which the patients also manifest concomitantly ulcerative colitis or other gastrointestinal disturbances. In fact, the history of colitis or a gastrointestinal disturbance often points to the diagnosis of the oral lesions.

Regional enteritis or regional ileitis, also known as *Crohn's disease*, is a granulomatous inflammation of the intestine of unknown etiology which is also recognized as one form of gastrointestinal disturbance that may be associated with pyostomatitis vegetans. This has been discussed by Cataldo and his associates, who illustrated a case in which the oral lesions ultimately led to the diagnosis of the intestinal disease.

Oral Manifestations. The oral lesions consist of large numbers of broad-based papillary projections, tiny abscesses or vegetations developing in areas of intense erythema (Fig. 6–12). These lesions may occur in any area of the oral cavity, although tongue involvement appears to be uncommon. These many small projections

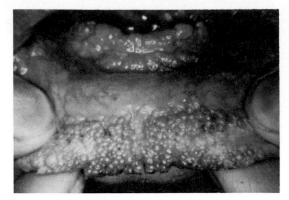

Figure 6–12. *Pyostomatitis vegetans.*
(Courtesy of Dr. Nathaniel H. Rowe.)

are red or pink in color, but careful examination may show tiny pustules beneath the epithelium which liberate purulent material when ruptured. These leave areas of ulceration which may coalesce into larger areas of necrosis.

The protean oral manifestations of 24 cases of Crohn's disease have been reviewed in detail by Bernstein and McDonald. They noted that the most frequently affected area was the buccal mucosa, which presented a "coblestone" appearance, while the vestibular lesions appeared as folds and ulcers, the lips were diffusely swollen and indurated, gingival and alveolar mucosal lesions were granular, and erythematous swellings and palatal lesions appeared as multiple aphthous ulcers.

Histologic Features. The papillary projections generally show an intact stratified squamous epithelium with an underlying loose connective tissue which is generally densely infiltrated by large numbers of plasma cells, lymphocytes, and occasional polymorphonuclear leukocytes, sometimes with a preponderance of eosinophils. Tiny areas of focal necrosis and microabscess formation, either intraepithelial or subepithelial, are common features of the lesions. In some instances, focal areas of degeneration and necrosis of the overlying epithelium are present.

Laboratory Findings. Bacteriologic studies are generally nonspecific, since only organisms of the normal oral microbial flora can be cultured from smears of the lesions.

Treatment. The treatment of pyostomatitis vegetans is not specific, since the oral lesions are usually refractory to antibiotic therapy. It has been found that the oral lesions tend to regress when the intestinal disturbance is brought under control. However, exacerbations of the gastrointestinal disease frequently result in exacerbation of the oral lesions as well.

VIRAL INFECTIONS

Viruses have been defined as submicroscopic entities which reproduce only within specific living cells and which can be introduced into these host cells from without. Viruses are almost infinite in distribution, affecting not only plants and animals, including man, but also insects and even bacteria. The size of viruses has been measured by various techniques and ranges between 10 millimicrons or less to more than 200 millimicrons. Some viruses have now been purified, crystallized and analyzed, and all have been found to contain a protein and either ribonucleic acid (RNA) or deoxyribonucleic acid (DNA). It has been suggested that viral-infected cells produce the nucleic acid characteristic of the virus and that, therefore, the susceptibility of cells to viral infection may depend upon the availability of suitable nucleic acid within the cell to sustain the virus.

Viruses have long been known to cause certain infectious diseases, and many of them produce a long-lasting immunity against reinfection by the same virus. In addition, there are many neoplasms in animals that have been transmitted by cell-free extracts of the tumor to other animals, establishing a viral etiology. More recent proof of the viral origin of certain animal leukemias has given impetus to the search for specific viruses in the cause of human cancer and the possibility of immunization against this disease.

The classification of viral diseases is difficult because of the size of viruses and their incompletely understood metabolic systems. However, their classification based on the biologic, chemical and physical properties of the animal viruses, separating them into groups according to the type of nucleic acid, and the size, shape and substructure of the particle, has been undertaken by the International Committee on Nomenclature of Viruses of the International Association of Microbiological Societies. This classification, with examples of human diseases in the various groups, is shown in Table 6–2.

HERPES SIMPLEX

(Acute Herpetic Gingivostomatitis; Herpes Labialis; Fever Blisters; Cold Sores)

Herpes simplex, an acute infectious disease, is probably the most common viral disease affecting man, with the exception of the viral respiratory infections. The tissues preferentially

Table 6–2. Classification of Major Virus Groups and Virus Diseases

I. RNA Viruses
   A. Orthomyxovirus
      1. Influenza
   B. Paramyxovirus
      1. Measles (rubeola)
      2. Mumps
   C. Rhabdovirus
      1. Rabies
      2. Hemorrhagic fever
   D. Arenavirus
      1. Lymphocytic choriomeningitis
      2. Lassa fever
   E. Calicivirus
   F. Coronavirus
      1. Upper respiratory infection
   G. Bunyavirus
   H. Picornavirus
      1. Poliomyelitis
      2. Coxsackie diseases
      3. Common cold
      4. Foot-and-mouth disease
      5. Encephalomyocarditis
   I. Reovirus
   J. Togavirus
      1. Rubella
      2. Yellow fever
      3. St. Louis encephalitis
   K. Retrovirus (RNA tumor virus)
II. DNA Viruses
   A. Herpesvirus
      1. Herpes simplex
      2. Varicella/herpes zoster
      3. Cytomegalic inclusion disease
      4. Epstein-Barr virus—infectious mononucleosis (?)
   B. Poxvirus
      1. Smallpox
      2. Molluscum contagiosum
   C. Adenovirus
      1. Pharyngoconjunctival fever
      2. Epidemic keratoconjunctivitis
   D. Parvovirus
   E. Iridovirus
   F. Papovavirus
      1. Human warts or papillomas
      2. Tumorigenic viruses in animals

After J. R. McGhee, S. M. Michalek, and G. H. Cassell: Dental Microbiology. Philadelphia, Harper & Row, Publishers, 1982.

involved by the herpes simplex virus (HSV), now often referred to as herpesvirus hominis, are derived from the ectoderm and consist principally of the skin, mucous membranes, eyes and central nervous system. There are two immunologically different types of HSV: type 1, usually affecting the face, lips, oral cavity and upper body skin; and type 2, usually affecting the genitals and skin of the lower body. Two other viruses that infect man also belong to the herpesvirus group: varicella-zoster virus and Epstein-Barr virus. A third virus, human cytomegalovirus, belongs to this same family of viruses but is in a separate genus. A recent in-depth summary of the structure, composition, growth cycle and cytopathogenic effects of HSV-1 has been published by Hicks and Terezhalmy.

Grüter was among the first to offer evidence that herpes simplex infection was caused by an infectious agent and that the fluid of vesicles from patients with herpes simplex would produce keratitis when inoculated on scarified rabbit cornea. Doerr also reported that the herpes virus would produce encephalitis in rabbits. Subsequently the virus has been found to multiply well on the chorioallantoic membrane of the chick embryo. Andrewes and Carmichael in 1930 found that neutralizing antibodies against the herpes simplex virus were present in the circulating blood of most normal adults and persisted throughout life, but that recurrent herpetic lesions frequently developed in these persons.

These and other studies have finally led to the established principle that two types of infection with the herpes simplex virus occur. The first is a *primary* infection in a person who is without circulating antibodies, and the second is a *recurrent* infection in persons who have such antibodies. It is impossible to differentiate clinically between the lesions of a primary and a recurrent attack, although the primary infection is accompanied more frequently by severe systemic manifestations and occasionally is fatal. It has been shown, however, that most adults have circulating antibodies in the blood, but have never exhibited a severe primary illness. Thus, it is reasoned, subclinical primary infections must be common. The relation between the primary and secondary forms of herpes simplex infection is shown in Figure 6–13.

Herpes genitalis, caused by HSV-2, is a relatively common disease of the uterine cervix, vagina, vulva and penis. The incidence of this form of the infection has increased precipitously in the United States within the past decade and, in fact, is now often termed the "new epidemic venereal disease," since it is transmitted through sexual contact. This virus differs immunologically from type 1 herpes virus, which is responsible for most cases of herpetic infection of the oral cavity. The type 2 virus of genital herpes is somewhat more virulent than type 1 and, significantly, has been associated repeatedly with carcinoma of the uterine cervix, thus suggesting a possible cause and effect

HOST-PARASITE RELATIONSHIP OF HERPES SIMPLEX VIRUS

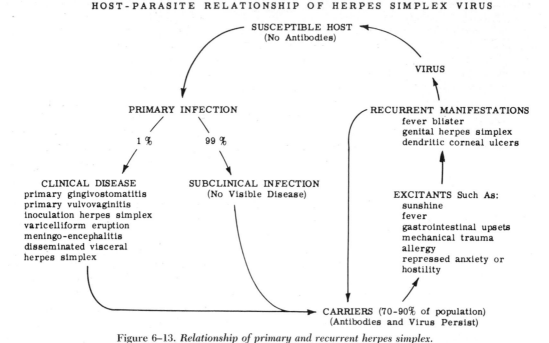

Figure 6–13. *Relationship of primary and recurrent herpes simplex.*
(Courtesy of Dr. Harvey Blank. From H. Blank and G. Rake: Viral and Rickettsial Diseases of the Skin, Eye and Mucous Membranes of Man. Boston, Little, Brown and Company, 1955.)

relationship. However, because of changing sexual practices in recent years, there has been rather widespread translocation in the usual habitats of type 1 and type 2 HSV. Thus, it is not unusual today to find HSV-2 on the lips or oral mucous membranes and HSV-1 on the genitalia.

Herpetic meningoencephalitis is a serious form of this infection, characterized by sudden fever and symptoms of increased intracranial pressure. Paralysis of various muscle groups occurs, while convulsions and even death may ensue. It is difficult to differentiate clinically between meningoencephalitis caused by the herpes virus and that produced by other viruses.

Herpetic conjunctivitis, or keratoconjunctivitis, is a rather common disease and is characterized by swelling and congestion of the palpebral conjunctiva, although keratitis and corneal ulceration also may occur. Herpetic vesicles of the eyelids are typical, but these eye lesions usually heal rapidly.

Herpetic eczema (Kaposi's varicelliform eruption) is an epidermal form of the herpetic infection superimposed upon a pre-existing eczema (possibly an example of anachoresis) and is characterized by diffuse vesicular lesions of the skin, usually of an extremely serious nature. In

addition to this atopic dermatitis, the herpetic infection may also be superimposed on severe seborrheic dermatitis, impetigo, scabies, Darier's disease and pemphigus vulgaris or foliaceus. It is most frequently due to the primary herpetic attack and may be fatal. The patients, usually children, exhibit a high fever coincident with the typical umbilicated vesicles as well as other systemic manifestations.

Disseminated herpes simplex of the newborn is a relatively uncommon disease in which the newborn infant acquires the infection during passage through the birth canal of a mother who is suffering from herpetic vulvovaginitis. However, occasional cases of transplacental infection by the virus have been reported. These infants usually manifest the disease by the fourth to seventh day of life, exhibit a wide variety of signs and symptoms of the disease and, with few exceptions, usually die on the ninth to twelfth day of life. Surviving infants frequently show residual neurologic involvement.

Primary Herpetic Stomatitis

Dodd and her co-workers reported in 1939 that the herpes simplex virus could be isolated from patients suffering from a gingivostomatitis with a particular clinical configuration. Burnet and Williams reported similar findings and, in addition, demonstrated that infants with this disease developed circulating antibodies during the convalescent period.

Clinical Features. Herpetic stomatitis is a common oral disease which develops in both children and young adults. However, it has been suggested by Sheridan and Herrmann that the primary form of the disease is probably more common in older adults than was once thought. It rarely occurs before the age of six months, apparently because of the presence of circulating antibodies in the infant derived from the mother. The disease occurring in children is frequently the primary attack and is characterized by the development of fever, irritability, headache, pain upon swallowing and regional lymphadenopathy. Within a few days the mouth becomes painful and the gingiva intensely inflamed. The lips, tongue, buccal mucosa, palate, pharynx and tonsils may also be involved. Shortly, yellowish, fluid-filled vesicles develop. These rupture and form shallow, ragged, extremely painful ulcers covered by a gray membrane and surrounded by an erythematous halo (Fig. 6–14). It is important to recognize that the gingival inflammation precedes the formation of the ulcers by several days. The ulcers vary considerably in size, ranging from very tiny lesions to lesions measuring several millimeters or even a centimeter in diameter. They heal spontaneously within 7 to 14 days and leave no scar. (See also Plate IV.)

Utilizing culture techniques, August and Nordlund found that HSV-1 could be isolated from facial, labial and oral herpetic lesions for a mean duration of 3½ days, with a range of 2 to 6 days, after the onset of the lesions, while HSV-2 could be isolated from genital lesions for a mean duration of 5½ days, with a range of 2 to 14 days, after onset. They also noted that viral persistence in lesions did not seem to differ between mild primary infection and recurrent infection. In addition, Turner and his colleagues have shown that HSV could survive for two to four hours on environmental surfaces such as cloth and plastic as well as on the skin of the hands contaminated by direct contact with labial or oral lesions.

It is now well established that the HSV does not remain latent at the site of the original infection in the skin or oral mucosa. Instead, the virus reaches nerve ganglia supplying the affected areas, presumably along nerve pathways, and remains latent there until reactivated. The usual ganglia involved are the trigeminal for HSV-1 and the lumbosacral for HSV-2. Viral DNA can be demonstrated in these ganglia. Unfortunately, this incorporation of viral DNA into host DNA insures a lifelong infection beyond the reach of antibody, cell-mediated immune responses or chemotherapy.

Histologic Features. The herpetic vesicle is an intraepithelial blister filled with fluid. Degenerating cells show "ballooning degeneration," while others characteristically contain intranuclear inclusions known as Lipschütz bodies. These are eosinophilic, ovoid, homogeneous structures within the nucleus which tend to displace the nucleolus and nuclear chromatin peripherally. The displacement of chromatin often produces a peri-inclusion halo. The subjacent connective tissue is usually infiltrated

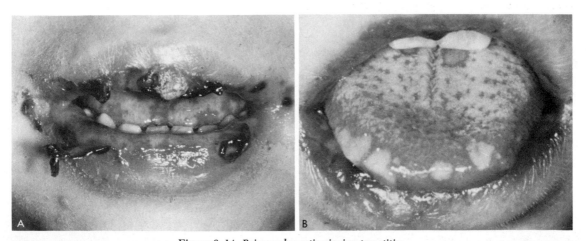

Figure 6–14. *Primary herpetic gingivostomatitis.*
The children in both cases exhibited severe involvement of the lips and oral cavity. (Courtesy of Drs. Warren B. Davis and John R. Mink.)

by inflammatory cells. When the vesicle ruptures, the surface of the tissue is covered by an exudate made up of fibrin, polymorphonuclear leukocytes and degenerated cells. The lesions heal by peripheral epithelial proliferation.

Mode of Transmission. The fact that the herpes virus may be recovered from the saliva of patients during the course of the disease leads to the assumption that transmission may occur by droplet infection, although some workers believe that direct contact is necessary. There is no animal reservoir for this virus. It has been reported in one series of patients that a history of contact with affected persons was present in nearly 50 per cent of the cases. After such contact, the incubation period appears to range from 2 to 20 days, with an average of 6 days before development of lesions. There also have been occasional epidemics of herpetic stomatitis, such as that reported by Hale and his associates in an orphanage nursery. In addition, it has been noted that primary herpetic eruptions are commonly associated with pneumonia, meningitis and the common cold.

Treatment. The treatment of primary herpetic infection is unsatisfactory. Of necessity, it is only supportive and symptomatic, since the course of the disease appears to be unalterable. Antibiotic therapy is of considerable aid in the prevention of secondary infection.

Recurrent, or Secondary, Herpetic Labialis and Stomatitis

Recurrent herpetic stomatitis is usually seen in adult patients and manifests itself clinically as an attenuated form of the primary disease. It has been reported by Nahmias and Roizman that between 80 and 100 per cent of adults in the lower socioeconomic levels have HSV-1 and/or HSV-2 circulating antibodies, whereas only 30 to 50 per cent of adults in the higher socioeconomic levels, including medical, dental and nursing personnel, have such antibodies. Those without antibodies are at higher risk of contact and infection, especially the latter groups because of the nature of their occupation. Also, as pointed out by Rowe and his co-workers, recurrent lesions of the fingers or hands (herpetic whitlow) and eyes may be encountered in these professional groups more frequently than in the general population. This variation in socioeconomic groups has not been explained.

The recurrent form of the disease is often associated with trauma, fatigue, menstruation, pregnancy, upper respiratory tract infection, emotional upset, allergy, exposure to sunlight or ultraviolet lamps, or gastrointestinal disturbances. The mechanism through which these various precipitating factors elicit an outbreak of lesions is unknown. The viruses, once they have been introduced into the body, appear to reside dormantly within the regional ganglia and, when reactivation is triggered, spread along the nerves to sites on the oral mucosa and skin where they destroy the epithelial cells and induce the typical inflammatory response with the characteristic lesions of recurrent infection.

Clinical Features. Recurrent herpes simplex infection may occur at widely varying intervals, from nearly every month in some patients to only about once a year or even less in others. The lesions may develop either on the lips (recurrent herpes labialis) or intraorally (Fig. 6–15 and Plate IV). In either location, the lesions are frequently preceded by a burning or tingling sensation and a feeling of tautness, swelling or slight soreness at the location in which the vesicles subsequently develop. These vesicles are generally small (1 mm. or less in diameter), tend to occur in localized clusters, and may coalesce to form somewhat larger lesions. These gray or white vesicles rupture quickly, leaving a small red ulceration, sometimes with a slight erythematous halo. On the lips, these ruptured vesicles become covered by a brownish crust. The degree of pain present is quite variable.

It has been emphasized by Weathers and Griffin that the recurrent intraoral herpetic lesions almost invariably develop on oral mucosa that is tightly bound to periosteum. Seldom do they occur on mobile mucosa, in contrast to the recurrent aphthous stomatitis (q.v.) which almost invariably occurs only on mobile mucosa. Thus, the most common sites for the recurrent intraoral herpetic lesions are the hard palate and attached gingiva or alveolar ridge. Interestingly, herpes labialis is seldom seen concurrently with intraoral lesions.

The lesions gradually heal within 7 to 10 days and leave no scar.

Histologic Features. A number of investigators, beginning with Blank and his associates, have shown that the Papanicolaou smear, using fresh scrapings from the base of a vesicle, is a reliable technique for the diagnosis of active herpes simplex infection if herpes zoster/varicella infection is ruled out, since no other conditions produce a similar cytopathic effect. "Ballooning degeneration," chromatin margination and typical Lipschütz bodies as described earlier are all seen in smears from these lesions,

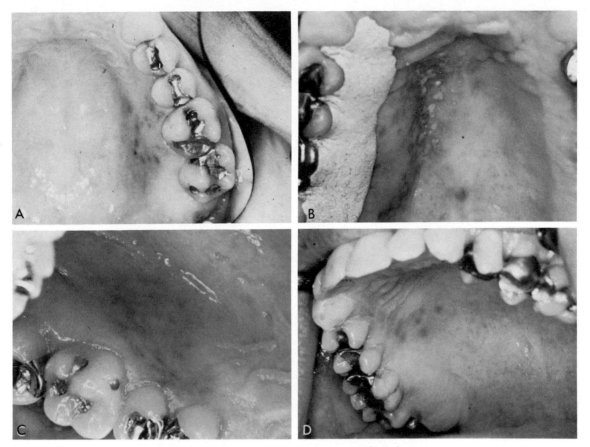

Figure 6–15. *Recurrent intraoral herpes simplex infection.*
(Courtesy of Dr. Dwight R. Weathers.)

as well as characteristic multinucleated giant cells originally observed by Tzanck (Fig. 6–16). Nowakovsky and her co-workers have thoroughly reviewed the manifestations of viral infections in exfoliated cells. The histologic findings in biopsy specimens from the recurrent lesions are identical to those described under the primary form of the disease.

Laboratory Findings. Isolation of herpes simplex virus can be accomplished in tissue culture, particularly in the early stages of the recurrent infection. According to Takumaru, the virus is easily isolated when there is a low production of γ-A globulin, but there is a rapid clearing of the virus, often within 1 day, after a rebound production of γ-A globulin. Similarly, smears would be positive for only a short time after the virus has cleared because of the rapid degeneration of affected cells.

Current diagnostic methods for herpes viral diagnosis have been reviewed by Burns. These have included (1) viral isolation and identification in various systems, including eggs and mice, as well as cell culture technique; (2) immunofluorescent staining of smears, impressions or cryostat sections with fluorescein-labeled HSV protein or antibody protein; (3) immunoperoxidase technique, which is reportedly far more sensitive than the immunofluorescence technique, is similar in basic principle but does not require fluorescence microscopy; and (4) serologic assays such as the complement fixation assay, radioimmunoassay (RIA) and enzyme-linked immunosorbent assay (ELISA).

Treatment. Until recently, little could be provided in the way of actual therapy except for symptomatic relief, although many drugs have been tested over the years.

Several specific antiviral chemotherapeutic agents are presently available for use under certain conditions and with certain forms of HSV infection. The most prominent of these are (1) acyclovir [9- (2-hydroxyethoxymethyl) guanine]; (2) vidarabine (adenine arabinoside); and (3) idoxuridine (5-iodo-2′-deoxyuridine). However, these must only be used according to prescribed indications and do not represent curative drugs for this disease. Many other

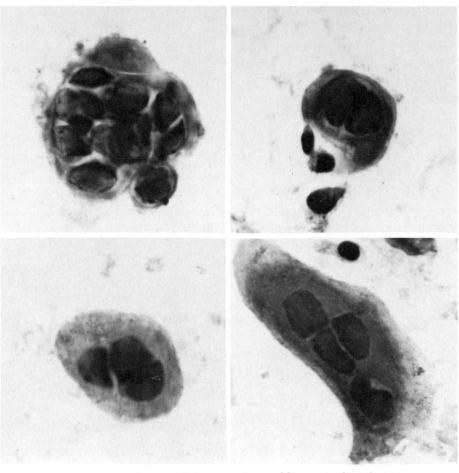

Figure 6–16. *Recurrent intraoral herpes simplex infection.*
Cytologic smear of lesions shows typical alterations in epithelial cells infected by herpes simplex virus.

modalities of treatment are occasionally of benefit in some forms of HSV infection.

Differential Diagnosis. A consideration of differential diagnosis is of great importance, since numerous diseases may bear some resemblance to herpes simplex. Thus some difficulty may be encountered in distinguishing herpes simplex particularly from the recurrent aphthous stomatitis (q.v.). Other conditions to be considered are herpes zoster, impetigo, erythema multiforme and related diseases, smallpox, pemphigus, epidermolysis bullosa, food or drug allergies and drug or chemical burns.

RECURRENT APHTHOUS STOMATITIS

(Aphthous Ulcers; Aphthae; Canker Sores)

Recurrent aphthous stomatitis is an unfortunately common disease characterized by the development of painful, recurring solitary or multiple ulcerations of the oral mucosa. Because of the similarity between this disease and herpes simplex infection with respect to precipitating factors leading to development of lesions, certain aspects of the clinical appearance of lesions, duration of lesions, chronic recurrence and general failure of response to any form of therapy, the two diseases have been generally confused until only a short time ago. A series of intense investigations over the past few years have conclusively established the fact that there is no etiologic relationship between recurrent aphthous stomatitis and herpes simplex infection; it is discussed in this section and at this point only because of its similarity to the viral disease.

Etiology. Numerous possible etiologic factors have been suggested in the interesting history of recurrent aphthous stomatitis and these have been adequately reviewed by Ship and his group and, more recently, in the Workshop on

Aphthous Stomatitis and Behçet's Syndrome at the National Institutes of Health in September 1977, co-chaired by Graykowski and Hooks. However, in light of present knowledge, it is obvious that there has been considerable confusion in the past between *etiologic* factors and *precipitating* factors.

BACTERIAL INFECTION. The work of Barile, of Graykowski and of Stanley a few years ago very strongly implicated a pleomorphic, transitional L-form of an α-hemolytic streptococcus, *Streptococcus sanguis*, as the causative agent of the disease. This organism has been consistently isolated from the lesions of patients with typical aphthous ulcers, and microorganisms morphologically consistent with the L-form streptococcus have been found histologically in the vast majority of aphthous lesions. Once again, it should be emphasized that the herpes simplex virus cannot be isolated from these aphthous ulcers.

The administration of this pleomorphic streptococcus to guinea pigs and rabbits has produced lesions of the skin and the oral mucosa which appear clinically and histologically similar to aphthous ulcers in the human. Finally, the work of Graykowski and his associates has shown that patients with recurrent aphthous ulcers, when tested with a Streptococcus vaccine, give a positive delayed type of hypersensitivity skin reaction in contrast to patients with no history of aphthae who give a less frequent and less severe response. Thus, there is some evidence for this disease being an immunologic hypersensitivity reaction to an L-form streptococcus.

IMMUNOLOGIC ABNORMALITIES. As an alternative etiologic factor, Lehner has proposed that the recurrent aphthous ulcer is the result of an autoimmune response of the oral epithelium. Utilizing a fluorescent antibody technique, he has shown both IgG and IgM binding by epithelial cells of the spinous layer of oral mucosa in patients suffering from recurrent aphthous ulcers, while the same cells in healthy control patients or patients with nonspecific ulcers show no such binding.

Normal levels of antinuclear factors and complement levels within normal limits in patients with this disease have been reported by Addy and Dolby and by Lehner. This has led Cohen to suggest that recurrent aphthous stomatitis is not an autoimmune disease arising from a central immunologic fault but rather represents a local immune response against an antigenically altered mucosa. He theorizes in this context

that the disease is the result of diffusion of bacterial toxins, foods and other substances acting as allergens or haptens which initiate an immune response. The same substances, he points out, could also react with epithelial cell surface antigens to produce a change resulting in an adverse inflammatory response.

Donatsky has found elevated gamma globulin levels against Streptococcus 2A and M5 by immunofluorescent studies in the serum of patients with recurrent aphthous stomatitis. The detected antibodies in these patients were able to bind serum complement. These investigations have led Antoon and Miller to conclude that the immune system appears actively involved in reaction to bacterial and autoimmune antigens and speculated that L-form streptococci might infect epithelium of the salivary ducts, stimulate formation of antibodies, fix complement and cause cytolysis. They believed that the disease might be further complicated by an autoimmune reaction to released antigens from epithelial tissues.

Thus, patients with recurrent aphthous stomatitis appear to have an altered immune response which is directed against both the nonpathogenic oral flora and the host oral tissue.

IRON, VITAMIN B_{12} OR FOLIC ACID DEFICIENCY. There has been some evidence that nutritional deficiencies might be of significance in the etiology of recurrent aphthous stomatitis. For example, a study has been reported by Wray and his colleagues in which a series of 330 patients with recurrent aphthae were screened for deficiencies of iron, folic acid, and vitamin B_{12}. A total of 47 deficient patients, or 14.2 per cent, was found: 23 patients were deficient in iron; 7 in folic acid; and 6 in vitamin B_{12}; and 11 had combined deficiencies. Thirty-nine of these patients were treated with the appropriate replacement therapy, and it was found that 23 had a complete remission of their ulcers, 11 were improved and 3 were not helped. While the results indicate that a small percentage of patients with recurrent aphthae do have certain nutritional deficiencies, the investigators pointed out that the prompt response to replacement therapy suggested a direct action on oral mucosa, but that it might be reasonably postulated that the presence of a deficiency allows the expression of an unrelated underlying tendency to ulceration and that the deficiency itself does not play a primary role. The failure of response in some patients also might indicate either that the deficiency was coincidental or that the therapy was inadequate.

In any event, the role of nutritional deficiencies in the etiology of this disease does not appear to be a major one.

Precipitating Factors. A variety of situations have been repeatedly identified immediately preceding the outbreak of aphthous ulcers in relatively large numbers of patients.

TRAUMA. Local trauma has been found to be the precipitating factor in nearly 75 per cent of cases in a series reported by Graykowski and his co-workers. The traumatic incidents included self-inflicted bites, oral surgical procedures, tooth brushing, dental procedures, needle injections and dental trauma.

ENDOCRINE CONDITIONS. It has been recognized for many years that a time relationship exists between the occurrence of the menstrual period and the development of aphthous ulcers. Most series show that the incidence of aphthae is greatest during the premenstrual period. Dolby has similarly shown that ulceration is maximal in the postovulation period and has related this to the blood level of progesterone.

It has also been reported that women may have remission of their aphthous lesions during pregnancy but show eruptions following parturition, sometimes very rapidly. On rare occasions, the onset of the disease has been associated with menarche and menopause.

PSYCHIC FACTORS. The role of psychic factors in certain oral diseases is well recognized. In cases of aphthous ulcers, acute psychologic problems appear many times to have precipitated attacks of the disease, although this is a difficult factor to analyze.

ALLERGIC FACTORS. Many patients with recurrent aphthous ulcers have a history of asthma, hay fever or food or drug allergies. This may be a purely fortuitous finding because of the high incidence of allergies in the general population. However, the outbreak of aphthae following the use of certain foods or drugs in the same patients has been reported so frequently that allergy must be considered a precipitating factor.

Classification. Recurrent aphthous stomatitis has been classified by many recent investigators into four chief varieties based upon the clinical manifestations: (1) *recurrent aphthous minor,* which is the most common form of the disease and the one referred to by the lay public as the "canker" sore; (2) *recurrent aphthous major,* which is now believed to be simply a more severe form of recurrent aphthous minor but which was thought at one time to represent a separate disease entity known as periadenitis mucosa necrotica recurrens (Mikulicz's scarring aphthae or Sutton's disease); (3) *recurrent herpetiform ulcerations,* which consist of clusters of ulcers resembling herpetic lesions but lacking evidence of the presence of viruses in patients with a low incidence of antibody to oral mucosa; and (4) *recurrent ulcers associated with Behçet's syndrome,* which will be considered separately.

Clinical Features. *Recurrent aphthous minor* occurs somewhat more frequently in women than in men, and the majority of patients report the onset of the disease between the ages of 10 and 30 years. However, it may commence much earlier in life or not begin until much later. Unfortunately, the disease typically persists with recurring attacks over a period of many years. It is believed that nearly 20 per cent of the general population is affected by this disease at one time or another. It is interesting that approximately 55 per cent of a large group of professional school students studied by Ship and his associates gave a positive history of recurrent aphthous ulcers. It is also of interest that a rather remarkable familial tendency for occurrence of the disease has been noted by many workers. For example, in the series of Graykowski and co-workers, over 80 per cent of the affected patients had an additional member or members of their families with a history of aphthae.

The frequency of outbreaks of the aphthae varies remarkably between patients. Some persons will have only one or two attacks a year, while others will have one or two attacks a month every month for prolonged periods, sometimes years. Occasional patients have continual, repeated outbreaks and are never free of lesions for extended intervals.

The onset of the disease may occur with a variety of manifestations which are not invariably present in all cases. These include the occurrence of one or more small nodules; generalized edema of the oral cavity, especially the tongue; paresthesia; malaise; low-grade fever; localized lymphadenopathy; and vesicle-like lesions containing mucus.

The aphthous ulcer begins as a single or multiple superficial erosion covered by a gray membrane (Fig. 6–17 and Plate IV). It generally has a well circumscribed margin surrounded by an erythematous halo. The lesion is typically very painful so that it commonly interferes with eating for several days. At one time it was thought that the aphthous ulcer begins with the formation of a vesicle as does the lesion of herpes simplex infection. The majority of the

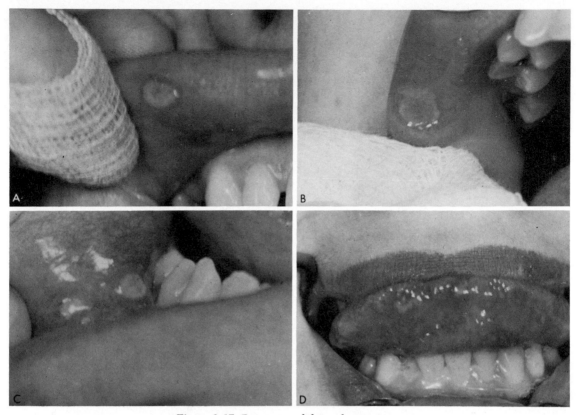

Figure 6–17. *Recurrent aphthous ulcers, minor.*

evidence now indicates that this is not the case; vesicle formation does not appear to be a stage in the development of the usual aphthous ulcer.

The number of lesions present in any one patient during a single outbreak may vary from one to over 100. However, according to Graykowski and his associates, over 90 per cent of patients have six lesions or less during a single outbreak. They vary in size from 2–3 mm. to over 10 mm. in diameter. The most common sites of occurrence are the buccal and labial mucosa, buccal and lingual sulci, tongue, soft palate, pharynx and gingiva, all locations of labile mucosa not bound to periosteum, in direct contrast to the sites of predilection of recurrent intraoral herpes simplex infection. The ulcers themselves generally persist for 7 to 14 days and then heal gradually with little or no evidence of scarring.

Recurrent aphthous major is characterized by the occurrence of large painful ulcers, usually one to ten in number, on the lips, cheeks, tongue, soft palate and fauces (Fig. 6–18). These ulcers occur at frequent intervals, and many patients with this disease are seldom free from

the presence of at least one ulcer. Unlike the typical ulcers of recurrent aphthous minor, these lesions may persist for up to 6 weeks and leave a scar upon healing. Not uncommonly, the ulcers recur in waves over a long period of time, so that eventually the oral mucosa may show a great deal of scarring. Patients with these severe major aphthae also occasionally show similar lesions of the vagina or penis, rectum and larynx, with associated rheumatoid arthritis or conjunctivitis.

According to the review of this disease by Hjørting-Hansen and Siemassen, there is no predilection for occurrence in any particular age group, although females are affected more frequently than males. An excellent discussion of the disease was published recently by Lehner.

Recurrent herpetiform ulcers are characterized by crops of multiple small, shallow ulcers, often up to 100 in number, which may occur at any site in the oral cavity. They were first described by Cooke in 1960, while Lehner as well as Brooke and Sapp have expanded our knowledge of this condition. Cooke pointed out

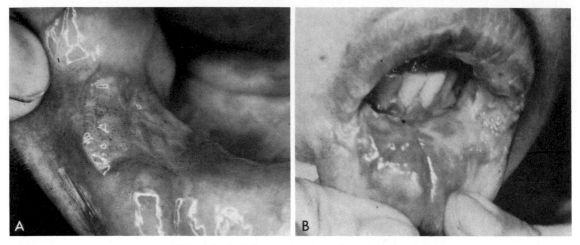

Figure 6–18. *Recurrent aphthous ulcers, major.*
Deep crateriform ulcer *(A)* and scars *(B)*. *(B*, Courtesy of Dr. T. H. Century.)

the clinical similarities of this disease to the lesions of herpes simplex and that the corresponding histologic changes were not similar, since these lesions resemble the recurrent aphthous ulcer rather than a viral lesion.

The characteristic clinical features of this uncommon condition known as herpetiform ulceration or recurrent herpetiform ulcers were listed by Brooke and Sapp as follows: (1) numerous, small lesions may be found on any intraoral mucosal surface; (2) lesions begin as small pinhead-sized erosions that gradually enlarge and coalesce; (3) lesions are more painful than would be suspected by their size; (4) lesions are present almost continuously for one to three years, with relatively short remissions; and (5) the patient receives immediate but temporary relief from symptoms with a 2 per cent tetracycline mouthwash. While these clinical features are very reminiscent of herpes simplex infection, Brooke and Sapp pointed out that laboratory tests show that (1) the herpes simplex virus cannot be cultured from the lesions or demonstrated by electron microscopy, although Sapp and Brooke have demonstrated nonviral intranuclear bodies in adjacent epithelial cells; (2) cytologic smears fail to reveal the typical multinucleated epithelial giant cells found in herpetic lesions; (3) the microscopic findings are nearly identical with those described for the recurrent aphthous ulcer; and (4) immunofluorescent and serologic techniques are negative for antibodies to herpes virus as well as to oral epithelium.

Although the exact nature of this disease is unknown, including its etiology and pathogen-

esis, it is considered appropriate by most investigators to include it as a variant of recurrent aphthous stomatitis and await further clarification.

Histologic Features. The minor aphthous ulcer of the oral mucous membrane exhibits a fibrinopurulent membrane covering the ulcerated area. Occasional superficial colonies of microorganisms may be present in this membrane. An intense inflammatory cell infiltration is present in the connective tissue beneath the ulcer, with considerable necrosis of tissue near the surface of the lesion, neutrophils predominating immediately below the ulcer but lymphocytes prevailing adjacent to this. Granulation tissue may be noted near the base of the lesion. Epithelial proliferation is present at the margins of the lesion, similar to that found in any nonspecific ulcer. Accessory salivary gland tissue, commonly present in areas of aphthae, will typically exhibit focal periductal and perialveolar fibrosis, ductal ectasia and mild chronic inflammation. These features may be present in even clinically normal mucosa of the aphthous patient. It has also been found that the aphthous ulcer itself, at least in some cases, begins immediately above the excretory duct of one of these minor glands where there is disruption of this ductal epithelium. The tissue involvement is generally superficial.

Lehner has shown that the histologic findings by light microscopy of the severe oral ulcers in recurrent aphthous major are identical with those described under the recurrent aphthous minor. Electron microscope studies have confirmed this similarity.

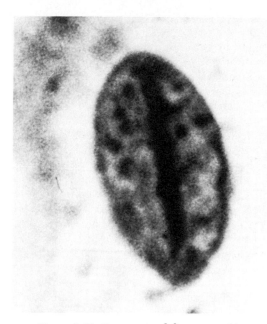

Figure 6–19. *Recurrent aphthous stomatitis.*
The typical Anitschkow cell in a cytologic smear from the margin of an aphthous ulcer.

The microscopic picture is nonspecific and, without a careful clinical history and description, does not permit the specific diagnosis of the disease.

Wood and his associates have described characteristic changes in the nuclei of epithelial cells taken by cytologic smear from around recurrent aphthous ulcers. These have been referred to as Anitschkow cells and consist of cells with elongated nuclei containing a linear bar of chromatin with radiating processes of chromatin extending toward the nuclear membrane (Fig. 6–19). They are quite abundant in patients with recurrent aphthous stomatitis but are not pathognomic of the disease, since they are also found in patients with sickle cell disease, megaloblastic anemias and iron-deficiency anemias, in children receiving chemotherapy for cancer and even in normal people. Their ultrastructure has been described by Haley and his associates, who found that the nuclear chromatin was made up of pleomorphic masses forming an irregular band along the long axis of the nucleus rather than being randomly dispersed.

Treatment. There is no specific treatment for recurrent aphthous ulcers although, over the years, many drugs have been advocated. The results of an excellent comparative clinical trial of a variety of drugs have been reported by Graykowski and his co-workers. Briefly, it was found that a tetracycline mouthwash (250 mg. per 5 ml.), used four times daily for 5 to 7 days, produced a good response in nearly 70 per cent of the patients tested by relieving the pain, reducing the size of the lesions and reducing the healing time. A steroid ointment, 1.5 per cent cortisone acetate, applied locally, and hydrocortisone acetate–antibiotic lozenges also showed some effectiveness but not as great as the tetracycline. Chemical cautery reduced pain but had no other beneficial effects. No significant improvement was found with the use of antihistaminics, gamma globulin, multiple smallpox vaccinations or a *Lactobacillus acidophilus-L. bulgaricus* preparation, all of which have variously been reported to be effective.

There has also been extensive clinical trial of levamisole, originally developed as an anthelmintic drug against nematodes in both man and animals, which has been found also to potentiate the immune response in a variety of ways. The results of a number of these studies in treating recurrent aphthous stomatitis have been reported, some showing a reduction in the duration of symptoms, some showing a decrease in the duration of lesions, some showing a diminished frequency of lesions, but others concluding that the drug had no significant effect on severity or incidence of lesions. It was concluded at the previously mentioned Workshop on Aphthous Stomatitis–Behçet's Syndrome, where a number of these reports were presented, that further clinical evaluation of this drug is necessary.

An excellent summary of the many drugs and chemicals which have been used to treat recurrent aphthous stomatitis over the years has been prepared by Antoon and Miller and is shown in Table 6–3. Unfortunately, despite any form of therapy, there is no known cure for the disease.

BEHÇET'S SYNDROME

Behçet's syndrome is a disease of uncertain etiology that may resemble an infectious disease and in the past has been suggested to be caused by pleuropneumonia-like organisms (PPLO) or, more frequently, by a virus. However, most of the evidence today favors an autoimmune etiology, since it has been shown by Oshima and his associates that these patients have a high incidence of autoantibodies against oral mucosa and also exhibit a rise in immunoglobulins in the oral mucosa and blood. Lehner has pointed out the similarity in immunologic features be-

Table 6–3.   Treatment Modalities for
Recurrent Aphthous Stomatitis

Immune enhancement
   Levamisole
   Vaccine

Immunosuppression, inflammatory suppression
   Prednisone
   Triamcinalone acetonide
   Betamethasone-17-benzoate
   Antihistamine
   (Tetracycline?)

Antibiotics
   Tetracycline suspension, topical
   Chloramphenicol
   Broad-spectrum antibiotics

Antiseptic
   Silver nitrate
   Coagulating agent, negatol
   Gentian violet
   (Lactobacillus?)

Diet supplementation
   Vitamin B-12, folic acid
   Iron
   Zinc sulfate

Symptomatic treatment
   Xylocaine/lidocaine
   Silver nitrate
   Benadryl, topical
   Camphor-phenol

From J. W. Antoon, and R. L. Miller: Aphthous ulcers—
a review of the literature on etiology, pathogenesis, diagnosis and treatment. J. Am. Dent. Assoc., *101*:803, 1980.

tween this disease and recurrent aphthous stomatitis, his studies suggesting that oral epithelium or some cross-reacting microorganism
could act as an antigen to stimulate humoral
antibody and cell-mediated immune responses.
According to Cohen, reviewing the etiology of
this disease in the Workshop on Aphthous Stomatitis–Behçet's Syndrome sponsored by the
National Institutes of Health in 1977, these
humoral antibody and cell-mediated immune
responses may act either jointly or independently upon the oral epithelium to cause the
pathologic lesion. The incidence is in favor of
cell-mediated immunity as the mechanism. The
immunologic competence and cytotoxic potential of lymphocytes to oral mucosa suggest that
these cells might cause the epithelial damage
which results in ulceration.

In this same workshop, Lehner reported that
while recurrent aphthous ulcers and Behçet's
syndrome cannot be distinguished by antibodies
and cell-mediated immune responses, human
leukocyte antigen (HLA) markers do seem to
differentiate the two. Nevertheless, the oral
lesions in the two diseases are similar if not
identical.

Clinical Features. The syndrome usually begins between 10 and 45 years of age, with a
mean age of 30 years, and is five to ten times
more common in males. It is characterized
chiefly by oral and genital ulcerations, ocular
lesions and skin lesions.

The first manifestation of the disease is usually the appearance of oral and/or genital lesions. The oral lesions are painful and very
similar in appearance to recurrent aphthous
ulcers. They occur in crops at any intraoral site
and consist of ulcers ranging in size from several
millimeters to a centimeter or more in diameter. These ulcers have an erythematous border
and are covered by a gray or yellow exudate.
The genital ulcers are small and located on the
scrotum, root of the penis or labia majora.

The ocular lesions, beginning as photophobia
and irritation, may range in severity from a
simple conjunctivitis to uveitis and finally hy-
popyon. The skin lesions are generally small
pustules or papules on the trunk or limbs and
around the genitalia. In addition to the various
forms of pyoderma, both erythema nodosum
and erythema multiforme have been reported
to occur. Arthralgia, thrombophlebitis and central nervous system involvement, as well as
cardiac or pulmonary involvement, are occasional complications of the disease.

While the oral ulcerations in recurrent
aphthous stomatitis and in Behçet's syndrome
appear clinically indistinguishable, the two diseases can be separated easily. In recurrent
aphthous stomatitis, the oral ulcers are the only
manifestation of disease. In Behçet's syndrome,
at least two of the classic triad of the disease
must be present: recurrent oral ulcers, recurrent genital ulcers and ocular inflammation.

Histologic Features. The intraoral ulcers are
entirely nonspecific and, according to Lehner,
are remarkably similar to recurrent aphthous
ulcers. Endothelial proliferation is reported in
the lesions of Behçet's disease but not in the
recurrent aphthous ulcer. Vasculitis also appears to be an essential lesion in Behçet's
disease.

Laboratory Findings. These patients frequently manifest a hypergammaglobulinemia,
leukocytosis with eosinophilia and elevated
sedimentation rate. Other findings are variable.

Treatment and Prognosis. There is no specific
treatment for the disease other than sympto-

matic or supportive measures. While Behcet's disease may undergo spontaneous remission after a variable period of months to years, it may progress to serious complications and even result in death.

REITER'S SYNDROME

Reiter's syndrome is a disease of unknown etiology, although there is evidence of an infectious origin. It is one of the most common complications of nonspecific urethritis and, in fact, clinically mimics gonorrhea, although the urethral discharge is negative for Neisseria. In recent years, pleuropneumonia-like organisms (PPLO) have been implicated and, even more recently, a Bedsonia group virus has been isolated from patients with the disease. Mycoplasmal and chlamydial species have also been suspected. There is an excellent review of the disease by Weinberger and his associates.

Clinical Features. Reiter's syndrome is almost totally confined to men, usually between 20 and 30 years of age. There is a typical tetrad of manifestations: urethritis, arthritis, conjunctivitis and mucocutaneous lesions. In any given case, however, the full tetrad is often not present.

The urethral discharge is usually associated with an itching, burning sensation. The arthritis is often bilaterally symmetrical and usually polyarticular. Conjunctivitis is often so mild as to be overlooked. The skin lesions are similar to those seen in keratoderma blennorrhagica and consist of red or yellow keratotic macules or papules which eventually desquamate. A possible relationship between Reiter's syndrome and psoriasis has been discussed by Perry and Mayne.

Oral Manifestations. Oral lesions occur in reported series of cases in from less than 5 per cent to about 50 per cent of patients with the disease. The lesions, described by Pindborg and his associates, appear as painless, red, slightly elevated areas, sometimes granular or even vesicular, with a white circinate border on the buccal mucosa, lips and gingiva. They may be mistaken for recurrent aphthous ulcers. The palatal lesions appear as small, bright red purpuric spots which darken and coalesce, while the lesions on the tongue closely resemble "geographic" tongue. Clinically, similar lesions occur on the glans penis, producing a circinate balanitis.

Histologic Features. The microscopic findings are not diagnostic. They consist of parakeratosis, acanthosis and polymorphonuclear leukocyte infiltration of epithelium, sometimes with microabscess formation. The connective tissue shows a lymphocyte and plasma cell infiltrate.

Laboratory Findings. The patients usually have a mild leukocytosis, an elevated sedimentation rate and pyuria.

Treatment and Prognosis. The disease may undergo spontaneous remission but has been treated by antibiotics and corticosteroids.

HERPANGINA

(Aphthous Pharyngitis; Vesicular Pharyngitis)

Herpangina is a specific viral infection which was described by Zahorsky in 1920 and later named by him. Studies by Huebner and coworkers proved that Coxsackie group A viruses are the cause of the disease, with types 1 through 6, 8, 10, 16 and 22, as well as other enteroviruses, being isolated at various times.

Clinical Features. Herpangina has been reported in many parts of the United States, frequently occurring in sporadic outbreaks. It is most commonly seen in young children; older children and adults are only occasionally affected. Herpangina is chiefly a summer disease, and many children may actually harbor the virus at this time without exhibiting clinical manifestations of the disease.

The clinical manifestations of herpangina are comparatively mild and of short duration. It begins with sore throat, low-grade fever, headache, sometimes vomiting, prostration and abdominal pain. The patients soon exhibit small ulcers, each showing a gray base and an inflamed periphery on the anterior faucial pillars and sometimes on the hard and soft palates, posterior pharyngeal wall, buccal mucosa and tongue (Fig. 6–20). These ulcers are preceded by the appearance of numerous small vesicles which are of short duration and are frequently overlooked by the examiner. The ulcers do not tend to be extremely painful, although dysphagia may occur. They generally heal within a few days to a week.

This disease appears to be transmitted from one person to another through contact, and multiple cases in a single household are common. The incubation period is probably 2 to 10 days. Children have been affected several times in one season by infection with different strains of the Coxsackie virus. A permanent immunity to the infecting strain usually develops rapidly,

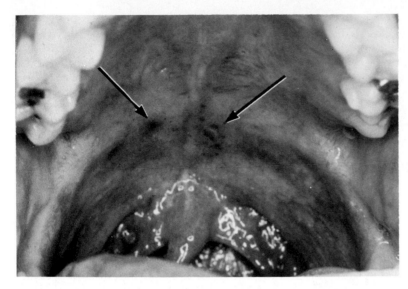

Figure 6–20. *Herpangina.* Small ulcers are shown on the soft palate and fauces.

and most adults have neutralizing antibodies against numerous strains.

Laboratory Findings. The Coxsackie virus can be isolated in suckling mice or hamsters by inoculation of scrapings from the throat lesions or stool specimens of nearly all patients who manifest clinical signs and symptoms of the disease or who have had contact with infected patients. Although there are distinct immunologic differences between various strains of herpangina virus, animal inoculation of any type produces the same manifestations—destruction of skeletal muscles followed by death. Even after disappearance of the clinical manifestations of the disease in the human patient, the virus may still be isolated from him for one to two months.

Treatment. No treatment is necessary, since the disease appears to be self-limiting and presents few complications. Those reported have consisted of acute parotitis, meningitis, hemolytic anemia and hemorrhagic diathesis.

ACUTE LYMPHONODULAR PHARYNGITIS

Acute lymphonodular pharyngitis is an acute febrile disease, first reported by Steigman and his co-workers in 1962, and caused by a strain of Coxsackie virus A10. The first recognized outbreak of the disease occurred in the vicinity of Louisville and Fort Knox, Kentucky, during the fall of 1960. Since then it has been recognized as occurring with a wide distribution. Delay in recognition of the disease as an entity

may have occurred because of the marked resemblance between this and herpangina.

Clinical Features. The disease affects predominantly children and young adults, although older adults are on occasion also involved. The chief complaints consist of sore throat, an elevation of temperature varying from 100° to 105° F., mild headache and anorexia. Typically, the patients do not manifest rhinorrhea, cough, tracheitis, gingivostomatitis, skin eruptions, arthralgia, otitis media, or lymphadenopathy.

The symptomatic course varies from 4 to 14 days and the local oral lesions resolve within 6 to 10 days, although a residual ring of fading erythema may sometimes be seen for several days, The estimated incubation period of the disease is 2 to 10 days.

Oral Manifestations. The lesions characteristic of the disease consist of raised, discrete, whitish to yellowish solid papules surrounded by a narrow zone of erythema (Fig. 6–21). The lesions are not vesicular and do not ulcerate. The lesions characteristically appear on the uvula, soft palate, anterior pillars and posterior oropharynx.

Laboratory Findings. Primary isolation of Coxsackie A10 virus can be established in suckling mice by inoculation of throat swab or fecal material. Serologic evidence of infection by this virus is also positive.

Histologic Features. The papular lesions consist of densely packed nodules of lymphocytes. In some cases the overlying epithelium has shown inclusion bodies which in some instances were intranuclear but in others, cytoplasmic.

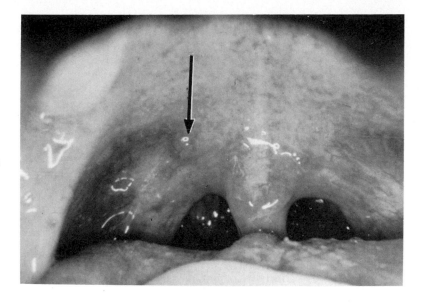

Figure 6–21. *Acute lymphonodular pharyngitis.*
Small papules are present on the soft palate and fauces.

Treatment. No specific treatment is necessary inasmuch as the disease is self-limiting. It has been found that antibiotic therapy is of no benefit.

HAND, FOOT AND MOUTH DISEASE

Hand, foot and mouth disease is an epidemic infection, first reported by Robinson and his co-workers in 1958, and caused by the enterovirus Coxsackie A16. It has been reported to be caused less frequently by types A5 and A6, and occasionally even by B2, B5 or enterovirus 71. This first recognized outbreak of the disease occurred in Toronto, Canada, but since then has appeared in many parts of the United States, with a large outbreak in Atlanta, Georgia, in 1964 and Baltimore, Maryland, in 1968, as well as in many other cities and other countries around the world. Despite the similarity in names, it bears no relationship to foot-and-mouth (hoof-and-mouth) disease, another viral disease with an animal vector.

Clinical Features. The disease is primarily one affecting young children, the majority of cases occurring between the ages of 6 months and 5 years. It is characterized by the appearance of maculopapular, exanthematous and vesicular lesions of the skin, particularly involving the hands, feet, legs, arms and occasionally the buttocks. The patients also commonly manifest anorexia, low-grade fever, coryza and sometimes lymphadenopathy, diarrhea, nausea and vomiting.

Oral Manifestations. A sore mouth with refusal to eat is one of the most common findings in the disease. This is due to the small, multiple vesicular and ulcerative oral lesions. In the series of cases reported by Adler and his associates, sore mouth was the principal symptom in 90 per cent of the patients, and oral lesions were present in 100 per cent of the patients. The most common sites for the oral lesions were the hard palate, tongue and buccal mucosa, with a much smaller percentage of patients showing involvement of the lips, gingiva and pharynx, including the tonsils. The tongue may also become red and edematous.

Laboratory Findings. Intracytoplasmic viral inclusions can sometimes be demonstrated in vesicular scrapings of the lesions. It has been found that these inclusions are indistinguishable from those found in vaccinia. In addition, viral isolates may usually be obtained from rectal or throat swabs from vesicular fluid itself. Finally, there is generally a remarkable rise in acute or convalescent serum antibody titer to Coxsackie A16. In a few patients there has been found to be a concomitant rise in herpes simplex virus antibody titer, but this is probably a fortuitous occurrence. Nevertheless, the clinical findings of hand, foot and mouth disease and of herpes simplex infection may be remarkably similar so that the two may be separated only with appropriate laboratory viral tests.

Treatment. No specific treatment is necessary since the disease is self-limiting and generally regresses within one to two weeks.

Differential Diagnosis. There is an obvious

similarity in the clinical appearance of the oral lesions of hand, foot and mouth disease and a variety of other conditions which may be encountered. In an excellent review of this disease, McKinney has listed several such conditions to be considered in the differential diagnosis, including herpetic gingivostomatitis, herpangina, erythema multiforme, recurrent aphthous ulcers and animal foot-and-mouth disease.

FOOT-AND-MOUTH DISEASE

(Aphthous Fever; Hoof-and-Mouth Disease; Epizootic Stomatitis)

Foot-and-mouth disease is a viral infection which only rarely affects man, but does affect hogs and sheep as well as cattle. Transmission of the disease occurs through contact with infected animals; in human beings this is usually through the use of milk from affected animals or through the handling of tissues from these animals. At present it is nearly nonexistent in the United States because of stringent cattle importation laws and effective domestic health laws. In fact, the virus itself cannot be imported legally into the United States even for experimental purposes. An excellent review of foot-and-mouth disease in human beings was published by Roset. This disease should not be confused in nomenclature with hand, foot and mouth disease, a Coxsackie virus infection previously discussed.

Clinical Features. When it is transmitted to the human, foot-and-mouth disease manifests itself clinically by fever, nausea, vomiting, malaise and the appearance of ulcerative lesions of the oral mucosa and pharynx. Development of vesicles on the skin also occurs in some cases. These vesicular lesions appear most commonly on the palms of the hands and soles of the feet.

Oral Manifestations. The lesions of the oral mucosa may occur at any site, although the lips, tongue, palate and oropharynx appear to be those chiefly affected. These lesions begin as small vesicles which rapidly rupture, but heal usually within two weeks.

MEASLES

(Rubeola; Morbilli)

Measles is an acute, contagious, dermatropic viral infection, primarily affecting children, and

occurring many times in epidemic form. Outbreaks are often cyclic in their appearance and are seen commonly at two- or three-year intervals. Spread of the disease occurs by direct contact with an affected person or by droplet infection, the portal of entry being the respiratory tract. However, widespread measles vaccination has greatly decreased the incidence of this disease in the United States and has, as a consequence, markedly altered many of its epidemiologic aspects within the last 20 years.

Clinical Features. The disease, which has an incubation period of 8 to 10 days, is characterized by the onset of fever, malaise, cough, conjunctivitis, photophobia, lacrimation and eruptive lesions of the skin and oral mucosa. The skin eruptions usually begin on the face, in the hair line and behind the ears, and spread to the neck, chest, back and extremities. These appear as tiny red macules or papules which enlarge and coalesce to form blotchy, discolored, irregular lesions which blanch upon pressure and gradually fade away in four to five days with a fine desquamation.

Oral Manifestations. The oral lesions are prodromal, frequently occurring two to three days before the cutaneous rash, and are pathognomonic of this disease. These intraoral lesions are called Koplik's spots and have been reported to occur in as high as 97 per cent of all patients with measles. In actual practice, they are seldom seen unless the affected child has had a known contact with measles and the dentist or parent watches carefully, since the child is often well at the time they appear. These characteristic spots, usually occurring on the buccal mucosa, are small, irregularly shaped flecks which appear as bluish, white specks surrounded by a bright red margin. These macular lesions increase in number rapidly and coalesce to form small patches. Palatal and pharyngeal petechiae as well as generalized inflammation, congestion, swelling and focal ulceration of the gingiva, palate and throat may also occur.

Complications. Measles is a disease which lowers the general body resistance and, for this reason, often leads to complications. These may include bronchial pneumonia, encephalitis, otitis media and, occasionally, noma. In addition, it has been recognized that measles has an immunosuppressive effect through impairment of cell-mediated immunity. Thus, while it may result in a delay in wound healing, it may also cause induction of remission of leukemia and Hodgkin's disease. The disease is rarely fatal except in the case of secondary complications.

RUBELLA

(German Measles)

Rubeola should not be confused with rubella or the so-called German measles. In rubella, Koplik's spots do not occur, and the oral mucous membranes are not usually inflamed, although the tonsils may be somewhat swollen and congested and red macules may appear on the palate. Complications following this disease are rare except when the disease occurs in women during the first trimester of pregnancy. In such cases there is in the offspring a high incidence of congenital defects such as blindness, deafness and cardiovascular abnormalities, if miscarriage does not occur.

Occasional reports in the literature have suggested that rubella affecting women during the first months of pregnancy can cause a number of developmental defects, including enamel hypoplasia, a high caries incidence and delayed eruption of deciduous teeth. However, a study by Grahnen provided some evidence that maternal rubella did not give rise to any clinically detectable defects in either the deciduous or permanent dentition of the offspring.

SMALLPOX

(Variola)

Smallpox is an acute viral disease which, before the discovery of vaccination by Jenner, was epidemic in nature and accounted for literally millions of deaths. For example, in Europe alone at the end of the eighteenth century, it is estimated that at least 400,000 people died of the disease each year.

The World Health Assembly in 1958 requested the Director General of the World Health Organization (WHO) to study the implications of a global smallpox eradication program and, in 1967, such a program was initiated. During 1967, 131,000 cases of smallpox were reported, although 10 to 15 million cases are estimated to have occurred in 33 countries with the endemic disease and 14 other countries reporting importations.

On December 9, 1979, the WHO Global Commission for the Certification of Smallpox Eradication declared:

1. Smallpox eradication has been achieved throughout the world.

2. There is no evidence that smallpox will return as an endemic disease.

This was officially endorsed by the World Health Assembly Meeting in Geneva on May 8, 1980, when, in Resolution 33.3, it "declares solemnly that the world and all its people have won freedom from smallpox . . . an unprecedented achievement in the history of public health . . .".

The last known patient in the world with "wild" or natural smallpox was a hospital cook in Somalia who developed the rash on October 26, 1977. Two other cases did occur in Birmingham, England, in 1978 as a result of a laboratory accident, but there have been no further cases, even though six laboratories throughout the world are known to be maintaining this virus.

Thus, there has been official international acceptance of the fact that, for the first time in history, a disease has been totally eliminated from this planet, an effort to which all future generations should pay tribute. The long eradication campaign is a fascinating documentation of public health officials carrying out a complex program with great technical, financial and administrative problems. Some of this information has been published by Breman and Arita and provides a fascinating insight into many aspects of this disease.

A discussion of the clinical and oral manifestations of smallpox is still maintained here inasmuch as all members of the United States overseas military forces still receive smallpox vaccinations, one complication of which is the development of the disease itself. Such vaccinations are still used because of the possibility of germ warfare, since controlled stocks of live virus are still maintained in certain countries.

Clinical Features. Smallpox, after an incubation period of seven to ten days, manifests itself clinically by the occurrence of a high fever, nausea, vomiting, chills and headache. The patient is extremely ill and may become comatose during this period.

The skin lesions begin as small macules and papules which first appear on the face, but rapidly spread to cover much of the body surface. Within a few days the papules develop into vesicles which themselves eventually become pustular. The pustules are small, elevated, and yellowish green with an inflamed border. They are secondarily infected and occasionally become hemorrhagic, a most serious portent. Desquamation marks the beginning of the healing phase of the disease. Severe pitting or pocking of the skin as a result of pustule formation is a common complication of smallpox.

Oral Manifestations. Ulceration of the oral

mucosa and pharynx is rather common, and similar involvement of other mucous membranes such as the trachea, esophagus and vagina also occurs. Multiple vesicles appear much like the cutaneous lesion but, instead of proceeding to the development of pustules, they rupture and form ulcers of a nonspecific nature. In some cases the tongue is swollen and painful, making swallowing difficult.

Complications. Complications are common in smallpox and are related to the secondary infection which often occurs. Thus the formation of abscesses and the development of septicemia sometimes occur, as well as respiratory infection, erysipelas and infections of the eye and ear.

MOLLUSCUM CONTAGIOSUM

Molluscum contagiosum is a disease caused by a virus of the pox group. The lesions, which only occur on skin or mucosal surfaces, are often considered tumorlike in nature because of the typical localized epithelial proliferation caused by the virus. The incidence of the condition is not reliably known.

Clinical Features. The infection is more common in children and young adults and manifests itself as single or, more frequently, multiple discrete elevated nodules, usually occurring on the arms and legs, trunk and face, particularly the eyelids. However, it is now recognized that the disease can be sexually transmitted, and lesions of the genitalia and pubo-abdominal area also occur with some frequency.

These lesions are hemispheric in shape, usually about 5 mm. in diameter with a central umbilication which may be keratinized, and are normal or slightly red in color. The disease appears to be spread by autoinoculation, by direct contact with an infected individual or by fomites with a reported incubation period of 14 to 50 days.

Oral Manifestations. Mucous membrane involvement, particularly the oral cavity, is not common. Cases have been reported, however, such as that of Barsh. The oral lesions, which occur most frequently on the lips, tongue and buccal mucosa, are similar to those on the skin.

Histologic Features. The lesion is quite characteristic, showing thickening and downgrowth of the epithelium with the formation of large eosinophilic intracytoplasmic inclusion bodies known as Henderson-Paterson inclusions or simply molluscum bodies, measuring approximately 25 microns in diameter. These bodies

characteristically accumulate in the crater formed by the distinctive central umbilication of the dome-shaped lesion.

Treatment. The lesions of molluscum contagiosum have been treated by surgical excision or by topical application of a wide variety of drugs such as podophyllin or cantharidin. In most cases, the lesions are self-limiting in 6 to 9 months but may persist for 3 to 4 years. There is some evidence that immunosuppressive drugs may evoke eruption of lesions.

CONDYLOMA ACUMINATUM
(Verruca Acuminata; Venereal Wart)

Condyloma acuminatum is an infectious disease caused by a virus which belongs to the same group of human papillomaviruses (HPV) as those associated with common and plantar warts, flat warts, cervical flat warts, pityriasislike lesions in patients with epidermodysplasia verruciformis and juvenile laryngeal papillomas. Howley, in an excellent discussion of the subject, has recently pointed out that there are 11 different human papillomaviruses now recognized and that very likely others will be described in the near future. The virus of anal, genital and presumably oral condyloma acuminata is known as HPV-6.

Clinical Features. This transmissible and autoinoculable viral disease presents as soft pink nodules which proliferate and coalesce rapidly to form diffuse papillomatous clusters of varying size. They occur most frequently on the anogenital skin or other warm, moist intertriginous areas.

Oral Manifestations. Oral lesions of condyloma acuminatum have been reported by Knapp and Uohara, as well as by Doyle and his associates and by Swan and his colleagues. These lesions have appeared as small, multiple, white or pink nodules which enlarge, proliferate and coalesce, or as papillomatous, bulbous masses scattered over or diffusely involving the tongue, especially the dorsum, buccal mucosa, palate, gingiva or alveolar ridge.

Histologic Features. The papillomatous projections making up the verrucoid lesion generally show a parakeratotic surface with marked underlying acanthosis. Vacuolated cells in the spinous layer are common, as are numerous mitotic figures. In some instances, the epithelial changes are sufficiently disturbing to be mistaken for carcinoma. The supporting connective tissue is usually edematous, with dilated capillaries and a chronic inflammatory cell infiltrate.

A case of oral condyloma acuminatum has been studied with both the light microscope and electron microscope by Shaffer and his associates, who found intranuclear viral inclusions in the lesional epithelial cells.

Treatment. Surgical excision is usually used to eradicate the lesions, although topical podophyllin has also been used.

CHICKENPOX

(Varicella)

Chickenpox is an acute viral disease, usually occurring in children and most common in the winter and spring months. The incubation period is approximately two weeks.

It has been stated by Sabin that the virus causing this disease is one of the most contagious and sooner or later infects everyone in the world. It rather closely resembles smallpox, but is far less severe. The virus is the same as that which causes herpes zoster, and the lesions of the two diseases have many features in common. The relationship between these two diseases is discussed under herpes zoster. The mode of transmission is by airborne droplets or direct contact with infected lesions, with the probable portal of entry being the respiratory tract.

Clinical Features. The disease is characterized by the prodromal occurrence of headache, nasopharyngitis and anorexia, followed by maculopapular or vesicular eruptions of the skin and low-grade fever. These eruptions usually begin on the trunk and spread to involve the face and extremities. They occur in successive crops so that many vesicles in different stages of formation or resorption may be found. The lesions of the skin eventually rupture, form a superficial crust and heal by desquamation. The disease runs its clinical course in a week to ten days, seldom leaving any after-effects. Occasionally, secondary infection of the vesicles results in the formation of pustules which may leave small pitting scars upon healing.

Oral Manifestations. Small blister-like lesions occasionally involve the oral mucosa, chiefly the buccal mucosa, tongue, gingiva and palate, as well as the mucosa of the pharynx (Fig. 6–22). The mucosal lesions, initially slightly raised vesicles with a surrounding erythema, rupture soon after formation and form small eroded ulcers with a red margin, closely resembling aphthous lesions. These lesions are not particularly painful. Typical cases have been reported by Badger.

Complications. Complications are not common, and the mortality rate is extremely low. Encephalitis or pneumonia occasionally occurs. However, children with chronic diseases, those receiving cortisone therapy or those with malignancies and receiving chemotherapy are prone to develop a severe or even fatal form of the disease.

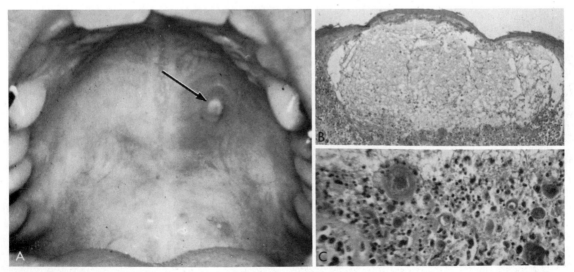

Figure 6–22. Chickenpox.
A single intraoral vesicle formed in association with the typical skin lesions (A). A vesicular lesion (B) showing typical viral inclusion bodies (C). (A, Courtesy of Dr. Stephen F. Dachi.)

HERPES ZOSTER

(Shingles; Zona)

Herpes zoster is an acute infectious viral disease of an extremely painful and incapacitating nature which is characterized by inflammation of dorsal root ganglia, or extramedullary cranial nerve ganglia, associated with vesicular eruptions of the skin or mucous membranes in areas supplied by the affected sensory nerves. The virus causing this disease is the same as that of varicella, or chickenpox (the V-Z virus), and occasionally the two diseases are clinically nearly indistinguishable. Similar eosinophilic intranuclear inclusion bodies, indicative of viral infection, occur in both diseases. It is now believed that herpes zoster is caused by reactivation of the latent V-Z virus which had been acquired during a previous attack of chickenpox. In essence, a primary infection by the V-Z virus results clinically in chickenpox, while a recurrent infection results clinically in herpes zoster. The fact that herpes zoster is sporadic in occurrence whereas varicella is seasonal further supports the belief that herpes zoster is not a result of a primary exogenous infection.

Clinical Features. The disease is most common in adult life and affects males and females with equal frequency. Although rare, it does occur in children. In 576 cases of herpes zoster in patients of all ages, 31 or 5.4 per cent were in children under 15 years of age according to Rogers and Tindall, but in this age group the disease has a very benign clinical course.

Initially, the adult patient exhibits fever, a general malaise, and pain and tenderness along the course of the involved sensory nerves, usually unilaterally. Often the trunk is affected. Within a few days the patient has a linear papular or vesicular eruption of the skin or mucosa supplied by the affected nerves. It is typically unilateral and dermatomic in distribution. After rupture of the vesicles, healing commences, although secondary infection may intervene and slow the process considerably. Occasionally, herpes zoster may resemble the lesions of herpes simplex, but the two diseases can be separated since the zoster virus cannot be transmitted to animals, e.g., the rabbit cornea, as can the simplex virus.

The triggering factors initiating the onset of an attack of herpes zoster are varied and may include trauma, development of malignancy or tumor involvement of dorsal root ganglia, local x-ray radiation or immunosuppressive therapy. It is a common infection in immunocompromised patients and those with certain malignan-

cies, including Hodgkin's disease and the malignant lymphomas, and can be life-threatening if the viscera become involved. However, many attacks begin for no apparent reason, and these have often been attributed to a decrease in host resistance due to age.

Oral Manifestations. Herpes zoster may involve the face by infection of the trigeminal nerve (Fig. 6–23). This usually consists of unilateral involvement of skin areas supplied by either the ophthalmic, maxillary or mandibular nerves. Lesions of the oral mucosa are fairly common, and extremely painful vesicles may be found on the buccal mucosa, tongue, uvula, pharynx and larynx (Fig. 6–24). These generally rupture to leave areas of erosion. One of the characteristic clinical features of the disease involving the face or oral cavity is the unilaterality of the lesions. Typically, when large, the lesions will extend up to the midline and stop abruptly.

A special form of zoster infection of the geniculate ganglion, with involvement of the external ear and oral mucosa, has been termed Hunt's syndrome (James Ramsay Hunt's syndrome). The clinical manifestations include facial paralysis as well as pain of the external auditory meatus and pinna of the ear. In addition, vesicular eruptions occur in the oral cavity and oropharynx with hoarseness, tinnitus, vertigo and occasional other disturbances.

Diagnosis. Herpes zoster can frequently be recognized by the characteristic distribution of the lesions, although there may be a similarity to the lesions of herpes simplex infection. Skin lesions and oral lesions in particular may be easily identified as viral diseases by cytologic smears and the finding of characteristic multinucleated giant cells (Tzanck test) and intranuclear inclusions. However, this does not differentiate between herpes zoster and herpes simplex. This can only be done by fluorescent antibody staining techniques, viral culture or serologic diagnosis.

Treatment. The newer anti-viral drugs are now under intensive clinical testing for potential effectiveness in treatment of herpes zoster. The preliminary results appear very promising.

CAT-SCRATCH DISEASE

(Cat-Scratch Fever; Benign Lymphoreticulosis; Benign Nonbacterial Regional Lymphadenitis)

Cat-scratch disease is a newly recognized disease, the first actual report being that of Debré and his co-workers in 1950. It is believed

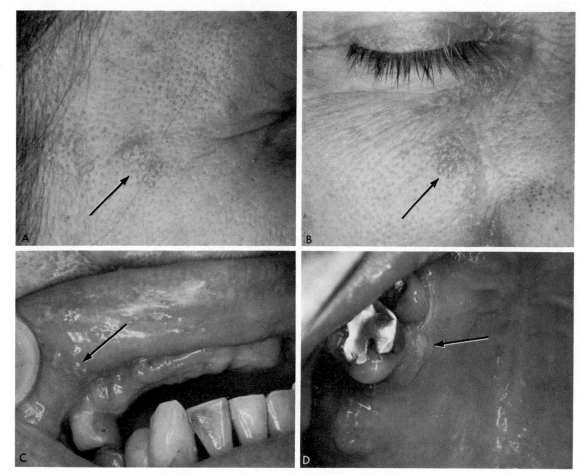

Figure 6–23. *Herpes zoster involving face and oral mucosa.*

to be viral in origin, although the actual agent has not been isolated. It is estimated that about 2000 cases occur annually in the United States. It has been possible to transmit this disease experimentally to monkeys as well as to human volunteers, although the disease is not contagious and the patients do not require isolation.

Clinical Features. This disease, occurring at any age, but predominantly in children and young adults, is thought to arise after a traumatic break in the skin due to the scratch or bite of the household cat. On rare occasions, dogs and monkeys have served as the vector. Actually, there is a definite history of scratches in only 55 to 60 per cent of patients, according to Rickles and Bernier, although 90 per cent of patients with the disease had recent contact with cats. Within a few days an indolent primary lesion, often a papule or vesicle, develops at the site of the injury. Within one to three

weeks later, a regional lymphadenitis without lymphangitis develops. The lymphadenopathy appears to be out of all proportion to the relatively innocuous skin wound. The cat apparently serves only as a carrier of the disease, since the animal is not ill and does not respond to the intradermal antigen test.

The lymphadenopathy is usually the cause for the patient's seeking professional advice. In a series of 115 patients with clinical cat-scratch disease reported by Margileth, 57 per cent had lymphadenopathy involving the extremities, and 43 per cent, the head and neck. The nodes are painful and may be several centimeters in diameter. The overlying skin may be inflamed. This lymphadenopathy may persist for one to six months and may be accompanied in the early stages of the disease by a low-grade fever, headache, chills, nausea, malaise or even abdominal pain. Other manifestations occasionally

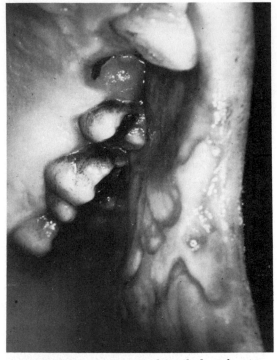

Figure 6–24. *Herpes zoster involving the buccal mucosa.*

seen include a nonpruritic macular or maculopapular rash, parotid swelling, conjunctivitis and grand mal seizures. Another unusual manifestation of the disease, reported by Carithers, is the oculoglandular syndrome of Parinaud. This consists of a localized granuloma of the eye and preauricular lymphadenopathy.

The lymph nodes gradually become soft and fluctuant, owing to necrosis and suppuration. The pus has been reported in numerous studies to be bacteriologically sterile. Occasionally an abscessed node will perforate the skin and drain.

If the preauricular, submaxillary or cervical chain of nodes is involved, the dentist may be consulted to rule out dental disease as an etiologic factor. Cat-scratch disease may also resemble more serious infectious granulomatous diseases such as tuberculosis or tularemia, lymphogranuloma venereum, infectious mononucleosis, Hodgkin's disease or lymphosarcoma.

The diagnosis is usually established by a positive intradermal skin test of antigen from a patient with proved cat-scratch disease. This test is not invariably positive, however.

Histologic Features. Early in the course of the disease the involved lymph nodes manifest reticuloendothelial hyperplasia; later, focal granulomas, suppuration and necrosis develop

with capsular thickening. Epithelioid cells and multinucleated giant cells are occasionally seen. The microscopic appearance is not particularly pathognomonic, but is certainly suggestive.

Prognosis. The prognosis is good, since the disease is self-limiting and regresses within a period of weeks or months. Incision and drainage of the involved node may be necessary. Antibiotic therapy is ineffective.

MUMPS

(Epidemic Parotitis)

Mumps is an acute contagious viral infection characterized chiefly by unilateral or bilateral swelling of the salivary glands, usually the parotid. The submaxillary and sublingual glands are occasionally involved, but seldom without parotid involvement also. Occasionally certain internal organs rather than the salivary glands are involved. Although it is usually a disease of childhood, mumps may also affect adults, and in such cases there is a greater tendency for complications to develop. Mumps has an incubation period of two to three weeks.

Clinical Features. The disease is usually preceded by the onset of headache, chills, moderate fever, vomiting, and pain below the ear. These symptoms are followed by a firm, somewhat rubbery or elastic swelling of the salivary glands, frequently elevating the ear, which usually lasts about one week. This salivary gland involvement produces pain upon mastication. Bilateral parotid involvement occurs in about 70 per cent of the cases.

It is of interest to note that the virus of epidemic parotitis is present in the saliva of affected persons. For this reason, droplet dissemination and infection are common. It is also reported that the papilla of the opening of the parotid duct on the buccal mucosa is often puffy and reddened.

Complications. Other organs of the body may be affected as a complication of the disease. These include the testes, ovaries, pancreas, mammary glands and occasionally the prostate, epididymis and heart. When mumps involves the adult male, orchitis is a great danger and ensues in approximately 20 per cent of the cases. This orchitis is usually unilateral, but occasionally complete sterility results. Involvement of the pancreas producing an acute pancreatitis often causes an elevation in serum lipase. Serum amylase is also elevated but this is regardless of pancreatic involvement. Meningoencephalitis, deafness and mastitis are also occasional complications.

The disease, though discomforting and often producing an acutely distressing condition, is seldom fatal.

The availability of live attenuated mumps virus vaccine, first licensed in 1968, has resulted in a marked decline in the incidence of the disease, with a corresponding decrease in cases of meningitis and encephalitis. Unfortunately, the vaccine is not protective to individuals already exposed to the virus and who are in the incubation stage of the disease.

NONSPECIFIC "MUMPS"

There are several "nonspecific" conditions characterized by enlargement of one or more of the major salivary glands that are not related etiologically to epidemic parotitis, or true mumps, but yet may produce considerable difficulty in diagnosis and differential separation from true mumps of viral origin. Banks has summarized a variety of these in his classification (Table 6–4) and discussion of parotid swellings. Although not all of these are of specific microbial origin, some of the more common conditions will be discussed here because of their clinical and occasional microscopic resemblance to epidemic parotitis, or mumps. These include (1) chronic nonspecific sialadenitis, (2) acute postoperative parotitis ("surgical mumps," retrograde sialadenitis), (3) nutritional "mumps," (4) chemical "mumps," and (5) miscellaneous.

CHRONIC NONSPECIFIC SIALADENITIS. Nonspecific chronic sialadenitis is an insidious inflammatory disease of the major salivary glands characterized by intermittent swelling of the glands which may lead to the development of clinically obvious fibrous masses. This condition has been reviewed by King and Koerner, and it was noted to be most common in adults, particularly males. A similar, and perhaps related, condition has been reported by Katzen and du Plessis under the term "recurrent parotitis" in children. They observed that the disease usually subsided spontaneously at puberty although David and O'Connell reported that it may extend into adult life. Brook has published an excellent review of this recurrent suppurative parotitis in children.

The most frequent cause of chronic sialadenitis is the occurrence of salivary duct calculi (q.v.) with subsequent pyogenic bacterial infec-

Table 6–4. Classification of Parotid Swellings

I. Neoplastic

II. Inflammatory
   A. Acute specific-virus infections
     1. Mumps
     2. Coxsackie A
     3. ECHO
     4. Lymphocytic choriomeningitis
   B. Chronic specific
     1. Tuberculosis
     2. Actinomycosis
     3. Sarcoidosis
   C. Acute suppurative parotitis
   D. "Recurrent subacute parotitis" and associated pathology

III. Hypersensitivity and drug reactions

IV. Metabolic
   A. Malnutrition, particularly protein deficiency
   B. Associated with alcoholic cirrhosis
   C. Diabetes mellitus and disturbed glucose tolerance

V. Miscellaneous
   A. Obstruction of duct
     1. Direct
       a. Papillary trauma
       b. Other traumatic stricture
       c. Impaction of foreign body (e.g., food particle)
       d. Congenital atresia
     2. Indirect
   B. Pneumoparotitis
   C. Functional hypersecretion

From P. Banks: Nonneoplastic parotid swellings: a review. Oral Surg., 25:732, 1968.

tion. But any condition which may result in salivary duct occlusion, such as tumors, foreign bodies or scar formation, may result in this form of the disease.

If the etiologic factor is removed, there is generally subsidence of the clinical manifestations of the disease. If untreated, the salivary gland may be replaced by fibrous tissue, which may be tumor-like in its extent.

ACUTE POSTOPERATIVE PAROTITIS. This condition has a long and interesting history that has been reviewed by Schwartz and his coworkers. Although originally ascribed to a variety of possible factors, it is now generally believed to be the result of a retrograde infection (one reaching the parotid gland by microorganisms ascending the parotid duct) in debilitated patients suffering from dehydration, suppression of salivary secretion, vomiting and/or mouth-breathing, after a surgical procedure. Thus it is felt that xerostomia, or dry mouth, is one of the most important factors, since the stagnation of salivary flow would allow the ascension of microorganisms through the duct into the gland.

The microorganisms involved are usually *Staphylococcus aureus, Staphylococcus pyogenes, Streptococcus viridans* and pneumococci.

The majority of patients involved are adults, of middle age or older. Bilateral parotid gland involvement is common, and the clinical signs and symptoms generally occur between the second and twentieth postoperative days. Any type of surgical procedure may be followed by the appearance of this condition, not just a local procedure in the area of the salivary glands, although the exact mechanism is not known.

The onset of the disease is rapid and is frequently accompanied by severe pain and rapid swelling of the parotid gland. The overlying skin may be reddened, and the associated edema may involve the cheek, periorbital area and neck. Trismus is present, as is a low-grade fever with headache, malaise and leukocytosis. A purulent discharge may be expressed from the parotid duct by digital pressure along the duct toward its orifice. Treatment of this condition is generally the administration of antibiotics.

NUTRITIONAL "MUMPS." Numerous investigators have reported a chronic, asymptomatic, bilateral enlargement of the parotid and/or submaxillary glands occurring endemically in populations suffering from malnutrition. Sandstead and his co-workers, as well as Duggan and Rothbell, have reviewed the literature pertaining to this condition and noted its worldwide distribution. The dietary factors specifically involved have not been identified, but the lesions occur most frequently in patients with multiple signs of nutritional deficiency such as hypoproteinemia, anemia, angular cheilosis, pellagroid pigmentation of the hands and face, and general underweight. A relation to either vitamin A or C deficiency has not been demonstrated.

The condition is a progressive one, but relatively slow to develop. It appears to be somewhat more common in young and middle-aged adults.

Histologic studies indicate that the salivary gland involvement is essentially noninflammatory. The enlargement of the salivary glands in the acute phase of the condition is due to hypertrophy of the individual acinar cells, but in the chronic phase, to a replacement of normal gland parenchyma with fat. There is apparently little interference with normal salivary gland function.

A clinically identical form of parotid swelling has been reported by Borsanyi and Blanchard in a series of patients suffering from Laennac's hepatic cirrhosis with a history of chronic alcoholism. This form of salivary gland disease is undoubtedly only one manifestation of the "nutritional mumps" discussed by Sandstead and his group.

CHEMICAL "MUMPS." Bilateral swelling of the salivary glands occasionally accompanies the administration of either inorganic or organic iodine, and this has frequently been referred to as "iodine mumps." This condition has been reviewed by Carter, who pointed out that this probably represents an iodine idiosyncrasy reaction. A similar form of salivary gland swelling has been reported by Albright and his co-workers to follow administration of triiodothyronine in the treatment of myxedema. These findings are of special interest in view of the long series of studies of Shafer and Muhler that have conclusively shown a close relation between the thyroid and salivary glands.

Another example of chemically induced experimental salivary gland swelling has been that following administration of isoproterenol to rats, reported by Selye and his group. In their studies the salivary glands increased approximately five times their normal size within 17 days after initiation of drug administration. In this case the glandular enlargement is due to a true hypertrophy of acinar cells.

MISCELLANEOUS FACTORS. There are numerous other situations in which salivary gland swelling may occur, and many of these have been discussed by Pearson and are described in more detail in other sections of this text. For example, salivary gland swelling is common in Sjögren's syndrome, Mikulicz's disease or benign lymphoepithelial lesion, salivary duct calculus, and allergic phenomena. In addition, swelling of the salivary glands was reported by Dobreff in 1936 to follow hypofunction of pancreatic islets and by Racine in 1939 to occur as a premenstrual phenomenon.

Fibrocystic disease (mucoviscidosis) of the pancreas is a hereditary defect of the secretory mechanism of most of the exocrine glands in the body, including the salivary glands. Bilateral enlargement of the submaxillary glands has been reported by Barbero and Sibinga in 92 per cent of a group of 106 children with fibrocystic disease as contrasted to similar enlargement in only 2 per cent of a group of 300 normal children. At necropsy these submaxillary glands from patients with fibrocystic disease were two to three times heavier than normal. These investigations suggested that cystic fibrosis is an important cause of chronic submaxillary gland enlargement in the pediatric age group.

Sarcoidosis has been reported by Greenberg and his associates to have caused enlargement of the parotid gland in 6 per cent of a series of 388 patients with this disease. The enlargement was bilateral in 83 per cent of the cases, and unilateral in 17 per cent.

Nevertheless, as in nearly every nonspecific condition of such an etiologically diverse nature, there is always an idiopathic group in which even careful evaluation of clinical, microscopic and laboratory findings fails to reveal the cause of the disease, and such is the case in noninfectious "mumps"; a certain percentage of these cases cannot be explained.

CYTOMEGALIC INCLUSION DISEASE

(Salivary Gland Virus Disease)

Salivary gland inclusion disease is a viral infection of interest since routine postmortem examinations have revealed that a considerable proportion of infants who die exhibit this disease, regardless of the cause of their death. Although it is frequently an inapparent infection, it is a cause of fetal encephalitis and may produce irreversible damage to the central nervous system. Smith and Vellios reported that in the majority of cases the patients are under two years of age, although the disease has been reported in a few adults. Some cases, reviewed by Amromin, have occurred widely disseminated in adults. There are no particular signs or symptoms of this disease, although some infants have been reported to have manifested hepatosplenomegaly, hemolytic anemia and a hemorrhagic tendency. It may be an incidental autopsy finding in patients who have died of blood dyscrasias, liver damage, pertussis, purpura, and other diseases. Transplacental infection may occur even without visible evidence of infection in the mother. In fact, approximately 50 per cent of women in the childbearing age group are seropositive for complement-fixing antibodies to this virus, while approximately 4 per cent of pregnant women excrete the virus in the urine. Occasional infants without an established diagnosis of generalized cytomegalic inclusion disease survive, although there may be some retardation of mental and motor development. In a review of cytomegalovirus as a major cause of birth defects, Marx has stated that it is the most common viral cause of mental retardation, surpassing even rubella virus.

Intranuclear and cytoplasmic inclusions in the cells of the salivary glands are a constant feature, while similar inclusions frequently occur in the kidneys, liver, pancreas, lungs, adrenals, intestine, brain and occasionally other organs. The diagnosis is frequently established in living infants by examination of urinary sediment and the demonstration of the inclusion bodies here. These inclusions have a distinctive morphologic appearance and are pathognomonic of the disease (Fig. 6–25).

There is evidence to suggest that disturbances of cellular metabolism such as those occurring in certain vitamin deficiencies may predispose to the viral infection or may possibly activate an existing subclinical infection. The widespread distribution of the virus is apparent from the fact that over 80 per cent of adults possess serum antibody against the virus. It is also now recognized, as reported by Cangir and Sullivan, that dissemination of the latent disease may occur in leukemia patients receiving antimetabolite therapy and in organ-transplantation patients or others receiving immunosuppressant drugs and subject to opportunistic infection.

Other interesting manifestations of this virus include: (1) cytomegalovirus mononucleosis, which may be very difficult to distinguish from infectious mononucleosis, since the clinical characteristics of the two may be nearly identical; and (2) its association with Kaposi's sarcoma in the acquired cellular immunodeficiency syndrome (q.v.).

POLIOMYELITIS

(Infantile Paralysis)

Poliomyelitis at one time was a very serious viral disease which has been almost totally eliminated, particularly the paralyzing form, as a result of the widespread use of the Salk and Sabin vaccines. Prior to this, poliomyelitis was of some significance in dentistry because of scattered reports which suggested that the exposed dental pulp might act as a portal of entry into the body for the virus. This no longer appears to be of any clinical significance.

FUNGUS INFECTIONS

Mycology, the study of fungal infections, has gained remarkable impetus in the past few

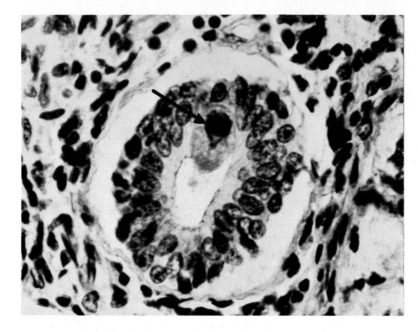

Figure 6–25. *Cytomegalic inclusion disease.*

The arrow points to the typical inclusion body in the parotid ductal epithelium. (Courtesy of Dr. Charles A. Waldron.)

decades, owing at least in part to the fact that fungal diseases are far more common than was previously suspected. Many erroneous conceptions of this branch of microbiology existed until only recently, but careful scientific investigation of various aspects of mycology, such as epidemiology, pathogenesis, immunology, diagnosis and treatment, has done much to eliminate the confusion. Furthermore, excellent monographs and reviews on certain of the fungal diseases, such as those on blastomycosis by Witorsch and Utz and by Sarosi and Davies, on coccidioidomycosis by Fiese and by Stevens, on cryptococcosis by Littman and Zimmerman, on histoplasmosis by Sweany and by Goodwin and his colleagues and on mucormycosis (phycomycosis) by Lehrer, have been valuable contributions to our understanding of these conditions.

NORTH AMERICAN BLASTOMYCOSIS
(Gilchrist's Disease)

North American blastomycosis is a mycotic infection caused by *Blastomyces dermatitidis* and may occur either in a cutaneous form or in a systemic form involving bones, liver, lungs, subcutaneous tissues and other organs. Experimental transmission to animals is only haphazardly successful and cannot be used as an aid in diagnosis, although spontaneous infection in dogs is quite common. The source of the infec-

tion in human beings is unknown, although affected persons commonly work or spend a great deal of time outdoors. It is becoming an important medical problem, particularly in central United States, as has been pointed out by Furcolow and his associates.

Clinical Features. North American blastomycosis is far more common in men than in women, and typically occurs in middle age. The skin lesions usually begin as small red papules which gradually increase in size and form tiny miliary abscesses or pustules which may ulcerate to discharge the pus through a tiny sinus. Crateriform lesions are typical, and these often exhibit indurated, elevated borders (Figs. 6–26, 6–27). The infection commonly spreads through the subcutaneous tissues and becomes disseminated through the blood stream. The systemic disease is characterized by fever, sudden weight loss and, in cases of lung involvement, a productive cough associated with other symptoms typical of pulmonary tuberculosis.

Oral Manifestations. Lesions of the oral cavity have been reported as occurring in blastomycosis and may resemble those of actinomycosis, although abscess formation is not usually as prominent. Tiny ulcers may be the chief feature. The oral infection may be either the primary lesion or secondary to lesions elsewhere in the body. In an extensive discussion of this disease, Witorsch and Utz have reported that 25 per cent of their group of patients had oral or nasal mucosal lesions. Bell and his co-

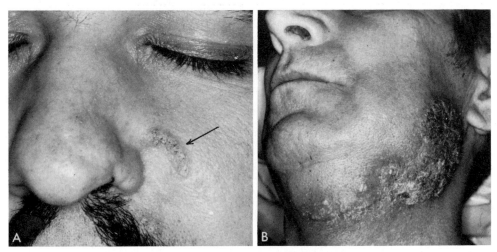

Figure 6–26. *North American blastomycosis.*
A, Early lesion; *B*, advanced lesion. (Courtesy of Dr. Stephen F. Dachi.)

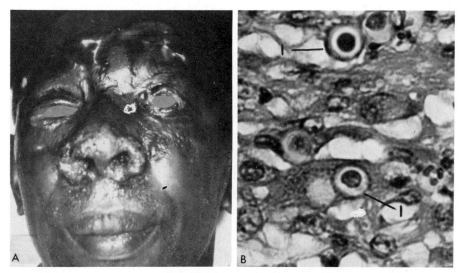

Figure 6–27. *North American blastomycosis.*
A, Advanced North American blastomycosis of the face. *B*, Photomicrograph of granulomatous lesion of blastomycosis, showing typical yeastlike organisms with doubly refractile capsule *(1)*. (*A*, Courtesy of Dr. Wilbur C. Moorman.)

workers have also pointed out that the oral lesions, which may be the first apparent manifestation of the disease, are probably more common than has been thought. In two cases reported by Page and his associates, the oral lesions bore enough resemblance to epidermoid carcinoma to warrant it as a consideration in the differential diagnosis.

Histologic Features. The microscopic features of North American blastomycosis are similar to those of other chronic granulomatous infections. The inflamed connective tissue shows occasional giant cells and macrophages and the typical round organisms, often budding, which appear to have a doubly refractile capsule (Fig. 6–27, B). The organisms, usually measuring between 5 and 15 microns in diameter, are common within giant cells. Microabscesses are frequently found. If the lesions are not ulcerated, overlying pseudoepitheliomatous hyperplasia may be prominent.

SOUTH AMERICAN BLASTOMYCOSIS

(Lutz's Disease; Paracoccidioidomycosis)

South American blastomycosis is related to the North American form of the disease and is caused by infection with *Blastomyces (Paracoccidioides) brasiliensis*. The systemic lesions are similar to those of North American blastomycosis.

Oral Manifestations. Bogliolo reported that the organisms may enter the body through the periodontal tissues and subsequently reach the regional lymph nodes, producing a severe lymphadenopathy. He has demonstrated the organisms in both the periodontal membrane and in a periapical granuloma and has cultivated them from these sites. The microorganisms also have been shown to penetrate the tissues and establish infection after extraction of teeth, producing papillary lesions of the oral mucosa. Widespread oral ulceration is also a common finding.

The chief difference between North American and South American blastomycosis is in the size of the causative organisms. The fungus in the South American form of the disease varies between approximately 10 and 60 microns in diameter, being considerably larger than that of the North American disease.

HISTOPLASMOSIS

(Darling's Disease)

Histoplasmosis is a generalized fungus infection caused by the organism *Histoplasma cap-*

sulatum. It is widespread in its distribution and endemic in the Mississippi Valley and northeastern United States, where up to 75 per cent of the population have had a primary but subclinical infection. It is estimated that 40 million people in the United States have been infected. It is usually acquired by inhalation of dust containing spores of the fungus, the contamination probably occurring from excreta of birds, such as pigeons, starlings and blackbirds.

Oral lesions are present in a high percentage of cases. Reports of 73 cases have been reviewed by Weed and Parkhill, who found that 24 of the cases, or 33 per cent, had oral lesions as part of the presenting complaint.

Clinical Features. The disease is characterized by a chronic low-grade fever, productive cough, splenomegaly, hepatomegaly and lymphadenopathy, since the organisms have a special predilection for the reticuloendothelial system and chiefly involve the spleen, liver, lymph nodes and bone marrow. Anemia and leukopenia also may be present. The infection by this organism may be extremely mild, manifesting only local lesions such as subcutaneous nodules or suppurative arthritis, and may produce no more serious effects than a positive histoplasmin skin reaction or calcified pulmonary nodules similar to those seen in tuberculosis. Histoplasmosis often terminates fatally, however, particularly the generalized form.

Oral Manifestations. The oral lesions of histoplasmosis have been reviewed by Levy and by Stiff. They appear as nodular, ulcerative or vegetative lesions on the buccal mucosa, gingiva, tongue, palate or lips (Fig. 6–28). The ulcerated areas are usually covered by a nonspecific gray membrane and are indurated. The organisms may be demonstrated in tissue sections in many, but not all, cases. Thus it is wise in suspected cases to preserve a piece of tissue at the time of biopsy for microbiologic examination. The organism may be readily isolated by inoculating the emulsified tissue onto blood agar containing penicillin and streptomycin. Occasionally cases have been mistaken for carcinoma or even Vincent's infection, while the lymphadenopathy has suggested Hodgkin's disease.

Histologic Features. Histoplasmosis appears basically to be a granulomatous infection which affects chiefly the reticuloendothelial system. Thus the organisms are found in large numbers in phagocytic cells and appear as tiny intracellular structures measuring little more than 1 micron in diameter (Fig. 6–28).

Treatment. Pulmonary histoplasmosis usually resolves spontaneously, while severe forms of the disease are usually treated by amphotericin B.

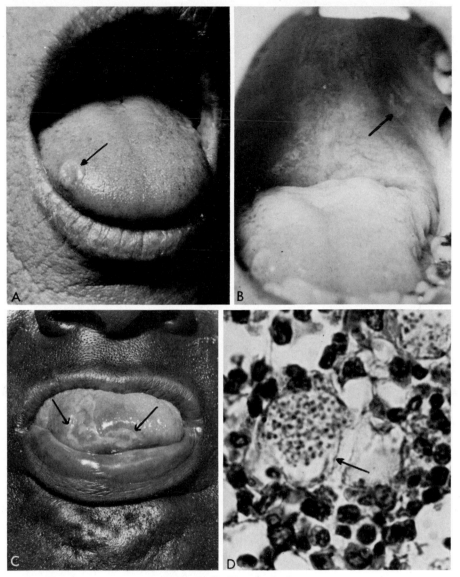

Figure 6–28. *Histoplasmosis.*
Lesions involving tongue (*A, C*) and palate (*B.*) The photomicrograph (*D*) of the bone marrow biopsy shows *Histoplasma capsulatum* within macrophages. (*A* and *B*, Courtesy of W. J. Bruins Slot: Arch. Dermatol., 76:4, 1957, and *C*, of Dr. Charles Newman.)

COCCIDIOIDOMYCOSIS

(Valley Fever; San Joaquin Valley Fever)

Coccidioidomycosis is now recognized as being a relatively common fungal disease endemic chiefly in the southwestern portion of the United States, chiefly in Arizona, California, Nevada, New Mexico, Texas and Utah. It is also known to occur in Mexico, Central and South America and occasionally Europe. In those areas where the disease is endemic, the vast majority of the population has at one time or another been infected by the organism, but usually this has been a subclinical infection. The disease appears to be transmitted to man and animals by inhalation of dust contaminated by the spores of the causative organism, *Coccidioides immitis*. This organism develops from an arthrospore into a nonbudding spherule, measuring between 10 and 80 microns in diameter, which is packed with endospores measuring approximately 5 microns in diameter.

When the spherules rupture, the endospores which are set free then develop into full-size spherules.

Clinical Features. There are two basic forms of the disease: primary nondisseminated and progressive disseminated coccidioidomycosis. In *primary* coccidioidomycosis, the patients generally develop manifestations suggestive of a respiratory disease such as cough, pleural pain, headache, and anorexia. In addition, about 20 per cent of the patients develop skin lesions, either erythema nodosum or erythema multiforme. This form of the disease is self-limiting and runs its course within 10 to 14 days. In a small percentage of cases, pulmonary cavitation, calcified nodules or pulmonary fibrosis may remain.

In the *disseminated* form of the disease which occurs in only about 1 per cent of the cases, there is a mortality rate of approximately 50 per cent. The disease usually runs a rapid course and the dissemination extends from the lung to various viscera, bones, joints and skin and to the central nervous system where meningitis is the most frequent cause of death. The dissemination to bone results in osteomyelitis in 10 to 50 per cent of cases.

Oral Manifestations. Lesions of the head and neck, including the oral cavity, occur with some frequency, as has been pointed out by Frauenfelder and Schwartz. The lesions of the oral mucosa and skin are proliferative granulomatous and ulcerated lesions that are nonspecific in their clinical appearance. These lesions tend to heal by hyalinization and scar. Marked chronicity is often a feature of these lesions. Lytic lesions of the jaws may also occur, and such a case has been reported by Igo and his associates.

Histologic Features. The tissue reaction in coccidioidomycosis is similar to that of many specific infectious granulomas. Large mononuclear cells, lymphocytes and plasma cells predominate, although epithelioid cells are not usually seen. Foci of coagulation necrosis are often found in the centers of the small granulomas, and multinucleated giant cells are scattered throughout the lesion. The organisms themselves are often found within the cytoplasm of the giant cells as well as lying free in the tissue. In tissue sections, the organisms will be found to vary greatly in size and generally show no budding. The endospores within the large spherules can usually be identified without difficulty.

Treatment. Amphotericin B has been found to provide effective chemotherapeutic control of the disease.

CRYPTOCOCCOSIS

(Torulosis; European Blastomycosis)

Cryptococcosis is a chronic fungal infection caused by *Cryptococcus neoformans (Torula histolytica)* and *Cryptococcus bacillispora*, and may present widespread lesions in the skin, oral mucosa, subcutaneous tissues, lungs, joints and particularly the meninges. The organisms are widespread and frequently found on the skin of healthy persons; for this reason, the exact mechanism of infection is not known. The organisms appear to be harbored by pigeons, but the actual infection of the human probably results from inhalation of airborne microorganisms. Since it is often an opportunistic infection, the disease has increased in incidence as immunosuppression has become more prevalent.

Clinical Features. The first evidence of infection by this organism is the presence of skin lesions from which bloodstream dissemination to other parts of the body frequently occurs. Nevertheless some authorities consider the respiratory tract colonization or visceral lesions to be the primary site, the skin lesions occurring secondarily. The skin lesions appear as multiple brown papules which ultimately ulcerate; the clinical picture is not specific. Most studies indicate a slight predilection for occurrence in middle-aged males.

The lesions of the lungs produce symptoms of a nonspecific pneumonitis, while the meningeal lesions produce a variety of neurologic signs and symptoms generally associated with increased intracranial pressure.

Cryptococcosis has been repeatedly reported in patients already suffering from some form of malignant lymphoma, evidence of the opportunistic nature of the disease.

Oral Manifestations. Occasional cases of oral cryptococcosis, almost invariably occurring in patients with other visceral or cutaneous lesions, have been reported. One of these reports was that of Newman and Rosenbaum, in which the oral lesions were the first evidence of the infection. Interestingly, their patient was also suffering from chronic lymphatic leukemia.

The oral lesions appear as simply nonspecific single or multiple ulcers which, in a patient known to have leukemia, may be mistaken for the widespread ulceration often seen in leukemic patients as a result of their inability to

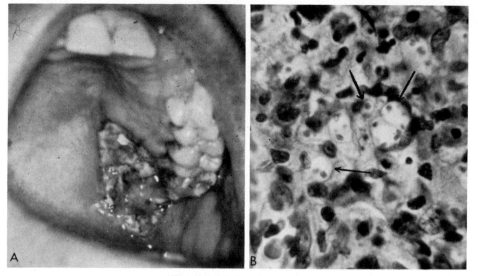

Figure 6–29. *Cryptococcosis.*
The large ulcer of the palatal mucosa *(A)* contained the typical organisms *(B)*, and these were subsequently cultured. (Courtesy of Dr. Charles W. Newman. From C. W. Newman and D. Rosenbaum: Oral cryptococcus. J. Periodontol., 33:266, 1962.)

react to a mild, nonspecific bacterial infection (Fig. 6–29).

Histologic Features. The causative organism is a gram-positive, budding, yeastlike cell with an extremely thick, gelatinous capsule. The cryptococcus measures 5 to 20 microns in diameter and, in tissue sections, appears as a small organism with a large clear halo, sometimes described as a "tissue microcyst" (Fig. 6–29,*B*). The capsule is colored intensely with the periodic acid-Schiff stain (PAS), and the organisms may be cultured on Sabouraud's glucose agar.

The tissue reaction is essentially a granulomatous one of the tuberculoid type, but focal necrosis is often absent and epithelioid cell proliferation minimal. Multinucleated giant cells are common, as is a chronic or subacute inflammatory cell infiltrate. The organisms with their characteristic halos are found singly or in groups scattered throughout the granuloma.

Treatment and Prognosis. The use of amphotericin B has been found to give excellent results. The ultimate prognosis of the patient is variable, however, and especially dependent upon the sites of involvement.

CANDIDIASIS

(Candidosis; Moniliasis; Thrush)

Candidiasis is a disease caused by infection with a yeastlike fungus, *Candida (Monilia) al-*

bicans, although other species may also be involved, such as *C. tropicalis, C. parapsilosis, C. stellatoidea* and *C. krusei.* It has been shown repeatedly that this microorganism is a relatively common inhabitant of the oral cavity, gastrointestinal tract and vagina of clinically unaffected persons. Thus it appears that the mere presence of the fungus is not sufficient to produce the disease. There must be actual penetration of the tissues, although such invasion is usually superficial and occurs only under certain circumstances. This disease is said to be the most opportunistic infection in the world. Its occurrence has increased remarkably since the prevalent use of antibiotics, which destroy the normally inhibitory bacterial flora, and immunosuppressive drugs, particularly corticosteroids and cytotoxic drugs. This is the chief cause of this disease in patients with leukemia, lymphoma or other tumors. In addition to affecting the oral cavity, monilial infection frequently involves the skin as well as the gastrointestinal tract, vaginal tract, urinary tract and lungs. Vaginal colonization appears to be increased by diabetes, pregnancy and oral contraceptive agents. Oral candidiasis, or thrush, usually remains a localized disease, but on occasion it may show extension to the pharynx or even to the lungs, often with a fatal outcome.

Clinical Features. Candidiasis is frequently classified into two major categories: (1) mucocutaneous candidiasis and (2) systemic candidiasis. The *mucocutaneous form* includes oral or oropharyngeal candidiasis (thrush), candidal esophagitis, intestinal candidiasis, candidal vulvovaginitis and balanitis, intertrigo and paronychia. One special group in this category is chronic mucocutaneous candidiasis, which is discussed later. The *systemic form* of the disease involves chiefly the eyes, the kidneys and the skin through hematogenous spread, although other visceral organs may also be involved.

Chronic mucocutaneous candidiasis is a group of different forms of this infection, some of which may have multiple features in common, although they can usually be separated as entities. Oral manifestations occur in numerous forms of candidiasis and these have been categorized most conveniently by Lehner, whose slightly modified classification is shown in Table 6–5, and includes the various forms of chronic mucocutaneous candidiasis. In general, chronic mucocutaneous candidiasis is characterized by chronic candidal involvement of the skin, scalp, nails and mucous membranes. As a group, the patients exhibit varying abnormalities in their immune system—impaired cell-mediated immunity, isolated IgA deficiency and reduced serum candidacidal activity—and they are usually resistant to the common forms of treatment. *Chronic familial mucocutaneous candidiasis* is an inherited disorder, probably an autosomal recessive characteristic, which occurs early in life, usually before the age of 5 years, and has an equal sex distribution. Oral lesions occur in these children. *Chronic localized mucocutaneous candidiasis* is a severe form of the disease also occurring early in life, but there is no genetic transmission. There is widespread skin involvement and granulomatous and horny masses on the face and scalp. There is an increased incidence of other fungal and bacterial

---

Table 6–5.   Classification of Oral Candidiasis

Acute
1. Acute pseudomembranous oral candidiasis (thrush)
2. Acute atrophic oral candidiasis

Chronic
1. Chronic hyperplastic oral candidiasis
2. Chronic mucocutaneous candidiasis
   (a) Chronic familial mucocutaneous candidiasis
   (b) Chronic localized mucocutaneous candidiasis
   (c) Candidiasis endocrinopathy syndrome
   (d) Chronic diffuse mucocutaneous candidiasis
3. Chronic atrophic oral candidiasis

Modified from T. Lehner: Oral candidosis. Dent. Pract., 17:209, 1967 and J. M. Higgs and R. S. Wells: Chronic mucocutaneous candidiasis; associated abnormalities of iron metabolism. Br. J. Derm., 86 (Suppl. 8):88, 1972.

---

infections. The mouth is the common primary site for the typical white plaques, and nail involvement is usually present. *Candidiasis endocrinopathy syndrome* is also a genetically transmitted condition characterized by Candida infection of the skin, scalp, nails and mucous membranes, classically the oral cavity, in association with either hypoadrenalism (Addison's disease), hypoparathyroidism, hypothyroidism, ovarian insufficiency or diabetes mellitus. It is recognized that the endocrine manifestations, which may be multiple, may not appear clinically for several years after the appearance of the thrush in the children. The oral findings in the autoimmune polyendocrinopathy-candidiasis syndrome, including the common finding of enamel hypoplasia, have been discussed by Myllärniemi and Perheentupa. *Chronic diffuse mucocutaneous candidiasis* is the least common form of the disease and appears to be of late onset, since all patients reported by Lehner were over 55 years of age. They exhibit extensive raised crusty sheets involving the limbs, groin, face, scalp and shoulders as well as mouth and nails. There is no familial history and usually the patients have no other abnormality.

Oral Manifestations.   The oral lesions in the different forms of candidiasis may have a different appearance and must be discussed separately (Table 6–5).

Acute pseudomembranous candidiasis is one of the more common forms of the disease. It may occur at any age but is especially prone to occur in the debilitated or the chronically ill, or in infants. The oral lesions are characterized by the appearance of soft, white, slightly elevated plaques most frequently occurring on the buccal mucosa and tongue, but also seen on the palate, gingiva and floor of the mouth (Figs. 6–30, 6–31,A). The plaques, which often have been described grossly as resembling milk curds, consist chiefly of tangled masses of fungal hyphae with intermingled desquamated epithelium, keratin, fibrin, necrotic debris, leukocytes and bacteria. The white plaque can usually be wiped away with a gauze, leaving either a relatively normal appearing mucosa or an erythematous area. In severe cases the entire oral cavity may be involved.

Acute atrophic candidiasis may occur either as a sequela to acute pseudomembranous candidiasis or it may originate de novo. The lesions in this form of the disease appear red or erythematous rather than white, thus resembling the pseudomembranous type in which the white membrane has been wiped off. It too may occur at any site. It is the only variety of oral candi-

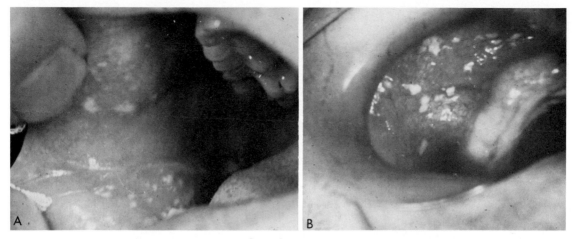

Figure 6–30. *Acute pseudomembranous oral candidiasis (thrush).*
(*B*, Courtesy of Dr. Robert J. Gorlin.)

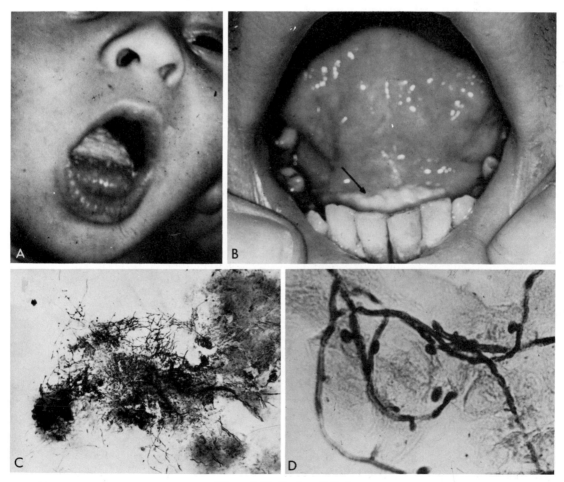

Figure 6–31. *Oral candidiasis.*

A, Acute pseudomembranous type in an infant; *B*, chronic hyperplastic type in floor of mouth in adult. *C*, *D*, Threadlike *Candida albicans* organisms having budding yeast cells are scattered along the pseudohyphae. (*C* and *D*, courtesy of Dr. Grant Van Huysen: Oral Surg., 9:970, 1956.)

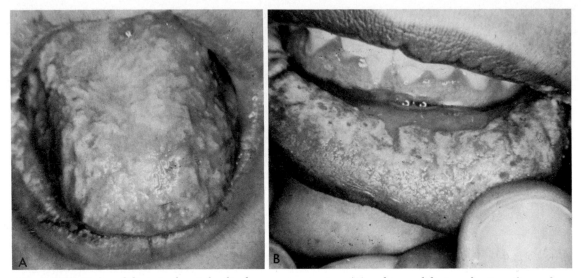

Figure 6–32. Oral candidiasis in chronic localized mucocutaneous type *(A)*; and in candidiasis endocrinopathy syndrome (diabetes) type *(B)*.

diasis which is consistently painful, according to Lehner.

Chronic hyperplastic candidiasis is often spoken of as the "leukoplakia" type of candidiasis. The oral lesions consist of firm, white persistent plaques, usually on the lips, tongue and cheeks (Fig. 6–31,*B*). These lesions may persist for periods of years.

In this regard, Roed-Petersen and his associates have reported a high incidence of Candida organisms present in the lesions of a series of 226 patients with true leukoplakia. In addition, they found a definite relationship between the presence of the organisms and the occurrence of cytologic epithelial atypia in the biopsied lesions of leukoplakia. Cawson and Binnie have presented data which indicate a definite relationship between chronic candidiasis and oral epidermoid carcinoma, basing this relationship on the finding that chronic candidiasis itself is a cause of leukoplakia and thus must be regarded as having possible premalignant potential.

Chronic mucocutaneous candidiasis presents oral lesions in all forms of the disease. In general, their clinical appearance is similar to the lesions described in chronic hyperplastic candidiasis and occur in the same intraoral locations (Fig. 6–32).

Chronic atrophic candidiasis is now considered to be synonymous with the condition better known as "denture sore mouth," a diffuse inflammation of the denture-bearing area, often occurring with angular cheilitis (Fig. 6–33,*A*).

There is no apparent age limit, and some studies show women affected more frequently than men.

Denture-related candidiasis may be the most common form of the oral disease. For example, in a recent study reported by Holbrook and Rodgers, they found that in nearly two-thirds of a group of 100 patients with candidiasis, dentures were the one "disorder" or situation predisposing or traceable to the development of the infection.

Histologic Features. Fragments of the plaque material may be smeared on a microscopic slide, macerated with 20 per cent potassium hydroxide and examined for the typical hyphae (Fig. 6–30, *C*, *D*). In addition, the organisms may be cultured in a variety of media, including blood agar, cornmeal agar and Sabouraud's broth, to aid in establishing the diagnosis.

Histologic sections of a biopsy from a lesion of oral candidiasis will show the presence of the yeast cells and hyphae or mycelia in the superficial and deeper layers of involved epithelium (Fig. 6–33,*B*). These are more easily visualized if the sections are stained with periodic acid-Schiff reagent (PAS) or methenamine silver, since the organisms are positive in both instances. Chlamydospores are seldom seen on oral smears or histologic sections.

Treatment. The development of new specific antifungal agents such as nystatin has been beneficial in the treatment of candidiasis. Suspensions of nystatin, held in contact with the

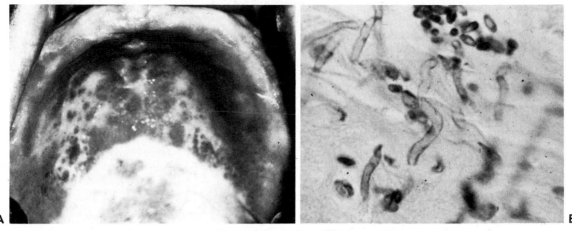

Figure 6–33. *Oral candidiasis.*
Chronic atrophic type in the edentulous patient with "denture sore mouth" in *A*; the hyphae and cells are seen in the epithelium in a biopsy specimen stained with periodic acid-Schiff (PAS) in *B*. (*A*, Courtesy of Dr. Birute Balciunas.)

oral lesion, have been successfully used in even chronic, severe cases of the disease. The use of tablets of the fungicide, prepared specifically for the treatment of intestinal thrush, are of little value in managing oral lesions, since the drug must make intimate contact with the organisms in order to be effective. Other drugs of value are chlortrimazoles, amphotericin B and iconazole.

It has been found that occasional cases of candidiasis have remained refractory to treatment by nystatin. These have frequently been associated with one of the endocrinopathies just described in connection with immunologic abnormalities.

GEOTRICHOSIS

Geotrichosis is a fungal disease similar to candidiasis in its clinical features, but caused by organisms of the Geotrichum species.

Clinical Features. The most common lesions are those of the lungs and oral mucosa, although cutaneous and intestinal tract lesions occur on occasion. The lung involvement produces symptoms of pneumonitis or bronchitis but the organisms can be detected in the sputum.

Oral Manifestations. The oral lesions are identical to those of candidiasis or thrush, being a white, velvety, patch-like covering of the oral mucosa, isolated or diffuse in distribution. The differentiation is made only by microscopic examination and/or culture of the organisms.

The development of the disease also parallels that of candidiasis, being seen frequently in

debilitated persons or as a secondary type of infection.

Histologic Features. The organisms are small, rectangular-shaped spores measuring approximately 4 by 8 microns, often with rounded ends. The tissue reaction is a nonspecific, acute inflammatory one.

Treatment. Treatment is nonspecific, and there are insufficient data on the effects on geotrichosis of drugs used in treating candidiasis.

PHYCOMYCOSIS

(*Mucormycosis*)

Phycomycosis is a fungus disease which has occurred in the United States with any significant incidence only within the past few decades, although a few sporadic cases have been reported for some years. A thorough review of this disease was published by Hutter, and more recently by Lehrer, and the craniofacial or rhinocerebral form discussed by Green and his co-workers as well as Landau and Newcomer, and Taylor and his associates. This is an opportunistic infection associated with debilitation and is becoming more frequently recognized as a secondary occurrence in cancer patients, especially those with any of the malignant lymphomas. It is also especially common in patients with diabetes mellitus, especially those with diabetic ketoacidosis; fully 75 per cent of patients with the rhinocerebral form of mucormycosis have the ketoacidosis. As might be expected, immunosuppressed patients are prone to develop this infection as well as patients with burns or open wounds. Cases have also been reported after administration of steroids and chemotherapeutic antimetabolites.

This disease may actually be caused by numerous Phycomycetes organisms of the Eumycetes (true fungi) class characterized by lack of septation (coenocytic). The three most important of these causing infection in man are *Rhizopus*, *Mucor* and *Absidia*.

Clinical Features. Two main types of phycomycosis infection occur in human beings: (1) superficial and (2) visceral, although it is also sometimes classified as localized and disseminated. The superficial infection includes involvement of the external ear, the fingernails and the skin. The visceral forms of phycomycosis are of three main types: (a) pulmonary, (b) gastrointestinal, and (c) rhinocerebral. Although all forms of phycomycosis are important, the rhinocerebral is of greatest interest to the dental profession, and only this variety will be discussed here.

Infections of the head by these organisms are characterized by the classical syndrome of uncontrolled diabetes, cellulitis, ophthalmoplegia and meningoencephalitis. The infection apparently enters the tissues through the nasal mucosa and extends to the paranasal sinuses, pharynx, palate, orbit and brain.

One early clinical manifestation of the disease is the appearance of a reddish-black nasal turbinate and septum with a nasal discharge. The necrosis may extend to the paranasal sinuses and orbital cavity, with the development of sinus tracts and sloughing of tissue.

Cases of phycomycosis involving the maxillary sinus may present clinically as a mass in the maxilla, resembling carcinoma of the antrum, and roentgenograms may support the latter diagnosis. Typical cases have been reported by Green and his associates, by Berger and his co-workers, and by Cruickshank and his colleagues. Surgical exploration, however, will reveal only masses of necrotic tissue in which the organisms can be demonstrated histologically. This involvement may occur at any age, cases having been reported in infants as well as adults.

Histologic Features. The tissue involved by this infection shows a variable amount of necrosis, some of which may be related to infarction brought about by thrombi consisting of the organisms. This fungus has an apparent predilection for blood vessels; it is able to penetrate their walls and thereby produce thromboses.

The organisms appear as large, nonseptate hyphae with branching at obtuse angles (Fig. 6-34). Round or ovoid sporangia are also frequently seen in tissue section. The organisms can be cultured.

Treatment and Prognosis. Treatment of the disease has been primarily (1) control of the predisposing factors such as diabetes, (2) surgical excision if the lesion is localized, and (3) amphotericin B, since it is the only drug with proven efficacy.

The majority of reported cases of phycomycosis have been diagnosed only at the time of autopsy. In recent years, however, numerous cases of even fulminating head and neck infection by this organism have been diagnosed, treated and cured. The current survival rate for

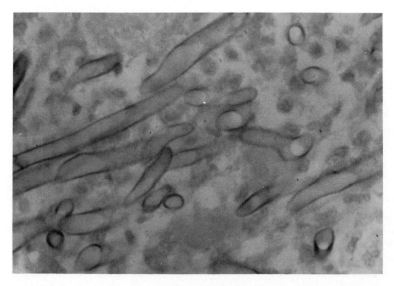

Figure 6–34. *Phycomycetes organisms.*

rhinocerebral disease in patients with no systemic disease is about 75 per cent; with diabetes, about 60 per cent; and with other underlying diseases, about 20 per cent. Pulmonary disease is almost uniformly fatal.

SPOROTRICHOSIS

Sporotrichosis is a fungal infection caused by *Sporotrichum schenckii* in which the portal of entry is not entirely understood. It has been reported to occur after (1) exposure to a wide variety of animals, both domestic and wild, (2) accidental injury from the thorns of some plants or bushes, and (3) accidental laboratory or clinical inoculation of hospital workers.

Clinical Features. The most common lesions of sporotrichosis involve the skin, subcutaneous tissues and oral, nasal and pharyngeal mucosa, although disseminated visceral involvement occasionally occurs. The skin lesions, often described as sporotrichotic "chancres," appear at the site of inoculation as firm, red to purple nodules which soon ulcerate. Neighboring nodules with regional lymphadenopathy generally develop soon, and both these subcutaneous nodules and involved lymph nodes may also ulcerate and drain.

Oral Manifestations. Nonspecific ulceration of the oral, nasal and pharyngeal mucosa also occurs in this disease, usually associated with regional lymphadenopathy. The lesions are described as healing by soft, pliable scars even though the organisms may still be present in the tissues.

Histologic Features. The fungus is a small, ovoid branching organism with septate hyphae, showing budding forms. It is only 3 to 5 microns in diameter and, because of the small size, is seldom recognized in the routine tissue sections. It can be cultured on Sabouraud's medium, however.

The tissue reaction is a granulomatous one with epithelioid cells, multinucleated giant cells of the Langhans type and lymphocytes, often surrounding a central area of purulent or caseous necrosis. Polymorphonuclear leukocytes are prominent in some cases. Asteroid bodies, radiate formations around the fungal spores in tissues, are commonly found in this disease as reported by Lurie. Pseudoepitheliomatous hyperplasia of the overlying epithelium of skin or mucosal lesions is also almost invariably present.

Treatment and Prognosis. There is no specific

treatment for the disease, most antibiotics being ineffective, but the prognosis is generally good, although chronic repetitive remissions and relapses are common. The chronic pulmonary form of the disease is often fatal.

RHINOSPORIDIOSIS

Rhinosporidiosis, caused by *Rhinosporidium seeberi*, is a fungal infection, rare in the United States, which affects chiefly the oropharynx and nasopharynx as well as the larynx, skin, eyes and genital mucosa. The mode of infection is not known.

Clinical Features. The skin lesions appear as small verrucae or warts which ultimately become pedunculated. Genital lesions resemble condylomas.

Oral Manifestations. The oronasopharyngeal lesions are often accompanied by a mucoid discharge and appear as soft red polypoid growths of a tumor-like nature which spread to the pharynx and larynx. The lesions are vascular and bleed readily. The oral lesions have been reviewed recently by Ramanathan and his coworkers. In addition, an unusual case involving the parotid duct has been reported by Topazian.

Histologic Features. The organisms appear as sporangia containing large numbers of round or ovoid endospores, each approximately 5 to 7 microns in diameter. In either smear preparations or tissue sections, these sporangia are characteristic in appearance. The surrounding tissue reaction itself is a nonspecific one consisting of a vascular granulation tissue with focal abscess formation and occasional multinucleated giant cells. Both acute and chronic inflammatory cells are present in variable number.

Treatment. There is no known specific treatment of the disease.

PARASITIC INFECTIONS

There is a considerable variety of protozoal and helminthic parasitic diseases which occasionally manifest oral involvement. The protozoa are unicellular animals which are usually divided into two subphyla: the Plasmodroma—protozoa which move by means of pseudopodia or flagella—and the Chilophora—protozoa which move by means of cilia.

The helminths are multicellular parasitic worms, often referred to as metazoa, and are generally divided into two phyla: the Nemathelminthes or roundworms and the Platyhelminthes or flatworms. Of the Nemathelminthes, those belonging to the class Nematoda (roundworms) are of medical importance, while of the Platyhelminthes, those belonging to the Cestoda class (tapeworms) and the Trematoda class (flukes) are important.

Of the more common protozoal diseases, it is recognized that the following may involve oral structures in some fashion: trypanosomiasis (Chagas' disease), leishmaniasis, trichomoniasis and toxoplasmosis.

Helminthic diseases may also involve oral structures with perhaps an even greater frequency than the protozoal diseases. Of the more common helminthic diseases, the following may manifest oral involvement: cysticercosis, trichinosis (trichiniasis), schistosomiasis (bilharziasis), echinococcus disease (hydatid disease), ascariasis, strongyloidiasis and myiasis.

The entire field of parasitology is becoming increasingly important since some parasitic infections, once restricted to certain parts of the world, are becoming worldwide in their distribution as a result of jet-age travel and military entanglements in countries which are parasite reservoirs. Nevertheless, the relative infrequency with which parasitic oral problems are encountered precludes a discussion of the individual diseases here. However, for pertinent discussions on the oral or paraoral manifestations of certain of these diseases, the reader is referred to the following authors, whose appropriate publications on the subject are listed in the references: (a) cysticercosis (Timosca and Gavrilita; Ostrofsky and Baker); (b) trichinosis (Moskow; Bruce); and (c) toxoplasmosis (Appel and associates; Dorfman and Remington; Stagno).

REFERENCES

Abbott, J. N., Briney, A. T., and Denaro, S. A.: Recovery of tubercle bacilli from mouth washings of tuberculous dental patients. J. Am. Dent. Assoc., 50:49, 1955.

Addy, M., and Dolby, A. E.: Aphthous ulceration: the antinuclear factor. J. Dent. Res., 51:1594, 1972.

Adler, J. L., Mostow, S. R., Mellin, H., Janney, J. H., and Joseph, J. M.: Epidemiologic investigation of hand, foot, and mouth disease. Am. J. Dis. Child., 120:309, 1970.

Albright, E. C., Larson, F. C., and Deiss, W. P.: Hypertrophy of salivary glands during treatment of myxedema with triiodothyronine. J. Lab. Clin. Med., 44:762, 1954.

Amromin, G.: Generalized salivary gland virus infection. Arch. Pathol., 56:323, 1953.

Andrewes, C. H.: Active immunisation in virus diseases. Br. Med. J., 2:1036, 1931; Lancet, 2:1241, 1931.

Angelopoulos, A. P.: Pyogenic granuloma of the oral cavity; statistical analysis of its clinical features. J. Oral Surg., 29:840, 1971.

Antoon, J. W., and Miller, R. L.: Aphthous ulcers—a review of the literature on etiology, pathogenesis, diagnosis, and treatment. J. Am. Dent. Assoc., 101:803, 1980.

Appel, B. N., Mendelow, H., and Pasqual, H. N.: Acquired toxoplasma lymphadenitis. Oral Surg., 47:529, 1979.

Arendorf, T. M., and Walker, D. M.: Oral candidal populations in health and disease. Br. Dent. J., 147:267, 1979.

Arita, I.: Virological evidence for the success of the smallpox eradication programme. Nature, 279:293, 1979.

August, M. J., Nordlund, J. J., and Hsiung, G. D.: Persistence of herpes simplex virus types 1 and 2 in infected individuals. Arch. Dermatol., 115:309, 1979.

Badger, G. R.: Oral signs of chickenpox (varicella): report of two cases. J. Dent. Child., 47:349, 1980.

Baker, M. A. A.: Oral cysticercosis: three case reports. J. Dent. Assoc. S. Afr., 30:535, 1975.

Baldridge, G. D.: Immunologic aspects of herpes simplex, herpes zoster, and vaccinia. Arch. Dermatol., 79:299, 1959.

Banks, P.: Nonneoplastic parotid swellings: a review. Oral Surg., 25:732, 1968.

Barbero, G. J., and Sibinga, M. S.: Enlargement of the submaxillary salivary glands in cystic fibrosis. Pediatrics, 29:788, 1962.

Barile, M. F., and Graykowski, E. A.: Primary herpes, recurrent labial herpes, recurrent aphthae and periadenitis aphthae. A review with some new observations. Dist. Columb. Dent. J., July, 1963.

Barile, M. F., Graykowski, E. A., Driscoll, E. J., and Riggs, D. B.: L form of bacteria isolated from recurrent aphthous stomatitis lesions. Oral Surg., 16:1395, 1963.

Barsh, L. I.: Molluscum contagiosum of the oral mucosa. Report of a case. Oral Surg., 22:42, 1966.

Baum, G. L., Schwarz, J., Bruins Slot, W. J., and Straub, M.: Mucocutaneous histoplasmosis. Arch. Dermatol., 76:4, 1957.

Bell, W. A., Gamble, J., and Garrington, G. E.: North American blastomycosis with oral lesions. Oral Surg., 28:914, 1969.

Berger, C. J., Disque, F. C., and Topazian, R. G.: Rhinocerebral mucormycosis: diagnosis and treatment. Oral Surg., 40:27, 1975.

Bernstein, M. L., and McDonald, J. S.: Oral lesions in Crohn's disease: report of two cases and update of the literature. Oral Surg., 46:234, 1978.

Binford, C. H., and Connor, D. H. (eds.): Pathology of Tropical and Extraordinary Diseases. An Atlas. Vols. 1 and 2. Washington, D.C., Armed Forces Institute of Pathology, 1976.

Binford, C. H., Meyers, W. M., and Walsh, G. P.: Leprosy. J.A.M.A., 247:2283, 1982.

Blank, H., and Rake, G.: Viral and Rickettsial Diseases of the Skin, Eye and Mucous Membranes of Man. Boston, Little, Brown and Company, 1955.

Blank, H., Burgoon, C. F., Baldridge, G. D., McCarthy, P. L., and Urbach, F.: Cytologic smears in diagnosis of herpes simplex, herpes zoster and varicella. J.A.M.A., 146:1410, 1951.

Blum, T.: Pregnancy tumors: a study of sixteen cases. J. Am. Dent. Assoc., 18:393, 1931.

Boffey, P. M.: Smallpox: outbreak in Somalia slows rapid progress toward eradication. Science, 196:1298, 1977.

Bogliolo, L.: South American blastomycosis (Lutz's disease). Arch. Dermatol. Syph., 61:470, 1950.

Borsanyi, S., and Blanchard, C. L.: Asymptomatic enlargement of the salivary glands. J.A.M.A., 174:20, 1960.

Bradlaw, R. V.: The dental stigmata of prenatal syphilis. Oral. Surg., 6:147, 1953.

Breman, J. G., and Arita, I.: The confirmation and maintenance of smallpox eradication. N. Engl. J. Med., 303:1263, 1980.

Brodsky, R. H.: Oral tuberculosis lesions. Am. J. Orthod., 28:132, 1942.

Brody, H. A., and Silverman, S., Jr.: Studies on recurrent oral aphthae. I. Clinical and laboratory comparisons. Oral Surg., 27:27, 1969.

Bronner, M., and Bronner, M.: Actinomycosis. Bristol, John Wright & Sons, Ltd., 1969.

Brook, A. H.: Recurrent parotitis in childhood. Br. Dent. J., 127:271, 1969.

Brooke, R. I.: Wegener's granulomatosis involving the gingivae. Br. Dent. J., 127:34, 1969.

Brooke, R. I., and Sapp, J. P.: Herpetiform ulceration. Oral Surg., 42:182, 1976.

Brown, J. R.: Human actinomycosis. A study of 181 subjects. Hum. Pathol, 4:319, 1973.

Bruce, K. W.: Tuberculosis of the alveolar gingiva. Oral Surg., 7:894, 1954.

Bruce, R. A.: Trichinosis associated with oral squamous cell carcinoma: report of three cases. J. Oral Surg., 33:136, 1975.

Brunell, P. A., Miller, L. H., and Lovejoy, F.: Zoster in children. Am. J. Dis. Child., 115:432, 1968.

Buchner, A.: Hand, foot, and mouth disease. Oral Surg., 41:333, 1976.

Burkwall, H. F.: Noma. Am. J. Orthod., Oral Surg., 28:394, 1942.

Burnet, F. M., and Williams, S. W.: Herpes simplex: a new point of view. Aust. Med. J., 1:637, 1939.

Burnett, G. W., and Scherp, H. W.: Oral Microbiology and Infectious Disease. 3rd ed. Baltimore, Williams & Wilkins Company, 1968.

Burns, J. C.: Diagnostic methods for herpes simplex infection: a review. Oral Surg., 50:346, 1980.

Cahn, L. R., Eisenbud, L., Blake, M. N., and Stern, D.: Biopsies of normal-appearing palates of patients with known sarcoidosis; a preliminary report. Oral Surg., 18:342, 1964.

Cangir, A., and Sullivan, M. P.: The occurrence of cytomegalovirus infections in childhood leukemia. J.A.M.A., 195:616, 1966.

Carithers, H. A.: Oculoglandular disease of Parinaud. A manifestation of cat-scratch disease. Am. J. Dis. Child., 132:1195, 1978.

Carpenter, A. M.: Studies on Candida. I. Identification of 100 yeastlike fungi isolated from children. Am. J. Clin. Pathol., 25:98, 1955.

Carter, J. E.: Iodide "mumps." N. Engl. J. Med., 264:987, 1961.

Idem: Gingival changes in Wegener's granulomatosis. Br. Dent. J., 118:30, 1965.

Cataldo, E., Covino, M. C., and Tesone, P. E.: Pyostomatitis vegetans. Oral Surg., 52:172, 1981.

Cawson, R. A., and Binnie, W. H.: Candida leukoplakia and carcinoma: a possible relationship; in I. C. Mackenzie, E. Dabelsteen and C. A. Squier: Oral Premalignancy. Iowa City, University of Iowa Press, 1980, p. 59.

Chu, F. T., and Fan, C.: Cancrum oris: a clinical study of 100 cases with special reference to prognosis. Chin. Med. J., 50:303, 1936.

Chue, P. W. Y.: Gonorrhea—its natural history, oral manifestations, diagnosis, treatment, and prevention. J. Am. Dent. Assoc., 90:1297, 1975.

Cobb, H. B., and Courts, F.: Chronic mucocutaneous candidiasis: report of case. J. Dent. Child., 47:352, 1980.

Cohen, L.: Etiology, pathogenesis and classification of aphthous stomatitis and Behçet's syndrome. J. Oral Pathol., 7:347, 1978.

Cooke, B. E. D.: Epithelial smears in the diagnosis of herpes simplex and herpes zoster affecting the oral mucosa. Br. Dent. J., 104:97, 1958.

Idem: Recurrent Mikulicz's aphthae. Dent. Pract., 12:116, 1961.

Cooper, P. H., McAllister, H. A., and Helwig, E. B.: Intravenous pyogenic granuloma. A study of 18 cases. Am. J. Surg. Pathol., 3:221, 1979.

Covel, E.: Boeck's sarcoid of mucous membrane: report of a case. Oral Surg., 7:1242, 1954.

Crowley, M. C.: Actinomyces in the normal mouth and in infectious processes. Am. J. Orthod., Oral Surg., 30:680, 1944.

Cruickshank, G., Vincent, R. D., Cherrick, H. M., and Derby, K.: Rhinocerebral mucormycosis. J. Am. Dent. Assoc., 95:1164, 1977.

D'Agostino, F. J.: A review of noma: report of a case treated with aureomycin. Oral Surg., 4:1000, 1951.

Daniels, W. B., and MacMurray, F. G.: Cat scratch disease. J.A.M.A., 154:1247, 1954.

David, R. B., and O'Connell, E. J.: Suppurative parotitis in children. Am. J. Dis. Child., 119:332, 1970.

Davis, M. I. J.: Analysis of forty-six cases of actinomycosis with special reference to its etiology. Am. J. Surg., 52:447, 1941.

Dawson, J.: Cancrum oris. Br. Dent. J., 79:151, 1945.

Debré, R., Lamy, M., Jamnet, M. L., Costil, L., and Mozziconacci, P.: Maladie des griffes de chat. Bull. Acad. Natl. Med. (Paris), 66:76, 1950.

DeRemee, R. A., McDonald, T. J., Harrison, E. G., Jr., and Coles, D. T.: Wegener's granulomatosis. Anatomic correlates, a proposed classification. Mayo Clin. Proc., 51:777, 1976.

Dobreff, M.: Compensatory hypertrophy of the parotid gland in presence of hypofunction of pancreatic islands. Dtsch. Med. Wochenschr., 62:67, 1936.

Dodd, K., Johnston, L. M., and Buddingh, G. J.: Herpetic stomatitis. J. Pediatr., 12:95, 1938.

Dolby, A. E.: Recurrent Mikulicz's oral aphthae. Their relationship to the menstrual cycle. Br. Dent. J., 124:359, 1968.

Dolby, A. E.: Recurrent aphthous ulceration, effect of sera and peripheral blood lymphocytes upon oral epithelial tissue culture cells. Immunology, 17:709, 1969.

Domonkos, A. N., Arnold, H. L., Jr., and Odom, R. B.: Andrews' Diseases of the Skin. 7th ed. Philadelphia, W. B. Saunders Company, 1982.

Donatsky, O.: Comparison of cellular and humoral immunity against streptococcal and adult human oral mucosa antigens in relation to exacerbation or recurrent aphthous stomatitis. Acta Pathol. Microbiol. Scand., 84:270, 1976.

Idem: Recurrent aphthous stomatitis, immunological aspects. A review. Thesis. Copenhagen, 1978.

Donatsky, O., and Dabelsteen, E.: Deposits of immunoglobulin G and complement C3 in recurrent aphthous ulcerations. Scand. J. Dent. Res., 85:419, 1977.

Dorfman, R. F., and Remington, J. S.: Value of lymphnode biopsy in the diagnosis of acute acquired toxoplasmosis. N. Engl. J. Med., 289:878, 1973.

Doyle, J. L., Grodjesk, J. E., and Manhold, J. H., Jr., Condyloma acuminatum occurring in the oral cavity. Oral Surg., 26:434, 1968.

Duggan, J. J., and Rothbell, E. N.: Asymptomatic enlargement of the parotid glands. N. Engl. J. Med., 257:1262, 1957.

Edwards, M. B., and Buckerfield, J. P.: Wegener's granulomatosis: a case with primary mucocutaneous lesions. Oral Surg., 46:53, 1978.

Edwards, M. B., Roberts, G. D. D., and Storrs, T. J.: Scleroma (rhinoscleroma) in a Nigerian maxillo-facial practice. Review and case reports. Int. J. Oral Surg., 6:270, 1977.

Enwonwu, C. O.: Epidemiological and biochemical studies of necrotizing ulcerative gingivitis and noma (cancrum oris) in Nigerian children. Arch. Oral Biol., 17:1357, 1972.

Epker, B. N., and Via, W. F., Jr.: Oral and preoral manifestations of leprosy. Report of a case. Oral Surg., 28:342, 1969.

Epstein, C. M., and Zeisler, E. P.: Chancre of the gingiva. J. Am. Dent. Assoc., 20:2228, 1933.

Eveson, J. W., and Slaney, A. E.: Non-healing midline granuloma. Br. J. Oral Surg., 20:102, 1982.

Farber, J. E., Friedland, E., and Jacobs, W. F.: Tuberculosis of the tongue. Am. Rev. Tuberc., 42:766, 1940.

Felber, T. D., Smith, E. B., Knox, J. M., Wallis, C., and Melnick, J. L.: Photodynamic inactivation of herpes simplex. Report of a clinical trial. J.A.M.A., 223:289, 1973.

Ferro, E. R., and Richter, J. W.: Oral lesions of granuloma inguinale: report of three cases. J. Oral Surg., 4:121, 1946.

Fiese, M. J.: Coccidioidomycosis. Springfield, Ill., Charles C Thomas, 1958.

Fiumara, N. J., and Lessell, S.: Manifestations of late congenital syphilis. Arch. Dermatol., 102:78, 1970.

Francis, T. C.: Recurrent aphthous stomatitis and Behçet's disease. Oral Surg., 30:476, 1970.

Frauenfelder, D., and Schwartz, A. W.: Coccidioidomycosis involving head and neck. Plast. Reconstr. Surg., 39:549, 1967.

Froeschle, J. E., Nahmias, A. J., Feorino, P. M., McCord, G., and Naib, Z.: Hand, foot and mouth disease (Coxsackie virus A16) in Atlanta. Am. J. Dis. Child., 114:278, 1967.

Furcolow, M. L., Balows, A., Menges, R. W., Pickar, D., McClellan, J. T., and Saliba, A.: Blastomycosis. An important medical problem in the central United States. J.A.M.A., 198:529, 1966.

Geist, R. M., Jr., and Mullen, W. H., Jr.: Roentgenologic aspects of lethal granulomatous ulceration of the midline facial tissues. Am. J. Roentgenol., 70:566, 1953.

Goodwin, R. A., Jr., Shapiro, J. L., Thurman, G. H., Thurman, S. S., and Des Prez, R. M.: Disseminated histoplasmosis: clinical and pathologic correlations. Medicine, 59:1, 1980.

Grahnen, H.: Maternal rubella and dental defects. Odontol. Revy, 9:181, 1958.

Graykowski, E. A., Barile, M. F., Lee, W. B., and Stanley, H. R.: Recurrent aphthous stomatitis, clinical, therapeutic, histopathologic and hypersensitivity aspects. J.A.M.A., 196:637, 1966.

Graykowski, E. A., and Hooks, J. J.: Aphthous stomatitis—Behçet's syndrome workshop. J. Oral Path., 7:341, 1978.

Green, W. H., Goldberg, H. I., and Wohl, G. T.: Mucormycosis infection of the cranio-facial structures. Am.

J. Roentgenol., Radium Ther. Nucl. Med., 101:802, 1967.

Greenberg, G., Anderson, R., Sharpstone, P., and James, D. G.: Enlargement of parotid gland due to sarcoidosis. Br. Med. J., 2:861, 1964.

Griffin, J. W.: Recurrent intraoral herpes simplex virus infection. Oral Surg., 19:209, 1965.

Gruhn, J. G., and Sanson, J.: Mycotic infections in leukemic patients at autopsy. Cancer, 16:61, 1963.

Grüter, W.: Experimentelle and klinische Untersuchungen über den sog. Herpes Corneae. Klin. Monasbl. Augenheilkd., 65:398, 1920.

Hale, B. D., Rendtorff, R. C., Walker, L. C., and Roberts, A. N.: Epidemic herpetic stomatitis in an orphanage nursery. J.A.M.A., 183:1068, 1963.

Haley, R. S., Kaplan, B. J., and Howell, R.: Ultrastructure of oral cells with bar-shaped nuclear chromatin. Acta Cytologica, 23:81, 1979.

Hamilton, M. K., Sherrer, E. L., and Schwartz, D. S.: Lethal midline granuloma. J. Oral Surg., 23:514, 1965.

Hamner, J. E., III, and Graykowski, E. A.: Oral lesions compatible with Reiter's disease: a diagnostic problem. J. Am. Dent. Assoc., 69:560, 1964.

Hicks, M. L., and Terezhalmy, G. T.: Herpesvirus hominis type 1: a summary of structure, composition, growth cycle, and cytopathogenic effects. Oral Surg., 48:311, 1979.

Higgs, J. M., and Wells, R. S.: Chronic mucocutaneous candidiasis; associated abnormalities of iron metabolism. Br. J. Dermatol., 86 (suppl. 8): 88, 1972.

Hillerup, S.: Diagnosis of sarcoidosis from oral manifestation. Int. J. Oral Surg., 5:95, 1976.

Hilming, F.: Gingivitis gravidarum. Oral Surg., 5:734, 1952.

Hjørting-Hansen, E., and Siemssen, S. O.: Stomatitis aphthosa recurrens cicatricans. Odontol. Tidskr., 69:294, 1961.

Hoffman, E. O.: The etiology of rhinoscleroma. Int. Pathol., 8:74, 1967.

Holbrook, W. P., and Rodgers, G. D.: Candidal infections: experience in a British dental hospital. Oral Surg., 49:122, 1980.

Hollander, L., and Goldman, B. A.: Syphilis of the oral mucosa. Dent. Dig., 40:135, 1934.

Honma, T.: Electron microscopic study on the pathogenesis of recurrent aphthous ulceration as compared to Behcet's syndrome. Oral Surg., 41:366, 1976.

Howley, P. M.: The human papillomaviruses. Arch. Pathol. Lab. Med., 106:429, 1982.

Huebner, R. J., Cole, R. M., Beeman, E. A., Bell, J. A., and Peers, J. H.: Herpangina. J.A.M.A., 145:628, 1951.

Huebsch, R. F.: Gumma of the hard palate, with perforation: report of a case. Oral Surg., 8:690, 1955.

Hughes, W. T.: Tularemia in children. J. Pediat., 62:495, 1963.

Hutter, R. V. P.: Phycomycetous infection (mucormycosis) in cancer patients: a complication of therapy. Cancer, 12:330, 1959.

Igo, R. M., Taylor, C. G., Scott, A. S., and Jacoby, J. K.: Coccidioidomycosis involving the mandible: report of a case. J. Oral Surg., 36:72, 1978.

Israelson, H., Binnie, W. H., and Hurt, W. C.: The hyperplastic gingivitis of Wegener's granulomatosis. J. Periodontol., 52:81, 1981.

Itakura, T.: The histo-pathological studies on teeth of lepers, especially on dental pulp and gingival tissues. Trans. Soc. Pathol. Jap., 30:357, 1940.

James, D. G., Neville, E., Siltzbach, L. E., and Turiaf, J.: A worldwide review of sarcoidosis. Am. N.Y. Acad. Sci., 278:321, 1976.

Jamsky, R. J.: Gonococcal tonsillitis. Oral Surg., 44:197, 1977.

Jansen, G. T., Dillaha, C. J., and Honeycutt, W. M.: Candida cheilitis. Arch. Dermatol., 88:325, 1963.

Jawetz, E., Melnick, J. L., and Adelberg, E. A.: Review of Medical Microbiology. 9th ed. Los Altos, Calif., Lange Medical Publications, 1970.

Katz, H. L.: Tuberculosis of the tongue. Q. Bull. Sea View Hosp., 6:239, 1941.

Katzen, M., and du Plessis, D. J.: Recurrent parotitis in children. S. Afr. Med. J., 38:122, 1964.

Kerr, D. A.: Granuloma pyogenicum. Oral Surg., 4:158, 1951.

Idem: Stomatitis and gingivitis in the adolescent and pre-adolescent. J. Am. Dent. Assoc., 44:27, 1952.

Kessel, L. J., and Taylor, W. D.: Chronic mucocutaneous candidiasis—treatment of the oral lesions with miconazole: two case reports. Br. J. Oral Surg., 18:51, 1980.

King, H. A., and Koerner, T. A.: Chronic sialadenitis. J.A.M.A., 167:1813, 1958.

Kirkpatrick, C. H., and Alling, D. W.: Treatment of chronic oral candidiasis with clotrimazole troches. A controlled clinical trial. N. Engl. J. Med., 299:1201, 1978.

Knapp, M. J., and Uohara, G. I.: Oral condyloma acuminatum. Oral Surg., 23:538, 1967.

Kornblut, A. D., Wolff, S. M., deFries, H. E., and Fauci, A. S.: Wegener's granulomatosis. Laryngoscope, 90:1453, 1980.

Kozinn, P. J., Taschdjian, C. L., and Wiener, H.: Incidence and pathogenesis of neonatal candidiasis. Pediatrics, 21:421, 1958.

Kulka, J. P.: The lesions of Reiter's syndrome. Arthritis Rheum., 5:195, 1962.

Kutscher, A. H., Mandel, I. D., Thompson, R. H., Jr., Wotman, S., Zegarelli, E. V., Fahn, B. S., Denning, C. R., Goldstein, J. A., Taubman, M., and Khotim, S.: Parotid saliva in cystic fibrosis. I. Flow rate. Am. J. Dis. Child., 110:643, 1965.

Landau, J. W.: Chronic mucocutaneous candidiasis: associated immunologic abnormalities. Pediatrics, 42:227, 1968.

Landau, J. W., and Newcomer, V. D.: Acute cerebral phycomycosis (mucormycosis). J. Pediatr., 61:363, 1962.

Laskin, R. S., and Potenza, A. D.: Cat scratch fever: a confusing diagnosis for the orthopaedic surgeon. Two case reports and a review of the literature. J. Bone Joint Surg., 53A:1211, 1971.

Lehner, T.: Pathology of recurrent oral ulceration and oral ulceration in Behçet's syndrome: light, electron and fluorescence microscopy. J. Pathol., 97:481, 1969.

Idem: Oral thrush, or acute pseudomembranous candidiasis. A clinicopathologic study of forty-four cases. Oral Surg., 18:27, 1964.

Idem: Chronic candidiasis. Br. Dent. J., 116:539, 1964.

Idem: Oral candidosis. Dent. Practit., 17:209, 1967.

Idem: Immunologic aspects of recurrent oral ulcers. Oral Surg., 33:80, 1972.

Idem: Immunological aspects of recurrent oral ulceration and Behçet's syndrome. J. Oral Pathol. 7:424, 1978.

Lehrer, R. I.: UCLA Conference—Mucormycosis (part I). Ann. Intern. Med., 93:93, 1980.

Levitt, H., and Levan, N. E.: Gumma of tongue. Arch. Dermatol. Syph., 63:405, 1951.

Levy, B. M.: Oral manifestations of histoplasmosis. J. Am. Dent. Assoc., 32:215, 1946.

Lighterman, I.: Oral moniliasis: a complication of aureomycin therapy. Oral Surg., 4:1420, 1951.

Littman, M. L., and Zimmerman, L. E.: Cryptococcosis. New York, Grune & Stratton, Inc., 1956.

Löwenstein, A.: Aetiologische Untersuchungen über den fieberhaften Herpes. Münch. Med. Wochenschr., 66:769, 1919.

Lurie, H. I.: Histopathology of sporotrichosis. Arch. Pathol., 75:421, 1963.

Maier, A. W., and Orban, B.: Gingivitis in pregnancy. Oral Surg., 2:334, 1949.

Margileth, A. M.: Cat scratch disease: nonbacterial regional lymphadenitis. Pediatrics, 42:803, 1968.

Marx, J. L.: Cytomegalovirus: a major cause of birth defects. Science, 190:1184, 1975.

McCarthy, F. P.: Pyostomatitis vegetans: report of 3 cases. Arch. Dermatol. Syph., 60:750, 1949.

McCarthy, P., and Shklar, G.: A syndrome of pyostomatitis vegetans and ulcerative colitis. Arch. Dermatol., 88:913, 1963.

McGhee, J. R., Michalek, S. M., and Cassell, G. H.: Dental Microbiology. Philadelphia, Harper & Row, Publishers, 1982.

McKinney, R. V.: Hand, foot, and mouth disease: a viral disease of importance to dentists. J. Am. Dent. Assoc., 91:122, 1975.

Meskin, L. H., Bernard, B., and Warwick, W. J.: Biopsy of the labial mucous salivary glands in cystic fibrosis. J.A.M.A., 188:82, 1964.

Meyer, I., and Shklar, G.: The oral manifestations of acquired syphilis. A study of eighty-one cases. Oral Surg., 23:45, 1967.

Miller, M. F., Garfunkel, A. A., Ram, C., and Ship, I. I.: Inheritance patterns in recurrent aphthous ulcers: twin and pedigree data. Oral Surg., 43:886, 1977.

Miller, M. F., Ship, I. I., and Ram, C.: A retrospective study of the prevalence and incidence of recurrent aphthous ulcers in a professional population, 1958–1971. Oral Surg., 43:532, 1977.

Miller, O. B., Arbesman, C., and Baer, R. L.: Disseminated cutaneous herpes simplex (Kaposi's varicelliform eruption). Arch. Dermatol. Syph., 62:477, 1950.

Moskow, B. S.: Trichinosis in oral musculature: report of case. J. Am. Dent. Assoc., 86:663, 1973.

Myllärniemi, S., and Perheentupa, J.: Oral findings in the autoimmune polyendocrinopathy-candidosis syndrome (APECS) and other forms of hypoparathyroidism. Oral Surg., 45:721, 1978.

Nahmias, A. J., and Roizman, B.: Infection with herpes-simplex viruses 1 and 2. N. Engl. J. Med., 289:781, 1973.

Naib, Z. M., Nahmias, A. J., Josey, W. E., and Kramer, J. H.: Genital herpetic infection. Association with cervical dysplasia and carcinoma. Cancer, 23:940, 1969.

Nally, F. F., and Ross, I. H.: Herpes zoster of the oral and facial structures. Report of five cases and discussion. Oral Surg., 32:221, 1971.

Nelson, R. N., and Albright, C. R.: Melioidosis. Oral Surg., 24:128, 1967.

Nessan, V. J., and Jacoway, J. R.: Biopsy of minor salivary glands in the diagnosis of sarcoidosis. N. Engl. J. Med., 301:922, 1979.

Newman, C. W., and Rosenbaum, D.: Oral cryptococcus. J. Periodontol., 33:266, 1962.

Norman, J. E. deB.: Cervicofacial actinomycosis. Oral Surg., 29:735, 1970.

Nowakovsky, S., McGrew, E. A., Medak, H., Burlakow, P., and Nands, S.: Manifestations of viral infections in exfoliated cells. Acta Cytol., 12:227, 1968.

Nutman, N. N.: A case of histoplasmosis with oral manifestations. Oral Surg., 2:1562, 1949.

Ord, R. J., and Matz, G. J.: Tuberculous cervical lymphadenitis. Arch. Otolaryngol., 99:327, 1974.

Page, L. R., Drummond, J. F., Daniels, H. T., Morrow, L. W., and Frazier, Q. Z.: Blastomycosis with oral lesions. Oral Surg., 47:157, 1979.

Pearson, R. S. B.: Recurrent swellings of the parotid gland. J. Br. Soc. Gastroenterol., 2:210, 1961.

Perry, H. O., and Mayne, J. G.: Psoriasis and Reiter's syndrome. Arch. Dermatol., 92:129, 1965.

Pindborg, J. J., Gorlin, R. J., and Asboe-Hansen, G.: Reiter's syndrome. Oral Surg., 16:551, 1963.

Pisanty, S., and Garfunkel, A.: Familial hypoparathyroidism with candidiasis and mental retardation. Oral Surg., 44:374, 1977.

Pollock, P. G., Meyers, D. S., Frable, W. J., Valicenti, J. F. Jr., Koontz, F. P., and Beavert, C. S.: Rapid diagnosis of actinomycosis by thin-needle aspiration biopsy. Am. J. Clin. Pathol., 70:27, 1978.

Popowich, L. and Heydt, S.: Tuberculous cervical lymphadenitis. J. Oral Maxillofac. Surg., 40:552, 1982.

Racine, W.: Le syndrome salivaire pre-menstrual. Schweiz. Med. Wochenschr., 69:1204, 1939.

Ramanathan, K., Omar-Ahmad, U. D., Kutty, M. K., Dutt, A. K., Balasegaram, M., Singh, H., and Keat, T. C.: Oral rhinosporidiosis in Malaysia. Dent. J. Malaysia Singapore, 9:No. 1, 1969.

Reichart, P.: Facial and oral manifestations in leprosy. Oral Surg., 41:385, 1976.

Reichart, P., Ananatasan, T., and Reznik, G.: Gingiva and periodontium in lepromatous leprosy. A clinical, radiological, and microscopical study. J. Periodont., 47:455, 1976.

Reichart, P. A., Srisuwan, S., and Metah, D.: Lesions of the facial and trigeminal nerve in leprosy. An evaluation of 43 cases. Int. J. Oral Surg., 11:14, 1982.

Reiches, A. J.: Antibiotic sensitivity and moniliasis. Arch. Dermatol. Syph., 64:604, 1951.

Renner, R. P., Lee, M., Andors, L., and McNamara, T. F.: The role of C. albicans in denture stomatitis. Oral Surg., 47:323, 1979.

Rickles, N. H., and Bernier, J. L.: Cat-scratch disease. Oral Surg., 13:282, 1960.

Ridley, D. S., and Jopling, W. H.: Classification of leprosy according to immunity. A five-group system. Int. J. Lep., 34:255, 1966.

Robbins, S. L., and Cotran, R. S.: Pathologic Basis of Disease. 2nd ed. Philadelphia, W. B. Saunders Company, 1979.

Robinson, C. R., Doane, F. W., and Rhodes, A. J.: Report of an outbreak of febrile illness with pharyngeal lesions and exanthem: Toronto, 1957, isolation of group A Coxsackie virus. Can. Med. Assoc. J., 79:615, 1958.

Robinson, H. B. G., and Ennever, J.: Etiology and diagnosis of actinomycosis. Oral Surg., 1:850, 1948.

Roed-Petersen, B., Renstrup, G., and Pindborg, J. J.: Candida in oral leukoplakias. Scand. J. Dent. Res., 78:323, 1970.

Rogers, R. S., III, and Tindall, J. P.: Herpes zoster in children. Arch. Derm., 106:204, 1972.

Rosebury, T.: The parasitic actinomycetes and other filamentous microorganisms of the mouth. Bacteriol. Rev., 8:189, 1944.

Roset, E. E.: Glosopeda Humana. An. Esp. Odontoestomatol., 21:927, 1962.

Rowe, N. H., Brooks, S. L., Young, S. K., Spencer, J., Petrick, T. J., Buchanan, R. A., Drach, J. C., and Shipman, C., Jr.: A clinical trial of topically applied 3 per cent vidarabine against recurrent herpes labialis. Oral Surg., 47:142, 1979.

Rowe, N. H., Heine, C. S., and Kowalski, C. J.: Herpetic whitlow: an occupational disease of practicing dentists. J. Am. Dent. Assoc., 105:471, 1982.

Sabin, A. B.: Varicella-zoster virus vaccine. J. Am. Med. Assoc., 238:1731, 1977.

Sanders, M., Kiem, I., and Lagunoff, D.: Cultivation of viruses: a critical review. Arch. Pathol., 56:148, 1953.

Sandstead, H. R., Koehn, C. J., and Sessions, S. M.: Enlargement of the parotid gland in malnutrition. Am. J. Clin. Nutr., 3:198, 1955.

Sapp, J. P., and Brooke, R. I.: Intranuclear inclusion bodies in recurrent aphthous ulcers with a herpetiform pattern. Oral Surg., 43:416, 1977.

Sarosi, G. A., and Davies, S. F.: Blastomycosis. State of the art. Am. Rev. Respir. Dis., 120:911, 1979.

Schmidt, H., Hjørting-Hansen, E., and Philipsen, H. P.: Gonococcal stomatitis. Acta Derm. Venereol., 41:324, 1961.

Schultz, E. W.: Some recent advances in the study of viruses and virus diseases. J. Am. Dent. Assoc., 26:434, 1939.

Schwartz, A. W., Devine, K. D., and Beahrs, O. H.: Acute postoperative mumps ("surgical mumps"). Plast. Reconstr. Surg., 25:51, 1960.

Scully, C.: Orofacial manifestations of chronic granulomatous disease of childhood. Oral Surg., 51:148, 1981.

Selye, H.: Effect of cortisone and somatotrophic hormone upon the development of a noma-like condition in the rat. Oral Surg., 6:557, 1953.

Selye, H., Veilleux, R., and Cantin, M.: Excessive stimulation of salivary gland growth by isoproterenol. Science, 133:44, 1961.

Shafer, W. G., and Muhler, J. C.: Endocrine influences upon the salivary glands. N.Y. Acad. Sci., 85:215, 1960.

Shaffer, E. L., Jr., Reimann, B. E. F., and Gysland, W. B.: Oral condyloma acuminatum. J. Oral Pathol., 9:163, 1980.

Shapiro, S., Olson, D. L., and Chellemi, S. J.: The association between smoking and aphthous ulcers. Oral Surg., 30:624, 1970.

Shengold, M. A., and Sheingold, H.: Oral tuberculosis. Oral Surg., 4:239, 1951.

Sheridan, P. J., and Hermann, E. C.: Intraoral lesions of adults associated with herpes simplex virus. Oral Surg., 32:390, 1971.

Ship, I. I., Ashe, W. K., and Scherp, H. W.: Recurrent "fever blister" and "canker sore." Tests for herpes simplex and other viruses with mammalian cell cultures. Arch. Oral Biol., 3:117, 1961.

Ship, I. I., Brightman, V. J., and Laster, L. L.: The patient with recurrent aphthous ulcers and the patient with recurrent herpes labialis: a study of two population samples. J. Am. Dent. Assoc., 75:645, 1967.

Ship, I. I., Pendleton, R. G., and White, C. L.: Effects of topical corticosteroids on aphthous ulcerations. Dent. Proc., 1:204, 1961.

Ship, I. I., Morris, A. L., Durocher, R. T., and Burket, L. W.: Recurrent aphthous ulcerations and recurrent herpes labialis in a professional school student population. Oral Surg., 13:1191, 1317, 1438, 1960; 14:30, 1961.

Siltzbach, L. E.: The Kveim test in sarcoidosis. A study of 750 patients. J.A.M.A., 178:476, 1961.

Silverman, S., Jr., and Beumer, J.: Primary herpetic gingivostomatitis of adult onset. Oral Surg., 36:496, 1973.

Small, I. A., and Kobernick, S.: Botryomycosis of the tongue. Oral Surg., 24:503, 1967.

Smith, M. G.: Propagation of a cytopathenogenic virus from salivary gland virus disease of infants in tissue cultures. Am. J. Pathol., 32:641, 1956.

Smith, M. G., and Vellios, F.: Inclusion disease of generalized salivary gland virus infection. Arch. Pathol., *50*:862, 1950.

Smith, M. J. A., and Myall, R. W. T.: Tetanus: review of the literature and report of a case. Oral Surg., *41*:451, 1976.

Southam, J. C., and Venkataraman, B. K.: Oral manifestations of leprosy. Br. J. Oral Surg., *10*:272, 1973.

Stagno, S.: Congenital toxoplasmosis. Am. J. Dis. Child., *134*:635, 1980.

Steigman, A. J., Lipton, M. M., and Braspennickx, H.: Acute lymphonodular pharyngitis: a newly described condition due to Coxsackie A virus. J. Pediatr., *61*:331, 1963.

Stenhouse, D., MacDonald, D. G., and MacFarlane, T. W.: Cervico-facial and intra-oral actinomycosis: a 5-year retrospective study. Br. J. Oral Surg., *13*:172, 1975.

Sternlicht, H. C.: Herpes zoster: report of a case. Oral Surg., *7*:60, 1954.

Stevens, D. A. (ed.): Coccidioidomycosis. A Text. New York, Plenum Medical Book Co., 1980.

Stewart, J. P.: Progressive lethal granulomatous ulceration of the nose. J. Laryngol. Otol., *48*:657, 1933.

Stiff, R. H.: Histoplasmosis. Oral Surg., *16*:140, 1963.

Sutton, R. L., Jr.: Recurrent scarring painful aphthae. J.A.M.A., *117*:175, 1941.

Swan, R. H., McDaniel, R. K., Dreiman, B. B., and Rome, W. C.: Condyloma acuminatum involving the oral mucosa. Oral Surg., *51*:503, 1981.

Taylor, C. G., Alexander, R. E., Green, W. H., and Kramer, H. S.: Mucormycosis (phycomycosis) involving the maxilla. Oral Surg., *27*:806, 1969.

Thompson, W. C.: Uveoparotitis. Arch. Intern. Med., *59*:646, 1937.

Timosca, G., and Gavrilita, L.: Cysticercosis of the maxillofacial region. A clinicopathologic study of five cases. Oral Surg., *37*:390, 1974.

Tokumaru, T.: A possible role of gamma-A-immunoglobulin in herpes simplex virus infection in man. J. Immunol., *97*:248, 1966.

Topazian, R. G.: Rhinosporidiosis of the parotid duct. Br. J. Oral Surg., *4*:12, 1966.

Trieger, N.: Cat-scratch fever. Oral Surg., *10*:383, 1957.

Tsokos, M., Fauci, A. S., and Costa, J.: Idiopathic midline destructive disease (IMDD). A subgroup of patients with the "midline granuloma" syndrome. Am. J. Clin. Path., *77*:162, 1982.

Turner, R., Shehab, Z., Osborne, K., and Hendley, J. O.: Shedding and survival of herpes simplex virus from "fever blisters." Pediatrics, *70*:547, 1982.

VanHale, H. M., Rogers, R. S., Doyle, J. A., and Schroeter, A. L.: Immunofluorescence microscopic studies of recurrent aphthous stomatitis. Arch. Dermatol., *117*:779, 1981.

van Maarsseveen, A. C. M. Th., van der Waal, I., Stam, J., Veldhuizen, R. W., and van der Kwast, W. A. M.: Oral involvement in sarcoidosis. Int. J. Oral Surg., *11*:21, 1982.

Weathers, D. R., and Griffin, J. W.: Intraoral ulcerations of recurrent herpes simplex and recurrent aphthae:

two distinct clinical entities. J. Am. Dent. Assoc., *81*:81, 1970.

Weed, L. A., and Parkhill, E. M.: The diagnosis of histoplasmosis in ulcerative disease of the mouth and pharynx. Am. J. Clin. Pathol., *18*:130, 1948.

Weichselbaum, P. K., and Derbes, V. J.: Chronic scarring aphthous ulcers of the mouth. Oral Surg., *10*:370, 1957.

Weinberger, H. W., Ropes, M. W., Kulka, J. P., and Bauer, W.: Reiter's syndrome, clinical and pathologic observations. Medicine, *41*:35, 1962.

Wesley, R. K., Osborn, T. P., and Dylewski, J. J.: Periapical actinomycosis: clinical considerations. J. Endocrinol., *3*:352, 1977.

Wheeler, C. E., Jr., and Huffines, W. C.: Primary disseminated herpes simplex of the newborn. J.A.M.A., *191*:455, 1965.

Williams, H. L.: Lethal granulomatous ulceration involving the midline facial tissue. Ann. Otol., Rhinol. Laryngol., *58*:1013, 1949.

Williams, H. L., and Hochfilzer, J. J.: Effect of cortisone on idiopathic granuloma of the midline tissues of the face. Ann. Otol., Rhinol. Laryngol., *59*:518, 1950.

Witorsch, P., and Utz, J. P.: North American blastomycosis: a study of 40 patients. Medicine, *47*:169, 1968.

Witzleben, C. L., and Driscoll, S. G.: Possible transplacental transmission of herpes simplex infection. Pediatrics, *36*:192, 1965.

Wolf, J. E., and Ebel, L. K.: Chronic granulomatous disease: report of case and review of the literature. J. Am. Dent. Assoc., *96*:292, 1978.

Wood, T. A., Jr., DeWitt, S. H., Chu, E. W., Rabson, A. S., and Graykowski, E. A.: Anitschkow nuclear changes observed in oral smears. Acta Cytol., *19*:434, 1975.

Woodburne, A. R.: Herpetic stomatitis (aphthous stomatitis). Arch. Dermatol. Syph., *43*:543, 1941.

Woods, J. W., Manning, I. H., Jr., and Patterson, C. N.: Monilial infections complicating the therapeutic use of antibiotics. J.A.M.A., *145*:207, 1951.

Wray, D., Ferguson, M. M., Hutcheon, A. W., and Dagg, J. H.: Nutritional deficiencies in recurrent aphthae. J. Oral Pathol., *7*:418, 1978.

Wyngaarden, J. B., and Smith, L. H., Jr.: Cecil Textbook of Medicine. 16th ed. Philadelphia, W. B. Saunders Company, 1982.

Wysocki, G. P., and Brooke, R. I.: Oral manifestations of chronic granulomatous disease. Oral Surg., *46*:815, 1978.

Young, S. K., Rowe, N. H., and Buchanan, R. A.: A clinical study of the control of facial mucocutaneous herpes virus infections. I. Characterization of natural history in a professional school population. Oral Surg., *41*:498, 1976.

Zahorsky, J.: Herpetic sore throat. South. Med. J., *13*:871, 1920.

Idem: Herpangina (a specific disease). Arch Pediatr., *41*:181, 1924.

Ziskin, D. E., Shoham, J., and Hanford, J. M.: Actinomycosis: a report of 26 cases. Am. J. Orthod. Oral Surg., *29*:193, 1943.

CHAPTER 7

Dental Caries

Dental caries is a microbial disease of the calcified tissues of the teeth, characterized by demineralization of the inorganic portion and destruction of the organic substance of the tooth. It is the most prevalent chronic disease affecting the human race. Once it occurs, its manifestations persist throughout life even though the lesion is treated. There are practically no geographic areas in the world whose inhabitants do not exhibit some evidence of dental caries. It affects persons of both sexes in all races, all socio-economic strata and every age group. It usually begins soon after the teeth erupt into the oral cavity. Persons who never develop carious lesions are designated "caries-free." No satisfactory explanation of their caries resistance has been found (Fig. 7–1).

Hundreds of dental research investigators for more than a century have studied various aspects of the dental caries problem. Despite this extensive investigation, many aspects of etiology are still obscure, and efforts at prevention have been only partially successful.

THE EPIDEMIOLOGY OF DENTAL CARIES

Dental caries may properly be considered a disease of modern civilization, since prehistoric man rarely suffered from this form of tooth destruction. Anthropologic studies of von Lenhossek revealed that the dolichocephalic skulls of men from preneolithic periods (12,000 B.C.) did not exhibit dental caries, but skulls from brachycephalic man of the neolithic period (12,000 to 3000 B.C.) contained carious teeth. In most instances the lesions were noted in older persons in teeth which showed severe attrition and impaction of food. The cervical areas were affected frequently.

Caries Incidence in Modern Societies. Extensive studies have been made of the incidence of dental caries. These have encompassed every part of the globe and serve to emphasize the worldwide distribution of this disease. Because the literature on the epidemiology of dental caries is so vast, only a summary review will be

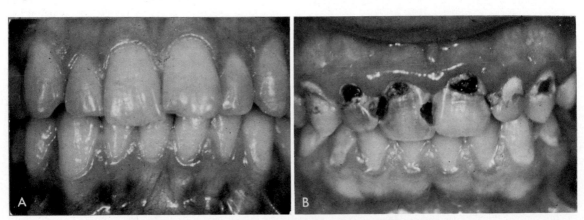

Figure 7–1. *The caries-resistant and caries-susceptible mouth.*

406

given. It will suffice to cite a number of studies from various geographic areas involving different races to illustrate the apparent influence of civilization on dental disease.

Mellanby in 1934 reviewed the literature on caries in existing primitive races and noted that the incidence was invariably less than that in modern man.

Eskimos living in native villages away from contact with so-called civilized man have a low incidence of carious lesions. Rosebury and Karshan found that among members of one isolated village 1.2 per cent of the teeth examined were carious, whereas in a village where a trader lived and dealt in processed foods, the incidence of carious teeth was 18.1 per cent. Price reported that Alaskan Eskimos living under isolated conditions exhibited a caries incidence of approximately 0.1 per cent, while Eskimos living in areas with access to processed foods showed an incidence of 13 per cent of the teeth examined.

A comparable effect of diet upon caries was demonstrated by Mellanby in studies on natives of Southern Rhodesia. About 5 per cent of the adults who had eaten European foods for only a short period had evidence of dental caries. On the other hand, about 20 per cent of the adolescents who had eaten such foods over a somewhat longer period of time had carious lesions. Of the children who had been in contact with European customs and foods for most of their lives, 50 per cent had carious teeth. Similar results have been reported in studies of native Samoans by Restarski, Maoris by Pickerill and Bedouins by Clawson.

These studies indicate that modern civilization and increased dental caries are constant in their association and that primitive isolated tribes are relatively caries-free. Although there may be a certain degree of racial resistance to dental caries, the dietary factor appears to be more significant, especially since the caries incidence is increased by contact with "civilized" foods.

Some studies show remarkable differences in caries experience between the various races. American blacks and whites, living in the same geographic area under similar conditions, offer an excellent opportunity for comparison. Investigations indicate that the black has fewer carious lesions than the white.

Thus, McRae reported that 74 per cent of 3188 white children in grades 1 to 6 in Tennessee had carious lesions, whereas only 41 per cent of 1096 blacks of the same age group in

this area were affected by caries. Brucker found that 20 per cent of 951 black boys and 26 per cent of 871 black girls were caries-free, while only 11 per cent of 3845 white boys and 9 per cent of 3602 white girls exhibited no cavities. In a study by Sebelius, the DMF (decayed, missing and filled teeth) average in a group of 2928 white children between the ages of 3 to 17 years was 4.0 teeth, while that of 2917 black children of the same ages was 3.1 teeth.

Most studies concerning other races have been relatively unsatisfactory because of complicating factors such as differences in diet or exposure to fluoride, which tend to mask any true differences due to racial background. Nevertheless there is some evidence to indicate that blacks, Chinese and East Indians average considerably less caries than American whites. The English have notoriously poor teeth and a higher caries incidence than Italians, Russians or Chinese.

CARIES INCIDENCE IN THE AMERICAN WHITE RACE. The incidence of dental caries among white persons in the United States varies with age, sex and geographic location. Numerous epidemiologic studies have been carried out to establish baselines of caries experience. These show that there are no areas in the United States which have been investigated where the people are totally free of caries. Caries in children of many localities begins shortly after eruption of the deciduous teeth and may continue to increase at a remarkable rate. The exposure of children during the period of tooth formation to a water supply containing either naturally occurring or artificially added fluoride greatly influences the prevalence of caries. This will be discussed later.

As children reach school age, they have an increasing incidence of carious lesions. In the United States, the caries increment averages approximately 1 DMF tooth and 2 DMF surfaces per child per year of school attendance. Klein, Palmer and Knutson examined the entire elementary school population of Hagerstown, Maryland—4416 children between the ages of six and 15 years—and reported the results in 1938. They found that 50 per cent of the boys and 56 per cent of the girls had dental caries in the permanent teeth by the age of eight years. By the age of 14, this caries experience rate had risen to 95 per cent in boys and 96 per cent in girls. The DMF index for the 14-year-old children, males and females combined, was 5.23 teeth. In contrast, Finn examined 5824 children in Newburgh and Kingston, New York, and found that the DMF index for the 14-year-old children, sexes combined, was 8.55 teeth. Approximately 98 per cent of the children of this age had decay experience. Thus there are some variations in the prevalence of dental caries among persons of the same age in different locations, but this difference is negligible with respect to over-all caries experience. Some differences between studies can be explained by the means used in examining the patients. Obviously, a far more thorough examination can be made with a mouth mirror, explorer and roentgenograms than by inspection with the aid of a tongue blade only. In fact, Blayney and Greco showed that over 50 per cent more proximal carious lesions were found through use of roentgenograms than by a thorough clinical examination with mirror and explorer.

One further variation in caries incidence, aside from age and geographic area, is that between the sexes. Studies indicate that the total caries experience in permanent teeth is greater in females than in males of the same age. Conversely, the caries experience in deciduous teeth is greater in males. It has been suggested that this apparent sex difference in caries prevalence is related to the difference in eruption times of teeth and to the length of exposure of the teeth to the oral environment. It is possible that other factors may also be important in this sex difference in caries.

Current Trends in Caries Incidence. Significant data have been presented since 1980 to substantiate the numerous observations that there has been marked improvement in dental health as measured by prevalence of dental caries, especially in children and young adults, not only in the United States but throughout the "civilized Western world" since approximately 1960. This trend has become so definitively established that the First International Conference on the Declining Prevalence of Dental Caries was held at the Forsyth Dental Center in Boston in June 1982 to evaluate "the evidence and the impact on dental education, dental research and dental practice." Its proceedings were edited by Glass and published in the Journal of Dental Research (1982).

Studies carried out under the National Caries Program in 1979–80 and reported by Brunelle and Carlos on 38,000 schoolchildren, aged 5 to 17 years, representative of approximately 48 million U.S. schoolchildren, revealed a substantial decrease in prevalence of dental caries in the last decade. Especially impressive was the increase in the percentage of children classified

as caries-free in their permanent dentitions; for example, in the 12–17 year group in the 1971–74 survey, 9.7 per cent of the children were caries-free, while in the 1979–80 survey, 17.2 per cent were caries-free. Just since the previous survey in 1971–74, the decayed, missing and filled permanent tooth surfaces in the 5–17 year age group declined from 7.06 to 4.77.

Glass reported trends in caries prevalence in 1775 children 7 to 13 years of age analyzed over a period of 20 years in Massachusetts. He similarly reported that dental caries prevalence had decreased by about 50 per cent and extractions due to caries decreased by 70 per cent. In addition, secondary caries had decreased to near zero. These changes had occurred in the absence of fluoridation and organized preventive programs. DePaola and his associates reported decreases of a similar magnitude in surveys on 9000 schoolchildren over a 30-year span.

It is significant and gratifying that such an improvement in dental health was not limited to those living in the United States. Data revealing a decline in caries prevalence also were reported at this conference by representatives from England, Denmark, Ireland, the Netherlands, New Zealand, Norway, Scotland and Sweden. Unfortunately, it was acknowledged that the prevalence of caries has been reported to be increasing in certain less-developed countries.

The causes for this widespread decline in the prevalence of dental caries is a matter of speculation but is almost certainly multifactorial. In some instances, communal water fluoridation has been present in the areas studied, but in other instances, it has not. Organized preventive dentistry programs had been available in some cases but not in others. However, the time period involved in most of these studies does coincide with the introduction and increased utilization of fluoride dentifrices and dietary fluoride supplements, as well as an increased awareness of the importance of oral health. Unfortunately, there have been no systematic studies of possible changes in oral microflora in recent years. However, the very limited studies available give no evidence that there is any change, for example, in the pervasiveness of *Streptococcus mutans* or any changes in dominant serotypes. Finally, dietary habits and eating patterns are difficult factors to study and analyze. However, there has been an obvious movement toward improved physical health through food and exercise in the past decade, although this has been directed more toward adults than children. Still, it is conceivable that a reduction in carbohydrate consumption might be related to this reduction of caries prevalence. Data from the United States Department of Agriculture in 1981, however, show no evidence of a reduction in the per capita consumption of sugar in this country during the past decade.

It now appears that the continued reduction of dental caries, from whatever combination of factors, coupled with the use of additional agents and techniques now in various stages of research and development, could result in the near total elimination of dental caries in the very forseeable future.

ECONOMIC IMPLICATIONS OF DENTAL CARIES

Surveys by the Bureau of Economic and Behavioral Research of the American Dental Association and by the Office of Health Research, Statistics, and Technology of the U.S. Department of Health and Human Services, from which the following data are derived, have been helpful in characterizing certain economic aspects of dental care in the United States. Statistical evaluation of such large surveys often delays reporting of results for several years, but the information gained is often crucial to future planning.

In 1976, ten billion dollars was spent in the United States for dental care. This represents 6.2 per cent of the total health expenditure, a gradual decline from 7.8 per cent of the total expenditure in 1950.

An estimated average of 107 million persons in the civilian noninstitutionalized population, or about 50 per cent of the population, had made at least one visit to a dentist in the year preceding 1978–79. This was a marked increase from 42 per cent in 1963–64, although since 1973 the percentage had remained rather constant.

There is a striking relationship between family income, education and percentage of persons visiting the dentist. It has been found that when the income was less than $5,000 per year, only 34 per cent of the persons visited the dentist in a given year, whereas with an income over $15,000 per year, 61.9 per cent visited the dentist during the same period. Of those with less than nine years of education, 30.2 per cent made a dental visit, but of those with more than

12 years of education, 64.1 per cent made such a visit. Furthermore, between 85 and 91 per cent of all practicing dentists in the United States (depending upon location, type of practice, age and a variety of other factors) are general practitioners whose major responsibility and service rendered are restorative fillings. Although no specific survey data are available since 1965, when in the United States the dentists' income from restorative fillings was approximately $1,224,000,000, obviously this total has been far surpassed today. In addition, insurance programs and prepayment plans are having an impact on dental economics. An increasing number of dental insurance programs permits an increasing number of people to avail themselves of dental care. Thus in 1976, a total of $1,609,300,000 was expended for dental care to approximately 46,500,000 beneficiaries.

These costs of primary dental care paid directly or indirectly to the dentist do not include the cost of oral hygiene products of all types sold in the marketplace. Data from Health Care Financing Review (1981) indicate that more than $1,350,000,000 is spent annually in the United States for oral hygiene products, including dentifrices (approximately 45 per cent of the total amount spent), denture products, toothbrushes, mouthwashes, and dental floss, at least some of which do contribute to oral health.

The increasing economic status of the population and their increasing educational status, the growing number of dental graduates, insurance programs, commercial pressures and governmental influences are just some of the factors that are changing the economic implications of treatment of dental caries. Nevertheless, the fact still remains that 45.5 per cent of the people over 64 years of age have both dental arches edentulous and that huge segment of the population is not being treated for dental diseases.

THE ETIOLOGY OF DENTAL CARIES

The etiology of dental caries is generally agreed to be a complex problem complicated by many indirect factors which obscure the direct cause or causes. There is no universally accepted opinion of the etiology of dental caries. However, two chief theories have evolved through years of investigation and observation: the acidogenic theory (Miller's chemico-parasitic theory), and the proteolytic theory. More recently a third theory, the proteolysis-chelation theory, has been proposed.

THE ACIDOGENIC THEORY

A number of investigators prior to Miller had made significant contributions to the problem of caries etiology. One of the earliest observations was that of Leber and Rotenstein, who, in 1867, reported finding microorganisms in carious lesions and suggested that dental caries was due to the activity of acid-producing bacteria. Clark (1871, 1879), Tomes (1873) and Magitot (1878) concurred in the belief that bacteria were essential to caries which was produced by acids, although they suggested an exogenous source of the acids. Underwood and Milles in 1881 found microorganisms in carious dentin and reported that caries was due primarily to bacteria which affected the organic portion of the tooth, liberating acid and dissolving the inorganic elements.

W. D. Miller, probably the best known of the early investigators of dental caries, published extensively on the results of studies, beginning in 1882. These culminated in the following hypothesis in which he stated: "Dental decay is a chemico-parasitic process consisting of two stages, the decalcification of enamel, which results in its total destruction and the decalcification of dentin, as a preliminary stage, followed by dissolution of the softened residue. The acid which affects this primary decalcification is derived from the fermentation of starches and sugar lodged in the retaining centers of the teeth." Miller found that bread, meat and sugar, incubated in vitro with saliva at body temperature, produced enough acid within 48 hours to decalcify sound dentin. The acid formation could be prevented by boiling, confirming the probable role of bacteria in its production. Subsequently he isolated numerous microorganisms from the oral cavity, many of which were acidogenic and some of which were proteolytic. Since a number of these bacterial forms were capable of forming lactic acid, Miller believed that caries was not caused by any single organism, but rather by a variety of microorganisms.

This theory has been accepted by the majority of investigators in a form essentially unchanged since its inception. The bulk of scientific evidence does implicate carbohydrates, oral microorganisms and acids, and for this reason these deserve further consideration.

The Role of Carbohydrates. Reference has been made previously to the finding that members of isolated primitive societies who have a relatively low caries index manifest a remarkable increase in caries incidence after exposure to "civilized" or refined diets. The presence of readily fermentable carbohydrates has been thought to be responsible for their loss of caries resistance. Numerous studies confirm this belief.

The early crude studies of Miller showed that when teeth were incubated in mixtures of saliva and bread or sugar, decalcification occurred. There was no effect on the teeth when meat or fat was used in place of the carbohydrate. Both cane sugar and cooked starches produced acid, but little acid was formed when raw starches were substituted. Volker and Pinkerton reported the production of similar quantities of acid from mixtures of either sucrose or starch incubated with saliva with no differences in acid production between raw and refined sugar cane.

In the United States, carbohydrates contribute from 50 to 60 per cent of the total daily caloric intake. Fermentable carbohydrates compose 25 to 50 per cent of this carbohydrate component. The cariogenic carbohydrates are dietary in origin, since uncontaminated human saliva contains only negligible amounts regardless of the blood sugar level. Salivary carbohydrates are bound to proteins and other compounds and are not readily available for microbial degradation. The cariogenicity of a dietary carbohydrate varies with the frequency of ingestion, physical form, chemical composition, route of administration and presence of other food constituents. Sticky, solid carbohydrates are more caries-producing than those consumed as liquids. Carbohydrates in detergent foods are less damaging to the teeth than the same substances in soft retentive foods. Carbohydrates which are rapidly cleared from the oral cavity by saliva and swallowing are less conducive to caries than those which are slowly cleared. Polysaccharides are less easily fermented by plaque bacteria than monosaccharides and disaccharides. Plaque organisms produce little acid from the sugar alcohols, sorbitol and mannitol. Glucose or sucrose, fed entirely by stomach tube or intravenously, does not contribute to decay as they are unavailable for microbial breakdown. Meals high in fat, protein or salt reduce the oral retentiveness of carbohydrates. Refined, pure carbohydrates are more caries-producing than crude carbohydrates complexed with other food elements capable of reducing enamel solubility or possessing antibacterial properties.

The Role of Microorganisms. The bacteriology of dental caries has a long and interesting history, but began in earnest scientifically only with the investigations of Miller. His work in isolating 22 different types of microorganisms from the oral cavity has already been mentioned. In 1900 Goadby isolated a gram-positive bacillus from carious dentin and termed it *B. necrodentalis*. Gies and Kligler, in 1915, made an extensive study of oral microorganisms and found high numbers in persons with caries. In the early stages of the disease, there was an alteration in abundance of certain forms in the oral cavity. Clarke, in 1924, described a new streptococcus species, *S. mutans*, which was almost invariably isolated from carious lesions in the teeth of British patients. Although the work was confirmed three years later by McLean, scientific interest in *S. mutans* lay dormant until its explosive rediscovery in the mid 1960's.

Many of the earlier workers focused attention on *L. acidophilus* because it was found with such frequency in caries-susceptible persons that it came to be regarded as of etiologic importance. Bunting, Nickerson and Hard carried out extensive studies on this organism and reported that it was almost universally absent in the mouths of caries-immune persons, but was usually present in the mouths of caries-susceptible persons. Similar findings were reported in 1927 by Jay and Voorhees, who also found that the presence of *L. acidophilus* in persons without active caries was often a portent of the development of cavities some months later. Bunting stated in 1928: "So definite is this correlation (between *B. acidophilus* and dental caries) that, in the opinion of this group, the presence or absence of *B. acidophilus* in the mouth constitutes a definite criterion of the activity of dental caries that is more accurate than any clinical estimation can be. Furthermore, it was noted that there was a spontaneous cessation of caries coincident with the disappearance of *B. acidophilus* from the mouth, either from prophylactic, therapeutic or dietetic control." Jay reported the isolation of 12 strains of Leptothrix in 1927, but doubted their importance in the carious process even though they produced acid from carbohydrates.

Between this period and the 1940's, numerous studies were carried out in attempts to confirm or deny the existence of a microorganism responsible for dental caries. Numerous workers such as Arnold and McClure and Becks, Jensen and Millarr reported a close correlation between the *L. acidophilus* counts and caries activity in large series of clinical patients. The latter group found that 88 per cent of 1250 persons with rampant caries had lactobacillus indices above 1000 colonies per ml of saliva when cultured on selective media, whereas 82 per cent of a group of 265 caries-free persons exhibited indices below 1000. Florestano, in 1942, cultured organisms from the saliva of carious and noncarious persons and studied their acidogenic potential. Aciduric streptococci and staphylococci were isolated from both groups of subjects. Their acid production and presence in large numbers suggested a role in dental caries equal to that of lactobacilli.

Bacteriologic studies in recent years have helped clarify the role of various organisms in the etiology of dental caries. Considerable emphasis has been placed on the various dieto-bacterial interactions which are involved in lesion development on different tooth surfaces. Specific microorganisms as well as combinations of organisms, including Lactobacillus, *Streptococcus mutans*, Actinomyces species and others, have been studied. Although there may be disagreement as to specifics, there is little doubt that bacteria are indispensable to the production of caries. The evidence does indicate that a number of organisms, including both streptococci and lactobacilli, are intimately associated with dental caries. The possibility exists that one or more organisms are implicated in the *initiation* of caries, while other distinctly different organisms may influence the *progression* of the disease. The two separate phases must be differentiated. Also, there is now good evidence that different dieto-bacterial interactions are involved in root surface and coronal caries, and they may represent two different diseases from the ecological and microbiological point of view.

In 1960, Keyes demonstrated that under certain laboratory conditions, dental caries in hamsters and rats could be considered an infectious and transmissible disease and therefore subject to those biologic principles which govern any infectious process. Fitzgerald and Keyes showed that even in a so-called caries-inactive strain of hamster, oral inoculation of certain pure cultures of streptococci isolated from hamster caries would induce the typical picture of active dental caries. The caries-inactive strain of hamster was found to have a noncariogenic microflora. These findings have led to interesting speculation about the importance of streptococci in the etiology of dental caries.

Confirmatory studies have been reported by Fitzgerald and his associates, who maintained gnotobiotic (germ-free) rats on a coarse-particle, high-sugar diet which produces dental caries in the normal animal. In these germ-free animals no caries developed until the animals were inoculated with a single strain of oral streptococcus isolated from a control rat on the same diet. The animals then suffered extensive cavitation of the molars which closely resembled that seen in the nongerm-free animals.

It is now recognized that the streptococcal organisms studied by Keyes and Fitzgerald were actually rodent strains of *Streptococcus mutans*, a very powerful and efficient cariogenic microorganism. The "rediscovery" surge of clinical and epidemiologic studies in many parts of the world has revealed that *S. mutans* is pandemic in its geographic distribution and is particularly prevalent in societies where sucrose consumption is high, such as England, the Scandinavian countries and the United States.

The Role of Acids. The exact mechanism of carbohydrate degradation to form acids in the oral cavity by bacterial action is not known. It probably occurs through enzymatic breakdown of the sugar, and the acids formed are chiefly lactic acid, although others such as butyric acid do occur. The fact that acid production appears to be dependent upon a series of enzyme systems has suggested a method of decreasing this acid formation by interference with certain of the enzymes. This will be considered at greater length in the section on Methods of Caries Control. The myth that acidic saliva causes tooth decay should be dispelled. It leads the patient to believe that little can be done to prevent dental caries.

The mere presence of acid in the oral cavity is of far less significance than the localization of acid upon the tooth surface. This suggests a mechanism for holding acids at a given point for relatively long periods. It is generally agreed that the structure known as the "dental plaque" fulfills this function.

The Role of the Dental Plaque. The dental plaque (microbial plaque or bacterial plaque) is a structure of vital significance as a contributing factor to at least the initiation of the carious lesion. It has been recognized for many years and was demonstrated in histologic preparations by Williams in 1897.

Although Miller emphasized the role of foods and the acids produced by bacterial degradation of them, he thought that the plaque protected the enamel against attack by the carious process. In contrast, G. V. Black regarded the plaque as important in the caries process and,

in 1899, described it thus: "The gelatinous plaque of the caries fungus is a thin, transparent film that usually escapes observation, and which is revealed only by careful search. It is not the thick mass of materia alba so frequently found upon the teeth, nor is it the whitish gummy material known as sordes, which is often prominent in fevers and often present in the mouth in smaller quantities in the absence of fever." He was confident of its importance in the carious process.

The dental plaque, or microcosm, as denoted by Arnim, is variable in both chemical and physical composition, but generally consists of such salivary components as mucin and desquamated epithelial cells and of microorganisms. It characteristically forms on tooth surfaces which are not constantly cleansed and appears as a tenacious, thin film which may accumulate to a perceptible degree in 24 to 48 hours (Fig. 7–2). An important component of dental plaque is *acquired pellicle*, which forms just prior to or concomitantly with bacterial colonization and may facilitate plaque formation. The pellicle is a glycoprotein that is derived from the saliva and is adsorbed on tooth surfaces. It is not dependent on bacteria but may serve as a nutrient for plaque microorganisms.

There is general agreement that enamel caries begins beneath the dental plaque. The presence of a plaque, however, does not necessarily mean that a carious lesion will develop at that point. Variations in caries formation have been attributed to the nature of the plaque itself, to the saliva or to the tooth. A fertile area for further investigation still exists.

Bibby (1931) emphasized that muco-bacterial films form on the surface of nearly all teeth, whether susceptible or resistant, so that the nature of the plaque must be important in the initiation of the carious lesion.

Extensive study of the bacterial flora of the dental plaque has indicated the heterogeneous nature of the structure. Most workers have stressed the presence of filamentous microorganisms, which grow in long interlacing threads and have the property of adhering to smooth enamel surfaces. Smaller bacilli and cocci then become entrapped in this reticular meshwork. Aciduric and acidogenic streptococci and lactobacilli are particularly numerous. Occasionally, strains of the filamentous organisms are actively acidogenic through carbohydrate fermentation, but this does not appear to be a general feature of this group.

Bibby (1940) studied the characteristics of

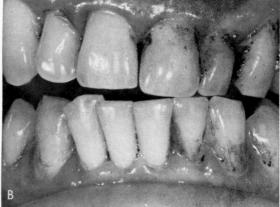

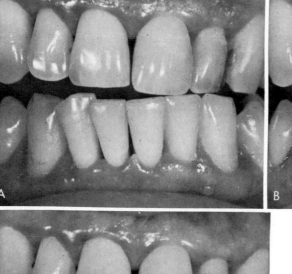

Figure 7–2. *Dental plaque.*
The appearance of the teeth in all quadrants is similar, although the teeth on one side were not brushed for three days *(A)*. The dental plaque on the unbrushed teeth becomes obvious after the application of a disclosing solution *(B)*. Brushing the teeth and reapplying disclosing solution reveals that the plaque, if in an accessible area, is readily removed by brushing. *(C)*.

different strains of filamentous organisms isolated from dental plaques and again noted their ability to adhere to smooth surfaces. Blayney and his associates (1942) studied plaque formation on teeth from the time of eruption until carious lesions were evident. They pointed out that the time required for the development of definite cavitation representing early caries in an intact enamel surface was several months. Hemmens and his co-workers (1946) believed that the dental plaque was the most likely starting point for investigation aimed at understanding the earliest stage of enamel caries. They examined numerous plaques from areas of children's teeth which became carious during the course of the investigation. The aciduric streptococci were the organisms most commonly isolated from plaques during the period of caries activity, being present in varying numbers in 86 per cent of the plaques. Alpha streptococci were isolated from slightly over 50 per cent of the plaques from carious surfaces and from 75 per cent of those from noncarious surfaces. The greatest incidence of occurrence

of lactobacilli in plaques was 57 per cent, but it was noted that these organisms increased in incidence during that period in which the carious lesions were developing.

It was once thought that the dental plaque, which is permeable to carbohydrates with the possible exception of starch, acted to hold the carbohydrate at a restricted site for a relatively long time. Stephan (1940) showed that this concept was incorrect and that carbohydrates permeating the plaque were degraded rapidly. He used an antimony microelectrode capable of measuring the pH in a dental plaque in situ. The pH of plaques in different persons varied, but averaged about 7.1 in caries-free persons to 5.5 in persons with extreme caries activity. Investigation of actual proximal cavities, opened mechanically, showed that the lowest pH varied from 4.6 to 4.1. Stephan also studied the pH in dental plaques after rinsing of the mouth with a 10 per cent glucose or sucrose solution. Within two to five minutes after the rinse, the pH in the plaque had fallen to between pH 4.5 and 5.0 and gradually returned to the initial pH

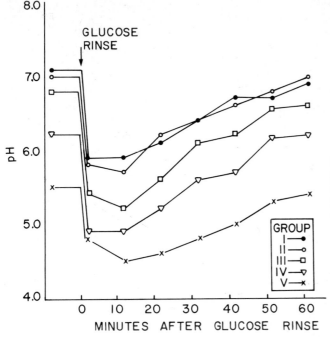

Figure 7–3. *The pH curves of plaques on labial surfaces of maxillary anterior teeth in different caries activity groups.*

Group I was caries-free; group II had previously had caries, but was caries-inactive during period of study; group III had slight caries activity; group IV had moderate caries activity; group V had extreme caries activity. (Courtesy of Dr. Robert M. Stephan: J. Dent. Res., 23:257, 1944.)

level within one to two hours (Fig. 7–3). Further studies indicated differences in reductions in pH in caries-free and caries-active subjects. The plaque pH in the caries-free group did not fall below 5.0 units after the glucose rinse, while the pH in the caries-active group fell below 5.0 units after the glucose rinse in over half the cases. The maxillary anterior teeth exhibited a greater pH drop in the plaque than the mandibular anterior teeth, indicating that the saliva influences plaque acid production. Brushing the teeth before the test carbohydrate rinse gave unsatisfactory plaque pH curves because of removal of plaque material.

Stralfors (1948) carried out studies similar to those of Stephan and in addition correlated the lowest level to which the plaque pH fell after the carbohydrate rinse with the lactobacillus count, utilizing this count as a test of caries activity. It was shown that persons with a higher pH minimum have a lower lactobacillus count and, presumably, lower caries activity. Stralfors also reported that the plaque has a much greater buffering capacity than saliva and that this is essentially due to the presence of bicarbonates and protein. Vratsanos and his colleagues studied plaque acidogenesis in caries-susceptible and caries-resistant patients both by in situ plaque pH measurement by antimony microelectrodes and through quantitative measurement of plaque acids by liquid chromatography. They found that plaque pH in caries-susceptible

persons was lower (6.1 ± 0.3) than in caries-resistant persons (7.3 ± 0.4) and that total plaque acid production was also significantly lower in the caries-resistant group.

Some studies have been devoted to investigation of substances capable of inhibiting the reduction in plaque pH after exposure to carbohydrate. Stephan and Miller (1943) applied several synthetic detergents and found at least partial inhibition of pH drop. One drawback is the penetration of the plaque by inhibitory substances. In thin plaques the inhibition is greater than in thick plaques. Application of urea has also been found effective by Stephan, apparently because of hydrolysis by bacterial urease, with the subsequent formation of ammonium carbonate.

Most investigations of the microbiology of the dental plaque have concluded that three basic groups of microorganisms predominate: streptococci, actinomyces and veillonellae. The major strains of streptococci present in plaque are *S. mutans, S. sanguis, S. mitior, S. milleri* and *S. salivarius* (uncommonly). Major actinomyces strains include *A. viscosus, A. naeslundi, A. israelii*, and *Rothia dentocariosa*. The veillonellae group are the anaerobic gram-negative cocci organisms, chiefly *V. parvula* and *V. alcalescens*. Of all these, *Streptococcus mutans* is considered today to be the chief etiologic agent in human dental caries.

An important discovery was the recognition

that certain cariogenic and highly acidogenic strains of streptococci, especially *S. mutans*, have the ability to metabolize dietary sucrose and synthesize glucan by cell-surface and extra-cellular glucosyltransferase. This enzyme is considered to be of special importance in the establishment of *S. mutans* in the dental plaque. This appears to occur through glucan on the *S. mutans* cell surface acting as the primary binding site for the enzyme, which then evokes new glucan synthesis from exogenous sucrose with subsequent adherence to the enamel surface. This glucan is an insoluble, sticky or slimy gel, relatively inert and resistant to bacterial hydrolytic enzymes, which causes plaque to adhere tenaciously to tooth surfaces and also appears to act as a barrier against the diffusion of salivary buffers which ordinarily would neutralize the acids formed in the plaque. The studies of Berman and Gibbons and of Jordan and Keyes in 1966 did much to clarify the role of this substance, while later studies by Gibbons and van Houte and by Loesche and his colleagues in 1975 have also added valuable information. In addition, Gibbons and Socransky demonstrated that certain cariogenic bacteria are capable of storing intracellular polysaccharides which may act as a reserve source of carbohydrate for fermentation and maintenance of acid production in the plaque during periods when the diet of the individual is sugar-free.

Both Bowen and Fitzgerald and his associates in 1968 studied dextranase, an enzyme produced by *Penicillium funiculosum* which hydrolyzes dextran (glucan) and found that it minimizes plaque formation and prevents smooth surface caries in experimental animals.

It is now generally and universally agreed that the accumulation of dental plaque, even on a clean tooth surface, can result in dental caries in an individual susceptible to the disease and consuming a diet conducive to the disease. This extremely important structure was reviewed in detail by Bilbiie and his associates, by Briner, and by Poole and Newman, in 1971. It was the object of an international conference held in 1969 in New York. More recently, excellent reviews of the nature of dental plaque have been published by Bowen (1976), role of the dental plaque in the etiology of caries and periodontal disease by Theilade and Theilade (1976), and immunologic aspects of dental plaque constituents in caries from a workshop sponsored by the National Institute of Dental Research, edited by Bowen, Genco and O'Brien (1976). Parenthetically, it may be pointed out

that plaque-forming streptococci, isolated from the gingival crevice, have been found to be morphologically and serologically similar to known cariogenic strains, thus suggesting a similar etiologic origin for both dental caries and periodontal disease.

A great deal of time and effort has been devoted to investigations of the microbial plaque. The limitations of classic techniques for study of the microorganisms from this structure have gradually been realized, and much remains to be learned about the plaque. The adaptation of newer techniques in research may aid in clarifying the problems.

THE PROTEOLYTIC THEORY

Although the evidence for the so-called acid theory of dental caries is considerable, it is still not accepted as conclusive because much is circumstantial in nature. Offered as an alternative explanation is the proteolytic theory.

Evidence has been accruing that the organic portion of the tooth may play an important role in the carious process. Some of the earlier workers, notably Heider and Wedl (1869), Bodecker (1878), Abbott (1879) and Heitzmann (1887) contributed significantly to our better understanding of the structure of teeth. Not only did they demonstrate certain of the enamel structures made up of organic material, such as enamel lamellae and enamel rod sheaths, but also Bodecker suggested that these lamellae may be important in the progress of dental caries, since they could serve as a pathway for microorganisms through the enamel. The continuity of the enamel cuticle with the enamel lamellae was also demonstrated by these early investigators.

Many other workers have since carried out intensive investigation of the tooth enamel, particularly the organic portion. It has been established that enamel contains approximately 0.56 per cent organic matter, of which 0.18 per cent is a type of keratin, 0.17 per cent a soluble protein, possibly a glycoprotein, and the remainder citric acid and peptides.

Both Baumgartner (1911) and Fleischmann (1914, 1921) demonstrated that microorganisms could invade the enamel lamellae and believed that acids produced by these bacteria were capable of destroying the inorganic portion of the enamel. Gottlieb (1944) and Gottlieb, Diamond and Applebaum (1946) postulated that caries is essentially a proteolytic process: the microorganisms invade the organic pathways and destroy them in their advance. They did admit that acid formation accompanied the proteolysis—lesser amounts in lamellar involvement, greater amounts in the case of rod sheath involvement. Gottlieb held that yellow pigmentation was characteristic of caries and that this was due to pigment production by proteolytic organisms. Dreizen and his co-workers reported that a similar type of pigmentation could be produced in vitro by the action of intermediary products of carbohydrate degradation on decalcified noncarious tooth crowns. A similar pigmentation has also been produced by exposing extracted caries-free teeth to pure cultures of lactobacilli in a synthetic medium containing glucose. If no glucose was present, no pigmentation occurred.

Frisbie, Nuckolls and Saunders (1944, 1947) were especially active in studying early carious lesions of the enamel and described a microscopic phase of caries in which microorganisms could be demonstrated beneath an apparently intact enamel surface or one in which there was no evidence of a break in continuity. In some cases a bacterial plaque was found in position on the overlying enamel surface. Definite early white or brown carious lesions in the enamel exhibited similar but more advanced changes in the enamel matrix. These early lesions extended laterally beneath the intact surface, thus explaining the phenomenon, described by Thewlis, Darling and others, of a radiopaque layer overlying early carious lesions. Fosdick and Hutchinson (1965) ascribed the radiopaque layer to a maturation process in the tooth surface following exposure to the oral environment, which renders the pathways of diffusion at or near the surface less reactive to acids. Under these circumstances, acids have to penetrate to a considerable depth before meeting acid-soluble apatite crystals. Minor variations in the organic and inorganic structures of the tooth presumably are important in determining the pattern and rate of progress of early caries. Thus, caries could penetrate either through enamel rods or along inter-rod areas; extension could occur along the course of a number of rods or could involve segments of numerous rods.

Caries of the dentin was demonstrated by Frisbie and Nuckolls (1945, 1947) to be similar to that occurring in enamel. These investigators also pointed out that there may be some softening of the dentin even though the overlying enamel appears hard and intact. They believed that acid would be neutralized before penetrating the full thickness of the enamel and therefore could not cause decalcification of less acid-soluble dentin.

Pincus (1948, 1949) proposed a somewhat different, albeit related, approach to the caries problem. He proposed that Nasmyth's membrane and other enamel proteins are mucoproteins, yielding sulfuric acid upon hydrolysis. Lending support to this theory has been the isolation from the oral cavity of gram-negative bacilli capable of producing the enzyme sulfatase. This enzyme releases the combined sulfuric acid from the mucoprotein, but only reluctantly unless the protein is first hydrolyzed to free the polysaccharide. Supposedly, the liberated acid then dissolves the enamel, combining with the calcium to form calcium sulfate. Interestingly, this compound has been found in carious enamel but not in sound enamel. Sognnaes and Wislocki (1949, 1950) demonstrated the presence of an acid mucopolysaccharide in the interprismatic organic matter of mature enamel, but pointed out that sulfatase has not been demonstrated at the site of a carious lesion. Furthermore, no enzyme systems capable of attacking keratin have been demonstrated in the oral cavity, although other enzymes such as collagenase, hyaluronidase, phosphatase and mucinase, capable of attacking less resistant proteins, have been found.

Manley and Hardwick (1951) attempted to reconcile the two chief theories concerning the etiology of dental caries. They pointed out that while the acidogenic and proteolytic mechanisms may be separate and distinct, they need not be. Thus, many bacteria produce acid from an appropriate carbohydrate substrate; some bacteria capable of producing acid from carbohydrate may even degrade protein in the absence of carbohydrate. On this basis it has been proposed that there may be two types of carious lesions. In one type, microorganisms invade enamel lamellae, attack the enamel and involve the dentin before there is clinical evidence of caries. In the other, no enamel lamellae are present, and there is alteration of the enamel prior to invasion by microorganisms. This alteration is produced through decalcification of the enamel by acids formed by bacteria in a dental plaque overlying the enamel. The early lesions produced are those typically described as "chalky" enamel.

THE PROTEOLYSIS-CHELATION THEORY

Certain minor flaws exist in both the acidogenic and proteolytic theories of dental caries that cannot be reconciled with the clinical and experimental findings in all instances. Although not of major significance, they have cast some shadow on the validity of these theories and, because of this, the proteolysis-chelation theory was advanced by Schatz and his co-workers to explain the cause of dental caries. Unfortunately, most of their publications have dealt with theoretic discussions of the dental disease and the chemical aspects of chelation, with little direct evidence given for proteolysis-chelation as a mechanism in the caries process. The role of chelation in certain other biologic mechanisms has assumed major proportions in recent years, however.

Chelation is a process involving the complexing of a metallic ion to a complex substance through a coordinate covalent bond which results in a highly stable, poorly dissociated or weakly ionized compound (*chelas:* claw). Two of the most widely occurring examples are: (1) that naturally occurring in the chlorophyll molecule of green plants when four pyrrole nuclei are linked by this type of bond to magnesium, and (2) that occurring in hemoglobin when four pyrrole nuclei are linked to iron by a similar bond. Chelation is independent of pH of the medium, so that removal of such metallic ions as calcium from even a biologic calcium-phosphorus system may occur at a neutral or even alkaline pH. Numerous naturally occurring biologic chelating agents exist, the most common of these being citrate. Amino acids are also known to act as chelators, as well as hydroxy and keto esters of the Meyerhof-Embden system of glycolysis; phosphorylated and nonphosphorylated compounds in the hexose monophosphate shunt; polyphosphates, including those involved in phosphorylation; carboxylates of the Krebs tricarboxylic acid cycle; certain antibiotics and fermentation products; some proteins, carbohydrates, lipids, nucleic acids and certain enzymes; amines, amidases and certain vitamins; and oxalates, tartrates, salicylate, polyhydric alcohols and even Dicumarol.

The *proteolysis-chelation theory of dental caries,* as proposed by Schatz, states that the bacterial attack on the enamel, initiated by keratinolytic microorganisms, consists in a breakdown of the protein and other organic components of enamel, chiefly keratin. This results in the formation of substances which may form soluble chelates with the mineralized component of the tooth and thereby decalcify the enamel at a neutral or even alkaline pH. Enamel also contains other organic components

besides keratin, such as mucopolysaccharides, lipid and citrate, which may be susceptible to bacterial attack and act as chelators.

The proteolysis-chelation theory resolves the arguments as to whether the initial attack of dental caries is on the organic or inorganic portion of enamel by stating that both may be attacked simultaneously. But several reconciliations must be made if the proteolysis-chelation theory is to be accepted. These include (1) the observation of increased caries incidence with increased sugar consumption, (2) the observation of increased lactobacillus counts with high caries activity, and (3) the observation of decreased caries incidence following topical or systemic administration of fluoride.

Increased caries incidence concomitant with increased carbohydrate consumption might occur through the action of the carbohydrate in (1) stimulating or increasing proteolysis, (2) producing conditions under which keratinous proteins are less stable, and (3) complexing calcium.

Increased caries incidence accompanying increased lactobacillus counts might be explained by the microorganism's being the *result* of the caries process, rather than its *cause*. Thus Schatz has suggested that (1) proteolysis may provide ammonia which prevents a pH drop that would tend to inhibit growth of the lactobacilli; (2) the release of calcium from hydroxyapatite by chelation might encourage the growth of lactobacilli, since calcium has been reported to produce this effect; and (3) calcium exerts a vitamin-sparing action on some lactobacilli.

Reduced caries incidence concomitant with administration of fluoride might occur through formation of fluorapatite, which strengthens the linkages between the organic and inorganic phases of the enamel, thereby preventing or reducing their complexing. Although this theory of Schatz is unique and reconciles some of the unexplained facets of the dental caries process, insufficient scientific data have been presented to permit sound evaluation. An excellent review of the proteolysis-chelation theory of dental caries and the supporting and contradicting evidence was published by Jenkins.

Several animal studies, such as those of Zipkin and of Larson and her associates, showed that the incorporation of a chelating agent, ethylene diamine tetra-acetic acid (EDTA), into the cariogenic diet resulted in an increase in severity of dental caries as well as a difference in the distribution pattern of the lesions. Although such evidence does not lend great strength to the proteolysis-chelation theory, at least it does not contradict it.

CONTRIBUTING FACTORS IN DENTAL CARIES

The fact that there is remarkable variation in the caries incidence between different persons of the same age, sex, race and geographic area, subsisting on similar diets under the same living conditions, underscores the complexity of the caries problem. The mere presence of microorganisms and a suitable substrate at a given point on a tooth surface is apparently insufficient to establish a carious lesion in all cases. It is reasonable to assume that variations in caries incidence exist because of a number of possible indirect or contributing factors.

A workshop conference on dental caries mechanisms and control techniques was held at the University of Michigan in 1947. At this meeting a concise evaluation of the available knowledge of certain aspects of dental caries was made. This group listed a number of indirect factors that might influence the etiology of caries, as follows:

A. Tooth
    1. Composition
    2. Morphologic characteristics
    3. Position
B. Saliva
    1. Composition
       a. Inorganic
       b. Organic
    2. pH
    3. Quantity
    4. Viscosity
    5. Antibacterial factors
C. Diet
    1. Physical factors
       a. Quality of diet
    2. Local factors
       a. Carbohydrate content
       b. Vitamin content
       c. Fluorine content

One additional factor also is important and warrants discussion in this section: the role of systemic conditions.

The Tooth Factor. The *composition of the tooth* has been investigated for many years to determine whether a relation to caries might exist. Actually, most studies have been concerned with the inorganic portion of the tooth, but not until recent years have techniques been sufficiently refined to allow detection of small differences in the physical aspects or chemical constituents which might be related to caries susceptibility or caries immunity.

In a number of studies on the relation of caries to the chemical composition of teeth, such as those of Armstrong and Malherbe and Ockerse, no differences were found in the calcium, phosphorus, magnesium and carbonate contents of enamel from sound and carious teeth. Significant differences in fluoride content of sound and carious teeth, however, have been reported by these same workers. Malherbe and Ockerse found the fluoride content of enamel and dentin from sound teeth to be 410 ppm and 873 ppm, respectively, but only 139 ppm and 223 ppm, respectively, in carious teeth. Armstrong reported that the enamel of sound teeth contained 0.0111 ± 0.0020 per cent fluoride, while that of carious teeth contained only 0.0069 ± 0.0011 per cent fluoride.

Studies of the chemical composition of enamel by Brudevold and his associates in 1965 indicate that surface enamel is more resistant to caries than subsurface enamel. Surface enamel is more highly mineralized and tends to accumulate greater quantities of fluoride, zinc, lead and iron than the underlying enamel. The surface is lower in carbon dioxide, dissolves at a slower rate in acids, contains less water and has more organic material than subsurface enamel. These factors apparently contribute to caries resistance and are partly responsible for the slower disintegration of surface enamel than of the underlying enamel in initial carious lesions.

The *morphologic characteristics of the tooth* have been suggested as influencing the initiation of dental caries. Mellanby contended that enamel hypoplasia predisposes to the development of dental caries and that the more severely a tooth is affected, the more extensive will be the caries. The studies upon which this hypothesis was predicated have been questioned, and the present consensus is that there is little evidence available to support the theory.

The only morphologic feature which conceivably might predispose to the development of caries is the presence of deep, narrow occlusal fissures or buccal or lingual pits. Such fissures tend to trap food, bacteria and debris, and since defects are especially common in the base of fissures, caries may develop rapidly in these areas. Conversely, as attrition advances, the inclined planes become flattened, providing less opportunity for entrapment of food in the fissures, and caries predisposition diminishes.

Table 7–1. Salivary Constituents and Factors Studied in Relation to Caries

INORGANIC CONSTITUENTS	ORGANIC CONSTITUENTS	ENZYMES, SOLIDS AND PHYSICAL FACTORS
Positive ions:	Carbohydrates:	Enzymes:
Calcium	Glucose	Carbohydrases:
Hydrogen:		Amylase
pH	Lipids:	Maltase
Buffering power	Cholesterol	Proteases:
Neutralizing power	Lecithin	Trypsin
Salivary factor		Oxidases:
Titratable alkalinity	Nitrogen:	Catalase
Magnesium	Nonprotein:	Oxidase
Potassium	Ammonia	
	Nitrites	Total solids
	Urea	
Negative ions:	Amino acids	Physical factors:
Carbon dioxide	Protein:	Conductivity
Carbonate	Globulin	Freezing point
Chloride	Mucin	Osmotic pressure
Fluoride	Total protein	Specific gravity
Phosphate		Surface tension
Thiocyanate	Miscellaneous:	Viscosity
Ash	Peroxide	

Modified from F. Krasnow: Biochemical analysis of saliva in relation to caries. Dent. Cosmos, 78:301, 1936.

All available evidence indicates that alteration of tooth structure by disturbances in formation or in calcification is of only secondary importance in dental caries. The rate of caries progression may be influenced, but initiation of caries is affected very little.

Tooth position may play a role in dental caries under certain circumstances. Teeth which are malaligned, out of position, rotated or otherwise not normally situated may be difficult to cleanse and tend to favor the accumulation of food and debris. This, in susceptible persons, would be sufficient to cause caries in a tooth which, under normal circumstances of proper alignment, would conceivably not develop caries. The position of the teeth seems to be a minor factor in the etiology of dental caries.

The Saliva Factor. The fact that the teeth are in constant contact with and bathed by the saliva would suggest that this "environmental" agent could profoundly influence the state of oral health of a person, including the dental caries process (Table 7–1). The complex nature of saliva and the great variation in its composition are premonitory of the difficulties involved in establishing which factors may directly influence dental health. The unusual nature of saliva makes study of even its "normal" constituents and physical activities difficult, while the range of "normal" values almost precludes establishing the point at which a pathologic state exists

(Table 7–2). Even more difficult is the correlation of such a state with a specific pathologic oral condition.

An exceedingly thorough review of the scientific literature dealing with saliva was published by Afonsky. This treatise, abstracting over 4000 references to work reported chiefly between the years 1930 and 1954, is an excellent authoritative source of information on the subject of saliva.

The *composition of saliva* varies between persons and exhibits no apparent constant relation to composition of the blood. One chief source of discrepancy lies in the expression of the composition in terms of "resting" and "stimulated" saliva. Stimulation of salivary flow would obviously influence the total volume secreted in a given period of time, so that expression of values of salivary constituents in terms of "milligrams per cent" are not particularly meaningful unless the exact conditions under which the saliva was collected are described. The term "resting" saliva is especially confusing, since many stimuli which influence salivary flow are insidious. The concept of Babkin that mixed saliva is of no fixed composition, but varies according to the circumstances under which the saliva is collected, is a most reasonable approach to this problem. Nevertheless, there have been many studies of the elementary composition of the saliva and the approximate

Table 7–2. Composition of Saliva*

Albumin	?	Fluorine	0.08-0.25 ppm
Amino acids:		Globulin	?
Alanine	0.22-0.91	Group-specific substances	.3
Arginine	0.00-0.35	Glutathione	15
Aspartic acid	0.05-0.49	Iodine	3.5-24.0 γ.%
β-Alanine	0.04-0.08	Iron	0.0-0.6 γ/gm.
Cystine	0.00-0.13	Lysozyme	Highest effective
Glutamic acid	0.16-0.92		dilution 1:300
Glycine	0.35-1.56	Magnesium	0.1-0.7
Histidine	0.27-1.25	Mucoids	?
Isoleucine	0.14-0.84	Nitrogen:	
Leucine	0.18-0.53	Total N	42-100
Lysine	0.72-1.37	Protein N	23-88
Methionine	0.00-0.07	Nonprotein N	6-40
Phenylalanine	0.26-0.49	Amino acid N	1-6
Proline	0.00-0.74	Ammonia N	0.27
Serine	0.09-0.31	Urea N	0-7
Taurine	0.20-0.67	Phosphorus:	
Threonine	0.07-0.38	Total	15-25
Tryptophan	0.00-0.26	Inorganic	6-22
Tyrosine	0.17-0.80	Organic:	
Valine	0.09-0.23	Total	0.5-10.0
Ammonia	1-25	Acid-soluble	1-8
Amylase	4.0 gm./L.	Acid-insoluble	±
Antibodies	?	Potassium	30-95
Apoerythein	55 milliunits/ml.	Proteins	140-640
Ash	55-370	Reducing substances	≈ 10-30 mg. glucose
Composition of ash:		Sex hormones	?
Calcium	5.01%	Sodium	1-65
Chlorine	18.35	Solids:	
Magnesium	0.15	Total	300-800
Phosphate	18.84	Organic	130-380
Potassium	45.71	Sulfur	3-20
Sodium	9.59	Thiocyanate	0-30
Sulfate	6.38	Urea	14-75
Calcium	3-11	Uric acid	0.5-4.0
Carbohydrates	3.5% of total solids	Vitamins:	
Chloride	30-145	B-Complex	?
Cholesterol	3-50	Biotin	0.008 μgm./ml.
Citrate	0-2	Folic acid	0.0001 μgm./ml.
Cobalt (stimulated)	0-12 μgm./%	Niacin	0.03 μgm./ml.
Copper (stimulated)	10-47 μgm./%	Pantothenic acid	0.08 μgm./ml.
Creatinine	0.5-2.0	Pyridoxine	0.6 μgm./ml.
Enzymes: (see Table 7–4)		Riboflavin	0.05 μgm./ml.
		Thiamine	0.2-1.4 γ %
		Vitamin B$_{12}$	0.00015-0.0005 γ/ml
		Vitamin C	0.0-0.4 mg. %
		Vitamin K	0.015 μgm./ml.

*Unless otherwise stated, the values are given in mg. per 100 ml. of unstimulated saliva.
(Courtesy of Dr. D. Afonsky. Modified from D. Afonsky: Saliva and Its Relation to Oral Health. A Survey of the Literature. Montgomery, Ala.: Univ. of Alabama Press, 1961.)

Table 7–3. Calcium and Phosphorus Content of Resting Saliva in 484 Individuals

	MG. %		MG./HR.	
	MEAN	RANGE	MEAN	RANGE
Total calcium*	5.71 ± 0.06	2.4 — 11.3	1.07 ± 0.04	0.12 — 6.28
Total inorganic phosphorus†	15.7 ± 0.24	6.4 — 64.0	2.94 ± 0.09	0.21 — 16.72

*H. Becks: Human saliva. XIV. Total calcium content of resting saliva of 650 healthy individuals. J. Dent. Res., 22:397, 1943.
†W. W. Wainwright: Human saliva. XV. Inorganic phosphorus content of resting saliva of 650 healthy individuals. J. Dent. Res., 22:403, 1943.

percentages under various circumstances, as well as of correlation with dental caries incidence.

The concentrations of inorganic calcium and phosphorus show considerable variation, depending upon the rate of flow. Becks and Wainwright did extensive studies on salivary calcium and phosphorus and noted that the values are greater in slow-flowing saliva and tend to be inversely related to the rate of flow. The calcium content of the saliva in a large group of subjects studied by Becks is shown in Table 7–3.

Karshan reported that the calcium and phosphorus content of saliva is low in caries-active persons, but most investigators have been unable to confirm this finding.

The inorganic phosphate content of the saliva has been investigated in conjunction with the calcium content in many studies and has been found to exhibit wide variation depending upon a number of factors. Exemplary values are shown in Table 7–3.

There are numerous other inorganic components of saliva such as sodium, magnesium, potassium, carbonate, chloride and fluoride. With the exception of fluoride, these substances have not been thoroughly investigated. Thiocyanate has also been isolated from saliva and at one time was thought to inhibit the microorganisms associated with dental caries. It is now conceded that thiocyanate probably has no effect either on the bacterial flora or on dental caries.

The organic constituents of saliva as a group have also been subjected to little more than a cursory examination. Salivary cholesterol was determined by Krasnow and Oblatt and reported as varying from 2.3 to 50.0 mg./100 ml. Its significance is unknown. Mucin content of saliva has also been determined, but its significance and the factors modifying its concentrations are likewise obscure.

The ammonia and urea content of saliva has been studied by many workers. Turkheim in 1925 noted that the saliva of caries-immune persons exhibited a greater ammonia content than saliva from persons with caries. The work of Grove and Grove in 1934 actually initiated an extensive series of investigations, which culminated in the preparation of ammonia-containing dentifrices compounded as a specific anticariogenic agent. Grove and Grove found that the only apparent difference between the saliva of caries-susceptible and caries-immune persons was in ammonia content. They reported that the ammonia nitrogen of saliva from caries-

susceptibles ranged from none to 8.0 mg./100 ml., while ammonia nitrogen in saliva from the caries-immunes ranged from 4.0 to 10.0 mg./100 ml. They suggested that a high ammonia concentration retarded plaque formation and neutralized acid, at least to some extent. White and Bunting, Youngberg and Karshan, among others, found no relation between salivary ammonia and dental caries.

Urea was reported in saliva by Stephan in an average concentration of 20 mg./100 ml. of resting saliva and 13 mg./100 ml. of stimulated saliva. Urea may be hydrolyzed to ammonium carbonate by urease, thus increasing the neutralizing power of the saliva.

The amino acids of saliva have also been suggested as a source of ammonia nitrogen, although Kirch and his co-workers could find no correlation between the amounts of amino acids in saliva and caries activity. The amino acids in saliva have been studied by Kesel and his associates and by Woldring. The work of Woldring on the concentration of the amino acids in stimulated saliva, determined by chromatographic analysis, is shown in Table 7–2.

The presence of a secreted carbohydrate in the saliva has been argued by various workers. Many investigators have been unable to isolate a reducing sugar in saliva that was not related to persistent carbohydrate from the diet. Young, in 1941, reported the presence of a reducing substance in saliva which he assumed to be glucose. This substance ranged from 11.3 to 28.1 mg./100 ml. in resting saliva and from 14.0 to 30.0 mg./100 ml. in stimulated saliva. It must be concluded that saliva is not rich in glucose.

A number of different enzymes have been isolated from saliva. As shown in Table 7–4, these enzymes are derived from both intrinsic and extrinsic sources. The presence of urease has already been mentioned, but this is probably derived from oral microorganisms.

The most prominent and important oral enzyme is amylase, or ptyalin, a substance responsible for the degradation of starches. Parotid saliva is always higher in amylase content than saliva from the other glands.

The relation between amylase activity and dental caries has been studied by numerous investigators with conflicting results. Bibby quoted a review by Afonsky in which "two of these studies found that high amylolytic activity was associated with low caries; three, that low activity occurred with low caries; and six, that there was no correlation." It is obvious that if

Table 7–4.   Salivary Enzymes

ENZYMES	SOURCES		
	Glands	*Microorganisms*	*Leukocytes*
Carbohydrases			
Amylase	X	O	O
Maltase	O	X	X
Invertase	O	X	O
β-Glucuronidase	X	X	X
β-D-galactosidase	O	X	X
β-D-glucosidase	O	X	O
Lysozyme	X	O	X
Hyaluronidase	O	X	O
Mucinase	O	X	O
Esterases			
Acid phosphatase	X	X	X
Alkaline phosphatase	X	X	X
Hexosediphosphatase	O	X	O
Aliesterase	X	X	X
Lipase	X	X	X
Acetylcholinesterase	X	O	X
Pseudocholinesterase	X	X	X
Chondrosulfatase	O	X	O
Arylsulfatase	O	X	O
Transferring enzymes			
Catalase	O	X	O
Peroxidase	X	O	X
Phenyloxidase	O	X	O
Succinic dehydrogenase	X	X	X
Hexokinase	O	X	X
Proteolytic enzymes			
Proteinase	O	X	X
Peptidase	O	X	X
Urease	O	X	O
Other enzymes			
Carbonic anhydrase	X	O	O
Pyrophosphatase	O	X	O
Aldolase	X	X	X

From H. H. Chauncey: Salivary enzymes. J. Am. Dent. Assoc., 63:360, 1961. Copyright by the American Dental Association. Reprinted by permission.

any true relation does exist, it must be a complex one to account for the differences in findings.

The *pH of the saliva* has been the subject of intensive investigation, partly because of the ease with which determinations may be made and partly because of the suspected relation of acid to dental caries. Nevertheless, the variation in techniques has given rise to conflicting data. One criticism of some workers has been the failure to collect the saliva under oil, thus reducing loss of carbon dioxide which would cause elevation of the pH.

The pH of the saliva shows far greater variation than the pH of the blood, but most persons fall within a rather narrow range.

Most of the studies dealing with the pH of the saliva and its relation to dental caries have shown no positive correlation (Table 7–5). Reported correlations are probably fortuitous and of no biologic significance.

The *quantity of saliva* secreted in a given period of time may, theoretically at least, influ-

ence caries incidence. This is especially evident in cases of salivary gland aplasia and xerostomia in which salivary flow may be entirely lacking, with rampant dental caries the typical result.

A certain amount of saliva is constantly being secreted by the salivary glands, and this constitutes the "resting" saliva. Many factors may affect the amount of secretion of "resting" saliva just as many factors may affect the basal metabolic rate, so that there is a considerable range of flow between different persons. Therefore the term "resting" saliva is arbitrary and somewhat nebulous, depending upon the conditions of "rest" imposed by the investigator.

The term "stimulated" or "activated" saliva is similarly poorly defined, since the means of stimulating flow, the rate of jaw movement, the substance chewed or administered systemically, the period of collection and other factors can influence the volume of saliva secreted. The importance of differentiating between the resting and stimulated saliva is obvious, since the composition is different, and conditions must

Table 7–5. Salivary pH

	NO. OF INDIVIDUALS	AGE (YRS.)	TYPE OF SALIVA	CARIES ACTIVITY	MEAN pH	pH RANGE
Karshan et al.[1]	44	19–25	Resting	Caries-free	7.03	6.7 –7.5
				Caries-active	6.90	6.6 –7.2
			Stimulated	Caries-free	7.54	7.3 –7.9
				Caries-active	7.39	7.3 –7.8
Hubbell[2]	32	9–16	Stimulated	Caries-free	7.3	6.9 –7.6
				Caries-active	7.1	6.8 –7.4
Brawley and Sedwick[3]	791	6–17	Resting		6.77	— —
			Stimulated		7.45	— —
Ericsson[4]	36	Adults (men 30 years)	Resting	Low caries	6.75	6.30–7.22
				High caries	6.47	5.64–6.86
			Stimulated	Low caries	7.25	6.99–7.45
				High caries	7.03	6.53–7.38
	23	Children (8–9 years)	Resting	Caries-free	6.95	6.53–7.41
				High caries	6.75	6.41–7.20
			Stimulated	Caries-free	7.44	7.13–7.77
				High caries	7.41	7.02–7.71

[1]M. Karshan, F. Krasnow, and L. E. Krejci: A study of blood and saliva in relation to immunity and susceptibility to dental caries. J. Dent. Res., *11*:573, 1931.

[2]R. B. Hubbell: The chemical composition of saliva and blood serum of children in relation to dental caries. Am. J. Physiol., *105*:436, 1933.

[3]R. E. Brawley, and J. H. Sedwick: Studies concerning the oral cavity and saliva. J. Dent. Res., *19*:315, 1940.

[4]Y. Ericsson: Enamel-apatite solubility. Investigations into the calcium phosphate equilibrium between enamel and saliva and its relation to dental caries. Acta Odontol. Scand., *8*(Suppl. 3):1, 1949.

be specified when reporting scientific data. It is impossible to list a "normal" salivary content of calcium or phosphorus, or any other component, as is done for blood, without specifying the exact conditions in which the determinations were carried out.

It has been found that the range of variation of resting saliva among different persons is greater than the range of stimulated saliva. Furthermore, when persons from a slow-flowing group and from a fast-flowing group are stimulated, the flow of activated saliva from the two groups exhibits little difference, the stimulation masking the natural difference.

The difficulties involved in studying salivary flow have complicated the problems involved in attempting to determine its role in dental caries experience. The few studies that have been reported have given conflicting and inconclusive results (Table 7–6). It seems probable that the rate of flow of saliva is simply one additional factor which helps contribute to caries susceptibility or caries resistance. Mild increases or decreases in flow may be of little significance; total or near-total reductions in salivary flow adversely affect dental caries in an obvious manner.

The *viscosity of saliva* has been suggested to be of some significance in accounting for differences in caries activity between different persons. This idea appears to have an empiric foundation rather than a scientific basis, as judged by the paucity of pertinent experimental studies reported in the scientific literature. Miller thought that salivary viscosity was not of great importance in the caries process, since numerous cases could be found in which saliva was extremely viscid and the patients were free of caries. The reverse has also been shown: patients with an abundant, thin, watery saliva often exhibit rampant caries. Occasional workers have reported, however, that a high caries incidence is associated with a thick, mucinous saliva. The viscosity of the saliva is due largely to the mucin content, derived from the submaxillary, sublingual and accessory glands, but the significance of this substance is not entirely clear.

The *antibacterial properties of saliva* have been investigated by numerous workers in an attempt to explain the wide variation in caries incidence among different persons. Clough in 1934 tested 41 different salivas for their effect on the growth of *L. acidophilus*, utilizing "wells" in seeded culture plates. Inhibition of growth was demonstrated by all salivas except one, although saliva which had been filtered showed no such inhibition. Clough was unable to correlate the caries experience of the patients from whom the saliva was taken with the degree of bacterial inhibition. Bibby and his co-workers carried out similar studies in 1938 and found

Table 7–6.   Salivary Flow

	NO. OF INDIVIDUALS	SEX	TYPE OF SALIVA	MEAN FLOW	RANGE
Brawley and Sedwick[1]	519	Male	Resting	0.51 cc./min.	—
	248	Female		0.35 cc./min.	—
	518	Male	Stimulated	1.41 cc./min.	—
	246	Female		1.07 cc./min.	—
Becks and Wainwright[2]	235	Male	Resting	20 cc./hr.	1–111 cc./hr.
	249	Female		19 cc./hr.	
McDonald[3]	30	Male	Stimulated	14.0 cc./15 min.	3–30 cc./15 min.
	38	Female		14.3 cc./15 min.	3–50 cc./15 min.
Shannon[4]	537	Male	Resting		
		Carious		5.46 cc./5 min.	—
		Resistant		5.55 cc./5 min.	—
		Restored		5.23 cc./5 min.	—

[1] R. E. Brawley and J. H. Sedwick: Studies concerning the oral cavity and saliva. J. Dent. Res., 19:315, 1940.

[2] H. Becks and W. W. Wainwright: Human saliva. XIII. Rate of flow of resting saliva of healthy individuals. J. Dent. Res., 22:391, 1943.

[3] R. E. McDonald: Human saliva: A study of the rate of flow and viscosity and its relationship to dental caries. M.S. Thesis, Indiana University, 1950.

[4] I. L. Shannon: Salivary sodium, potassium and chloride levels in subjects classified as to dental caries experience. J. Dent. Res., 37:401, 1958.

that growth of air- and water-borne organisms was inhibited to a greater extent than that of oral organisms. Van Kesteren and associates found that the saliva probably contains at least two antibacterial substances, one of which resembles lysozyme, the other being distinctly different.

Using *L. acidophilus* as the test organism, Hill in 1939 found that saliva from caries-free persons had a greater inhibiting effect than saliva from caries-active persons.

The significance of antibacterial factors in saliva has been questioned by many workers, including Bibby (1956), who pointed out that regardless of the quality of the saliva, including the relative presence or absence of inhibitory principles, saliva always appears to contain bacteria capable of producing caries if carbohydrates are present.

A bacteriolytic factor in the saliva of caries-immune persons which was absent in saliva from caries-susceptible ones was reported by Green. This factor was active against lactobacilli and streptococci and appeared to exert its lytic effect on cells commencing the process of division. Further studies indicated that the factor was a protein substance associated with the globulin fraction of saliva. Since it resembles some antibacterial factors in serum, it is apparently different from other reported salivary antibacterial substances.

The *buffer capacity of the saliva* is another factor that has received considerable attention because of its potential effect on acids in the oral cavity. The acid-neutralizing power of saliva is not necessarily reflected by the pH of the saliva, which may account for some of the observed differences between salivary pH and caries incidence. Karshan and his associates (1931) pointed out that titratable alkalinity is a better indication of buffer capacity than is the pH, but they found that saliva from caries-immune and caries-susceptible persons exhibited essentially the same titratable alkalinity. White and Bunting in 1936 studied the carbon dioxide capacity of resting and stimulated saliva in caries-free and caries-susceptible children. Although the values for stimulated saliva were much higher than those for resting saliva, no remarkable differences were noted in the mean values. The carbon dioxide capacity of stimulated saliva was studied in 1936 by Karshan, who found a significant difference between a caries-free group and a caries-active group. The respective means for the two groups were: caries-free, 31.1 ml./100 ml. of saliva; caries-active, 19.5 ml./100 ml. of saliva.

Sellman in 1949 studied the buffer capacity

of saliva and its relation to dental caries and found that the total amount of acid needed to reduce the salivary pH to a given pH level (6.0, 5.0, 4.0 and 3.0) was always greater for saliva from caries-resistant persons. Sullivan and Storvick in 1950 also reported a significant inverse correlation between the DMF teeth and the buffer capacity of saliva in 574 college students.

The relation between buffer capacity of saliva per se and dental caries activity is not as simple as might be supposed. The acid production, significant in the caries process, occurs at a localized site on the tooth. This site, particularly in the early stages of caries, is protected by the dental plaque, which appears to act as an osmotic membrane preventing a completely free exchange of ions. Thus, even though buffer ions are present in the saliva, these may not be totally available at those specific sites where they are needed on the tooth surface. The entire problem of the buffer capacity of saliva and its relation to dental caries requires further investigation.

The Diet Factor. The role of the diet and nutritional factors deserves special consideration because of the often observed differences in caries incidence of various populations who subsist on dissimilar diets. Although many clinical studies have been carried out in an attempt to study certain components of the diet with regard to caries, a number of variable factors have usually clouded the results. The use of experimental animals which are susceptible to a destruction of the teeth similar to human dental caries has greatly aided the study of dietary considerations, as has the purification of animal diets so that an otherwise adequate diet can be prepared that varies in only one component (Fig. 7–4).

The *physical nature of the diet* has been suggested as one factor responsible for the difference in caries experience between primitive and modern man. The diet of the primitive man consisted generally of raw unrefined foods containing a great deal of roughage, which cleanses the teeth of adherent debris during the usual masticatory excursions. In addition, the presence of soil and sand in incompletely cleaned vegetables in the primitive diet induced severe attrition of both occlusal and proximal surfaces of the teeth, the flattening causing a reduction in the probability of decay.

In the modern diet, soft refined foods tend to cling tenaciously to the teeth and are not removed because of the general lack of rough-

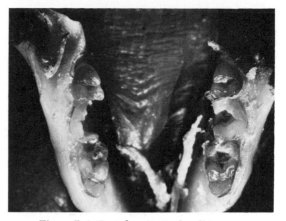

Figure 7–4. *Dental caries in the albino rat.*
Occlusal caries has led to severe destruction of several molars. (Courtesy of Dr. Joseph C. Muhler.)

age. Augmenting this collection of debris on the teeth is the reduction of mastication due to the softness of the diet. The detrimental effect of this decreased function on the periodontal apparatus should be obvious.

It has been demonstrated that mastication of food dramatically reduces the number of culturable oral microorganisms. Since those areas of teeth that are exposed to the excursions of food are usually immune to caries, mechanical cleansing by detergent foods may have some value in caries control.

The *carbohydrate content of the diet* has been almost universally accepted as one of the most important factors in the dental caries process and one of the few factors which may be voluntarily altered as a preventive dentistry measure. In spite of the overwhelming evidence relating carbohydrate intake to dental caries, enough exceptions have been noted (e.g., in India among certain segments of the population there may be a high carbohydrate intake, but a very low caries incidence) to make it obvious that this is not a simple problem. A complicating factor, and one which has slowed the resolution of this problem, has been the difficulty in obtaining data from human feeding studies under controlled experimental conditions.

As an indication of the increase in carbohydrate consumption over the past years, Day and his co-workers (1935) reported that the per capita consumption of sugar in the United States increased from 11 pounds in 1800 to 115 in 1930, although it is somewhat lower at present.

Becks and his associates (1944) studied the effect of carbohydrate restriction on the *L. acidophilus* index and caries experience in a group of 1250 persons with rampant caries and in 265 caries-free persons. Replacement of refined dietary carbohydrate with meat, eggs, vegetables, milk and milk products resulted in an 82 per cent reduction in the lactobacillus index and in clinical evidence of extensive arrest of caries. The observation was made that some persons consumed large amounts of carbohydrate without acquiring caries, while others had rampant caries even though consuming very little carbohydrate. These workers were prompted to suggest that, in addition to excessive amounts of refined carbohydrates, other factors undoubtedly have a bearing on the disease.

The DMF rates of 3905 persons of all ages from four Italian cities were reported by Schour and Massler in 1947. They found that the prevalence of caries was approximately two to seven times lower than that in the United States and suggested that this was due to the lower per capita consumption of sugar in Italy.

Bransby and Knowles in 1949 reported that examination of children of Guernsey and Jersey Islands in 1945 after the German occupation, and in 1947 after a return to a prewar diet, including an increase in consumption of "sugar, jam and confectionery," revealed an increased caries rate over this two-year period.

Significant data were also accumulated during and after World War II from several European countries in which the sugar consumption was remarkably reduced during the German occupation. Sognnaes in 1948 reported that the reduction in refined carbohydrate consumption in Norway during the occupation did not result in a reduction in caries during this period. Rather, there was a delay of several years after carbohydrate restriction before the caries reduction was noted (Fig. 7–5). Sognnaes thought that this finding could best be explained by an indirect favorable influence on the development and maturation of the teeth and not by a change in the oral environment alone. Toverud (1949) also studied the change in caries incidence in Norwegian children during the war and related it to differences in consumption of refined carbohydrates. The mechanism of this beneficial "delayed action" effect on the teeth is not known.

Many animal studies have been carried out in attempting to clarify some of the perplexing problems of dental caries. Some of these have dealt with the cariogenic effect of different carbohydrates, and it has been found that not all sugars have the same cariogenicity. Further-

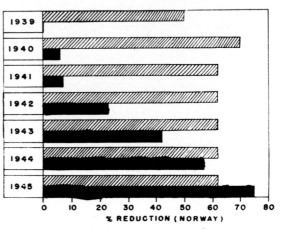

Figure 7–5. *Time lag between wartime reduction in sugar consumption and in dental caries experience in Norwegian children.*

Solid bars indicate carious permanent teeth of seven-year-olds (i.e., effect on the newly erupted teeth). Cross-hatched bars denote sugar consumption (i.e., change in oral environment). Groups of seven-year-old children during each year of the war are compared. Their permanent teeth *after eruption* were exposed to a similar sugar concentration in the oral environment. Significant caries reduction is seen in the teeth of those groups (1943-45) whose teeth had the longest "exposure" to the wartime diet *before eruption*, i.e., during development and final maturation. (Courtesy of Dr. Reidar F. Sognnaes: Science, *106*:448, 1947.)

more, the studies carried out at the University of Notre Dame on animals born and raised entirely germ-free revealed that even when the animals were fed a cariogenic diet, dental caries did not develop in the absence of microorganisms.

On a sound scientific basis, it is difficult to draw definite conclusions about the relation between dental caries and refined carbohydrates. The difficulties involved in direct observations have necessitated compromises in methods of study. Nevertheless, the bulk of the available evidence indicates that a positive relation exists, even though many other factors are also important.

The *vitamin content of the diet* has been reported by many workers to have a significant effect on dental caries incidence.

Vitamin A deficiency has definite effects on developing teeth in animals and presumably in human beings as well, although only a few reports on dental disturbances in vitamin A deficiency in humans are in the literature. There are no human studies relating vitamin A, excess or deficiency, to dental caries experience.

Vitamin D has probably been investigated with greater thoroughness in relation to dental caries than any other vitamin. There is general agreement on the necessity of vitamin D for the normal development of the teeth. Malformation, particularly enamel hypoplasia, has been described in the deficiency state by many workers, the most prominent being Lady May Mellanby.

The relation of rickets to dental caries is not well defined, however. The only possible way in which infantile rickets could influence dental caries incidence is through an alteration in tooth structure which makes the teeth more susceptible to caries. The pertinent clinical studies are not in agreement. Many of the early studies are particularly confusing because of inaccurate reporting of data.

Hess and Abramson in 1931 studied a group of 71 rachitic children, five to nine years old, and compared their caries incidence with that of a control group of 24 children. They noted that a higher rate of dental caries of the deciduous teeth was present in the rachitic group. Subsequent studies on the permanent teeth showed no differences in caries incidence between the rachitic and control groups.

Shelling and Anderson in 1936 found that the average caries incidence of 126 children in Baltimore with roentgenographic evidence of rickets in infancy or early childhood was five lesions. The average caries incidence of a control group of 150 children receiving sufficient vitamin D to protect them against rickets was 7.5 carious lesions. Because a far greater number of children in the rachitic group were blacks (93 per cent) as compared to the control group (28 per cent), the significance of the data is questionable because of the probable inherent racial differences in dental caries incidence.

Day in 1944 studied 200 boys in India and observed no relation between the incidence of rickets and the average number of carious lesions present or the occurrence of enamel hypoplasia.

In spite of the fact that children who have suffered from rickets may exhibit a slightly higher caries experience, other local factors appear to be of greater importance.

The effect of vitamin D supplement on dental caries experience has also been studied to determine whether this might be of significant benefit. Agnew and associates in 1933 studied 350 children divided into three groups receiving, respectively, an institutional diet, the same diet supplemented with vitamin D, and the diet supplemented by both vitamin D and phosphorus. In the vitamin D group a reduction in the dental caries increment was found, as well as an arrest in existing carious lesions.

Brodsky and his co-workers (1941, 1942) studied the effect of massive doses of vitamin D on dental caries incidence in hospitalized tuberculous children. The control group consisted of 33 children receiving the hospital diet, but no supplements. This group had an average of 1.18 new carious lesions per child during the year of the study. The 33 children in the group receiving a supplement of 305,000 U.S.P. units of vitamin D and 2,445,000 U.S.P. units of vitamin A at the beginning of the study had an average increase of only 0.39 cavity per child. A third group of 35 children received 600,000 U.S.P. units of vitamin D and had only an average of 0.17 new carious lesion per child.

The evidence indicates that vitamin D supplements may reduce the dental caries increment, particularly in children who may not be receiving adequate vitamin D. Ingestion of vitamin D in excess of adequate metabolic requirements has only a questionable effect on caries experience. Although the effect of vitamin D on dental caries experience is uncertain, its effect on forming dental structures cannot be overemphasized.

Related to the effect of vitamin D on dental caries has been a series of reports dealing with the relation between caries and exposure to sunshine. Several investigators have denied such a correlation, although others have presented substantiating evidence for it. The difficulty of eliminating other complicating factors must be appreciated.

East studied this problem extensively (1939, 1940, 1941, 1942) and noted a close correlation between the mean annual number of hours of sunlight and the dental caries incidence. Although his data appear sound, most of them are based upon United States Public Health Service figures collected in some instances by persons not particularly qualified to determine caries extent, such as physicians and school nurses. Nevertheless the possibility does exist that there is a correlation.

Vitamin K has been tested as a possible anticaries agent by virtue of its enzyme-inhibiting activity in the carbohydrate degradation cycle. This will be discussed in the section dealing with the control of caries. There are no known effects of vitamin K deficiency on dental caries incidence.

Vitamin B complex and its relation to dental

caries has been the object of a few clinical studies. Mann and associates in 1947 reported that the average of DMF tooth surfaces in a group of 124 malnourished patients was 4.54, while the average of DMF tooth surfaces in 99 well-nourished patients was 14.94. The malnourished patients comprised "34 patients with evidence of pellagra, 84 with riboflavin deficiency, 29 with the initial nervous syndrome, 15 with nutritional macrocytic anemia, 27 with clinical evidence of thiamin deficiency, 11 with vitamin A deficiency and 17 with clinical scurvy." Sixty-two of these patients displayed clinical evidence of multiple deficiency diseases operating simultaneously, which Spies, Bean and Ashe (1939) showed to be the rule rather than the exception in cases of prolonged malnutrition.

Dreizen and his co-workers (1947) studied the effect of these deficiency diseases on dental caries in children. The malnourished children presented a remarkably lower caries increment than the group of well-nourished children. The data suggest that vitamin B complex deficiency may exert a caries-protective influence on the tooth, since several of the B vitamins are essential growth factors for the oral acidogenic flora and also serve as components of the coenzymes involved in glycolysis.

Vitamin B_6 (pyridoxine) has been proposed as an anticaries agent on the hypothetical ground that it selectively alters the oral flora by promoting the growth of noncariogenic organisms which suppress the cariogenic forms (Strean, 1957). Slight to significant reductions in the caries increment of children and pregnant women have been reported following the use of pyridoxine-containing lozenges after each meal. These studies have been limited in both duration and number of subjects.

Vitamin C deficiency is well recognized as producing severe changes in the periodontal tissues and pulps of the teeth. A few studies have also been carried out to determine whether scurvy might be related to dental caries incidence or whether ascorbic acid supplements might prevent dental caries. The available scientific evidence indicates that there is no relation between scurvy and increased caries incidence in the human being. Furthermore, there is no evidence to indicate that vitamin C supplements would in any way protect against dental caries.

The *calcium and phosphorus dietary intake* has been popularly related to dental caries experience, although the scientific evidence for this correlation is lacking. Disturbance in calcium and phosphorus metabolism during the period of tooth formation may result in severe enamel hypoplasia and defects of the dentin. But a calcium disturbance occurring after tooth formation has been completed results in no changes in the tooth substance itself. Albright and his associates in 1934 studied 16 cases of human hyperparathyroidism and noted that even though there was severe loss of calcium from the bone, the teeth remained intact.

The effect on caries experience of increasing the calcium and phosphorus intake was studied by Malan and Ockerse in 1941 in a group of South African schoolchildren. The control group consisted of 85 children receiving their typical diet containing an average of 0.43 gm. of calcium and 0.79 gm. of phosphorus. The experimental group contained 97 children receiving the same diet plus one tablet daily of 0.5 gm. each of calcium and phosphorus. The dental caries increment over a three-year period revealed no differences between the two groups in either the deciduous or the permanent dentition. On the other hand, evidence was presented by Boyd and associates (1933) that calcium and phosphorus retention is related to dental caries. Thus the daily values of calcium and phosphorus retention per kilogram in a group of 28 caries-free children were 17 and 15 mg., respectively, while the calcium and phosphorus retention values in a group of 38 children with active dental caries were 10 and 9 mg., respectively.

The literature is replete with studies which show that phosphates are effective cariostatic agents when added to diets cariogenic for laboratory rodents (Nizel and Harris, 1964). Their effectiveness depends on the anions and cations with which they are combined and on the foodstuffs with which they are fed. The caries reduction in rodents given supplemental phosphates involves a mechanism which operates after the teeth have erupted. The results of clinical tests of phosphate additives for the express purpose of controlling human caries have been equivocal.

The available evidence indicates that there is no relation between dietary calcium and phosphorus and dental caries experience. Furthermore, as Robinson (1943) concluded in a review of the literature on the value of calcium therapy in dentistry, there is no known effect of calcium supplementation on caries incidence. There is some evidence that calcium and phosphorus retention may be related to inactivity or arrest of dental caries. Finally, there is no demonstrable relation between the concentration of calcium and phosphorus in the blood and the incidence of dental caries.

The fluorine content of the diet and of specific foodstuffs in particular has been investigated by numerous workers. Varying amounts of fluoride are found in a good many plant substances, depending to some extent upon the fluoride content of the soil in which they were grown. In general, the leaves of plants contain more fluoride than the stems, and the skin of fruit contains more than the pulp.

There has been little attempt made to study the dietary fluoride in relation to dental caries as has been done for the fluoride content of drinking water. Some workers believe that dietary fluoride is relatively unimportant compared to fluoride in the drinking water because of its metabolic unavailability. Fluoride in the water and its relation to caries will be considered at length in the section on Methods of Caries Control.

The effect of two additional trace minerals, selenium and vanadium, present in the drinking water and food in certain localities, has been investigated for possible effects on dental caries by Tank and Storvick. Their studies indicate that the dental caries rates were significantly higher in permanent teeth of persons residing in seleniferous areas than in nonseleniferous areas, but that a decrease in dental caries rates of permanent teeth was observed with increasing vanadium concentrations. The signficance of these findings has not been clarified.

Systemic Factors. There are certain factors, dissociated from the local environment or at least not intimately associated with it, which have been related to dental caries incidence and which may be conveniently discussed under this general heading. It should not be inferred that these systemic factors are not operating through some local mechanism, for such may be the case.

Heredity has been linked with the dental caries incidence in the scientific literature for many years. In 1899 G. V. Black wrote: "When the family remains in one locality, the children living under the conditions similar to those of the parents in their childhood, the susceptibility to caries will be very similar in the great majority of cases. This will hold good even to the particular teeth and localities first attacked, the order of occurrence of cavities, and the particular age at which they occur."

The racial aspects of caries susceptibility and caries immunity have been previously discussed. This racial tendency for high caries or low caries incidence, in some instances at least, appears to follow hereditary patterns. The fact that local factors may easily alter this caries tendency (e.g., exposure to a highly refined diet inducing high caries experience) would indicate that heredity does not exert a strong influence in determining individual caries susceptibility. That it is a factor, however, cannot be denied. Even in the experimental animal, definite caries-susceptible and caries-immune strains of rats and hamsters have been developed.

Some of the earlier studies aimed primarily at confirming this heredity-caries relation were carried out on different races living in the same geographic areas. Unfortunately, in any such study there are uncontrollable factors which cannot be compensated. The dietary habits, food likes and dislikes, cooking habits and even such toilet habits as toothbrushing frequency and methods are all often passed down from generation to generation, parents to offspring, and confuse the pure effects of heredity. In 1909 Bunting reported that black children exhibited less dental caries than a comparable group of white children over 10 years of age in Detroit. Blackerby (1939) reported similar differences in caries experience based upon study of 1117 black children and 11,674 white children in schools in different sections of the United States. Approximately 80 per cent of the white children in this study were in need of dental care and averaged 5.18 defective teeth, while only 68 per cent of the black children needed dental care, and this group averaged 3.39 defective teeth.

A greater similarity in caries incidence between siblings than between unrelated children was reported by Klein and Palmer in 1940, based upon study of 488 siblings and 301 unrelated children. They, too, pointed out the difficulties encountered in attempting to separate hereditary from environmental factors.

One of the most significant studies is that reported by Klein in 1946 on the results of examination of 5400 persons in 1150 families of Japanese ancestry. In this study the DMF was established for each individual, and 30 per cent of the fathers with the lowest DMF rate were designated arbitrarily as "low DMF." The 30 per cent with the highest DMF were designated as "high DMF," while the middle 40 per cent were classed as "middle DMF." The same groupings were used for the mothers and for

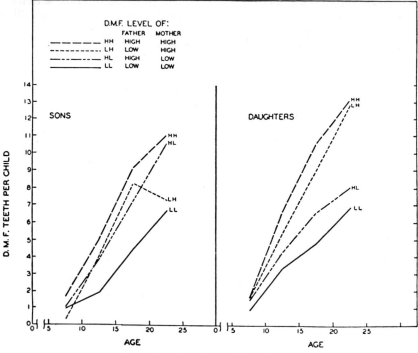

Figure 7–6. *Heredity and dental caries.*
The relation between DMF levels of sons and daughters and DMF levels of fathers and mothers, by age of offspring, is illustrated. (From H. Klein: The family and dental disease. IV. Dental disease (DMF) experience in parents and offspring. J. Am. Dent. Assoc., 33:735, 1946.)

the sons and daughters of these parents. It was found that a "high DMF" father and "high DMF" mother produced offspring, both sons and daughters, with a high DMF rate. On the other hand, if the father and mother were both "low DMF," the children also were in a low DMF group. The differences between these two extremes became more pronounced with increasing age, but the results were so consistent that this investigator found it difficult to exclude the view that dental caries in children involves strong familial vectors, probably with a genetic basis, perhaps sex-linked (Fig. 7–6).

An interesting study of genetic factors has been reported by Mansbridge, who studied the caries incidence in 224 pairs of like-sex twins, both identical and fraternal. Of this group, 96 pairs were identical and 128 pairs were fraternal twins. Comparisons of the caries experience between each set of twins indicated that there is a greater resemblance between identical twins than between fraternal twins, while unrelated pairs of children showed less resemblance than either type of twin. Mansbridge concluded from his study that environmental factors clearly have greater influence, although genetic factors also contribute to the causation of dental caries.

There is still no incontrovertible evidence that heredity per se has a definite relation to dental caries incidence. The possibility exists that if there is any such relation, it may be mediated through inheritance of tooth form or structure which predisposes to caries immunity or susceptibility. The problem is of such complexity that more intensive investigation is necessary before any positive conclusions can be drawn.

Pregnancy and lactation have been so thoroughly related to dental caries in the minds of the general public that it is difficult to believe that such a prevailing opinion is not based upon scientific fact. The saying "A tooth for every child" has been quoted widely for many years. It is, as will be pointed out, a misconception. It should also be remembered that there is no mechanism for the physiologic withdrawal of calcium from teeth as there is from bone, so that a developing fetus cannot calcify at the expense of the mother's teeth.

Ziskin in 1926 examined a group of 599 pregnant women, most of whom were in the later months of pregnancy, and a group of 205 nulliparous women. He found that the caries experience of the pregnant women increased with the age of the patients at a rate comparable to that of the women who had never borne children. He found no relation between dental caries experience and pregnancy per se or between caries and the number of pregnancies. He even pointed out that the slightly lower caries value in the pregnant group as compared to that of the nulliparous controls suggested a slight protection against caries. In 1937 Ziskin and Hotelling reported the results of a similar study which also indicated that pregnancy tended to prevent caries.

Deakins (1943) and Deakins and Looby (1943) studied the specific gravity of dentin as an indication of its mineral content and found that there were no significant differences in dentin samples from carious teeth of pregnant and nonpregnant women. They concluded that there was no calcium withdrawal from sound dentin during pregnancy. A similar study was carried out by Dragiff and Karshan in 1943, utilizing direct analysis of ash. They reported that no differences were observed in calcium and phosphorus content of root dentin from teeth of pregnant and nonpregnant women.

Hunscher in 1930 studied calcium and phosphorus metabolism of three women during two successive lactations and, in addition, carried out complete oral examinations. She found no changes in caries activity during lactation.

It is a fairly common clinical observation that a woman during the later stages of pregnancy or shortly after delivery will manifest a signifi-cant increase in caries activity. In nearly all cases thorough questioning will reveal that the woman has neglected her ordinary oral care because of the press of other duties attendant to the birth of the baby. Thus the increased caries incidence, though indirectly due to the pregnancy, may actually be a local problem of neglect.

The available evidence indicates that preg-nancy does not cause increased caries. Studies relating lactation and caries incidence are too few to contribute any significant data for clari-fying this problem.

CLINICAL ASPECTS OF DENTAL CARIES

Clinical Classification of Caries. Dental caries has been classified in a number of ways, de-pending upon the clinical features which char-acterize the particular lesion. Dental caries may be classified according to location on the indi-vidual tooth as (1) pit or fissure caries and (2) smooth surface caries. Sometimes it is advisable to classify dental caries according to the rapidity of the process as (1) acute dental caries and (2) chronic dental caries.

Caries may also be classified according to whether the lesion is a new one attacking a previously intact surface (Fig. 7–7) or whether it is occurring around the margins of a restora-tion (Fig. 7–8): (1) primary (virgin) caries and (2) secondary (recurrent) caries.

PIT OR FISSURE CARIES. Pit or fissure caries of the primary type develops in the occlusal sur-

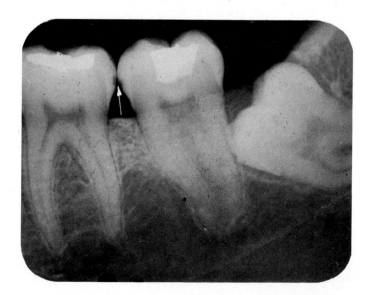

Figure 7–7. *Primary caries of interproximal surfaces.*

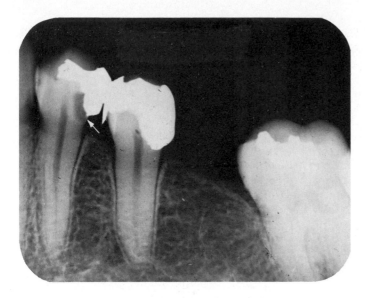

Figure 7–8. *Recurrent caries beneath a faulty restoration.*

face of molars and premolars, in the buccal and lingual surface of the molars and in the lingual surface of the maxillary incisors. Pits or fissures with high steep walls and narrow bases are those most prone to develop caries. These deep pits or fissures are sometimes considered developmental faults, particularly since the enamel in the extreme depth is often very thin or even occasionally absent and thus allows exposure of dentin. Deep narrow pits and fissures favor the retention of food debris and microorganisms, and caries may result from fermentation of this food and the formation of acid.

Pits and fissures affected by early caries may appear brown or black and will feel slightly soft and "catch" a fine explorer point. The enamel directly bordering the pit or fissure may appear opaque bluish white as it becomes undermined. This undermining occurs through lateral spread of the caries at the dentino-enamel junction, and it may be a rapid process if the enamel in the base of the pit or fissure is thin.

The lateral spread of caries at the dentino-enamel junction as well as penetration into the dentin along the dentinal tubules may be extensive without fracturing away the overhanging enamel. Thus, there may be a large carious lesion with only a tiny point of opening. This undermined enamel may suddenly give way under the stress of mastication, or the dentist may suddenly open into a large cavity when excavating the pit or fissure. This phenomenon was the origin of the mistaken idea of "internal caries," the view that a tooth may decay from inside outward. Needless to say, a point of penetration is always present. It should not be inferred that all pit and fissure caries begins with a narrow penetration point and develops a large cavitation with overhanging enamel. In many cases the lesion begins as an open cavity and becomes progressively larger, nearly the full extent of the cavity being exposed to the oral environment. In this latter type of caries the progress of the disease is usually much slower, and pulp involvement is often delayed.

SMOOTH SURFACE CARIES. Smooth surface caries of the primary type is caries that develops on the proximal surfaces of the teeth or on the gingival third of the buccal and lingual surfaces. Seldom does caries occur on other areas of the teeth, except in cases of malposed or malformed teeth, because of the self-cleansing properties of these areas. Unlike pit or fissure caries, which is not dependent upon the development of a definite, grossly recognizable plaque for the initiation of caries, smooth surface caries is generally preceded by the formation of a microbial or dental plaque. This ensures the retention of carbohydrate and microorganisms on the tooth surface in an area not habitually cleansed, and the subsequent formation of acid to initiate the caries process.

Proximal caries usually begins just below the contact point, and appears in the early stage as a faint white opacity of the enamel without apparent loss of continuity of the enamel surface (Fig. 7–9). In some cases it appears as a yellow or brown pigmented area, but in either event is usually rather well demarcated. The early white chalky spot becomes slightly roughened,

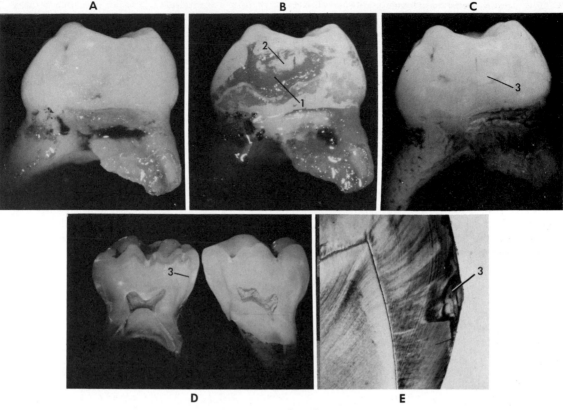

Figure 7–9. *Smooth surface caries.*
The bacterial plaque is difficult to see *(A)* unless stained by a disclosing solution *(B)*. The plaque *(1)* is disclosed by aqueous basic fuchsin. Note the absence of the plaque at the contact point *(2)*. *C,* The plaque is mechanically removed, revealing the chalky white spot of early enamel caries *(3)*. *D,* The tooth is split to show the extent of the carious lesion. *(3)*. *E,* Photomicrograph of a ground section through the carious lesion *(3)*.

owing to superficial decalcification of the enamel.

As the caries penetrates the enamel, the enamel surrounding the lesion assumes a bluish white appearance similar to that seen sometimes around carious pits or fissures. This is particularly apparent as lateral spread of caries at the dentino-enamel junction occurs. The more rapid type of caries usually produces a small area of penetration; the slower forms an open, shallow cavity. It is not uncommon for proximal caries to extend both buccally and lingually, but seldom does the cavity encroach upon areas accessible to excursion of food or to the toothbrush.

Cervical caries occurs on buccal, lingual or labial surfaces and usually extends from the area opposite the gingival crest occlusally to the convexity of the tooth surface marking the self-cleansing portion of this surface. It extends laterally toward the proximal surfaces and, on occasion, extends beneath the free margin of the gingiva. Thus the typical cervical carious

lesion is a crescent-shaped cavity beginning, as does proximal caries, as a slightly roughened chalky area which gradually becomes excavated. Cervical caries is almost always an open cavity and does not present the narrow point of penetration seen commonly in pit or fissure caries and proximal caries. This form of caries occurs on any tooth without predilection and is directly related to lack of oral hygiene. Of all forms of dental caries on different areas of the tooth, there is least excuse for cervical caries, since it can be prevented in nearly every instance by proper hygiene.

ACUTE DENTAL CARIES. Acute dental caries is that form of caries which runs a rapid clinical course and results in early pulp involvement by the carious process. It occurs most frequently in children and young adults, presumably because the dentinal tubules are large and open and show no sclerosis. The process is usually so rapid that there is little time for the deposition of secondary dentin.

The initial entrance of the carious lesion

remains small, while the rapid spread of the process at the dentino-enamel junction and diffuse involvement of the dentin produce a large internal excavation. It has been suggested that saliva does not easily penetrate the small opening to the carious lesion, so that as acids are formed there is little opportunity for buffering or neutralization. In acute caries the dentin is usually stained a light yellow rather than the darker brown of chronic caries (Fig. 7–10). Pain is more apt to be a feature of acute caries than of chronic caries, but this is not an invariable finding.

Nursing bottle caries, also called nursing caries, baby bottle syndrome, and bottle mouth syndrome, is an interesting and unfortunate form of rampant caries affecting the deciduous dentition. It has been variously attributed to prolonged use of (1) a nursing bottle containing milk or milk formula, fruit juice or sweetened water, (2) breast feeding, or (3) sugar or honey-sweetened pacifiers. Almost invariably, there is habitual use of one of the above after one year of age, usually as an aid for sleeping at night or at naptime. The disease has been reviewed recently by Kammerman and Starkey.

The disease presents clinically as widespread carious destruction of deciduous teeth, most commonly the four maxillary incisors, followed by the first molars and then the cuspids if the habit is prolonged. It has been emphasized that it is the absence of caries in the mandibular incisors which distinguishes this disease from ordinary rampant caries. The carious process in affected teeth may be so severe that only root stumps remain.

When milk or other forms of carbohydrate are cleared rapidly from the mouth, they are not highly cariogenic. However, if they pool in the mouth when the baby falls asleep, the repetitious act soon leads to severe caries. The mandibular incisors usually escape because they are covered and protected by the tongue. It is essential that parents be made aware of this condition.

CHRONIC DENTAL CARIES. Chronic dental caries is that form which progresses slowly and tends to involve the pulp much later than acute caries. It is most common in adults. The entrance to the lesion is almost invariably larger than that of acute caries. Because of this there is not only less food retention, but also greater access of saliva. The slow progress of the lesion allows sufficient time for both sclerosis of the dentinal tubules and deposition of secondary dentin in response to the adverse irritation. The carious dentin is often stained deep brown.

Although there is considerable surface destruction of tooth substance, the cavity is generally a shallow one with a minimum of softening of the dentin. There is little undermining of enamel and only moderate lateral spread of caries at the dentino-enamel junction. Pain is not a common feature of chronic caries because of the protection afforded the pulp by secondary dentin.

RECURRENT CARIES. Recurrent caries is that type which occurs in the immediate vicinity of a restoration. It is usually due to inadequate extension of the original restoration, which favors retention of debris, or to poor adaptation of the filling material to the cavity, which produces a "leaky margin." In either event, the renewed caries follows the same general pattern as primary caries.

It has been thought that recurrent caries occurs beneath restorations if all the carious dentin is not removed before inserting the filling. The fallacy of this idea is apparent if one recalls that caries is dependent upon the presence not only of microorganisms, but also of substrate, carbohydrate. In cases of recurrent caries beneath restoration, it can usually be shown that the restoration has poor margins which permitted leakage and the entrance of both bacteria and substrate. Besic in 1943 studied the fate of bacteria sealed in dentinal tubules and noted that lactobacilli died out, while streptococci persisted.

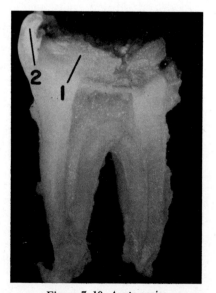

Figure 7–10. *Acute caries.*
There is accumulation of soft, necrotic dentin *(1)* and undermined enamel *(2)*.

ARRESTED CARIES. Arrested caries has been described as caries which becomes static or stationary and does not show any tendency for further progression. It is relatively uncommon, occurring in only 0.6 per cent of all teeth examined, according to a report of the Medical Research Council of Great Britain. However, other reports show a much higher percentage of teeth with arrested caries. Much of the confusion is due to the lack of agreement on the clinical diagnosis of arrested caries.

The deciduous and permanent dentitions are both affected by this condition. It occurs almost exclusively in caries of occlusal surfaces and is characterized by a large open cavity in which there is lack of food retention and in which the superficially softened and decalcified dentin is gradually burnished until it takes on a brown-stained, polished appearance and is hard. This has been referred to as "eburnation of dentin" (Fig. 7–11). Sclerosis of dentinal tubules and secondary dentin formation commonly occur in cases of arrested caries.

Another form of arrested caries is that sometimes seen on the proximal surfaces of teeth in cases in which the adjacent approximating tooth has been extracted, revealing a brown-stained area at or just below the contact point of the retained tooth. This represents very early caries which, in many cases, is arrested following the extraction because of the formation of a self-cleansing area.

Caries arrest following the topical application

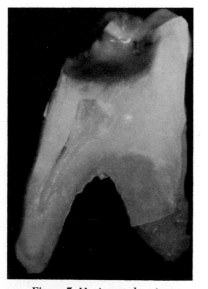

Figure 7–11. Arrested caries.
The dentin is dark brown, hard and shiny. The enamel is not appreciably undermined.

of stannous fluoride solution has been reported by Muhler in as high as 22 to 25 per cent of tooth surfaces originally diagnosed as carious. When areas that had been considered incipient carious areas, demineralized areas, etchings, or frank carious lesions were treated with the stannous fluoride solution, subsequent clinical examination showed the areas to be apparently sound, but manifesting certain typical acquired characteristics: (1) the presence of brown pigmentation, (2) the change from a soft to a hard texture, (3) the change from a chalky whiteness to light brown, (4) no increase in the size of the lesion, and (5) no further progress of the lesion as long as the pigmentation remained. Muhler stated that the smaller the size of the lesions at the time of the initial application of stannous fluoride, the greater the chance of caries arrest.

ENAMEL CARIES REMINERALIZATION. This process, also described under the terms "caries reversibility" and "consolidation" of the early enamel carious lesion, has received increased attention in recent years, chiefly due to recognition of its more common occurrence than formerly believed.

Several early studies had suggested the possibility of such a phenomenon. For example, Anderson in 1938 had noted that the early white lesions of enamel caries could become arrested and rehardened under certain oral conditions. Muhler in 1961 also described reversals of some of his diagnoses of early carious lesions in his studies on the topical application of stannous fluoride solution in children when lesions previously charted appeared to have subsequently healed or disappeared, as discussed previously, but referred to this as arrested caries. Backer-Dirks reported similar occurrences in 1966. Koulourides and his co-workers in related studies in 1961 utilized actual surface hardness testing to study the rehardening of tooth surfaces that had been previously softened by exposure to acid solutions. They found that exposure of a softened tooth to calcium phosphate solution would cause hardening of the surface but that the exposure of similarly softened teeth to solutions containing 1.0 ppm fluoride would cause an acceleration in the rate of rehardening compared to solutions without fluoride. This entire phenomenon has been reviewed and discussed at length by Silverstone in 1977 and 1982, and clinical evidence for the remineralization phenomenon occurring in vivo is well documented. It is also well established that this can only take place if cavitation has not occurred.

The results of research investigations now indicate that a natural biologic remineralizing process exists in the mouth which is responsible for the maintenance of tooth surfaces by precipitation of mineral salts from saliva. It is further suggested that the fluoride ion plays a role in stimulating the remineralization process through increasing the rate of deposition of calcium phosphate, and enhancing the degree of remineralization achieved, and then—itself becoming incorporated into the mineral—produces a remineralized enamel with a reduced acid solubility.

Small enamel lesions, representing early stage carious lesions, cannot be detected by conventional clinical or radiographic techniques, according to Silverstone, since the alteration consists of a limited zone of demineralization below the surface without cavitation. It is these areas, appearing clinically normal, which become remineralized with fluoride-containing salts and which may be maintained in this state indefinitely until some alteration in the balance occurs, and the lesion enlarges and becomes the usual clinically and roentgenographically detectable carious lesion.

Caries Susceptibility of Jaw Quadrants, Individual Teeth and Tooth Surfaces. A good many clinical studies have been devoted to determination of caries rates of individual jaw quadrants, individual teeth and individual tooth surfaces. Such information is extremely important and useful in contributing to a more thorough understanding of the caries process.

Caries susceptibility of the jaw quadrants has been shown by numerous investigators to exhibit a bilateral distribution between the right and left quadrants of both maxillary and mandibular arches. Although unilateral caries is found in some persons, it occurs with a random distribution. In a relatively large sample of the population the right and left sides of the mouth are involved with equal frequency. This horizontal relation is closer than either a vertical or a diagonal one. It was reported by Scott in 1944, for example, that bilateral caries was found in over 95 per cent of a group of 300 persons whose dental roentgenograms were studied.

There is general acceptance of the numerous reports that the maxillary arch is more frequently involved by caries than the mandibular arch. This appears to hold true despite the extremely high incidence of carious mandibular first molars, since this is compensated for by the general immunity of mandibular anterior teeth. Day and Sedwick (1935), in a study of 433 13-year-old children, reported that 60 per cent of all caries was in the maxillary arch. Healey and Cheyne in 1943, studying caries activity in University of Minnesota and Indiana University students, reported that in the former institution 44.4 per cent and 47.5 per cent of the maxillary teeth were involved in men and women respectively, compared to 33.1 per cent and 34.4 per cent of the mandibular teeth in the respective sexes. At Indiana University 40.0 per cent and 42.9 per cent of the maxillary teeth in men and women respectively were carious, and only 31.0 per cent and 32.9 per cent of the mandibular teeth in the respective sexes were carious.

The reason for the difference between the arches in caries susceptibility is not well documented. It may relate to gravity and the fact that saliva with its buffering action would tend to drain from the upper teeth and collect around the lower. It is of interest that in the laboratory rat, mandibular caries far surpasses maxillary caries.

Caries susceptibility of individual teeth has been studied by numerous investigators, and it has been found that, generally speaking, there is a definite order of caries attack for the different teeth of both the deciduous and the permanent dentitions.

Brekhus in 1931 studied a group of 3711 students at the University of Minnesota and reported the following caries susceptibility incidence of the teeth:

Upper and lower first molars	95%
Upper and lower second molars	75%
Upper second bicuspids	45%
Upper first bicuspids and lower second bicuspids	35%
Upper central and lateral incisors	30%
Upper cuspids and lower first bicuspids	10%
Lower central and lateral incisors and lower cuspids	3%

Klein and Palmer in 1941 studied the problem of individual tooth susceptibility, pointing out that the teeth farthest back in the mouth are most frequently carious and that these are the teeth with the pits, fissures and broadest contact points.

The posteruptive tooth age has been plotted against caries attack rate by Healey and Cheyne. They concluded that this posteruptive tooth age is important, but probably minor

Table 7–7. Carious Surfaces per 100 Teeth

	LINGUAL	BUCCAL	MESIAL	DISTAL	OCCLUSAL
Maxillary teeth	7.33	3.46	16.17	13.09	45.66
Mandibular teeth	0.73	11.18	4.96	4.47	37.98
All teeth	4.21	6.93	10.82	8.98	41.65

From T. P. Hyatt and A. J. Lotka: How dental statistics are secured in the Metropolitan Life Insurance Company. J. Dent. Res., 9:411, 1929.

compared to other factors such as tooth morphology, structure and position in the mouth.

Caries susceptibility of individual tooth surfaces has been found to exhibit considerable variation depending upon the morphology, location and posteruptive age.

Hyatt and Lotka in 1929 studied carious involvement of various tooth surfaces in 2943 patients under 25 years of age. Their findings are shown in Table 7–7. These data indicate that occlusal surfaces are by far the most commonly affected, followed by the mesial, distal, buccal and lingual surfaces in descending order.

Comparable studies have been carried out by Day and Sedwick (1935) and Klein and his associates (1938). The former studied 433 13-year-old children, while Klein and his associates reported on 23,753 surfaces in elementary school children. Their data, presented in terms of total percentage of involved surfaces, are shown in Table 7–8.

The various studies indicate that the occlusal cavity is the most prevalent type of lesion in both the deciduous and permanent dentitions. Occlusal caries appears to start earlier in life than proximal caries. In general, mesial caries is more common than distal caries, while buccal caries is more common than lingual in the mandibular molars. In maxillary molars, lingual cavities occur more frequently than buccal cavities.

THE HISTOPATHOLOGY OF DENTAL CARIES

Dental caries is a most interesting but difficult process to study microscopically because of the technical problems involved in preparation of the tissue for examination. The principal manner in which caries of the enamel has been studied is through the use of ground sections of teeth. The decalcification process necessary for cutting thin sections usually results in complete loss of enamel unless special methods are used. This has materially impeded the investigation of dental caries at the microscopic level, although surprising advances have been made in the face of adverse conditions.

The recent application of transmission and scanning electron microscopy to the study of dental caries has added greatly to our understanding of this disease, as has utilization of other techniques, including histochemical studies and the use of radioactive isotopes. For ease of understanding, the histopathology of dental caries will be considered under the general headings of caries of enamel, of dentin and of cementum.

Caries of the Enamel. Caries of the enamel is believed by most investigators to be preceded by the formation of a microbial (dental) plaque. The process varies slightly, depending upon the occurrence of the lesion on smooth surfaces or

Table 7–8. Total Percentage of Carious Surfaces

	LINGUAL (%)	BUCCAL (%)	MESIAL (%)	DISTAL (%)	OCCLUSAL (%)
Klein et al.[1]	13	13	17	14	43
Day and Sedwick[2]	9	7	16	10	57

[1]H. Klein, C. E. Palmer, and J. W. Knutson: Studies on dental caries. I. Dental status and dental needs of elementary school children. U.S. Public Health Rep. 53:751, 1938.

[2]C. D. M. Day and H. J. Sedwick: Studies on the incidence of dental caries. Dent. Cosmos, 77:442, 1935.

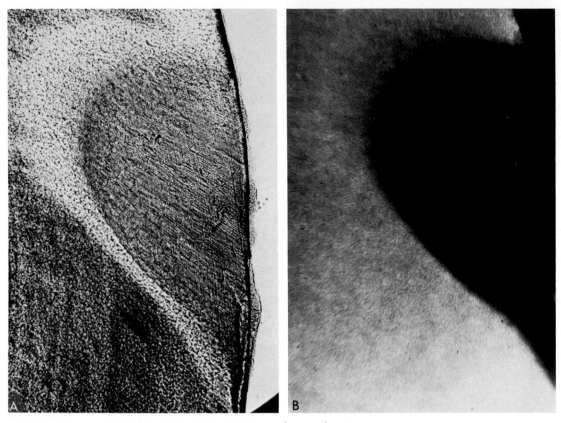

Figure 7–12. *Early enamel caries.*
A photomicrograph through a chalky area of enamel *(A)* shows demonstrable change without actual cavitation. The Grenz-ray picture *(B)* shows loss of mineral in this area. (Courtesy of Dr. Edmund Applebaum.)

in pits or fissures. For this reason it is best to discuss enamel caries under these two headings.

SMOOTH SURFACE CARIES. The surface of the enamel, at least in newly erupted teeth, is covered by a membrane composed of the primary and secondary cuticle. The significance of this membrane in forestalling the development of a carious lesion is not known, but it is probably not clinically important because it is lost early in posteruptive life.

The earliest manifestation of incipient caries of the enamel is the appearance beneath the dental plaque of an area of decalcification which resembles a smooth chalky white area (Figs. 7–9, 7–12). That this is a critical point in the development of this disease is underscored by the convening of a symposium, "Incipient Caries of Enamel," which was held at the University of Michigan in November 1977 and edited by Rowe. Study of early lesions by the transmission electron microscope, particularly by Scott and his associates, has revealed that the first change is usually a loss of the interprismatic

or inter-rod substance of the enamel with increased prominence of the rods. In some instances the initial change seems to consist of roughening of the ends of the enamel rods, suggesting that the prism may be more susceptible to early attack. (Fig. 7–13). The work of Sognnaes and Wislocki on the mucopolysaccharide present in the interprismatic organic substance of the enamel revealed that the degradation of this substance occurred very early in the caries process. Very early in the process, also, there is the appearance of transverse striations of the enamel rods, dark lines or bands occurring at right angles to the enamel prisms, suggesting segments. These striations are probably due to changes occurring in the rods between calcospherites and actually can be produced in vitro by the exposure of a ground section of tooth to dilute acid.

Another change in early enamel caries is the accentuation of the incremental striae of Retzius (Fig. 7–14). This conspicuous appearance of the calcification lines is an optical phenomenon due

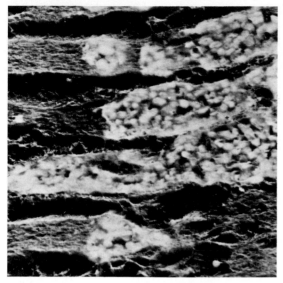

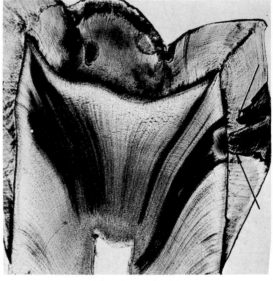

Figure 7–13. *Early enamel caries.*
Electron photomicrograph of demineralized enamel showing microorganisms apparently localized within prisms in early stage of caries. The specimen was cut from a tooth slice and demineralized 18 hours in 5 per cent trichloracetic acid. Original magnification: × 7500. (Courtesy of Dr. David B. Scott; from D. B. Scott and J. T. Albright: Oral Surg., 7:64, 1954.)

Figure 7–15. *Advanced enamel caries with early involvement of dentin.*
The typical pyramidal shape of the proximal enamel lesion is apparent.

to loss of minerals which causes the organic structures to appear more prominent.

As this process advances and involves deeper layers of enamel, it will be noted that smooth surface caries, particularly of proximal surfaces, has a distinctive shape. It forms a triangular or actually a cone-shaped lesion with the apex toward the dentino-enamel junction and the base toward the surface of the tooth (Fig. 7–15).

There is eventual loss of continuity of the enamel surface, and the surface feels rough to the point of an explorer. This roughness is caused by the disintegration of the enamel prisms after decalcification of the interprismatic substance and the accumulation of debris and microorganisms over the enamel rods (Fig. 7–16).

Before complete disintegration of the enamel, several zones can be distinguished, beginning on the dentinal side of the lesion:

Zone 1: The translucent zone lies at the advancing front of the enamel lesion. It is not always present. By means of polarized light it has been shown that this zone is slightly more porous than sound enamel, having a pore volume of 1 per cent compared with 0.1 per cent in sound enamel.

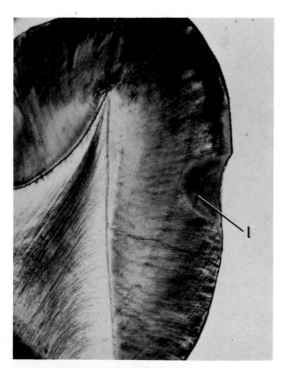
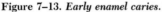

Figure 7–14. *Early enamel caries.*
Accentuation of a stria of Retzius (1) as it crosses the carious lesion is illustrated.

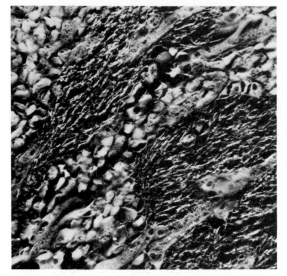

Figure 7–16. *Advanced enamel caries.*
Electron photomicrograph of demineralized enamel showing the presence of matrix fibrils in advanced stage of caries. A tooth slice was demineralized 11 days in 5 per cent formic acid, and the specimen was cut from the demineralized enamel. Original magnification: × 10,000. (Courtesy of Dr. David B. Scott; from D. B. Scott and J. T. Albright: Oral Surg., 7:64, 1954.)

Zone 2:   The dark zone lies adjacent and superficial to the translucent zone. It has been referred to as the positive zone, because it is usually present. This zone is formed as a result of demineralization.

Zone 3:   The body of the lesion lies between the relatively unaffected surface layer and the dark zone. It is the area of greatest demineralization. In polarized light the zone shows a pore volume of 5 per cent in spaces near the periphery to 25 per cent in the center of the intact lesion.

Zone 4:   The surface zone, when examined by the polarizing microscope and microradiography, appears relatively unaffected. The greater resistance of the surface layer may be due to a greater degree of mineralization and/or a greater concentration of fluoride in the surface enamel.

There has been some attempt at implication of enamel lamellae as pathways of invasion of proteolytic microorganisms and the subsequent development of caries, but there is no direct evidence to indicate that enamel lamellae play

any significant role in the development of caries. Some investigators do think that if lamellae occur at areas on the tooth surface where caries is apt to arise, caries is more likely to develop than if the lamellae were not present.

Scott and Wyckoff reported that there is no direct relation between the occurrence of enamel lamellae and smooth surface caries on the basis of electron microscope studies. They have pointed out that in those cases in which lamellae appear to be associated with caries, the association is by chance (Fig. 7–17).

PIT AND FISSURE CARIES. The carious process in pits and fissures does not differ in nature from smooth surface caries except as the variations in anatomic and histologic structure dictate. Here too the lesion begins beneath a bacterial plaque with decalcification of the enamel (Fig. 7–18).

Pits and fissures are often of such depth that food stagnation with bacterial decomposition in the base is to be expected. Furthermore, the enamel in the bottom of the pit or fissure may be very thin, so that early dentin involvement frequently occurs. On the other hand, some pits and fissures are shallow and have a relatively thick layer of enamel covering their base. In both types the enamel rods flare laterally in the bottom of the pits and fissures. When caries occurs here, it follows the direction of the enamel rods and characteristically forms a tri-

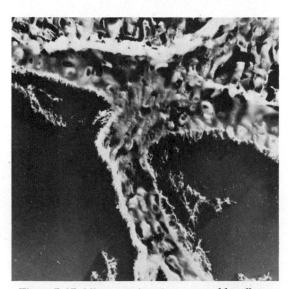

Figure 7–17. *Microorganisms in an enamel lamella or "defect" isolated by acid-flotation from clinically noncarious enamel.*
Original magnification: × 13,000. (Courtesy of Dr. David B. Scott; from D. B. Scott and J. T. Albright: Oral Surg., 7:64, 1954.)

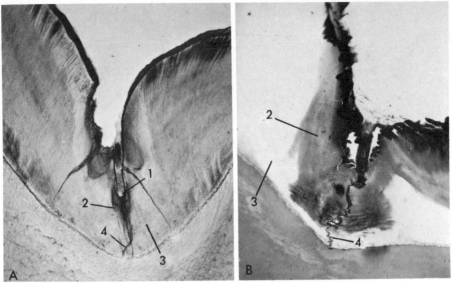

Figure 7–18. *Fissure caries of enamel.*
Ground section of tooth *A)* shows the bacterial plaque *(1)*, carious enamel *(2)* and noncarious enamel *(3)*. The decalcified section *(B)* illustrates that the carious enamel *(2)* is not lost during preparation of the section as is noncarious enamel *(3)*. Enamel lamella is shown at *(4)*.

angular or cone-shaped lesion with its apex at the outer surface and its base toward the dentino-enamel junction (Fig. 7–19). It should be noted that the general shape of the lesion here

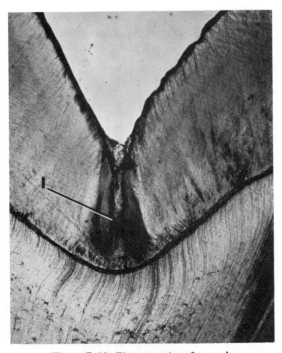

Figure 7–19. *Fissure caries of enamel.*
The lesion is pyramidal in shape and generally follows the direction of the enamel rods. Note the depth of the actual fissure *(1)*.

is just the opposite of that occurring on smooth surfaces. Because of this shape, there is almost invariably a greater number of dentinal tubules involved when the lesion reaches the dentino-enamel junction. Pit and fissure caries, particularly of occlusal surfaces, usually produces greater cavitation than proximal smooth surface caries.

The carious lesion is more apt to be stained with a brown pigment in pits and fissures and generally tends to produce more undermining of the enamel because of the difference in shape of the cavity. Occasionally, enamel lamellae are found in the base of pits and fissures, and here too this occurrence has suggested to some investigators that they may be important as a caries pathway (Fig. 7–20).

Caries of the Dentin. Caries of the dentin begins with the natural spread of the process along the dentino-enamel junction and the rapid involvement of great numbers of dentinal tubules, each of which acts as a tract leading to the dental pulp along which the microorganisms may travel at a variable rate of speed, depending upon a number of factors (Fig. 7–21). In some instances carious invasion appears to occur through an enamel lamella so that little if any visible alteration in the enamel occurs. Thus, when lateral spread at the dentino-enamel junction occurs with involvement of underlying dentin, a cavity of considerable size may actually form with only slight clinically evident changes

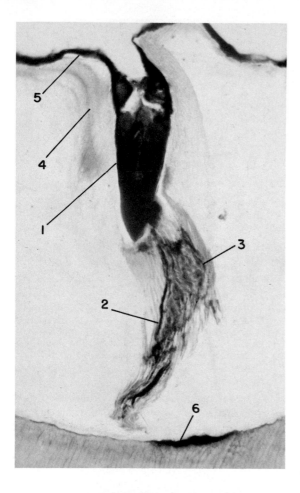

Figure 7–20. *Fissure caries.*
Decalcified section of a tooth demonstrating a bacterial plaque *(1)*, enamel lamella *(2)*, carious enamel *(3)*, accentuated striae of Retzius *(4)*, enamel cuticle *(5)* and early caries of dentin *(6)*. (Courtesy of Dr. Edmund Applebaum.)

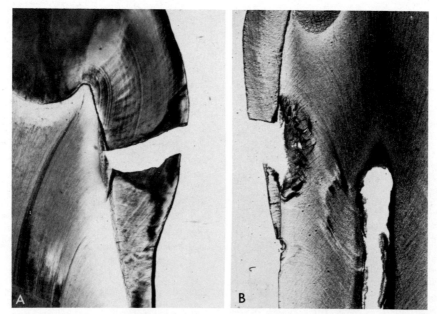

Figure 7–21. *Early caries of dentin.*
There is lateral spread of caries at the dentino-enamel junction.

in the overlying enamel except for its undermining.

EARLY DENTINAL CHANGES. The initial penetration of the dentin by caries may result in alterations in the dentin previously described as dentinal sclerosis, or "transparent dentin." This dentinal sclerosis is a reaction of vital dentinal tubules and a vital pulp in which there results a calcification of the dentinal tubules that tends to seal them off against further penetration by microorganisms. The formation of sclerotic dentin is minimal in rapidly advancing caries and is most prominent in slow chronic caries. The term "transparent dentin" has been applied because of the peculiar transparent appearance of the tooth structure when a ground section is viewed by transmitted light. By reflected light sclerotic dentin appears dark.

The appearance of fatty degeneration of Tomes' dentinal fibers, with the deposition of fat globules in these processes, precedes even the early sclerotic dentinal changes. This can be demonstrated only by the application to fresh dentin of special stains such as Sudan red, which selectively stains fat. The significance of this phenomenon is not known, although it has been suggested that the fat contributes to the impermeability of the dentinal tubules. Beust showed in 1933, however, that "transparent" dentin remains impenetrable to dyes even though the tooth is treated with alcohol and ether to remove the fatty material. Fatty degeneration may be a predisposing factor favoring sclerosis of the tubules.

Except in unusual cases of arrested caries, continued destruction of dentin inevitably occurs despite the attempts at walling off on the part of the tooth. The rate at which the carious destruction progresses tends to be slower in older adults than in young persons because of the generalized dentinal sclerosis that occurs as a part of the aging process. Close examination of the dentin behind a zone of sclerosis formed in response to caries will reveal decalcification of the dentin, which appears to occur slightly in advance of the bacterial invasion of the tubules. In the earliest stages of caries when only a few tubules are involved, microorganisms may be found penetrating these tubules before there is any clinical evidence of the carious process (Figs. 7–22, 7–23). These have been termed "pioneer bacteria."

This initial decalcification involves the walls of the tubules, allowing them to distend slightly as they become packed with masses of microorganisms (Fig. 7–24). Careful study of individual tubules will usually show almost pure forms

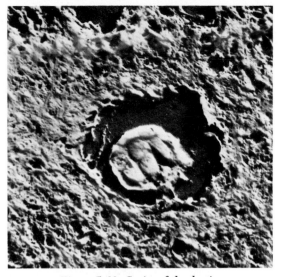

Figure 7–22. *Caries of the dentin.*
Electron photomicrograph of demineralized carious dentin showing bacteria in a dentinal fiber. Specimen cut from tooth slice and demineralized 3 days in 5 per cent trichloracetic acid. Original magnification: × 16,500. (Courtesy of Dr. David B. Scott; from D. B. Scott and J. T. Albright: Oral Surg., 7:64, 1954.)

of bacteria in each one. Thus one tubule may be filled with coccal forms, while the adjacent tubules may contain only bacilli or thread forms (Fig. 7–25).

It is evident that these microorganisms, as

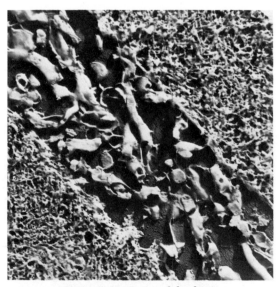

Figure 7–23. *Caries of the dentin.*
Electron photomicrograph of demineralized carious dentin showing bacteria in a dentinal tubule. Specimen cut from tooth slice and demineralized 3 days in 10 per cent lactic acid. Original magnification: × 10,000. (Courtesy of Dr. David B. Scott; from D. B. Scott and J. T. Albright: Oral Surg., 7:64, 1954.)

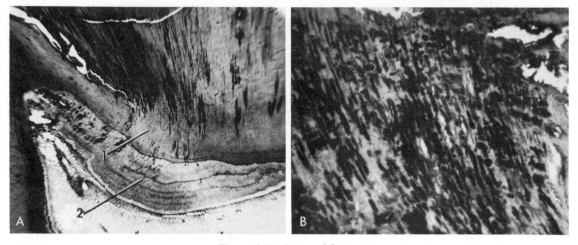

Figure 7–24. *Caries of dentin.*

The low-power photomicrograph *(A)* shows involvement of both primary *(1)* and secondary dentin *(2)* by the carious process. In the high-power photomicrograph *(B)* the dentinal tubules are seen packed with microorganisms.

they penetrate farther and farther into the dentin, become separated more and more from the carbohydrate substrate upon which the bacteria responsible for the *initiation* of the disease depend. The high protein content of the dentin would favor the growth of those microorganisms which have the ability to utilize this protein in their metabolism. Thus proteolytic organisms would appear to predominate in deeper caries of the dentin, while acidogenic forms are more prominent in early caries. The observation that the morphologic type of the bacteria in deep carious dentin is different from that of the bacteria in initial caries substantiates the hypothesis that *initiation* and *progression* of dental caries are two distinct processes and must be differentiated. The evidence indicates that the organisms responsible for the initiation of caries

are subsequently replaced by others as the environmental conditions occasioned by the advancing carious lesion are altered. Nevertheless, many microorganisms do have both acidogenic and proteolytic properties.

ADVANCED DENTINAL CHANGES. The decalcification of the walls of the individual tubules leads to their confluence, although the general structure of the organic matrix is maintained for some time. A thickening and swelling of the sheath of Neumann may sometimes be noted

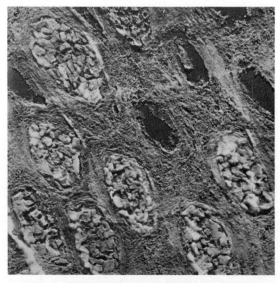

Figure 7–26. *Caries of dentin.*

Electron photomicrograph of demineralized carious dentin shows packing by bacteria of dentinal tubules cut in cross section. Original magnification: × 10,000. (Courtesy of Dr. David B. Scott.)

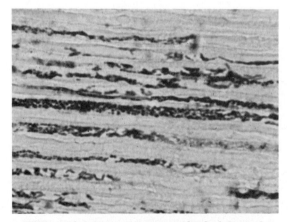

Figure 7–25. *Microorganisms in individual dentinal tubules. (Gram stain.)*

at irregular intervals along the course of involved dentinal tubules, in addition to the increase in diameter of the dentinal tubules due to packing of the tubules by microorganisms (Fig. 7–26). Tiny "liquefaction foci," described by Miller, are formed by focal coalescence and breakdown of a few dentinal tubules (Fig. 7–27). This "focus" is an ovoid area of destruction, parallel to the course of the tubules and filled with necrotic debris which tends to increase in size by expansion. This produces compression and distortion of adjacent dentinal tubules so that their course is bent around the "liquefaction focus." In areas of globular dentin, decalcification and confluence of tubules occur rapidly. The presence of considerable amounts of globular dentin accounts for the rapid spread of caries in so-called malacotic or soft teeth.

It has been pointed out that acidogenic organisms are apparently responsible for the initial decalcification of the dentin occurring in the caries process, but that another mechanism must be necessary for the ultimate destruction of the remaining organic matrix. The most logical explanation is that this matrix is destroyed by the action of proteolytic enzymes produced

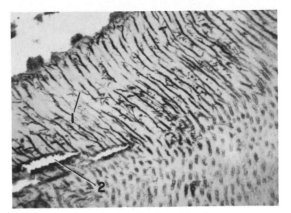

Figure 7–28. *Caries of dentin.*
Lateral branches of the dentinal tubules (1) are filled with microorganisms. Note the typical transverse clefts (2).

by microorganisms deep in the cavity. This enzymatic digestion is of maximal activity only when the organic matrix is decalcified; there is little effect on intact dentin.

The destruction of dentin through a process of decalcification followed by proteolysis occurs at numerous focal areas which eventually coalesce to form a necrotic mass of dentin of a leathery consistency. Clefts are rather common in this softened dentin, although they are rare in chronic caries, since the formation of a great deal of softened necrotic dentin is unusual. These clefts extend at right angles to the dentinal tubules and appear to be due to extension of the carious process along the lateral branches of the tubules or along the matrix fibers which run in this direction (Fig. 7–28). These clefts parallel the contour lines of the dentin, which are due to alternating resting periods during the calcification of the dentin. The clefts account for the manner in which carious dentin often can be excavated by peeling away thin layers with hand instruments.

As the carious lesion progresses, various zones of carious dentin may be distinguished which grossly tend to assume the shape of a triangle with the apex toward the pulp and the base toward the enamel. Beginning pulpally at the advancing edge of the lesion adjacent to the normal dentin, these zones are as follows:

Zone 1: Zone of fatty degeneration of Tomes' fibers.

Zone 2: Zone of dentinal sclerosis characterized by deposition of calcium salts in dentinal tubules.

Zone 3: Zone of decalcification of dentin, a narrow zone, preceding bacterial invasion.

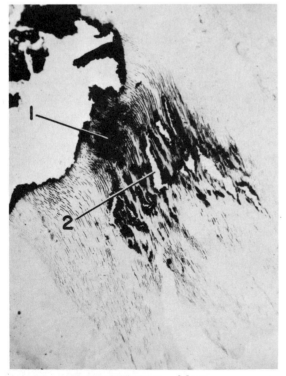

Figure 7–27. *Caries of dentin.*
The tubules contain microorganisms. There are liquefaction necrosis (1) and clefts (2) in the carious dentin. (Periodic acid–Schiff stain.)

Zone 4: Zone of bacterial invasion of decalcified but intact dentin.

Zone 5: Zone of decomposed dentin.

SECONDARY DENTIN INVOLVEMENT. The carious involvement of secondary dentin does not differ remarkably from involvement of the primary dentin, except that it is usually somewhat slower because the dentinal tubules are fewer in number and more irregular in their course, thus delaying penetration of the invading microorganisms. Sooner or later, however, involvement of the pulp results with ensuing inflammation and necrosis. Occasionally caries will spread laterally at the junction of the primary and secondary dentin and produce a separation of the two layers.

Root Caries. The carious lesion discussed prior to this point has been limited chiefly to coronal caries, and the process has involved basically the enamel and dentin of that portion of the tooth. Another form of the disease does exist which is known as root caries or root surface caries. At one time, it was also referred to as "caries of cementum." Excellent investigations of root caries, including a review of the literature with clinical, histopathologic and microradiographic descriptions, have been published by Hazen and his associates and by Westbrook and his colleagues.

There are few published studies on the prevalence of root caries. However, it is generally recognized that the longer lifespan of persons today, with the retention of teeth into the later decades of life, has increased the number of the population exhibiting gingival recession with clinical exposure of cemental surfaces and thereby probably increasing the prevalence of root caries. The root surface must be exposed to the oral environment before caries can develop here.

There are four different destructive lesions which may affect the root surface of a tooth: (1) abrasion, (2) erosion, (3) idiopathic resorption, and (4) caries. Our concern here is only with root caries, which has been defined by Hazen and his colleagues as "a soft, progressive lesion that is found anywhere on the root surface that has lost connective tissue attachment and is exposed to the oral environment. Enamel may become secondarily involved if it is undermined during the progression of the lesion. Dental plaque and microbial invasion are an essential part of the cause and progression of this lesion." However, there is some evidence that the microorganisms involved in root caries are different from those involved in coronal caries, being filamentous rather than coccal.

Microorgansims appear to invade the cementum either along Sharpey's fibers or between bundles of fibers, in a manner comparable to invasion along dentinal tubules. Since cementum is formed in concentric layers and presents a lamellated appearance, the microorganisms tend to spread laterally between the various layers. Irregular mineralization on this cemental surface may often be seen at the same time, probably representing beginning calculus formation. After decalcification of the cementum, destruction of the remaining matrix occurs similar to the process in dentin, with ultimate softening and destruction of this tissue. As the caries process continues, there is invasion of microorganisms into underlying dentinal tubules, subsequent matrix destruction and finally pulpal involvement.

Most investigators have felt that once caries involves the dentin, the process is identical with coronal dentinal caries, according to Westbrook and his associates. However, it has been pointed out that since there are more dentinal tubules per unit area in the crown than in the root of the tooth, one might expect differences in the rate of caries progression and the amount of dentinal sclerosis present.

One excellent investigation of the prevalence and distribution of root caries in the adult population has been reported by Katz and his associates. Their study, involving 473 persons between 20 and 64 years of age, revealed a root caries index rate of 11.4 per cent, which indicated that approximately one in nine tooth surfaces exhibiting gingival recession had developed root caries. Significantly, there was an 18-fold increase in the average number of surfaces with root caries per subject between ages 20 and 64. The intraoral distribution patterns for root caries were also studied, and it was found that the teeth most frequently affected were first the mandibular molars, next the mandibular premolars, and then the maxillary cuspids. The mandibular incisors were the least frequently attacked teeth. It was also of interest that the interproximal surfaces were affected most frequently in the maxillary arch, while the buccal surfaces were attacked most frequently in the mandibular arch.

Methods of caries control will be discussed later. However, it may be pointed out here that there is one report dealing with the effect of fluoride on root caries. This is an investigation by Stamm and Banting, who compared the

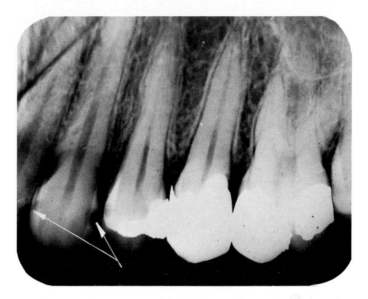

Figure 7–29. *Interproximal caries.*

prevalence of root surface caries in 502 adult lifelong residents of a naturally fluoridated (1.6 ppm F) Canadian community to that of 465 similar adults in a nonfluoridated community. They found a mean of 0.48 root surfaces decayed and another 0.16 filled in the fluoridated population in contrast to a mean of 0.99 root surfaces decayed and 0.37 filled in the nonfluoridated community. The differences were statistically significant, and the authors concluded that the lifelong consumption of fluoridated water is capable of significantly reducing the prevalence of root surface caries, which may itself be a growing dental public health problem in the adult population.

ROENTGENOGRAPHIC DIAGNOSIS OF DENTAL CARIES

The roentgenogram is a necessary adjunct to a complete oral examination by the dentist. Although many carious lesions are accessible and visible for easy diagnosis, there is a great percentage of lesions, chiefly interproximal in location, which are not found by the routine examination with mouth mirror and explorer. It has been pointed out previously that studies have indicated that the use of roentgenograms may reveal 50 per cent more cavities than may be found by visual examination alone.

The interproximal carious lesion is most easily

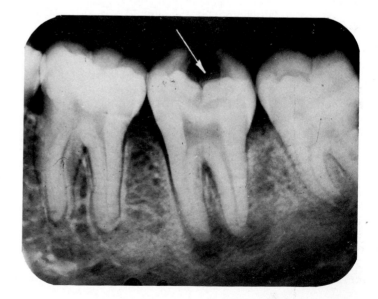

Figure 7–30. *Occlusal caries (with periapical involvement.)*

recognized on the roentgenogram and appears in early lesions as a small, triangular radiolucent area of the enamel, and later of the dentin, occurring approximately at the contact point (Fig. 7–29). The roentgenogram is of little value in the diagnosis of occlusal cavities, until they become so large that the use of the film is unnecessary, because of the irregularity of the surface and the superimposition of cusps (Fig. 7–30). The roentgenogram is similarly unsuited for use in the detection of small cavities in buccal or lingual pits or at the cervical margin.

METHODS OF CARIES CONTROL

The control of dental caries presents one of the greatest challenges that must be met today by the dental profession. It is not sufficient that we try to perfect techniques to repair damage to the dental apparatus once it has occurred. It has been a general failing of the healing professions that the treatment of disease has been overemphasized and prevention minimized. Kauffman has stated that "the supreme ideal of the dental profession should be to eliminate the necessity for its own existence." Although this Utopian suggestion can probably never be realized, it does emphasize the necessity for a more forceful approach to the problem of preventing dental caries.

Research in dentistry, particularly that aimed at a better understanding of the carious process, has not been lacking. Although the ideal has not been reached or even approached, there have been definite accomplishments in the field of caries control. Methods are at hand for producing a substantial reduction in dental caries experience, provided the patient can be properly educated.

The most promising methods of caries control will be discussed in this section, along with the experimental evidence upon which their use has been predicated. These suggested methods of control may be classified into three general types: (1) chemical measures, (2) nutritional measures, and (3) mechanical measures.

CHEMICAL MEASURES OF CARIES CONTROL

A vast number of chemical substances have been proposed for the purpose of controlling dental caries. The use of some of these has been based upon sound experimental evidence; the use of others has been purely empiric and without scientific foundation. These chemicals include: (1) substances which alter the tooth surface or tooth structure, (2) substances which interfere with carbohydrate degradation through enzymatic alterations, and (3) substances which interfere with bacterial growth and metabolism. In the light of our present knowledge, each of these theoretically may be of benefit in controlling caries. Final proof, however, depends upon thorough clinical trial.

Substances Which Alter the Tooth Surface or Tooth Structure

Of the chemical substances falling within this category, fluorine appears to be the most promising and hence has been the most widely tested.

Fluorine. The history of fluorine and dental caries dates from the recognition by G. V. Black and Frederick S. McKay that teeth with even a severe degree of mottled enamel have a greater immunity to dental caries than normal teeth.

Fluorine has been administered principally in two ways: through the communal water supply and by topical application.

FLUORIDATION OF WATER SUPPLIES. The studies of Dean and other members of the United States Public Health Service were instrumental in establishing the inverse relation between the fluorine content of the communal water supply and dental caries experience (Table 7–9). These studies have been carried out in numerous cities throughout the United States and have generally indicated that persons residing for their entire lives in an area where significant amounts of fluorine are naturally present in the drinking water exhibit less caries than persons born and raised in fluoride-free areas (Fig. 7–31). If persons are born in a fluoride area, but are removed from exposure to fluoride-containing water at variable times after birth, their caries experience increases proportionately.

Dean and his associates (1941) studied this problem in children in Bauxite, Arkansas, where the drinking water had a fluoride content of 14 ppm until the water supply was changed to a fluoride-free source. Children born in this area and exposed to the high fluoride water for a sufficient period to exhibit mottled enamel had a low caries attack rate compared to children born in the area after the change in water supply. The percentages of children who were caries-free in the two groups were 27 and 15 per cent, respectively. In the high fluoride

Table 7–9. Relation of Fluorine in Drinking Water to Caries Experience and Mottled Enamel in 12- to 14-Year-Old Children

CITY	NO. OF CHILDREN EXAMINED	FLUORINE CONTENT OF WATER (PPM)	CARIES EXPERIENCE PER 100 CHILDREN			INCIDENCE MOTTLED ENAMEL (%)
			TOTAL	CARIOUS UPPER INCISOR SURFACES	1ST MOLAR MORTALITY	
Colorado Springs, Colo.	404	2.55	246	0.31	4.7	73.8
Joliet, Ill.	447	1.30	321	1.30	19.5	25.3
Kewanee, Ill.	123	0.90	343	1.40	29.3	12.2
Marion, Ohio	263	0.43	556	3.30	25.1	6.1
Zanesville, Ohio	459	0.19	733	11.40	99.8	1.5
Waukegan, Ill.	423	0.00	810	17.70	79.9	0.2

Adapted from H. T. Dean, F. A. Arnold and E. Elvove: Domestic water and dental caries. V. Additional studies of the relation of fluoride domestic waters to dental caries experience in 4,425 white children, aged 12 to 14 years, of 13 cities in 4 states. U.S. Public Health Rep., 57:1155, 1942.

Distribution of Communities With 0.7 PPM or More Natural Fluoride in Community Water Supply Systems, 1969

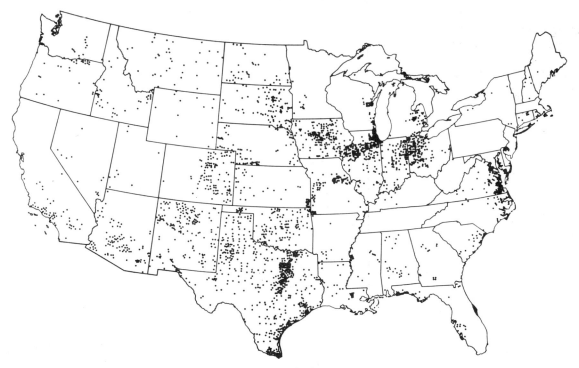

Figure 7–31.
This map of the United States shows those towns using naturally fluoridated water, i.e., water containing 0.7 ppm or more of fluoride, according to information gathered by the United States Public Health Service, Department of Health, Education, and Welfare, and is published through the courtesy of the Division of Dental Health, Bureau of Health Manpower Education of the National Institutes of Health (1969).

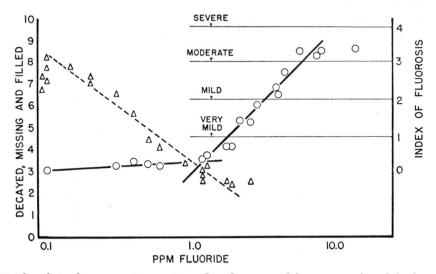

Figure 7–32. *The relation between caries experience, fluoride content of the water supply and the degree of dental fluorosis.*

There appears to be a precise relation between the index of dental fluorosis and the logarithm of the ppm F in the drinking water. The intersection of the index-of-fluorosis line with the DMF (caries incidence) line at 1 ppm F gives this concentration the significance of maximal tooth health with minimal hazard. On the basis of the available evidence from human studies, a twofold factor of safety exists between levels of fluoride producing enamel hypoplasia and the level of 1 ppm. (Courtesy of Dr. Harold C. Hodge; from H. C. Hodge and F. A. Smith: Some public health aspects of water fluoridation; in J. H. Shaw (ed.): Fluoridation as a Public Health Measure. Washington, D. C., American Association for the Advancement of Science, 1954.)

group, only 39 per cent of the first molars were carious, while in the group not exposed to fluoride 65 per cent of the first molars were carious.

The many clinical studies reported indicate that a reduction in caries experience is not necessarily dependent upon the presence of mottled enamel. Hodge and Smith clearly showed the relation between the fluoride content of water, the index of dental fluorosis and the DMF rate based upon public health data in Figure 7–32. This demonstrates diagrammatically the level of ppm of fluoride in the drinking water which produces the maximal amount of protection against caries with the minimal hazard of fluorosis. These workers have pointed out that a twofold factor of safety exists between the protective level of 1 ppm of fluoride and the level necessary to produce significant clinical fluorosis.

The natural occurrence of fluoride in the drinking water and the attendant reduced caries incidence suggested that the artificial addition of fluoride to the communal water supply might result in a similar reduction in caries. In addition, the studies of Armstrong, among others, indicated that the fluoride content of caries-free teeth is higher than that of carious teeth.

One of the first experimental clinical studies of artificial fluoridation was that carried out in two cities in New York, Kingston and Newburgh, at the proposal of Ast and supported by the New York State Board of Health. These two cities were selected because they had similar populations and were geographically close. The water supply of Kingston was low in fluoride (less than 0.15 ppm); so Kingston served as the control city. Sufficient fluoride was added to the water of Newburgh to raise the level to 1.0 to 1.2 ppm. This fluoridation was begun in 1945.

The results of caries examinations completed eight to nine years after initiation of fluoridation in Newburgh were reported by Ast and his co-workers. The data were based upon 756 children six to ten years of age, 374 in Kingston and 382 in Newburgh, including only those children in the latter city who had been exposed to the Newburgh water supply continuously since fluoridation was begun. The study is summarized in Table 7–10 and indicates that the DMF rate among Newburgh children was 60 per cent lower than that among Kingston children. The DMF rate of the first permanent molars in the Newburgh children was only about 50 per cent of that among Kingston

Table 7–10. Effect of Fluoridation on Caries Experience in the
Kingston-Newburgh Study

AGE	NO. OF CHILDREN EXAMINED		NO. OF DMF TEETH		DMF TEETH PER 100 ERUPTED PERMANENT TEETH			DMF TEETH PER 100 CHILDREN WITH PERMANENT TEETH		
	KINGS-TON	NEW-BURGH	KINGS-TON	NEW-BURGH	KINGS-TON	NEW-BURGH	DIFFER-ENCE (%)	KINGS-TON	NEW-BURGH	DIFFER-ENCE (%)
6	113	74	42	8	8.3	2.1	—74.7	45.2	12.7	—71.9
7	71	94	107	47	18.6	5.9	—68.3	155.1	50.0	—67.8
8	89	80	230	91	24.1	10.1	—58.1	258.4	113.8	—56.0
9	59	73	237	97	30.3	10.3	—66.0	401.7	132.9	—66.9
10	42	61	229	153	30.4	14.9	—51.0	545.2	250.8	—54.0
Total	374	382	845	396	23.7	9.8	—58.6	240.1	106.7	—55.6
Adjusted rate	—	—	—	—	23.7	9.4	—60.3	240.1	94.1	—60.8

Modified from D. B. Ast, A. Bushel, B. Wachs, and C. Chase: Newburgh-Kingston caries-fluorine study. VIII. Combined clinical and roentgenographic dental findings after 8 years of fluoride experience. J. Am. Dent. Assoc., 50:680, 1955.

children. There was not a single missing first permanent molar in Newburgh children even though approximately 7 per cent of the first permanent molars were missing in the 9- and 10-year-old children residing in Kingston. Newburgh children in the 6- to 9-year-old age range exhibited over three times as many caries-free deciduous teeth as the Kingston group.

A similar controlled study was carried out in the cities of Grand Rapids and Muskegon, Michigan, by the United States Public Health Service, the Michigan Department of Health and the University of Michigan. Both cities obtain their domestic water supply from Lake Michigan. These cities were chosen because considerable caries data had already been collected on children using domestic water from Lake Michigan and because this general area was known to be one in which caries experience was high. In addition, the city of Aurora, Illinois, was selected for inclusion in this study to establish a "caries expectancy curve," since this city has had a water supply containing 1.2 ppm of natural fluoride for many years. The fluoridation of the Grand Rapids water supply with 1.0 ppm fluoride was begun in January, 1945. No change was made in the water supply of Muskegon, and the fluoride content remained at less than 0.2 ppm of fluoride.

The effects of this fluoridation on caries experience in the test city are shown in Table 7–11. The Grand Rapids children manifested a reduction in dental caries experience in the permanent teeth ranging from 76 per cent in 6-year-old children to 51 per cent in the 10-year-old age group. The deciduous teeth also showed

reductions in caries. The caries rate in Muskegon, the control city, remained constant over the entire period of study. The investigators also concluded that a comparison of the caries rates in Grand Rapids and Aurora indicated that, as far as can be determined, artificially fluoridated water gives the same beneficial effects as water containing natural fluoride at the same concentration.

A number of other cities began fluoridation of the communal water supply at approximately the same times as Grand Rapids and Newburgh and have carefully followed the dental caries rate since the initiation of fluoridation. The results in these cities have been summarized by Ast and his associates in Table 7–11. Literally hundreds of cities in the United States today are adding fluoride to the communal water supply, although opposition to fluoridation has developed in some areas because of the supposed systemic effects of fluoride (Fig. 7–33). As of November 30, 1982, according to the Dental Disease Prevention Activity of the Department of Health and Human Services, Public Health Service, Centers for Disease Control at Atlanta, 112,282,896 persons out of the total United States population of 229,837,916, or 48.9 per cent, were receiving either naturally occurring or adjusted (added) fluoride in their water supply (Fig. 7–34).

Good reviews of the subject of fluoridation and caries prevention have been published by Ericsson (1977) and Fejerskov and co-workers in 1981. Cariostatic mechanisms of fluorides were also the subject of a workshop organized by the American Dental Association and the

Table 7–11. Dental Caries Reductions as a Result of Fluoridation of
Water Supply in Eight Areas

CITY	DATE STARTED	REPORT PERIOD	AGE GROUP	REDUCTION IN DENTAL DECAY	
				PERMANENT (%)	PRIMARY (%)
Brantford, Ontario[1]	June, 1945	After 10 years	5	—	61
			6	65	56
			7	51	48
			8	52	37
			9	52	46
			10	43	61
			11	44	10
			12	42	
			13	44	
			14	32	
Evanston, Illinois[2, 4]	February, 1947	After 12 to 23 months	6	50	
			7	33	
			8	22	
		After 59 to 70 months	12	22	
			13	21	
			14	13	
Grand Rapids, Michigan[4]	January, 1945	After 9 years	6	76	
			7	62	
			8	52	
			9	53	
			10	51	
Lewiston, Idaho[2]	June, 1947	After 4 years, 9 months	6	77	
			7	52	
			8	59	
			9	46	
Madison, Wisconsin[2]	June, 1948	After 3½ years	Kindergarten		48
Marshall, Texas[2]	May, 1946	After 29 months	6	47	
			All school ages	23	
Newburgh, New York[2, 3] (compared with control city of Kingston)	May, 1945	After 7 years	5	—	59
			6	56	47
			7	69	35
			8	43	17
			9	57	
			10	47	
			11	47	
			12	39	
		After 10 years	6– 9	57	
			10–12	52	
			13–14	48	
			16	41	
Sheboygan, Wisconsin[2]	March, 1946	After 5½ years	5– 6		54
			9–10	30	
			12–14	23	

[1]Report to the Minister of Health, Province of Ontario, on the Brantford fluoridation experiment. J. Can. Dent. Assoc., 22:342, 1956.

[2]D. B. Ast and H. C. Chase: The Newburgh-Kingston caries fluorine study. IV. Dental findings after six years of water fluoridation. Oral Surg., 6:114, 1953.

[3]D. B. Ast, D. J. Smith, B. Wachs, and K. T. Cantwell: Newburgh-Kingston caries-fluorine study. XIV. Combined clinical and roentgenographic dental findings after ten years of fluoride experience. J. Am. Dent. Assoc., 52:314, 1956.

[4]H. T. Dean: Fluorine in the control of dental caries. J. Am. Dent. Assoc., 52:1, 1956.

DISTRIBUTION OF COMMUNITIES SERVED WITH CONTROLLED FLUORIDATED WATER, 1969

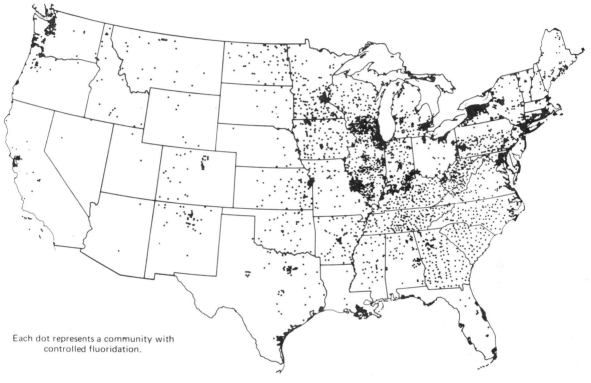

Each dot represents a community with controlled fluoridation.

Figure 7–33.

This map of the United States shows those towns artificially fluoridating their water supply. This map was prepared by the United States Public Health Service, Department of Health, Education, and Welfare, and is published through the courtesy of the Division of Dental Health, Bureau of Health Manpower Education of the National Institutes of Health (1969).

This is the latest map available indicating individual fluoridated communities and is presented only to illustrate the widespread nature of controlled fluoridation. Since the preparation of this map, there has been an estimated 25 to 30 per cent increase in the number of communities benefiting from controlled fluoridation throughout the United States.

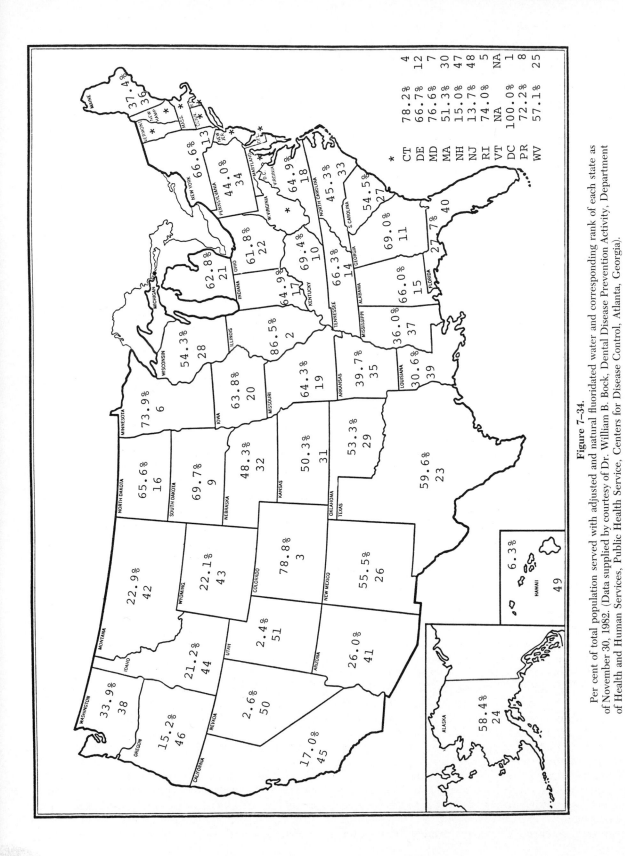

Figure 7-34.

Per cent of total population served with adjusted and natural fluoridated water and corresponding rank of each state as of November 30, 1982. (Data supplied by courtesy of Dr. William B. Bock, Dental Disease Prevention Activity, Department of Health and Human Services, Public Health Service, Centers for Disease Control, Atlanta, Georgia).

National Institute of Dental Research, with the proceedings published in Caries Research (1977) and edited by Brown and König. Careful studies of chronic toxicity by many workers have failed to reveal the slightest detrimental effect caused by fluoridation of the water supply. Blood cell counts, hemoglobin determinations and urinalyses have always been within normal limits, and there has been no evidence of alterations in development of bones. It must be concluded that fluoridation of water is not only an absolutely safe procedure, but also a highly beneficial one because of its caries-protective action.

Mechanism of Action of Ingested Fluoride. The mechanism of action of fluoride in the drinking water has been discussed by many workers, and several theories have been proposed. Since fluoride inhibits enzymes by inactivating the co-enzyme portion of the enolase system, and specifically by inhibiting the conversion of 2-phosphoglyceric acid to (enol) phosphopyruvic acid, it has been thought to protect against caries by preventing carbohydrate degradation. But the level of fluoride taken in is so low, the dilution factor by saliva is so great and the oral clearance is so rapid that this mechanism is generally dismissed as insignificant. Studies by McClure of amylolytic activity of saliva indicated that this enzyme is unaffected by the fluoride content of the water supply.

The *L. acidophilus* counts of saliva of patients in cities with varying amounts of fluoride in the drinking water received considerable attention by the United States Public Health Service workers in the earlier studies. The scientific consensus based upon these studies is that the *L. acidophilus* counts are more closely associated with caries activity than with the fluoride content of the water supply. Thus the mechanism of action of fluoride does not appear to be through inhibition of microorganisms.

The most widely accepted theory on the mechanism of action of ingested fluoride is that of alteration of the structure of the developing tooth through systemic absorption of the element. Such a mechanism would explain the clinical observation of greater caries protection of children residing in fluoride areas during tooth formation as compared to caries experience of children moving into such an area after tooth crown formation has been completed. The exact means whereby fluoride would alter the tooth structure to resist caries has not been completely established, but it is probably through incorporation of fluorine in the crystal lattice structure of the enamel, with the formation of a fluorapatite producing a less acid-soluble enamel.

TOPICAL APPLICATION OF FLUORIDE. The second manner in which fluoride is used for the prevention of dental caries is by topical or local application to the teeth. The first suggestion that such a technique might be effective was contained in the work of Volker and his associates when they reported that the exposure of powdered enamel to solutions of sodium fluoride resulted in a reduction in the solubility of the enamel. Subsequent work indicated that the enamel adsorbed fluoride onto its surface. Although the exact mechanism is not known, it appears that there is formed either a calcium fluoride or a calcium fluorapatite.

Numerous laboratory studies have been carried out to improve the means of decreasing enamel solubility. Thus various fluoride compounds have been tested at varying pH levels. Although early studies dealt with sodium fluoride, it was subsequently found that potassium, ammonium and even lead fluoride were effective in reducing enamel solubility. Muhler and Van Huysen found that tin fluoride was an even more effective fluoride compound.

It was only natural that some attempt would be made to decrease the solubility of "whole" enamel in vivo by exposing it to a relatively concentrated fluoride solution, thereby adsorbing some of the material onto the surface. This, theoretically, should result in a greater resistance of the tooth to acid decalcification. A great many clinical studies have been carried out, and the majority have conclusively demonstrated the benefit of topical application of fluoride.

Many problems had to be investigated in the early studies, such as the number of applications necessary to derive maximal benefit in caries reduction, the appropriate interval between applications and the optimal concentration of fluoride solution. One of the earliest studies was that of Bibby, who applied a 0.1 per cent solution of sodium fluoride to one mouth quadrant of a group of children from 10 to 12 years old after a dental prophylaxis. During the first year three applications at intervals of four months were carried out. At the end of the first year there were 33 new carious lesions in the treated quadrants, but there were 61 such lesions in the untreated quadrants. This represented a caries reduction of approximately 46 per cent in the treated quadrants.

Knutson and Armstrong reported a similar

study in which 8 to 15 applications of a 2 per cent solution of sodium fluoride were made to the teeth of one side of the mouth in a group of 289 children aged 7 to 15 years. After a period of one year the reduction in the caries rate of the treated teeth was found to be approximately 40 per cent. A good many other topical application studies have also been reported in the scientific literature, and the results are similar. The evidence indicates that the topical application of sodium fluoride to the teeth of children has a significant beneficial effect in reducing the dental caries incidence.

More recently, a great many clinical studies on the effectiveness of topical application of stannous fluoride in reducing the incidence of dental caries have been reported. For example, Muhler treated the teeth of a group of 232 children, 6 to 17 years of age, with a single topical application of an 8 per cent solution of stannous fluoride; 228 children of a similar age were treated with distilled water and served as controls. All children in this study had resided for their entire lifetime in an area in which fluoride had been added to the communal water supply, and thus the experiment tested an additional beneficial anticariogenic effect of topical fluoride under optimal communal fluoride conditions. At the end of 12 months Muhler found a 35 per cent reduction in DMF teeth in the stannous fluoride-treated group, thus indicating an extension of benefit of fluoride therapy in children already benefiting from communal water fluoridation.

A five-year clinical study was reported by Gish and his associates, who tested the effectiveness on permanent teeth of a single yearly application of an 8 per cent solution of stannous fluoride against a conventional series of four applications each three years of a 2 per cent solution of sodium fluoride. At the end of the five-year period the stannous fluoride children showed 30 per cent fewer DMF teeth and 35 per cent fewer DMF surfaces than the sodium fluoride group, thus indicating the anticariogenic effectiveness of a single yearly application of stannous fluoride. The cumulative annual caries data also showed that there was no loss of effectiveness in anticariogenicity under the stannous fluoride reapplication schedule during the five-year period.

A similar study reported by Mercer and Muhler tested the effectiveness of a single application of a 2 per cent solution of sodium fluoride as contrasted to a single application of an 8 per cent solution of stannous fluoride. At

the end of one year the 151 children treated with sodium fluoride exhibited no reduction in either DMF teeth or DMF surfaces as compared to the control group of 152 children treated only with distilled water. But the 154 children receiving the single topical application of stannous fluoride exhibited a 50 per cent reduction in DMF teeth and a 51 per cent reduction in DMF surfaces. A similar study reported by Salter and his associates confirmed the findings of Mercer and Muhler. Another previous investigation in preschool children by Compton and his co-workers also reported a reduction in caries increment after a single application of 8 per cent stannous fluoride.

The effectiveness of a single topical application on the caries incidence in adults also was studied by Muhler in a group of 500 university students between the ages of 18 and 35 years. The application of a 10 per cent solution of stannous fluoride resulted in a 24 per cent decrease in DMF teeth and a 16 per cent decrease in DMF surfaces after a period of one year. A similar study on a young male adult group of military personnel between 17 and 21 years of age was reported by Protheroe. In the first 12 months after a single application of a 10 per cent stannous fluoride solution there was an average 54 per cent reduction in the increment of DMF surfaces.

Many other studies testing the clinical anticariogenic effectiveness of topical stannous fluoride solution have been reported in the literature, and the results are generally uniform in their findings of benefit of this compound.

Acidulated fluoride-phosphate solutions and gels also have received considerable attention since the work of Brudevold and his associates in which it was shown that topical application of an acidulated sodium fluoride-phosphate (AFP) mixture increased the uptake of fluoride in enamel. While numerous clinical studies have been carried out to test this system, the reports generally have failed to show more than a moderate reduction in caries incidence in children not receiving fluoride in the communal water supply. For example, the report of DePaola and his co-workers (1968) showed a reduction of 20.6 per cent in DMF surfaces in children 6 to 11 years of age, one year after initial application of the AFP solution, but only a 12.8 per cent reduction after 3 years. Similarly, Cons and Janerich (1969) reported a reduction of 18 per cent in PMF surfaces after three years in a similar study.

Englander and his associates (1967) reported

a 75 to 80 per cent reduction in DMF surface increments in a study in which an AFP gel or neutral sodium fluoride gel was applied in a group of school children, with no loss of effective protection after nearly two years. Enamel of teeth treated by the AFP gel showed greater fluoride uptake than the neutral fluoride group.

Two studies by Muhler and his associates (1965), using a stannous fluoride-phosphate system, found exceptional reductions in caries incidence, and it appeared that this modality is more effective than either stannous fluoride alone or the acidulated sodium fluoride-phosphate mixture.

Another method for the topical application of fluoride to prevent dental caries, suggested by Bibby and his associates, is that it might be used in a prophylactic paste. Only very limited data are available on the results of studies utilizing sodium fluoride in such a paste, and in these, caries reduction has been quite limited. There are numerous studies, however, in which stannous fluoride has been incorporated in a prophylactic paste with either a lava pumice or silex base. In general, it has been reported that stannous fluoride in a prophylactic paste provides caries reductions of between 30 and 40 per cent in both children and adults in the presence or absence of fluoride in the communal water supply. For example, Gish and Muhler (1965) reported a reduction of 39.2 per cent in DMF surfaces in a three-year study of a group of children 6 to 14 years of age, who were receiving stannous fluoride prophylaxis treatment.

Also tested was a stannous fluoride-zirconium silicate paste used as a patient-applied treatment procedure. Muhler (1968) reported a 63 per cent reduction in DMF surfaces after one year in a limited group of children 10 to 13 years of age applying the fluoride-zirconium paste themselves, while Gish and Mercer (1969) reported a 25 per cent reduction in DMF surfaces in a comparable study. The fact that this treatment procedure is patient-applied may make it a practical tool in the field of preventive dentistry.

FLUORIDE DENTIFRICES. Still another method of applying fluoride is through the medium of a dentifrice. Although fluoride-containing mouthwashes, lozenges and chewing gum have all been suggested, and in some cases tested, there is no evidence to indicate that their use produces any beneficial effect. Fluoride dentifrices have been extensively tested.

Muhler reported the effect of a stannous fluoride dentifrice on caries experience after 36 months of unsupervised use by a group of 343 children, divided between a control group of 169 and an experimental group of 174 patients. The mean DMF teeth increment in the control group was 5.17 and that in the experimental group was 4.02, a 22 per cent reduction in DMF teeth. A similar reduction was found for DMF surfaces. On the basis of caries data obtained by examination of patients every six months throughout the three-year test period, Muhler concluded that the stannous fluoride dentifrice produced a benefit which increased linearly in relation to time.

Jordan and Peterson also reported that the use of a stannous fluoride-containing dentrifice in 609 school children, 8 to 11 years of age, resulted in a reduction of 35 per cent DMF teeth and 34 per cent DMF surfaces after one year as compared to a control group of children. At the end of the second year there were 16 per cent fewer DMF teeth and 21 per cent fewer DMF surfaces in the children brushing at school with the test dentifrice than in the control children brushing under similar conditions.

A study of the effect of stannous fluoride dentifrice used under controlled brushing habits, at least two minutes per brushing three times a day, in a group of 311 military schoolboys ranging in age from 10 to 19 years has been reported by Peffley and Muhler. At the end of 10 months they found a 93 per cent reduction in DMF teeth and a 57 per cent reduction in DMF surfaces. The comparatively high caries reduction was thought to be related to the greater frequency of usage of the dentifrice in this study than in previously reported studies.

It is generally recognized that the most effective mass reduction in dental caries is afforded by communal fluoridation. This procedure is unavailable, however, in many communities and impractical in rural areas. Therefore it is possible that the use of more than one of the other effective anticariogenic agents may produce cumulative effects. Muhler tested this hypothesis in a three-year clinical test conducted in a nonfluoride area on a group of 314 children between the ages of 6 and 15 years. The experimental group of 156 patients received single topical applications of an 8 per cent solution of stannous fluoride each six months and in addition used a stannous fluoride dentifrice. The 158 control patients received topical applications of distilled water and used a similar but nonfluoride dentifrice. At the end of a the 36-month period the experimental group showed a 57 per cent reduction in DMF teeth and a 63 per cent reduction in DMF surfaces. The most new decayed surfaces in any treated child during the entire three-year study was 14, while in the control group it was 50. Furthermore, Muhler reported that the carious lesions in the stannous fluoride group failed to increase in size as rapidly as those in the control group. He concluded that these findings strongly suggest that the use of "multiple principles of preventive dentistry" are not only practical, but also very highly effective.

Hill reviewed the investigations dealing with the clinical use of fluoride dentifrices and concluded that, although some variation exists in results between individual studies, the one thing constant is that all the studies have shown some degree of control of caries.

The beneficial anticariogenic effects reported in the numerous clinical investigations of a stannous fluoride dentifrice prompted official recognition and acceptance of one commercial dentifrice as a caries-preventive agent by the Council on Dental Therapeutics of the American Dental Association in August, 1960, the first dentifrice ever accepted as such. Since that time, a number of other commercial dentifrices have received approval for their therapeutic value against dental caries. There can be no doubt that the basic investigations on topical application of stannous fluoride and the development of an accepted stannous fluoride dentifrice have added immeasurably to those concrete measures available for prevention of dental caries and improvement of oral health.

FLUORIDE MOUTHWASHES OR RINSES. There has been extensive clinical trial of mouthwashes or rinses containing fluoride used either as a mouthwash to flush the oral cavity or, in a few instances, by application with a toothbrush in efforts to prevent dental caries. These studies, whose different regimens and results have been summarized in a thorough review of the literature by the Council on Dental Therapeutics of the American Dental Association (1975) and more recently by Ripa (1981), have demonstrated conclusively that rinsing is a simple and inexpensive method of utilizing fluoride to inhibit dental caries. This has been proven so unequivocally that the Council on Dental Therapeutics of the American Dental Association has now recognized neutral sodium fluoride and acidulated phosphate-fluoride rinses as effective caries-preventive agents (1975) as well as stan-

nous fluoride rinse (1980). Since the rinsing can be performed as an individual caries-preventive measure at home or as a school-based group preventive program, the dentist must be familiar with the different techniques involved, because they vary considerably with the different circumstances and objectives.

One of the earliest large scale successful clinical trials was that reported by Torell and Ericsson in 1965. They undertook a two-year study in Göteborg, Sweden, to evaluate the caries-reducing effects of various methods of local application of fluorides. Of six experimental groups each containing approximately 200 children, 10 years of age, several groups developed significantly less caries compared with control groups that included: (1) a group with daily unsupervised mouthwashing with a 0.05 per cent sodium fluoride solution, and (2) a group with supervised mouthwashing once every two weeks with a 0.2 per cent sodium fluoride solution, as well as several other groups receiving topical fluoride application and using fluoride dentifrices.

This study was soon followed by many others, such as those of Englander and his associates (1967), who reported an 80 per cent reduction in DMF surfaces following the daily use of sodium fluoride mouthwash rinse in a group of children ranging in age from 11 to 14 years, and of Conchie and his associates (1969) who reported a reduction of 25 per cent in DMF surfaces in a three-year study of supervised toothbrushing with a fluoride-phosphate solution in a group of 12- to 13-year-old children.

The vast majority of succeeding studies were aimed not at continuously proving the value of fluoride mouthrinses as a caries-preventive agent, but rather at defining the best technical methods to use in achieving the desired result. Thus, many different fluoride concentrations were tested, ranging from 0.01 per cent NaF to 0.66 per cent NaF, and many rinsing frequencies tried, ranging from twice a day to three or four times a year. These studies are too numerous to review individually, but they have basically given rise to the two chief techniques used today: (1) the low potency/high frequency technique, usually recommended for home use and (2) the high potency/low frequency technique, usually recommended for school-based programs.

The extreme importance of fluoride rinsing as a caries-inhibiting technique mandates periodic thorough review and update of these procedures by all practicing dentists.

Bis-biguanides. Chlorhexidine and alexidine have received the most attention as potential anticaries agents, since they have been shown to be effective antiplaque agents. It has been shown by in vitro studies that chlorhexidine is adsorbed onto tooth surfaces and salivary mucins, then is released very slowly in an active form.

The effect of chlorhexidine on growth of human dental plaque has been studied by Harrap in persons using a chlorhexidine gluconate dentifrice. He found highly significant reductions in plaque growth that were related to the concentrations of the drug. In contrast, Johansen and his colleagues could find no effect on plaque index as a result of the use of chlorhexidine dentifrice by a group of dental students, although possible favorable effects on caries were noted. Unfortunately, chlorhexidine has a bitter taste, produces a brownish discoloration of hard and soft tissues and may produce a painful desquamation of mucosa.

More research and clinical trials with these agents will decide their true effectiveness.

Silver Nitrate. Silver nitrate impregnation of teeth was used clinically for many years to prevent or arrest dental caries. The earlier workers believed that the silver "plugged" the enamel, either the organic invasion pathways such as the enamel lamellae or the inorganic pathways, combining with the soluble inorganic portion of enamel to form a less soluble combination.

A group of 700 children, ranging in age from 5 to 12 years, was used in a study by Klein and Knutson to investigate the effect of ammoniacal silver nitrate on caries experience. Over a period of three and one-half years they treated the maxillary right and mandibular left first molars once a year with silver nitrate, while the opposing untreated first molars served as controls. The results indicated that there were no significant differences in caries attack rate between treated and untreated teeth. Carious lesions present at the time of silver nitrate treatment had extended to approximately the same degree in both treated and control teeth.

This study is in contrast to one of Younger, who applied silver nitrate precipitated with calcium chloride to the teeth of 25 children 5 to 12 years of age, after first restoring all carious lesions. After one year these 25 children manifested 11 new cavities, or an average of 0.44 per child. The control group of 5 children had a total of 21 new cavities, an average of 4.2 per child. By the end of the second year of observation the experimental group averaged 0.65 new cavity per child; the control group, 5.2 new cavities. In a later study Younger reported a similar reduction in caries in a group of children who were 8 to 13 years of age. After one year the group treated with silver nitrate exhibited an average of 0.6 new carious lesion, while the controls had an average of 4.5 new cavities. Crawford found that a group of 81 patients averaged 3.09 cavities per person during the year preceding treatment with silver nitrate and an average of only 0.54 new cavity in the year after treatment.

Zinc Chloride and Potassium Ferrocyanide. Gottlieb, in accordance with his theories of the importance of the protein matrix of the enamel in the dental caries process, proposed that the use of a solution of zinc chloride and potassium ferrocyanide would effectively impregnate the enamel and seal off caries invasion pathways.

Ast and his associates tested the effect of these substances in a group of children 12 to 15 years of age. The teeth on one side of the mouth were impregnated, while those on the opposite side served as controls. After one year no significant differences were noted between the two sides in the number of new carious surfaces. A similar study was carried out by Pelton on a group of 100 children ranging from 8 to 14 years of age. He found that the number of teeth which became carious after application of zinc chloride and potassium ferrocyanide was essentially the same as that of untreated teeth. Finally, a study of Anderson and Knutson on 299 children ranging in age from 7 to 15 years in whom half the mouth had been treated with these compounds revealed that the total new decayed or filled surfaces after approximately one year were essentially the same for treated and untreated teeth.

The available evidence indicates that the use of substances to impregnate the enamel and thus block organic pathways of caries is of little clinical value.

Substances Which Interfere with Carbohydrate Degradation through Enzymatic Alterations

There are many substances known which have the ability to interfere with enzyme systems responsible for carbohydrate degradation and the subsequent formation of acid. If such an inhibitor is to be effective in the clinical prevention of dental caries, it must reach the susceptible areas of the mouth in sufficient concentration at the time at which the sugar is undergoing breakdown.

Vitamin K. Synthetic vitamin K (2-methyl-1,4-naphthoquinone) was suggested by Fosdick and his co-workers to be of potential value in the prevention of caries on the basis of certain studies in vitro. In these studies the vitamin K was found to prevent acid formation in incubated mixtures of glucose and saliva. Many of the quinones have been found to have a similar action, but none is superior to synthetic vitamin K.

The clinical effectiveness of this vitamin K was tested by Burrill and his associates. A group of students received a chewing gum containing the synthetic vitamin K and sodium bisulfite and were instructed to chew this gum for at least 10 minutes after eating any food. The control group received the same chewing gum without the vitamin K. The occurrence of new cavities was determined at 12- and 18-month intervals, at which time it was found that the incidence of new carious lesions was decreased by 48 per cent and 42 per cent respectively for the two intervals in the experimental group. Thus there is evidence to indicate that the naphthoquinones may be of value in preventing caries.

Sarcoside. A method of screening potential anticariogenic compounds was suggested by Fosdick and his co-workers in 1953, based on the ability of some compounds to penetrate the dental plaque and prevent the pH fall below a level of 5.5 after a carbohydrate rinse. They tested several hundred compounds and noted that two of these were promising enzyme inhibitors or "antienzymes": sodium N-lauroyl sarcosinate and sodium dehydroacetate.

Brudevold and Little continued investigation of this sarcoside in patients who brushed their teeth with solutions of the material and then measured the fall in pH of plaque material from proximal surfaces after a sugar rinse. The effectiveness of a toothpaste containing sodium lauroyl sarcoside and dehydroacetic acid was also studied. All tests were negative, and it was concluded that the sarcoside did not reduce acid production in subsurface material of bulky plaque.

The effect of sodium lauroyl and palmitoyl sarcosinate in reducing the solubility of powdered enamel was studied by Volker and his associates. The palmitoyl compound was found to be better than the lauroyl, and in concentrations of 0.01 per cent to 1.0 per cent was as effective as sodium fluoride in reducing enamel solubility in the presence of acids.

Fosdick presented the results of a limited clinical study of patients who brushed their teeth with a dentifrice containing 2 per cent sodium N-lauroyl sarcosinate. The patients in this study were a group consisting chiefly of students at several universities and employees of a publishing firm, all of whom were under 35 years of age. The results indicated that the number of new carious surfaces developing in the controls varied somewhat from group to group, but averaged 0.63 in 628 patients of the random control group who brushed their teeth throughout the one-year period with their own dentifrice. In the group of 686 patients who brushed with a placebo dentifrice which was furnished them, the average number of new carious surfaces was 0.72. The 700 patients who brushed their teeth with the sarcosinate dentifrice morning and night exhibited only 0.27 new carious surface, while the 251 patients who brushed with the sarcosinate dentifrice after each meal averaged 0.35 new carious surface. Combining test and control groups, the average numbers of new carious surfaces were, respectively, 0.29 and 0.67, indicating a caries reduction of 57 per cent in patients who brushed with the experimental dentifrice.

Substances Which Interfere with Bacterial Growth and Metabolism

An alternative method for preventing enzymatic degradation of carbohydrates to acids is the prevention of, or at least interference with, bacterial growth and metabolism. There are, of course, great numbers of bactericidal or bacteriostatic agents, but the number of these which are compatible with the oral mucous membranes and with continued good health is small.

Urea and Ammonium Compounds. Urea and ammonium compounds have been tested extensively for use in the oral cavity as anticariogenic agents, the former after the preliminary report of Wach and his associates that a quinine-urea solution prevented acid formation in tests in vitro on carbohydrate-saliva mixtures. They also noted that the oral bacteria count was decreased after the use of a quinine-urea mouthwash and that the salivary pH generally increased to a value over 8 and remained high for approximately an hour.

Stephan continued the study of urea and found that a 40 to 50 per cent solution of urea applied to dental plaques for several minutes prevented the typical pH fall following a carbohydrate rinse for periods up to 24 hours. The evidence indicated that urea, upon degradation by urease, releases ammonia, which acts to neutralize acids formed through carbohydrate digestion and also interferes with bacterial growth.

The original observation of Grove and Grove in 1935 that a high salivary ammonia content was correlated with a relative immunity to dental caries provided impetus to the investigation of the ammonium compounds and urea. Kesel and his associates reported that dibasic ammonium phosphate in both a mouthwash and a dentifrice caused a reduction in oral lactobacillus counts. Studies in vitro indicated that the combination of 5 per cent dibasic ammonium phosphate and 3 per cent urea was even more effective as a bacteriostatic agent and in preventing acid formation than either substance alone.

Other workers, such as Jenkins and Wright, have indicated that the ammonium ion plays no specific role in inhibiting growth of acidogenic microorganisms. The ammonium ion failed to inhibit the growth of lactobacilli in the studies of Kirchheimer and Douglas, while the work of Ludwick and Fosdick showed no relation between the ammonia content of the oral cavity and caries immunity.

Several clinical studies have been carried out to evaluate the effectiveness of ammoniated dentifrices. Henschel and Lieber (1949) tested a dentifrice containing 27.5 per cent active ammonium compounds (22.5 per cent carbamide and 5.0 per cent dibasic ammonium phosphate) on a group of patients averaging 37.5 years of age. There was no attempt at supervision of home care. It was found that the experimental group, after using the therapeutic dentifrice for an average of 34.3 months, averaged 37.5 per cent reduction of DMF teeth as compared to the control group of the same approximate age, and a 35.2 per cent reduction in DMF teeth as compared to an auto-control pretest period averaging 7.8 years.

Kerr and Kesel reported on a group of children using a dentifrice containing 5 per cent dibasic ammonium phosphate and 3 per cent urea and found that over a two-year period, brushing with the ammoniated dentifrice resulted in a reduction of 21 per cent in the number of teeth attacked, as compared to a control group of children who did not brush their teeth in school under supervision. A group who brushed under supervision with a non-ammoniated dentifrice manifested a 9 per cent reduction in the number of teeth attacked as compared to the unsupervised control group. The authors concluded that the results of this study showed a trend indicating the usefulness both of good oral hygiene and of ammoniated dentifrices.

Cohen and Donzanti reported the results of a similar study on a group of 169 children using a dentifrice containing 13 per cent urea and 3 per cent diammonium phosphate and 137 children using a similar dentifrice without these two ingredients. Brushing was supervised in the schools twice daily. At the end of one year the mean number of new carious teeth was 1.01 in the control group, but only 0.78 in the experimental group, a 23 per cent reduction in caries incidence. By the end of the second year the number of new carious teeth in the control group was 2.27 and in the experimental group 1.70, a reduction of 25 per cent in caries incidence.

Hawes and Bibby reported the results of a study on 372 children between the ages of 7 and 13 who brushed their teeth for a period of one year under supervision with a dentifrice containing 12 per cent urea (carbamide) and a urease. Bacteriologic studies showed that the lactobacillus counts of the children using the therapeutic dentifrice were not affected to any greater extent than those of the children using the cosmetic dentifrice. The 177 children in the control group exhibited an average increase of 9.01 total tooth surfaces decayed and filled, while the test group, composed of 196 children, presented an average of 9.33 surfaces decayed and filled during the test period. The difference between the two groups was approximately 4 per cent and indicates that the urea dentifrice failed to produce any significant reduction in occurrence of new caries under the conditions of this study.

Although there are some studies to indicate that ammoniated dentifrices are capable of producing some reduction in dental caries incidence, the magnitude of this reduction, particularly in persons whose toothbrushing habits are not controlled or supervised, is not so great as to justify recommending them for widespread use as an anticariogenic agent.

Chlorophyll. Chlorophyll, the green pigment of plants, has been proposed as an anticariogenic agent on the basis of a number of in vitro studies and animal studies. Shafer and Hein reported that a water-soluble form of chlorophyll, sodium copper chlorophyllin, was capable of preventing or reducing the pH fall in carbohydrate-saliva mixtures in vitro. The same workers found that the incidence of experimental caries in hamsters was reduced when a chlorophyllin solution was substituted for the drinking water of these animals, but that the lactobacillus counts were not affected. Other workers, such as Griffiths and Rapp and Nevin and Bibby, have reported that chlorophyll is bacteriostatic with respect to many oral microorganisms, including lactobacilli, streptococci and micrococci.

There have been no clinical studies reported testing the effect of water-soluble chlorophyll on dental caries experience. A number of short-term clinical studies have suggested that this compound may be of some use in reducing mouth odors and allaying gingivitis. Results are inconclusive, however.

Nitrofurans. Nitrofurans are derivatives of furfural, which itself is derived from pentoses. They have been found to exert a bacteriostatic and bactericidal action on many gram-positive and gram-negative organisms and, on this basis, have been tested by Dreizen and his associates for their ability to inhibit acid production. A number of different nitrofuran compounds were utilized in this study, and it was reported that, even in low concentrations, acid production in saliva from caries-active persons was prevented in nearly all cases.

Hufstader and his associates tested the effect of Furacin (2-nitro-5-furaldehyde semicarbazone) incorporated in a chewing gum on the oral lactobacillus counts of a group of students. During the 10-day test period during which only a sugar-coated gum was chewed, the lactobacillus counts were definitely increased in the majority of patients. Chewing gum containing Furacin did not reduce the oral lactobacillus count.

The effectiveness of Furadroxyl (5-nitro-2-furaldehyde-2-hydroxyethyl semicarbazone) in preventing dental caries was tested clinically by Dreizen and Spies through use of the compound incorporated in a chewing gum. Three groups of patients, ranging from 6 to 38 years of age, were studied: one group received the medicated chewing gum (30 persons); a second group received the same gum without the nitrofuran compound (25 persons); and the third group received no chewing gum (25 persons). The study lasted for a period of 12 months. Only 25 new carious surfaces developed in the entire experimental group receiving Furadroxyl, or an average of 0.9 per person, compared to a total of 82 new carious surfaces, or an average of 3.3 new surfaces per person, in the group receiving the nonmedicated gum. The third group, which received no chewing gum, had a total of 106 new carious surfaces, an average of 4.2 per person. Although the number of patients in each group was relatively small, the data indicated that the nitrofuran compound significantly reduced the dental caries experience and that this substance may have potential use as an anticariogenic agent.

Penicillin. Penicillin has been tested as an anticariogenic compound because of its antibiotic property, which is the ability of the product of an organism to inhibit the normal biologic processes of other organisms. The effect on oral lactobacillus counts of a dentifrice containing 1000 units of penicillin per gram was studied by Hill in a group of 10 students. A remarkable reduction from an average of 72,000 colony count to an average of 300 was found after use of the dentifrice for five weeks. After discontinuing use of the dentifrice, the count stayed low for three months and then returned to the same high level. This was again reduced by a return to use of the penicillin dentifrice, but the reduction was considerably slower. A second study was carried out by Hill on a group of orphanage children, and though full cooperation was doubtful, there was some tendency for reduction in lactobacillus counts in the group who brushed their teeth with a penicillin dentifrice. White and her associates reported that small amounts of penicillin did not greatly alter the balance of the normal oral flora, although larger doses resulted in an increase of gram-negative organisms of the genera Aerobacter and Escherichia, apparently owing to their replacing that part of the flora destroyed by the penicillin.

The effect of prolonged use of a penicillin dentifrice was studied by Fitzgerald and his associates. Their results indicated that after use of the dentifrice for eight months or longer, there were no changes in the lactobacillus counts attributable to the penicillin. However, there was no increase in numbers of penicillin-fast lactobacilli.

Studies of Zander and Bibby indicated that penicillin effectively interfered with the production of acid in carbohydrate-saliva mixtures even in quantities as low as 10 units in 5 ml. of total solution. These investigators also reported the effect of brushing the teeth of hamsters with a penicillin dentifrice. In a group of control animals whose teeth were not brushed, an average of 19.0 cavities was found, whereas in the group whose teeth were brushed with a control tooth paste, an average of only 5.87 cavities occurred. Brushing with a penicillin toothpaste resulted in a remarkable reduction in caries, this group averaging only 0.86 cavity. McClure and Hewitt reported complete inhibition of caries in rats by administering penicillin to the experimental animals in the food and drinking water.

A clinical study was designed by Hill and Kniesner to determine the effect of a penicillin dentifrice on dental caries experience in the human being under uncontrolled conditions of oral hygiene. Examination of the children after one year revealed no significant differences in new carious surfaces between control and experimental groups even though there was a reduction in lactobacillus counts in the experimental group. Such a finding only emphasizes the difficulty in attempting to relate caries susceptibility or caries activity with the lactobacillus count.

Another clinical study was carried out by Zander on a group of children who brushed their teeth with a penicillin dentifrice under supervision during a 2-year period. The children ranged in age from 6 to 14 years and were distributed into an experimental group of 235 children who used the dentifrice containing 500 units of potassium penicillin per gram, and a control group of 174 children who used a nontherapeutic dentifrice. Compared to those of the control group, the permanent teeth in the experimental group showed a 58 per cent reduction in new carious surfaces at the end of the first year and a 60 per cent reduction by the end of the second year. The use of a dentrifice containing 600 units of potassium penicillin per gram by a group of school children for 18 months has been reported by Lunin and Mandel. They found no statistically significant differences in the caries incidence between control and experimental groups.

The results appear to indicate that penicillin is not a particularly effective anticariogenic agent. The wisdom of using this material for such a purpose has been further questioned by many because of the possibility of development of penicillin-resistant pathogenic microorganisms and sensitization.

Other Antibiotics. A variety of other antibiotics have been tested, in both experimental animal and clinical trials, for potential use as anticaries agents. These, along with other chemotherapeutic agents, have been reviewed by Johnson and Rozanis with special reference to plaque control. These investigators also pointed out some of the problems in using these drugs in humans: the possible induction of resistant strains of microorganisms, the possibility of allergic reactions, the occurrence of side-effects such as nausea and diarrhea, and the expense of long-term use. They also characterized the "ideal" antibiotic for use as an anticaries agent as being one which has a very narrow spectrum directed toward plaque-forming microorganisms, is not in general use against systemic diseases, is neither toxic nor allergenic and is retained in the tissue in an active state for a prolonged period with a predilection for the oral cavity.

Erythromycin was tested by Lobene and his associates, who reported a 35 per cent decrease in plaque formation after a seven-day test period of rinsing then swallowing the agent four times a day. This effect was lost rapidly when the drug was withdrawn in three of four patients and, in addition, all developed diarrhea as a side effect.

Kanamycin has been evaluated by Loesche and his associates for its effects on dental plaque in a small low-caries group when the antibiotic was applied topically for a few weeks and for one year. While there was some improvement in gingivitis scores, plaque scores were not changed despite some physicochemical changes in the plaque.

Spiramycin was noted by Keyes and his colleagues to be the most effective of nine antibacterial agents tested in hamsters for controlling dental plaque, caries and periodontal lesions. However, the clinical trials have been somewhat conflicting as to the beneficial effects of the drug on dental plaque. It would appear that any benefits derived are considerably less than highly significant.

Tetracycline was reported by Löe and his co-workers to decrease plaque scores when used as an 0.5 per cent mouthwash three times a day for five days in place of mechanical oral hygiene. However, there is little additional information available concerning its potential use as an anticaries agent.

Tyrothricin was reported by Shiere to be responsible for a 35 per cent reduction in the incidence of new decayed and filled permanent tooth surfaces in children 7 to 14 years of age after one year and for a 26 per cent reduction in the incidence of such surfaces after two years during a controlled clinical trial of brushing with an 0.05 per cent tyrothricin toothpaste.

Vancomycin has been reported by DePaola and his associates to temporarily suppress *Streptococcus mutans* when applied to the teeth of children as a 15 per cent gel on five successive days. The microorganism generally could not be detected on teeth for one week following the cessation of treatment. A similar diminution in *S. mutans* was found following testing with a 1 per cent vancomycin paste. DePaola and his colleagues also conducted a one-year clinical trial on the effect of topically applied vancomycin on dental caries increment in 268 children aged 9 to 11 years. They found a statistically significant reduction in dental caries experience in fissures but not on smooth surfaces in the experimental groups. Furthermore, they found that caries reduction was significant in newly erupting teeth but not in teeth already present in the mouth at the initiation of the study. Thus, this antibiotic also does not appear to satisfy sufficient criteria for universal use as an anticaries agent.

Caries Vaccine. Interest in a vaccine for dental caries protection dates back to a period when the lactobacilli were thought to be of paramount importance in the initiation of dental caries. By means of immunization with a homologous lactobacillus vaccine, in 1944 Williams was partially successful in reducing the number of lactobacilli in human saliva. More recently, the recognition of the important role that *Streptococcus mutans* plays in the initiation of caries has led to a reawakening of interest in the vaccine approach, as evidenced by the numerous experimental attempts to control caries immunologically in laboratory animals such as the rat and monkey. Although results have not always been encouraging, development of a caries vaccine is considered a highly desirable goal because of the potentially important public health implications. Considering the properties of *S. mutans*, which are associated with its cariogenicity, an antibody (immunologic) approach to caries control could theoretically be accomplished by a number of mechanisms, including (1) interfering with adherence, colonization and dissemination of the organism in the oral cavity, (2) reducing its "stickiness" by altering its polysaccharide metabolism, or (3) altering the ability of the microorganism to produce acid. Although recent studies have shown that antibody can reach the oral environment via saliva or gingival crevicular fluid, much more research will be necessary before a caries vaccine becomes available to the general public. Many important unanswered questions remain about the effectiveness of mode and route of immunogen administration, dosages and schedules of immunization, types of immunogen and adjuvants, possible adverse reactions and cross-reactivity of immunogens, and effectiveness in monitoring the immune response to immunization procedures. An excellent review on immunologic aspects of dental caries was published in 1976 by Bowen, Genco and O'Brien.

NUTRITIONAL MEASURES FOR CARIES CONTROL

The control of dental caries through nutritional or dietary means is impossible to achieve on the basis of a mass prevention program and, for this reason, is relatively unimportant in public health preventive dentistry in contrast to fluoridation of water supplies. It is important, however, for the dentist in private practice to understand the significance of controlling caries in the individual patient by dietary measures. In many persons, particularly those suffering from rampant caries, every means at the disposal of the dentist must be utilized to preserve the dentition.

The chief nutritional measure advocated for the control of dental caries is restriction of refined carbohydrate intake. Only the most cooperative patient will adhere rigidly to the type of diet designed to reduce sugar consumption drastically. For this reason clinical studies on large groups of patients for the purpose of ascertaining the extent of caries reduction that would occur with restriction of sugar consumption are difficult to carry out. Because of the apparent relation between the oral lactobacillus count and carbohydrate intake, this count frequently has been used to study sugar restriction. This does not necessarily imply that a causative relation exists between the lactobacillus and dental caries activity.

One of the best known studies dealing with the effect of dietary carbohydrate restriction on dental caries incidence is that of Becks and his co-workers. This project was designed to investigate the association of dental caries and the *L. acidophilus* indices in patients with rampant caries and in caries-free persons, as well as the effect of carbohydrate reduction on the lactobacillus count and on subsequent caries experience in a group of patients with rampant caries.

A close correlation between caries activity and the lactobacillus index was found in this study. In a group of 1250 cases of rampant caries, 1096, or 87.7 per cent, had lactobacillus indices over 1000. Conversely, of 265 caries-free patients, 218, or 82.3 per cent, had lactobacillus indices below 1000. The sharp reduction in refined carbohydrate intake resulted in a reduction of the lactobacillus index in 1000 of 1228 patients (81.7 per cent) with rampant caries within a few weeks. Most important, it was found that 62.3 per cent of 790 cases of rampant caries were completely arrested during the year of the study, while an additional 17.7 per cent had only one or two new cavities during this period.

Gustafsson and his associates from Vipeholm, Sweden, reported a study dealing with the general correlation between sugar intake and dental caries. One of their chief concerns was investigation of various forms of carbohydrates, since different forms may have different retention periods in the oral cavity. The results of this study, which extended over a period of five years, indicated that the addition of sugar to the diet resulted in an increase in caries activity and that this was maximal if the form of the sugar favored retention in the mouth. For example, sticky candies such as taffies and cookies which cling tenaciously to the teeth were especially harmful. Another important observation was that removal of carbohydrate results in a prompt return to the caries rate experienced before the experiment was begun. This appears to indicate that there exists for each person an inherent caries susceptibility which is difficult to alter.

Phosphated Diets. The results of clinical tests of dietary phosphate additions for the express purpose of controlling human dental caries are as yet inconclusive. Stralfors mixed 2 per cent dibasic calcium phosphate into the bread, flour, and sugar used in a school lunch program in Sweden and obtained a significant reduction in caries incidence in the maxillary incisors over a two-year period. Ship and Mickelsen found no meaningful reduction in the caries attack rate of children consuming a diet in which flour used in the preparation of bakery products was supplemented with 2 per cent calcium acid phosphate for three years. Similarly, Averill and Bibby, and Averill, Freire and Bibby failed to influence the initiation or progress of caries when 2 per cent dicalcium phosphate was incorporated in flour and sugar fed to children in upstate New York for 24 months, and in mandioca eaten by Brazilian children for 30 months.

Stookey, Carroll and Muhler reported that fortification of presweetened ready-to-eat breakfast cereal with 1 per cent sodium dihydrogen phosphate lowered the incidence of dental caries in 500 school-age children by approximately 30 per cent over a two-year feeding period. The cariostatic superiority of sodium dihydrogen phosphate over calcium acid phosphate was attributed to the greater systemic action of the sodium salt as demonstrated by radiophosphorus uptake studies on sound and carious enamel. The possibility that dicalcium phosphate may be caries inhibitory in the human, if permitted to remain in the oral cavity long enough, has lately been demonstrated by Finn and Jamison, who had children chew a sugar-containing gum supplemented with 225 mg. dicalcium phosphate per stick for 20 minutes five times daily. After 30 months on this regimen, there was a significant reduction in caries increment compared to that of a group using an unphosphated sugar gum.

In Australia, Harris and Beveridge obtained a 30 per cent reduction in caries in 1400 children restricted to a diet in which calcium sucrose phosphate was added to the carbohydrate component at levels ranging from 0.2 to 1.0 per cent. They hypothesized that the calcium sucrose phosphate penetrates the surface crystalline layers of enamel, tightening the attachment between crystals. This reinforcing action protects enamel from disintegration by acids formed during the microbial degradation of carbohydrates.

Despite the apparent importance of caries control through nutritional measures, there is a remarkable dearth of controlled studies by which one may judge the value of such procedures. This attests to the difficulties which would be involved in imposing such measures on large groups of patients.

MECHANICAL MEASURES FOR CARIES CONTROL

The control of dental caries by mechanical measures refers to procedures specifically designed for and aimed at removal of plaque from tooth surfaces. Although the saying "A clean tooth does not decay" is not based upon sound scientific evidence, it seems reasonable that a tooth surface free from the accumulation of microorganisms and carbohydrate substances could not become carious.

There are numerous means of cleansing the tooth mechanically, and these were reviewed and classified by Hine in a discussion of caries control measures as (1) prophylaxis by the dentist, (2) toothbrushing, (3) mouth rinsing, (4) use of dental floss or toothpicks, and (5) incorporation of detergent foods in the diet. To these might be added the use of chewing gum. He pointed out that although most investigators writing about caries control have stressed the importance of maintaining oral hygiene in preventing dental caries, no evidence is cited to support these statements. Experienced clinicians know that filthy teeth do not always decay and that, conversely, "clean" teeth often become carious. Thus, although complete scientific evidence is not available for the actual value of mechanical cleansing of the tooth, the possibility must be considered.

Dental Prophylaxis. In the control of periodontal disease the value of routine scaling and polishing of the teeth at periodic intervals of three or six months cannot be denied. Yet since dental plaque formation occurs within a matter of hours to a day or two after complete removal of the structure, there is probably little if any value in prophylaxis for the control of dental caries. Hine pointed out that the careful polishing of roughened tooth surfaces and the correction of faulty restorations is probably of more importance than the mechanical cleansing of the tooth by prophylaxis. These procedures might conceivably reduce the retention of food debris and decrease the formation of bacterial plaques, thereby reducing the development of new carious lesions. There are no studies in the scientific literature with sufficient data to establish definitely the value of dental prophylaxis in the control of caries.

Toothbrushing. The value of toothbrushing in the control of dental caries has been argued by many authorities. It cannot be denied that there are some persons who have never used a toothbrush and yet are free of caries. These persons are certainly exceptional and probably prove only that the inherent caries resistance of the individual may be of greater importance than local factors.

On the other hand, there are many persons who conscientiously brush their teeth at least twice a day and yet suffer from a serious amount of dental caries. Since most persons delay brushing their teeth after meals for varying periods of time and since, as Stephan has shown, acid production in the dental plaques occurs within a matter of minutes after the ingestion of carbohydrate, a high caries incidence despite persistent toothbrushing is at least understandable.

Another factor in the explanation of the failure of toothbrushing to prevent dental caries lies in the difficulty of reaching with the brush all exposed surfaces of teeth upon which plaques may form. The majority of patients do not reach all areas with their toothbrushing technique. Indeed, it is ironic that most patients spend the greatest amount of time brushing buccal, labial and lingual surfaces, which are not as prone to decay as the more inaccessible interproximals and the deep fissures of occlusal surfaces into

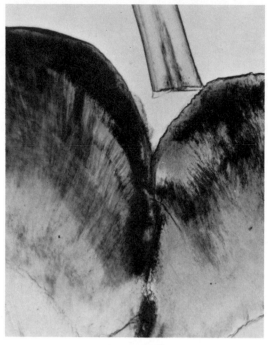

Figure 7–35.

A ground section of a tooth shows the relative size of an occlusal fissure compared with a single bristle from a standard toothbrush to illustrate the difficulty which may be encountered in attempting to cleanse the depth of these fissures.

which toothbrush bristles will not reach (Fig. 7–35).

A number of studies have indicated that toothbrushing will reduce the number of bacteria in the oral cavity; but in view of the countless millions of microorganisms remaining in the oral cavity, the significance of removing a certain but undoubtedly small percentage is probably negligible.

There are several studies on the effect of toothbrushing on the incidence of experimental dental caries in animals. In a study testing the effect of a penicillin dentifrice on caries in hamsters, Zander and Bibby found that simply brushing the teeth of animals with a control nonmedicated toothpaste resulted in a 69 per cent reduction in caries as compared to a group in which the teeth were not brushed. Subsequent studies in other animals have demonstrated similar results.

There have been few controlled studies of the effects of toothbrushing on the incidence of caries in the human. Fosdick in 1950 studied a group of 523 persons who were instructed to brush their teeth within 10 minutes after eating with a neutral dentifrice or to rinse their mouths well with water. The control group consisted of 423 persons who were allowed to continue with their usual brushing habits, in most cases morning and night brushing. Clinical examination at the end of one year revealed that the control group had an average of 2.21 new carious surfaces while the experimental group averaged only 0.82 new carious surface. Over a two-year period the average number of new carious surfaces was 2.53 in the controls, but only 1.49 for the experimental group. The reduction in caries due to the toothbrushing technique was 62 per cent in the first year, 26 per cent in the second year and 41 per cent over the two-year period.

Weisenstein and his associates reported a study of 150 children 9 to 14 years of age, equally divided between a control and an experimental group. The experimental group brushed their teeth immediately after each meal, whereas the controls were uninstructed. After six months the test group exhibited 28 per cent fewer new DMF surfaces than the controls, although during the second six-month period both groups demonstrated 43 per cent fewer new DMF surfaces than during the first period. Hein found in a limited study that there was no appreciable effect on dental caries in a group of 60 males who brushed once or twice a day. Although a group of females who brushed four times a day showed somewhat less caries than groups who brushed once, twice or three times a day, the frequency of brushing in a group of 155 males had little effect on caries. Thus, although toothbrushing would seem to be important, not all clinical studies completely support this idea.

Mouth Rinsing. The use of a mouthwash for the benefit of its action in loosening food debris from the teeth has been suggested to be of value as a caries control measure. There is no scientific evidence to confirm this suggestion, and mouthwashes would appear to be of only limited value except for the fluoride mouthwashes previously discussed (q.v.).

Dental Floss. As early as 1819, Levi Parmly wrote of dental floss, "It is to be passed through the interstices of the teeth, between their necks and arches of the gums to dislodge that irritating matter which no brush can remove and which is the real source of disease."

Dental flossing has been shown to be effective in removing plaque from an area gingival to the contact areas on proximal surfaces of teeth, an area impossible to reach with the toothbrush. There is general agreement that flossing is necessary if interproximal gingival health is to be maintained, but opinions differ as to the value of flossing in preventing dental caries. The research findings regarding control or prevention of dental caries by flossing are contradictory. Most of the studies involved children, and thus digital aptitude in manipulating the dental floss is an important variable. Nevertheless, Wright and his associates reported a 50 per cent reduction in dental caries when trained personnel flossed the interproximal surfaces of a group of young children.

The use of dental floss is of prime importance in patient education programs. In light of what is understood regarding remineralization of incipient enamel lesions, it is reasonable to expect arrest and prevention of enamel lesions when smooth surfaces are kept free of plaque. Those involved and interested in attaining and maintaining oral health will find that using floss is mandatory.

Oral Irrigators. The custom of flushing the mouth for therapeutic purposes dates from antiquity. However, the use of flushing devices was first reported in the early 1900's, and authors have written of their experiences in treating dental infection by flushing since that time.

Most of these reports are concerned with the beneficial effects of oral irrigation on gingival infections. No reports have referred to the effect of irrigation on the control of dental caries.

Detergent Foods. Some workers have related the high caries incidence among modern civilized races to the unrestrained use of soft, sticky, refined foods, which tend to adhere to the teeth. The softness of the diet was thought to be due to removal of the natural fibers in foods, either in preparation or in cooking. It has been stated that fibrous foods in the diets prevent lodging of food in pits and fissures of teeth and, in addition, act as a detergent.

A number of studies have indicated that the act of eating removes a relatively large number of microorganisms from the oral cavity. Crowley and Rickert reported that after eating there was a reduction of as high as 78 per cent in the number of bacteria that could be recovered from the mouth. It is logical that hard, fibrous food would be more beneficial in mechanically cleansing the oral cavity than soft, sticky food. It also appears reasonable that the adherence of soft foods to the teeth would predispose to the development of more caries than would be found in a mouth kept relatively clean by a fibrous diet. Yet despite recommendations that the eating of fibrous foods, either as a part of the diet or simply after meals, is beneficial as a caries control measure, there is no scientific evidence based upon controlled studies in human beings to indicate that this is true.

Chewing Gum. It has been suggested that the chewing of gum would tend to prevent dental caries by its mechanical cleansing action. But most chewing gums contain a considerable amount of carbohydrate, and this might actually increase caries susceptibility.

Volker studied the effect of gum chewing on the incidence of caries in a group of young adults. The gum was chewed for at least ten minutes after the morning and evening meals. After 18 months no significant differences were found in the caries experience between the experimental group and those in the control group who did not chew gum. Neither did gum chewing have any influence on gingival inflammation or on the formation of calculus. As might be expected, the gum did remove a great deal of residual oral debris.

The evidence indicates that chewing gum in moderate amounts has neither a harmful nor a beneficial effect on the teeth or supporting tissues.

Pit and Fissure Sealants. Pits and fissures of occlusal surfaces are among the most difficult areas on teeth to keep clean and from which to remove plaque. For this reason, occlusal caries, beginning in these pits and fissures, is the most prevalent type of this disease. Because of this, it was suggested many years ago that prophylactic odontotomy, the preparation of cavities in these areas and their restoration by some material such as amalgam before extensive decay had developed, be carried out. In this way, these caries-susceptible pit and fissure areas would be made less susceptible to subsequent caries.

In the 1960's sealants were developed for these pits and fissures which may be placed in these areas without the need for cavity preparation. The pit and fissure sealants, generally used in conjunction with an acid pretreatment to enhance their retention, contain either cyanoacrylate, polyurethane or the adduct of bisphenol A and glycidyl methacrylate as major components. Cueto and Buonocore (1967) reported that a cyanoacrylate sealant, applied every six months, resulted in an 86 per cent reduction in caries after one year. Ripa and Cole, utilizing the same type of sealant, reported that 85 first permanent molars had 84.3 per cent less occlusal caries than an equal number of controls after one year. Buonocore

tested 60 patients using bisphenol A-glycidyl methacrylate containing benzoin methyl ether, making the curing process sensitive to ultraviolet light. He reported that there was a caries reduction of 100 per cent after one year, and 99 per cent after two years in the permanent molars. In deciduous teeth tested, he reported an 87 per cent protection.

More recently, Boudreau and Jerge (1976) have reviewed the literature dealing with this technique and concluded that all available evidence demonstrated that sealants were effective in preventing occlusal decay, although they emphasized that most investigators suggested that occlusal sealants should be but one component of a multiple approach to a preventive dentistry program. Several years later, Brooks and his associates (1979) published the three-year results of a comparative study of two different sealants on dental caries in the first permanent molars in a group of 254 children. The sealants ranged between 39 per cent and 69 per cent in their effectiveness in preventing occlusal caries for three years after a single application.

A conference on various aspects of usage of pit and fissure sealants also was convened by the Council on Dental Materials, Instruments and Equipment of the American Dental Association on May 11, 1981. In addition to confirming the safety and effectiveness of pit and fissure sealants in preventing dental caries, other discussions involved their acceptance and use by the educators and the practitioners, and their cost effectiveness.

Thus, the evidence is accruing that pit and fissure sealants are an additional aid in the prevention of one form of dental caries.

REFERENCES

Abbott, F.: Caries of human teeth. Dent. Cosmos, 21:113, 177, 184, 1879.

Afonsky, D.: Saliva and Its Relation to Oral Health. A Survey of the Literature. Montgomery, Ala.: Univ. of Alabama Press, 1961.

Agnew, M. C., Agnew, R. G., and Tisdall, F. F.: The production and prevention of dental caries. J. Am. Dent. Assoc., 20:193, 1933; J. Pediatr., 2:190, 1933.

Albright, F., Aub, J. C., and Bauer, W.: Hyperparathyroidism: a common and polymorphic condition as illustrated by seventeen proved cases from one clinic. J.A.M.A., 102:1276, 1934.

American Association for the Advancement of Science: Fluorine and Dental Health. Washington, D.C., Am. Assoc. Adv. Sci., 1942.

American Dental Association, Bureau of Economic Research and Statistics: 1950 survey of the dental profession. J. Am. Dent. Assoc., *41*:253, 376, 505, 625, 761, 1950; *42*:196, 444, 1951.

Idem: Survey of needs for dental care. J. Am. Dent. Assoc., *45*:706, 1952; *46*:200, 562, 1953; *47*:206, 340, 572, 1953.

Idem: 1959 survey of dental practice. J. Am. Dent. Assoc., *60*:498, 750, 791, 1960; *61*:128, 373, 520, 749, 1960; *62*:116, 220, 453, 627, 764, 1961.

Idem: The 1977 Survey of Dental Practice. Chicago, 1977.

American Dental Association, Council on Dental Therapeutics: Evaluation of Crest Toothpaste. J. Am. Dent. Assoc., *61*:272, 1960.

Idem: Council classifies fluoride mouthrinses. J. Am. Dent. Assoc., *91*:1250, 1975.

Anderson, B. G.: Clinical study of arresting dental caries. J. Dent. Res., *17*:443, 1938.

Anderson, R. W., and Knutson, J. W.: Effect of topically applied zinc chloride and potassium ferrocyanide on dental caries experience. Public Health Rep., *66*:1064, 1951.

Armstrong, W. D.: Biochemical and nutritional studies in relation to the teeth. Ann. Rev. Biochem., *11*:441, 1942.

Idem: An evaluation of the role of vitamins and minerals in the control of caries; in K. A. Easlick (ed.): Dental Caries, Mechanism and Present Control Technics as Evaluated at the University of Michigan Workshop. St. Louis, C. V. Mosby Company, 1948.

Idem: Fluorine content of enamel and dentin of sound and carious teeth. J. Biol. Chem., *119*:v-vi, 1937.

Arnim, S. S.: Thoughts concerning cause, pathogenesis, treatment and prevention of periodontal disease. J. Periodontol, *29*:217, 1958.

Idem: Microcosms of the human mouth. J. Tenn. Dent. Assoc., *39*:3, 1959.

Idem: Dental caries. Minneap. Dist. Dent. J.: 91, 1953.

Arnold, F. A., Jr.: An evaluation of the effectiveness as caries control measures of ingested fluorides in water, food, bone flour, and proprietary preparations; in K. A. Easlick (ed.): Dental Caries, Mechanism and Present Control Technics as Evaluated at the University of Michigan Workshop. St. Louis, C. V. Mosby Company, 1948.

Idem: The production of carious lesions in the molar teeth of hamsters *(C. auratus)*. Public Health Rep., *57*:1599, 1942.

Arnold, F. A., Jr., and McClure, F. J.: A study of the relationship of oral Lactobacillus acidophilus and saliva chemistry of dental caries. Public Health Rep., *56*:1495, 1941.

Arnold, F. A., Jr., Dean, H. T., and Knutson, J. W.: Effect of fluoridated public water supplies on dental caries prevalence. Public Health Rep., *68*:141, 1953.

Ast, D. B., and Chase, H. C.: The Newburgh-Kingston caries-fluorine study. IV. Dental findings after six years of water fluoridation. Oral Surg., *6*:114, 1953.

Ast, D. B., Bushel, A., and Chase, H. C.: A clinical study of caries prophylaxis with zinc chloride and potassium ferrocyanide. J. Am. Dent. Assoc., *41*:437, 1950.

Ast, D. B., Finn, S. B., and Chase, H. C.: Newburgh-Kingston caries-fluorine study. III. Further analysis of dental findings, including the permanent and deciduous dentitions after four years of water fluoridation. J. Am. Dent. Assoc., *42*:188, 1951.

Ast, D. B., Bushel, A., Wachs, B., and Chase, H. C.: Newburgh-Kingston caries-fluorine study. VIII. Combined clinical and roentgenographic dental findings after 8 years of fluoride experience. J. Am. Dent. Assoc., *50*:680, 1955.

Ast, D. B., Smith, D. J., Wachs, B., and Cantwell, K. T.: Newburgh-Kingston caries-fluorine study. XIV. Combined clinical and roentgenographic dental findings after ten years of fluoride experience. J. Am. Dent. Assoc., *52*:314, 1956.

Averill, H. M., and Bibby, B. G.: A clinical test of additions of phosphate to the diet of children. J. Dent. Res., *43*:1150, 1964.

Averill, H. M., Freire, P. S., and Bibby, G. G.: The effect of dietary phosphate supplements on dental caries incidence in tropical Brazil. Arch. Oral Biol., *11*:315, 1966.

Babkin, B.: The physiology of the salivary glands; in S. M. Gordon (ed.): Dental Science and Dental Art. Philadelphia, Lea & Febiger, 1938, p. 219.

Backer-Dirks, O.: Posteruptive changes in dental enamel. J. Dent. Res., *45*:503, 1966.

Baumgartner, E.: Über das wesender Zahnkaries mit besonderer Berücksichtigung der Histologie des gesunden und kariosen Zahnschmelzes. Dtsch. Mschr. Zahnheilk., *29*:322, 1911.

Becks, H.: Human saliva. XIV. Total calcium content of resting saliva of 650 healthy individuals. J. Dent. Res., *22*:397, 1943.

Idem: The physical consistency of food and refined carbohydrate restrictions—their effect on caries; in K. A. Easlick (ed.): Dental Caries, Mechanism and Present Control Technics as Evaluated at the University of Michigan Workshop. St. Louis, C. V. Mosby Company, 1948.

Becks, H., and Wainwright, W. W.: Human saliva. XVIII. Rate of flow of resting saliva of healthy individuals. J. Dent. Res., *22*:391, 1943.

Becks, H., Jensen, A. L., and Millarr, C. B.: Rampant dental caries: prevention and prognosis; a five year clinical survey. J. Am. Dent. Assoc., *31*:1189, 1944.

Becks, H., Wainwright, W. W., and Young, D. H.: Further studies of the calcium and phosphorus content of resting and activated saliva of caries-free and caries-active individuals. J. Dent. Res., *22*:139, 1943.

Bellinger, W. R.: The dental implications of fluorine: a review of the literature. J. Am. Dent. Assoc., *34*:719, 1947.

Bergeim, O., and Barnfield, W. F.: Lack of correlation between dental caries and salivary amylase. J. Dent. Res., *24*:141, 1945.

Berman, K. S., and Gibbons, R. J.: Iodophilic polysaccharide synthesis by human and rodent oral bacteria. Arch. Oral Biol., *11*:533, 1966.

Besic, F. C.: The fate of bacteria sealed in dental cavities. J. Dent. Res., *22*:349, 1943.

Beust, T. B.: Reactions of dentine to advancing caries. J. Am. Dent. Assoc., *20*:631, 1933.

Bibby, B. G.: New approach to caries prophylaxis. Tufts Dent. Outlook, *15*:4, 1942.

Idem: Fluoride mouthwashes, fluoride dentifrices, and other uses of fluorides in control of caries; in K. A. Easlick (ed.): Dental Caries, Mechanism and Present Control Technics as Evaluated at the University of Michigan Workshop. St. Louis, C. V. Mosby Company, 1948.

Idem: A study of a pigmented dental plaque. J. Dent. Res., *11*:855, 1931.

Idem: Saliva and dental caries; in J. C. Muhler and M. K. Hine (eds.): A Symposium on Preventive Dentistry. St. Louis, C. V. Mosby Company, 1956.

Idem: Studies on dental caries. Tufts Dent. Outlook, *14*:4, 1940.

Idem: The use of fluorine in the prevention of dental caries. J. Am. Dent. Assoc., *31*:228, 1944.

Bibby, B. G., Hine, M. K., and Clough, O. W.: The

antibacterial action of human saliva. J. Am. Dent. Assoc., 25:1290, 1938.

Bibby,B. G., Zander, H. A., McKelleget, M., and Labunsky, B.: Preliminary reports on the effect on dental caries of the use of sodium fluoride in a prophylactic cleaning mixture and in a mouthwash. J. Dent. Res., 25:207, 1946.

Bilbiie, V., Steiber, C., and Popescu, A.: The bacterial dental plaque as an ecologic system. Int. Dent. J., 21:322, 1971.

Black, G. V.: Susceptibility and immunity to dental caries. Dent. Cosmos., 41:826, 1899.

Black, G. V., and McKay, F. S.: Mottled teeth; an endemic developmental imperfection of the enamel of the teeth heretofore unknown in the literature of dentistry. Dent. Cosmos, 58:129, 1916.

Blackerby, P. E., Jr.: Comparative analysis of dental conditions among white and negro children of rural and semirural communities. J. Am. Dent. Assoc., 26:1574, 1939.

Blayney, J. R., and Greco, J. F.: The Evanston dental caries study. IX. The value of roentgenological vs. clinical procedures for the recognition of early carious lesions on proximal surfaces of teeth. J. Dent. Res., 31:341, 1952.

Blayney, J. R., Bradel, S. F., Harrison, R. W., and Hemmens, E. S.: Continuous clinical and bacteriologic study of proximal surfaces of premolar teeth before and after the onset of caries. J. Am. Dent. Assoc., 29:1645, 1942.

Bodecker, C. F.: Preliminary communication upon a method of decalcifying structures containing minute quantities of organic matter, with special reference to the enamel. Dent. Rev., 19:448, 1905.

Idem: Die Bakterien im Schmelzgewebe als ursache karioser Vorgange. Vjschr. Zahnheilk., 44:242, 1928.

Bodecker, C. F. W.: Distribution of living matter in human dentine, cementum and enamel. Dent. Cosmos., 20:582, 645; 21:7, 1878–79.

Boudreau, G. E., and Jerge, C. R.: The efficacy of sealant treatment in the prevention of dental caries: a review and interpretation of the literature. J. Am. Dent. Assoc., 92:383, 1976.

Bowen, W. H.: Nature of plaque. Oral Sci. Rev., 9:3, 1976.

Bowen, W. H., Genco, R. N., and O'Brien, T. C.: Immunologic Aspects of Dental Caries. Special Supplement to Immunology Abstracts. Washington, D.C., Information Retrieval Inc., 1976.

Boyd, J. D., and Wessels, K. E.: Epidemiologic studies in dental caries. III. The interpretation of clinical data relating to caries. Am. J. Public Health, 41:976, 1951.

Boyd, J. D., Drain, C. L., and Stearns, G.: Metabolic studies of children with dental caries. J. Biol. Chem., 103:327, 1933.

Bransby, E. R., and Knowles, E. M.: A comparison of the effect of enemy occupation and postwar conditions on the incidence of dental caries in children in the Channel Islands in relation to diet and food supplies. Br. Dent. J., 87:236, 1949.

Brawley, R. E.: Studies of the pH of normal resting saliva. II. Diurnal variation. J. Dent. Res., 15:79, 1935–36.

Brawley, R. E., and Sedwick, J. H.: Studies concerning the oral cavity and saliva. J. Dent. Res., 19:315, 1940.

Brekhus, P. J.: A report of dental caries in 10,445 university students. J. Am. Dent. Assoc., 18:1350, 1931.

Briner, W. W.: Plaque in relation to dental caries and periodontal disease. Int. Dent. J., 21:293, 1971.

Brodsky, R. H., Schick, B., and Vollmer, H.: Prevention of dental caries by massive doses of vitamin D. Am. J. Dis. Child., 62:1183, 1941.

Brooks, J. D., Mertz-Fairhurst, E. J., Della-Giustiana, V. E., Williams, J. E., and Fairhurst, C. W.: A comparative study of two pit and fissure sealants: three-year results in Augusta, Georgia. J. Am. Dent. Assoc., 99:42, 1979.

Brown, W. E., and König, K. G.: Cariostatic Mechanisms of Fluoride. Proceedings of a workshop organized by the American Dental Association Health Foundation and the National Institute of Dental Research. Caries Res., 11 (Suppl. 1):1977.

Brucker, M.: Studies on the incidence and cause of dental defects in children. V. Freedom from caries. J. Dent. Res., 22:469, 1943.

Brudevold, F., and Little, M. F.: Effect of certain antienzymes on acid production in plaque. J. Dent. Res., 33:703, 1954.

Brudevold, F., Little, M. F., and Rowley, J.: Acid-reducing effect of "antienzymes" in the mouth. J. Am. Dent. Assoc., 50:18, 1955.

Brudevold, F., McCann, H. G., and Gron, P.: Caries resistance as related to the chemistry of the enamel; in G. E. W. Wolstenholme and M. O'Connor (eds.): Caries Resistant Teeth. Boston, Little, Brown & Company, 1965.

Brudevold, F., Savory, A., Gardner, D. E., Spinelli, M., and Speirs, R.: A study of acidulated fluoride solutions. I. In vitro effects on enamel. Arch. Oral Biol., 8:167, 1963.

Brunelle, J. A., and Carlos, J. P.: Changes in the prevalence of dental caries in U.S. schoolchildren, 1961–1980. J. Dent. Res., 61:1346, 1982.

Bunting, R. W.: Report of the examination of the mouths of 1500 school children in the public schools of Ann Arbor, Michigan. Dent. Cosmos, 51:310, 1909.

Idem: Studies of the relation of bacillus acidophilus to dental caries. J. Dent. Res., 8:222, 1928.

Bunting, R. W., Nickerson, G., and Hard, D. G.: Further studies of the relation of bacillus acidophilus to dental caries. Dent. Cosmos, 68:931, 1926.

Buonocore, M. G.: Adhesive sealing of pits and fissures for caries prevention, with use of ultraviolet light. J. Am. Dent. Assoc., 80:324, 1970.

Idem: Caries prevention in pits and fissures sealed with an adhesive resin polymerized by ultraviolet light: a two-year study of a single adhesive application. J. Am. Dent. Assoc., 82:1090, 1971.

Burrill, D. Y., Calandra, J. C., Tilden, E. B., and Fosdick, L. S.: The effect of 2-methyl-1,4-naphthoquinone on the incidence of dental caries. J. Dent. Res., 24:273, 1945.

Chauncey, H. H.: Salivary enzymes. J. Am. Dent. Assoc., 63:360, 1961.

Cheyne, V. D., and Horne, E. V.: The value of the roentgenograph in the detection of carious lesions. J. Dent. Res., 27:59, 1948.

Clark, F. Y.: Bacteremia. Johnston's Dental Miscellany, 6:447, 1879.

Idem: Report of the committee on dental therapeutics. Trs. South. D.A., 3rd Annual Meeting, 1871, p. 40.

Clarke, J. K.: On the bacterial factor in the aetiology of dental caries. Br. J. Exp. Path., 5:141, 1924.

Clawson, M. D.: The Shammar Bedouin dental survey. Dent. Mag. Oral Topics, 53:117, 1936.

Clough, O. W.: Inhibition of bacterial growth by human saliva. J. Dent. Res., 14:164, 1934.

Cohen, A., and Donzanti, A.: Two year clinical study of

caries control with high-urea ammoniated dentifrice. J. Am. Dent. Assoc., 49:185, 1954.

Compton, F. H., Burgess, R. C., Mondrow, T. G., Grainger, R. M., and Nikiforuk, G.: The Riverdale preschool dental project. J. Can. Dent. Assoc., 25:478, 1959.

Conchie, J. M., McCombie, F., and Hole, L. W.: Three years of supervised toothbrushing with a fluoride-phosphate solution. J. Public Health Dent., 29:11, 1969.

Cons, N. C., and Janerich, D. T.: Albany topical fluoride study: 2 year preliminary report. I.A.D.R. Abstract 545, 1969.

Cox, G. J., Matuschak, M. C., Dixon, S. F., Dodds, M. L., and Walker, W. E.: Experimental dental caries. IV. Fluorine and its relation to dental caries. J. Dent. Res., 18:481, 1939.

Crabb, H. S. M.: Enamel caries: observations on the histology and pattern of progress of the approximal lesion. Br. Dent. J., 121:115, 167, 1966.

Idem: Observations on the histology of the carious attack on enamel and related developmental faults. Adv. Fluor. Res. Dent. Caries Prevent., 4:225, 1966.

Crawford, H. M.: Clinical results of impregnation. Texas D. J., 67:52, 1949.

Crowley, M. C., and Rickert, U. G.: A method for estimating the bacterial content of the mouth by direct count. J. Bacteriol., 30:395, 1935.

Cueto, E. I., and Buonocore, M. G.: Sealing of pits and fissures with an adhesive resin: its use in caries prevention. J. Am. Dent. Assoc., 75:121, 1967.

Cushman, F. H., Etherington, J. W., and Thompson, G. E.: Quantitative relationship between saliva and caries in an adolescent group. J. Dent. Res., 19:298, 1940.

Davies, G. N., and King, R. M.: The effectiveness of an ammonium ion toothpowder in the control of dental caries. J. Dent. Res., 30:645, 1951.

Day, C. D. M.: Nutritional deficiencies and dental caries in Northern India. Br. Dent. J., 70:115, 143, 1944.

Day, C. D. M., and Sedwick, H. J.: Studies on the incidence of dental caries. Dent. Cosmos, 77:442, 1935.

Day, C. D. M., Draggs, R. G., and Sedwick, H. J.: High sugar diets and dental caries in the white rat. J. Am. Dent. Assoc., 22:913, 1935.

Deakins, M.: Effect of pregnancy on the mineral content of dentin of human teeth. J. Dent. Res., 22:198, 1943.

Deakins, M., and Looby, J.: Effect of pregnancy on mineral content of human teeth. Am. J. Obstet. Gynecol., 6:265, 1943.

Dean, H. T.: Fluorine and dental caries. Am. J. Orthod. Oral Surg., 33:49, 1947.

Idem: Fluorine in the control of dental caries. J. Am. Dent. Assoc., 52:1, 1956.

Dean, H. T., Arnold, F. A., and Elvove, E.: Domestic water and dental caries. V. Additional studies of the relation of fluoride domestic waters to dental caries experience in 4,425 white children, aged 12 to 14 years, of 13 cities in 4 states. Public Health Rep., 57:1155, 1942.

Dean, H. T., McKay, F. S., and Elvove, E.: Mottled enamel survey of Bauxite, Arkansas, ten years after a change in the common water supply. Public Health Rep., 53:1736, 1938.

Dental Manpower Fact Book. U.S. Dept. of Health, Education and Welfare, Publication (HRA) 79–14. Washington, D.C., Government Printing Office, 1979.

DePaola, P. F., Wellock, W. D., Maitland, A., and Brudevold, F.: The relationship of cariostasis, oral hygiene, and past caries experience in children receiving three sprays annually with acidulated phosphate-fluoride: three-year results. J. Am. Dent. Assoc., 77:91, 1968.

DePaola, P. F., Jordan, H. V., and Berg, J.: Temporary suppression of Streptococcus mutans in humans through topical application of vancomycin. Arch. Oral Biol., 53:108, 1974.

DePaola, P. F., Jordan, H. V., and Soparkar, P. M.: Inhibition of dental caries in school children by topically applied vancomycin. Arch. Oral Biol., 22:187, 1977.

DePaola, P. F., Soparkar, P. M., Tavares, M., Allukian, M., Jr., and Peterson, H.: A dental survey of Massachusetts schoolchildren. J. Dent. Res., 61:1356, 1982.

Dietz, V. H., Williams, N. B., and Lawton, W. E.: Relationship between blood agglutinins for oral lactobacilli, salivary counts and caries. J. Am. Dent. Assoc., 30:385, 1943.

Dragiff, D. A., and Karshan, M.: Effect of pregnancy on the chemical composition of human dentin. J. Dent. Res., 2:261, 1943.

Dreizen, S. Diet and dental decay. Postgrad. Med., 43:233, 1968.

Dreizen, S., and Spies, T. D.: Decalcification and discoloration of intact non-carious human tooth crowns. Oral Surg., 4:388, 1951.

Idem: Effectiveness of a chewing gum containing nitrofuran in the prevention of dental caries. J. Am. Dent. Assoc., 43:147, 1951.

Dreizen, S., Greene, H. I., and Spies, T. D.: In vitro studies of the dental caries inhibiting properties of some selected nitrofuran compounds. J. Dent. Res., 28:288, 1949.

Dreizen, S., Mann, A. W., Spies, T. D., and Skinner, T. A.: Prevalence of dental caries in malnourished children: a clinical study. Am. J. Dis. Child., 74:265, 1947.

Easlick, K. A. (ed.): Dental Caries, Mechanism and Present Control Technics as Evaluated at the University of Michigan Workshop. St. Louis, C. V. Mosby Company, 1948.

East, B. R.: Mean annual hours of sunshine and the incidence of dental caries. Am. J. Public Health, 29:777, 1939.

Idem: Relationship of dental caries in city children to sex, age, and environment. Am. J. Dis. Child., 61:494, 1941.

East, B. R., and Kaiser, H.: Relation of dental caries in rural children to sex, age, and environment. Am. J. Dis. Child., 60:1289, 1940.

Eisenbrandt, L. L.: Studies of the pH of saliva. J. Dent. Res., 23:363, 1944.

Englander, H. R., Keyes, P. H., Gestwicki, M., and Suitz, H. A.: Clinical anticaries effect of repeated topical sodium fluoride applications by mouthpieces. J. Am. Dent. Assoc., 75:638, 1967.

Ericsson, Y.: Enamel-apatite solubility. Investigations into the calcium phosphate equilibrium between enamel and saliva and its relation to dental caries. Acta Odontol. Scand., 8(Suppl. 3):1, 1949.

Idem: Cariostatic mechanisms of fluorides: Clinical observations. Caries Res., 11(Suppl. 1):2, 1977.

Fejerskov, O., Thylstrup, A., and Larsen, M. J.: Rational use of fluorides in caries prevention: a concept based on possible cariostatic mechanisms. Acta Odontol. Scand., 39:241, 1981.

Finn, S. B., and Jamison, H. C.: The effect of a dicalcium phosphate chewing gum on caries incidence in children: 30-month results. J. Am. Dent. Assoc., 74:987, 1967.

Fitzgerald, D. B., Stevens, R., Fitzgerald, R. J., and

Mandel, I. D.: Comparative cariogenicity of *Streptococcus mutans* strains isolated from caries-active and caries-resistant adults. J. Dent. Res., 56:894, 1977.

Fitzgerald, R. J.: The microbial ecology of plaque in relation to dental caries; in H. Stiles, W. Loesche, and T. O'Brien (eds.): Microbial Aspects of Dental Caries. Suppl. Microbiol. Abstr., 3:849, 1976.

Fitzgerald, R. J., Jordan, H. V., and Stanley, H. R.: Experimental caries and gingival pathologic changes in the gnotobiotic rat. J. Dent. Res., 39:923, 1960.

Fitzgerald, R. J., and Keyes, P. H.: Demonstration of the etiologic role of streptococci in experimental caries in the hamster. J. Am. Dent. Assoc., 61:9, 1960.

Fitzgerald, R. J., Zander, H. A., and Jordan, H. U.: The effects of a penicillin dentifrice on oral lactobacilli. J. Am. Dent. Assoc., 4:62, 1950.

Fleischmann, L.: The etiology of dental caries. Dent. Cosmos, 66:1379, 1914.

Idem: Zur Pathogenese der Zahnkaries. Z. Stomatol., 19:153, 1921.

Florestano, H. J.: Acidogenic properties of certain oral microorganisms. J. Dent. Res., 21:263, 1942.

Florestano, H. J., Faber, J. E., and James, L. H.: Studies of the relationship between diastatic activity of saliva and incidence of dental caries. J. Am. Dent. Assoc., 28:1799, 1941.

Fosdick, L. S.: The degradation of sugars in the mouth and the use of chewing gum and vitamin K in the control of dental caries. J. Dent. Res., 27:235, 1948.

Idem: A preliminary clinical report on the effectiveness of sodium N-lauroyl sarcosinate in the control of dental caries. Northwestern Univ. Bull., 54:20, 1953.

Idem: The reduction of the incidence of dental caries. I. Immediate toothbrushing with a neutral dentifrice. J. Am. Dent. Assoc., 40:133, 1950.

Fosdick, L. S., Fancher, O. E., and Calandra, J. C.: The effect of synthetic vitamin K on the rate of acid formation in the mouth. Science, 96:45, 1942.

Fosdick, L. S., Calandra, J. C., Blackwell, R. Q., and Burrill, J. H.: A new approach to the problem of dental caries control. J. Dent. Res., 32:486, 1953.

Fosdick, L. S., and Hutchinson, A. P. W.: The mechanism of caries of dental enamel. Ann. N.Y. Acad. Sci., 131:758, 1965.

Frisbie, H. E.: Caries of the dentin. J. Dent. Res., 24:195, 1945.

Frisbie, H. E., and Nuckolls, J.: Caries of the enamel. J. Dent. Res., 26:181, 1947.

Frisbie, H. E., Nuckolls, J., and Saunders, J. B. de C. M.: Distribution of the organic matrix of the enamel in the human tooth and its relation to the histopathology of caries. J. Am. Coll. Dent., 11:243, 1944.

Gibbons, H. J., and Socransky, S. S.: Intracellular polysaccharide storage by organisms in dental plaque, its relation to dental caries and microbial ecology of the oral cavity. Arch. Oral Biol., 7:73, 1962.

Gibbons, R. J., and Van Houte, J.: Bacterial adherence in oral microbial ecology. Ann. Rev. Microbiol., 29:19, 1975.

Gies, W. J., and Kligler, I. J.: Chemical studies of the relations of oral microorganisms to dental caries. 2. A biochemical study and differentiation of oral bacteria with special reference to dental caries. J. Allied Dent. Soc., 10:141, 282, 445, 1915.

Gish, C. W., and Mercer, V. H.: Child self-application of a zirconium silicate-stannous fluoride anticariogenic paste: clinical results after 1 and 2 years. I.A.D.R. Abstract 552, 1969.

Gish, C. W., and Muhler, J. C.: Effect on dental caries in children in a natural fluoride area of combined use of three agents containing stannous fluoride: a prophylactic paste, a solution and a dentifrice. J. Am. Dent. Assoc., 70:914, 1965.

Gish, C. W., Muhler, J. C., and Howell, C. L.: A new approach to the topical application of fluorides for the reduction of dental caries in children: results at the end of five years. J. Dent. Child., 29:65, 1962.

Glass, R. L. (ed.): The First International Conference on the Declining Prevalence of Dental Caries. J. Dent. Res., 61:1301, 1982.

Glass, R. L.: Secular changes in caries prevalence in two Massachusetts towns. J. Dent. Res., 61:1352, 1982.

Goadby, K. W.: Micro-organisms in dental caries. J. Br. Dent. Assoc., 21:65, 1900.

Gottlieb, B.: Untersuchungen über die organische Substanz im Schmelz menschlicher Zahne. Ost.-Ung. Vjschr. Zahnheilk, 31:19, 1915.

Idem: Dental caries. J. Dent. Res., 23:141, 1944.

Idem: Histopathology of enamel caries. J. Dent. Res., 23:169, 1944.

Idem: New concept of the caries problem and its clinical application. J. Am. Dent. Assoc., 31:1482, 1489, 1598, 1944.

Gottlieb, B., Diamond, M., and Applebaum, E.: The caries problem. Am. J. Orthod. Oral Surg., 32:365, 1946.

Green, G. E.: A bacteriolytic agent in salivary globulin of caries-immune human beings. J. Dent. Res., 38:262, 1959.

Griffiths, B., and Rapp, G. W.: The effect of water-soluble chlorophyll on mouth organisms. J. Dent. Res., 29:690, 1950 (Abst.).

Grove, C. T., and Grove, C. J.: The biochemical aspect of dental caries. Dent. Cosmos, 76:1029, 1934.

Idem: Chemical study of human saliva indicating that ammonia is an immunizing factor in dental caries. J. Am. Dent. Assoc., 22:247, 1935.

Gustafsson, B. E., Quensel, C. E., Lanke, L. S., Lundqvist, C., Grahnen, H., Bonow, B. E., and Krasse, B.: Vipeholm dental caries study. The effect of different levels of carbohydrate intake on caries activity in 436 individuals observed for 5 years. Acta Odontol. Scand., 11:232, 1954.

Hadden, W. C.: Basic data on health care needs of adults ages 25–74 years, United States, 1971–75. Vital and health statistics: Series 11, Data from the National Health Survey; no. 218. DHHS publication no. (PHS) 81-1668. Washington, D.C., Government Printing Office, 1980.

Hardwick, J. L., and Manley, E. B.: Caries of enamel. II. Acidogenic caries. Br. Dent. J., 92:225, 1952.

Harrap, G. J.: Assessment of the effect of dentifrices on the growth of dental plaque. J. Clin. Periodontol., 1:166, 1974.

Harris, R., and Beveridge, J.: Report to the Australian Dental Congress. Dent. Abstr., 12:1967.

Harrison, R. W., and Opal, Z. Z.: Comparative studies on lactobacilli isolated from the mouth and intestine. J. Dent. Res., 23:1, 1944.

Hartzell, T. B., and Henrici, A. T.: The pathogenicity of mouth streptococci and their role in the etiology of dental diseases. J. Natl. Dent. Assoc., 4:477, 1917.

Harvey, C. R., and Kelly, J. E.: Decayed, missing and filled teeth among persons 1–74 years, United States 1971–74. Vital and health statistics: Series 11, Data from the National Health Survey; no. 223. DHHS publication no. (PHS) 81-1673. Washington, D.C., Government Printing Office, 1981.

Hawes, R. R., and Bibby, B. G.: Evaluation of a dentifrice

containing carbamide and urease. J. Am. Dent. Assoc., *46*:280, 1953.

Hazen, S. P., Chilton, N. W., and Mumma, R. D., Jr.: The problem of root caries. I. Literature review and clinical description. J. Am. Dent. Assoc., *86*:137, 1973.

Healey, H. J., and Cheyne, V. D.: Comparison of caries prevalence between freshman students in two midwestern universities. J. Am. Dent. Assoc., *30*:692, 1943.

Heider, M., and Wedl, C.: Atlas to the Pathology of the Teeth. Leipzig, Arthur Felix, 1869.

Hein, J. W.: A study of the effect of frequency of toothbrushing on oral health. J. Dent. Res., *33*:708, 1954.

Hein, J. W., and Shafer, W. G.: Chlorophyll as a potential caries-preventive agent. Pa. Dent. J., (Harrisb.), *16*:221, 1949.

Heitzmann, C., and Bodecker, C. F.: Contribution to the history of development of the teeth. Indep. Pract. (D), 8:225, 281; 9:1, 57, 112, 169, 225, 285, 344, 1887–88.

Helmcke, J.-G.: Dental caries in the light of electron microscopy. Int. Dent. J., *12*:322, 1962.

Hemmens, E. S., Blayney, J. R., and Bradel, S. F.: The microbic flora of the dental plaque in relation to the beginning of caries. J. Dent. Res., 25:195, 1946.

Henderson, P.: An investigation into the health of 1,530 preschool children. Arch. Dis. Child., *12*:157, 1937.

Henschel, C. J., and Lieber, L.: Caries incidence reduction by unsupervised use of 27.5 per cent ammonium therapy dentifrice. J. Dent. Res., 28:248, 1949.

Hess, A. F., and Abramson, H.: The etiology of dental caries. Dent. Cosmos., 73:849, 1931.

Hill, I. N., Blayney, J. R., and Wolf, W.: The Evanston dental caries study. XI. The caries experience rates of 12-, 13- and 14-year-old children after exposure to fluoridated water for fifty-nine to seventy months. J. Dent. Res., *34*:77, 1955.

Hill, T. J.: A salivary factor which influences the growth of *L. acidophilus* and is an expression of susceptibility or resistance to dental caries. J. Am. Dent. Assoc., 26:239, 1939.

Idem: A Textbook of Oral Pathology. 4th ed. Philadelphia, Lea & Febiger, 1949, pp. 153–64.

Idem: Therapeutic dentifrices: panel discussion. J. Am. Dent. Assoc., *48*:1, 1954.

Idem: The use of penicillin in dental caries control. J. Dent. Res., 27:259, 1948.

Idem: Fluoride dentifrices. J. Am. Dent. Assoc., 59:1121, 1959.

Hill, T. J., and Kniesner, A. H.: Penicillin dentifrice and dental caries experience in children. J. Dent. Res., 28:263, 1949.

Hill, T. J., Sims, J., and Newman, M.: The effect of penicillin dentifrice on the control of dental caries. J. Dent. Res., *32*:448, 1953.

Hine, M. K.: Prophylaxis, toothbrushing, and home care of the mouth as caries control measures; in K. A. Easlick (ed.): Dental Caries, Mechanism and Present Control Technics as Evaluated at the University of Michigan Workshop. St. Louis, C. V. Mosby Company, 1948.

Hodge, H. C., and Smith, F. A.: Some public health aspects of water fluoridation; in J. H. Shaw (ed.): Fluoridation as a Public Health Measure. Washington, D.C., American Association for Advancement of Science, 1954.

Hoppert, C. A., Webber, P. A., and Canniff, T. L.: The production of dental caries in rats fed an adequate diet. Science, *74*:77, 1931.

Howell, C. L., Gish, G. W., Smiley, R. D., and Muhler, J. C.: Effect of topically applied stannous fluoride on dental caries experience in children. J. Am. Dent. Assoc., *50*:14, 1955.

Hubbell, R. B.: The chemical composition of saliva and blood serum of children in relation to dental caries. Am. J. Physiol., *105*:436, 1933.

Hufstader, R. D., Anderson, V. J., Phatak, N., and Snyder, M. L.: Effect of a selected nitrofuran, furacin, on the oral lactobacillus count. J. Dent. Res., *29*:794, 1950.

Hunscher, H. A.: Metabolism of women during reproductive cycle. II. Calcium and phosphorus utilization in two successive lactation periods. J. Biol. Chem., *86*:37, 1930.

Hunt, H. R., Hoppert, C. A., and Erwin, W. G.: Inheritance of susceptibility to caries in albino rats (*Mus norvegicus*). J. Dent. Res., *23*:385, 1944.

Hyatt, T. P., and Lotka, A. J.: How dental statistics are secured in the Metropolitan Life Insurance Company. J. Dent. Res., *9*:411, 1929.

Jay, P.: An anaerobe isolated from dental caries. J. Bacteriol, *14*:385, 1927.

Jay, P., and Voorhees, R. S.: *B. acidophilus* and dental caries. Dent. Cosmos, *69*:977, 1927.

Jay, P., Hadley, F. P., Bunting, R. W., and Koehne, M.: Observations on relationship of *L. acidophilus* to dental caries in children during experimental feeding of candy. J. Am. Dent. Assoc., *23*:846, 1936.

Jenkins, G. N.: A critique of the proteolysis-chelation theory of caries. Brit. Dent. J., *111*:311, 1961.

Jenkins, G. N., and Wright, D. E.: The role of ammonia in dental caries, Part II. Br. Dent. J., *90*:117, 1951.

Johansen, J. R., Gjermo, P., and Eriksen, H. M.: Effect of 2 years' use of chlorhexidine-containing dentifrices on plaque, gingivitis and caries. Scand. J. Dent. Res., 83:288, 1975.

Johnson, R. H., and Rozanis, J.: A review of chemotherapeutic plaque control. Oral Surg., *47*:136, 1979.

Jordan, H. V., and Keyes, P. H.: In vitro methods for the study of plaque formation and carious lesions. Arch. Oral Biol., *11*:793, 1966.

Jordan, W. A., and Peterson, J. K.: Caries-inhibiting value of a dentifrice containing stannous fluoride: first year report of a supervised toothbrushing study. J. Am. Dent. Assoc., *54*:589, 1957.

Idem: Caries-inhibiting value of a dentifrice containing stannous fluoride: final report of a two year study. J. Am. Dent. Assoc., *58*:42, 1959.

Kammerman, A. M., and Starkey, P. E.: Nursing caries: a case history. J. Ind. Dent. Assoc., *60*:7, 1981.

Karshan, M.: Factors in human saliva correlated with the presence and activity of dental caries. J. Dent. Res., *15*:383, 1935–36.

Idem: Do calcium and phosphorus in saliva differ significantly in caries-free and active-caries groups? J. Dent. Res., *21*:83, 1942.

Karshan, M., Krasnow, F., and Krejci, L. E.: A study of blood and saliva in relation to immunity and susceptibility to dental caries. J. Dent. Res., *11*:573, 1931.

Katz, R. V.: Root caries: clinical implications of the current epidemiologic data. Northwest Dent., *60*:306, 1981.

Katz, R. V., Hazen, S. P., Chilton, N. W., and Mumma, R. D., Jr.: Prevalence and distribution of root caries in an adult population. Caries Res., *16*:265, 1982.

Kauffmann, J. H.: The prevention concept: its critical significance. Bull. N. Y. State Soc. Dent. Child., *6*:1, 1955.

Kerr, D. W., and Kesel, R. G.: Two-year caries control study utilizing oral hygiene and an ammoniated dentifrice. J. Am. Dent. Assoc., *42*:180, 1951.

Kesel, R. G.: The effectiveness of dentifrices, mouthwashes, and ammonia-urea compounds in the control of dental caries; in K. A. Easlick (ed.): Dental Caries, Mechanism and Present Control Technics as Evaluated at the University of Michigan Workshop. St. Louis, C. V. Mosby Company, 1948.

Kesel, R. G., O'Donnell, J. F., Kirch, E. R., and Wach, E. C.: The biological production and therapeutic use of ammonia in the oral cavity in relation to dental caries prevention. J. Am. Dent. Assoc., 33:695, 1946.

Keyes, P. H.: The infectious and transmissible nature of experimental dental caries. Arch. Oral Biol., 1:304, 1960.

Idem: Questions raised by the infectious and transmissible nature of experimental caries. Conf. on Oral Biol. J. Dent. Res., 39:1086, 1960 (Abst. 9).

Keyes, P. H., and Shourie, K. L.: Dental caries in the Syrian hamster. V. The effect of 3 different fluoride compounds on caries activity. J. Dent. Res., 28:138, 1949.

Keyes, P. H., Rowberry, S. A., Englander, H. R., and Fitzgerald, R. J.: Bio-assays of medicaments for the control of dentobacterial plaque, dental caries, and periodontal lesions in Syrian hamsters. J. Oral Ther. Pharm., 3:157, 1966.

Kirch, E. R., Kesel, R. G., O'Donnell, J. F., and Wach, E. C.: Amino acids in human saliva. J. Dent. Res., 26:297, 1947.

Kirchheimer, W. F., and Douglas, H. C.: The failure of ammonium ions to inhibit the growth of oral lactobacilli. J. Dent. Res., 29:320, 1950.

Klein, H.: The family and dental disease. IV. Dental disease (DMF) experience in parents and offspring. J. Am. Dent. Assoc., 33:735, 1946.

Klein, H., and Knutson, J. W.: Studies on dental caries. XIII. Effect of ammoniacal silver nitrate on caries in the first permanent molar. J. Am. Dent. Assoc., 29:1420, 1942.

Klein, H., and Palmer, C. E.: Dental caries in brothers and sisters of immune and susceptible children. Milbank Mem. Fund Q., 18:67, 1940.

Idem: Studies on dental caries. XIII. Comparison of the caries susceptibility of the various morphological types of permanent teeth. J. Dent. Res., 20:203, 1941.

Klein, H., Palmer, C. E., and Knutson, J. W.: Studies on dental caries. I. Dental status and dental needs of elementary school children. Public Health Rep., 53:751, 1938.

Kligler, I. J.: A biochemical study and differentiation of oral bacteria, with special reference to dental caries. J. Am. Dent. Soc., 10:141, 282, 445, 1915.

Knutson, J. W.: An evaluation of the effectiveness as a caries control measure of the topical application of solutions of fluorides; in K. A. Easlick (ed.): Dental Caries, Mechanism and Present Control Technics as Evaluated at the University of Michigan Workshop. St. Louis, C. V. Mosby Company, 1948.

Knutson, J. W., and Armstrong, W. D.: The effect of topically applied sodium fluoride on dental caries experience. III. Report of findings for the third study year. Public Health Rep., 61:1683, 1946.

Koulourides, T., Ceuto, H., and Pigman, W.: Rehardening of softened enamel surfaces of human teeth by solutions of calcium phosphates. Nature, 189:226, 1961.

Krasnow, F.: Biochemical studies of dental caries. J. Dent. Res., 12:530, 1932.

Idem: Biochemical analysis of saliva in relation to caries. Dent. Cosmos, 78:301, 1936.

Krasnow, F., and Oblatt, A. B.: Salivary cholesterol. J. Dent. Res., 16:151, 1937.

Kronfeld, R.: Histopathology of the Teeth. 4th ed. (P. E. Boyle, ed.): Philadelphia, Lea & Febiger, 1955, pp. 150–158.

Larson, R. H.: The effect of EDTA on the pattern of caries development and its association with biologic changes in the rat. J. Dent. Res., 38:1207, 1959.

Larson, R. H., Zipkin, I., and Rubin, M.: Effect of administration of EDTA by various routes on dental caries in the rat. Arch. Oral Biol., 5:49, 1961.

Lazansky, J. P., Robinson, L., and Radofsky, L.: Factors influencing the incidence of bacteremias following surgical procedures in the oral cavity. J. Dent. Res., 28:533, 1949.

Leber, T., and Rottenstein, J. B.: Investigations on Caries of the Teeth. Berlin, 1867, p. 94. (Translated by T. H. Chandler. Philadelphia, Lindsay and Blakiston, 1873.)

Lenhossek, M. von: Die Zahn-caries einst und jetz. Arch. Anthropol., 17:44, 1919.

Lobene, R. R., Brion, M., and Socransky, S. S.: Effect of erythromycin on dental plaque and plaque-forming microorganisms. J. Periodontol., 40:287, 1969.

Löe, H., Theilade, E., Jensen, S. B., and Schiött, C. R.: Experimental gingivitis in man. III. The influence of antibiotics on gingival plaque development. J. Periodont. Res., 2:282, 1967.

Löe, H, von der Fehr, F. R., and Schiött, C. R.: Inhibition of experimental caries by plaque prevention. The effect of chlorhexidine mouthrinses. Scand. J. Dent. Res., 80:1, 1972.

Loesche, W. J.: Chemotherapy of dental plaque infections. Oral Sci. Rev., 9:65, 1976.

Loesche, W. J., and Nafe, D.: Reduction of supragingival plaque accumulations in institutionalized Down's syndrome patients by periodic treatment with topical kanamycin. Arch. Oral Biol., 18:1131, 1973.

Loesche, W. J., Hockett, R. N., and Syed, S. A.: Reduction in proportions of dental plaque streptococci following a 5-day kanamycin treatment. J. Periodont. Res., 12:1, 1977.

Loesche, W. J., Rowan, J., Straffon, L. H., and Loos, P. J.: The association of Streptococcus mutans with human dental decay. Infect. and Immunol., 11:1252, 1975.

Ludwick, L. S., and Fosdick, L. S.: The ammonia content of the mouth. J. Dent. Res., 29:38, 1950.

Lunin, M., and Mandel, I. D.: Clinical evaluation of a penicillin dentifrice. J. Am. Dent. Assoc., 51:696, 1955.

Magitot, E.: Treatise on Dental Caries; Experimental and Therapeutic Investigations. Translated by T. H. Chandler. Boston, Houghton, Osgood and Company, 1878.

Malann, A. L., and Ockerse, T.: The effect of the calcium-phosphorus intake of school children upon dental caries, body weights and heights. S. Afr. Dent. J., 15:153, 1941.

Malherbe, M., and Ockerse, T.: Dental caries in a high and low incidence area in South Africa; a study of possible contributory factors with special reference to diet. S. Afr. J. Med. Sci., 9:75, 1944.

Mandel, I. D.: Histological, histochemical and other aspects of caries initiation. J. Am. Dent. Assoc., 51:432, 1955.

Idem: Dental caries. Am. Sci., 67:680, 1979.

Manley, E. B., and Hardwick, J. L.: Caries of enamel. I. The significance of enamel lamellae. Br. Dent. J., 91:36, 1951.

Mann, A. W., Dreizen, S., Spies, T. D., and Hunt, F. M.: A comparison of dental caries activity in malnourished and well-nourished patients. J. Am. Dent. Assoc., 34:244, 1947.

Mansbridge, J. N.: Heredity and dental caries. J. Dent. Res., 38:337, 1959.

Matsumiya, S.: Recent advances in dental caries research by electron microscopy. Int. Dent. J., 12:433, 1962.

McClure, F. J.: Effect of fluorides on salivary amylase. Public Health Rep., 54:2165, 1939.

Idem: Cariostatic effect of phosphates. Science, 144:1337, 1964.

McClure, F. J., and Hewitt, W. L.: The relation of penicillin to induced rat dental caries and oral lactobacillus. J. Dent. Res., 25:441, 1947.

McDonald, R. E.: Human saliva: a study of the rate of flow and viscosity and its relationship to dental caries. M. S. Thesis, Indiana University, 1950.

McHugh, W. D. (ed.): Dental Plaque. Edinburgh and London, E. & S., Livingstone Ltd., 1970.

McIntosh, J., James, W. W., and Lazarus-Barlow, P.: An investigation into the aetiology of dental caries. I. The nature of the destructive agent and the production of artificial caries. Br. Dent. J., 43:728, 1922.

McKay, F. S.: The relation of mottled enamel to caries. J. Am. Dent. Assoc., 15:1429, 1928.

McRae, L. J.: Tooth conditions among white and negro children. J. Am. Dent. Assoc., 20:1917, 1933.

Mellanby, M.: Effect of diet on the resistance of teeth to caries. Proc. R. Soc. Med., 16, pt. 3:74, 1923.

Idem: The relation of caries to the structure of the teeth. Br. Dent. J., 44:1, 1923.

Idem: Diet and the teeth: an experimental study. III. The effect of diet on dental structure and disease in man. Med. Research Council, Special Rept., Series No. 191, London, 1934.

Mercer, V. H., and Muhler, J. C.: Comparison of a single application of stannous fluoride with a single application of sodium fluoride or two applications of stannous fluoride. J. Dent. Child., 28:84, 1961.

Messner, C. T., Gafafer, W. M., Cady, F. C., and Dean, H. T.: Dental survey of school children, ages 6–14 years, made in 1933–34 in 26 states. Public Health Bull. No. 226, 1936, p. 248.

Miller, W. D.: Die Mikroorganismen des Mundhohle. Leipzig, 1889.

Idem: Microorganisms of the Human Mouth. Philadelphia, S. S. White Publishing Company, 1890.

Idem: New theories concerning decay of teeth. Dent. Cosmos, 47:1293, 1905.

Mills, C. A.: Factors affecting the incidence of dental caries in population groups. J. Dent. Res., 16:417, 1937.

Moulton, F. R. (ed.): Dental Caries and Fluorine, Washington, D.C., American Association for the Advancement of Science, 1946.

Muhler, J. C.: The effect of a single topical application of stannous fluoride on the incidence of dental caries in adults. J. Dent. Res., 37:448, 1958.

Idem: The effectiveness of stannous fluoride in children residing in an optimal communal fluoride area. J. Dent. Child., 27:51, 1960.

Idem: Stannous fluoride enamel pigmentation evidence of caries arrestment. J. Dent. Child., 27:157, 1960.

Idem: A practical method for reducing dental caries in children not receiving the established benefits of communal fluoridation. J. Dent. Child., 28:5, 1961.

Idem: Effect of a stannous fluoride dentifrice on caries reduction in children during a three-year study period. J. Am. Dent. Assoc., 64:216, 1962.

Idem: Mass treatment of children with a stannous fluoride-zirconium silicate self-administered prophylactic paste for partial control of dental caries. J. Amer. Coll. Dent., 35:45, 1968.

Muhler, J. C., and Day, H. G.: Effect of stannous fluoride, stannous chloride and sodium fluoride on the incidence of dental lesions in rats fed a caries-producing diet. J. Am. Dent. Assoc., 41:528, 1950.

Muhler, J. C., and Hine, M. K. (eds.): A Symposium on Preventive Dentistry. St. Louis, C. V. Mosby Company, 1956.

Muhler, J. C., and Van Huysen, G.: Solubility of enamel protected by sodium fluoride and other compounds. J. Dent. Res., 26:119, 1947.

Muhler, J. C., Radike, A. W., Nebergall, W. H., and Day, H. G.: The effect of a stannous fluoride-containing dentifrice on caries reduction in children. J. Dent. Res., 33:606, 1954.

Idem: Effect of a stannous fluoride-containing dentifrice on caries reduction in children. II. Caries experience after one year. J. Am. Dent. Assoc., 50:163, 1955.

Idem: The effect of a stannous fluoride-containing dentifrice on dental caries in adults. J. Dent. Res., 35:49, 1956.

Muhler, J. C., Stookey, G. K., and Bixler, D.: Evaluation of the anticariogenic effect of mixtures of stannous fluoride and soluble phosphates. J. Dent. Child., 3:154, 1965.

Mummery, J. R.: On the relations which dental caries, as discovered amongst the ancient inhabitants of Britain and amongst existing aboriginal races, may be supposed to hold to their food and social condition. Trans. Odontol. Soc., 2:7, 1870.

National Center for Health Statistics, C. S. Wilder: Dental visits, volume and interval since last visit, United States, 1978–1979. Vital and Health Statistics. Series 10, No. 138, DHHS Pub. No. (PHS) 82-1566. Washington, D.C., Government Printing Office, 1982.

Nevin, T. A., Bibby, G. B.: The effect of water-soluble chlorophyll on pure cultures of organisms commonly found in the oral cavity. J. Dent. Res., 30:469, 1951 (Abst.).

Newbrun, E.: Cariology. 4th ed. Baltimore, Williams & Wilkins, 1976.

Nigel, A. E., and Harris, R. S.: The effects of phosphates on experimental dental caries: a literature review. J. Dent. Res., 43:1123, 1964.

Nolte, W. A. (ed.): Oral Microbiology with Basic Microbiology and Immunology. 4th ed. St. Louis, C. V. Mosby Company, 1982.

Orland, F. J., Blayney, J. R., Harrison, R. W., Reynier, J. A., Trexler, P. C., Ervin, R. F., Gordon, H. A., and Wagner, M.: Experimental caries in germfree rats inoculated with enterococci. J. Am. Dent. Assoc., 50:254, 1955.

Parmly, L.: Practical Guide to Management of the Teeth. Philadelphia, Collins and Croft, 1819.

Peffley, G. E., and Muhler, J. C.: The effect of a commercial stannous fluoride dentifrice under controlled brushing habits on dental caries incidence in children: preliminary report. J. Dent. Res., 39:871, 1960.

Pelton, W. J.: The effect of zinc chloride and potassium ferrocyanide as a caries prophylaxis. J. Dent. Res., 29:756, 1950.

Pickerill, H. P., and Champtaloup, S. T.: The bacteriology of the mouth in Maori children, being part of an investigation into the cause of immunity to dental disease in the Maori of the Uriwera country, New Zealand. Brit. Med. J., 2:1482, 1913.

Pincus, P.: Further tests on human enamel protein. Biochem. J., 42:219, 1948.

Idem: Production of dental caries. Br. Med. J., 2:358, 1949.

Poole, D. F. G., and Newman, H. N.: Dental plaque and oral health. Nature, 234:329, 1971.

Price, W. A.: Eskimo and Indian field studies in Alaska and Canada. J. Am. Dent. Assoc., 23:417, 1936.

Protheroe, D. H.: A study to determine the effect of topical application of stannous fluoride on dental caries in young adults. R. Can. Dent. Corps Q., 3:20, 1962.

Read, T. T., and Knowles, E. M.: A study of the diet and habits of school children in relation to freedom from or susceptibility to dental caries. Br. Dent. J., 64:185, 1938.

Restarski, J. S.: Incidence of dental caries among pure-blooded Samoans. U. S. Naval Med. Bull., 41:1713, 1941.

Ripa, L. W.: Fluoride rinsing: what dentists should know. J. Am. Dent. Assoc., 102:477, 1981.

Ripa, L. W., and Cole, W. W.: Occlusal sealing and caries prevention: results 12 months after a single application of adhesive resin. J. Dent. Res., 49:171, 1970.

Ripa, L. W., Leske, G. S., Sposato, A. L., and Rebich, T., Jr.: Supervised weekly rinsing with a 0.2% neutral NaF solution: results of a demonstration program after four school years. J. Am. Dent. Assoc., 102:482, 1981.

Robinson, H. B. G.: Dental caries and the metabolism of calcium. J. Am. Dent. Assoc., 30:357, 1943.

Idem: The effect of systemic disease on the caries process: pregnancy, endocrinopathies, osteomalacia, emotional disturbances, and others; in K. A. Easlick (ed.): Dental Caries, Mechanism and Present Control Technics as Evaluated at the University of Michigan Workshop. St. Louis, C. V. Mosby Company, 1948.

Rodriguez, F. E.: Studies in the specific bacteriology of dental caries. Milit. Dent. J., 5:199, 1922.

Rosebury, T., and Karshan, M.: Dietary habits of Kuskok-wim Eskimos, with varying degrees of dental caries. J. Dent. Res., 16:307, 1937.

Rowe, N. H. (ed.): Proceedings of Symposium on Incipient Caries of Enamel. University of Michigan School of Dentistry, Ann Arbor, 1977.

Russell, B. G., and Bay, L. M.: Oral use of chlorhexidine gluconate toothpaste in epileptic children. Scand. J. Dent. Res., 86:52, 1978.

Salter, W. A. T., McCombie, F., and Hole, L. W.: The anticariogenic effects of one and two applications of stannous fluoride on the deciduous and permanent teeth of children age 6 and 7. J. Can. Dent. Assoc., 28:363, 1962.

Sampson, W. E. A.: Dental examination of the inhabitants of the Island of Tristan da Cunha. Br. Dent. J., 53:397, 1932.

Schatz, A., and Martin, J. J.: Keratin utilization by oral microflora. Proc. Pa. Acad. Sci., 29:48, 1955.

Idem: Destruction of bone and tooth by proteolysis-chela-tion: its inhibition by fluoride and application to dental caries. N. Y. J. Dent., 30:124, 1960.

Idem: The proteolysis-chelation theory of dental caries. J. Am. Dent. Assoc., 65:368, 1962.

Schatz, A., Karlson, K. E., and Martin, J. J.: Destruction of tooth organic matter by oral keratinolytic microorganisms. N. Y. State Dent. J., 21:438, 1955.

Schatz, A., Karlson, K. E., Martin, J. J., and Schatz, V.: The proteolysis-chelation theory of dental caries. Odontol Revy, 8:154, 1957.

Schatz, A., Karlson, K. E., Martin, J. J., Schatz, V., and Adelson, L. M.: Some philosophical considerations on the proteolysis-chelation theory of dental caries. Proc. Pa. Acad. Sci., 32:20, 1958.

Schour, I., and Massler, M.: Dental caries experience in postwar Italy (1945). I. Prevalence in various age groups. J. Am. Dent. Assoc., 35:1, 1947.

Schwartz, J.: The teeth of the Massai. J. Dent. Res., 25:17, 1946.

Scott, D. B.: A study of the bilateral incidence of carious lesions. J. Dent. Res., 23:105, 1944.

Scott, D. B., and Albright, J. T.: Electron microscopy of carious enamel and dentine. Oral Surg., 7:64, 1954.

Sebelius, C. L.: Variations in dental caries: rates among white and Negro children. J. Am. Dent. Assoc., 31:544, 1944.

Sellman, S.: The buffer value of saliva and its relation to dental caries. Acta Odontol. Scand., 8:244, 1949.

Shafer, W. G., and Hein, J. W.: Further studies on the effect of chlorophyllin on experimental dental caries. J. Dent. Res., 29:666, 1950 (Abst.).

Idem: Further studies on the inhibition of experimental caries by sodium copper chlorophyllin. J. Dent. Res., 30:510, 1951 (Abst.).

Shannon, I. L.: Salivary sodium, potassium and chloride levels in subjects classified as to dental caries experience. J. Dent. Res., 37:401, 1958.

Shelling, D. H., and Anderson, G. M.: Relation of rickets and vitamin D to the incidence of dental caries, enamel hypoplasia and malocclusion in children. J. Am. Dent. Assoc., 23:840, 1936.

Ship, I. I., and Mickelsen, O.: The effects of calcium acid phosphate on dental caries in children: a controlled clinical trial. J. Dent. Res., 43:1144, 1964.

Shiere, F. R.: The effectiveness of a tyrothricin dentifrice in the control of dental caries. J. Dent. Res., 36:237, 1957.

Silverstone, L. M.: The primary translucent zone of enamel caries and of artificial caries-like lesions. Br. Dent. J., 120:461, 1966.

Idem: Remineralization phenomena. Caries Res., 11(Suppl. 1):59, 1977.

Idem: The effect of fluoride in the remineralization of enamel caries and caries-like lesions in vitro. J. Pub. Health Dent., 42:42, 1982.

Sognnaes, R. F.: An analysis of a war-time reduction of dental caries in European children, with special regard to observations from Norway. Am. J. Dis. Child., 75:792, 1948.

Idem: Advances in Experimental Caries Research. Washington, D.C., American Association for the Advancement of Science, 1955.

Sognnaes, R. F., and Wislocki, G. B.: Histochemical observations on enamel and dentine undergoing carious destruction. Oral Surg., 3:1283, 1950.

Spies, T. D., Bean, W. B., and Ashe, W. F.: Recent advances in the treatment of pellagra and associated deficiencies. Ann. Intern. Med., 12:1830, 1939.

Stack, M. V.: Organic constituents of enamel. J. Am. Dent. Assoc., 48:297, 1954.

Stallard, R. E.: A Textbook of Preventive Dentistry. 2nd ed. Philadelphia, W. B. Saunders Company, 1982.

Stamm, J. W., and Banting, D. W.: Comparison of root caries prevalence in adults with lifelong residence in fluoridated and non-fluoridated communities. J. Dent. Res., 59:405, 1980 (Abst.).

Starr, H. E.: Studies of mixed human saliva. II. Variations

in the hydrogen ion concentration of human mixed saliva. J. Biol. Chem., *54*:55, 1922.

Stephan, R. M.: Relative importance of polysaccharides, disaccharides and monosaccharides in the production of caries. J. Am. Dent. Assoc., *37*:530, 1938.

Idem: Changes in H-ion concentration on tooth surfaces and in carious lesions. J. Am. Dent. Assoc., *27*:718, 1940.

Idem: Two factors of possible importance in relation to the etiology and treatment of dental caries and other dental diseases. Science, *92*:578, 1940.

Idem: The effect of urea in counteracting the influence of carbohydrates on the pH of dental plaques. J. Dent. Res., *22*:63, 1943.

Idem: Intra-oral hydrogen-ion concentrations associated with dental caries activity. J. Dent. Res., *23*:257, 1944.

Idem: Some local factors in the development of cavities: plaques, acidity, aciduric bacteria, proteolytic bacteria; in K. A. Easlick (ed.): Dental Caries, Mechanism and Present Control Technics as Evaluated at the University of Michigan Workshop. St. Louis, C. V. Mosby Company, 1948.

Stephan, R. M., and Miller, B. F.: The effect of synthetic detergents on pH changes in dental plaques. J. Dent. Res., *22*:53, 1943.

Stevens, R. H., and Mandel, I. D.: *Streptococcus mutans* serotypes in caries-resistant and caries-susceptible adults. J. Dent. Res., *56*:1044, 1977.

Stookey, G. K., Carroll, R. A., and Muhler, J. C.: The clinical effectiveness of phosphate-enriched breakfast cereals on the incidence of dental caries in children: results after 2 years. J. Am. Dent. Assoc., *74*:752, 1967.

Stralfors, A.: The acid fermentation in the dental plaques in situ compared with lactobacillus count. J. Dent. Res., *27*:576, 1948.

Idem: The effect of calcium phosphate on dental caries in school children. J. Dent. Res., *43*:1137, 1964.

Strean, L. F.: Vitamin B$_6$ und Zahnkaries. Schweiz. Mschr. Zahnheilk., *67*:981, 1957.

Suk, V.: Eruption and decay of permanent teeth in whites and Negroes, with comparative remarks on other races. Am. J. Phys. Anthropol., *2*:351, 1919.

Sullivan, J. H., and Storvick, C. A.: Correlation of saliva analyses with dental examinations of 574 freshmen at Oregon State College. J. Dent. Res., *29*:165, 1950.

Sumnicht, R. W.: Research in preventive dentistry. J. Am. Dent. Assoc., *79*:1194, 1969.

Taber, L. B. (ed.): Sugar and dental caries, a symposium. J. Calif. Dent. Assoc., *26*:No. 3, May-June, 1950.

Tank, G., and Storvick, C. A.: Effect of naturally occurring selenium and vanadium on dental caries. J. Dent. Res., *39*:473, 1960.

Theilade, E., and Theilade, J.: Role of plaque in the etiology of periodontal disease and caries. Oral Sci. Rev., *9*:23, 1976.

Thewlis, J.: The structure of teeth. Br. Dent. J., *53*:655, 1932.

Idem: X-ray analysis of teeth. Br. J. Radiol., *5*:353, 1932.

Idem: X-ray examination of teeth. Br. Dent. J., *57*:457, 1934.

Tomes, J. A.: A System of Dental Surgery. 2nd ed. London, Lindsay and Blakiston, 1873.

Torell, P., and Ericsson, Y.: Two-year clinical tests with different methods of local caries-preventive fluorine

applications in Swedish school-children. Acta Odont. Scand., *23*:287, 1965.

Toverud, G.: Decrease in caries frequency in Norwegian children during World War II. J. Am. Dent. Assoc., *39*:127, 1949.

Turkheim, H.: Salivary content of mucin, ammonia, sodium chloride and calcium. D. Monat. Zahnh., *43*:897, 1925.

Turner, J. G., and Bennett, F. J.: Some specimens of caries from ancient Egyptian teeth. Dent. Surg., *9*:475, 1913.

Turner, N. C., and Crowell, G. E.: Dental caries and tryptophane deficiency. J. Dent. Res., *26*:99, 1947.

Underwood, A. S., and Milles, W. T.: An investigation into the effects of organisms upon the teeth and alveolar portions of the jaws. Trans. Int. Med. Congr., 7th Session, *3*:523, 1881.

Van Kesteren, M., Bibby, B. G., and Berry, G. P.: Studies on the antibacterial factors of human saliva. J. Bacteriol, *43*:573, 1942.

Volker, J. F.: Effect of fluorine on solubility of enamel and dentin. Proc. Soc. Exp. Biol. Med., *42*:725, 1939.

Idem: Solubility of fluorosed enamel and dentin. Proc. Soc. Exp. Biol. Med., *43*:643, 1940.

Idem: The effect of chewing gum on the teeth and supporting structures. J. Am. Dent. Assoc., *36*:23, 1948.

Volker, J. F., and Pinkerton, D. M.: Acid production in saliva-carbohydrate mixtures. J. Dent. Res., *26*:229, 1947.

Volker, J. F., Fosdick, L. S., Manahan, R..D., and Manly, R. S.: Effect of sodium N-palmitoyl sarcosinate on tooth enamel solubility. Proc. Soc. Exp. Biol. Med., *87*:332, 1954.

Volker, J. F., Hodge, H. C., Wilson, H. J., and van Voorhis, S. M.: The absorption of fluorides by enamel, dentin, bone, and hydroxyapatite as shown by the radioactive isotope. J. Biol. Chem., *134*:543, 1940.

Vratsanos, S. M., Abelson, D. C., and Mandel, I. D.: Plaque acidogenesis and caries resistance. J. Dent. Res., *58*:425, 1979 (Abst.).

Wach, E. C., O'Donnell, J. F., and Hine, M. K.: Effects of a mouth rinse on oral acidogenic bacteria. J. Am. Dent. Assoc., *29*:61, 1942.

Wainwright, W. W.: Human saliva. XV. Inorganic phosphorus content of resting saliva of 650 healthy individuals. J. Dent. Res., *22*:403, 1943.

Weisenstein, P., Radike, A., and Robinson, H. B. G.: Clinical studies of dental caries in small groups of children; dentifrice, brushing and participation effects. J. Dent. Res., *33*:690, 1954 (Abst.).

Westbrook, J. L., Miller, A. S., Chilton, N. W., Williams, F. L., and Mumma, R. D., Jr.: Root surface caries: a clinical, histopathologic and microbiographic investigation. Caries Res., *8*:249, 1974.

White, B. J., Kniesner, A. H., and Hill, T. J.: Effect of small amounts of penicillin on the oral bacterial flora. J. Dent. Res., *28*:267, 1949.

White, J., and Bunting, R. W.: An investigation into the possible relationship of ammonia in the saliva and dental caries. J. Am. Dent. Assoc., *22*:468, 1935.

Idem: A comparison of the chemical composition of stimulated and resting saliva of caries-free and caries-susceptible children. Am. J. Physiol., *117*:529, 1936.

Williams, J. L.: A contribution to the study of pathology of enamel. Dent. Cosmos., *39*:169, 269, 353, 1897.

Williams, N. B.: Immunization of human beings with oral lactobacilli. J. Dent. Res., *23*:403, 1944.

Wislocki, G. B., and Sognnaes, R. F.: The organic elements of the enamel. V. Histochemical reactions of the organic matter in undecalcified enamel. J. Dent. Res., 28:678, 1949.

Woldring, M. G.: Free amino acids of human saliva: a chromatographic investigation. J. Dent. Res., 34:248, 1955.

Wright, C. Z., Banting, D. W., and Feasby, W. H.: The Dorchester dental flossing study: final report. Clin. Prev. Dent., 1:23, 1979.

Young, D.: Past and present methods and results of sugar analysis of saliva. J. Dent. Res., 20:597, 1941.

Youngburg, G. E.: Salivary ammonia and its relation to dental caries. J. Dent. Res., 15:247, 1935–36.

Younger, H. B.: Clinical results of caries prophylaxis by impregnation. Tex. Dent. J., 67:96, 1949.

Zander, H. A.: The effectiveness of the topical application of silver salts in the control of caries; in K. A. Easlick (ed.): Dental Caries, Mechanism and Present Control Technics as Evaluated at the University of Michigan Workshop. St. Louis, C. V. Mosby Company, 1948.

Idem: Effect of a penicillin dentifrice on caries incidence in school children. J. Am. Dent. Assoc., 40:469, 1950.

Zander, H. A., and Bibby, B. G.: Penicillin and caries activity. J. Dent. Res., 26:365, 1947.

Zipkin, I.: Caries potentiating effect of ethylene diamine tetraacetic acid in the rat. Proc. Soc. Exp. Biol. Med., 82:80, 1953.

Ziskin, D. E.: The incidence of dental caries in pregnant women. Am. J. Obstet. Gynecol., 12:710, 1926.

Ziskin, D. E., and Hotelling, H.: Effect of pregnancy, mouth acidity, and age on dental caries. J. Dent. Res., 16:507, 1937.

CHAPTER 8

Diseases of the Pulp and Periapical Tissues

DISEASES OF THE DENTAL PULP

The dental pulp is a delicate connective tissue liberally interspersed with tiny blood vessels, lymphatics, myelinated and unmyelinated nerves, and undifferentiated connective tissue cells. Like other connective tissues throughout the body, it reacts to bacterial infection or to other stimuli by an inflammatory response. Certain anatomic features of this specialized connective tissue, however, tend to alter the nature and the course of this response. The enclosure of the pulp tissue within the calcified walls of the dentin precludes the excessive swelling of tissue that occurs in the hyperemic and edematous phases of inflammation in other tissues. The fact that the blood vessels supplying the pulp tissue must enter the tooth through the tiny apical foramina precludes the development of an extensive collateral blood supply to the inflamed part. The proceedings of a conference on the biology of the human dental pulp and many aspects of its pathology were edited by Siskin and published in 1973. The interested reader is referred to this publication for a detailed review.

The diseases of the dental pulp to be considered in this section are those occurring chiefly as sequelae of dental caries. Those reactions following various mechanical, thermal, and chemical injuries are discussed in Chapter 10. The sequential conditions are almost exclusively inflammatory and do not differ basically from inflammation elsewhere in the body.

Etiologic Factors in Pulp Disease. Most cases of pulpitis are primarily a result of dental caries in which bacterial invasion of the dentin and pulp tissue occurs. However, Brännström and Lind, among others, have reported that changes in the pulp may occur even with very early dental caries represented by demineralization limited to the enamel alone, appearing as white spots without actual cavitation. Occasionally there is bacterial invasion in the absence of caries, as in cases of tooth fracture that expose the dental pulp to the oral fluids and microorganisms or as a result of a bacteremia. Robinson and Boling reported that bacteria circulating in the blood stream tend to settle out or accumulate at sites of pulpal inflammation, such as that which might follow some chemical or mechanical injury to the pulp. They termed this particular phenomenon "anachoretic pulpitis." Although anachoresis represents a distinct mechanism for bacterial infection of an intact pulp, it probably occurs in a clinically insignificant number of cases of pulpitis, compared with the number of cases occurring as a result of dental caries.

The significance of microorganisms in the etiology of pulpitis has been confirmed by Kakehashi and his associates, who produced surgical pulp exposures in germ-free rats. It was found that no devitalized pulps or periapical infections developed even when gross food impactions existed. By contrast, conventional animals rapidly developed complete pulpal necrosis.

Pulpitis may also arise as a result of chemical irritation of the pulp. This may occur not only in an exposed pulp to which some irritating medicament is applied but also in intact pulps beneath deep or moderately deep cavities into which some irritating filling material is inserted. This is undoubtedly a result of penetration of the irritating substances into the pulp tissue via the dentinal tubules. In many instances, however, the pulp may respond to the irritation by forming reparative dentin.

479

Severe thermal change in a tooth may also produce pulpitis. This is most common in teeth with large metallic restorations, particularly when there is inadequate insulation between the filling material and the pulp. Heat and more particularly cold are transmitted to the pulp, often producing pain and, if the stimulus is prolonged and severe, actual pulpitis. Mild thermal changes are most apt to stimulate only the formation of reparative dentin, and this is a relatively common phenomenon.

Robertson and co-workers reported a histologic study of the effects on the pulp of an electrosurgical current applied to a metallic restoration in rhesus monkey teeth. Teeth subjected to brief application of electrosurgical current on cervical restorations showed histologic evidence of major damage to both the pulp and the periodontal tissues. Twenty-four hours following the application of the current, coagulation necrosis of the pulp tissue was observed adjacent to the restoration. By the end of one week, the coronal portion of the pulp was necrotic. A sharply demarcated line separated necrotic from vital pulp tissue. Focal areas of necrosis with mineralized tissue resorption were also seen in the furcations of multirooted teeth. At eight weeks, necrosis involved the entire pulp. Loss of periodontal ligament and osteoclastic resorption of interradicular bone was a common finding in multirooted teeth, and periapical granulomatous inflammation was noted involving several teeth. The effect on the pulp was apparently the result not of high temperature but rather of transmission of electrosurgical current through the dentin interposed between the amalgam restoration and the pulp.

A condition clinically simulating pulpitis by the occurrence of odontalgia, or toothache, was reported during World War II in flying personnel at high altitudes and has been called aerodontalgia. It is relatively uncommon and is associated particularly with recently filled teeth. The work of Orban and Ritchey suggests that the pain in decompression does not usually occur in normal pulps. Interestingly, aerodontalgia reportedly may be delayed for hours or even days after decompression or ascent to high altitudes. Apparently the same condition may occur in submarine crews and in astronauts. Some cases of pain localized to the dental area and resembling aerodontalgia have been reported to represent aerosinusitis and not to be related to the teeth.

It is apparent that pulpitis may be caused by a variety of circumstances, each producing a deleterious effect on the dental pulp. This effect is nonspecific, but the nature of the etiologic agent or agents can usually be found through study of the clinical or microscopic features of the condition or both.

Classification of Pulp Disease. Pulp disease of an inflammatory nature has been classified in a variety of ways, the simplest being a division into *acute* and *chronic pulpitis*. Furthermore, some investigators classify both acute and chronic pulpitis in several different ways. There may be a *partial pulpitis* or a *subtotal pulpitis*, depending upon the extent of involvement of the pulp. If the inflammatory process is confined to a portion of the pulp, usually a portion of the coronal pulp such as a pulp horn, the condition has been called *partial* or *focal pulpitis*. If most of the pulp is diseased, the term *total* or *generalized pulpitis* has been used.

Another classification of both acute and chronic pulpitis is based upon the presence or absence of a direct communication between the dental pulp and the oral environment, usually through a large carious lesion. The term *open pulpitis* (pulpitis aperta) has been used to describe those cases of pulpitis in which the pulp obviously communicates with the oral cavity, whereas the cases in which no such communication exists are described as *closed pulpitis* (pulpitis clausa). In both the clinical and the histologic features of open and closed pulpitis, differences do exist that are referable to the presence or absence of drainage. The basic process is the same in each case, but the classification has been used as an aid in understanding the variations in clinical features that occur in different cases.

PULPITIS

In this section, pulpitis will be discussed under the two chief types of the disease: *acute* and *chronic*. In addition, attention will be drawn to those differences in clinical and histologic features that are dependent upon the extent of the inflammation and upon whether drainage can occur. No classification of pulpitis will be made beyond that dependent upon the duration of the process.

Focal Reversible Pulpitis

One of the earliest forms of pulpitis is the condition known as *focal reversible pulpitis*. At one time, this was often referred to as *pulp hyperemia*. However, it is known that vascular dilatation can occur artefactually from the "pumping" action during tooth extraction as well as pathologically as a result of dentinal and pulpal irritation. Therefore, this early mild transient pulpitis, localized chiefly to the pulpal ends of irritated dentinal tubules, is now known as focal reversible pulpitis.

Clinical Features. A tooth with focal pulpitis is sensitive to thermal changes, particularly to cold. The application of ice or cold fluids to the tooth results in pain, but this disappears upon removal of the thermal irritant or restoration of the normal temperature. It will be found also that such a tooth responds to stimulation by the electric pulp tester at a lower level of current, indicating a lower pain threshold (or a greater sensitivity) than that of adjacent normal teeth.

Teeth in which this condition exists usually show deep carious lesions, large metallic restorations (particularly without adequate insulation), or restorations with defective margins.

Histologic Features. Focal pulpitis is characterized microscopically by dilatation of the pulp vessels (Fig. 8–1). Edema fluid may collect because of damage to the capillary walls, allowing actual extravasation of red blood cells or some diapedesis of white blood cells. Slowing of the blood flow and hemoconcentration due to transudation of fluid from the vessels conceivably could cause thrombosis. The belief has prevailed also that self-strangulation of the pulp may occur as a result of increased arterial pressure occluding the vein at the apical foramen.

Boling and Robinson argued that this belief is incorrect because the pulp may have several afferent and efferent vessels and several foramina, making self-strangulation unlikely.

Treatment and Prognosis. Focal pulpitis is generally regarded as a reversible condition, provided the irritant is removed before the pulp is severely damaged. Thus, a carious lesion should be excised and restored or a defective filling replaced as soon as it is discovered. If the primary cause is not corrected, extensive pulpitis eventually results, with subsequent "death" of the pulp.

Acute Pulpitis

Extensive acute inflammation of the dental pulp is a frequent immediate sequela of focal reversible pulpitis, although it may also occur as an acute exacerbation of a chronic inflammatory process. Significant differences in both the clinical and microscopic features are found between acute and chronic pulpitis.

Clinical Features. Acute pulpitis usually occurs in a tooth with a large carious lesion or a restoration, commonly a defective one around which there has been "recurrent caries." Even in its early stages when the inflammatory reaction involves only a portion of the pulp, usually that area just beneath the carious lesion, relatively severe pain is elicited by thermal changes, particularly those caused by ice or cold drinks. Characteristically, this pain persists

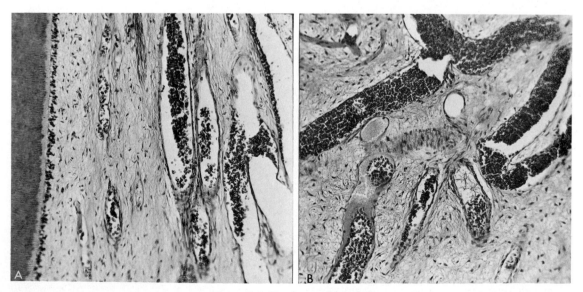

Figure 8–1. *Focal reversible pulpitis.*
The photomicrographs show vasodilatation but as yet no extravasation of red or white blood cells.

even after the thermal stimulus has disappeared or been removed. However, a clinicopathologic study by Mitchell and Tarplee provided evidence that evaluation of the type or degree of pulpitis present by sensitivity to either heat or cold is fallacious, since in their study most patients with any type of pulpitis exhibited increased sensitivity to *both* heat and cold. This has been confirmed by Seltzer and his associates, who have also shown that the severity of the pain is only partially related to the severity of the inflammatory response. Other factors include whether there has been establishment of drainage, the patient's previous experiences, emotions, and so forth.

As a greater proportion of the pulp becomes involved with intrapulpal abscess formation, the pain may become even more severe and is often described as a lancinating type. It may be continuous, and its intensity may be increased when the patient lies down. The application of heat may cause an acute exacerbation of pain. The tooth reacts to the electric pulp vitality tester at a lower level of current than adjacent normal teeth, indicating increased sensitivity of the pulp. When necrosis of the pulp tissue occurs, this sensitivity is lost.

Severe pain is more apt to be present when the entrance to the diseased pulp is not wide open. Pressure increases because of lack of escape of inflammatory exudate, and there is rapid spread of inflammation throughout the pulp with pain and necrosis. Until this inflammation or necrosis extends beyond the pulp tissue within the root apex, the tooth is not particularly sensitive to percussion. When a large open cavity is present, there is no opportunity for a build-up of pressure. Thus the inflammatory process does not tend to spread rapidly throughout the pulp. In such a case the pain experienced by the patient is a dull, throbbing ache, but the tooth is still sensitive to thermal changes.

The patient with a severe acute pulpitis is extremely uncomfortable and at least mildly ill. He is usually apprehensive and desirous of immediate attention.

Histologic Features.   Early acute pulpitis is characterized by the continued vascular dilatation seen in focal reversible pulpitis, accompanied by the accumulation of edema fluid in the connective tissue surrounding the tiny blood vessels. The pavementing of polymorphonuclear leukocytes becomes apparent along the walls of these vascular channels, and these leukocytes rapidly migrate through the endothelium-lined structures in increasing numbers. Soon great collections of white blood cells may

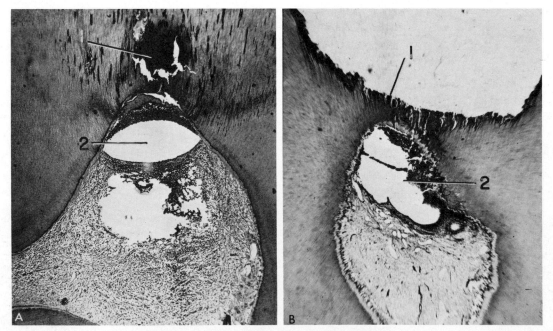

Figure 8–2. *Acute pulpitis with pulp abscess formation.*
There is diffuse inflammation of the pulp chamber in *A* beneath the carious lesion *(1)* with the formation of a circumscribed focus of suppuration, a pulp abscess *(2)*. In *B*, the carious lesion *(1)* has evoked only a focal inflammation of the pulp with abscess formation *(2)*.

be found, especially beneath an area of carious penetration. By this stage, the odontoblasts in this area have usually been destroyed.

Early in the course of the disease, the polymorphonuclear leukocytes are confined to a localized area, and the remainder of the pulp tissue appears relatively normal. Even at this period there may be localized destruction of pulp tissue and the formation of a small abscess, known as a *pulp abscess*, containing pus arising from breakdown of leukocytes and bacteria as well as from digestion of tissue (Fig. 8–2). In tissue section, because of loss of the liquid pus, this abscess frequently appears as a small void surrounded by a dense band of leukocytes (Fig. 8–3). Abscess formation is most apt to occur when the entrance to the pulp is a tiny one and there is lack of drainage.

Eventually, in some cases in only a few days, the acute inflammatory process spreads to involve most of the pulp so that neutrophilic leukocytes fill the pulp. The entire odontoblastic layer degenerates. If the pulp is closed to the outside, there is considerable pressure formed, and the entire pulp tissue undergoes rather rapid disintegration. Numerous small abscesses may form, and eventually the entire pulp undergoes liquefaction and necrosis. This

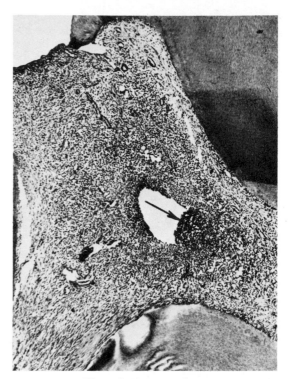

Figure 8–4. *Acute pulpitis.*
The entire pulp is involved (total pulpitis), and a focal area of suppuration is present.

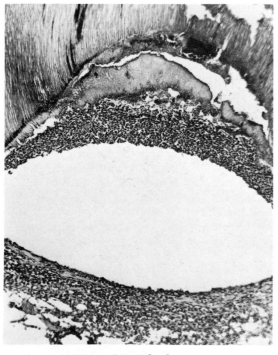

Figure 8–3. *Pulp abscess.*
The high-power photomicrograph of Figure 8–2, *A*, shows the void caused by the loss of the suppurative contents of the abscess and the limiting band of leukocytes.

is sometimes referred to as *acute suppurative pulpitis* (Fig. 8–4).

The pulp, especially in the later stages of pulpitis following carious invasion, contains large numbers of bacteria. These microorganisms are usually a mixed population and consist essentially of those found normally in the oral cavity.

Treatment and Prognosis. There is no successful treatment of an acute pulpitis involving most of the pulp that is capable of preserving the pulp. Once this degree of pulpitis occurs, the damage is irreparable. Occasionally, acute pulpitis—especially with an open cavity—may become quiescent and enter a chronic state. This is unusual, however, and appears to occur most frequently in persons who have a high tissue resistance or in cases of infection with microorganisms of low virulence.

In very early cases of acute pulpitis involving only a limited area of tissue, there is some evidence to indicate that pulpotomy (removal of the coronal pulp) and placing a bland material that favors calcification, such as calcium hydroxide, over the entrance to the root canals may result in survival of the tooth. This technique is also used in cases of mechanical pulp exposures without obvious infection (Fig. 8–5).

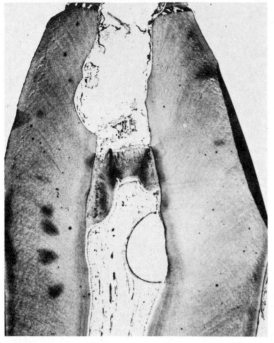

Figure 8–5. *Healing of a pulp exposure by a dentinal bridge.*

Calcium hydroxide placed over the mechanically exposed pulp stimulated the production of a dentinal bridge over the pulp. The circumscribed space in the pulp is an artefact and not a pulp abscess.

Teeth involved with acute pulpitis may be treated by filling the root canals with an inert material, provided the pulp chamber and root canals can be sterilized. When the pulp is initially opened to evacuate any pus, a drop of yellowish fluid frequently escapes, and if the operation is performed without anesthesia, the patient is afforded immediate relief from pain. A considerable number of techniques are available for successful root canal therapy.

Chronic Pulpitis

Chronic pulpitis may arise on occasion through quiescence of a previous acute pulpitis, but more frequently it occurs as the chronic type of disease from the onset. As in most chronic inflammatory conditions, the signs and symptoms are considerably milder than those in the acute form of the disease.

This form of pulpitis has also been classified into both an open and a closed form, but, as in acute pulpitis, the classification is artificial. Minor differences do exist in the clinical and histologic features, but these are readily explained on a purely physical basis. A special form of chronic pulpitis is recognized that presents such characteristic features that its separation is deemed warranted. This is known as *chronic hyperplastic pulpitis* and will be described separately.

Clinical Features. Pain is not a prominent feature of chronic pulpitis, although sometimes the patient complains of a mild, dull ache, which is more often intermittent than continuous. The reaction to thermal change is dramatically reduced in comparison to that in acute pulpitis. Because of the degeneration of nerve tissue in the affected pulp, the threshold for stimulation by the electric pulp vitality tester is often increased, in contrast to cases of acute pulpitis, in which it is usually decreased.

The general features of chronic pulpitis are not distinctive, and serious involvement of the pulp may be present in the absence of significant symptoms. Even in cases of chronic pulpitis with wide-open carious lesions and with exposure of the pulp to the oral environment, there is relatively little pain. The exposed pulp tissue may be manipulated by a small instrument, but though bleeding may occur, pain is often absent. As Selzer and his associates have emphasized, pulps may become totally necrotic without pain.

Histologic Features. Chronic pulpitis is characterized by infiltration of the pulp tissue by varying numbers of mononuclear cells, chiefly lymphocytes and plasma cells (Fig. 8–6). Capillaries are usually prominent; fibroblastic activity is evident; and collagen fibers are seen, often gathered in bundles.

There is sometimes an attempt by the pulp to wall off the infection through deposition of collagen about the inflamed area. The tissue reaction may resemble the formation of granulation tissue. When this occurs on the surface of the pulp tissue in a wide-open exposure, the term *ulcerative pulpitis* has been applied. With bacterial stains, microorganisms may be found in the pulp tissue, especially in the area of a carious exposure. In some cases the pulpal reaction vacillates between an acute and a chronic phase. This holds true not only for diffuse inflammation but also for that form of pulp disease characterized by pulp abscess formation. Thus a pulp abscess may become quiescent and be surrounded by a fibrous connective tissue wall.

In nearly all cases the pulp is eventually involved in its entirety by the chronic inflammatory process, although this may take a long time and present few clinical symptoms.

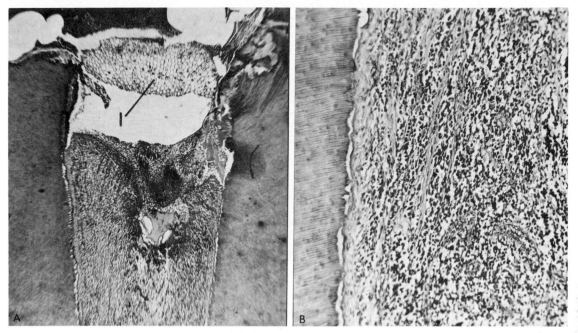

Figure 8–6. *Chronic pulpitis.*

A, The pulp of this tooth shows diffuse involvement by chronic inflammatory cells. The entrance to the pulp chamber is wide open (open pulpitis), but contains food debris *(1). B,* In the high-power photomicrograph there is seen diffuse infiltration of lymphocytes and plasma cells with fibrosis and loss of the odontoblastic layer.

Treatment and Prognosis. The treatment of chronic pulpitis does not differ dramatically from that of acute pulpitis. The integrity of the pulp tissue is lost sooner or later, necessitating either root canal therapy or extraction of the tooth.

Chronic Hyperplastic Pulpitis

(Pulp Polyp)

This form of chronic pulp disease is uncommon and occurs either as a chronic lesion from the onset or as a chronic stage of a previously acute pulpitis.

Clinical Features. Chronic hyperplastic pulpitis is essentially an excessive, exuberant proliferation of chronically inflamed dental pulp tissue. It occurs almost exclusively in children and young adults and involves teeth with large, open carious lesions. A pulp so affected appears as a pinkish-red globule of tissue protruding from the pulp chamber and often filling the entire cavity (Fig. 8–7). Because the hyperplastic tissue contains few nerves, it is relatively insensitive to manipulation. However, Southam and Hodson have found that sometimes innervation of polyps may be quite rich and have

stated that the number of nerve fibers in pulp polyps cannot be presumed to be directly related to the sensory acuity found on clinical examination. They have even noted innervation of the epithelium in epithelized polyps in some instances. The lesion may or may not bleed readily, depending upon the degree of vascularity of the tissue.

The teeth most commonly involved by this phenomenon are the deciduous molars and the first permanent molars. These have an excellent blood supply because of the large root opening, and this, coupled with the high tissue resistance and reactivity in young persons, accounts for the unusual proliferative property of the pulp tissue. On occasion the gingival tissue adjacent to a broken-down, carious tooth may proliferate into the carious lesion and superficially resemble an example of hyperplastic pulpitis. In such cases the distinction can be made by careful examination of the tissue mass to determine whether the connection is with pulp or gingiva.

Histologic Features. The hyperplastic tissue is basically granulation tissue made up of delicate connective tissue fibers interspersed with variable numbers of small capillaries (Fig. 8–7). Inflammatory cell infiltration, chiefly lymphocytes and plasma cells, sometimes admixed with

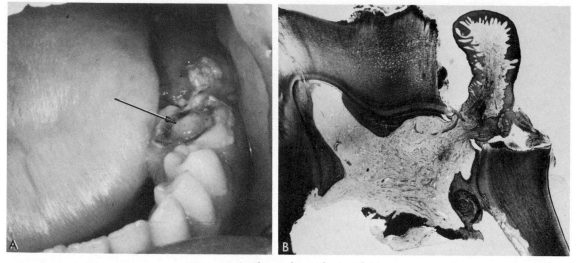

Figure 8–7. *Chronic hyperplastic pulpitis.*
A, There is a mass of tissue protruding from the pulp chamber into the carious lesion. *B,* In the photomicrograph this is seen to be continuous with the pulp and covered by stratified squamous epithelium.

polymorphonuclear leukocytes, is common. In some instances fibroblast and endothelial cell proliferation is prominent.

This granulation tissue commonly becomes epithelized as a result of implantation of epithelial cells on its surface. The epithelium is stratified squamous in type and closely resembles the oral mucosa, even to the extent of developing well-formed rete pegs. The grafted epithelial cells are thought to be normally desquamated cells carried to the surface of the pulp by the saliva. In some instances the buccal mucosa may rub against the hyperplastic tissue mass, and epithelial cells become transplanted directly. Southam and Hodson have reported that polyps from deciduous teeth were epithelized far more frequently (82 per cent of 56 polyps) than those of permanent teeth (44 per cent of 77 polyps).

It should be appreciated that the tissue reaction here is an inflammatory hyperplasia and does not differ from inflammatory hyperplasia occurring elsewhere in the oral cavity as well as in other parts of the body.

Treatment and Prognosis. Chronic hyperplastic pulpitis may persist as such for many months or even several days. The condition is not reversible and may be treated by extraction of the tooth or by pulp extirpation.

Gangrenous Necrosis of Pulp

Untreated pulpitis, either acute or chronic, will ultimately result in complete necrosis of the pulp tissue. Since this is generally associated with bacterial infection, the term *pulp gangrene* has sometimes been applied to this condition, gangrene being defined as necrosis of tissue due to ischemia with superimposed bacterial infection. Although many attempts have been made to associate pulp gangrene with a specific organism, obviously it may be caused by any saprophytic organism that invades the tissue.

Pulp gangrene should not be considered a specific form of pulp disease but simply the most complete end result of pulpitis in which there is total necrosis of tissue.

A type of gangrene known as *dry gangrene* sometimes occurs when the pulp dies for some unexplained reason. The nonvital pulp maintains its general histologic characteristics, being nonpurulent. This condition may be due to some traumatic injury or infarct.

DISEASES OF THE PERIAPICAL TISSUES

Once infection has become established in the dental pulp, spread of the process can be in only one direction—through the root canals and into the periapical region. Here a number of different tissue reactions may occur, depending upon a variety of circumstances.

It is important to realize that these periapical lesions do not represent individual and distinct entities, but rather that there is a subtle transformation from one type of lesion into another type in most cases. Furthermore, it should be appreciated that a certain degree of reversibility is possible in some lesions. The interrelations between the types of periapical infection must be clearly understood, and the schematic diagram shown in Figure 8–8 will aid in clarification of this.

PERIAPICAL GRANULOMA

(Apical Periodontitis)

The periapical granuloma is one of the most common of all sequelae of pulpitis. It is essentially a localized mass of chronic granulation tissue formed in response to the infection (Fig. 8–9).

It should be pointed out here that the spread of pulp infection is usually, but not always, in a periapical direction. The presence of lateral or accessory root canals opening on the lateral surface of the root at any level is a well-recognized anatomic deviation along which the infection may spread. This would give rise to a "lateral" granuloma or related inflammatory lesion. The significance of this occurrence, particularly in endodontic therapy, has been discussed by Nicholls.

Clinical Features. The first evidence that infection has spread beyond the confines of the tooth pulp may be a noticeable sensitivity of the involved tooth to percussion, or mild pain occasioned when biting or chewing on solid food. In some cases the tooth feels slightly elongated in its socket and may actually be so. The sensitivity is due to hyperemia, edema,

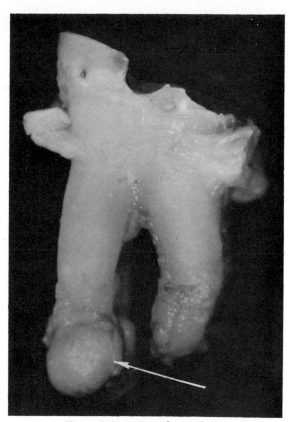

Figure 8–9. *Periapical granuloma.*
The granuloma often remains attached to the root when the tooth is extracted.

and inflammation of the apical periodontal ligament.

The early or even the fully developed chronic periapical granuloma seldom presents any more severe clinical features than those just described. Actually, many cases are entirely asymptomatic. There is usually no perforation of overlying bone and oral mucosa with the formation of a fistulous tract unless the lesion undergoes an acute exacerbation.

Roentgenographic Features. The earliest periapical change in the periodontal ligament appears as a thickening of the ligament at the root apex (Fig. 8–10). As proliferation of granulation tissue and concomitant resorption of bone continue, the periapical granuloma appears as a radiolucent area of variable size seemingly attached to the root apex (Fig. 8–11). In some cases this radiolucency is a well-circumscribed lesion, definitely demarcated from the surrounding bone. In these instances a thin radiopaque line or zone of sclerotic bone may sometimes be seen outlining the lesion. This indicates that the periapical lesion is a slowly progressive one of long standing that has probably not undergone an acute exacerbation.

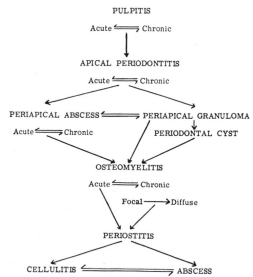

Figure 8–8. *Interrelationships of periapical infection.*

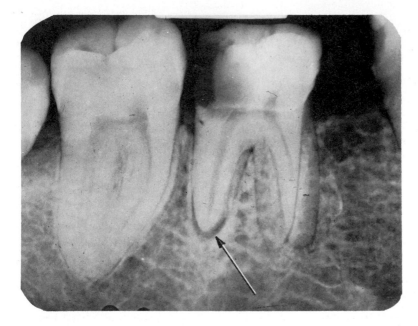

Figure 8–10. *Early apical periodontitis.*
There is roentgenographic evidence of thickening of the apical periodontal membrane as a result of the large carious lesion involving the dental pulp.

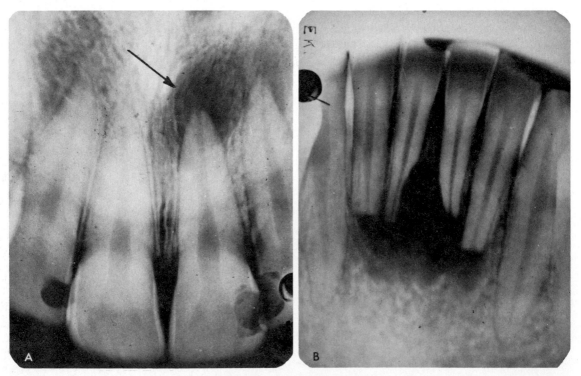

Figure 8–11. *Periapical granuloma.*
The periapical radiolucencies signify destruction of bone and replacement by granulation tissue. The maxillary central incisor (A) has a carious lesion of the distal surface that involves the pulp. The mandibular incisors (B) have sustained traumatic injury with loss of pulp vitality and subsequent formation of diffuse periapical granulomata.

The periphery of granulomas in other instances appears on the roentgenogram as a diffuse blending of the radiolucent area with the surrounding bone. This difference in roentgenographic appearance cannot be used to distinguish between different forms of periapical disease. Although the diffuse radiolucency might suggest a more acute phase of disease or a more rapidly expanding lesion, this is not necessarily the case. In addition, some degree of root resorption is occasionally observed.

Histologic Features. The periapical granuloma that arises as a chronic process from the onset and does not pass through an acute phase begins as a hyperemia and edema of the periodontal ligament with infiltration of chronic inflammatory cells. The inflammation and locally increased vascularity of the tissue are associated with resorption of the supporting bone adjacent to this area. Occasionally, microscopic or even macroscopic resorption of the root apex occurs, but this is not usually an early finding. As the bone is resorbed, there is proliferation of both fibroblasts and endothelial cells and the formation of more tiny vascular channels as well as numerous delicate connective tissue fibrils

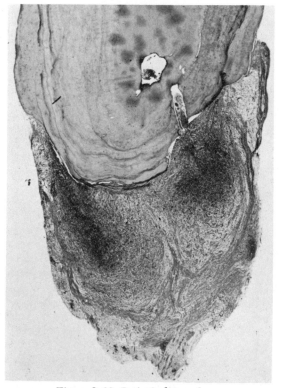

Figure 8–12. *Periapical granuloma.*
The mass attached to the root is composed of granulation tissue.

(Figs. 8–12, 8–13). The new capillaries are usually lined by swollen endothelial cells. It is a relatively homogeneous lesion composed predominantly of macrophages, lymphocytes, and plasma cells, thus qualifying as an immune-type granuloma. As Athanassiades and Spears and Page and his associates have pointed out, immune granulomas have more lymphocytes and plasma cells than nonimmune granulomas, which are relatively pure collections of macrophages and giant cells with only a rare plasma cell.

Because innumerable histopathologic studies have failed to provide definitive data concerning the numeric distribution of inflammatory and reactive cellular elements in periapical granulomas, Stern and his associates undertook a quantitative analysis of some 25 periapical granulomas and 8 periapical cysts. In addition, they established both the proportions of immunoglobulin-positive B lymphocytes and plasma cells according to immunoglobulin class and the immunoglobulin distribution in periapical granulomas and cysts. They found that macrophages constituted 24 per cent, lymphocytes 16 per cent, plasma cells 7 per cent, neutrophils 4 per cent, fibroblasts 40 per cent, vascular elements 6 per cent, and epithelial cells 5 per cent of all lesional cells. The inflammatory cells, which made up approximately 52 per cent of the formed elements in the lesions, consisted of macrophages (46 per cent), lymphocytes (32 per cent), plasma cells (13 per cent), and neutrophils (8 per cent). The vast majority of the small lymphocytes (81 per cent) were not associated with immunoglobulin production and were designated non-B lymphocytes. Nineteen per cent of the lymphocytes contained immunoglobulins, of which the majority (74 per cent) produced IgG. IgA was found in 20 per cent of the lymphocytes, while IgE and IgM were found in 4 per cent and 2 per cent, respectively. Many of the plasma cells contained Russell bodies, some of which were subsequently extruded and could be found extracellularly in the granulomatous tissue, either singly or in discrete collections. The non-B lymphocytes are probably the T cells of the cellular arm of the immune system, thus making the lesion an expression of delayed type hypersensitivity. There is ample evidence to indicate that T-cell activity could account for much of the bone and tooth resorption through the production of osteoclast activating factor (OAF). Since T cells also produce various cytotoxic lymphokines, collagenase, and other enzymes and destructive

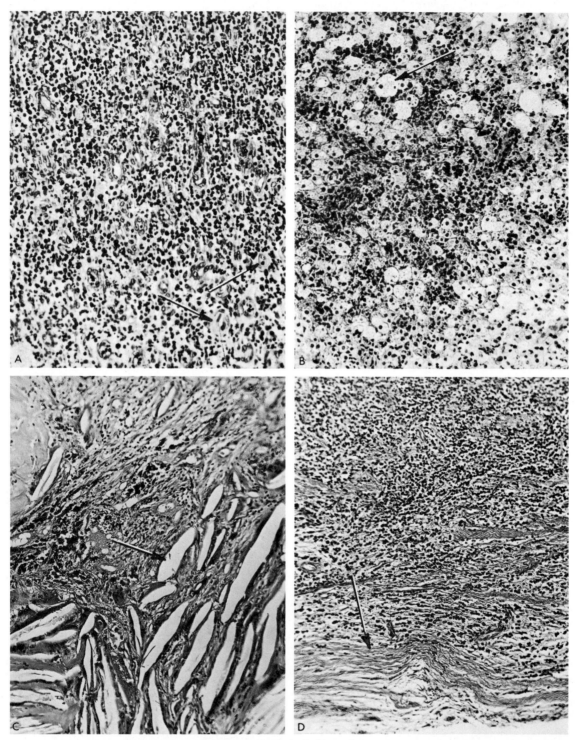

Figure 8–13. *Periapical granuloma.*

The photomicrographs represent various histologic features, although all such features need not be present in a single granuloma. The typical periapical granuloma shows the delicate fibrillar stroma with intense lymphocytic and plasma cell infiltration and sometimes polymorphonuclear leukocytes as well as many small capillaries *(A)*, collections of macrophages that are often filled with lipoid material *(B)*, and cholesterol slits in the tissue *(C)*. The typical granuloma is usually surrounded by a connective tissue "capsule" *(D)*.

lymphokines, they may be responsible for much of the destructive potential of the periapical lesion. On the other hand, the presence of antibody-producing lymphocytes and plasma cells in periapical granulomas is very important because antibodies are known to be modulators of disease activity. In addition, their specificity may provide clues to the antigens and thus to the causes of periapical granulomas and cysts.

Macrophages and other mononuclear phagocytes are the hallmarks of granulomatous inflammation, a specific form of chronic inflammation. Compared with granulomatous inflammation, banal chronic inflammation lacks organization. Rather it is a diffuse heterogeneous collection of cells, usually dominated by mononuclear cells other than macrophages, as Adams has noted. The cause of differentiation from solid to cystic periapical lesions cannot be deduced from alterations in the inflammatory cell populations of granulomas and cysts. There were no differences in inflammatory cell composition, immunoglobulin production, or immunoglobulin distribution between granulomas and cysts.

In some granulomas, large numbers of phagocytes will ingest lipid material and become collected in groups, forming sheets of so-called foam cells (Fig. 8–13, B). Abundant mast cells may be found also. Cholesterol crystals also may accumulate in the tissue and appear microscopically as clear needle-like spaces or clefts owing to the dissolving of the contained cholesterol by the agents used in the preparation of the tissues for histologic examination (Fig. 8–13, C). These are most common in lesions in which there has been epithelial proliferation and actual cyst formation and are almost invariably associated with multinucleated giant cells of the foreign body type.

Connective tissue activity is usually most prominent on the periphery of the granuloma, and the bundles of collagen become condensed there, apparently as a result of the slow expansion of the soft-tissue mass, to form a continuous capsule separating the granulation tissue from the bone (Fig. 8–13, D).

One other important feature noted in the chronic periapical granuloma is the presence of epithelium. This epithelium originates in nearly all cases from the epithelial rests of Malassez, although in some instances it arises from (1) respiratory epithelium of the maxillary sinus in cases in which the periapical lesion perforated the sinus wall, (2) oral epithelium growing in through a fistulous tract, or (3) oral epithelium proliferating apically from a periodontal pocket,

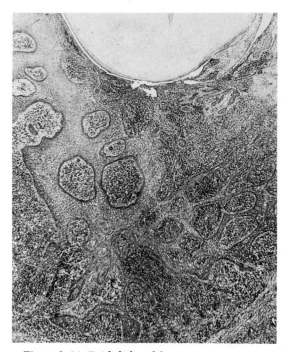

Figure 8–14. *Epithelial proliferation in a periapical granuloma attached to the tooth root.*
Sheets of proliferating epithelial cells are derived from the epithelial rests of Malassez.

or bifurcation or trifurcation involvement by periodontal disease also with apical proliferation. In early periapical granulomas the epithelium is confined to the immediate vicinity of the periodontal ligament. Eventually, however, the proliferation of this epithelium, stimulated by the inflammatory process, becomes extensive, and sheets of stratified squamous epithelial cells as well as anastomosing cords are common (Fig. 8–14). It is this epithelium that gives rise to the apical periodontal cyst, and a sharp dividing line between granuloma and cyst cannot always be drawn because of the tendency for degeneration of individual epithelial cells that could be considered precystic (Fig. 8–15).

That epithelium is uniformly present in all periapical granulomas has been substantiated by numerous workers. Its demonstration is dependent in many cases upon serial section of the tissue specimens, but this procedure will reveal its presence. Thus every periapical granuloma may potentially form a periodontal cyst if it is left undisturbed and if the inflammatory reaction persists to stimulate the epithelium.

One additional interesting finding in occasional periapical granulomas is a condition described by Dunlap and Barker as *giant-cell*

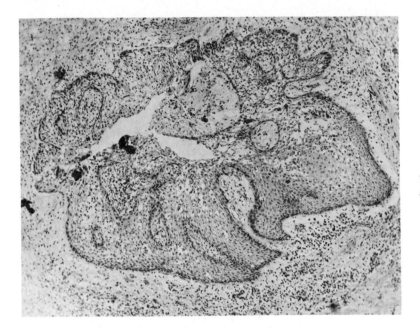

Figure 8–15. *Precystic epithelial proliferation in a periapical granuloma.*
A lumen has just formed and may be considered the beginning of an apical periodontal cyst.

hyalin angiopathy. This consists of inflammatory cell infiltration, collections of foreign body type giant cells, and the presence of ringlike structures composed of an eosinophilic material resembling hyalinized collagen. There may also be seen fragments of foreign material, sometimes resembling vegetable matter such as legumes, which suggested the use of the term "pulse granuloma" for this lesion by King and by Mincer and his co-workers. Dunlap and Barker believed that the earliest change was an acute vasculitis with subsequent thickening and hyalinization of vessel walls. This tissue finding is not confined to periapical granulomas but has also been reported in granulomas in edentulous jaws, in a nasopalatine duct cyst, and in chronic periostitis. This has been studied by both electron microscopy and immunoperoxidase procedure by Chen and his colleagues, who concluded that the hyaline bodies are probably endogenous in origin. The true nature of this lesion still remains uncertain but is of little apparent clinical significance.

Bacteriologic Features. There has been surprisingly little sound scientific study of the periapical tissues of infected teeth reported in the dental literature. One of the factors that has made this a difficult area of investigation is the inability of the dentist to extract a tooth without bacteriologically contaminating the periapical area or the granuloma. The majority of studies have been based upon bacteriologic cultures taken after extraction of the tooth. Pre-extraction cultures have been made in a few instances through the root canal or the alveolar plate, and these have been relatively free of actual contamination. The microorganisms that have been isolated by such techniques, e.g., in the studies of Burket, were those generally found in the oral cavity, such as *Streptococcus viridans, Str. hemolyticus,* nonhemolytic streptococci, *Staphylococcus aureus, Staph. albus, Escherichia coli,* and pneumococci (Table 8–1).

The evidence available indicates that many but certainly not all teeth with infected pulps and periapical lesions yield positive bacteriologic cultures from these periapical areas. Seldom can microorganisms actually be demonstrated intracellularly in the periapical granuloma. Some investigators have even suggested that the dental granuloma is usually a sterile lesion. It has not been possible to associate particular types of microorganisms with specific periapical lesions, based upon either clinical or histologic evaluation.

Treatment and Prognosis. The treatment of the periapical granuloma consists in extraction of the involved teeth or, under certain conditions, root canal therapy with or without subsequent apicoectomy. If left untreated, the periapical granuloma may ultimately undergo transformation into an apical periodontal cyst through proliferation of the epithelial rests in the area.

Table 8–1. Occurrence of Microorganisms of 206 Periapical Areas

	PURE AND MIXED CULTURES		PURE CULTURES	
	(NO.)	(%)	(NO.)	(%)
Streptococcus viridans	127	61.2	58	28.0
Streptococcus hemolyticus	21	10.2	4	2.0
Nonhemolytic streptococcus	35	17.0	3	1.4
Staphylococcus aureus	66	32.0	31	15.0
Staphylococcus albus	4	2.0	2	1.0
Bacillus coli	9	4.4	8	3.9
Pneumococcus	6	2.9	4	2.0
Gram-negative coccus	9	4.4		
Gram-positive bacillus	5	2.4	3	1.4
Pseudomonas pyocyanea	4	2.0	4	2.0
Gram-negative bacillus	4	2.0	1	0.5
Bacillus typhosus	2	1.0	2	1.0
Diphtheroids	1	0.5	1	0.5
Hemophilus influenzae	1	0.5	1	0.5
Gram-positive coccus	1	0.5		
Micrococcus tetragenus	1	0.5	1	0.5

From L. W. Burket: Recent studies relating to periapical infection, including data obtained from human necropsy studies. J. Am. Dent. Assoc., 25:260, 1938.

APICAL PERIODONTAL CYST

(Radicular Cyst; Periapical Cyst; Root End Cyst)

The apical periodontal cyst is a common but not inevitable sequela of the periapical granuloma originating as a result of bacterial infection and necrosis of the dental pulp, nearly always following carious involvement of the tooth. It is a true cyst, since the lesion consists of a pathologic cavity that is lined by epithelium and is often fluid-filled (Fig. 8–16). The epithelial lining is derived from the epithelial rests of Malassez, which proliferate as a result of the in-

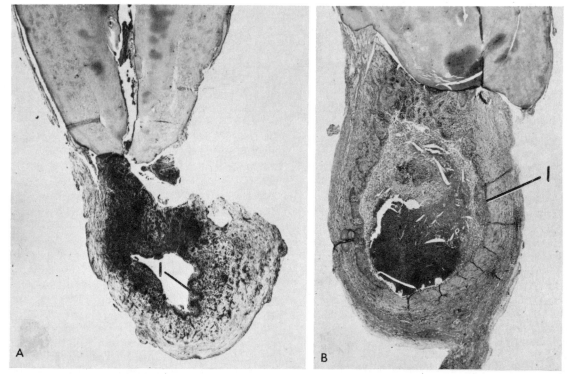

Figure 8–16. *Apical periodontal cyst.*
This may be a small sac *(A)* or a large sac *(B)* lined by epithelium *(1)* attached to the root apex.

flammatory stimulus in a pre-existing granuloma. As pointed out in the section on the periapical granuloma, the epithelium may be derived in some cases from (1) respiratory epithelium of the maxillary sinus when the periapical lesion communicates with the sinus wall, (2) oral epithelium from a fistulous tract, or (3) oral epithelium proliferating apically from a periodontal pocket.

Pathogenesis. This type of periodontal cyst exhibits a lumen that is almost invariably lined by stratified squamous epithelium, while the wall is made up of condensed connective tissue. Although the stimulus for the proliferation of epithelium in the periodontal cyst is recognized to be the inflammation in the periapical granuloma, the reason that all such granulomas do not eventually develop into cysts is not known. This is particularly puzzling, since rests of Malassez are universally present in the periodontal membrane areas of all teeth. It might be that if all periapical granulomas persisted for a sufficiently long time, they would eventuate in cysts.

The actual mode of development of the apical periodontal cyst is an interesting phenomenon. The initial reaction leading to cyst formation is a proliferation of the epithelial rests in the periapical area involved by the granuloma. This epithelial proliferation follows an irregular pattern of growth and occasionally presents a frightening picture because of the pseudo-invasiveness and inflammatory-altered appearance of the cells (Fig. 8–14). As this proliferation continues with the epithelial mass increasing in size by division of the cells on the periphery, corresponding to the basal layer of the surface epithelium, the cells in the central portion of the mass become separated further and further from their source of nutrition, the capillaries and tissue fluid of the connective tissue. As these central cells fail to obtain sufficient nutrients, they eventually degenerate, become necrotic, and liquefy (Fig. 8–15). This creates an epithelium-lined cavity filled with fluid, the apical periodontal cyst.

It is conceivable also that a cyst may form through proliferation of epithelium to line a pre-existing cavity formed through focal necrosis and degeneration of connective tissue in a periapical granuloma. But the finding of epithelium or epithelial proliferation near an area of necrosis is not common, so that the formation of a cyst in this manner is presumably uncommon.

Clinical Features. The majority of cases of apical periodontal cysts are asymptomatic and present no clinical evidence of their presence. The tooth is seldom painful or even sensitive to percussion. This type of cyst is only infrequently of such a size that it destroys much bone, and even more rarely does it produce expansion of the cortical plates.

The apical periodontal cyst is a lesion that represents a chronic inflammatory process and develops only over a prolonged period of time. In some cases such a cyst of long standing may undergo an acute exacerbation of the inflammatory process and develop rapidly into an abscess that may then proceed to a cellulitis or form a draining fistula. The cause of such a sudden flareup is not known, but it may be a result of loss of local or generalized tissue resistance.

Roentgenographic Features. The roentgenographic appearance of the apical periodontal cyst is identical in most cases with that of the periapical granuloma. Since the lesion is a chronic progressive one developing in a pre-existing granuloma, the cyst may be of greater size than the granuloma by virtue of its longer duration, but this is not invariably the case (Fig. 8–17).

Priebe and his co-workers showed that it is impossible to distinguish between a periapical granuloma and a cyst by roentgenographic means alone. These workers reported that the oral surgeon and radiologist were able to diagnose correctly only 13 per cent of a group of 55 cases of periodontal cysts by means of roentgenograms alone. Of the group of 46 periapical granulomas and abscesses, 59 per cent were correctly diagnosed. The actual diagnoses were established by histologic examination of the tissue after its removal (Table 8–2). Occasionally the apical periodontal cyst exhibits a thin, radiopaque line around the periphery of the radiolucent area, and this indicates a reaction of the bone to the slowly expanding mass. The granuloma also presents such a phenomenon in many instances.

This study of Priebe and his associates indicates the fallacy of attempting to distinguish between the granuloma and the cyst, although such a distinction may have important endodontic implications. Thus periapical radiolucent areas will fill in with bone, apparently healing, after root canal therapy of some teeth. In other instances, even after clinically identical treatment, healing does not take place. The latter cases may represent examples of periodontal cysts, which would, of course, heal slowly if at all after endodontic therapy.

Histologic Features. The epithelium lining

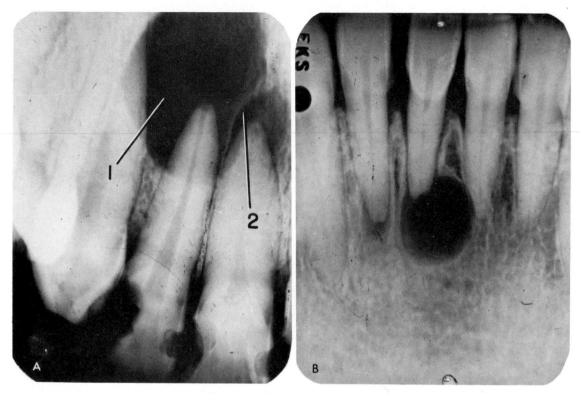

Figure 8–17. *Apical periodontal cyst.*

A, This cyst *(1)* developed in a pre-existing periapical granuloma such as that involving the apex of the maxillary central incisor *(2)*. The two conditions cannot be differentiated by the roentgenogram—only histologically. *B,* This cyst developed after traumatic injury to the mandibular incisors with loss of pulp vitality. There is mild apical root resorption associated with the development of the periapical lesion.

Table 8–2. Interpretation of Cysts and Granulomas from the Roentgenogram

	CYSTS		ABSCESS-GRANULOMAS	
	(NO.)	(%)	(NO.)	(%)
Total	55	54.5	46	45.5
Correct interpretations*	7	12.7	27	58.7
Incorrect interpretations*	29	52.7	1	2.2
Disputed interpretations	19	34.6	18	39.1

From W. A. Priebe, J. P. Lazansky and A. H. Wuehrmann: The value of the roentgenographic film in the differential diagnosis of periapical lesions. Oral Surg., 7:979, 1954.

*By all observers on basis of microscopic evidence.

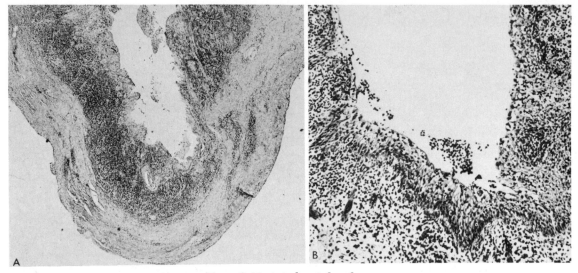

Figure 8–18. *Apical periodontal cyst.*
The epithelium lining the cavity is relatively thin and distorted by the inflammation but is recognizable as stratified squamous type.

the apical periodontal cyst is usually stratified squamous in type (Fig. 8–18). The only exception to this is in those rare cases of periapical lesions of maxillary teeth that involve the maxillary sinus. In occasional instances the cyst may then be lined with a pseudo-stratified ciliated columnar or respiratory type of epithelium.

The usual squamous epithelium seldom exhibits keratin formation. This lining epithelium varies remarkably in thickness from case to case. It may be only a few cells thick, or exceedingly thick with a great deal of proliferation into the adjacent connective tissue. Actual rete peg for-

mation sometimes occurs. The epithelial lining many times is discontinuous, frequently being missing over areas of intense inflammation. Despite the presence of long-standing inflammation, alterations in individual epithelial cells, such as dyskeratosis, are uncommon (Fig. 8–19). Shear has reported that there is no apparent relationship between the degree of inflammation present, either in the connective tissue wall or within the epithelium itself, and the thickness of the epithelial lining of the cyst.

In rare instances, carcinoma has been reported developing from the lining epithelium

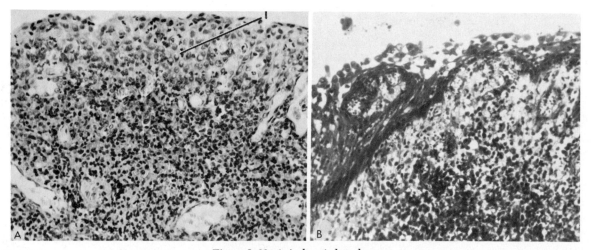

Figure 8–19. *Apical periodontal cyst.*
The epithelium (*1*) sometimes shows considerable reaction to the underlying inflammation.

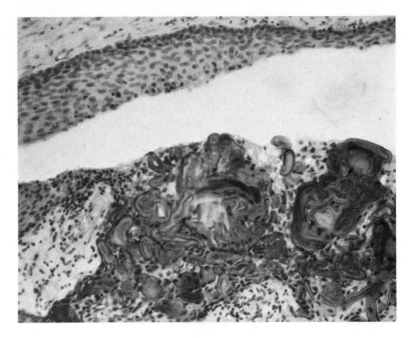

Figure 8–20. *Apical periodontal cyst with numerous hyaline (Rushton) bodies.*

of odontogenic cysts, including the apical periodontal cyst. These have been reviewed by Gardner.

An interesting and peculiar structure, originally described by Rushton and subsequently reported by Molyneux, Medak and Weinmann, and Shear, is the hyaline body or Rushton body, often found in great numbers in the epithelium of apical periodontal or residual cysts. These hyaline bodies are tiny linear or arc-shaped bodies, generally associated with the lining epithelium, that appear amorphous in structure, eosinophilic in reaction, and brittle in nature, since they evidence fracture in some cases (Fig. 8–20). Their frequency of occurrence in cyst linings ranges between 2.6 and 9.5 per cent of cysts, according to a review by Allison. The etiology, pathogenesis, and significance of these structures are unknown. However, Sedano and Gorlin have reported a marked morphologic and histochemical similarity between these bodies and red blood cells, suggesting that they arise from thrombus formation in small capillaries, being formed chiefly from these red blood cells—a rouleau phenomenon. Nevertheless, even by electron microscopic study of these hyaline bodies, Allison was unable to shed any further light on their etiology.

The connective tissue that makes up the wall of the apical periodontal cyst is composed of parallel bundles of collagen fibers that often appear compressed. Variable numbers of fibroblasts and small blood vessels are also present.

A characteristic feature is the almost universal occurrence of an inflammatory infiltrate in the connective tissue immediately adjacent to the epithelium. This infiltrate varies in its composition but generally is made up of lymphocytes and plasma cells, with some admixed polymorphonuclear leukocytes, depending partially upon the intensity of the infection. In some lesions, collections of cholesterol slits with associated multinucleated giant cells are found in the wall of the lesion. This mass of cholesterol frequently erodes through the lining epithelium and is extruded into the cyst lumen. The source of this cholesterol is not known, although there are numerous theories as reviewed by Shear. It appears that local tissue damage is a prerequisite for the cholesterol accumulation. In other instances, collections of lipid-filled macrophages or even macrophages containing hemosiderin are present.

The lumen of the cyst usually contains a fluid with a low concentration of protein that stains palely eosinophilic. Occasionally the lumen may contain a great deal of cholesterol, and in rare instances limited amounts of keratin are present. Blood is a rare finding except when associated with the surgical procedure involved in removing the cyst. Whitten has reported that cytologic smears on aspirated material from cysts and cystlike lesions of the jaws, including the apical periodontal cyst, frequently permit a provisional diagnosis of the nature of the lesion.

The apical periodontal cyst is histologically

identical with the periapical granuloma, from which it is actually derived, except for the presence of the epithelium-lined lumen.

Treatment and Prognosis. The treatment of this type of cyst is similar to that of the periapical granuloma. The involved tooth may be removed and the periapical tissue carefully curetted. Under some conditions root canal therapy may be carried out with apicoectomy of the cystic lesion.

The cyst does not recur if surgical removal is thorough. If the cystic sac is badly fragmented, leaving epithelial remnants, or if a periapical granuloma is incompletely removed with epithelial rests remaining, a *residual cyst* may develop in this area months or even years later.

The apical periodontal cyst does not seem to have the marked propensity for ameloblastomatous transformation that is present in the dentigerous cyst. As indicated earlier, epidermoid carcinoma may develop from the lining epithelium, but this is rare.

If untreated, the periodontal cyst slowly increases in size at the expense of the surrounding bone. The bone undergoes resorption, but seldom is there a remarkable compensating expansion of the cortical plates, as is frequently seen in the case of the dentigerous cyst.

PERIAPICAL ABSCESS

(Dento-alveolar Abscess; Alveolar Abscess)

The periapical abscess is an acute or chronic suppurative process of the dental periapical region. It usually arises as a result of infection following carious involvement of the tooth and pulp infection, but it does occur also after traumatic injury to the teeth, resulting in necrosis of the pulp, and in cases of irritation of the periapical tissues either by mechanical manipulation or by the application of chemicals in endodontic procedures.

This abscess may develop directly as an acute apical periodontitis following an acute pulpitis, but more commonly it originates in an area of chronic infection, the periapical granuloma.

Clinical Features. The acute periapical abscess presents the features of an acute inflammation of the apical periodontium. The tooth is extremely painful and is slightly extruded from its socket. As long as this abscess is confined to the immediate periapical region, there are seldom severe systemic manifestations, although regional lymphadenitis and fever may be pres-

ent. However, rapid extension to adjacent bone marrow spaces frequently occurs, producing an actual osteomyelitis, but this is sometimes still considered clinically to be a dento-alveolar abscess. In such cases the clinical features may be severe and serious.

The chronic periapical abscess generally presents no clinical features, since it is essentially a mild, well-circumscribed area of suppuration that shows little tendency to spread from the local area (Fig. 8–21).

Roentgenographic Features. The acute periapical abscess is such a rapidly progressive lesion that, except for slight thickening of the periodontal membrane, there is usually no roentgenographic evidence of its presence. The chronic abscess, developing in a periapical granuloma, presents the radiolucent area at the apex of the tooth described previously.

Histologic Features. The area of suppuration is composed chiefly of a central area of disintegrating polymorphonuclear leukocytes surrounded by viable leukocytes and occasional lymphocytes. There is dilatation of the blood vessels in the periodontal ligament and adjacent marrow spaces of the bone. These marrow spaces also show an inflammatory cell infiltrate. The tissue around the area of suppuration contains a serous exudate.

Treatment and Prognosis. The principle of treatment of the periapical abscess is the same as for any abscess: drainage must be established. This can be accomplished by either opening the pulp chamber or extracting the tooth. Under some circumstances the tooth may be retained and root canal therapy carried out if the lesion can be sterilized.

If the periapical abscess is not treated, it may lead to serious complications through spread of the infection. These include osteomyelitis, cellulitis, and bacteremia and the ultimate formation of a fistulous tract opening on the skin or oral mucosa. Cavernous sinus thrombosis has also been reported.

OSTEOMYELITIS

Osteomyelitis, an inflammation of bone and bone marrow, may develop in the jaws as a result of odontogenic infection as well as in a variety of other situations. The disease may be either acute, subacute, or chronic and presents a different clinical course, depending upon its nature.

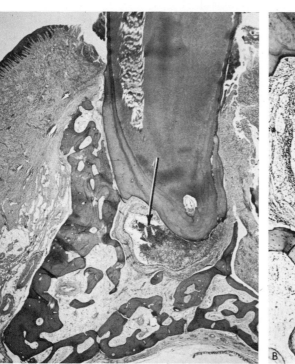

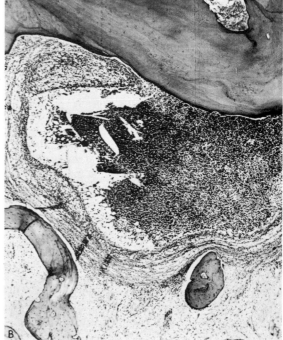

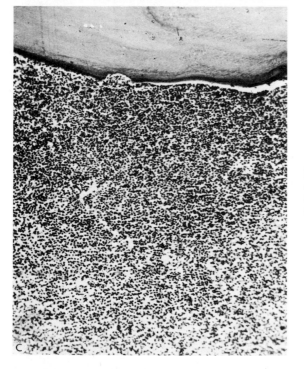

Figure 8–21. *Chronic periapical abscess.*
The periapical destruction of bone in *A* is shown in the high-power photomicrograph *(B)* to be caused by a circumscribed area of suppuration. This area of suppuration *(C)* consists entirely of inflammatory cells in various stages of disintegration.

Acute Suppurative Osteomyelitis

Acute suppurative osteomyelitis of the jaw is a serious sequela of periapical infection that often results in a diffuse spread of infection throughout the medullary spaces, with subsequent necrosis of a variable amount of bone. The clinical features of this form of osteomyelitis, which arises from a dental infection, are the same as those present after infection due to a fracture of the jaw, a gunshot wound, or even hematogenous spread. For this reason the disease and its clinical aspects will be considered a single entity.

Dental infection is the most frequent cause of acute osteomyelitis of the jaws, but osteomyelitis is not a particularly common disease. It may be a rather well-localized infection or one involving a great volume of bone. A periapical infection (usually an abscess), if it is a particularly virulent one and not walled off, may spread spontaneously throughout the bone. In other instances a chronic periapical infection such as a granuloma, or even a cyst that is walled off, may undergo an acute exacerbation, especially if the area is traumatized or surgically disturbed without establishing and maintaining drainage.

Different types of organisms may be cultured from these lesions, although the most common are *Staphylococcus aureus* and *Staph. albus*, various streptococci, or, in some instances, mixed organisms. Cases of specific infectious osteomyelitis in tuberculosis, syphilis, actinomycosis, and so forth, are considered in the discussions of these diseases.

Clinical Features. Acute or subacute suppurative osteomyelitis may involve either the maxilla or the mandible. In the maxilla the disease usually remains fairly well localized to the area of initial infection. In the mandible, bone involvement tends to be more diffuse and widespread.

The disease may occur at any age. A particular form of acute osteomyelitis in infants and young children is a well-recognized entity that is fortunately becoming extremely uncommon because of the antibiotic drugs. In some instances this osteomyelitis of infants is of hematogenous origin, but at other times it seems to be a result of local oral infection following some minor injury or abrasion. Infants so affected are seriously ill and may not survive the disease. In some cases the source of the infecting organism cannot be discovered. A series of 24 such cases of maxillary osteomyelitis in infants was reported by Cavanagh, while Nørgaard and

Pindborg reviewed the literature and discussed the dental implications of this disease.

The adult afflicted with acute suppurative osteomyelitis is usually in rather severe pain and manifests an elevation of temperature with regional lymphadenopathy. The white blood cell count is frequently elevated. The teeth in the area of involvement are loose and sore so that eating is difficult if not impossible. Paresthesia or anesthesia of the lip is a common development in cases of mandibular involvement. Until periostitis develops, there is no swelling or reddening of the skin or mucosa.

Roentgenographic Features. Acute osteomyelitis progresses rapidly and demonstrates little roentgenographic evidence of its presence until the disease has developed for at least one to two weeks. At this time diffuse lytic changes in the bone begin to appear. Individual trabeculae become fuzzy and indistinct, and radiolucent areas begin to appear (Fig. 8–22,A).

Histologic Features. The medullary spaces are filled with an inflammatory exudate that may or may not have progressed to the actual formation of pus (Fig. 8–22, B). The inflammatory cells are chiefly neutrophilic polymorphonuclear leukocytes but may show occasional lymphocytes and plasma cells. The osteoblasts bordering the bony trabeculae are generally destroyed, and depending upon the duration of the process, the trabeculae may lose their viability and begin to undergo slow resorption.

Treatment and Prognosis. The general principles of treatment demand that drainage be established and maintained and that the infection be treated with antibiotics to prevent further spread and complications.

When the intensity of the disease becomes attenuated, either spontaneously or under treatment, the bone that has lost its vitality begins to separate from the living bone. Each separated fragment of dead bone is called a *sequestrum*, and these sequestra, if small, may gradually be spontaneously exfoliated or sequestrated through the mucosa. If a large sequestrum forms, its surgical removal may be necessary, since its removal by normal processes of bone resorption would be extremely slow. Sometimes an *involucrum* forms when the sequestrum becomes surrounded by new living bone.

Unless proper treatment is instituted, acute suppurative osteomyelitis may proceed to the development of periostitis, soft-tissue abscess, or cellulitis (Fig. 8–23). Pathologic fracture occasionally occurs because of weakening of the jaw by the destructive process.

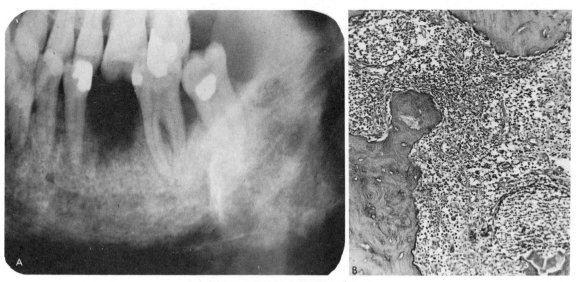

Figure 8–22. *Acute osteomyelitis*.

The diffuse destruction of bone is evident on the roentgenogram in a case of acute osteomyelitis of several weeks' duration. Note the raggedness of the inferior border of the mandible in *A*. The inflammatory process in *B* shows both a polymorphonuclear and a lymphocyte and plasma cell response. There is also irregular resorption of bone.

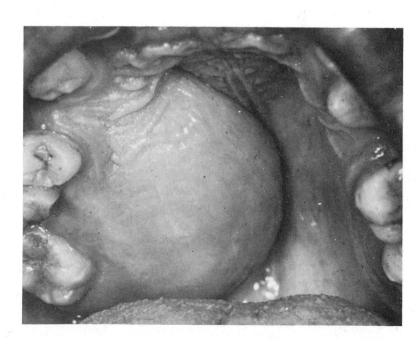

Figure 8–23. Palatal abscess following periapical infection of maxillary second bicuspid.

Chronic Suppurative Osteomyelitis

Chronic suppurative osteomyelitis may develop after the acute phase of the disease has subsided, or occasionally it may arise from a dental infection without a preceding acute stage. The clinical features are similar to those of acute osteomyelitis except that all signs and symptoms are milder. The pain is less severe; the temperature is still elevated, but only mildly; and the leukocytosis is only slightly greater than normal. The teeth may not be loose or sore, so that mastication is at least possible even though the jaw may not be perfectly comfortable.

Acute exacerbations of the chronic stage may occur periodically, and these present all features of acute suppurative osteomyelitis. The suppuration may perforate the bone and overlying skin or mucosa to form a fistulous tract and empty on the surface. This form of the disease should be treated on the same principles as its acute counterpart.

Chronic Focal Sclerosing Osteomyelitis

(Condensing Osteitis)

Chronic focal sclerosing osteomyelitis is an unusual reaction of bone to infection, occurring in instances of extremely high tissue resistance or in cases of a low-grade infection.

Clinical Features. This form of osteomyelitis arises almost exclusively in young persons before the age of 20 years. The tooth most commonly involved is the mandibular first molar, which presents a large carious lesion. There may be no signs or symptoms of the disease other than mild pain associated with an infected pulp.

Roentgenographic Features. The periapical roentgenogram demonstrates the pathognomonic, well-circumscribed radiopaque mass of sclerotic bone surrounding and extending below the apex of one or both roots (Fig. 8–24). The entire root outline is nearly always visible, an important feature in distinguishing it from the benign cementoblastoma (q.v.) that it roentgenographically may closely resemble. The border of this lesion, abutting the normal bone, may be smooth and distinct or appear to blend into the surrounding bone. In either case the radiopacity stands out in distinct contrast to the trabeculation of the normal bone.

Chronic focal sclerosing osteomyelitis is basically a reaction of bone to a mild bacterial infection entering the bone through a carious tooth in persons who have a high degree of tissue resistance and tissue reactivity. In such instances the tissues react to the infection by proliferation rather than destruction, since the infection acts as a stimulus rather than as an irritant.

Histologic Features. Histologic examination reveals only a dense mass of bony trabeculae with little interstitial marrow tissue (Fig. 8–25). If interstitial soft tissue is present, it is generally fibrotic and infiltrated only by small numbers of lymphocytes. Osteoblastic activity may have completely subsided at the time of microscopic study.

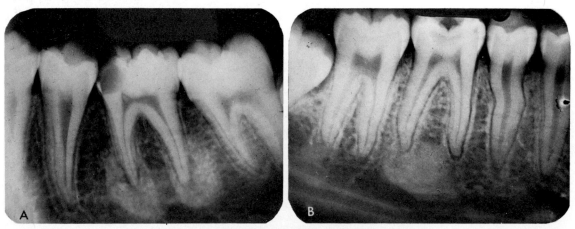

Figure 8–24. *Chronic focal sclerosing osteomyelitis.*
The apical sclerosis involves both roots of the first molar in *A*. Only the distal root of the first molar is involved in *B*, while the mesial root shows thickening of the apical periodontal membrane. Note the large carious lesions in the teeth associated with this focal sclerosing osteomyelitis.

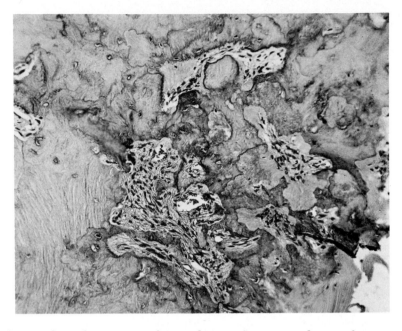

Figure 8–25. *Chronic focal sclerosing osteomyelitis.*
The lesion consists of dense, irregular bone with some intermingled fibrous tissue.

Treatment and Prognosis. The tooth with which this specific lesion is associated may be treated endodontically or extracted, since the pulp is infected and the infection has spread past the immediate periapical area. The sclerotic bone constituting the osteomyelitis is not attached to the tooth and remains after the tooth is removed. This dense area of bone is sometimes not remodeled but in many cases may be recognized on the roentgenogram even years later (Fig. 8–26). For example, Boyne has reported finding 38 cases of such focal osteosclerotic areas in a review of 927 full-mouth roentgenograms of male patients between the ages of 22 and 56 years, an incidence of 4 per cent. This incidence is somewhat higher than previously supposed.

Since the condition is actually an indication that the body has been able to deal effectively with the infection, surgical removal of the sclerotic lesions should not be attempted unless symptomatic.

Chronic Diffuse Sclerosing Osteomyelitis

Chronic diffuse sclerosing osteomyelitis is a condition analogous to the focal form of the disease and also apparently represents a prolif-

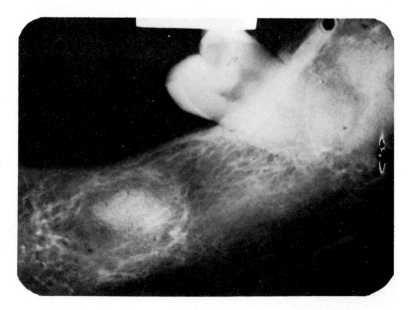

Figure 8–26. *Residual chronic focal sclerosing osteomyelitis ("bone scar").*

erative reaction of the bone to a low-grade infection. In many of these cases, the portal of entry for the infection is not through a carious lesion with subsequent pulp infection, as in chronic focal sclerosing osteomyelitis but rather through diffuse periodontal disease. The basic nature of this condition has been discussed by Shafer and by Bell.

Clinical Features. The diffuse type of sclerosing osteomyelitis, in contrast with the focal type, may occur at any age, but is most common in older persons, especially in edentulous mandibular jaws or edentulous areas. Most reported cases have occurred in blacks, especially in older females, but the disease may be seen in any race. Often the disease is of such an insidious nature that it presents no clinical indications of its presence. On occasion there is an acute exacerbation of the dormant chronic infection, and this results in mild suppuration, many times with the spontaneous formation of a fistula opening onto the mucosal surface to establish drainage. In such instances the patient may complain of vague pain and a bad taste in the mouth, but other features are usually lacking.

Roentgenographic Features. The roentgenographic appearance of chronic diffuse sclerosing osteomyelitis is, as the name suggests, that of a diffuse sclerosis of bone (Fig. 8–27). This radiopaque lesion may be extensive and is sometimes bilateral. In occasional cases there is bilateral involvement of both the maxilla and the mandible in the same patient. Because of the diffuse nature of the disease, the border between the sclerosis and the normal bone is often indistinct. The pattern may actually mimic

that of the jaws in osteitis deformans or Paget's disease of bone, which has been described as having a "cotton-wool" appearance.

Histologic Features. Microscopic study of tissue taken from the lesion shows dense, irregular trabeculae of bone, some of which are bordered by an active layer of osteoblasts (Fig. 8–28). Focal areas of osteoclastic activity are sometimes seen. The bone in some lesions shows a pronounced "mosaic" pattern, indicative of repeated periods of resorption followed by repair. The soft tissue between the individual trabeculae is fibrous and shows proliferating fibroblasts and occasional small capillaries as well as small focal collections of lymphocytes and plasma cells. Polymorphonuclear leukocytes may be present, particularly if the lesion is undergoing an acute phase. In some lesions, the inflammatory component is completely "burned out," leaving only sclerotic bone and fibrosis, but this does not contravene a diagnosis of chronic sclerosing osteomyelitis.

Treatment and Prognosis. The treatment of chronic diffuse sclerosing osteomyelitis is a difficult problem. The lesion is usually too extensive to be removed surgically, yet it frequently undergoes acute exacerbations. The most reasonable approach to this disease is a conservative one of treatment of the acute episodes by antibiotic administration, but no other intervention. Although the lesion may be slowly progressive, it is not particularly dangerous, since it is not destructive and seldom produces any complications.

If a tooth is present in one of these sclerotic areas and must be extracted, the probability of infection and protracted healing must be rec-

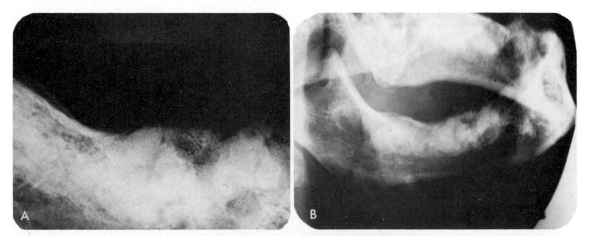

Figure 8–27. *Chronic diffuse sclerosing osteomyelitis.*
The periapical roentgenogram *(A)* shows osteosclerosis in a diffuse pattern. The extent of this sclerosis is seen on the lateral jaw film *(B)*.

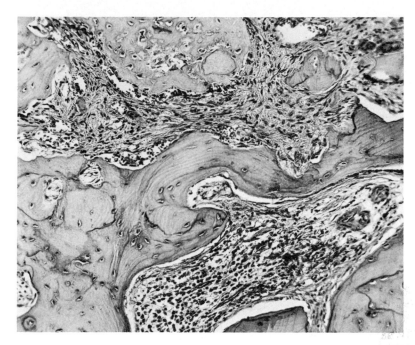

Figure 8–28. *Chronic diffuse sclerosing osteomyelitis.* The reactive nature of the lesion is evident from the presence of both formation and destruction of bone. A mild inflammatory cell infiltration is present in the fibrous stroma.

ognized. Sclerotic bone is relatively avascular and responds poorly to any bacterial infection. Bell has recommended tooth extraction only as a last resort, utilizing a surgical approach with removal of liberal amounts of bone to facilitate extraction and increase bleeding.

Sclerotic Cemental Masses

A series of 38 cases of lesions of the jaws with striking similarities to those lesions described as chronic diffuse sclerosing osteomyelitis has been reported by Waldron and his co-workers under the term "sclerotic cemental masses of the jaws."

Clinical Features. Just as in chronic diffuse sclerosing osteomyelitis, the majority of cases reported by Waldron and his associates occurred in older black females, who often presented with multiple, symmetric lesions that sometimes produced pain, drainage, or localized expansion. The roentgenographic appearance was also similar to that of diffuse sclerosis.

Histologic Features. The only significant difference between the two diseases, described in one case as sclerosing osteomyelitis and in the other as sclerotic cemental masses, was in the microscopic appearance of the radiopaque lesional tissue. In sclerosing osteomyelitis, the tissue was essentially sclerotic bone, while in the cemental masses, the tissue usually was

interpreted as cementum. In some instances, this cementum was in the form of large solid masses with smooth, lobulated margins, often with a globular accretion pattern. In other cases, variable amounts of bone were admixed.

The remarkable similarities between the two diseases suggest very strongly that these represent two closely related facets of the same basic disease process. Supporting this concept, in addition to the clinical and roentgenographic similarities, is the fact that lesions are commonly seen that exhibit the microscopic features of both diseases in the same lesional tissue: sclerotic bone and sclerotic cementum. For this reason, it appears more appropriate to understand the nature of the reaction of the tissues to injury rather than to adhere to rigid standards of nomenclature.

Florid Osseous Dysplasia

Another disease that appears very closely related to both chronic diffuse sclerosing osteomyelitis and sclerotic cemental masses is that described by Melrose and his associates under the term "florid osseous dysplasia."

The clinical and roentgenographic features, as well as the microscopic findings, are virtually identical with those described under the former two diseases. However, Melrose and his co-workers did describe one additional feature that had not been reported previously: the simultaneous occurrence of simple bone "cysts" in approximately 40 per cent of their series of 34 cases of florid osseous dysplasia.

It appears that the term florid osseous dysplasia has been used to imply rather broad parameters of an "exuberant variant of osseous dysplasia, defined by Robinson to be an abnormal reaction of bone to irritation or stimulation," according to Melrose and his associates, and includes chronic diffuse sclerosing osteomyelitis and sclerotic cemental masses.

Chronic Osteomyelitis with Proliferative Periostitis

(Garré's Chronic Nonsuppurative Sclerosing Osteitis; Periostitis Ossificans)

This distinctive type of chronic osteomyelitis was first described in 1893 by Garré as a focal gross thickening of the periosteum of long bones, with peripheral reactive bone formation resulting from mild irritation or infection. It is essentially a periosteal osteosclerosis analogous to the endosteal sclerosis of chronic focal and diffuse sclerosing osteomyelitis.

Clinical Features. This sclerosing osteomyelitis occurs almost entirely in young persons before the age of 25 years and most frequently involves the anterior surface of the tibia. The lesion in this location has been recognized for many years by orthopedic surgeons and pathologists. It was generally overlooked as a distinctive entity affecting the jaws also until the report of Pell and his associates. Since there is probably greater opportunity for infection to enter the bone of the maxilla and the mandible than any other bone of the body, because of the peculiar anatomic arrangement of the teeth situated in and protruding from the bone, it is surprising that the disease has not been described more frequently as a dental complication. A review of the literature in 1980 by Lichty and his associates revealed 22 reported cases involving the jaws.

The condition in the jaws occurs almost exclusively in children or young adults and shows a definite predilection for the mandible. Seldom is the maxilla affected, although the reason for this is not clear. The patient usually presents complaining of a toothache or pain in the jaw and a bony hard swelling on the outer surface of the jaw. This mass is usually of at least several weeks' duration.

Occasionally, this reactive periostitis may develop not as a result of a central dental infection of the jaw that perforates outward but as a result of an overlying soft-tissue infection or cellulitis that subsequently involves the deeper periosteum. Three such cases, all in infants under 2 years of age, have been reported by Suydam and Mikity. In addition, a most unusual case of the condition occurring simultaneously in four quadrants of the jaws in an 11-year-old child has been reported by Eisenbud and his co-workers.

Roentgenographic Features. Intraoral roentgenograms will often reveal a carious tooth opposite the hard bony mass (Fig. 8–29). An

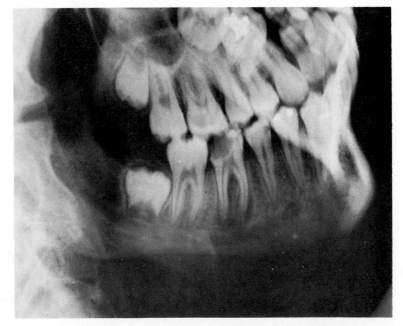

Figure 8–29. *Chronic osteomyelitis with proliferative periostitis.*
There are caries and periapical involvement of the mandibular first molar, but the periosteal reaction is not evident on the lateral jaw roentgenogram.

occlusal roentgenogram shows a focal over-growth of bone on the outer surface of the cortex, which may be described as a duplication of the cortical layer of bone (Fig. 8–30). This

mass of bone is smooth and rather well calcified and may itself show a thin but definite cortical layer.

Histologic Features. This supracortical but

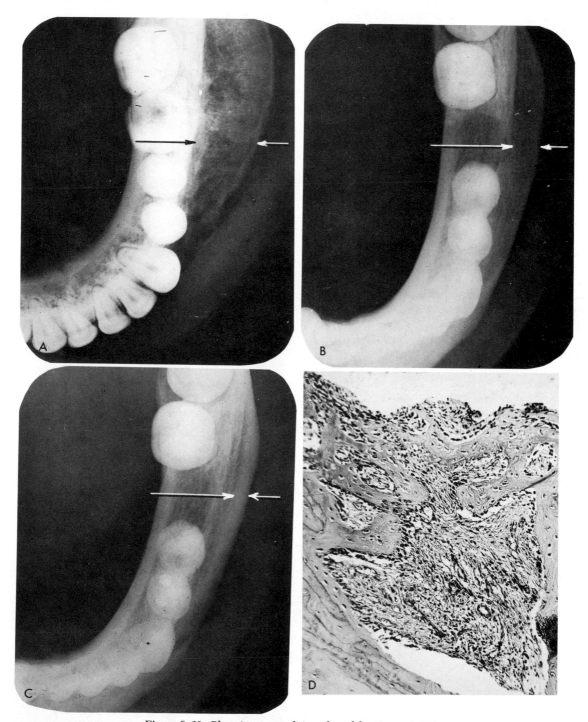

Figure 8–30. *Chronic osteomyelitis with proliferative periostitis.*
The intense periosteal reaction is seen on the occlusal film (A). The second occlusal film (B) was taken three months after extraction of the first molar, while the third film (C) was taken one year after the extraction and demonstrates the remarkable remodeling that occurred without other treatment. The photomicrograph (D) shows reactive new periosteal bone formed in response to the mild chronic inflammation present.

subperiosteal mass is composed of much reactive new bone and osteoid tissue, with osteoblasts bordering many of the trabeculae. These trabeculae often are oriented perpendicular to the cortex, with the trabeculae arranged parallel to each other or in a retiform pattern. The connective tissue between the bony trabeculae is rather fibrous and shows a diffuse or patchy sprinkling of lymphocytes and plasma cells (Fig. 8–30, D).

The periosteal reaction is a result of the infection from the carious tooth perforating the cortical plate and becoming attenuated, stimulating the periosteum rather than producing the usual suppurative periostitis.

Treatment and Prognosis. Chronic osteomyelitis with a proliferative periostitis is best treated by removal of the carious infected tooth, with no surgical intervention for the periosteal lesion except for biopsy to confirm the diagnosis. Pell and his co-workers reported that after extraction of the involved tooth, gradual remodeling of the jaws occurs, restoring the original facial symmetry (Fig. 8–30, C).

Periosteal new bone formation, or neoperiostosis, may occur in a variety of other conditions, and care must be taken to exclude them from the diagnosis. These include infantile cortical hyperostosis (Caffey's disease), hypervitaminosis A, syphilis, leukemia, Ewing's sarcoma, metastatic neuroblastoma, and even a fracture callus. This differential diagnosis has been discussed by Eversole and his associates in their review of this disease.

REFERENCES

Adams, D. O.: The granulomatous inflammatory response. Am. J. Pathol., 84:164, 1976.

Aison, E. L.: Osteomyelitis of the jaw. J. Am. Dent. Assoc., 25:1261, 1938.

Allison, R. T.: Electron microscopic study of 'Rushton' hyaline bodies in cyst linings. Brit. Dent. J., 137:102, 1974.

Athanassiades, T. J. and Speirs, R. S.: Granuloma induction in the peritoneal cavity: a model for the study of inflammation and plasma-cytopoiesis in nonlymphatic organs. J. Reticuloendothel. Soc. 11:60, 1972.

Bell, W. H.: Sclerosing osteomyelitis of the mandible and maxilla. Oral Surg., 12:391, 1959.

Besic, F.: Fate of bacteria sealed in dental cavities. J. Dent. Res., 22:349, 1943.

Blair, V. P., Brown, J. B., and Moore, S.: Osteomyelitis of the jaws. Int. J. Orthod., 17:168, 1931.

Boling, L. R., and Robinson, H. B. G.: Vascular changes in inflamed dental pulp. J. Dent. Res., 17:310, 1938.

Idem: The anachoretic effect in pulpitis. Arch. Pathol., 33:477, 1942.

Boulger, E. P.: Histologic study of a hypertrophied pulp. J. Dent. Res., 11:256, 1931.

Bourgoyne, J. R., and Quinn, J. H.: The periapical abscess. J. Oral Surg., 7:320, 1949.

Boyle, P. E.: Intracellular bacteria in a dental granuloma. J. Dent. Res., 14:297, 1934.

Boyne, P. J.: Incidence of osteosclerotic areas in the mandible and maxilla. J. Oral Surg., 18:486, 1960.

Brannstrom, B., and Lind, P. O.: Pulpal response to early dental caries. J. Dent. Res., 44:1045, 1965.

Buchanan, J. C.: Oral abscesses and granuloma. Dent. Cosmos, 72:605, 1930.

Burket, L.: Recent studies relating to periapical infection, including data obtained from human necropsy studies. J. Am. Dent. Assoc., 25:260, 1938.

Cahn, L. R.: The role of the pulp in dental caries: a clinicopathological study. Dent. Cosmos, 74:1164, 1932.

Cavanagh, F.: Osteomyelitis of the superior maxilla in infants. Br. Med. J., 1:468, 1960.

Chen, S-Y., Fantasia, J. E., and Miller, A. S.: Hyaline bodies in the connective tissue wall of odontogenic cysts. J. Oral Path. 10:147, 1981.

Cohen, M.: Osteomyelitis of the mandible in the newborn. Oral Surg., 2:50, 1949.

Cook, T. J.: Dental granuloma. J. Am. Dent. Assoc., 14:2231, 1927.

Dachi, S. F.: The relationship of pulpitis and hyperemia to thermal sensitivity. Oral Surg., 19:776, 1965.

de Campos Vidal, B.: Histochemistry of the dental granuloma. Ann. Histochem., 8:35, 1963.

Dunlap, C. L., and Barker, B. F.: Giant-cell hyalin angiopathy. Oral Surg., 44:587, 1977.

Durbeck, W. E.: Mandibular osteomyelitis: its diagnosis and treatment. J. Oral Surg., 4:33, 1946.

Eisenbud, L., and Klatell, J.: Acute alveolar abscess; a review of 300 hospitalized cases. Oral Surg., 4:208, 1951.

Eisenbud, L., Miller, J., and Roberts, I. L.: Garré's proliferative periostitis occurring simultaneously in four quadrants of the jaws. Oral Surg., 51:172, 1981.

El-Labban, N. G., and Kramer, R. H.: The nature of the hyaline rings in chronic periostitis and other conditions: an ultrastructural study. Oral Surg., 51:509, 1981.

Eversole, L. R., Leider, A. S., Corwin, J. O., and Karian, B. K.: Proliferative periostitis of Garré: its differentiation from other neoperiostoses. J. Oral Surg., 37:725, 1979.

Fabe, S. S.: Acute hematogenous osteomyelitis of the mandible. Oral Surg., 3:22, 1950.

Fish, E. W.: The pathology of the dentin and dental pulp. Br. Dent. J., 53:351, 1932.

Freeman, N.: Histopathological investigations of the dental granuloma. J. Dent. Res., 11:175, 1931.

Frey, H.: A contribution to the histopathology of pulp "polypi" especially of temporary teeth. Br. Dent. J., 85:225, 1948.

Frithiof, L., and Hagglund, G.: Ultrastructure of the capsular epithelium of radicular cysts. Acta Odontol. Scand., 24:23, 1966.

Fullmer, H. M.: Observations on the development of oxytalan fibers in dental granulomas and radicular cysts. A. M. A. Arch. Pathol., 70:59, 1960.

Gardner, A. F.: The odontogenic cyst as a potential carcinoma: a clinicopathologic appraisal. J. Am. Dent. Assoc., 78:746, 1969.

Harris, R., and Griffin, C. J.: Histogenesis of the fibroblasts in the human dental pulp. Arch. Oral Biol., 12:459, 1967.

Hasler, J. F., and Mitchell, D. F.: Analysis of 1628 cases of odontalgia: a corroborative study. J. Indianap. Dist. Dent. Soc., 17:23, 1963.

Herbert, W. E.: Correlation of clinical signs and symptoms and histologic conditions of pulps of 52 teeth. Br. Dent. J., 78:161, 1945.

Hill, T. J.: The epithelium in dental granuloma. J. Dent. Res., 10:323, 1930.

Idem: Experimental granulomas in dogs. J. Am. Dent. Assoc., 19:1389, 1932.

Idem: Pathology of the dental pulp. J. Am. Dent. Assoc., 21:820, 1934.

James, W. W., and Counsell, A.: A histological study of the epithelium associated with chronic apical infection of the teeth. Br. Dent. J., 53:463, 1932.

Kader, M. I., and Christmas, B. H.: Generalized suppurative osteomyelitis of the mandible. Oral Surg., 4:732, 1951.

Kakehashi, S., Stanley, H.R., and Fitzgerald, R. J.: The effects of surgical exposure of dental pulps in germ-free and conventional laboratory rats. Oral Surg., 20:340, 1965.

Kreshover, S. J., and Bevelander, G.: Histopathology of the dental pulp of dogs following exposure. J. Dent. Res., 27:467, 1948.

Leonard, E. P., Lunin, M., and Provenza, D. V.: On the occurrence and morphology of Russell bodies in the dental granuloma. Oral Surg., 38:584, 1974.

Lichty, G., Langlais, R. P., and Aufdemorte, T.: Garré's osteomyelitis. Oral Surg., 50:309, 1980.

Lundy, T., and Stanley, H. R.: Correlation of pulpal histopathology and clinical symptoms in human teeth subjected to experimental irritation. Oral Surg., 27:187, 1969.

Lutz, J., Cimasoni, G., and Held, A. J.: Histochemical observations on the epithelial lining of radicular cysts. Helv. Odontol. Acta, 9:90, 1965.

McConnell, G.: The histopathology of dental granuloma. J. Am. Dent. Assoc., 8:390, 1921.

McMillan, M. D., Kardos, T. B., Edwards, J. L., Thorburn, D. N., Adams, D. B., and Palmer, D. K.: Giant cell hyalin angiopathy or pulse granuloma. Oral Surg., 52:178, 1981.

Mathiesen, A.: Preservation and demonstration of mast cells in human apical granulomas and radicular cysts. Scand. J. Dent. Res., 81:218, 1973.

Medak, H., and Weinmann, J. P.: Hyaline bodies in dental cysts. Br. Dent. J., 109:312, 1960.

Melrose, R. J., Abrams, A. M., and Mills, B. G.: Florid osseous dysplasia. Oral Surg., 41:62, 1976.

Mincer, H. H., McCoy, J. M., and Turner, J. E.: Pulse granuloma of the alveolar ridge. Oral Surg., 48:126, 1979.

Mitchell, D. F., and Tarplee, R. E.: Painful pulpitis. Oral Surg., 13:1360, 1960.

Molyneux, G.: Hyaline bodies in the wall of dental cysts. Aust Dent. J., 2:155, 1957.

Morse, D. R.: Immunologic aspects of pulpal-periapical diseases. Oral Surg., 43:436, 1977.

Nicholls, E.: Lateral radicular disease due to lateral branching of the root canal. Oral Surg., 16:839, 1963.

Nørgaard, B., and Pindborg, J. J.: Acute neonatal maxillitis. Acta Ophthalmol., 59:52, 1959.

Orban, B.: Contribution to histology of dental pulp and periodontal membrane with special reference to cells of defense of those tissues. J. Am. Dent. Assoc., 16:695, 1929.

Orban, B., and Ritchey, B. T.: Toothache under conditions simulating high altitude flight. J. Am. Dent. Assoc., 32:145, 1945.

Padgett, E. C.: Osteomyelitis of jaws: analysis of 59 patients. Surgery, 8:821, 1940.

Page, R. C., Davies, P., and Allison, A. C.: Pathogenesis of the chronic inflammatory lesion induced by Group A streptococcal cell walls. Lab. Invest., 30:568, 1974.

Pell, G. J., Shafer, W. G., Gregory, G. T., Ping, R. S., and Spear, L. B.: Garré's osteomyelitis of the mandible. J. Oral Surg., 13:248, 1955.

Priebe, W. A., Lazansky, J. P., and Wuehrmann, A. H.: The value of the roentgenographic film in the differential diagnosis of periapical lesions. Oral Surg., 7:979, 1954.

Reeves, R., and Stanley, H. R.: The relationship of bacterial penetration and pulpal pathosis in carious teeth. Oral Surg., 22:59, 1966.

Robertson, P. B., Lüscher, B., Spangberg, L. S., and Levy, B. M.: Pulpal and periodontal effects of electrosurgery involving cervical metallic restoration. Oral Surg., 46:702, 1978.

Robinson, H. B. G.: Pathology of periapical infection. Oral Surg., 4:1044, 1951.

Robinson, H. B. G.: Osseous dysplasia—Reaction of bone to injury. J. Oral Surg., 16:483, 1958.

Robinson, H. B. G., and Boling, L. R.: Diagnosis and pathology of anachoretic pulpitis. I. Bacteriologic studies. J. Am. Dent. Assoc., 28:268, 1941.

Rushton, M. A.: Hyaline bodies in the epithelium of dental cysts. Proc. R. Soc. Med., 48:407, 1955.

Russell, W.: An address on a characteristic organism of cancer. Brit. Med. J., 2:1356, 1890.

Sedano, H. O., and Gorlin, R. J.: Hyaline bodies of Rushton: some histochemical considerations concerning their etiology. Oral Surg., 26:198, 1968.

Seltzer, S., and Bender, I. B.: The Dental Pulp. Biologic Considerations in Dental Procedures. 2nd ed. Philadelphia, J. B. Lippincott Company, 1975.

Seltzer, S., Bender, I. B., and Ziontz, M.: The dynamics of pulp inflammation: correlations between diagnostic data and actual histologic findings in the pulp. Oral Surg., 16:846, 969, 1963.

Seltzer, S., Soltanoff, W., and Bender, I. B.: Epithelial proliferation in periapical lesions. Oral Surg., 27:111, 1969.

Shafer, W. G.: Chronic sclerosing osteomyelitis. J. Oral Surg., 15:138, 1957.

Shear, M.: Cholesterol in dental cysts. Oral Surg., 16:1465, 1963.

Idem: Inflammation in dental cysts. Oral Surg., 17:756, 1964.

Idem: The hyaline and granular bodies in dental cysts. Br. Dent. J., 110:301, 1961.

Shroff, F. R.: Observations on the reactions of the pulp and dentin to advancing caries. N. Z. Dent. J., 40:103, 1944.

Siskin, M. (ed.): The Biology of the Human Dental Pulp. St. Louis, C. V. Mosby Company, 1973.

Southam, J. C., and Hodson, J. J.: Neurohistology of human dental pulp polyps. Arch. Oral Biol., 18:1255, 1973.

Southam, J. C., and Hodson, J. J.: The growth of epithelium, melanocytes, and Langerhans cells on human and experimental dental pulp polyps. Oral Surg., 37:546, 1974.

Stanley, H. R.: The cells of the dental pulp. Oral Surg., 15:849, 1962.

Stephan, R. M.: Correlation of clinical tests with microscopic pathology of the dental pulp. J. Dent. Res.,
16:267, 1937.

Stern, M. H., Dreizen, S., Mackler, B. F., and Levy, B.
M.: Antibody-producing cells in human periapical
granulomas and cysts. J. Endod., *7*:447, 1981.

Idem: Isolation and characterization of inflammatory cells
from the human periapical granuloma. J. Dent. Res.,
61:1408, 1982.

Stern, M. H., Dreizen, S., Mackler, B. F., Selbst, A. G.,
and Levy, B. M.: Quantitative analysis of cellular
composition of human periapical granuloma. J. Endod.
7:117, 1981.

Suydam, M. J., and Mikity, V. G.: Cellulitis with underlying inflammatory periostitis of the mandible. Am. J.
Roentgenol., Radium Ther. Nucl. Med., *106*:133,
1969.

Thoma, K. H.: A histologic study of the dental granuloma
and diseased root apex. J. Am. Dent. Assoc., *4*:1075,
1917.

Idem: The condition of the bone in cases of dental granuloma. Dent. Items Interest, *40*:421, 1918.

Idem: The histologic pathology of alveolar abscesses and
diseased root ends. Dent. Cosmos, *60*:13, 1918.

Idem: A practical discussion of pulp disease based on
microscopic study. Dent. Items Interest, *47*:637, 1925.

Idem: The infected vital dental pulp. J. Dent. Res., *8*:529,
1928.

Thoma, K. H., and Kalil, F. H.: Chronic osteomyelitis of
the mandible. Am. J. Orthod. Oral Surg., *29*:536,
1943.

Toller, P. A.: Experimental investigation into factors concerning the growth of cysts of the jaws. Proc. R. Soc.
Med., *41*:681, 1948.

Torabinejad, M., and Bakland, L. K.: Immunopathogenesis
of chronic periapical lesions. Oral Surg., *46*:685, 1978.

Waldron, C. W.: Osteomyelitis of the jaws. J. Oral Surg.,
1:317, 1943.

Waldron, C. A., Giansanti, J. S., and Browand, B. C.:
Sclerotic cemental masses of the jaws (so-called chronic
sclerosing osteomyelitis, sclerosing osteitis, multiple
enostosis, and gigantiform cementoma). Oral Surg.,
39:590, 1975.

Weine, F. S.: Endodontic Therapy. 2nd ed. St. Louis, C.
V. Mosby Company, 1976.

Wellings, A. W.: Early inflammatory reactions of the tooth
pulp to bacterial invasion of the dentinal tubules. Br.
Dent. J., *68*:510, 1940.

Whitten, J. B., Jr: Cytologic examination of aspirated
material from cysts or cystlike lesions. Oral Surg.,
25:710, 1968.

CHAPTER 9

Spread of Oral Infection

An oral infection may originate in the dental pulp and extend through the root canals and into the periapical tissues, or it may originate in the superficial periodontal tissues and subsequently become dispersed through the spongy bone. Thence it may perforate the outer cortical bone and spread in various tissue spaces or discharge onto a free mucous membrane or skin surface. It may become localized or extend diffusely. The spread of the disease depends upon a variety of factors and circumstances which may alter its course at any point. If the infection escapes from the confines of the bone of the maxilla or mandible, an infinitely more dangerous situation exists, although even the intrabony confined infection is serious.

The type of organism or organisms influences the degree of spread of the infection, since some agents tend to remain localized, while others spread rapidly and diffusely throughout the tissues. The physical state of the patient also affects the extent and rapidity of spread of the infection. Certain anatomic features determine to a large extent the actual direction which the infection may take (Fig. 9–1). Drainage by perforation of a bony plate occurs along lines of least resistance, so that, other circumstances being equal, perforation of a thin cortex occurs before that of a thick cortex. The attachment of muscles may determine the route which an infection will take, channeling the infection into certain tissue spaces. The distribution and the interrelations of the many potential tissue spaces in the facial and cervical regions must be appreciated to understand the ease with which infection may spread throughout this area and even into distant areas.

CELLULITIS

(Phlegmon)

Cellulitis is a diffuse inflammation of soft tissues which is not circumscribed or confined to one area, but which, in contradistinction to the abscess, tends to spread through tissue spaces and along fascial planes. This type of reaction occurs as a result of infection by micro-

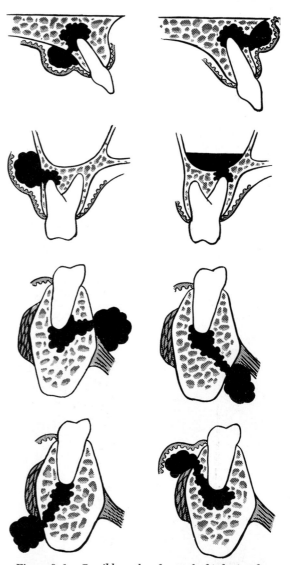

Figure 9–1. *Possible paths of spread of infection from acute periapical abscess.*

organisms that produce significant amounts of hyaluronidase (the spreading factor of Duran-Reynals) and fibrinolysins which act to break down or dissolve, respectively, hyaluronic acid, the universal intercellular cement substance, and fibrin. Streptococci are particularly potent producers of hyaluronidase and are therefore a common causative organism in cases of cellulitis. The less common hyaluronidase-producing staphylococci are also pathogenic and frequently give rise to cellulitis.

Cellulitis of the face and neck most commonly results from dental infection, either as a sequela of an apical abscess or osteomyelitis, or following periodontal infection. The pericoronal infection or *pericoronitis* (operculitis) occurring around erupting or partially impacted third molars and resulting in cellulitis and trismus is an especially common clinical condition. Sometimes cellulitis of the face or neck will occur as a result of infection following a tooth extraction, injection either with an infected needle or through an infected area, or following jaw fracture.

Clinical Features. The patient with cellulitis of the face or neck originating from a dental infection is usually moderately ill and has an elevated temperature and leukocytosis. There is a painful swelling of the involved soft tissues which is firm and brawny (Fig. 9–2). The skin

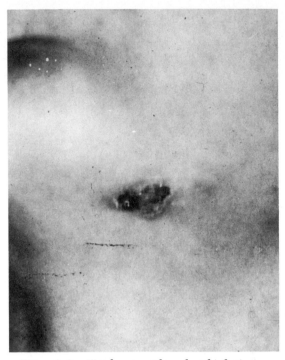

Figure 9–3.   *Fistulous tract from dental infection opening on skin.*

is inflamed, sometimes even purplish, if the superficial tissue spaces are involved. In the case of inflammatory spread of infection along deeper planes of cleavage, the overlying skin may be of normal color. In addition, regional lymphadenitis is usually present.

Infections arising in the maxilla perforate the outer cortical layer of bone above the buccinator attachment and cause swelling initially of the upper half of the face. The diffuse spread, however, soon involves the entire facial area. When infection in the mandible perforates the outer cortical plate below the buccinator attachment, there is a diffuse swelling of the lower half of the face which then spreads superiorly as well as cervically.

As the typical facial cellulitis persists, the infection frequently tends to become localized, and a facial abscess may form. When this happens, the suppurative material present seeks to "point" or discharge upon a free surface (Fig. 9–3). If early treatment is instituted, resolution usually occurs without drainage through a break in the skin.

Histologic Features. A microscopic section through an area of cellulitis shows only a diffuse exudation of polymorphonuclear leukocytes and occasional lymphocytes, with considerable serous fluid and fibrin causing separation of connective tissue or muscle fibers (Fig. 9–4). Cel-

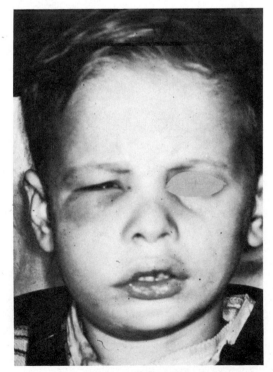

Figure 9–2.   *Cellulitis of the face.*

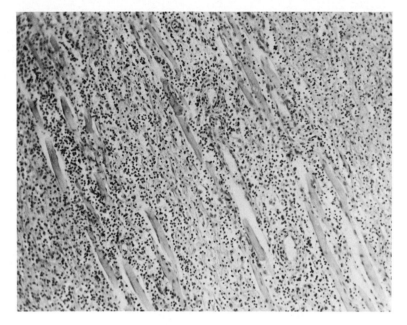

Figure 9–4. *Cellulitis.* An acute inflammatory exudate separates the muscle fibers.

lulitis presents only a nonspecific picture of diffuse acute inflammation.

Treatment and Prognosis. Cellulitis is treated by the administration of antibiotics and the removal of the cause of the infection. Although this condition is extremely serious, resolution is usually prompt with adequate treatment, and untoward sequelae are uncommon.

INFECTIONS OF SPECIFIC TISSUE SPACES

Tissue spaces, or fascial spaces, are potential spaces situated between planes of fascia which form natural pathways along which infection may spread, producing a cellulitis, or within which infection may become localized with actual abscess formation. A knowledge of these fascial spaces, their boundaries, contents and relation to other structures is a necessity for the dentist because of the propensity for their involvement by spread of dental infection.

Infratemporal Space. The infratemporal space is bounded anteriorly by the maxillary tuberosity; posteriorly by the lateral pterygoid muscle, the condyle and temporal muscle; laterally by the tendon of the temporal muscle and the coronoid process; and medially by the lateral pterygoid plate and inferior belly of the lateral pterygoid muscle. The inferior portion of the infratemporal space is called the *pterygomandibular space* and lies between the internal pterygoid muscle and the ramus of the mandible. Extending anteromedially from the infratemporal space and considered a part of it is the *postzygomatic space.*

The infratemporal space contains the pterygoid plexus, the internal maxillary artery, the mandibular, mylohyoid, lingual, buccinator and chorda tympani nerves and the external pterygoid muscle.

Infection in this space is often difficult to diagnose. The patient may exhibit trismus and sometimes swelling of the eyelids, especially if there is involvement of the postzygomatic fossa. The involvement of the pharynx may cause dysphagia and severe pain or a feeling of pressure in the general area of the infection.

Infection in the pterygomandibular space may arise through extension from a pericoronitis of a mandibular third molar and has occurred in cases of injection of local anesthetic solution into this space. Severe trismus results from infection in this location and extreme radiating pain is common. There is no clinical facial swelling evident, although swelling of the lateral posterior portion of the soft palate may occur. Injection of the maxillary tuberosity with an infected needle or solution has also caused infection of the infratemporal fossa.

Lateral Pharyngeal Space. The lateral pharyngeal space, one of the parapharyngeal spaces, is bounded anteriorly by the buccopharyngeal aponeurosis, the parotid gland and the pterygoid muscles, posteriorly by the pre-

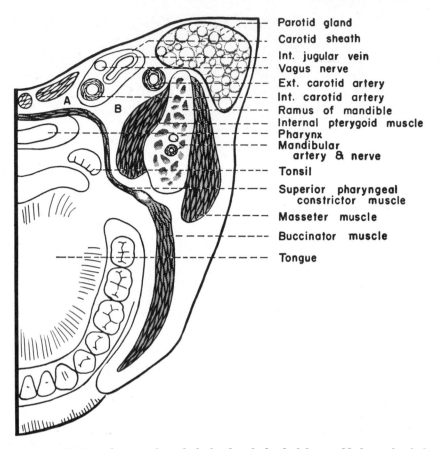

Parotid gland
Carotid sheath
Int. jugular vein
Vagus nerve
Ext. carotid artery
Int. carotid artery
Ramus of mandible
Internal pterygoid muscle
Pharynx
Mandibular
    artery & nerve
Tonsil
Superior pharyngeal
    constrictor muscle
Masseter muscle
Buccinator muscle
Tongue

Figure 9–5. *Horizontal section through the head at the level of the mandibular occlusal plane.* The parapharyngeal spaces are indicated: (A) retropharyngeal space, (B) lateral pharyngeal space.

vertebral fascia, laterally by the carotid sheath and medially by the lateral wall of the pharynx (Fig. 9–5).

Infection of this space with abscess formation may impinge on the pharynx, causing difficulty in swallowing and even in breathing. Trismus is usually present. The source of the infection is most frequently a third molar, sometimes a second molar, particularly by way of infection in the submandibular space or by direct extension from the tooth. The lateral pharyngeal space communicates with the mediastinum by the prevertebral fascia, so that infection may reach this area by direct extension.

Retropharyngeal Space. The retropharyngeal space is bounded anteriorly by the wall of the pharynx, posteriorly by the prevertebral fascia, and laterally by the lateral pharyngeal space and carotid sheath.

Infection here may result from medial extension of infection in the lateral pharyngeal space, and an abscess may form, displacing or pressing the buccopharyngeal fascia forward and imping-

ing on the pharynx. Since the prevertebral fascia extends inferiorly to the posterior mediastinum, it is possible for infection in this retropharyngeal space to spread down to the mediastinum.

Parotid Space. The parotid space contains the parotid gland and all invested associated structures, including the facial nerve, the auriculotemporal nerve, the posterior facial vein, and the external carotid, internal maxillary and superficial temporal arteries. The gland itself is situated outside of the masseter muscle, extending posteriorly behind the ramus of the mandible and medially between the masseter and internal pterygoid muscles.

Infection in the parotid space, often reaching the gland from the lateral pharyngeal space or by retrograde extension along the parotid duct, typically points medially or inferiorly and opens into the neck or oral cavity. Primary infections of the parotid space break into the lateral pharyngeal space readily because the fascia is thin over the deep portion of the parotid space.

Spread of infection superiorly to the temporal fossa may also occur.

Space of the Body of the Mandible. The space of the body of the mandible is enclosed by a layer of fascia derived from the outer layer of the deep cervical fascia, which attaches to the inferior border of the mandible and then splits to enclose the body of the mandible. Superiorly it becomes continuous with the alveolar mucoperiosteum and muscles of facial expression which have their attachment on the mandible. The space contains the mandible anterior to the ramus as well as the covering periosteum, fascia, muscle attachments, blood vessels, nerves, teeth and periodontal structures. Shapiro pointed out that infections in this space may be dental, periodontal or vascular in origin, or may arise from fractures or by direct extension from infection in the masticator or lateral pharyngeal spaces.

When infection originating from incisor, cuspid or bicuspid teeth involves the space of the body of the mandible, there is induration or fluctuation of the labial sulcus if the outer cortical plate is involved. When the inner cortical plate is involved, the infection is restricted to the floor of the mouth.

Infection originating from the molar teeth and involving the outer cortical plate results in a swelling in the oral vestibule if the infection perforates the bone above the external oblique line, the buccinator attachment. If perforation is below this line, the infection may point on the skin. Lingual spread from infected bicuspid or molar teeth is into the floor of the mouth when perforation of the bone is above the level of attachment of the mylohyoid muscle. Below the mylohyoid, infection extends into the submaxillary space or medially and posteriorly into the lateral pharyngeal space.

Submasseteric Space. The submasseteric space is situated between the masseter muscle and the lateral surface of the mandibular ramus. The masseter attaches to the ramus at three sites: the deep part on the lateral surface of the coronoid process, the middle part in a linear pattern on the lateral surface of the ramus extending upward and backward, and the superficial part close to the angle of the mandible. The submasseteric space is a narrow space which parallels the middle attachment by extending upward and backward between the middle and deep attachments. The posterior boundary of this space is the parotid gland, and anteriorly it adjoins the retromolar fossa (Fig. 9–6).

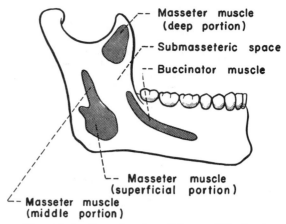

Figure 9–6. *Lateral surface of the mandible showing the location of the submasseteric space.* (Redrawn from G. M. Bransby-Zachary: The submasseteric space. Br. Dent. J., *84*:10, 1948).

Infection of this space usually occurs from a mandibular third molar, the infection passing through the retromolar fossa and into the submasseteric space. The patient may suffer from severe trismus and pain, and there may be facial swelling. The patient is often seriously ill.

Submandibular Spaces. There are three chief spaces in the submandibular region: the submaxillary, sublingual and submental spaces. Each is in anatomic continuity with the other as well as with its mate of the opposite side, and infection may spread contralaterally by extension anterior to the hyoglossus muscle (Fig. 9–7).

SUBMAXILLARY SPACE. The submaxillary space is located medial to the mandible and below the posterior portion of the mylohyoid muscle. It is bordered medially by the hyoglossus and digastric muscles and laterally by superficial fascia and skin. This space encloses the submaxillary salivary gland and lymph nodes.

Infection of the submaxillary space usually orginates from the mandibular molars and produces a swelling near the angle of the jaw. It is one of the most commonly involved of all facial and cervical tissue spaces. Because of the anatomic proximity, there is usually involvement of the submaxillary gland and nodes also, with resulting sialadenitis and lymphadenitis. The infection, in addition to spreading locally to involve the other submandibular spaces, may extend to the lateral pharyngeal space, carotid space, cranial fossa or even the mediastinum. Involvement of the pharynx and larynx may even necessitate tracheotomy.

SUBLINGUAL SPACE. The sublingual space is

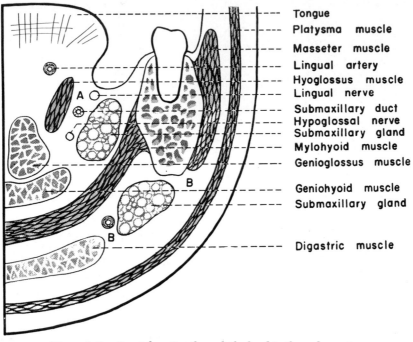

Figure 9–7. *Frontal section through the head in the molar region.*
The sublingual space *(A)* and the submaxillary space *(B)* are illustrated.

bounded superiorly by the mucosa of the floor of the mouth, inferiorly by the mylohyoid muscle, anteriorly and laterally by the body of the mandible, medially by the median raphe of the tongue and posteriorly by the hyoid bone. This space is situated above the submaxillary space, and infection here sometimes involves the tongue also. The infection may arise directly from perforation of the lingual cortical plate above the mylohyoid attachment or by extension from other spaces, primarily the submaxillary space.

Infection in the sublingual space produces an obvious swelling in the floor of the mouth and may cause both dyspnea and dysphagia. Extension of the infection takes the same paths as infection of the submaxillary space.

SUBMENTAL SPACE. The submental space extends from the anterior border of the submaxillary space to the midline and is limited in depth by the mylohyoid muscle.

Infection in this area presents as an anterior swelling in the submental area. This may cause dyspnea and dysphagia. The spread of infection is similar to that in the submaxillary and sublingual spaces.

LUDWIG'S ANGINA

Ludwig's angina is a severe cellulitis beginning usually in the submaxillary space and secondarily involving the sublingual and submental spaces as well. The disease is not usually considered to be true Ludwig's angina unless all submandibular spaces are involved. The chief source of infection is involvement of a mandibular molar, either periapical or periodontal, but it may result also from a penetrating injury of the floor of the mouth, such as a gunshot or stab wound, or from osteomyelitis in a compound jaw fracture.

The second and third molars are the teeth most commonly cited as the source of infection. The study of Tschiassny showed that of 30 teeth involved in 24 cases of Ludwig's angina, 20 per cent were first molars, 40 per cent were second molars, and 40 per cent were third molars. The explanation for this phenomenon lies in the fact that when an infection perforates bone to establish drainage, it seeks the path of least resistance. Since the outer cortical plate of the mandible is thick in the molar region, the lingual plate is the one most frequently perforated.

Initial infection of the submaxillary space, particularly in cases of the second and third molars, is due to the fact that the apices of these teeth are situated below the mylohyoid ridge in 65 per cent of cases, according to the studies of Tschiassny. He also noted that because the apices of the roots of the first molar are above this ridge in about 60 per cent of the cases, infection of the sublingual space is most common in cases of infection of this tooth.

Clinical Features. The patient with Ludwig's angina manifests a rapidly developing boardlike swelling of the floor of the mouth and consequent elevation of the tongue. The swelling is firm, painful and diffuse, showing no evidence of localization. There is difficulty in eating and swallowing as well as in breathing. Patients usually have a rather high fever, rapid pulse and fast respiration. A moderate leukocytosis is also found.

As the disease continues, the swelling involves the neck, and edema of the glottis may occur. This carries the serious risk of death by suffocation. Next, the infection may spread to the parapharyngeal spaces, to the carotid sheath or to the pterygopalatine fossa. Cavernous sinus thrombosis with subsequent meningitis may be a sequela to this type of spread of the infection.

Laboratory Findings. Most cases of Ludwig's angina are a mixed infection, but streptococci are almost invariably present. Fusiform bacilli and spiral forms, various staphylococci, diphtheroids and many other microorganisms have been cultured on different occasions.

There are apparently no specific organisms associated with the etiology of this disease. It appears to be a nonspecific mixed infection.

Treatment and Prognosis. Before the advent of antibiotics the disease carried an exceedingly high mortality rate due primarily to asphyxiation and severe sepsis. Most studies reported a death rate of 40 to 50 per cent. The antibiotics have greatly reduced the occurrence of cases of Ludwig's angina, and the seriousness of those which do arise is attenuated by the antibiotic therapy. The edema of the glottis, which may develop rapidly, often necessitates emergency tracheotomy to prevent suffocation.

INTRACRANIAL COMPLICATIONS OF DENTAL INFECTION

A variety of intracranial complications may occur as a direct result of dental infection or dental extraction. Haymaker reviewed a series of 28 fatal infections occurring after tooth extraction, noting that the infecting process proceeded along fascial planes to the base of the skull and then, traversing the skull by one or more routes, spread to the intracranial cavity despite combative measures. The specific complications included:

	NO. OF CASES
Subdural empyema	1
Suppurative encephalitis and ependymitis	1
Transverse myelitis	1
Subdural empyema and brain abscess	2
Leptomeningitis	2
Leptomeningitis and brain abscess	2
Brain abscess	8
Sinus thrombosis	11

The majority of these cases occurred after extraction of maxillary teeth. Interestingly, only 8 of the 28 cases occurred in patients whose mouths were classfied as being in poor hygienic condition. Furthermore, in 19 of the 28 cases the dental extraction involved only a single tooth.

CAVERNOUS SINUS THROMBOSIS OR THROMBOPHLEBITIS

Cavernous sinus thrombophlebitis is a serious condition consisting in the formation of a thrombus in the cavernous sinus or its communicating branches. Infections of the head, face and intraoral structures above the maxilla are particularly prone to produce this disease. There are many routes by which the infection may reach the cavernous sinus. Infection from the face and lip is carried by the facial and angular veins, while dental infection is carried by way of the pterygoid plexus. It has been emphasized by Mazzeo that infection spreading by the facial or external route is very rapid with a short fulminating course because of the large, open system of veins leading directly to the cavernous sinus. In contrast, infection spreading through the pterygoid or internal route reaches the cavernous sinus only through many small, twisting passages and has a much slower course, often with a lack of obvious symptoms early in the disease.

Clinical Features. The patient with cavernous sinus thrombophlebitis is extremely ill and manifests the characteristic features of exophthalmos with edema of the eyelids as well as chemosis. Paralysis of the external ocular muscles is reported, along with impairment of vision and sometimes photophobia and lacrimation. There are also usually headache, nausea and vomiting, pain, chills and fever.

Treatment and Prognosis. The disease was once almost invariably fatal, death occurring as a result of brain abscess or meningitis. The use of antibiotics has decreased this mortality, but the condition is still serious.

MAXILLARY SINUSITIS

Maxillary sinusitis, an acute or chronic inflammation of the maxillary sinus, is often due to direct extension of dental infection, but originates also from infectious diseases such as the common cold, influenza and the exanthematous diseases; from local spread of infection in the adjoining frontal or paranasal sinuses; or from traumatic injury of the sinuses with a superimposed infection. The occurrence of maxillary sinusitis as a result of the extension of dental infection is dependent to a great extent upon the relation and proximity of the teeth to the sinus. When sinusitis is secondary to dental infection, the microorganisms associated with the sinusitis are the same as those associated with the dental infection.

ACUTE MAXILLARY SINUSITIS

Acute sinusitis may result from an acute periapical abscess or acute exacerbation of a chronic inflammatory periapical lesion which involves the sinus through direct extension. In some cases a latent chronic sinusitis may be awakened by extraction of a maxillary bicuspid or molar and perforation of the sinus.

Clinical Features. Patients with acute maxillary sinusitis suffer moderately severe pain with swelling overlying the sinus. Pressing over the maxilla increases the pain. Often the painful sensation is one of pressure. Pain may be referred to various areas, including the teeth and ear.

The patient may complain of a discharge of pus into the nose and often a fetid breath. Fever and malaise are usually present. The diagnosis of acute maxillary sinusitis from clinical manifestations alone is frequently difficult.

Histologic Features. The lining of the maxillary sinus may show a typical acute inflammatory infiltrate with edema of the connective tissue and often hemorrhage. Sometimes squamous metaplasia of the specialized ciliated columnar epithelium occurs.

Treatment and Prognosis. The prime objective of treatment is removal of the infecting locus. This is particularly efficacious if the infection is of dental origin. Because of infection present, antibiotics should also be administered; when this is done, healing is usually uneventful.

CHRONIC MAXILLARY SINUSITIS

Chronic sinusitis may develop as an acute lesion subsides or may represent a chronic lesion from the onset.

In cases of acute or chronic maxillary sinusitis, the possibility of phycomycosis infection (q.v.) must always be considered, especially in diabetic patients.

Clinical Features. Clinical symptoms of chronic sinusitis may be generally lacking, and the condition may be discovered only during routine examination. Sometimes vague pain is present, or there is a stuffy sensation on the affected side of the face. There may be a mild discharge of pus into the nose and a fetid breath.

Histologic Features. The mucosa lining the maxillary sinus may show remarkable thickening and the development of numerous sinus "polyps." These polyps are simply hyperplastic granulation tissue with lymphocytic and sometimes plasma cell infiltration. This tissue, which is usually covered by ciliated columnar epithelium, tends to fill the sinus and obliterate it. In some instances there is no remarkable proliferation of granulation tissue; rather, there is only a mild lymphocytic infiltration of the lining tissue with squamous metaplasia of the epithelium.

Roentgenographic Features. Sinusitis can be seen on the roentgenogram as a clouding of the sinus due to the hyperplastic tissue or fluid present. Films of both sinuses should be compared before a diagnosis is attempted.

Treatment and Prognosis. The treatment for chronic maxillary sinusitis consists in removal of the cause of the disease, if this can be determined, and removal of the affected lining membrane. The prognosis is good, particularly if the disease is due to dental infection which can be eliminated. Infection from other sites may be difficult to eradicate.

FOCAL INFECTION

Oral foci of infection have been related to general health since the very inception of the theory of focal infection early in the twentieth century. This theory, originating during the infancy of microbiology as a science, was based chiefly upon clinical observation with but little foundation in scientifically determined fact. The enthusiastic acceptance of this concept by the medical and dental professions soon after its promulgation has gradually waned, but it is still of sufficient importance to warrant detailed consideration. A complete review of this subject cannot be made here because of the extensive literature. For greater detail, the evaluations of the effects of dental foci of infection on health prepared by Easlick and by Mitchell and Helman should be consulted.

Definition. *Focus of infection* refers to a circumscribed area of tissue which is infected with exogenous pathogenic microorganisms and which is usually located near a mucous or cutaneous surface. This should be carefully distinguished from *focal infection*, which refers to the metastasis from the focus of infection of organisms or their toxins that are capable of injuring tissue.

Mechanism of Focal Infection. There are two generally accepted mechanisms in the possible production of focal infection. In one instance there may be a metastasis of microorganisms from an infected focus by either hematogenous or lymphogenous spread. Secondly, toxins or toxic products may be carried, through the blood stream or lymphatic channels, from a focus to a distant site where they may incite a hypersensitive reaction in the tissues.

The spread of microorganisms through vascular or lymphatic channels is a recognized phenomenon, as is their localization in tissues. Thus certain organisms have a predilection for isolating themselves in specific sites in the body. This localization preference is probably an environmental phenomenon rather than an inherent or developed feature of the microorganisms.

The production of toxins by microorganisms and their dissemination by vascular channels are also recognized occurrences. One of the most dramatic examples is in scarlet fever, the remarkable cutaneous features of the disease being due to the erythrogenic toxin liberated by the infecting streptococci.

Rheumatic fever is an example of an important disease which probably develops as a result of an altered reactivity or hypersensitization of tissues to hemolytic streptococci. High concentrations of antibodies to antigens of the group of hemolytic streptococci are found in many patients with rheumatic fever. But the fact that microorganisms cannot be cultured from the blood or from any of the tissues involved in the disease indicates that this is not a direct bacterial infection. The importance of the oral cavity as a source for streptococci is obvious and will be discussed presently.

Oral Foci of Infection. A variety of situations exist in the oral cavity which are at least theoretical sources of infection and which may set up distant metastases. These include (1) infected periapical lesions such as the periapical granuloma, cyst, and abscess, (2) teeth with infected root canals, and (3) periodontal disease with special reference to tooth extraction or manipulation.

Infected periapical lesions, particularly those of a chronic nature, are usually surrounded by a fibrous capsule which effectively walls off or separates the area of infection from the adjacent tissue but does not prevent absorption of bacteria or toxins. The periapical granuloma has been described as a manifestation of a vigorous body defense and repair reaction, while the cyst appears to be merely a progressive form of the granuloma. The abscess may be considered a reaction occurring where the reparative or defensive phase is minimal.

The mere presence of a periapical granuloma does not necessarily mean that bacteria are present in this site. Bacteriologic studies are difficult to evaluate because of the constant probability of contamination with mouth organisms. Nevertheless, utilizing an aseptic technique of entrance through the root canal in situ, Sommer and Crowley cultured 14 teeth in which there was roentgenographic evidence of periapical granuloma formation and found that 10 of these were bacteriologically sterile. Streptococci were recovered from the other 4 teeth. In a similar study Ostrander and Crowley found that 46 cases (38.6 per cent) of a total of 119 periapical lesions were bacteriologically negative. Studies of Morse and Yates yielded similar results. Burket tabulated the bacterial population of the periapical region from cultures taken at postmortem examination, and his findings are shown in Table 8–1 (p. 493).

The majority of investigations indicate that

an unusually high percentage of periapical granulomas are bacteriologically sterile, and for this reason the possibility that such lesions give rise to focal infection is minimal.

Teeth with infected root canals without the actual formation of a periapical granuloma are a potential source of dissemination of both microorganisms and toxins. Many teeth, however, never yield a positive culture during routine root canal treatment. In the 265 cases reported by Morse and Yates, during the treatment of which 2202 cultures were carried out, 77 cases, or 29 per cent, yielded no positive cultures at any time. A somewhat higher proportion of noninfected root canals was reported by Ostrander and Crowley—40.4 per cent in a series of 859 teeth cultured during routine root canal treatment.

It has been pointed out that one of the most striking features of the cultures from teeth during root canal therapy is the relative infrequency of occurrence of hemolytic streptococci, since these are regarded as most important etiologically in rheumatoid arthritis and rheumatic fever, systemic diseases that are particularly related in the literature to dental foci of infection.

Periodontal disease is equally significant as a potential focus of infection, and the pertinent literature has been reviewed by Mitchell and Helman. The mechanisms involved in the production of the focal infection are the same as those previously described.

Bacteremia has been found to be closely related to the severity or degree of periodontal disease present after manipulation of the gingiva or, more commonly, after tooth extraction. As early as 1932 Richards had demonstrated that simple massage of inflamed gingiva resulted in a transitory bacteremia in 3 of 17 patients. Okell and Elliott reported that a transitory bacteremia developed in 75 per cent of a group of 40 patients who had severe periodontal disease after tooth extraction, but in only 34 per cent of 38 patients with "no noticeable pyorrhea." The usual organism recovered was *Streptococcus viridans*. In 110 cases of periodontal disease in this same study, 11 per cent of patients showed a bacteremia at the time of examination regardless of the operative procedure, but no positive blood cultures were found in a group of 68 patients who had no obvious gingival disease.

The "rocking" of teeth in their sockets by forceps before extraction has been shown by Elliott to favor bacteremia in patients who have periodontal disease. Thus 86 per cent of patients with severe periodontal disease had positive blood cultures under the foregoing conditions, while only 25 per cent of patients with no demonstrable gingival disease showed a bacteremia. That the "pumping" action occurring during dental extraction may force microorganisms from the gingival crevice into the capillaries of the gingiva as well as into the pulp of the tooth has been shown by Fish and Mac-Lean. In their study, two teeth were extracted after cauterization of the periodontal pockets, and two others were extracted without bacteriologic precautions. Organisms were readily cultured from the pulp and periodontal tissues of the untreated teeth, but not from those with cauterized pockets. Burket and Burn utilized a tracer microorganism, *Serratia marcescens*, to demonstrate the forcing of microorganisms into the blood stream by "rocking" the teeth during extraction. This microorganism was cultured from the blood of 60 per cent of 37 patients who had a suspension of the bacteria painted on the gingival margin before extraction.

Lazansky, Robinson, and Rodofsky studied the occurrence of bacteremia in 221 operations in the oral cavity involving 125 patients. Transient streptococcal bacteremias were found in 22 cases, or 10 per cent of the operations. A positive blood culture was found in 16 cases, or 17 per cent of a group of 92 multiple extractions, but only once in 56 single extractions. It is of considerable interest that a positive blood culture was found in five cases of a group of 72 patients receiving simple periodontal scalings.

Even oral prophylaxis may be followed by bacteremia, as was demonstrated by De Leo and his associates in a group of 39 children between 7 and 12 years of age. Of these patients, 5 per cent were found to have a preprophylaxis bacteremia, but 28 per cent had a postprophylaxis bacteremia. On the basis of these findings, they concluded that it was mandatory that prior to dental prophylaxis, antibiotic premedication—as advocated by the American Heart Association—be employed for those children diagnosed as having rheumatic or congenital heart disease, because of the possible serious consequences of bacterial endocarditis.

A great many other excellent pertinent studies dealing with tooth extraction or manipulation and bacteremia have been reported, some of which are summarized in Table 9–1. The evidence overwhelmingly indicates that the extraction of teeth, and sometimes even more

Table 9–1. Summary of Results of Studies on Bacteremia
Following Oral Procedures

TYPE OF OPERATION	INVESTIGATOR	NO. OF CASES	NO. OF POSTOPERATIVE CULTURES CONSIDERED POSITIVE BY INVESTIGATOR	NO. OF POSTOPERATIVE CULTURES CONSIDERED POSITIVE FOR PATHOGENIC MICROORGANISMS*
Single extractions	Okell et al.	10	1	1
	Burket et al.	182	44	19
	Glaser et al. (control group)	16	10	10
Total		208	55	30 (14%)
Multiple extractions only	Okell et al.	128	83	83
	Bender et al. (control group)	30	25	25
	Glaser et al. (control group)	24	17	17
Total		182	125	125 (69%)
One or more extractions	Marseille	100	42	42
	Northrop et al. (control group)	99	16	16
	Hopkins	108	18	18
	Hirsh et al. (control group)	65	22	19
	Rhoads et al. (control group)	68	24	24
Total		440	122	119 (27%)
All extractions		830	302	274 (33%)
Rocking; chewing; gingival massage	Elliott	41	23	23
	Richards	17	3	3
	Round et al.	10	2	2
	Murray et al.	336	185	0
Total		404	214	28 (7%)
Irritation of dental foci		1232	515	302 (25%)

From L. Robinson, F. W. Kraus, J. P. Lazansky, R. E. Wheeler, S. Gordon, and V. Johnson: Bacteremias of dental origin. I. A review of the literature. Oral Surg., 3:519, 1950.

*Included here are pure or mixed cultures containing streptococci, *Staphylococcus aureus*, pneumococci, actinomyces. Excluded are cultures not containing any of the mentioned, but showing growth of *Staph. albus*, diphtheroids, unspecific diplococci, sarcinae, gram-negative cocci and rods, and fusiform bacilli.

minor oral procedures, may produce a transient bacteremia. This bacteremia seldom persists for over 30 minutes in the majority of patients.

Significance of Oral Foci of Infection. There have been a vast number of reports, based chiefly on clinical evidence alone, purporting to show that oral foci of infection either cause or aggravate a great many systemic diseases. The diseases most frequently mentioned are (1) arthritis, chiefly of the rheumatoid and rheumatic fever types, (2) valvular heart disease, particularly subacute bacterial endocarditis, (3) gastrointestinal diseases, (4) ocular diseases, (5) skin diseases, and (6) renal diseases.

Arthritis of the rheumatoid type is a disease of unknown etiology, but probably represents only one manifestation of a generalized systemic disease. It bears close resemblance to many features of rheumatic fever, and though micro-

organisms cannot be cultured from the joints, the patients frequently have a high antibody titer to group A hemolytic streptococci. This has suggested a tissue hypersensitivity reaction as the cause for the basic inflammatory reactions.

It was only logical that dental infection would be implicated because of the occurrence of streptococcal infection in the mouth. The "Ninth Rheumatism Review" (Hench) emphasized several points in favor of the septic foci theory of the etiology of rheumatoid arthritis. These include the following:

1. Streptococcal infections of the throat, tonsils, or nasal sinuses may precede the initial or recurrent attacks.

2. Dramatic improvement sometimes follows removal of a septic focus.

3. The pathologic and anatomic features of

lymphoid tissue in tonsillar infection, sinus infection, and root abscess suggest that toxic products can be absorbed into the circulation.

4. A temporary bacteremia may occur immediately after tonsillectomy or tooth extraction or after vigorous massage of the gums.

Against this theory are the following points:

1. Often no infectious focus can be found.

2. Usually when a focus has been extirpated, no dramatic results are produced.

3. Many persons who are in good health or are suffering from a disease other than rheumatoid arthritis may have septic foci in the same situations and of the same magnitude as patients who are suffering from rheumatoid arthritis.

4. Sulfonamides, antibiotics, and vaccines have failed to produce a beneficial effect.

The failure of removal of oral foci to result in improvement of rheumatoid arthritis has proved the wisdom of the advice of Freyberg, who stated that two conditions should govern the management of foci of infection: (1) Just as a patient without rheumatic disease should have abscessed teeth or infected tonsils removed, so should the patient with rheumatoid arthritis, and (2) by removal of such infected tissues, the patient's general health might be improved, and thereby his ability to combat the arthritis might be indirectly facilitated. He stresses that the patient should be warned that removal of such foci may not be of direct value as treatment for his arthritic disease.

Subacute bacterial endocarditis (or "infective endocarditis") can without doubt be related to oral infection, since (1) there is a close similarity in most instances between the etiologic agent of the disease and the microorganisms in the oral cavity, in the dental pulp, and in periapical lesions; (2) symptoms of subacute bacterial endocarditis have been observed in some instances shortly after extraction of teeth; and (3) transient bacteremia frequently follows tooth extraction.

This disease is generally recognized as being due to the accretion of bacterial vegetations on heart valves that are predisposed to the development of the condition, usually by rheumatic fever or congenital heart disease. Although streptococci of the viridans type once caused the majority of the subacute cases of bacterial endocarditis, the advent of the antibiotics has resulted in the drug-resistant microorganisms assuming a more important role.

Numerous studies have already been cited indicating that tooth extraction is often followed by a streptococcal bacteremia of the type usually associated with subacute bacterial endocarditis. In addition, many reports have indicated that the appearance of this form of endocarditis is sometimes preceded by tooth extraction. Elliott, for example, reported that 13 of 56 patients, or 23 per cent, gave a history of recent dental operations preceding the occurrence of infective endocarditis. Geiger noted that the beginning of subacute bacterial endocarditis among 50 patients was specifically related to tooth extraction in 12 cases. Bay reported that in a series of 26 cases of subacute bacterial endocarditis, 6 patients had had dental extraction, while Barnfield reported 6 of 92 cases to be associated with tooth extraction. In a series of 250 cases reported by Kelson and White, the predisposing cause in 1 of each 4 cases of bacterial endocarditis was found to be some dental procedure, usually tooth extraction.

The majority of cases of subacute bacterial endocarditis reported in the literature as following tooth extraction have occurred within a few weeks to a few months after the dental procedure. It is now recognized that the premedication of patients with various antibiotics will prevent the transient bacteremias that follow dental manipulations, and that this prophylactic measure is an *absolute necessity* in patients who have a past history of rheumatic fever or other evidence of known valvular damage.

Gastrointestinal diseases have been periodically related to oral foci of infection. Gastric and duodenal ulcers have reportedly been produced experimentally by the injection of streptococci. Some workers have proposed that the constant swallowing of microorganisms might lead to a variety of gastrointestinal diseases. In most instances, however, the low pH of the gastric secretions is an adequate defense against such infection.

The lack of either clinical or experimental evidence of a relation between oral foci of infection and gastrointestinal diseases suggests that such a relation is highly questionable.

Ocular diseases have often been attributed in the ophthalmologic literature to primary foci of infection such as those associated with the teeth, tonsils, sinuses, genitourinary tract, and so forth. A study was carried out by Guyton and Woods on 562 patients hospitalized with iritis, cyclitis, choroiditis, and generalized uveitis. Definite evidence of foci of infection as the etiologic factor was found in 31, or 5.5 per cent, of the patients, and presumptive evidence of the same etiologic factor in 116, or 20.6 per cent, of the patients. But when this group of patients was compared with a control group of 517 persons without uveitis, the percentages of foci of infection were almost identical. This would indicate that the role of foci of infection in this situation is questionable at the very least.

Woods evaluated the role of foci of infection in ocular disease and, as pointed out by Easlick, listed the factors supporting the hypothesis as follows:

1 Many ocular diseases occur in which no systemic cause other than the presence of remote foci of infection can be demonstrated.

2. Numerous instances of prompt and dramatic healing of ocular diseases are reported to have followed the removal of these foci.

3. Sudden transient exacerbations occasionally are observed after the removal of teeth or tonsils and often are accepted as an indication of a relationship.

4. Some reports indicate the presence of blood stream infection in the early stages of ocular disease.

5. In animal experiments iritis may be produced by the intravenous injection of microorganisms, especially streptococci.

6. Meager evidence is available that some microorganisms may have a special predilection for ocular tissue.

There are objections to these points, however, and they may be listed as follows:

1. Many otherwise healthy people can be found who have focal infection, but no ocular disease.

2. Spontaneous cures frequently occur if nothing is done.

3. The exacerbations following surgery may also be explained as simple examples of the Shwartzman phenomenon, the flaring of an inflammatory focus through absorption of nonspecific protein, or on the basis of allergic shock to specifically sensitized tissue.

4. Positive blood cultures and cultures of the aqueous humor are rare in cases of acute iritis, and few secondary infections of the uveal tract follow the common transient streptococcal or staphylococcal bacteremias in patients.

5. Although lesions do occur in the eyes of laboratory animals after intravenous injection of microorganisms, lesions also occur with equal frequency in other organs, and the eye lesions are usually purulent, only occasionally simulating the clinical lesions of the iris and uveal tract.

6. Scientific proof that ocular disease of unclear etiology may be caused by bacteria from remote foci of infection appears to be missing, and the acceptance of the conclusion must be based largely on faith; however, a strong possibility exists (on a research, not clinical basis) that sensitization to secondary metastatic products from a focus may be related to ocular disease.

Studies with ACTH and cortisone in ocular disease suggest that in many such cases the ophthalmologist may be dealing with an abnormal metabolism rather than with a reaction to a focus of infection. Scientific evidence establishing dental foci of infection as the etiologic agent in ophthalmic disease is scanty. If such a relationship does exist, the most probable mechanism is sensitization.

Skin diseases have been suggested by some dermatologists to be related to foci of infection in occasional instances. Fox and Shields discussed dermatologic lesions and stated that the 10 most common skin diseases are: (1) acne, (2) seborrheic dermatitis, (3) tinea (fungus infection of the scalp, body, groin, hands, feet, nails), (4) eczema (eczematous dermatitis, nummular eczema, infectious eczematoid dermatitis, and atopic dermatitis), (5) dermatitis venenata (eczematous contact type dermatitis, occupational dermatitis), (6) impetigo, (7) scabies, (8) urticaria, (9) psoriasis, and (10) pityriasis rosea. Of these diseases, only some forms of eczema and possibly urticaria can conceivably be related to oral foci of infection.

A few other dermatoses have been related to focus of infection, although there is little scientific proof for this association. These diseases include erythema multiforme, pustular dermatitis, lupus erythematosus, lichen planus, and pustular acrodermatitis. If the relationship does exist, the mechanism is probably sensitization rather than metastatic spread of microorganisms.

Renal diseases of certain types are sometimes blamed on foci of infection. The microorganism most commonly involved in urinary infections is *Escherichia coli*, although other staphylococci and streptococci also may be cultured. Of the streptococci, *Streptococcus hemolyticus* seems to be most common. This streptococcus is an uncommon inhabitant of dental root canals or periapical and gingival areas. Since the microorganisms commonly involved in oral infection are only infrequently involved in renal infections, it appears that there is little relation between the two and that oral foci of infection play a small role even when the possibility exists of superimposition on a damaged urinary tract.

REFERENCES

Barnfield, W. F; Subacute bacterial endocarditis and dental procedures. Am. J. Orthod. Oral Surg., 31:55, 1945.

Bauer, W. H.: Maxillary sinusitis of dental origin. Am. J. Orthod., 29:133, 1943.

Bay, E. B.: Teeth as a portal of entry for systemic disease, especially subacute bacterial endocarditis. Ann. Dent., 3:64, 1944.

Bender, I. B., and Pressman, R. S.: Factors in dental bacteremia. J. Am. Dent. Assoc., 32:836, 1945.

Berger, A.: Pterygomandibular abscess. Dent. Items Interest, 74:722, 1952.

Bransby-Zachary, G. M.: The submasseteric space. Br. Dent. J., 84:10, 1948.

Burket, L. W., and Burn, C. G.: Bacteremias following dental extractions: demonstration of source of bacteria by means of a nonpathogen (Serratia marcescens). J. Dent. Res., 16:521, 1937.

Cobe, H. M.: Transitory bacteremia. Oral Surg., 7:609, 1954.

Cogan, M. I. C.: Necrotizing mediastinitis secondary to descending cervical cellulitis. Oral Surg., 36:307, 1973.

De Leo, A. A., Schoenknecht, F. D., Anderson, M. W., and Peterson, J. C.: The incidence of bacteremia following oral prophylaxis on pediatric patients. Oral Surg., 37:36, 1974.

Dingman, R. O.: The management of acute infections of the face and jaw. Am. J. Orthod. Oral Surg., 25:780, 1939.

Doherty, J.: Ludwig's angina. J. Am. Dent. Assoc., 28:588, 1941.

Easlick, K. A. (ed.): An evaluation of the effect of dental foci of infection on health. J. Am. Dent. Assoc., 42:617, 1951.

Elliott, S. D.: Bacteraemia and oral sepsis. Proc. R. Soc. Med., 32:747, 1939.

Ennis, L. M.: Roentgenographic variations of the maxillary sinus and the nutrient canals of the maxilla and mandible. Am. J. Orthod. 23:173, 1937.

Fish, E. W., and MacLean, I.: The distribution of oral streptococci in the tissues. Br. Dent. J., 61:336, 1936.

Fox, E. C., and Shields, T. L.: Résumé of skin diseases most commonly seen in general practice. J.A.M.A., 140:763, 1949.

Fox, S. L., and West, G. B.: Thrombosis of the cavernous sinus. J.A.M.A., 134:1452, 1947.

Frankl, Z.: The submandibular and parapharyngeal spaces: their topography and importance in oral surgery. Oral Surg., 2:1131, 1270, 1949.

Freyberg, R. H.: "Focal infection" in relation to rheumatic diseases: a critical appraisal. J. Am. Dent. Assoc., 33:1101, 1946.

Geiger, A. J.: Relation of fatal subacute bacterial endocarditis to tooth extraction. J. Am. Dent. Assoc., 29:1022, 1942.

Gerrie, J. W.: The floor of the maxillary antrum. J. Am. Dent. Assoc., 22:731, 1935.

Gregory, G. T.: Infections in infratemporal fossa. J. Oral Surg., 2:19, 1944.

Grodinsky, M.: Ludwig's angina. Surgery, 5:678, 1939.

Grodinsky, M., and Holyoke, E. A.: The fascia and fascial spaces of the head, neck, and adjacent regions. Am. J. Anat., 63:367, 1938.

Guyton, J. S., and Woods, A. C.: Etiology of uveitis: a clinical study of 562 cases. Arch. Ophthalmol., 26:983, 1941.

Haymaker, W.: Fatal infections of the central nervous system and meninges after tooth extraction. Am. J. Orthod. Oral Surg., 31:117, 1945.

Hench, P. S.: Rheumatism and arthritis: review of American and English literature of recent years (ninth rheumatism review). Ann. Intern. Med., 28:66, 309, 1948.

Herd, R. H., and Hall, J. F.: Ludwig's syndrome. Oral Surg., 4:1523, 1951.

Job, T. T., and Fouser, R. H.: Relationship of the teeth to the mandibular canal and the maxillary sinus. J. Am. Dent. Assoc., 14:1072, 1927.

Jones, I. H.: Anatomy and pathology of the spread of infection from dental foci. Dent. Gazette, 9:106, 1942.

Kay, L. W.: Investigations into the nature of pericoronitis. I, II. Br. J. Oral Surg., 3:188, 4:52, 1966.

Kelson, S. R., and White, P. D.: Notes on 250 cases of subacute bacterial (streptococcal) endocarditis, studied and treated between 1927 and 1939. Ann. Intern. Med., 22:40, 1945.

Kent, H. A.: Cellulitis. Am. J. Orthod. Oral Surg., 25:172, 1939.

Krogh, H. W.: Extraction of teeth in the presence of acute infections. J. Oral Surg., 9:136, 1951.

Lazansky, J. P., Robinson, L., and Rodofsky, L.: Factors influencing the incidence of bacteremias following surgical procedures in the oral cavity. J. Dent. Res., 28:533, 1949.

Lederer, F. L., and Fishman, L. Z.: Phlegmons, including fascial sheath infections of the face and neck of dental origin. J. Am. Dent. Assoc., 27:1439, 1940.

Mazzeo, V. A.: Cavernous sinus thrombosis. J. Oral Med., 29:53, 1974.

Mitchell, D. F., and Helman, E. Z.: The role of periodontal foci of infection in systemic disease: an evaluation of the literature. J. Am. Dent. Assoc., 46:32, 1953.

Morse, F. W., Jr., and Yates, M. F.: Follow-up studies of root-filled teeth in relation to bacteriologic findings. J. Am. Dent. Assoc., 28:956, 1941.

Mustian, W. F.: The floor of the maxillary sinus and its dental, oral and nasal relations. J. Am. Dent. Assoc., 20:2175, 1933.

O'Brien, G. R., and Rubin, L. B.: One hundred and one cases of infections of the face and neck following oral pathology. Am. J. Surg., 55:102, 1942.

Okell, C. C., and Elliott, S. D.: Bacteraemia and oral sepsis, with special reference to the aetiology of subacute endocarditis. Lancet, 2:869, 1935.

Ostrander, F. D., and Crowley, M. C.: The effectiveness of clinical treatment of pulp-involved teeth as determined by bacteriological methods. J. Endodontia, 3:6, 1948.

Pace, E.: Thrombosis of the cavernous sinus. Arch. Otolaryngol., 63:216, 1941.

Richards, J. H.: Bacteremia following irritation of foci of infection. J.A.M.A., 99:1496, 1932.

Robinson, L., Kraus, F. W., Lazansky, J. P., Wheeler, R. E., Gordon, S., and Johnson, V.: Bacteremias of dental origin. I. A review of the literature. Oral Surg., 3:519, 1950.

Robinson, L., Kraus, F. W., Lazansky, J. P., Wheeler, R. E., Gordon, S., and Johnson, V.: Bacteremias of dental origin. II. A study of the factors influencing occurrence and detection. Oral Surg., 3:923, 1950.

Shapiro, H. H., Sleeper, E. L., and Guralnick, W. C.: Spread of infection of dental origin. Oral Surg., 3:1407, 1950.

Shaw, R. E.: Cavernous sinus thrombophlebitis: a review. Br. J. Surg., 40:40, 1952.

Sommer, R. F., and Crowley, M. C.: Bacteriologic verification of roentgenographic findings in pulp involved teeth. J. Am. Dent. Assoc., 27:723, 1940.

Taffel, M., and Harvey, S. C.: Ludwig's angina; analysis of 45 cases. Surgery, 11:841, 1942.

Topazian, R. G., and Goldberg, M. H.: Management of Infections of the Oral and Maxillofacial Regions. Philadelphia, W. B. Saunders Company, 1981.

Tschiassny, K.: Ludwig's angina: anatomic study of role of lower molar teeth in its pathogenesis. Am. J. Orthod. Oral Surg., 30:133, 1944.

Wakefield, B. G.: Maxillary antrum complications in exodontia. J. Oral Surg., 1:51, 1948.

White, I. L.: Postoperative parotitis-paraparotid space infection. Arch. Otolaryngol., 79:88, 1964.

Woods, A. C.: Focal infection. Am. J. Ophthalmol., 25:1423, 1942.

Zeff, S.: Some relations of the lymphatic system to surgery of the mouth and jaws. Oral Surg., 2:189, 1949.

SECTION III

INJURIES AND REPAIR

CHAPTER 10

Physical and Chemical Injuries of the Oral Cavity

INJURIES OF THE TEETH ASSOCIATED WITH REPAIR OF DENTAL CARIES

The teeth, particularly the dental pulp, may be injured not only from dental caries, but also from those procedures necessary for the repair of carious lesions. These latter injuries may be associated either with the physical methods designed for the actual preparation of the cavity by some form of cutting instrument or with the various medicaments and filling materials which are inserted in the prepared cavity.

THE EFFECT OF CAVITY PREPARATION

The effect upon the dental pulp of cavity preparation alone is difficult to assess except in the sound tooth, since the carious lesion itself produces demonstrable changes in both the dentin and the pulp. Even when cavities are prepared in sound teeth, care must be taken in observing the effects to separate those which are due solely to the cutting of the cavity from those which are due to the filling material inserted in the cavity.

Effect of Steel Bur. The reaction of the dental pulp to cutting of dentin with a dental bur has been studied by Fish in both dogs and monkeys. He had previously demonstrated by diffusion experiments that when dentin is injured, there is stasis of the contents of the dentinal tubules, which lose their fluid communication with the pulp because of the formation of secondary dentin. Calcium is also deposited in the communicating dentinal tubules, so that the involved tract of dentin is separated physiologically from the rest of the tooth.

The cavities prepared by Fish in the teeth of dogs or monkeys were cut with steel burs which were kept wet to prevent the complication of heat-induced damage to the pulp. In some cases the cavities were then filled with copper oxyphosphate cement and in other instances they were left open and exposed to the oral fluids. The animals were sacrificed after varying periods of time, and sections of the filled teeth were prepared for microscopic study. Three general reactions to cavity preparation were noted: (1) the production of secondary dentin, (2) changes in the odontoblasts associated with injured tubules, and (3) general changes in the pulp. Fish carefully pointed out that the reaction of the tooth with the formation of a calcified barrier and secondary dentin production is always strictly confined to the pulp surface of the injured tract of dentinal tubules. There is never overlap of uninjured tubules, and for this reason the changes may be regarded as a specific reaction to injury of the dentinal tubules.

The pulp reaction to superficial injury of the dentin varies in degree of severity, depending partially upon the depth of the prepared cavity and partially upon the elapsed time between cutting the cavity and extraction of the tooth for study. In mild reactions the odontoblasts become distorted and reduced in number. Small vacuoles may appear between them, probably lymph exudate. Capillaries in the damaged area may be prominent. In more severe injuries there may be complete disorganization of and hemorrhage in the odontoblastic layer (Fig. 10–1). The bulk of the pulp tissue away from the cut tubules may exhibit little or no reaction.

In more serious injuries there is a greater infiltration of the injured locus by polymor-

528

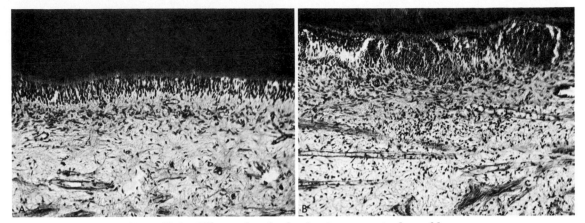

Figure 10–1. *Effect on dental pulp of cavity preparation by steel bur.*
Cavities were prepared in human teeth and filled with gutta-percha. A section of pulp from an intact normal tooth is shown in *A*, while the injured area in the pulp six days after cavity preparation is seen in *B*. (Courtesy of Drs. David F. Mitchell and J. H. Jensen: J. Am. Dent. Assoc., 55:57, 1957.)

phonuclear leukocytes, which gradually become replaced by lymphocytes. The majority of the severe pulp injuries are probably associated with irritation brought about by the open cavities, with the sudden exposure of large numbers of open dentinal tubules to oral fluids and bacteria. The findings of other investigators have generally confirmed those of Fish.

Even after such severe injuries the majority of damaged pulps undergo spontaneous healing or at least enter a quiescent phase and produce no signs or symptoms of persisting damage (Fig. 10–2). The factors responsible for the determination of the reversibility of this phenomenon, especially from the clinical aspect, are unknown.

Effect of Heat. The reaction of the dental pulp to heat is an important clinical problem because of the extraordinary amount of heat that may be generated by the revolving cutting and grinding instruments used in operative dentistry. Actually, temperatures over 700° F. have been recorded on the cutting surfaces of stones and burs under abusive conditions. This general problem has been particularly studied by Henschel and by Peyton and Vaughn.

Thermal change may be influenced by (1) the size, shape and composition of the bur or stone, (2) the speed of the bur or stone, (3) the amount and direction of pressure on the cutting instrument, (4) the amount of moisture in the field of operation, (5) the length of time that the bur or

Figure 10–2. *Effect of cavity preparation by steel bur on dental pulp.*

A calciotraumatic line (*1*) and reparative dentin (*2*) are found beneath the cavity nine weeks after preparation. (Courtesy of Drs. David F. Mitchell and J. H. Jensen: J. Am. Dent. Assoc., 55:57, 1957.)

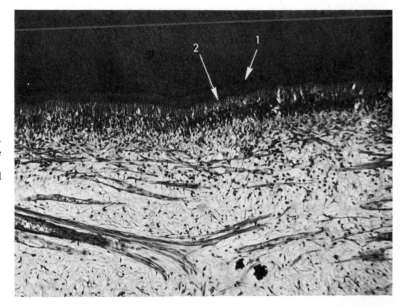

stone is in contact with the tooth, and (6) the type of tissue being cut, enamel or dentin. Of further significance is the heat generated during the setting of various filling materials, particularly the direct resins. In in vitro experiments, Wolcott and his associates showed that the temperature at the dentin-resin junction may reach 212° F., and they recorded a temperature of 133° F. in the pulp chamber.

The effects of measured temperatures on the dental pulp of dogs' teeth were studied by Lisanti and Zander after applying heat for variable periods of time and using a thermocouple inserted into the vital pulp. It was found that the application of 150° F. of heat to the base of a prepared cavity for ten seconds resulted in separation of the odontoblastic layer, edema, hyperemia, and inflammatory cell infiltration of the pulp within four hours. The application of 200° F. for one minute resulted in destruction of the odontoblasts opposite the site of the heat within four hours, as well as inflammatory reaction in the pulp. This reaction subsided within one month, and the odontoblastic layer was repaired. Similar findings were noted after applying 300° F. for ten seconds. The application of 600° F. for ten seconds resulted in extensive destruction and blister formation in the pulp, but even this severe injury healed with irregular dentin formation after two months.

It appears that dentin has a heat-dissipating action which reduces the temperature increase within the pulp to only a fraction of the actual temperature applied to the tooth. This is due to the low thermal conductivity of dentin, which acts as an effective insulating medium. Nevertheless *the application of heat to a dental pulp already injured from a carious lesion of the dentin,* but not an actual pulp exposure, *may be sufficient to affect adversely the repair or healing of the pulp* even though an apparently successful restoration is placed in the tooth. The preparation of cavities under the constant application of water to cool the cutting instrument and tooth will prevent many of the serious consequences due to heat, and this procedure is strongly recommended. For example, Swerdlow and Stanley have shown that cavity preparation by a diamond stone at 20,000 rpm and continuous water spray resulted in only mild pulpal reactions after varying intervals of time and that evidence of pulpal repair indicated an increase of recovery potential in these human teeth. In contrast, they found that identical cavity preparations without water spray resulted in extensive pulpal damage or even abscess formation.

Effect of Airbrasive Technique. In the airbrasive technique, aluminum oxide sprayed under pressure is used as an abrasive for the preparation of cavities. The effect on the dental pulp of the use of this instrument in cavity preparation has been studied in human teeth by James and her co-workers and compared to the effects produced by the conventional steel bur. The cavities were filled with gutta-percha, a fact which the investigators recognized did not permit study of the effect of cavity preparation alone on the pulp, since this filling material is an irritating agent because of imperfect sealing, pressure, and heat involved in its application. It is significant that no differences could be found in the pulpal response between the use of the steel bur and the airbrasive technique. This suggests that the *mode* of injury of the dentinal tubules and their enclosed cytoplasmic processes is not important with respect to pulpal response; only the fact that injury does occur and the degree of this injury are the deciding factors.

Effect of Ultrasonic Technique. The use of ultrasonic equipment for cutting cavities in teeth has been advocated because it involves less heat, noise, and vibration in contrast to the more conventional methods utilizing rotating instruments. Essentially, the technique consists in the conversion of electrical energy into mechanical energy in the form of vibration of a tiny cutting tip, approximately 29,000 vibrations per second with an amplitude of about 0.0014 inch. An aluminum oxide abrasive in a liquid carrier is washed across this tip, and the vibration of the particles in turn results in a rapid cutting of tooth substance.

The effects of this technique, as used in cavity preparation, on the tooth and dental pulp have been evaluated by a number of investigators whose results are in essential agreement. Zach and Brown, Healey and his co-workers, and Lefkowitz among others have found that there are no remarkable differences in the reaction of the dental pulp to the preparation of cavities by the steel bur, the diamond stone or the ultrasonic instrument. This again emphasizes that only the dentinal injury itself is important, not how this injury is produced.

Mitchell and Jensen, studying the effect of steel bur and ultrasonic cavity preparation on the human tooth, also reported that no differences could be observed in the reaction of the pulp to these two techniques. Mild hyperemia, hemorrhage and a slight neutrophilic and lymphocytic infiltration of the pulp tissue immediately below the cut dentinal tubules were noted

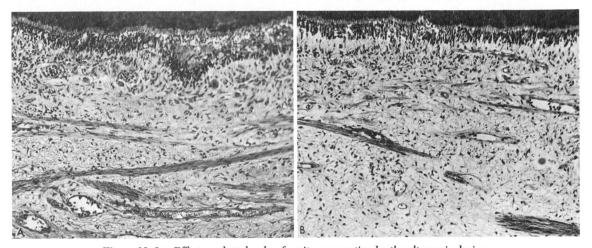

Figure 10–3. *Effect on dental pulp of cavity preparation by the ultrasonic device.*
The injured area of pulp beneath the ultrasonic cavity six days after preparation is comparable to changes occurring beneath a cavity prepared by a steel bur (A). The pulp beneath the ultrasonic cavity, twelve days after preparation, has largely recovered (B). (Courtesy of Drs. David F. Mitchell and J. H. Jensen: J. Am. Dent. Assoc., 55:57, 1957.)

during the 6- to 12-day period following cavity preparation by either means (Fig. 10–3). After several weeks the late reaction consisted in slight, irregular secondary dentin deposition and the formation of a "calciotraumatic" line, a hematoxyphilic line between the regular dentin and the postoperative dentin apparently representing a disturbance in dentin formation at the time of the operative procedure. Butt and his associates studied in the teeth of monkeys cavities that were also prepared by steel burs and by the use of ultrasonic technique. Their findings were essentially identical with those of Mitchell and Jensen in the human being.

Knapp and Bernier found similar mild reactions in the pulps of dogs' teeth after cavity preparation by an ultrasonic machine and noted no changes in either the oral soft or hard tissues from which recovery was not possible.

Effect of High-Speed Instrumentation. The development of high-speed dental engines and hand-pieces necessitated investigation of the possible effects which their use might have on pulp tissue, and numerous reports of such studies have been published.

The first complete report comparing pulp responses to conventional low-speed (6000 rpm) and high-speed (50,000 rpm) cavity preparation was that of Langeland in 1957. After cavities had been prepared in human teeth by both techniques, the teeth were extracted twenty minutes later and subsequently studied microscopically. The only change noted was odontoblastic displacement with both instruments, but even this finding was minimized if cooling by water-spray was done.

Another study of high-speed instrumentation was reported by Bernier and Knapp, utilizing various speeds up to 100,000 rpm. They found evidence of mild pulpal damage, but, in addition, observed a new type of lesion which they termed the "rebound response." This consisted variously in (1) an alteration in ground substance, (2) edema, (3) fibrosis, (4) odontoblastic disruption, and (5) reduced predentin formation in a region directly across the pulp opposite the cavity site or at a distant pulpal site, and thought to be caused by waves of energy transmitted to the pulp focused into a certain region by the pulpal walls. The significance of this phenomenon is still not clear.

Swerdlow and Stanley studied pulpal effects in human teeth in which cavities had been prepared with equipment at 150,000 rpm and found *less* severe damage than at lower speeds, even though the average thickness of dentin remaining over the pulp was less. In a subsequent study on 450 human teeth using eight operative techniques ranging up to 200,000 rpm, Stanley and Swerdlow found that speeds over 50,000 rpm with coolants were less injurious to the pulp than lower speeds. They concluded that the combination of high speed, controlled temperature and light load produced minimal pathologic pulpal alteration. When heavy loads were used, even coolants did not minimize inflammatory responses. Extending this investigation to 13 operative techniques, Diamond and his co-workers found that the 300,000 rpm air-water spray—No. 35 carbide bur technique—provided all the cutting efficiency of a high-speed instrument without producing extended or burn lesions and caused the highest incidence of reparative dentin formation, a favorable protective reaction. A speed of 250,000 rpm with water coolant was reported by Nygaard-Østby to produce even less pulpal reaction than the conventional (6000 rpm) machine without water-spray.

The practicability of use of accelerated handpiece speeds has been accurately summarized by Stanley and Swerdlow, who stated: *"In principle, high speed techniques approach the ideal but at the same time these methods can be easily abused. . . . Properly used, ultraspeed is an extremely safe and efficient method of reducing tooth structure."*

A conference of representative investigators interested in the effects of operative dentistry on the dental pulp was held at Ohio State University in 1956. It was concluded on the basis of the evidence presented that the only irreparable damage to pulps of teeth of limited growth, such as those of dogs, monkeys and human beings, under the conditions of the various experiments which have been carried out, was on human teeth subjected to the preparation of cavities by high-speed rotating instruments without a water coolant. Cavity preparations by high-speed rotating instruments using a water coolant, by ultrasonic techniques, or by airbrasive techniques produced no significant lesions in the dental pulps of dogs, monkeys or human beings.

An excellent, authoritative review of the literature dealing with the history and evaluation of the many forms of cavity preparation, compiled at the request of the Council on Dental Research of the American Dental Association, was reported by Stanley, and every practitioner of dentistry should be thoroughly familiar with these studies. Stanley has also detailed the methods and criteria to be used in the evaluation of future dentin and pulp response investigations.

The Effect of Filling Materials

The dentist has at his disposal a great many materials prepared commercially for insertion into cavities to restore the original contour of the tooth attacked by dental caries. Furthermore, new materials are constantly becoming available to make the choice even greater. The dentist must be familiar with the advantages and disadvantages of each material from the point of view of its physical properties and its

ability to fulfill the purpose for which it is intended. In addition, he must be acquainted with the biologic effects of the filling material on the tooth, especially on the dental pulp. The reader is referred to the textbook on dental materials by Phillips for a current and in-depth discussion of these materials, including their biologic properties and effects on tissues.

A great many experimental studies have been carried out to investigate the effects of the different filling materials on the dental pulp, and today such testing is routine before new filling materials are released by ethical manufacturers for use by dentists. It should be obvious that a filling material inserted into a prepared cavity is in contact with more than just a block of inert calcified material. The dentinal tubules, containing odontoblastic processes which have been freshly cut, form a series of passageways leading directly to the dental pulp through which a fluid or soluble material may reach the pulp tissue. If this material is irritating, it may lead to serious injury. For this reason a comparison of the effects of the various common filling materials is important.

Much of the experimental work has been carried out on laboratory animals because of the inordinately greater possibility of accurately controlling experimental factors and of obtaining specimens in large numbers. Since most human teeth are carious before restorations are placed, it is difficult to separate the effect of the filling material from that of the carious lesion. Using sound teeth in experimental animals eliminates this complication, but presents another: the difficulty of separating and evaluating pulpal responses to the filling material from those responses due to cavity preparation alone.

Zinc Phosphate (Oxyphosphate) Cement. This particular cement is widely used in dentistry both as a protective base in deep cavities before the insertion of the restoration and also in cementing cast inlays, crowns, and other similar restorations. The majority of investigators have reported significant deleterious effects on the pulp when the material is placed in cavities, the actual injurious agent supposedly being the phosphoric acid.

Gurley and Van Huysen prepared cavities in teeth of young dogs and filled them with zinc phosphate cement. After approximately 1½ months they found hyperemia and inflammatory cell infiltration of the pulp with disarrangement of the odontoblastic layer. Secondary dentin had formed under the shallower cavities. The more severe pulpal reactions occurred under the deeper cavities. Similar findings were reported in Lefkowitz, Seelig and Zachinsky in monkeys.

Studies on human teeth, such as those by Manley, by Shroff and by Kramer and McLean, show that hyperemia or hemorrhage with inflammatory cell infiltration of the pulp accompanied by reduction in the size and number of the odontoblasts occurs after placement of this cement in prepared cavities.

The studies generally indicate that zinc oxyphosphate cement is an irritant when placed in the base of a deep cavity, particularly in bulk, although the human pulp may be able to localize this reaction in most instances. When this cement is used in shallow cavities, it is relatively innocuous and reportedly serves a useful function in the stimulation of secondary dentin formation.

Silicate Cement. The silicate cement is generally considered to be an extremely injurious filling material, but it is still widely used in the dental profession. It finds particular use in restoration of proximal cavities in anterior teeth, but here death of the pulp with subsequent darkening of the tooth is most distressing.

Palazzi in 1923 and Fasoli in 1924 first demonstrated severe pulp damage attendant to placing silicate cement in a prepared cavity. Subsequent studies by Manley and by Zander and his co-workers on dogs showed that this cement, when placed in a prepared cavity, invoked an intense inflammatory reaction of the pulp with hyperemia, destruction of odontoblasts and even formation of pulp abscesses in some cases.

Studies on human beings by Manley, Shroff, Zander and his associates and Lefkowitz and his co-workers are in essential agreement on the serious damage to the pulp brought about by silicate cement. In these human investigations a mild to severe pulpitis with varying degrees of degeneration, necrosis and destruction of odontoblasts was found and was particularly severe under deep cavity preparations restored with the silicate. A cavity liner of varnish was found to be of no benefit in preventing these changes. Dachi and his co-workers have reported that prednisolone, topically applied to the cavity preparation prior to the insertion of a silicate cement restoration, was more effective in reducing thermal sensitivity and resulted in a milder inflammatory pulp reaction than an inert placebo.

The phosphoric acid is reputedly the injurious agent in the silicate cement. It differs in reaction from that of the zinc phosphate cement only because of the mixing technique, which allows more free acid in the silicate.

Copper Cement. This cement has been used widely, especially as a temporary filling material in children's teeth, because of its supposed but exaggerated germicidal property. Like the other cements, it also produces severe pulp damage.

Fish, Manley, and Gurley and Van Huysen have all reported that copper cement placed in prepared cavities of teeth of dogs, monkeys, and human beings produced inflammatory cell infiltration, hemorrhage, and necrosis with destruction of odontoblasts in the pulp. This was particularly notable under deep cavities.

It has been suggested that the severe effects of the copper cements, both red and black, on the dental pulp may be due to the soluble copper ions which are dissolved in the acid, since heavy metals are deleterious to most tissues.

Amalgam. Amalgam is the filling material most widely used in dentistry. Despite this, there are few studies available dealing with the effect of this substance on the dental pulp.

The investigations of Manley and of Shroff in both dogs and human beings have suggested that amalgam is an innocuous material, particularly in shallow cavities. Beneath deep cavities filled with amalgam Manley found a decrease in the number of odontoblasts, as well as mild inflammatory cell infiltration of the pulp. The complication of thermal shock transmitted by deep amalgam restorations is difficult to evaluate, but is a source of potential damage.

In contrast, Swerdlow and Stanley studied the pulpal responses in 73 intact human teeth with cavities prepared at speeds of 20,000 to 300,000 rpm and filled with either amalgam or zinc oxide and eugenol. They reported that the amalgam increased the intensity of mild pulpal response to cavity preparation and that this appeared to be due, in part at least, to the mechanical aspects of amalgam condensation. Brännström studied the effect of amalgam restorations on pulp tissue and concluded that any damage to the pulp was due to leakage around the restoration, not to the filling material itself. Dachi and his co-workers have found that the topical application of prednisolone to cavity preparations, preceding the placement of silver amalgam restorations, was more effective in reducing thermal sensitivity and resulted in a slightly milder inflammatory reaction in the pulp than an inert placebo.

Gutta-percha. Gutta-percha is used extensively as a temporary filling material because of its ease of manipulation and its stability. But Gurley and Van Huysen showed that placing gutta-percha in prepared cavities of dogs' teeth resulted in a chronic productive inflammation. Similar results have been noted in human teeth by Rovelstad and St. John and by James and co-workers.

The mode of action of gutta-percha is probably not a chemical one, since the material is inert. Because it is necessary to heat gutta-percha in order to insert it into the cavity, it is possible that the pulp reaction is a thermal injury. Furthermore, gutta-percha provides a poor seal of the cavity margins, and the leakage of saliva and bacteria may contribute to the irritation of the pulp. These qualities suggest that gutta-percha is not a satisfactory temporary filling material.

Zinc Oxide and Eugenol. There is almost universal agreement that zinc oxide and eugenol is the least injurious of all filling materials to the dental pulp. Not only is there no irritation produced by this substance, but actually it exerts a palliative and sedative effect on the mildly damaged pulp. It seems to be such a bland substance that it may lack even the necessary irritating properties requisite to the stimulation of secondary dentin formation.

Manley, Gurley and Van Huysen, and Zander have specifically emphasized the innocuous nature of zinc oxide and eugenol when placed in prepared cavities of both dog and human teeth. In addition, Shroff and Kramer and McLean showed that zinc oxide and eugenol, when used as a base, protects the dental pulp against the irritating action of silicate cement and self-curing resins. In view of these findings, zinc oxide and eugenol is the material of choice for use over injured pulps or as a base in deep cavity preparations.

Self-Polymerizing Acrylic Resin. Self-curing resins are extensively used as filling materials, particularly in anterior teeth, because of certain properties, chiefly physical, which render them superior to silicate cements. There is evidence to indicate, however, that these resins may cause serious damage to the dental pulp. Still, not all investigations are in complete agreement.

Lefkowitz and his associates, working with monkeys, as well as Zander and Coy and his co-workers, working on dogs, demonstrated a mild inflammatory reaction of the pulp after insertion of self-curing resins in prepared cavities of teeth. Numerous studies on the teeth of

human beings have also been carried out, such as those of Kramer and McLean and of Nygaard-Østby. The results generally indicated that these resins provoked odontoblastic damage and inflammatory cell infiltration of the pulp which was more severe under the deeper cavities. Pulp necrosis was a variable finding. Grossman, on the basis of clinical observation alone, reported four times as many pulpal deaths under acrylic resin restorations as under silicate cements.

It has been suggested that the injurious agent of the resin is the monomer. But since all acrylic resins undergo remarkable shrinkage and thus exhibit leakage of the margins of the restorations, it is equally plausible that the saliva and bacteria which penetrate along the marginal defect may be responsible for the pulp reaction. Kramer reported that acrylic resins containing methacrylic acid result in the formation of edema-blisters of the pulp. Most investigators believe that some cavity-lining material is desirable before placement of a self-polymerizing acrylic resin as an aid in preventing pulp damage.

Conventional Composite Resins. These are restorative materials developed chiefly because methyl methacrylate or unfilled acrylic resins have restrictive characteristics such as low hardness and strength, a high coefficient of thermal expansion and a lack of adhesion to tooth structure. The resin matrix is a compromise between epoxy and methacrylate resins. This resin is combined with a filler of dispersed particles of varying types in relatively high concentration. While most conventional composite resins are chemically activated, some are now marketed whose cure is based on light activation.

The biologic properties of the composite resins show the same irritational characteristics as the unfilled acrylic resins. For this reason, the same measures should be taken to protect the pulp from possible injury, especially when the cavity preparation is deep. A calcium hydroxide base is preferable to a zinc oxide and eugenol base because of the possible interaction of eugenol and resin.

Microfilled Composite Resins. These are a newer group of resins which contain the same resin matrix as the conventional composite resins but differ in that the size of the filler is much smaller than in the conventional resin. The diameter of the filler particles in the conventional resin averages about 500 times greater than that of particles in the microfilled resin.

The biologic properties of the microfilled

resins, including their irritational effects on the pulp, are comparable to those of the conventional composite resins. Thus, some pulpal protection is necessary under deep cavities.

———————

The many experimental studies cited would indicate superficially that the majority of cavity-filling materials used in dentistry today are dangerous because of the serious effects on the dental pulp which they often induce. It is true that many of these materials are potentially injurious. Nevertheless, literally millions of restorations with these substances are placed each year, and clinical experience has shown that, unless actual pulp exposure has occurred, the death rate of dental pulps directly attributable to the filling material is extremely low. Even the occurrence of clinical symptoms of pulp injury is uncommon. Although this seems contradictory to experimental evidence, it should be appreciated that most cavities prepared by the dentist in which these materials are inserted are to repair a destructive carious lesion. The presence of this carious lesion, in contrast to the experimental cavities prepared in sound human and animal teeth, has usually induced the deposition of secondary dentin and has caused a certain amount of dentinal sclerosis, and these reactions offer considerable protection to the pulp. It is on this basis that the dentist is justified in continuing to use these filling materials. There is a need, however, for continued study of this general problem.

The Effect of Cement Bases, Cavity Liners, Varnishes and Primers

A variety of materials commonly used in dental practice are inserted in a cavity preparation between the tooth and the restoration. These are generally used for one or more of the following purposes: (1) to serve as a bacteriostatic agent; (2) to provide thermal insulation, particularly under metallic restorations; (3) to provide electrical insulation under metallic restorations; (4) to prevent discoloration of tooth structure adjacent to certain types of restorative materials; (5) to prevent the penetration of deleterious constituents of restorative materials into the dentin and pulp; and (6) to improve the marginal seal of certain restorative materials by preventing microleakage and the ingress of saliva and debris along the tooth-restoration interface. These materials, reviewed in detail by Going, are generally classified as cement bases, cavity liners, cavity varnishes and cavity primers, and they are important because of their possible effects on the dental pulp.

Cement Bases. A cement base is a layer of cement commonly used beneath a permanent dental restoration either to encourage recovery of the injured pulp or to protect the pulp against the injuries just described. Intermediary base materials that are commonly used under permanent restorations include zinc phosphate cement, zinc oxide-eugenol cement and calcium hydroxide cement. Ideally, a cement base should be biologically compatible with the dental pulp and such is the case with zinc oxide-eugenol and calcium hydroxide. However, zinc phosphate cement, when placed against dentin, acts as an irritant to the dental pulp because of the acid content which varies between pH 3.5 and 6.6, as discussed previously.

Polycarboxylate or polyacrylate cements are a newer type of material which have properties comparable to those of the phosphate cements, but have a low degree of pulpal irritation similar to that of the zinc oxide-eugenol cements.

Glass ionomer cements are polyacrylate based and are similarly biocompatible materials. No agent is required in deep cavities for protection of the pulp. Furthermore, they appear to have some anticariogenic properties, and with their use the acid solubility of enamel in contact with the cement is reduced.

It is generally agreed that if the cavity depth is shallow, with 2.0 mm. or more of primary dentin remaining between the floor of the cavity preparation and the dental pulp, dentin probably provides its own insulation against traumatic, thermal or restorative material irritation. However, if the remaining thickness of primary dentin is less than 2.0 mm., it is necessary that a cement base of one type or another be utilized.

Cavity Liners. Cavity liners are aqueous or volatile organic liquid suspensions or dispersions of zinc oxide or calcium hydroxide that can be applied in a relatively thin film to the surface of a cavity. They may also be solutions of resins in an organic solvent to which have been added calcium hydroxide or zinc oxide, or aqueous suspensions of calcium hydroxide in methylcellulose. The cavity liner provides the beneficial effects of zinc oxide and calcium hydroxide as thin films in shallow cavities and, in addition, neutralizes the free acid of zinc phosphate and silicate cements. The cavity liners themselves have no effect on dental pulp and, in fact, actually form a chemical barrier to provide reliable protection for the pulp under certain deep restorations.

Stanley has compared the protective effect of reparative dentin with man-made cavity liners and bases, and generally concluded that: (1) pulpal tissue beneath preoperatively formed reparative dentin is safe from most subsequent procedures; (2) cavity liners and/or bases, should be employed since the completeness of the reparative dentin barrier cannot be ascertained; (3) the unrestored tooth being utilized as an abutment lacks reparative dentin and is more subject to the damaging effects of chemical agents because of patent dentinal tubules; (4) although 2.0 mm. of primary dentin between the floor of the cavity preparation and the dental pulp is usually a sufficient protective barrier, the condensation of amalgam or gold foil, as well as the chemical irritation of cements and self-curing resins, may render this thickness of protection insufficient; (5) age changes in the tooth, with the production of reparative dentin in the involved area, are of no recognizable benefit regarding pulp protection; (6) high-speed, water-cooled cutting techniques produce an average incidence of reparative dentin formation of under 20 per cent; even less reparative dentin formation is produced if more than 1 mm. of primary dentin remains beneath the cavity preparation; (7) if reparative dentin does not form within the first 50 days following a restorative procedure, then there will be none; (8) nearly 20 postoperative days are required for new odontoblasts to differentiate and produce reparative dentin, and it has been shown that an average of 100 productive days of matrix formation is required to produce a reparative dentin barrier of 0.15 mm.; (9) final cementation of restorations need not be delayed in allowing time for reparative dentin to form, since the use of cavity-lining materials is a reasonable substitute; and (10) cavity varnish and calcium hydroxide lining materials appear capable of protecting dental pulp if used appropriately.

Cavity Varnishes. Cavity varnishes are solutions of one or more resins from natural gums, synthetic resins and rosin in organic solvents. It is generally agreed that varnishes may be of aid in reducing postoperative sensitivity, but their film thickness is insufficient to provide thermal insulation. This film also acts as a semipermeable membrane so that certain types of ions penetrate it while others do not. It has been found also that varnishes are effective in reducing the microleakage of fluids around the margins of restorations. For example, Brännström and Söremark have reported that a cavity varnish either prevented or greatly reduced the penetration of Na^{22}-labeled saline around amalgam restorations, compared to uninsulated controls.

While cavity varnishes themselves appear to have no significant effect upon a dental pulp, neither do they have a sedative effect. Therefore, in deep restorations, it may be advisable to utilize calcium hydroxide or zinc oxide-eugenol cements first, then apply the varnish over this base.

Cavity Primers. Cavity primers are materials which are placed in a cavity preparation to increase the adaptation of methyl methacrylate filling materials to cavity walls and to aid in producing a marginal seal. The effect of cavity primers on dental pulp has not been widely tested.

THE EFFECT OF CAVITY-STERILIZING AGENTS

Cavity-sterilizing agents are frequently used as a final step in routine cavity preparation and also in an attempt to sterilize discolored, infected dentin in the base of deep carious lesions when this dentin cannot be completely removed without risk of pulp exposure. It has been suggested that cavity sterilization is unnecessary, since microorganisms persisting in the dentinal tubules after a restoration has been placed do not flourish but, rather, die or exist in an inactive state. Furthermore, should the dentin be carious so near the pulp that exposure is feared were it all to be removed, the pulp tissue by this time would almost certainly have become infected, and attempts at sterilization would be worthless.

The studies of Kraus and of Besic showed that bacteria may die out under restorations, but only if the cavity is hermetically sealed by the filling material. Since such a seal is almost impossible to attain even with present-day materials, one must admit that though a cavity is sterilized at the time of preparation, it cannot long remain sterile after placement of the restoration. In this regard, Armstrong and Simon showed that all the commonly used filling materials are poorly adapted to cavity margins and allow penetration of ions there. They prepared cavities in teeth, restored these with amalgam, gold foil, gold inlay, zinc oxyphosphate cement, silicate cement and acrylic resin, and soaked these teeth in a solution of radioactive calcium, Ca⁴⁵, for 48 hours. After the preparation of radioautographs, the radiocalcium was found to have penetrated the margins of all the filling materials used but in somewhat varying amounts (Fig. 10–4). On the basis of these findings, the soundness of the principles of cavity sterilization may be questioned.

The efficacy of sterilizing agents has also been questioned, since it would depend upon pene-

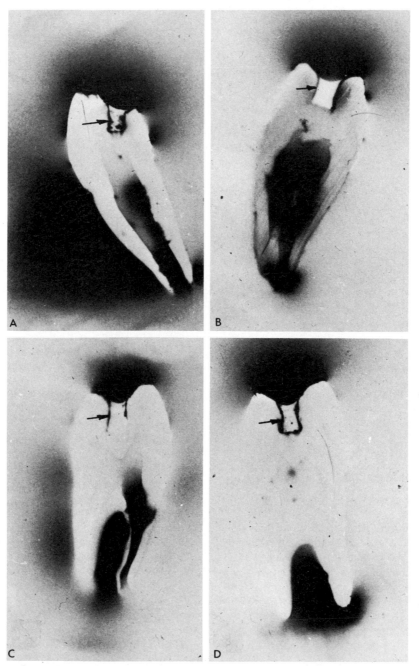

Figure 10–4. Radioautographs of typical examples of microleakage, as shown by penetration of radioactive calcium (Ca⁴⁵), with four different restorative materials: amalgam (A), gold inlay (B), gold foil (C) and self-cured resin (D). The penetration can be seen as a black line around the wall of the cavity preparations. Although the results of these studies in vitro cannot be directly transferred to the clinical restoration, it is probable that a certain amount of leakage does occur in vivo with most restorations. (Courtesy of Prof. Ralph W. Phillips and Marjorie L. Swartz.)

tration of the dentinal tubules to destroy the microorganisms. Numerous studies have been carried out on a wide variety of antibacterial agents used in cavity sterilization, including alcohol, phenol, silver nitrate, Metaphen, beechwood creosote, thymol, iodine solution, chlorphenol and hexylresorcinol. The results generally indicate that when these compounds are applied to the floor of a cavity for the usually accepted time, two to three minutes, there is only surface sterilization of the dentin. It has been demonstrated that in order to sterilize dentin, the agent must be sealed in the cavity for 24 to 48 hours.

Since practically all materials studied show little tubular penetration after their application for purposes of sterilization, it might be predicted that the dental pulp usually escapes injury after their use. This is actually the case. Thomas and Kramer and McLean have reported essentially no effect on the dental pulp in the human being after the application of phenol to prepared cavities. The essential oils also were reported by Barker and by Hardwick to be without effect on the dental pulp. The use of silver nitrate in cavity sterilization has been reported by Barker, Hardwick, and Zander and his co-workers to cause little serious damage to the dental pulp. It should be obvious, however, that any such chemical sterilizing agent, if applied to the base of deep cavities, may cause damage to the pulp if there is insufficient dentin between the floor of the cavity and the pulp to prevent its shallow penetration.

PHYSICAL INJURIES OF THE TEETH

BRUXISM

("Night-grinding"; Bruxomania)

Bruxism is the habitual grinding of the teeth, either during sleep or as an unconscious habit during waking hours. This term is generally applied both to the clenching habit, during which pressure is exerted on the teeth and periodontium by the actual grinding or clamping of the teeth, and also to the repeated tapping of the teeth. The incidence of bruxism has been variously reported as between 5 per cent and 20 per cent.

Etiology. In a review of the subject by Nadler, and more recently by Meklas, the causes of bruxism have been described as (1) local, (2) systemic, (3) psychologic, and (4) occupational.

Local factors are generally associated with some form of mild occlusal disturbance which produces mild discomfort and chronic, even though unrecognized, tension. It has been suggested that in many cases bruxism becomes a firm habit as a result of an unconscious attempt by the patient to establish a greater number of teeth in contact or to counteract a local irritating situation. In children the habit is frequently associated with the transition from the deciduous to the permanent dentition and may result from an unconscious attempt to place the individual tooth planes so that the musculature will be at rest.

Systemic factors have been proposed as etiologically significant, but the role of most of these is difficult to assess. Gastrointestinal disturbances, subclinical nutritional deficiencies, and allergy or endocrine disturbances have all been reported as causative factors. A hereditary background has been described in some cases.

Psychologic factors are believed by some investigators to be the most common cause of bruxism. Emotional tension may be expressed through a number of nervous habits, one of which may be bruxism. Thus, when a person suffers from fear, rage, rejection or a variety of other emotions which he is unable to express, these become hidden in the subconscious but are expressed periodically by numerous means. It has been observed that bruxism is common in mental institutions. Bruxism is a manifestation of nervous tension in children also and may be related to chronic biting or chewing of toys.

Occupations of certain types favor the development of this habit. Athletes engaged in physical activities often develop bruxism, although the exact reason for this is uncertain. Occupations in which the work must be unusually precise, such as that of the watchmaker, are prone to cause bruxism. Voluntary bruxism is also recognized in those persons who habitually chew gum, tobacco or objects such as toothpicks or pencils. Although voluntary, this too is a nervous reaction and may lead eventually to involuntary or subconscious bruxism.

Clinical Features. The person who engages in bruxism performs the typical grinding or clenching motions during sleep or subconsciously when awake. These may be associated with a grinding or grating noise. The symptomatic effects of this habit have been reviewed by Glaros and Rao, who have divided them into six major categories: (1) effects on the dentition, (2) effects on the periodontium, (3) effects on the masticatory muscles, (4) effects on the temporomandibular joint, (5) head pain, and (6) psychologic and behavioral effects.

When the habit is firmly established, severe wearing or attrition of the teeth may occur, not only occlusal wear, but also interproximal wear. On both surfaces actual facets may be worn in the teeth.

As the bruxism continues, there may be loss of integrity of the periodontal structures, resulting in loosening or drifting of teeth or even gingival recession with alveolar bone loss. Temporomandibular joint disturbances are also reported to occur as a result of the traumatic injury of continuous tooth impact without normal periods of rest. Hypertrophy of the masticatory muscles, particularly the masseter muscle, may interfere with maintenance of the rest position, cause trismus, and alter occlusion and the opening and closing pattern of the jaws.

Finally, while it has been suggested that bruxism may give rise to facial pain and headache as well as psychologic and behavioral effects, these are very difficult manifestations to evaluate and correlate. Although such assumptions may prove founded, substantiation awaits further research.

Treatment and Prognosis. If the underlying cause of the bruxism is an emotional one, the nervous factor must be corrected if the disease is to be cured. Removable splints to be worn at night may be constructed to immobilize the jaws or to guide the movement so that periodontal damage is minimal. If the disease is left untreated, severe periodontal and/or temporomandibular disturbances may result.

FRACTURES OF TEETH

Tooth fracture is a common injury which may arise in a variety of situations, the most frequent of which is sudden severe trauma. This is usually a fall, a blow, an automobile accident or any of a large number of incidents in which children especially are frequently involved. Some cases of fracture occur when a tooth is weakened as by a large restoration, leaving thin walls or unsupported cusps which give way under the stress of mastication. A similar weakening and subsequent fracture occur also in cases of internal resorption of teeth. Teeth which have had root canal therapy are often described as being somewhat brittle and susceptible to fracture. The etiology and pathogenesis of these traumatic dental injuries have been discussed by Andreasen.

Clinical Features. Although fracture of teeth may occur at any age, children are especially prone to sustain this type of injury. The prevalence of tooth fracture is difficult to assess or evaluate, particularly since minor chipping of teeth is common. Some studies indicate that among large groups of children up to 5 per cent may show such injuries. A study by Schützmannsky reported that 13 per cent of examined schoolchildren, at the age of 18 years, had been exposed to dental injuries during adolescence. As might be expected, boys are more frequently involved than girls. There is a definite predilection for involvement of maxillary teeth, with between 75 and 90 per cent of fractures occurring there (Fig. 10–5).

There are several classifications of fractured teeth, the simplest being only whether or not the fracture line involves the pulp. A more detailed classification is that of Ellis, who divides all traumatized anterior teeth (for these constitute the vast majority of such injuries) into nine classes:

Class 1. Simple fracture of the crown, involving little or no dentin.

Class 2. Extensive fracture of the crown, involving considerable dentin but not the dental pulp.

Class 3. Extensive fracture of the crown, involving considerable dentin and exposing the dental pulp.

Class 4. The traumatized tooth becomes nonvital, with or without loss of crown structure.

Class 5. Teeth lost as a result of trauma.

Class 6. Fracture of the root, with or without loss of crown structure.

Class 7. Displacement of a tooth, without fracture of crown or root.

Class 8. Fracture of the crown en masse and its replacement.

Class 9. Traumatic injuries to deciduous teeth.

The clinical manifestation as well as the treatment and prognosis of the fractured tooth depend chiefly upon whether the dental pulp is pierced by the fracture and whether the crown or the root of the tooth is involved. If there is crown fracture without pulp involvement, vitality of the tooth is usually maintained, although there may be mild pulp hyperemia even when the overlying dentin is relatively thick. If the dentin over the pulp is exceedingly thin, bacteria may penetrate the dentinal tubules, infect the pulp and produce pulpitis, leading to death of the pulp. When vitality is maintained, usually a layer of secondary dentin is deposited over the involved dentinal tubules. The tooth may be sore and slightly loose because of the traumatic injury, but severe pain is usually absent.

A fractured tooth crown which exposes the pulp is a more serious problem, but pulp exposure does not necessarily imply that death of

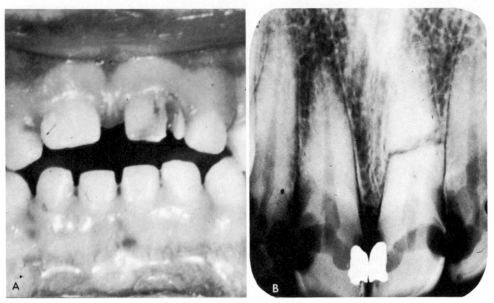

Figure 10–5. *Fractured teeth after traumatic injury.*
A, Fracture of crown with pulp exposure; B, root fracture.

the pulp will occur. In some cases the exposure can be capped by calcium hydroxide, and a dentinal bridge will form as a part of the healing reaction. Pulpotomy or pulpectomy may often be necessary, however, since the pulp becomes infected almost immediately after the injury.

Root fractures are somewhat uncommon in young children, since their tooth roots are not completely formed and the teeth have some resilience in their sockets. When fracture does occur, the tooth is loose and sore and there may be displacement of the coronal portion of the tooth.

Histologic Features. Healing in such cases may be of several types. The most satisfactory form of healing is the union of the two fragments by calcified tissue, and this is analogous to the healing of a bony fracture. The clot between the root fragments is organized, and this connective tissue is subsequently the site of new cementum or bone formation. There is nearly always some resorption of the ends of the fragments, but these resorption lacunae ultimately are repaired. If the apposition between the two fragments is not close, the union is by connective tissue alone. It appears likely that the repair process can be organized from connective tissue cells in both the pulp and the periodontal ligament. The root fracture and its repair were discussed at length by Pindborg, who also reviewed the literature, and by Andreasen and Hjørting-Hansen.

TOOTH ANKYLOSIS

Ankylosis between tooth and bone is an uncommon phenomenon in the deciduous dentition and even more rare in permanent teeth. The condition of deciduous tooth ankylosis ("submerged" tooth) has been described in Chapter 1.

Ankylosis ensues when partial root resorption is followed by repair with either cementum or bone that unites the tooth root with the alveolar bone. It must not be inferred that root resorption invariably leads to ankylosis. Actually, it is an uncommon sequela, and the cause for this sporadic happening is unknown. Ankylosis does occur rather frequently after a traumatic injury to a tooth, particularly occlusal trauma, but it is also seen as a result of periapical inflammation subsequent to pulp infection. Periapical inflammation is a well-recognized cause of root resorption. Ankylosis sometimes also follows root canal therapy if the apical periodontal ligament is irritated or seriously damaged.

Clinical Features. Ankylosis of the permanent tooth seldom manifests clinical symptoms unless there is a concomitant pulp infection which may be the underlying cause. If there is an extensive area of the root surface involved, the tooth may give a dull, muffled sound on percussion rather than the normal sharp sound. The fact that this condition exists may become apparent only at the time of extraction of the tooth, when considerable difficulty will be encountered, sometimes necessitating surgical removal.

Roentgenographic Features. If the area of ankylosis is of sufficient size, it may be visible on the roentgenogram as a loss of the normal thin radiolucent line that represents the periodontal ligament, with a mild sclerosis of the bone and apparent blending of the bone with the tooth root.

Histologic Features. Microscopic examination reveals an area of root resorption which has been repaired by a calcified material, bone or cementum, which is continuous with the alveolar bone. The periodontal ligament is completely obliterated in the area of the ankylosis (Fig. 10–6).

Treatment and Prognosis. There is no treatment for ankylosis, although any infection present should be treated by appropriate measures. Ankylosed teeth have a good prognosis and, unless removed for some other reason, should serve well indefinitely.

PHYSICAL INJURIES OF THE BONE

TRAUMATIC CYST

(Solitary Bone Cyst; Hemorrhagic Cyst; Extravasation Cyst; Unicameral Bone Cyst; Simple Bone Cyst; Idiopathic Bone Cavity)

The traumatic cyst is an unusual lesion which occurs with considerable frequency in the jaws as well as in other bones of the skeleton. The term "cyst" is actually a misnomer, since these intrabony cavities are not lined by epithelium.

Etiology. The etiology of the solitary bone cyst is unknown, although a number of theories have been proposed and at least one has been rather widely accepted. Howe and also Sieverink have carried out extensive reviews of the literature and pointed out the wide acceptance of the theory of origin from intramedullary hemorrhage following traumatic injury. Hemorrhage occurring within the medullary spaces of bone after trauma heals in most cases by organization of the clot and eventual formation of connective tissue and new bone. According to the traumatic theory, however, it is suggested that after injury to an area of spongy bone containing hemopoietic marrow enclosed by a layer of dense cortical bone, there is failure of organization of the blood clot and, for some unexplained reason, subsequent degeneration

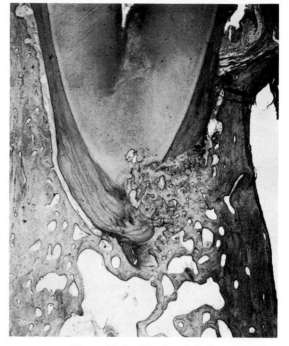

Figure 10–6. *Tooth ankylosis.*
Resorption of a portion of the root with repair unites the root and alveolar bone.

of the clot that eventually produces an empty cavity within the bone. In the development of the lesion, the trabeculae of bone in the involved area become necrotic after degeneration of the clot and the bone marrow, although some viable marrow tissue must persist to initiate resorption of the involved trabeculae. The lesion then appears to increase in size by a steady expansion produced by a progressive infiltrating edema on the basis of restriction of venous drainage. This expansion tends to cease when the cystlike lesion reaches the cortical layer of bone, so that expansion of the involved bone is not a common finding in the solitary bone cyst. It is not at all unusual, however, for the patient to be unable to recall any traumatic injury to the jaw. This may indicate that an injury so mild that the patient would not be aware of it or remember it is sufficient to cause this lesion to develop. In the series reported by Howe, only slightly over 50 per cent of the patients gave a history of trauma, the time lag between injury and discovery of the lesion varying from one month to 20 years. However, the frequency with which a history of trauma may be elicited varies remarkably between different series of cases. For example, in a group of 30 cases of traumatic cyst of the jaws reported by Beasley, only 27 per cent of the patients gave a history of trauma, while in a series of 66 cases reported by Hansen and his co-workers, approximately 80 per cent of the patients indicated a preceding traumatic episode.

Other theories of origin, reviewed by Whinery, have included (1) origin from bone tumors that have undergone cystic degeneration, (2) a result of faulty calcium metabolism such as that induced by parathyroid disease, (3) origin from necrosis of fatty marrow due to ischemia, (4) the end result of a low-grade chronic infection, and finally (5) a result of osteoclasis resulting from a disturbed circulation caused by trauma creating an unequal balance of osteoclasis and repair of bone.

Clinical Features. The traumatic cyst occurs most frequently in young persons, the median age being 18 years in a series of 45 cases reviewed and reported by Gardner and Stoller. According to Howe, over 75 per cent of cases occur in the second decade of life. Males are affected somewhat more frequently, probably because they are exposed to traumatic injuries more often than females, the ratio being about 3:2. Although it has been stated that the posterior portion of the mandible is more commonly involved than the anterior, numerous cases have been reported in the incisor region, since in the young person this area contains hemopoietic marrow. The maxilla has been known to develop the solitary bone cyst, but only on extremely rare occasions. Surprisingly, in the series reported by Hansen and his associates approximately 32 per cent of the lesions were in the maxilla. In some cases enlargement of the mandible has been observed, but often

the lesion is discovered during routine roentgenographic examination of the patient. For example, in the series of Howe, only 35 per cent of cases showed expansion, and this was the most common complaint causing patients to seek treatment. In the majority of cases the pulps of the teeth in the involved area are vital, and this is important to ascertain, because the vital teeth should not be sacrificed. When the cavity is opened surgically, it is found to contain either a small amount of straw-colored fluid, shreds of necrotic blood clot, fragments of fibrous connective tissue or nothing. The dentist is frequently astonished to open into an empty space in bone and find that it has no clinically demonstrable membrane. It was reported by Toller in one case that the hydrostatic intracystic pressure was exceptionally low and comparable with capillary pressure, quite unlike that in other cysts of the jaw.

Roentgenographic Features. Roentgenographic examination usually reveals a rather smoothly outlined radiolucent area of variable size, sometimes with a thin sclerotic border, depending upon the duration of the lesion. Some traumatic cysts may measure only a centimeter in diameter (Fig. 10–7), whereas others may be so large that they involve most of the molar area of the body of the mandible as well as part of the ramus. When the radiolucency appears to involve the roots of the teeth, the cavity may have a lobulated or scalloped appearance extending between the roots of these teeth (Fig. 10–8). Seldom is there any displacement of teeth and, in many cases, the lamina dura will appear intact.

Care must be taken to differentiate the small

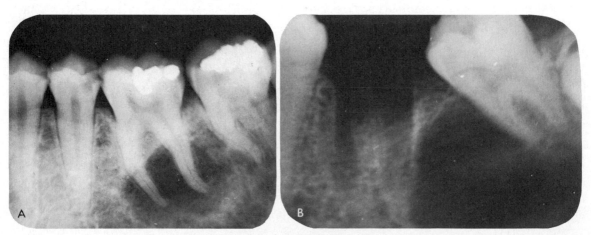

Figure 10–7. *Traumatic bone cyst.*
The radiolucent area in both cases was entirely empty and devoid of any lining. The molar teeth were vital.

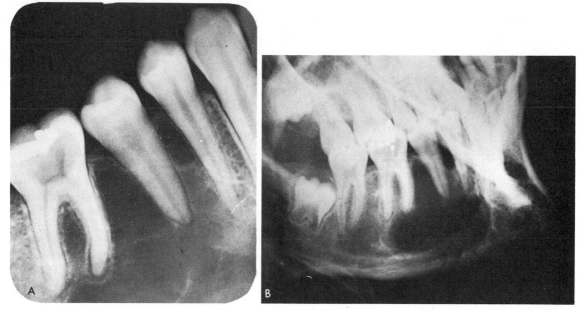

Figure 10–8. *Traumatic bone cyst.*
This large empty space in bone extended between the roots of the teeth. Periapical film (A) and lateral jaw film (B).

solitary traumatic cyst occurring in the molar area and appearing as a round or ovoid radiolucent area associated with vital teeth from the lingual salivary gland depression of the mandible (q.v.) which has a similar roentgenographic appearance. However, the latter lesion is usually located below the mandibular canal, whereas the traumatic cyst usually lies above it.

The greater frequency of detection of asymptomatic traumatic bone cysts through panoramic roentgenography has been stressed by Morris and his associates.

Histologic Features. Histologic examination of the solitary bone cyst may reveal a thin connective tissue membrane lining the cavity, but no other significant features. Sometimes no such membrane is demonstrable. Waldron had the opportunity to study a solitary bone cyst in toto in a resected mandible. His case exhibited a thin connective tissue membrane and, in

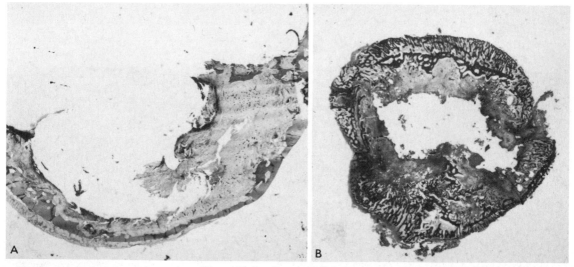

Figure 10–9. *Traumatic bone cyst.*
Traumatic cyst of mandible (A) and fibula (B). Only a thin shell of the cortical plates of the jaw remain with limited peripheral osteophyte reaction. The fibula shows a similar empty central cavity and thinning of the cortex, although osteophyte reaction is pronounced. (A, Courtesy of Dr. Charles A. Waldron and B, of Dr. William G. Sprague.)

addition, an extensive osteophytic reaction on the outer surface of the cortical plate (Fig. 10–9).

Treatment and Prognosis.   Since the definitive diagnosis of the solitary bone cyst cannot be established without surgical exploration, the dentist usually opens into the cavity, attempts to enucleate a lining and, in the course of manipulation, re-establishes bleeding into the lesion. If the cavity is then closed, it has been found that healing and filling of the space by bone occur in most cases in 6 to 12 months. Seldom is a second surgical procedure necessary. If the space is a large one, bone chips have been used to aid in filling the defect with good results.

The extreme rarity of these lesions in older patients would suggest that not only may they be self-limiting, but at least some are capable of complete and spontaneous remission.

FOCAL OSTEOPOROTIC BONE-MARROW DEFECT OF THE JAW

The focal osteoporotic bone-marrow defect of the jaw is a lesion which has been described by Standish and Shafer, by Crawford and Weathers, and by Barker and his associates. Although hematopoietic marrow occurs normally in the jaws at the angle of the mandible, the maxillary tuberosity and occasionally other areas, its occurrence as a focal radiolucent defect is unusual. It is well recognized that bone marrow may be stimulated in response to unusual demands for increased blood cell production and that this hyperplastic marrow may extend between adjacent trabeculae of bone, producing roentgenographically obvious osteoporosis and even thinning of the cortex. Bone resorption associated with red marrow hyperplasia has been demonstrated by Box in human jaw material and in mandibles of rabbits made anemic by repeated bleedings.

Clinical Features.   In the three reported series of cases, approximately 75 per cent of the focal osteoporotic bone-marrow defects of the jaws occurred in women, and they involved the mandible in approximately 85 per cent of the cases. In nearly every instance the lesions were asymptomatic and discovered only during routine roentgenographic examination.

Roentgenographic Features.   This lesion, which has a predilection for the mandibular molar area, generally appears as a radiolucency of variable size, a few millimeters to a centimeter or more, with a poorly defined periphery indicative of lack of reactivity of adjacent bone (Fig. 10–10). The lesions are most common in edentulous areas, and this suggests that they result from failure of normal bone regeneration after tooth extraction, at least in some cases.

Histologic Features.   The tissue removed from these defects consists of either normal red marrow, fatty marrow or a combination of the two (Fig. 10–10, B). The trabeculae of bone usually present in the sections are long, thin, irregular, and devoid of an osteoblastic layer.

Treatment.   The roentgenographic appearance of these lesions is not sufficiently characteristic to permit diagnosis with certainty, and for this reason they must be investigated surgically. Once the diagnosis has been established, no additional treatment is necessary.

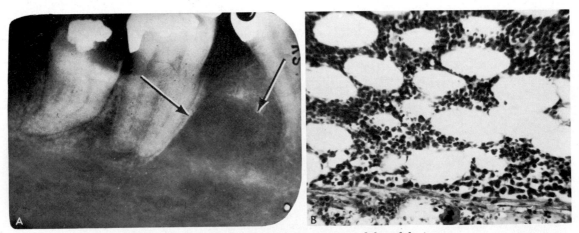

Figure 10–10.   *Focal osteoporotic bone-marrow defect of the jaw.*
The obvious radiolucency in *A* was filled with normal hematopoietic bone marrow (*B*).

Differential Diagnosis. The roentgenographic appearance of the focal osteoporotic bone-marrow defect of the jaws is not unlike that of residual dental infections, central neoplasms or even the traumatic cyst of bone.

SURGICAL CILIATED CYST OF MAXILLA

The surgical ciliated cyst of the maxilla, originally reported by Gregory and Shafer, is a cyst which develops after surgical entry into the maxillary sinus, usually a Caldwell-Luc operation. Basically, it is an implantation type of cyst in which epithelium of the maxillary sinus becomes entrapped along the line of surgical entry into the sinus and subsequently proliferates to form a true cystic cavity, anatomically separated from the sinus. A series of 71 cases has been reported recently by Kaneshiro and his associates and confirms the observations in the original study.

Clinical Features. The majority of patients with this type of lesion are middle-aged or older and present with a complaint of a nonspecific, poorly localized pain, tenderness, or discomfort in the maxilla. Extraoral or intraoral swelling is also frequently evident. Careful questioning of the patient usually reveals a history of some type of surgical procedure involving the maxilla and maxillary sinus, frequently 10 to 20 years previously. Interestingly, it has been emphasized by Ohba and his associates among others that this lesion is more common in Japan than in America or Europe, possibly because of the higher incidence of maxillary sinusitis in Japan.

Roentgenographic Features. Roentgenographic examination shows a well-defined radiolucent area closely related to the maxillary sinus, often appearing to encroach upon the sinus but anatomically separate from it, as may be demonstrated by injection of the sinus with a radiopaque material. A filling defect of the cyst can then be seen (Fig. 10–11).

Histologic Features. The surgical cyst is lined by pseudostratified ciliated columnar epithelium identical with that of the maxillary sinus (Fig. 10–11, B). If infection or inflammation is present, squamous metaplasia may be found. The wall of the cyst is composed of fibrous connective tissue with or without inflammatory cell infiltration.

Treatment. The treatment of this lesion consists in enucleation of the cyst. It does not tend to recur.

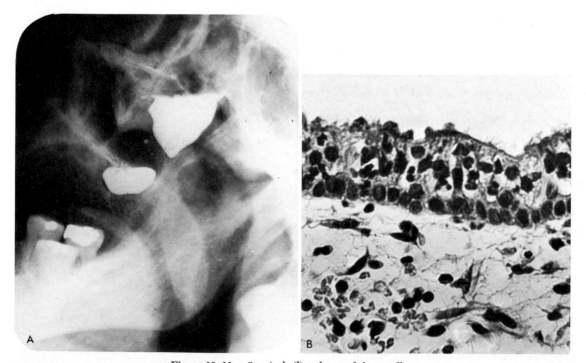

Figure 10–11. *Surgical ciliated cyst of the maxilla.*
The two anatomically separated cavities, the maxillary sinus and surgical cyst, were injected with radiopaque material (A). The cyst lining was respiratory in type (B).

EFFECTS OF ORTHODONTIC TOOTH MOVEMENT

The science of orthodontics is based upon the ability of teeth to be moved through bone, without their subsequent extrusion or loss, by the application of pressure or tension under appropriate and controlled circumstances. Although the exact biologic mechanism responsible for this phenomenon is unknown, it is generally agreed that bone under pressure responds by resorbing, whereas the application of tension results in deposition of new bone. The periodontal ligament mediates this pressure or tension and, for this reason, is particularly important in the movement of teeth by orthodontic appliances.

Investigation of the tissue changes occurring during orthodontic tooth movement has been hampered by the difficulty in obtaining human material. For this reason, most studies utilizing controlled conditions have been restricted to tooth movement in animals, chiefly the dog and monkey. The earliest scientific studies were those of Sandstedt (1904) and Oppenheim (1911).

Sandstedt applied force to the maxillary incisors of a dog, moving them lingually by means of a labial arch wire, and described the histologic findings of bone resorption, with numerous associated osteoclasts, on the pressure side of the teeth and formation of new bone on the tension side. He noted no tooth resorption, although necrosis or at least hyalinization of the periodontal ligament was found in the areas of pressure. The extensive work of Oppenheim on monkeys is classic for his thorough examination of the tissue changes incident to a great variety of orthodontic movements such as labial and lingual tipping of the tooth and elongation and depression of the tooth.

Since the contributions of these investigators, other researchers have published the results of detailed studies dealing with other features of tooth movement. Johnson, Appleton and Rittershofer studied tooth movement in the monkey, concerning themselves particularly with changes in the area of the tooth apex. These workers were the first to record the amount of force and the distance through which it was active. In 1932 Herzberg reported the first histologic studies of human tissue subjected to tooth movement by orthodontic forces, and the results confirmed earlier work in the experimental animal. During this same period Schwartz reported on numerous experiments in which known forces were applied to the teeth of dogs.

Many workers, such as Grubrich and Gubler, also became interested in the phenomenon of root resorption associated with orthodontic tooth movement in both human beings and animals. This problem was studied extensively by Marshall from 1930. He fed various diets to monkeys subjected to orthodontic movements in attempting to relate root resorption to nutrition. Tooth root resorption has been discussed in Chapter 5.

Not all the studies dealing with the tissue changes incident to the application of orthodontic forces are in complete accord. Slight differences in technique or in the experimental conditions account for some of the disparities. In other instances the lack of agreement is due essentially to interpretation of results. It is impossible and inadvisable to provide here a full account of the orthodontic literature dealing with tissue changes following tooth movement, particularly since important studies are still in progress which may help clarify the problems. A brief summary of the general tissue changes will be cited with no attempt at separation of human and animal studies, since the basic tissue reactions appear to be identical.

Tipping Movement. The exact movements which a tooth will undergo and the exact position it will assume after the application of orthodontic force will depend upon the degree and direction of the force and the position of

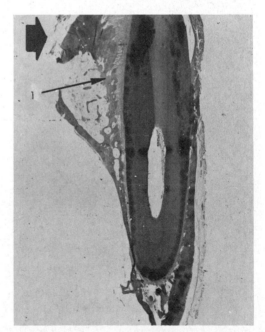

Figure 10–12. *Tipping tooth movement.*
Force was applied to this dog's tooth in the direction of the arrow, and even at this magnification, widening of the periodontal ligament space (*1*) is noted.

the fulcrum around which the force acts. The general statement can be made, however, that pressure upon a tooth results in the resorption of bone in the direction of the application of force and compensatory new bone formation on the opposite side of the tooth, the tension side (Fig. 10–12).

The initial reaction on the pressure side is a compression of the periodontal ligament which, if excessive and prolonged, may result in ischemia with hyalinization and/or actual necrosis of tissue (Fig. 10–13, B). On the opposite side under excessive force there may be actual tearing of the periodontal fibers and small capillaries with hemorrhage into the area. With reasonable forces, the periodontal ligament on the tension side of the tooth demonstrates stretching and widening of the periodontal space. Within a matter of hours or at the most a few days, large numbers of osteoclasts make their appearance along the surface of the bone under pressure, and resorption begins. This continues until the force of the pressure has been entirely dissipated.

New trabeculae of bone on the tension side become evident early and appear as thin, elongated spicules arranged parallel to the periodontal fibers and confluent with them at their bony attachment (Fig. 10–13, A). These spi-

cules show evident osteoblastic activity along the sides and the end adjacent to the tooth, but usually there is intense osteoclastic activity at the ends of the spicules away from the tooth. As stabilization occurs, the alveolar bone gradually assumes its compact pattern that existed before movement occurred.

A secondary but most important occurrence is the deposition of new spicules of bone on the outer surface of the labial plate in instances of pressure in the labial direction. This serves to maintain the thickness of the already thin labial plate and prevent its perforation by the tooth. It is not entirely certain why resorption of even compact bone occurs before resorption of cementum and the tooth root. It is known that resorption of calcified tissues is favored by increased local vascularity, and the hypothesis has been advanced in explanation that the bone of the alveolus is in a more vascular environment than the tooth cementum when orthodontic pressure is applied, particularly since ischemia of the periodontal ligament adjacent to the cementum is the usual situation.

It is generally recognized that the teeth of young persons respond much more rapidly and with less applied force to orthodontic movements than do the teeth of older adults. Although differences do exist in the chemical

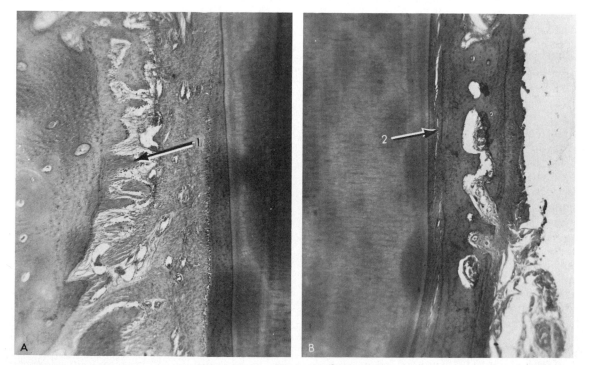

Figure 10–13. *Tipping tooth movement.*
There is widening of the periodontal ligament with formation of new spicules of bone (*1*) on the tension side of the tooth (A) and compression of the periodontal ligament (*2*) on the pressure side (B).

constitution of bone at varying ages, the difference in orthodontic response is probably due to variation in general tissue reactivity and local vascularity. Although bone retains the ability to undergo resorption throughout life, the degree of the stimulus needed to evoke this response shows dramatic differences between the various age groups.

Extrusive Movement. Extrusion of a tooth by an orthodontic appliance is similar to normal tooth eruption. The tissue changes induced by this form of movement consist in deposition or apposition of new bone spicules at the alveolar crest and at the fundus of the alveolus arranged in a direction parallel to the direction of force. The direction of the spicules then is parallel to the long axis of the tooth and tends to increase the height of the alveolar crest. The normal width of the apical periodontal ligament is maintained by the new bony spicules here formed in the same direction. The relation between the tooth and the alveolus tends to remain constant.

Depressive Movement. The application of orthodontic force in such a manner as to cause depression of a tooth results in tissue changes that are the opposite of those found during extrusion, or elongation. In tooth depression, resorption of bone occurs at the apical area and around the alveolar margin. New bone formation is actually minimal.

Tissue Reactions During Retention Period. Discontinuance of the active phase of orthodontic force signals the beginning of alterations in the bone characteristic of the retention period. During this period there is gradual reformation of the normal dense pattern of the alveolar bone by apposition of bone around the bony spicules until they meet, fuse and gradually remodel. The studies of Oppenheim indicated that this reformation is slower around teeth held in position during the retention period by a retaining appliance as compared to teeth which remained free during this time. In any event, the final remodeling and the attainment of absolute bone-tooth equilibrium following orthodontic movements involve an extremely slow process, and a breakdown in this process is probably one of the most important contributing factors in cases of orthodontic failure due to relapse during the retention period.

Effect of Deciduous Tooth Movement Upon Permanent Tooth Germs. The result of orthodontic movement of deciduous teeth with particular reference to its effect on the permanent tooth germ was studied by Breitner and Tischler in young monkeys. They found that when a deciduous tooth was moved, the associated permanent tooth germ followed this movement.

Whenever a deciduous tooth was moved away from a tooth germ, the permanent tooth germ quickly followed. If a deciduous tooth was moved toward a permanent tooth germ, this germ moved in the same direction as the deciduous tooth.

These studies offered suggestive evidence that the form of the permanent dental arch may be modified by altering the deciduous arch through orthodontic treatment of the deciduous dentition.

PHYSICAL INJURIES OF SOFT TISSUES

TRAUMATIC ULCER

(Decubitus Ulcer)

The traumatic ulcer of the oral mucous membranes is a lesion that is caused by some form of trauma. This may be an injury such as biting the mucosa, denture irritation, toothbrush injury, exposure of the mucous membrane to a sharp tooth or carious lesion, or it may be injury to the mucosa by some other external irritant. The "cotton roll injury," an iatrogenic injury, is a common reaction when the dry cotton roll placed by the dentist is roughly removed and the mucosa adhering to it is torn (Fig. 10–14).

The traumatic ulcer often occurs in such sites as the lateral border of the tongue, usually after injury in which the patient severely bites the tongue (Figs. 10–15, 10–16). These ulcers are also seen, however, on the buccal mucosa, on the lips and occasionally on the palate. Although in most instances of injury to the oral mucous membrane healing is rapid and uneventful, occasional injuries persist for a long time without healing. This is particularly true of the traumatic ulcer of the tongue, which may bear considerable clinical resemblance to carcinoma and which sometimes is repeatedly biopsied in an attempt to establish a diagnosis of neoplasm. It is interesting, however, that many times the traumatic ulcer which has persisted for a matter of weeks or even months without healing will heal promptly after a minor surgical procedure such as an incisional biopsy.

FACTITIAL INJURIES

Factitial injuries are accidentally self-induced injuries on the basis of habit with a frequent psychogenic background. As such, these overlap with a number of physical and chemical injuries to be discussed in this section. Thus factitial injuries originate as the result of such

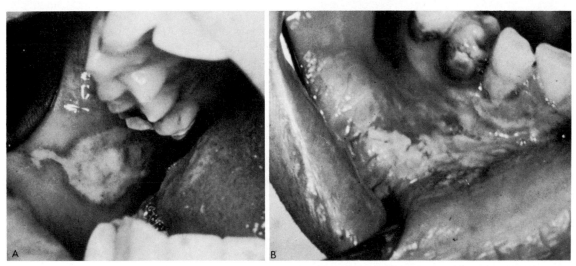

Figure 10–14. *Iatrogenic injuries.*

The lesion on the buccal mucosa (A) is a burn produced by a handpiece used injudiciously by a dentist. The lesion in the mucobuccal fold (B) represents macerated mucosa torn by a cotton roll which had dried and adhered to the surface and was removed carelessly by a dentist. (A, Courtesy of Dr. Stephen F. Dachi.)

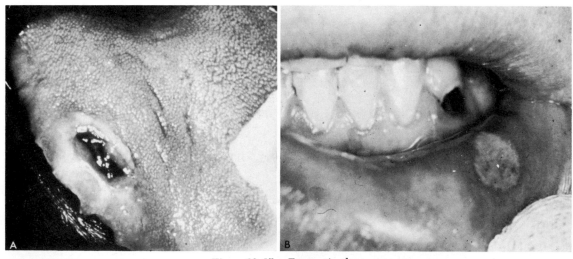

Figure 10–15. *Traumatic ulcer.*

The ulcer of the tongue (A) occurred during an epileptic seizure as a result of the patient's biting himself. The ulcer of the lip (B) resulted from injury of the lip by rubbing against the large gingival carious lesion on the cuspid. The ulcer healed promptly after restoration of the carious lesion. (A, Courtesy of Dr. Stephen F. Dachi.)

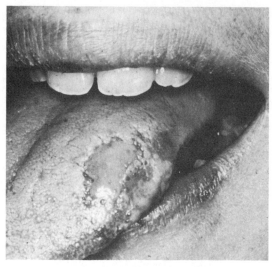

Figure 10–16. *Traumatic ulcer.*
Traumatic ulcer of tongue. The lesion occurred in a
patient who had received a mandibular injection of local
anesthesia for restorative work and was not cautioned by
the dentist against inadvertently biting the tissue before
the anesthesia had disappeared. (Courtesy of Dr. Stephen
F. Dachi.)

habits as lip-biting (*morsicatio labiorum*),
cheek-biting (*morsicatio buccarum*), unconscious gingival trauma, and so forth (Fig. 10–
17). These biting habits, also referred to as
pathomimia mucosae oris, have been analyzed
and discussed by Hjørting-Hansen and Holst
and by Sewerin.

The factitial injuries constitute a group of
lesions that are related only in the manner in
which they are produced, with no particular
anatomic, etiologic or even microscopic similarities.

DENTURE INJURIES

The oral mucosa is subject to a variety of
injuries as a result of the wearing of artificial
dentures. These may be manifested specifically
as (1) traumatic ulcer, (2) generalized inflammation, (3) inflammatory hyperplasia, (4) papillary hyperplasia of palate, and (5) denture base
(acrylic or vulcanite) intolerance or allergy.

Traumatic Ulcer

(*"Sore Spots"*)

The traumatic ulcer caused by denture irritation is the same type of ulcer that may be
produced by a variety of other physical injuries.
This lesion has been discussed in the preceding
section.

Clinical Features. The denture ulcer, one
or more, commonly develops within a day or
two after the insertion of a new denture. This
may be a result of over-extension of the flanges,
sequestration of spicules of bone under the
denture or a roughened or "high" spot on the
inner surface of the denture.

These ulcers are small, painful, irregularly
shaped lesions usually covered by a delicate
gray necrotic membrane and surrounded by an
inflammatory halo. If treatment is not instituted, there sometimes may be beginning proliferation of tissue around the periphery of the
lesion on an inflammatory basis.

Histologic Features. The traumatic ulcer is
a nonspecific ulcer and microscopically shows
loss of continuity of surface epithelium with a
fibrinous exudate covering the exposed connec-

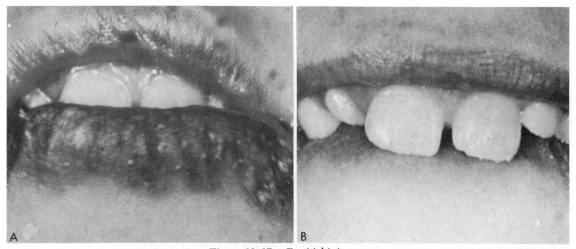

Figure 10–17. *Factitial injury.*
Severe maceration of the lip had occurred as a result of a biting habit. (Courtesy of Dr. Ralph E. McDonald.)

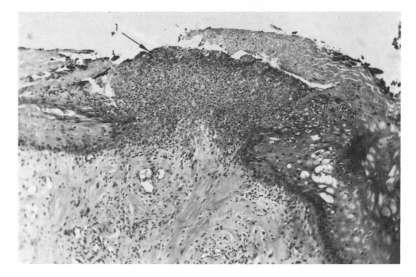

Figure 10–18. *Traumatic ulcer.* The area of the ulceration is covered by a fibrinous exudate (*1*).

tive tissue (Fig. 10–18). The epithelium bordering the ulcer usually demonstrates proliferative activity. There is infiltration of polymorphonuclear leukocytes in the connective tissue, particularly beneath the area of ulceration, although in chronic lesions these may be replaced by lymphocytes and plasma cells. Capillary dilatation and proliferation may also be evident. Fibroblastic activity is sometimes prominent, and macrophages may be present in moderate numbers.

Treatment and Prognosis. The treatment for the traumatic denture ulcer consists in correction of the underlying cause: relief of the flange, removal of a tiny sequestrum or relief of high spots. When this is accomplished, the ulcer usually heals promptly.

Generalized Inflammation

(*"Denture Sore Mouth"; Denture Stomatitis*)

The "denture sore mouth" is an uncommon condition occurring in patients who may or may not have a new set of dentures. The condition is not due to a true allergy, since patch testing with the denture material gives negative results. Some cases appear to be due to an infection with *Candida albicans*, although the typical white patches of thrush (q.v.) do not usually develop, according to Cahn and Bartels. Lehner has classified the condition as chronic atrophic candidiasis. Newton has suggested that denture sore mouth may be related to the "sweat retention syndrome," in which keratin plug formation of the sweat glands or accessory salivary glands forces sweat or saliva into the adjacent tissues

with subsequent inflammation. This concept has not been accepted widely, however.

More recently, Budtz-Jørgensen and Bertram studied denture stomatitis in considerable detail. They demonstrated that yeastlike fungi of *C. albicans* type could be cultivated from 90 per cent of patients with denture stomatitis, but from only 40 per cent of patients with dentures but without stomatitis. They also showed that poor denture cleanliness was associated with severe inflammation.

Renner and his associates emphasized that this condition is a multifaceted disease entity in which parasitism by *C. albicans* may be an extremely important factor often in association with other major contributions from denture trauma and continual denture wearing, poor oral hygiene habits and possibly dietary and systemic alterations.

Clinical Features. The mucosa beneath the denture becomes extremely red, swollen, smooth or granular and painful. Multiple pinpoint foci of hyperemia, usually involving the maxilla, frequently occur. A severe burning sensation is common. The redness of the mucosa is rather sharply outlined and restricted to the tissue actually in contact with the denture.

Treatment and Prognosis. Treatment of this condition may not be successful. However, Budtz-Jørgensen and Bertram have reported significant therapeutic effects on denture stomatitis by antifungal therapy. Nystatin tablets, 500,000 units, were allowed to dissolve in the mouth three times a day for 14 days. Bergendal and Isacsson reported similar results by treating denture stomatitis with nystatin powder placed on the fitting surface of the denture three times a day for 14 days. In addition, when the dentures fit poorly, construction of new appliances and instruction on hygienic care of the dentures aid in correcting the situation. If new dentures are not constructed, the old dentures must be sterilized daily by soaking in a nystatin solution overnight during the treatment period. Rebasing dentures with soft-tissue conditioners is also reported of benefit in conjunction with nystatin.

Inflammatory (Fibrous) Hyperplasia

(*"Denture Injury Tumor"; Epulis Fissuratum; Redundant Tissue*)

One of the most common tissue reactions to a chronically ill-fitting denture is the occurrence of hyperplasia of tissue along the denture borders. Such hyperplasia of oral mucosa is not restricted to this location but occurs in many areas where chronic irritation of any type exists, such as on the gingiva, buccal mucosa and angle of the mouth.

Clinical Features. Inflammatory fibrous hyperplasia as a result of denture injury is characterized by the development of elongated rolls of tissue in the mucolabial or mucobuccal fold area into which the denture flange conveniently fits (Figs. 10–19, 10–20). This proliferation of tissue is usually slow in developing and probably is as much a result of the resorption of the alveolar ridge as of the trauma of the loose dentures.

This excess fold of tissue is not usually highly inflamed clinically, although there may be irritation or even ulceration in the base of the fold into which the denture flange fits. The lesion is firm to palpation. (See also Plate V.)

Histologic Features. The hyperplastic mass of tissue is composed of an excessive bulk of fibrous connective tissue covered by a layer of stratified squamous epithelium which may be of normal thickness or show acanthosis (Fig. 10–20). Pseudoepitheliomatous hyperplasia is often found. Hyperorthokeratosis or parakeratosis is frequently present. The connective tissue is composed chiefly of coarse bundles of collagen fibers with few fibroblasts or blood vessels unless there is an active inflammatory reaction present. Such a reaction is frequently seen, however, in the base of the fissure adjoining the denture flange, especially if the tissue is superficially ulcerated. Cutright reported the histopathologic findings in 583 cases of inflammatory fibrous hyperplasia and discussed their significance.

One additional histologic finding often seen in the surface epithelium of inflammatory fibrous hyperplasia is *mucopolysaccharide keratin dystrophy*, also referred to as "plasma pooling," first described by Toto. Its occurrence is not confined to inflammatory hyperplasia but may also be found in oral epithelium under a wide variety of other conditions, especially those involving irritated epithelium. This mucopolysaccharide keratin dystrophy consists histologically of homogeneous, eosinophilic pools of material in the superficial spinous layer of epithelium, where it appears to have replaced individual cells. Its significance is not known.

Treatment and Prognosis. Inflammatory fibrous hyperplasia should be surgically excised, and either new dentures constructed or the old dentures rebased to provide adequate retention. If the denture is replaced or repaired, the lesion should not recur. Complete regression, even after construction of new dentures, will not occur, although subsidence of the inflammatory reaction may produce some clinical improvement of the condition.

Inflammatory Papillary Hyperplasia

(*Palatal Papillomatosis*)

Papillary hyperplasia is an unusual condition involving the mucosa of the palate. It is of unknown etiology but may be considered a form of inflammatory hyperplasia associated in most instances with ill-fitting dentures, which permit frictional irritation and a poor state of oral hygiene. Since many persons who have what might be described as poor-fitting dentures never acquire papillomatosis, however, there must be some as yet unidentified predisposing factors present in those persons who develop the lesion.

Clinical Features. Papillary hyperplasia occurs predominantly in edentulous patients with dentures, but is seen on rare occasions in patients with a full complement of teeth and no prosthetic appliance. In a series of 5892 dental patients, Guernsey reported an incidence of 2.9 per cent in denture wearers but only 0.2 per cent in nondenture wearers. However, Bhaskar and his associates have stated that approximately 20 per cent of all patients who wear dentures 24 hours a day show papillary hyperplasia, while among all denture wearers, the prevalence is 10 per cent. Ettinger, studying the etiology and incidence of papillary hyperplasia, reported a similar occurrence of 97 af-

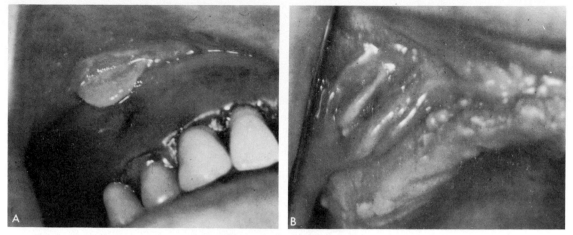

Figure 10–19. *Inflammatory hyperplasia.*
The redundant tissue forming at the border of the poorly fitting denture (A) is actually made up of several folds into which the denture seats (B). (Courtesy of Dr. Grant Van Huysen.)

Figure 10–20. *Inflammatory hyperplasia.*
Some cases of redundant tissue exhibit extremely large rolls of fibrous tissue around the denture. (B, Courtesy of Dr. Grant Van Huysen.)

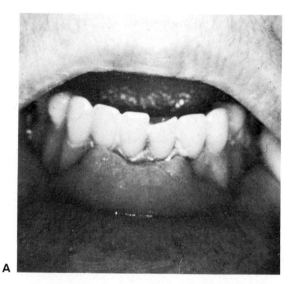

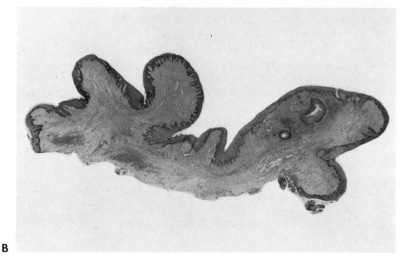

PLATE V

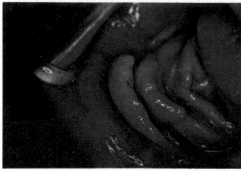
Inflammatory hyperplasia (redundant tissue)

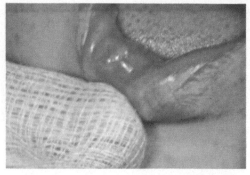
Salivary gland retention phenomenon (mucocele)

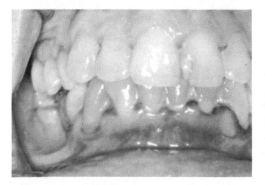
Bismuth gingivitis

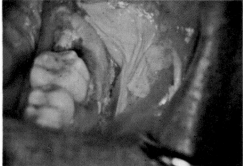
Aspirin burn

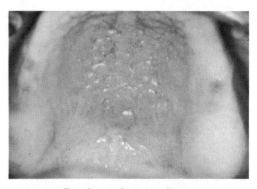
Papillary hyperplasia (papillomatosis)

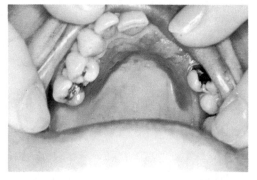
Acrylic allergy

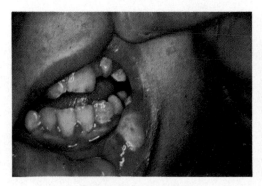
Traumatic ulcer (lip bite after
mandibular injection)

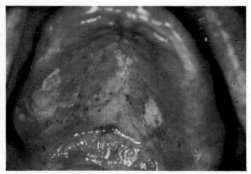
Radiation mucositis

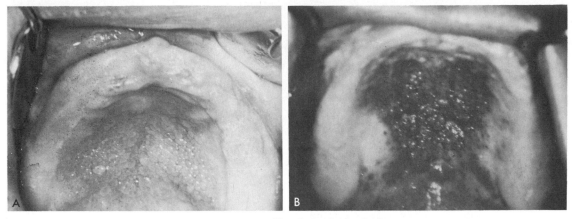

Figure 10–21. *Papillary hyperplasia of palate.*
The many small projections are confined to the palatal area and may be free of inflammation (*A*) or may be highly inflamed (*B*). (*A*, Courtesy of Dr. R. L. Trueblood; *B*, courtesy of Dr. Grant Van Huysen.)

fected patients, or 13.9 per cent, in a series of 700 denture wearers. He concluded that constant wearing of the denture was one of the most important factors associated with the condition. When an appliance is present, the site of the lesion corresponds to the denture base, sometimes only to the relief chamber. It may arise at any age in the adult and has no definite sex predilection.

The lesion presents itself as numerous, closely arranged, red, edematous papillary projections, often involving nearly all of the hard palate and imparting to it a warty appearance. The lesions may extend onto the alveolar mucosa, and mandibular alveolar mucosa involvement occasionally occurs. The individual papillae are seldom over a millimeter or two in diameter. The tissue exhibits varying degrees of inflammation, but seldom is there ulceration (Fig. 10–21; see also Plate V).

Histologic Features. The microscopic section of papillomatosis shows numerous, small vertical projections each composed of paraker-

atotic or sometimes orthokeratotic stratified squamous epithelium and a central core of connective tissue (Fig. 10–22). Pseudoepitheliomatous hyperplasia, in varying degrees, is seen in the vast majority of cases; this is sometimes so severe as to be interpreted by the inexperienced as epidermoid carcinoma. However, most authorities now agree that true epithelial dysplasia and malignant transformation do not occur in palatal papillomatosis. Relatively severe inflammatory cell infiltration is nearly always present in the connective tissue, as is chronic sialadenitis in the accessory palatal glands. In the latter instance, metaplastic changes in acinar and ductal epithelium may mimic neoplastic transformation. Cutright has discussed the morphogenesis of these lesions in detail.

Treatment and Prognosis. There is no well-recognized and accepted course of therapy for this condition. Discontinuing the use of the ill-fitting dentures or construction of new dentures without surgical removal of the excess tissue

Figure 10–22. *Papillary hyperplasia of palate.*
The lesion is composed of numerous small papillary projections.

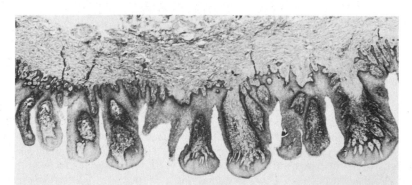

will generally result in regression of the edema and inflammation, but the papillary hyperplasia persists. Preferably, surgical excision of the lesion prior to new denture construction will return the mouth to a normal state. The use of a tissue conditioner to rebase an old denture often results in some improvement of the lesion, but seldom complete regression unless it is in an early stage.

Denture Base Intolerance or Allergy

A true allergy to denture base material is extremely rare. Occasional cases have been reported, and studies have suggested that these were due to sensitivity to the monomer, both regular and self-curing types. Some investigators believe that methyl methacrylate in any form can produce a reaction in susceptible persons. However, Turrell has reviewed this entire problem and concluded that a well-processed new resin denture is not in itself likely to provide a source of allergens, although absorbed fluids may be allergenic. The problem of contact dermatitis from acrylic compounds, among dentists and dental technicians as well as others, has been pointed out by Rycroft, with special emphasis on the light-sensitive acrylates.

Clinical Features. The clinical features of cases of true acrylic allergy are similar to those of the simple generalized inflammations, or "denture sore mouth," and for this reason the diagnosis depends upon a positive patch test (see Plate V). The patch test is carried out by strapping the entire denture to the forearm for 48 hours or scraping off shavings of acrylic from the denture and applying them to the forearm by adhesive tape. A strip of tape without acrylic must also be used because of the sensitivity of some persons to adhesive tape alone. When using the entire denture as the test sample, an occasional positive reaction will occur, owing to a pressure phenomenon rather than an allergic sensitization.

Cobalt-chromium alloy base materials in dentures on very rare occasions cannot be tolerated by patients. In such cases, it is usually the nickel present in the alloy to which the patient is sensitive. One such case has been reported by Wood, in which the patient gave a positive skin patch test for nickel as well as for the cobalt-chromium alloy.

Vulcanite dentures have also been thought to evoke allergic sensitization in some patients, possibly because of sulfur in the base material. The infrequent use of this material now renders such an occurrence clinically insignificant.

Occasional cases, such as that of Samuels, are reported in which acute reactions to denture base materials are manifested, disappearing upon removal of the base material, although sensitivity patch tests are *negative*. These cases probably represent only exaggerated examples of "denture sore mouth."

General allergic sensitization of the oral mucosa is discussed elsewhere in this section.

PERLÈCHE

(Angular Cheilitis; Angular Cheilosis)

Perlèche is a clinical description of a lesion in whose development several predisposing factors may play an important role. Finnerud brought together the prevailing theories on the underlying causes of perlèche and reconciled the protean features of the condition.

It has long been considered a lesion caused by microorganisms, and numerous studies variously have reported that pure cultures of certain microorganisms, particularly *Candida albicans,* but also staphylococci and streptococci, were obtained from the fissures.

The suggestion has also been made, however, that many cases of perlèche are due to overclosure of the jaws such as occurs in edentulous patients or in patients with artificial dentures which lack proper vertical dimension. In this event, a fold is produced at the corners of the mouth in which saliva tends to collect, and the skin becomes macerated, fissured and secondarily infected by these organisms. Many such cases are reported to have been corrected by increasing the vertical height of the dentures— i.e., by opening the bite.

Cawson has evaluated a series of patients with "denture sore mouth" (q.v.) many of whom also had perlèche or angular cheilitis. He was able to isolate *Candida albicans* or related organisms from the major percentage of these, and suggested that the angular cheilitis in many cases appeared to be due to intraoral infection by *Candida.*

Another theory of the etiology of perlèche is that it represents a riboflavin deficiency with a superimposed fungal or bacterial infection. In human patients ariboflavinosis will induce circumoral lesions which are prone to become infected, and when this happens, the lesions are indistinguishable from the perlèche of other causes. Some of these cases can be cured by administration of the vitamin B complex.

Clinical Features. Perlèche occurs in both young children and adults and is characterized

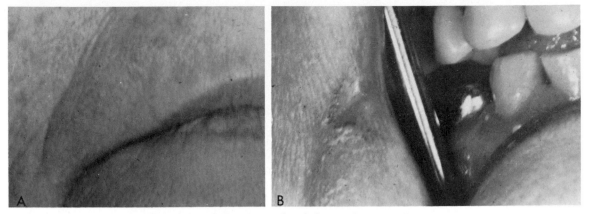

Figure 10–23. *Perlèche associated with decreased intermaxillary space.*
A, Mouth closed, showing deep fissure at angle of mouth, *B*, Mouth opened, showing typical lesions.

symptomatically by a feeling of dryness and a burning sensation at the corners of the mouth. Clinically, the epithelium at the commissures appears wrinkled and somewhat macerated. In time the wrinkling becomes more pronounced to form one or more deep fissures or cracks which appear ulcerated, but which do not tend to bleed, although a superficial exudative crust may form (Fig. 10–23). These fissures do not involve the mucosal surface of the commissures inside the mouth, but stop at the mucocutaneous junction. If the lesions are not treated, they often show a tendency for spontaneous remission. Subsequent exacerbation is common, however, and only rarely do the lesions completely disappear.

Treatment. The treatment of perlèche is empirical at best because of the apparently varied etiology. It should be remembered that the infection present is secondary and that, unless the primary cause is corrected, treatment of the infection will not produce a permanent cure.

MUCOUS RETENTION PHENOMENON

(Mucocele; Mucous Retention Cyst)

The mucous retention phenomenon, which is generally conceded to be of traumatic origin, is a lesion involving salivary glands and their ducts.

Etiology and Pathogenesis. The mucous retention phenomenon is a common lesion, although only a few studies have been reported that describe its detailed features. Many authorities formerly believed that this type of lesion resulted from obstruction of the duct of a minor or accessory salivary gland, but exper-

imental investigations on mice by Bhaskar and his associates and on rats by Standish and Shafer failed to produce the mucous retention phenomenon by ligation of the submaxillary and sublingual gland ducts. The studies of Bhaskar and co-workers have shown instead that if the salivary duct was severed so that a continuous pooling of saliva occurred in the tissues, a well-demarcated cavity developed which was histologically identical with the natural mucocele.

These investigations appear to indicate that traumatic severance of a salivary duct, such as that produced by biting the lips or cheek or pinching the lip by extraction forceps, precedes the development of the retention phenomenon. It is also possible that a chronic partial obstruction of a salivary duct, in contrast to the acute total obstruction experimentally produced by ligation in mice and rats, may be of etiologic importance. Such a partial obstruction could result from a small piece of intraductal calculus or even from contraction of developing scar connective tissue around a duct after a traumatic injury. Occasional cases of calculus in the ducts of accessory salivary glands, or sialolithiasis (q.v.), have been reported, but are rather uncommon. Thus, mucoceles often have been classified as (1) an extravasation mucocele, or (2) a retention mucocele (or true retention cyst). The extravasation type is far more common than the retention type. These two forms have been discussed by Harrison.

Clinical Features. The retention phenomenon involving accessory salivary gland structures occurs most frequently on the lower lip, but may also occur on the palate, cheek, tongue (involving the glands of Blandin-Nuhn), and floor of the mouth. In the series of cases re ported by Standish and Shafer, nearly 45 per cent of the 97 mucoceles occurred on the lower lip. No cases were found in their series on the upper lip. In addition, there was no predilection for any age group, the lesions being rather equally divided among all decades of life, from lesions present at birth to the ninth decade. An equal distribution in occurrence between males and females was also noted in their study. In a more recent study of 125 cases of mucocele, Robinson and Hjørting-Hansen reported similar findings except for the age predilection. They found that nearly 65 per cent of their cases occurred within the first three decades of life. Ramanathan and his co-workers, in their series of 250 cases of mucoceles, found that nearly 85 per cent occurred in the same time span.

Clinically, the lesion may lie fairly deep in the tissue or be exceptionally superficial and, depending upon the location, will present a variable clinical appearance (Fig. 10–24; Plate V). The superficial lesion appears as a raised, circumscribed vesicle, several millimeters to a centimeter or more in diameter, with a bluish, translucent cast. The deeper lesion is manifested also as a swelling but because of the thickness of the overlying tissue, the color and surface appearance are those of normal mucosa.

It is interesting and significant that the mucous retention phenomenon is restricted almost entirely to the lower lip, seldom found on the upper lip, while accessory salivary gland neoplasms of the lips are almost universally found on the upper lip and only rarely on the lower lip. This could imply that trauma plays no role in the development of salivary gland tumors in this location.

The mucous retention phenomenon often arises within a few days, reaches a certain size and may persist as such for months unless treated. If the contents of the cyst are liberated, they usually are found to consist of a thick, mucinous material. Some lesions regress and enlarge periodically and may disappear after traumatic injury which results in their evacuation. They almost invariably recur, however.

Histologic Features. The majority of mucoceles, being of the extravasation type, consist of a circumscribed cavity in the connective tissue and submucosa, producing an obvious elevation of the mucosa with thinning of the epithelium as though it were stretched (Fig. 10–25). The cavity itself is not lined by epithelium and is, therefore, not a true cyst. Instead, its wall is made up of a lining of compressed fibrous connective tissue and fibroblasts. Sometimes these cells may be mistaken for flattened epithelial cells. Not uncommonly the connective tissue wall is essentially granulation tissue, but in any event it usually shows infiltration by abundant numbers of polymorphonuclear leukocytes, lymphocytes and plasma cells. The lumen of the cystlike cavity is filled with an eosinophilic coagulum containing variable numbers of cells, chiefly leukocytes and mononuclear phagocytes.

Occasional mucoceles demonstrate an intact, flattened epithelial lining. It is probable that this simply represents the portion of the excretory duct bordering the line of severance, if severance is actually the manner in which these lesions develop. The flattened epithelial lining has been referred to as epithelium of the "feeder duct." In other instances, the epithelium-lined mucocele represents a lesion of the retention type.

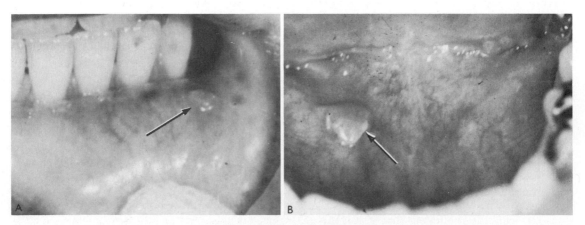

Figure 10–24.   *Retention cyst.*
The typical lesion appears as a small vesicle on the lip (A) and floor of the mouth (B).

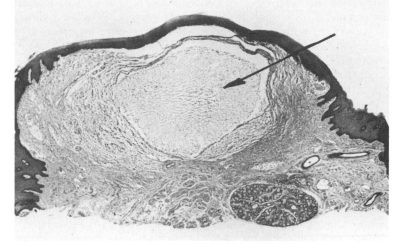

Figure 10–25. *Mucous retention phenomenon.*
The photomicrograph shows the circumscribed lesion containing mucoid material.

The salivary gland acini which lie adjacent to the area of the mucocele and are associated with the involved duct often show alterations. These may consist of interstitial inflammation or sialadenitis, dilatation of intralobular and interlobular ducts with collection of mucus, and breakdown of individual acinar mucous cells resulting in the formation of tiny areas of pooled mucus.

Treatment and Prognosis. Treatment of the mucous retention phenomenon is excision. If the lesion is simply incised, its contents will be evacuated, but it will be rapidly filled again as soon as the incision heals. There is occasional recurrence after excision, but this possibility is less likely if the associated salivary gland acini are removed also.

Ranula

The ranula is a form of mucocele which specifically occurs in the floor of the mouth in association with the ducts of the submaxillary or sublingual gland. The etiology and pathogenesis appear to be essentially the same as for the mucous retention phenomenon involving accessory glands, although some workers believe that it may arise through duct blockage or through the development of a ductal aneurysm.

Clinical Features. This lesion, which is rare compared to the usual mucocele, develops as a slowly enlarging painless mass on one side of the floor of the mouth (Fig. 10–26). Since the lesion is usually a deep-seated one, the overlying mucosa is normal in appearance. If the

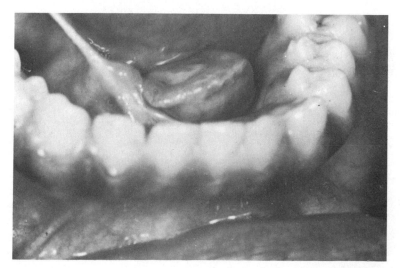

Figure 10–26. *Ranula.*
This form of retention cyst manifests itself as a mass in the floor of the mouth.

lesion is superficial, the mucosa may have a translucent bluish color. A rare, plunging, suprahyoid type which has herniated through the mylohyoid muscle is also described. A thorough review of the literature on the plunging or cervical ranula has been reported by van den Akker and his associates, who also described four typical cases.

Histologic Features. The microscopic appearance is similar to that of the smaller mucocele except that a definite epithelial lining is sometimes present. Because of this finding, most investigators consider the ranula to be a true retention cyst, probably occurring as a partial blockade phenomenon, although a salivary duct stone is often not demonstrable.

Treatment and Prognosis. The treatment and prognosis are also the same except that some operators prefer only to unroof the lesion rather than to excise it totally. Occasionally the lesion recurs. Some prefer initially to excise the entire sublingual gland.

RETENTION CYST OF MAXILLARY SINUS

(Secretory Cyst of Maxillary Antrum; Mucocele of Maxillary Sinus; Mucosal Cyst of Maxillary Sinus)

The retention cyst of the maxillary sinus is an uncommon variant of the mucous retention phenomenon most frequently encountered as an incidental finding in dental roentgenograms. It should be recognized, however, because of the possibility of confusing it with a variety of other lesions occurring in the same location.

This lesion appears to represent a retention phenomenon of the mucous glands associated with the lining of the maxillary sinus. The cause of development of the cystlike lesion is unknown, although traumatic injury associated with tooth extraction may be of etiologic significance. In some cases, however, the lesion develops in dentulous areas with no history of a surgical procedure. Other suggested causative factors include sinusitis, allergy and sinus infection, but these are without firm support.

Clinical Features. Most retention cysts of the maxillary sinus are completely asymptomatic and are discovered only during routine roentgenographic examination of the jaws. Occasionally, discomfort in the cheek or maxilla may be present. Pain and soreness of the face and teeth and numbness of the upper lip were described by Wright in about 10 per cent of his series of 78 cases. Buccal expansion of the maxillary antrum has also been reported. There is no clear-cut age or sex predilection for occurrence of the lesion. Additional series of cases have been reported by Casamassimo and Lilly (73 cases in 4546 patients, or 1.6 per cent), Myall and his co-workers (75 cases in 1469 patients, or 5.1 per cent) and Halstead (45 cases in 2325 patients, or 1.9 per cent).

Roentgenographic Features. In the dental periapical roentgenogram, the lesion appears as a well-defined, homogeneous, dome-shaped or hemispheric radiopacity, varying in size from a tiny lesion to one completely filling the antrum, arising from the floor of the antrum and superimposed on it (Fig. 10–27). This radiopacity

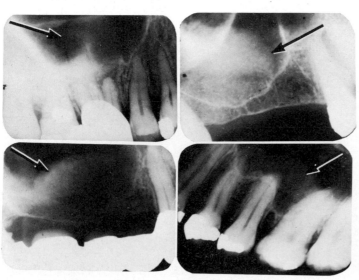

Figure 10–27. *Retention cyst of maxillary sinus.*
Four examples of this soft-tissue opacity in association with the maxillary sinus are shown.

appears as a soft tissue mass rather than a calcified area, so that medial and lateral landmarks can generally be visualized through the lesion. In some instances the lesion appears more radiolucent than radiopaque. In the various reported series, between 10 and 20 per cent of the cases have occurred bilaterally.

Histologic Features.   Some of these retention cysts are analogous to the mucous retention phenomenon inasmuch as they consist of the accumulation of fluid within connective tissue spaces and have no definite lining. This type has sometimes been referred to as a *non-secretory* cyst. In other instances the lesion may be lined by a respiratory type of epithelium, and this has sometimes been described as the *secretory* type of antral cyst. In either case inflammatory cell infiltration in the connective tissue wall of the specimen is common.

Treatment.   The majority of these cysts either persist unchanged or disappear spontaneously within a relatively short period, and for this reason it has been suggested that no treatment is necessary.

Differential Diagnosis.   Care must be taken to differentiate this lesion from apical periodontal cysts of teeth in close association with the maxillary sinus, from fibro-osteomas of this area, and especially from the surgical ciliated cyst of the maxilla. Although etiologically different from the last lesion, the antral mucocele may be related to it pathogenetically.

SIALOLITHIASIS

(Salivary Duct Stone; Salivary Duct Calculus)

Sialolithiasis is the occurrence of calcareous concretions in the salivary ducts or glands. They form by deposition of calcium salts around a central nidus which may consist of desquamated epithelial cells, bacteria, foreign bodies or products of bacterial decomposition.

Clinical Features.   Many patients with sialolithiasis involving a duct of a major salivary gland complain of moderately severe pain, particularly just before, during and after meals, owing to psychic stimulation of salivary flow, associated with swelling of the salivary gland. The occlusion of the duct prevents the free flow of saliva, and this stagnation or accumulation of saliva under pressure produces the pain and swelling. In some instances this swelling is diffuse and simulates a cellulitis. Occasionally the stone presents no remarkable symptoms, and the only evidence may be a firm mass palpable in the duct or gland. In some cases

large numbers of individual small stones may be found occluding the duct system.

Stones, particularly in the more peripheral portion of the duct, may often be palpated if they are of sufficient size. They may also be demonstrated on the dental roentgenogram when appropriately located, particularly by the use of sialography (Fig. 10–28). Sialography is the retrograde injection of a radiopaque material into the duct system of a salivary gland and the study of its distribution by a roentgenogram.

Sialolithiasis may occur at any age, but is most common in middle-aged adults. Wakely reported that the occurrence of sialolithiasis in a large group of cases shows the following distribution: submaxillary gland and duct, 64 per cent; parotid gland and duct, 20 per cent; and sublingual gland and duct, 16 per cent. In a series of 180 cases reported by Levy and his associates, the gland distribution was 80 per cent, 19 per cent and 1 per cent, respectively. The common involvement of the submaxillary gland and duct is thought to be due to the tenacity of the submaxillary saliva, which, because of its high mucin content, adheres to any foreign particle. The submaxillary duct is also long and irregular in its course.

Sialolithiasis involving ducts of the minor or intraoral accessory salivary glands sometimes also is seen. A review of 55 cases involving the accessory glands was reported by Pullon and Miller, and an additional series of 47 cases was presented by Jensen and his associates. The majority of these sialoliths are found in the upper lip, with only slightly fewer in the buccal mucosa, together accounting for nearly 90 per cent of all cases. Occasional cases are reported in the buccal sulcus, lower lip, palate and tongue. They usually present as solitary, firm, freely movable, small masses or nodules and may or may not be symptomatic.

Chemical and Physical Features.   The sialolith may be round, ovoid or elongated. It may measure just a few millimeters or 2 cm. or more in diameter. The involved duct may contain a single stone or many stones. They are usually yellow. Wakeley reported the average composition of the apatite structure as follows:

$Ca_3(PO_4)_2$ 74.3%
$CaCO_3$................................. 11.1
Soluble salts 6.2
Organic matter......................... 6.2
Water 2.2

Treatment and Prognosis.   Small calculi may sometimes be removed by manipulation. The

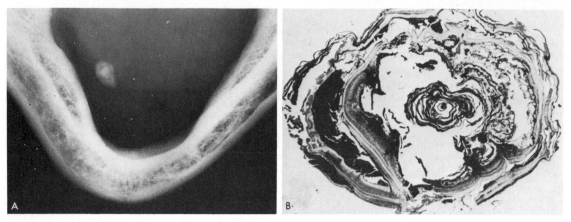

Figure 10–28.   *Sialolithiasis.*
A piece of calculus in the submaxillary duct is shown in the occlusal roentgenogram (**A**). The laminated structure of the stone is obvious in the photomicrograph (**B**).

larger stones almost always require surgical exposure for removal. If they are present near or in the substance of the gland itself, particularly if multiple, surgical extirpation of the gland may be necessary. The solitary sialolith does not usually recur, although occasional cases have presented chronic multiple recurrences.

Maxillary Antrolithiasis

(Antral Rhinolith)

Maxillary antrolithiasis is a relatively rare condition which is defined as a complete or partial calcific encrustation of an antral foreign body, either endogenous or exogenous, which serves as a nidus. An endogenous nidus may consist of a dental structure such as a root tip or may simply be a fragment of soft tissue, bone, blood or mucus. Exogenous nidi are uncommon, but may consist of such materials as snuff or paper. This condition has been discussed by Karges and his associates.

Clinical Features.   The antrolith may occur at any age in either sex. There may be a complete absence of symptoms, although some cases are marked by pain, sinusitis, nasal obstruction, and/or foul discharge and epistaxis.

Some cases, according to Blaschke and Brady, are discovered accidentally during roentgenographic examination in which an opaque mass is evident in the sinus.

Treatment.   The antrolith should be surgically removed.

Rhinolithiasis

Rhinolithiasis is a condition analogous to antrolithiasis, except that the calcification of the foreign body occurs intranasally. Literally hundreds of cases of this condition have been reported in the literature, occurring with such frequency presumably because of the ease with which small objects may be inserted in the nasal cavity. This condition has been discussed by Schwartz, who pointed out that the rhinolith may be present for years and frequently gives rise to odorous discharge and symptoms of nasal obstruction as well as pain and epistaxis. At least one case of an antrorhinolith, a "stone" partially in the nasal passage and partially in the antrum, has also been reported.

X-Ray Radiation

The general term "radiation" is applied to two different forms of energy: (1) that derived from electromagnetic radiation, and (2) that derived from particle radiation. Electromagnetic radiation consists of a continuous spectrum of varying wavelengths ranging from long electrical and radiowaves down through infra-red, visible light, ultraviolet light, roentgen rays and gamma rays. Particle radiation is generated through spontaneous decay of various natural and artificial radioactive materials, Particles may also be generated by accelerating deuterons, electrons, and so forth, in devices such as the cyclotron and betatron.

Certain natural radioactive elements such as radium and thorium give off radiant energy spontaneously in their decay process. A portion of this is electromagnetic or gamma (γ) rays, but most of the radiation consists of alpha (α) and beta (β) particles. Alpha particles, which are helium nuclei in rapid motion, have little ability to penetrate tissues and thus give up their energy in a very short distance. Beta particles, which are negatively charged electrons in rapid motion, have a greater penetrating power than alpha particles, but lose their energy in a few millimeters of tissue. Alpha and beta particles actually have little use in medical therapy and are important chiefly as hazards.

Radioactive isotopes of most of the known elements have been prepared. The half-life of these isotopes ranges from a fraction of a second to centuries (Table 10–1). The majority of the isotopes produce only beta radiation, although some produce alpha particles and gamma rays. In recent years many of these radioactive isotopes have found use in medicine as tracer substances, therapeutic agents and diagnostic agents, as well as in many areas of research.

These different types of radiant energy or radiation are sometimes spoken of as "ionizing radiation." This term refers to rays which carry enough energy to produce ionization in materials which absorb them, including living tis-sues. The most commonly used unit of measure of x-ray and gamma ray exposure is the roentgen (r). This is defined as the amount of x-rays or gamma rays which, on passing through 1 cc. of dry atmospheric air at 0°C. and 760 mm. of mercury, causes emission from atoms of this air of electrons which, when they give up all their energy in the production of ions in air, produce 2.095×10^9 ion pairs, or one electrostatic unit. Another important unit of radiation measurement is the rad or radiation absorbed dose. The rad, a unit of *absorbed* dose rather than exposure, is a measure of the energy imparted to matter by ionizing radiation per unit mass of irradiated material at the point of interest, and is 100 ergs per gram. A roentgen and a rad are roughly equivalent, although they can vary markedly depending upon the type of tissue or material involved. In contrast to these precise *physical* measures of exposure and absorbed dose, there is no adequate unit of *biologic* measurement of dosage, the most closely approaching this being the "skin erythema dose" (S.E.D.). This is often used to indicate the exposure just sufficient to produce reddening of the skin. Unfortunately, it varies widely among different persons.

General Effects of Radiation on Tissue. The exact means by which radiation exerts its effect on cells and tissues is unknown. Most investi-

Table 10–1. Table of Common Radioisotopes

ELEMENT	ISOTOPE	HALF-LIFE	ELEMENT	ISOTOPE	HALF-LIFE
Arsenic	As^{76}	26.7 hr.	Plutonium	*Pu^{239}	24.3×10^3 yr.
Bromine	Br^{82}	36 hr.		Pu^{241}	13 yr.
Calcium	Ca^{41}	1×10^5 yr.		Pu^{242}	3.8×10^5 yr.
	Ca^{45}	160 days	Potassium	*K^{40}	1×10^9 yr.
	Ca^{47}	4.7 days	Radium	*Ra^{226}	16.2×10^2 yr.
Carbon	*C^{14}	5.6×10^3 yr.	Radon	*Rn^{222}	3.82 days
Chlorine	Cl^{36}	3×10^5 yr.	Silver	Ag^{110}	24 sec.
Cobalt	Co^{58}	71 days		Ag^{111}	7.5 days
Copper	Cu^{64}	12.8 hr.	Sodium	Na^{22}	2.6 yr.
Gold	Au^{198}	2.69 days		Na^{24}	15 hr.
Hydrogen	*H^3	12.3 yr.	Strontium	Sr^{85}	64 days
Iodine	I^{129}	1×10^7 yr.		Sr^{89}	51 days
	I^{131}	8.05 days		Sr^{90}	28 yr.
Iron	Fe^{55}	2.9 yr.	Sulfur	S^{35}	87 days
	Fe^{59}	45 days	Thorium	Th^{228}	1.91 yr.
Lead	Pb^{202}	1×10^5 yr.		*Th^{232}	1.4×10^{10} days
	*Pb^{210}	19.4 yr.	Tin	Sn^{113}	119 days
Mercury	Hg^{197}	65 hr.	Uranium	U^{233}	1.6×10^5 yr.
	Hg^{203}	47 days		*U^{234}	2.5×10^5 yr.
Molybdenum	Mo^{99}	67 hr.		*U^{235}	7.1×10^8 yr.
Nickel	Ni^{59}	8×10^4 yr.		*U^{238}	4.5×10^9 yr.
	Ni^{63}	125 yr.	Zinc	Zn^{65}	245 days
Phosphorus	P^{32}	14.2 days			

*Naturally occurring radioactive isotopes.

gators believe that it is related to the mechanism of ionization, localized injuries being produced in single cells. The cellular injury has been postulated to be due to a number of possible factors. These include (1) toxic effect of protein breakdown products, (2) inactivation of enzyme systems, (3) coagulation or flocculation of protoplasmic colloids, or (4) denaturation of nucleoproteins.

There is great variation in the radio-sensitivity of different types of living cells despite the fact that it is possible to kill any living thing with sufficiently large doses of radiation (Table 10–2). In general, embryonic, immature or poorly differentiated cells are more easily injured than differentiated cells of the same type. Once these cells are injured, however, they usually show greater recovery properties, although there are many exceptions to this rule. Significantly, all cells show increased vulnerability to radiation injury at the time of mitotic division. Furthermore, if cells are irradiated during the resting phase, mitosis is delayed or inhibited.

Latent tissue injury is one of the most unusual phenomena related to x-ray or gamma radiation

Table 10–2. Radiosensitivity of Normal Cells and Tissues

1. *Radiosensitive* (2500 r or less kills or seriously injures many cells)
   Lymphocytes and lymphoblasts
   Bone marrow (myeloblastic and erythroblastic cells)
   Epithelium of intestine and stomach
   Germ cells (ovary and testis)
2. *Radioresponsive* (2500–5000 r kills or seriously injures many cells)
   Epithelium of skin and skin appendages
   Endothelium of blood vessels
   Salivary glands
   Bone and cartilage (growing)
   Conjunctiva, cornea and lens of eye
   Collagen and elastic tissue (fibroblasts themselves are resistant)
3. *Radioresistant* (over 5000 r necessary to kill or injure many cells)
   Kidney
   Liver
   Thyroid
   Pancreas
   Pituitary
   Adrenal and parathyroid glands
   Mature bone and cartilage
   Muscle
   Brain and other nervous tissue

In part from S. Warren: Effects of radiation of normal tissues. Arch. Path., *34*:443, 562, 749, 917, 1070, 1942; 35:121, 304, 1943.

and refers to residual tissue damage after the initial radiation reaction has subsided. Although frequently no residual injury can be detected by ordinary means, the tissues will retain for years an increased susceptibility to injury if again radiated. Furthermore, repeated exposure to small doses of radiation, no one of which is sufficient to evoke a perceptible reaction, may in the aggregate produce serious latent damage. Thus the biologic effects of radiation are cumulative, but show incomplete summation.

Effects of Radiation on Oral and Paraoral Tissues. The common treatment of neoplasms in and about the oral cavity by x-ray radiation with inadvertent radiation of adjacent structures necessitates an understanding of the possible forms of damage which may result. Actually, radiation effects are dependent upon a great number of factors such as the source of the radiation, the total amount of radiation administered, the period of time over which the radiation was administered (fractionation), the type of filtration used and the total area of tissue irradiated. The changes to be described here are those frequently seen after delivery of local therapeutic doses of x-ray radiation in the treatment of neoplasms about the head and neck. They are in no way related to the use of the diagnostic x-ray machine. No attempt will be made to describe the effects of total body radiation, such as those occurring after detonation of the various nuclear bombs, because of the lack of significant clinical application of such information.

However, adult patients with acute leukemia in relapse, whose disease has become refractory to all known chemotherapeutic drugs, may receive bone marrow transplantation following total body radiation in an attempt to prolong their lives. The oral changes in 35 patients following 850 to 950 rads of total body x-ray radiation were detailed by Dreizen and his associates in 1979. Almost every patient exhibited bilateral parotitis, partial xerostomia, and oral mucositis following total body radiation. The parotitis resembled mumps that resolved spontaneously in 24 to 48 hours. Saliva production during the first week after radiation was noticeably reduced in amount and was thicker, ropier and more mucoid than usual. The mucositis, which lasted two to three weeks, began as swelling, soreness and whitening of the oral mucosa. Within 48 to 72 hours, the lips, tongue and/or entire oral cavity showed an intense reddening of the oral mucosa. Pain and denudation accompanied the mucositis. After two or three weeks there was a whitening of the oral mucosa, which has been attributed to impaired mitotic activity and prolonged retention of the superficial epithelial cells, leading to an abnormally high degree of keratinization. Palliation of the transient radiation mucositis was achieved with warm salt water or sodium bicarbonate mouthrinses. Administration of lidocaine-hydrochloride in a viscous solution, oxethazaine (Oxaine M), diphenhydramine hydrochloride (Benadryl), or Kaopectate was also effective in some patients.

Evidence is accumulating that cobalt-60 radiation therapy, as contrasted with conventional orthovoltage radiation, may have significant skin- and bone-sparing qualities. Thus, this technique may reduce the incidence of radiation complications so frequently seen in the past. Animal studies, comparing tissue healing and infection following irradiation by cobalt-60 and orthovoltage, have been reported by Meyer and his co-workers, who have also discussed the possible future significance of this sparing effect.

EFFECTS ON SKIN. The effects of heavy therapeutic doses of x-ray radiation on the skin are well documented, although variable among patients. Erythema is the earliest visible reaction and begins within a few days after irradiation. The original erythema fades quickly, only to reappear within two to four weeks. The secondary erythema fades slowly, often leaving the skin permanently pigmented a light tan shade. After heavy irradiation the secondary erythema may be accompanied by edema with desquamation of epithelial cells resulting in denudation of the surface. Re-epithelization occurs in 10 to 14 days. These early effects are caused by direct injury of the radiated cells and tissues, while the later effects are brought about chiefly by changes in the vascular bed and in the intercellular material.

Alterations in the sebaceous gland activity, evidenced by a reduction in secretion with dryness of the skin, may occur within a week after the beginning of irradiation. The hair follicles are also sensitive to this type of radiation, and epilation, either temporary or permanent, may be produced. The sweat glands are similarly disturbed so that their absence of secretion contributes to the dryness and scaling of the skin.

Eventually the epithelium becomes thin and atrophic, and the superficial blood vessels become telangiectatic or occluded. The telangiec-

tasis may persist for months or even years as evidence of the effect of x-rays. Other evidence of vascular damage includes thickening of the intima and, in some cases, thrombosis. Some veins and arteries show subintimal fibrosis with thickening of the wall at the expense of the lumen. Endophlebitis and phlebosclerosis may be particularly evident. Both early and delayed radiation injuries in skin have been reviewed in detail recently by Fajardo and Berthrong.

EFFECTS ON ORAL MUCOSA. The changes occurring in the oral mucosa after x-ray radiation are essentially the same as those in the skin and are related to the dose and the duration of therapy. The erythema may develop at a somewhat lower dose of x-ray, and the mucositis which occurs after therapeutic radiation is evoked somewhat earlier than the analogous dermatitis (Fig. 10–29; see also Plate V).

Dreizen and his co-workers studied the effects of radiotherapy for oral cancer on the oral mucosa. They found that the mucosa in the path of radiation first appeared hyperemic and edematous. As treatment continued, the mucosa became denuded, ulcerated and covered with a fibrinous exudate. Great discomfort, which was intensified by contact with coarse or highly seasoned foods, was commonly present. The mucositis persisted throughout radiotherapy and for several weeks thereafter. Unless secondary infection occurred, spontaneous remission followed termination of the radiation therapy. In many patients, a lidocaine mouthrinse before mealtimes was necessary to produce topical anesthesia so that eating was possible. When pain and dysphasia could not be controlled with local anesthetics and analgesics, nasogastric tube feeding was necessary.

Patients undergoing radiotherapy for oral cancer also quickly lost their sense of taste, probably because of damage to the microvilli and outer surface of the taste cells. The effect was usually transitory, and taste acuity was restored within 60 to 120 days after completion of the radiotherapy.

EFFECTS ON SALIVARY GLANDS. Xerostomia, or dryness of the mouth, is one of the earliest and most universal of complaints of patients receiving therapeutic radiation about the head and neck. Alterations in the salivary glands, characterized by diminution or even complete loss of secretion, may occur within a week or two after the beginning of radiation. It is interesting that the morphologic changes do not particularly mirror the physiologic changes which occur. There is some obvious damage of

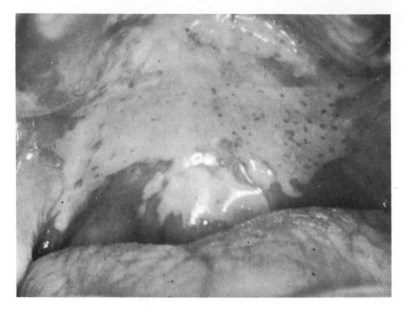

Figure 10–29. *Radiation mucositis of palate.*
The seven-day postradiation reaction consisted of a yellowish-white necrotic exudate which disappeared within an additional 14 days.

the acinar cells, chiefly a decrease in the number of secretory granules present, with congestion, edema and inflammatory cell infiltration of the interstitial connective tissue. There are no remarkable changes in the ducts of the salivary glands.

One interesting feature of acute postirradiation sialadenitis is the elevation of serum and urinary amylase, the source of this amylase being the salivary glands. This is one of the few biochemical changes that occurs early and consistently following irradiation. Kashima and his associates have discussed this finding, as well as other clinical and histopathologic features of postirradiation sialadenitis, concluding that direct exposure of the salivary glands is necessary to provoke this change and that the serum amylase response is related to the dose of irradiation. Fajardo and Berthrong have recently written a review of radiation injuries to the salivary glands.

The loss of secretion may be a permanent sequela of the radiation, or there may be a gradual return of salivation, usually only after many months.

EFFECTS ON TEETH. Erupted teeth are often affected in patients who have received x-ray radiation about the head and neck, but the damage may not appear for several years after the radiation. The most common manifestation of the injury is a peculiar destruction of tooth substance, resembling dental caries and sometimes called "radiation caries," which often begins at the cervical area of the teeth. The lesion

resembles a demineralization more than it does true caries because of its pattern or the manner in which it sweeps across the tooth, sometimes causing amputation of the tooth crown at its neck. Teeth often seem brittle, and pieces of the enamel may fracture away from the tooth (Fig. 10–30).

The primary cause of the condition lies in alterations of the saliva induced by either direct or indirect radiation of the salivary glands. Although physical and chemical changes in the saliva following salivary gland irradiation have been postulated, there is no evidence for such changes other than the direct observation that the saliva often becomes somewhat thicker and more tenacious after irradiation. The xerostomia of varying degrees certainly favors the collection of debris on the teeth and ensuing caries. Perhaps related to this problem are findings reported by Brown and his co-workers that radiation-induced xerostomia in humans produced pronounced shifts in the oral microbial population, with cariogenic microorganisms gaining prominence at the expense of noncariogenic ones. These changes occurred prior to the onset of clinical caries and were irrespective of the use of a topical fluoride gel as a caries-preventive measure.

Close cooperation between the radiotherapist, the dentist, and the patient is essential in promoting oral care for these patients. As Dreizen and his associates pointed out in 1977, xerostomia also deprives the teeth of an important natural defense against dental decay. There

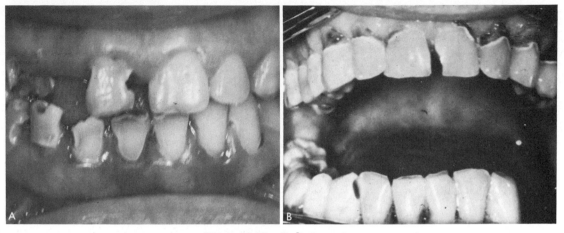

Figure 10–30. *Radiation caries.*
In *A*, the salivary glands on the side showing the caries were radiated during the course of treatment of an intraoral neoplasm; the radiation produced a xerostomia on that side and the ultimate caries. In *B*, the typical destruction of tooth substance at the cervical margins of the teeth is well illustrated. (*B*, Courtesy of Dr. Charles A. Waldron.)

is a sharp decrease in the total daily output of caries-protective salivary electrolytes and immunoproteins. Patients with xerostomia change their eating habits to include frequent, nondetergent, high carbohydrate meals. The microbial, chemical, immunologic and dietary changes produce an enormous increase in the caries challenge.

Regardless of the patient's previous caries history, the development of xerostomia is inevitably followed by rampant dental decay unless stringent protective steps are taken. Cariogenesis is so greatly accelerated that frank lesions may appear within three months after radiotherapy. However, the ravages of dental decay in the radiated patient can be almost completely prevented with one daily application of a 1 per cent sodium fluoride gel containing a red, plaque-disclosing dye. This protocol was developed by Daly and Drane in 1972. The gel is applied for at least five minutes by means of custom fabricated flexible plastic carriers. When the carriers are removed and the gel is rinsed off, the plaque is stained red and can be removed by brushing and flossing. To be maximally effective, the program must be instituted at the beginning of radiotherapy and continued every day. Such a regimen can also arrest caries caused by xerostomia in previously unprotected patients. Because of the ever-present risk of caries in xerostomic patients, only diligent, lifelong cooperation will assure prevention.

Developing teeth are also particularly sensitive to x-ray radiation, as was pointed out ex-

perimentally by Tribondeau and Recamier in 1905. Later work extended their observations, and both Leist and Smith demonstrated that irradiation of developing teeth in rats resulted in a disorganization of the odontoblasts and the formation of atypical dentin. Ameloblasts appear to be considerably more resistant to radiation than odontoblasts, although Burstone demonstrated in mice that, after sufficient radiation there was cessation of ameloblastic histogenesis and metaplasia of ameloblasts to a less differentiated type of cell. Similar interference with tooth formation in rats has been reported by English and his co-workers. Medak and his associates confirmed earlier reports that x-ray radiation in animals retards or, in high doses, entirely inhibits tooth eruption. It is not established whether this is due to a direct local injury in the odontogenic area or is secondary to pituitary damage induced by the radiation.

Radiation of developing teeth in human beings sometimes occurs, and if it is at a sufficiently young age, manifestations of the injury may be obvious. Such radiation is usually administered for the treatment of a tumor about the head and neck, frequently a hemangioma. Depending upon the age of the patient at the time of the irradiation, there may be complete cessation of odontogenesis resulting in anodontia in the involved area or simply a stunting of the teeth (Fig. 10–31). Poyton has discussed the effects of radiation on both developing and fully formed teeth, and examples have been cited recently by Carl and Wood.

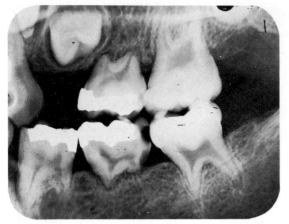

Figure 10–31. *Radiation damage to teeth.*
There is stunting of the roots of the teeth due to x-ray radiation of the dental area during the time of tooth formation. (Courtesy of Dr. John Mink.)

EFFECTS ON BONE. Bone itself is relatively resistant to x-ray radiation, although osteoblasts are sensitive. If the radiation has been sufficiently intense, the normal balance between bone formation and bone resorption is disturbed; general bone vitality is decreased, and localized osteoporosis may result.

The greatest clinical significance of bone which has been irradiated lies in the inability of this bone to react in the normal fashion to infection. This is related, at least in part, to the damage of the vascular bed with subsequent disturbance of the typical inflammatory response. There is little actual danger to the patient except in a situation in which infection may enter the bone with little difficulty and spread widely. This may occur in the maxilla and mandible.

An experimental study of the effects of radiation on extraction wound healing in rats has been reported by Stein and co-workers. They found that when radiation shortly followed tooth extraction, there was retardation of surface closure of the wound, leaving an open pathway for tissue infection. The healing response was poor and slow. As the interval between tooth extraction and radiation was increased, impairment of healing decreased. Frandsen has reported similar findings. These studies confirm most clinical observations that healing of sockets in human beings is more retarded the earlier the radiation is begun after tooth extraction. The possibility of such a detrimental occurrence must always be tempered, however, with the expediency of beginning therapy in any patient with a malignant neoplasm. In general, the longer the in-

terval between tooth extraction and initiation of radiation, the less possibility is there of healing complications. Unfortunately, achieving optimum conditions is not always possible under the circumstances.

Osteoradionecrosis is that pathologic process which sometimes follows heavy radiation of bone and is characterized by a chronic, painful infection and necrosis accompanied by late sequestration and sometimes permanent deformity.

Histologically, there is destruction of osteocytes, absence of osteoblasts, and lack of new bone or osteoid formation. The walls of the regional blood vessels are thickened by fibrous connective tissue. They are also the seat of endarteritis and periarteritis. The loose connective tissue which usually replaces the bone marrow is infiltrated by lymphocytes, plasma cells and macrophages. The devitalized bone may undergo sequestration, although there is no clear line of demarcation between vital and nonvital bone. The necrotic process may extend throughout the radiated bone. Although the exact pathogenesis is not completely understood, it is generally agreed that there are three factors involved: radiation, trauma, and infection.

The mandible is affected by osteoradionecrosis far more frequently than the maxilla. The cause for this is unknown, but may be related to the difference in blood supply between the two bones. After the infection has gained entry to the bone, following traumatic injury, extraction, pulp infection or even severe periodontitis, there is a relatively diffuse spread of the process. There is minimal localization of the infection, and there may be necrosis of a considerable amount of bone, periosteum, and overlying mucosa (Fig. 10–32). Sequestration eventually occurs, but this may be delayed for many months or several years, during which time the patient usually suffers intense pain.

The occurrence of osteoradionecrosis is unpredictable, and it may arise even without gross infection or trauma. Watson and Scarborough reported that 13 per cent of a series of 1819 patients with intraoral carcinoma or allied diseases treated with radiation suffered osteoradionecrosis. Of even greater importance is the fact that 5 per cent of these patients died as a result of this bone disease without evidence of their original cancer.

Meyer also reviewed the problem of osteoradionecrosis and found that only 5 per cent of his series of 491 patients had this disease. This

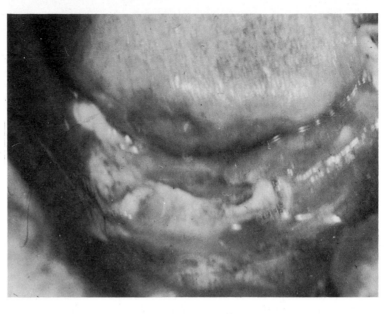

Figure 10–32. *Osteoradionecrosis.* This lesion followed heavy x-ray irradiation for epidermoid carcinoma in this area.

lower incidence figure is probably due to improved methods of radiotherapy in recent years. Similarly, Morrish and his associates reported recently that when they treated patients for cancer of the oral cavity, oropharynx and nasopharynx with doses of radiation less than 6500 rads, the risk of osteoradionecrosis of the jaw was minimal (less than 4 per cent). However, they found that when they attempted to improve their cure rate by more aggressive radiation therapy over 7500 rads, osteoradionecrosis became a significant problem (a 22 per cent rate of occurrence). They concluded that the most important risk factor for the development of osteoradionecrosis was the radiation dose to bone.

Because patients that ultimately developed osteoradionecrosis of the jaws seemed to have many characteristics in common, Daly and Drane were able to formulate a bone necrosis profile. The more factors present, the greater the chance of necrosis. Factors leading to osteoradionecrosis were listed as (1) irradiation of an area of previous surgery before adequate healing had taken place, (2) irradiation of lesions in close proximity to bone, (3) a high dose of irradiation with or without proper fractionation, (4) use of a combination of external radiation and intraoral implants, (5) poor oral hygiene and continued use of irritants, (6) poor patient cooperation in managing irradiated tissues or fulfilling home care programs, (7) surgery in the irradiated area, (8) indiscriminate use of prosthetic appliances following radiation therapy,

(9) failure to prevent trauma to irradiated bony areas, and (10) presence of numerous physical and nutritional problems prior to therapy. Patients are most vulnerable to osteoradionecrosis of the jaws in the two years following radiotherapy.

LASER RADIATION

The laser is an electro-optical device which, upon stimulation, can convert jumbles of light waves into an intense, concentrated, uniform, narrow beam of monochromatic light with an energy source of great intensity and exceptional flexibility. The radiation may be continuous or modulated, or the emission may occur in short pulses. This high-intensity radiation can be focused on an extremely small area, approximately 1 micron in diameter, because of the small angle of divergence and coherency of the beam. The term "laser" is derived from the first letters of the full name "light amplification by stimulated emission of radiation."

Applications of lasers to biology and medicine began shortly after 1960, while the laser effects on tissues and materials related to dentistry began shortly thereafter.

Effects on Teeth. The effects of laser on teeth were first reported by Stern and Sognnaes, who found that exposure of intact dental enamel caused a glasslike fusion of the enamel, whereas dentin exposed to laser exhibited a definitive charred crater. Chalky spots, craters, or small holes in enamel may also be produced under other conditions, and these have been described by a variety of workers including Kinersly and his associates, Lobene and Fine, Peck and Peck, and, in the experimental animal, by Taylor and his associates.

An excellent review of the literature on the use of the laser in dentistry has been compiled by Stern.

Effects on Pulp. The pulps of teeth in animals subjected to laser radiation have been described by Taylor and his associates as showing severe pathologic changes, including hemorrhagic necrosis with acute and chronic inflammatory cell infiltration. The odontoblastic layer also underwent coagulation necrosis, although the severity of the response varied with the amount of radiation.

Effect on Soft Tissue. When directed at soft tissue, laser radiation has the ability to produce nonspecific ulceration of the epithelium with acute purulent inflammation. This finding was reported by Taylor and his associates when laser radiation was directed at the tongue of experimental animals.

Whether any significant uses of laser radiation in dentistry will be found cannot be answered at present. Although it has been shown that selective deep destruction of carious tooth substance can be accomplished, the practicality of its use in removing carious lesions is still questionable. Bleaching of stained teeth has also been accomplished by lasing.

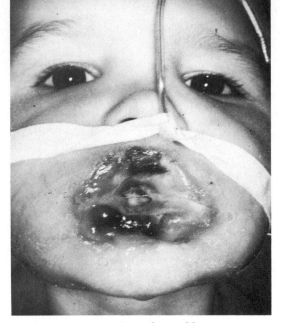

Figure 10–33.   *Electrical burn.*
This severe burn resulted when the child bit an electrical cord carrying a current.

ELECTRICAL BURNS

Electrical burns of the oral cavity are seen with an unpleasant frequency in children. This unfortunate injury has been discussed in detail by Gormley and his associates, who also reported 22 cases. They invariably result from an accident in which the child chews on an electrical cord, breaks the insulation and contacts the bare wire or sucks on the socket end of an extension cord.

The resulting burn of the lips, and sometimes of the gingiva and tongue, usually causes destruction and necrosis of a considerable amount of tissue (Fig. 10–33). Developing tooth germs or buds are often destroyed in the accident with permanent cosmetic disfigurement. This type of wound heals relatively slowly.

It has been emphasized by Needleman and Berkowitz in a thorough review of electric trauma to the oral tissues of children that the nature of the wounds frequently requires inter-

disciplinary efforts and very comprehensive care because of the variety of potential problems which ultimately may develop.

CERVICOFACIAL EMPHYSEMA

Emphysema is a swelling due to the presence of gas or air in the interstices of the connective tissue. There have been numerous cases of emphysema reported involving the cervicofacial and even mediastinal areas following a variety of dental and oral procedures—e.g., tooth extraction; blowing of compressed air into a root canal during endodontic treatment, or into a periodontal pocket; blowing of air from a high-speed-air-rotor machine; following middle-face fractures; or spontaneously as a result of the patient's breathing actions following some type of surgical procedure, with a break in the tissue permitting air to enter connective tissue spaces. Such cases have been reported and discussed by Lantz, by Rhymes and by Noble.

Clinical Features. The emphysema manifests itself as a unilateral swelling of the tissues of the face and/or neck which occurs very rapidly and is generally somewhat painful, particularly during the first few days (Fig. 10–34). Not infrequently, the patient will complain of a

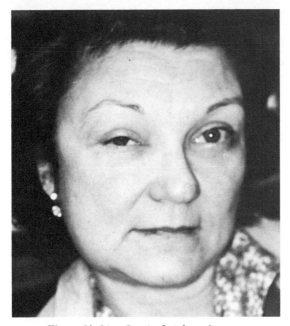

Figure 10–34. *Cervicofacial emphysema.*
The swelling of the facial soft tissues occurred within a few hours following a dental extraction.

"bubbling" sensation when palpating this tissue and of difficulty in breathing.

Treatment and Prognosis. Unfortunately, venous air embolism is an unusual but often fatal complication of this condition. For example, Longenecker has reported that, of six cases of venous air embolism occurring during head and neck surgery, five terminated fatally. If the entrance of air into the venous circulation can be recognized promptly, resuscitation may prevent death. A second complicating factor is the possibility of bacterial infection in the emphysematous connective tissue, microorganisms being carried into the tissues with the air. In such instances, antibiotic therapy is recommended. Aside from this, there is no particular treatment indicated and the condition will generally resolve within a week.

HUMAN BITE

(Morsus Humanus)

The human bite is a potentially serious injury which may occur in a variety of situations including quarrels, children's play, child abuse, mental derangements, and sexual assaults or related activities. While the bite may involve any part of the body, the extremities are most frequently involved and, according to a series of approximately 900 cases of human bite inju-

ries reported by Boyce in 1942, about 8 per cent involved the head and neck region. Laskin and Donohue have reported 14 cases, all involving the lips, while Weinstein and his coworkers have reviewed the dental literature on the subject and presented an additional case.

There is great potential for serious infections as well as for marked disfigurement from the human bite. The infections are usually of mixed types of microorganisms and can be difficult to treat, especially since patients frequently delay seeking treatment for several days after the incident because of the embarrassing circumstances involved.

The human bite also has assumed a very important role in forensic medicine and forensic dentistry, especially in murder, rape, or assault cases in which legal identification of the guilty party has been made through a set of characteristic tooth imprints in bite marks on a breast, neck or other smooth skin surface.

FELLATIO

Changes in sexual behavior and increasing sexual permissiveness in recent years have contributed to the recognition of an intraoral lesion that has become relatively common and of diagnostic importance.

The lesion consists of palatal erythema, petechiae, and ecchymoses following fellatio, or oral intercourse, apparently as a result of the physical trauma to the area and/or the negative pressure occurring at the site from the irrumation. There are usually multiple lesions, which are most often found at the junction of the hard and soft palate. They heal without treatment within seven to ten days. Typical examples have been reported by Schlesinger and his associates and by Giansanti and his co-workers.

The differential diagnosis is extremely important, since identical lesions at the same site may occur also in infectious mononucleosis, thrombocytopenic purpura or a variety of similar dyscrasias including leukemia in which a secondary thrombocytopenia may exist, and diseases of capillary fragility, among others.

CHEMICAL INJURIES OF THE ORAL CAVITY

The oral cavity frequently manifests a serious reaction to a wide variety of drugs and chemicals, although the mechanism of this reaction may be dissimilar in different cases. In some instances the tissue reaction is that of a local response to a severe irritant or even a caustic used injudiciously. In other cases the drug or chemical is administered systemically, but manifests an oral reaction of a particular type. One of the most common reactions to drugs or chemicals is the allergic phenomenon, the two main types that are of dental interest being (1) drug allergy, or stomatitis medicamentosa, and (2) contact stomatitis, or stomatitis venenata. Angioneurotic edema is still another allergic phenomenon which will be considered separately.

NONALLERGIC REACTION TO DRUGS AND CHEMICALS USED LOCALLY

The materials used locally which induce a nonallergic reaction are chiefly irritants or caustics, many of which are used by the dentist in various therapeutic or technical procedures. Some of these substances also constitute occupational hazards, but these will be considered separately.

Aspirin (Acetylsalicylic Acid)

Aspirin tablets are used mistakenly by many people as a local obtundent, especially for the relief of toothache. Although efficacious if used systemically, they are particularly harmful to the oral mucosa if applied locally. The usual mode of local use is to place the tablet against the offending tooth, allowing the cheek or lip to hold it in position, and to let it dissolve slowly. Within a few minutes a burning sensation of the mucosa will be noted, and the surface becomes blanched or whitened in appearance (Fig. 10–35). The caustic action of the drug causes separation and sloughing of the epithelium and frequently bleeding, especially if the area is traumatized. The healing of the painful "aspirin burn" usually takes a week or more. (See also Plate V.)

Sodium Perborate

Sodium perborate has been widely used as a mouthwash and in a dentifrice because of its supposed therapeutic effect on gingival disease. Clinical studies reveal, however, that the compound may produce an erythema of the oral mucosa which may even progress to sloughing of the tissues. Studies in dogs by Glickman and Bibby confirmed the clinical findings that gingivitis is not alleviated by application of sodium perborate. In some instances the inflammation was aggravated, and edema and ulceration of mucosa frequently occurred. The lesions healed spontaneously with cessation of treatment.

The fact that this compound has no definitive therapeutic value in the treatment of oral disease and that it is potentially capable of injuring the mucosa precludes recommending its use in the oral cavity.

Phenol

Phenol is widely used in dentistry as a cavity sterilizing agent as well as a cauterizing agent in various procedures. It is extremely caustic

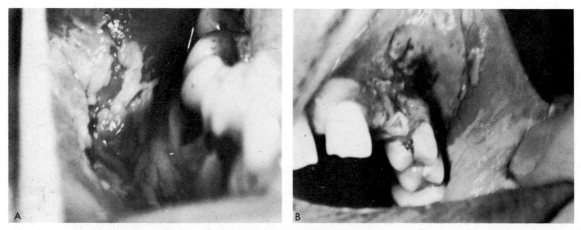

Figure 10–35. *Aspirin reaction.*
Blanching and sloughing of the epithelium are evident in *A* after the local application of an aspirin tablet; bleeding occurred in the case illustrated in *B*.

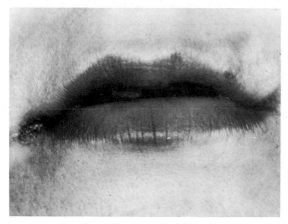

Figure 10–36. *Phenol burn.*
Injudicious handling of phenol resulted in severe burns of the lips.

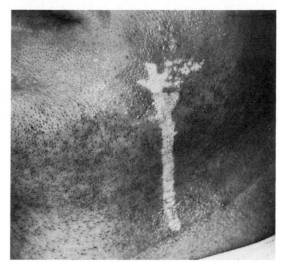

Figure 10–37. *Pyrazone "burn" of the face.*

and if used carelessly may produce severe painful burns of the oral mucosa and skin which heal slowly (Fig. 10–36).

Silver Nitrate

This material is also used extensively in dentistry as a cavity sterilizing agent, topically as a caries-preventive agent and as a chemical cautery. Injudicious or overzealous use may produce painful burns of the oral mucous membranes.

Trichloroacetic Acid

Trichloroacetic acid is used in dentistry as a cauterizing agent, particularly to cauterize gingival tissue when preparing a proximal or gingival cavity, placing a band or taking an impression of a cavity. Because of its extremely caustic nature, this acid may cause serious injury to the mucosa or skin if it is used carelessly.

Volatile Oils

A number of volatile oils such as oil of cloves, oil of wintergreen and eucalyptus oil are used in dentistry and can produce mild burns of the mucous membranes.

Miscellaneous Drugs and Chemicals

The various drugs and chemicals listed above constitute only an infinitesimal number of those substances which are of potential danger if used injudiciously in the oral cavity and are included for exemplary purposes only. Any strong acid, alkali, germicidal agent, strong counter-irritant, or even certain plant and animal irritants (Figs. 10–37, 10–38) may produce injury.

NONALLERGIC REACTIONS TO DRUGS AND CHEMICALS USED SYSTEMICALLY

The systemic administration of various drugs and chemicals frequently evokes an oral reaction which is not on the basis of an allergy or sensitivity. This reaction is often a part of a generalized epidermal reaction, but other times it occurs as a specific phenomenon apparently

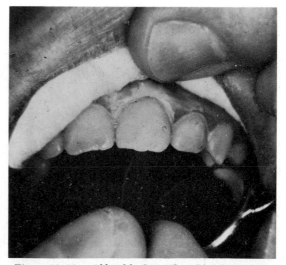

Figure 10–38. *Chloral hydrate "burn" of the gingiva.*

due to the anatomic peculiarities of the oral cavity.

Arsenic

Arsenic in both organic and inorganic forms is sometimes used therapeutically and may produce symptoms of either acute or chronic poisoning. Many cases of arsenic poisoning occur as an occupational hazard because of the wide use of this metal in industry.

Oral Manifestations. The oral mucous membranes may become intensely inflamed, and severe gingivitis may develop. The tissues may be painful. Local contact with arsenic trioxide often produces ulceration. Systemic arsenic poisoning also produces excessive salivation.

Bismuth

Bismuth was formerly used widely in the treatment of syphilis, but it has been replaced in recent years by the antibiotics. The use of this metal is still common in treating certain dermatologic disorders as well as various other diseases, so that oral signs are still sometimes seen.

Oral Manifestations. Bismuth pigmentation of the oral mucosa, particularly of the gingiva and buccal mucosa, is the most common oral feature of bismuth therapy and is reported to occur in a high proportion of patients receiving preparations containing the metal.

The pigmentation appears as a "bismuth line," a thin blue-black line in the marginal gingiva which is sometimes confined to the gingival papilla (Fig. 10–39). There may also be the same type of pigmentation of the buccal mucosa, the lips, the ventral surface of the tongue, or in any localized area of inflammation such as around partially erupted third molars or around the periphery of an ulcer as an anachoretic phenomenon (Fig. 10–40).

This pigment represents precipitated granules of bismuth sulfide produced by the action of hydrogen sulfide on the bismuth compound in the tissues. The hydrogen sulfide is formed through bacterial degradation of organic material or food debris and is most common in sites of food retention. The bismuth line occurs in the majority of patients receiving prolonged bismuth treatment and is more frequent in unclean mouths. Cruikshank reported that oral pigmentation occurred in 75 per cent of a large group of patients receiving bismuth therapy who had poor oral hygiene, but in only 7 per cent of a group who had good oral hygiene.

Patients receiving this metal also complain occasionally of a burning sensation of the mucosa and a metallic taste in the mouth.

Histologic Features. The granules of the sulfide are seen in the tissue section as small, irregular black collections of pigment, sometimes perivascular in location, but other times diffuse without apparent arrangement (Fig. 10–41). The material may be present in endothelial cells or in mononuclear phagocytes in the tissue, but it usually is in the intercellular tissue. It provokes no foreign body response and may be present even in the absence of inflammation.

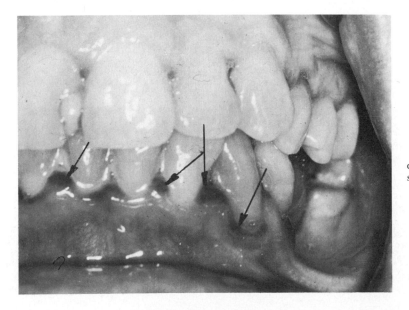

Figure 10–39. *Bismuth pigmentation.*
The gingiva shows the black line caused by the deposition of bismuth salts.

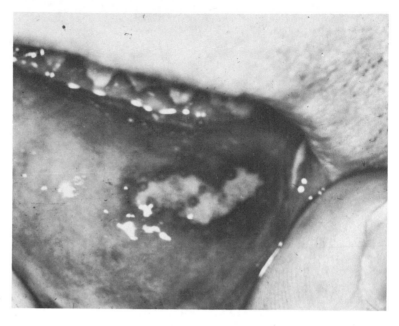

Figure 10–40. *Bismuth pigmentation.*
Deposition of bismuth around the periphery of this ulcer has produced a black "halo" effect. Gingival pigmentation is also present.

Treatment and Prognosis. There is no specific treatment for the bismuth line once it is established, although it reportedly can be bleached by concentrated hydrogen peroxide. Its prevention by scrupulous oral hygiene during therapy is recommended. The prognosis of the condition is good. If untreated, the line will gradually disappear over a long period of time if use of the bismuth compound is discontinued.

Dilantin Sodium

Dilantin sodium (sodium diphenylhydantoinate) is an anticonvulsant drug extensively used in the control of epileptic seizures. An unfortunate side effect of its use is fibrous hyperplasia of the gingiva. Most clinicians expect this hyperplasia to occur in less than half the cases, but if good oral hygiene is maintained, the incidence may be less than 10 per cent. Why proliferation of fibrous tissue occurs in one case and not in another is not known, nor is it understood why Dilantin stimulates overgrowth of gingival fibrous tissue. Nuki and Cooper have shown experimentally in cats that in the presence of local irritants in the form of orthodontic bands on the teeth and in the absence of brushing to remove plaque and debris, inflammation was produced and gingival enlargement occurred after diphenylhydantoin administration. However, when no bands were present and the teeth were brushed so that there was

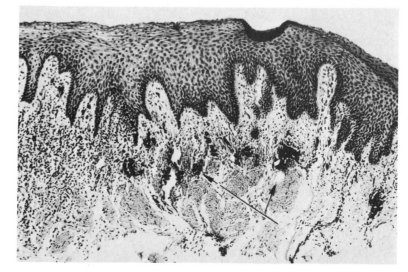

Figure 10–41. *Bismuth pigmentation.*
Collections of black amorphous material, the bismuth salts, are seen in the photomicrograph of a section through the gingiva.

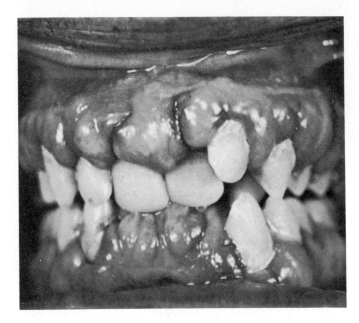

Figure 10–42. *Dilantin hyperplasia of gingiva, demonstrating remarkable gingival enlargement.*

no irritation, the administration of the drug produced no gingival enlargement. In addition, studies of Shafer and his associates have shown stimulation of wound healing in experimental animals treated with Dilantin, presumably as a result of stimulation of fibroblastic proliferation and increased collagen synthesis. In other studies Shafer has also shown remarkable stimulation of growth of human gingival fibroblasts in a tissue culture system after exposure to Dilantin. Interestingly, this drug appeared to be cell-specific in his studies, since there was no similar stimulation of other types of cells.

Oral Manifestations. Gingival hyperplasia may begin as early as two weeks after Dilantin therapy has been instituted, although usually it takes two to three months. The first change noted is a painless increase in the size of the gingiva, starting with the enlargement of one or two interdental papillae. The surface of the gingiva shows an increased stippling and finally a cauliflower, warty or pebbled surface. As enlargement increases, the gingival tissue becomes lobulated, and clefts remain between each enlarged gingiva in many cases (Fig. 10–42). Palpation reveals that the tissue is dense,

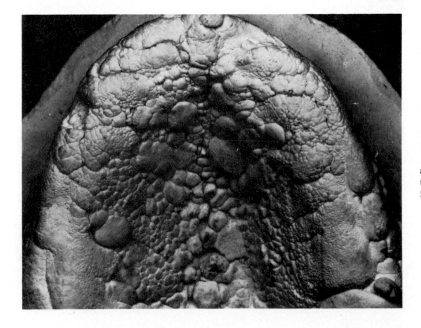

Figure 10–43. *Dilantin hyperplasia in an edentulous patient, an uncommon situation.*
In this case the denture probably acted as a contributing irritating factor. (Courtesy of Drs. Frank R. Shroff and B. Dallas.)

resilient and insensitive. It shows little tendency to bleed.

The hyperplasia of oral mucosa is almost entirely confined to the gingival tissues surrounding the teeth. In cases in which a patient is dentulous, but has a few edentulous areas, the gingival tissues around the teeth may show extreme hyperplasia, while the edentulous regions are generally normal in appearance. On rare occasions hyperplasia may occur in localities apart from the gingiva, such as the palate in patients wearing a prosthetic appliance, a probable source of chronic irritation (Fig. 10–43).

Histologic Features. Microscopic study of the gingival tissue reveals a suggestive but not pathognomonic appearance. The stratified squamous epithelium covering the tissue is thick and has a thin keratinized layer. The rete pegs are extremely long and thin, sometimes called "test-tube" pegs, with considerable confluence, but mitotic figures are seldom seen. The bulk of the tissue is made up of large bundles of collagen fibers interspersed with fibroblasts and fibrocytes (Fig. 10–44). Vascularity is not a prominent feature of the lesion. If chronic inflammation is superimposed on this hyperplasia, plasma cells and leukocytes will be found.

Treatment and Prognosis. No treatment is necessary until the enlargement becomes esthetically objectionable. If the hyperplasia interferes with function, surgical excision is recommended, but the hyperplasia will often recur. Discontinuing use of the drug will result in a gradual diminution of the bulk of the gingiva. Most patients, however, prefer to continue use of the drug and suffer with the hyperplasia rather than resort to some other, less effective drug for the prevention of the epileptic seizures.

Lead

Lead poisoning (plumbism) occurs chiefly as an occupational hazard today, but occasionally occurs because of some other accidental exposure of either an acute or chronic nature. In adults the chief means of poisoning is through inhalation of lead vapor or dust. In infants most cases result from ingestion by the child while chewing on wood painted with lead-containing paint. Many other unusual sources of lead may also result in poisoning. It appears that there have been increasing environmental levels of lead in recent years and that much of the increase is related to industry. An extremely comprehensive review of lead poisoning and its oral manifestations has been published by Gordon and his associates.

Clinical Features. Lead intoxication is manifested by serious gastrointestinal disturbances which include nausea, vomiting, colic and constipation. A peripheral neuritis also develops which may produce the characteristic wrist-drop or foot-drop. Encephalitis may also occur. Blood changes are those of a hypochromic anemia with basophilic stippling of the red blood cells. Skeletal changes due to deposition of lead in growing bone occur in children and are demonstrable on the roentgenogram.

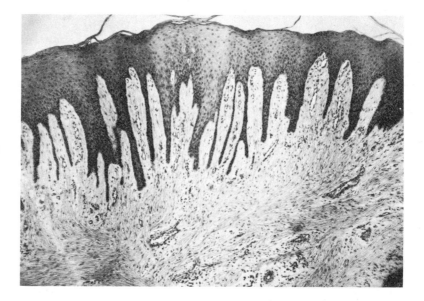

Figure 10–44. *Dilantin hyperplasia.*

Oral Manifestations. The formation of a "lead line" similar to the "bismuth line" occurs in lead poisoning. This gray or bluish black line of sulfide pigmentation occurs in the gingiva, but is somewhat more diffuse than that of bismuth. It is also found occasionally in other areas of the oral cavity. Ulcerative stomatitis is an additional reported finding.

Excessive salivation and a metallic taste are also common complaints in this condition, as is swelling of the salivary glands.

It is reported by Altshuller and his associates that lead is deposited in the deciduous teeth of children suffering from lead poisoning, and that these teeth may serve as an index of the body burden of lead.

Treatment and Prognosis. Treatment of the oral lesions is secondary to systemic treatment, and the prognosis depends upon the systemic condition of the patient.

Mercury

Mercury poisoning may be acute or chronic, but the systemic reactions in the acute form are so serious that the oral features need not be considered. Chronic mercurialism occurs after prolonged contact with mercurial compounds in a variety of situations, including therapeutic use of these compounds and as an occupational hazard.

Clinical Features. Chronic mercurialism is characterized by gastric disturbances, diarrhea, excitability, insomnia, headache, and mental depression. The patients frequently have fine tremors of the fingers and limbs as well as of the lips and tongue. In addition, a desquamative dermatitis occurs in some persons. Nephritis is common in acute mercurial poisoning, but does not occur in severe form in the chronic type.

Oral Manifestations. The oral cavity suffers seriously in mercurialism and evidences numerous characteristic but not necessarily pathognomonic signs and symptoms. There is a remarkably increased flow of saliva (ptyalism), and a metallic taste in the mouth due to excretion of mercury in the saliva. The salivary glands may be swollen, and the tongue is also sometimes enlarged and painful. Hyperemia and swelling of the gingiva are occasionally seen.

The oral mucosa is prone to ulcerations on the gingiva, palate and tongue. In severe cases pigmentation of the gingiva similar to the bismuth and lead lines may occur as a result of deposition of the dark sulfide compound. Loosening of the teeth, even leading to exfoliation, has been reported.

A toxic reaction from absorption of mercury in dental amalgam has been reported on a number of occasions. Frykholm, after a thorough review of the literature and numerous studies on the absorption and excretion of mercury, concluded that the amount of estimated exposure to mercury from dental amalgam is not sufficient to cause mercury poisoning in the conventional sense. Nevertheless this exposure may suffice to bring about allergic manifestations in patients sensitive to the mercury, as in the case reported by Fernström and his associates.

Treatment and Prognosis. The treatment of the oral lesions in chronic mercurialism is supportive only and is secondary to the treatment of the poisoning itself. The prognosis is usually good, although severe periodontal destruction and loss of teeth may occur.

Acrodynia
(Pink Disease; Swift's Disease)

Acrodynia is an uncommon disease with striking cutaneous manifestations. Until recent years, its etiology was unknown, but the work of Warkany and Hubbard established the cause of the disease as a mercurial toxicity reaction, either an actual mercury poisoning or, more likely, an idiosyncrasy to the metal. The source of the mercury is usually a teething powder, ammoniated mercury ointment, calomel lotion or bichloride of mercury disinfectant.

Clinical Features. Acrodynia occurs most frequently in young infants before the age of two years, although children are occasionally affected up to the age of five or six years. The skin, particularly of the hands, feet, nose, ears and cheeks, becomes red or pink and has a cold, clammy feeling. The appearance has been described as resembling raw beef. The skin over the affected areas peels frequently during the course of the disease. The patients also have a maculopapular rash which is extremely pruritic. Severe sweating is an almost constant feature of acrodynia. Other features are a state of extreme irritability, photophobia with lacrimation, muscular weakness, tachycardia, hypertension, insomnia, gastrointestinal upset and stomatitis. The children will frequently tear their hair out in patches (Fig. 10–45).

The excretion of mercury from the body appears to be a variable phenomenon. For this reason the recovery of unusual amounts of mercury from the urine is not always possible.

Oral Manifestations. Patients with acro-

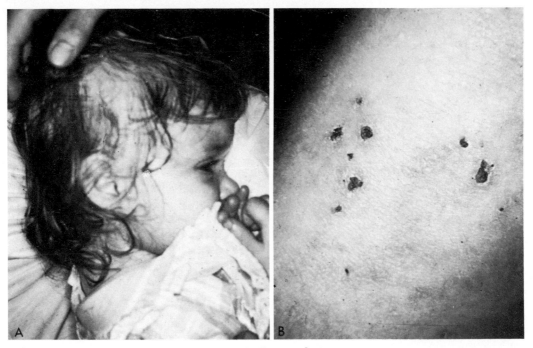

Figure 10–45. *Acrodynia.*
The child shows patchy loss of hair and numerous lesions of the skin which are scabbed from the scratching due to the severe pruritus. Premature exfoliation of numerous deciduous teeth had also occurred. (Courtesy of Dr. Nathaniel Rowe.)

dynia exhibit profuse salivation and often much "dribbling." The gingiva becomes extremely sensitive or painful and may exhibit ulceration. Bruxism is a common finding, and loosening and premature shedding of teeth often occur; many times the child will extract loose teeth with his fingers. Mastication is difficult because of the pain.

Treatment and Prognosis. The discontinuance of possible exposure to mercury is a necessity, and the administration of BAL (British anti-lewisite; dimercaprol) has proved successful in most cases unless the disease is of long duration. Although recovery is the common outcome, patients occasionally die of this disease.

Silver

(Argyria; Argyrosis)

Chronic exposure to silver compounds may occur as an occupational hazard or as the result of therapeutic use of silver compounds such as silver arsphenamine or silver nitrate. It results in a permanent pigmentation of the skin and mucous membranes. In this instance the pigmentation is due to reduction of the silver compound in the tissues and appears bluish gray. The pigmentation of the oral mucous membrane is diffusely dispersed throughout the oral cavity. There are usually no other signs or symptoms, either local or systemic, associated with argyria.

Amalgam tattoo of oral mucous membrane is a relatively common finding in dental practice, generally occurring in one of four ways, according to Buchner and Hansen: (1) from condensation in gingiva during amalgam restorative work, (2) from particles entering mucosa lacerated by revolving instruments during removal of old amalgam restorations, (3) from broken pieces introduced into a socket or beneath periosteum during tooth extraction, or (4) from particles entering a surgical wound during root canal treatment with a retrograde amalgam filling. The most common locations for amalgam tattoos, as evidenced by 268 cases reported by Buchner and Hansen, were gingiva (28 per cent), buccal mucosa (23 per cent) and alveolar mucosa (19 per cent).

This tattoo has frequently been mistaken for a melanin-pigmented lesion, and in some cases biopsy is necessary to differentiate if the amalgam fragments are too small or diffuse to be visible on the dental roentgenogram. When the amalgam fragments are embedded within bone, they may be mistaken for a variety of other foreign bodies (Fig. 10–46).

Microscopically, the dental amalgam fragments frequently show no tissue reaction to their presence, even no inflammatory response (Fig. 10–47). Such was the case in 45 per cent of the 268 cases reported by Buchner and Hansen. However, in 38 per cent of the cases there was a chronic inflammatory response, usually manifesting as a foreign body granuloma with either foreign body giant cells or Langhans' giant cells. In 17 per cent of the cases there was a macrophagic reaction of some type, with or without a chronic inflammatory cell response.

The amalgam fragments appear as black or olive-brown granules or even as macroscopic pieces of material which can be seen plainly in the paraffin-embedded specimen as silver-gray flecks in the tissue. These granules are prominently arranged in a linear fashion along collagen fibers and around blood vessels. In addition, they are found around nerve sheaths and striated muscle fibers and along the basement membrane of mucosal epithelium.

Harrison and his associates have studied these tattoos by electron microscopy and electron probe analysis and found that the original mercury-silver-tin amalgam undergoes eventual

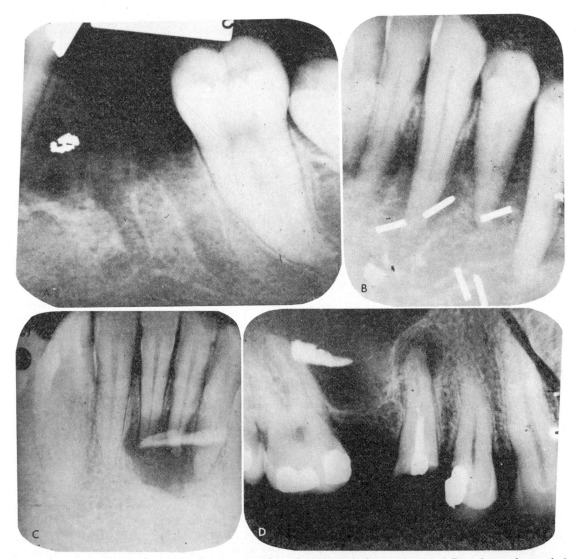

Figure 10–46. Amalgam in bone (A). This is compared to other foreign bodies seen occasionally such as radon seeds for radiation of a tumor (B), embedded glass after an automobile accident (C), and a bomb-shell fragment (D). (B, Courtesy of Dr. Henry M. Swenson; C, Dr. G. Thaddeus Gregory; and D, Dr. Raymond Price.)

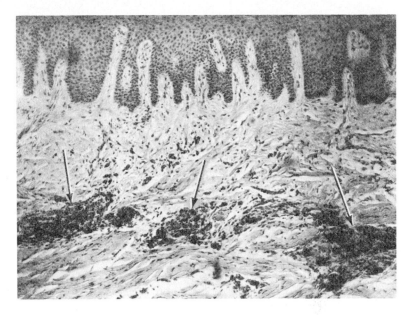

Figure 10–47. *Amalgam tattoo.* The black deposits of amalgam exhibit no surrounding tissue reaction.

corrosion, leaving chiefly silver in the extracellular sites.

Tetracycline

Discoloration of either deciduous or permanent teeth may occur as a result of tetracycline deposition during prophylactic or therapeutic regimens instituted either in the pregnant female or postpartum in the infant. Tetracycline and its homologues have a selective affinity for deposition in bone and tooth substance, possibly through the formation of a complex with calcium ions in the surface of the microcrystals of hydroxyapatite, according to Urist and Ibsen.

That portion of the tooth stained by tetracycline is determined by the stage of tooth development at the time of drug administration. Since tetracycline does cross the placental barrier, it may involve those deciduous teeth developing antepartum, although the discoloration itself depends upon the dosage, the length of time over which administration occurred, and the form of the tetracycline. Moffitt and his coworkers have emphasized that the critical period for tetracycline-induced discoloration in the deciduous dentition (the period of mineralization of the first millimeter of dentin nearest the dentinoenamel junction) is four months in utero to three months postpartum for maxillary and mandibular incisors and five months in utero to nine months postpartum for maxillary and mandibular canines. The period for permanent maxillary and mandibular incisors and

canines is three to five months postpartum to about seven years of age. The age at which tetracycline administration occurred can easily be pinpointed by reference to a chart on the chronology of odontogenesis.

According to Grossman and his associates, the use of oxytetracycline, or possibly doxycycline, may diminish tooth discoloration if tetracycline therapy is indicated in the pregnant female or during the first six to seven years of life. After this age, the probability of discoloration need not be considered since the cosmetically important anterior teeth have completed their formation.

Clinical Features. The teeth affected by tetracycline appear to have a yellowish or brownish-gray discoloration which is most pronounced at the time of eruption of the teeth. This discoloration gradually becomes more brownish after exposure to light. Tetracycline itself fluoresces under ultraviolet light and, accordingly, the teeth involved by its discoloration also fluoresce a bright yellow under ultraviolet light. However, in time this fluorescence gradually diminishes. It has been shown by Wallman and Hilton and by Zussman that the dentin is more heavily stained than the enamel.

Cancer Chemotherapeutic Agents

A chemically very diverse group of drugs and agents has come into recent use for the treatment of certain malignant neoplastic diseases. Their chief function is the destruction of malignant cells. Most of these cytotoxic agents exert their effect preferentially against cells in mitosis. Unfortunately, in addition to neoplastic cells, which undergo rapid division, certain normal cells—including the cells of the oral and gastrointestinal mucosa, bone marrow and skin—also exhibit a similar degree of mitotic activity and are especially prone to manifest the toxic and damaging effects of the antineoplastic agents. The specific reactions of the mucocutaneous tissues have been reviewed by Adrian and his associates.

Clinical Features. The major groups of cancer chemotherapeutic agents are shown in Table 10–3. Because the major effect of these materials on cells and tissues is similar, regardless of each agent's specific mechanisms of action, there are a few general manifestations of the

Table 10–3. Cancer Chemotherapeutic Agents

ALKYLATING AGENTS
    Busulfan (Myleran)
    Chlorambucil (Leukeran)
    Cyclophosphamide (Cytoxan)
    Melphalan (Alkeran; L–PAM)
    Triethylenethiophosphoramide (Thio-TEPA)

ANTIMETABOLITES
    Arabinosylcytosine (Ara-C)
    Adenine arabinoside (Ara-A)
    6-Mercaptopurine (6-MP)
    6-Thioguanine (6-TG)
    Methotrexate (MTX)
    5-Fluorouracil (5-FU)

ANTITUMOR ANTIBIOTICS
    Actinomycin-D (Dactinomycin)
    Bleomycin (Blenoxane)
    Daunorubicin (Daunomycin)
    Doxorubicin (Adriamycin)
    Mithramycin (Mithracin)
    Mitomycin-C (Mutamycin)

PLANT ALKALOIDS
    Vinblastine (Velban)
    Vincristine (Oncovin)

NITROSOUREAS (HALOGENATED N-ALKYL-N-NITROSOUREAS)
    Carmustine (BCNU)
    Lomustine (CCNU)
    Semustine (Methyl-CCNU)

ENZYMES
    L-Asparaginase (Elspar)

MISCELLANEOUS
    Dacarbazine (DTIC-Dome)
    Hydroxyurea (Hydrea)
    Procarbazine (Matulane)
    Cis-diamminedichloroplatinum (Platinol)
    Hexamethylmelamine (HMM)

---

group as a whole that can be emphasized. These are (1) alopecia, due to arrest of mitosis of the rapidly germinating hair roots, (2) stomatitis, which may take a variety of forms, and (3) radiation recall or radiation sensitization, a reactivation of radiation reaction within the field of radiation following administration of certain of the antineoplastic agents.

Oral Manifestations. The most common oral reaction is mucosal erosion and ulceration, frequently diffuse and multiple, often related to the neutropenia produced by the drug but occasionally occurring in its absence. This may occur anywhere in the mouth but is most likely to be seen on the lips, tongue, and buccal mucosa. Hemorrhage is also a common manifestation resulting from the thrombocytopenia secondary to the drug therapy. These reactions do not occur following use of all cancer chemotherapeutic agents but are especially common with the alkylating, antimetabolite and antitumor antibiotic groups.

Another oral finding in patients undergoing this type of therapy is the presence of any one of a variety of specific or nonspecific infections (commonly herpes simplex infection, Candida infection or infection by staphylococcal or streptococcal organisms), especially since many of these patients are also immunosuppressed.

Finally, hyperpigmentation of oral mucosa has been reported occasionally, especially in patients receiving alkylating agents and antitumor antibiotics.

Treatment. There is no specific treatment for the oral lesions which, although severe, must be considered of only secondary importance to the patient's major problem.

ALLERGIC REACTIONS TO DRUGS AND CHEMICALS

"Allergy" is a broad term used generally to encompass the hypersensitive state acquired by exposure to a specific material and the altered capacity of the living organism to react upon re-exposure to this allergen. Nearly all cases of allergy depend upon the combination of an antigen, usually but not always a protein or a polysaccharide, with an antibody produced by the host almost invariably as a result of previous exposure to the antigen.

There are two general types of allergic reactions, although great diversity of appearance of the various phenomena exists in each group. One type of reaction, the so-called immediate reaction, is that associated with antibodies circulating in the serum of the allergic person and includes anaphylaxis, hay fever and asthma, serum sickness, angioneurotic edema and the wheal-and-erythema skin reaction. The second type of reaction, or delayed reaction, is generally not associated with circulating antibodies, since the causative agents are not strictly antigens, but rather attain antigenic properties by combining with the tissues of the individual. In contrast to the immediate reaction, which develops as soon as the allergenic substance is absorbed, the delayed reaction is not manifested clinically for several hours after exposure. Reactions of the latter type include drug allergies, allergies of certain infections and contact reactions to a vast variety of materials.

Angioneurotic Edema

(Angioedema; Quincke's Edema; Giant Urticaria)

Angioneurotic edema is a rather common form of edema occurring in both hereditary and nonhereditary forms. It appears to be closely related to general urticaria. The "neurotic" implication has persisted since the original description of the disease by Quincke in 1882, and there is no doubt that many patients do present psychologic problems which seem to contribute to the disease. Some cases of the nonhereditary form of angioneurotic edema are seemingly due to a food allergy, but seldom can the specific food be determined by the usual methods of allergen skin testing. In some cases it is thought that drugs, an endocrine disturbance, or a focal infection plays an important etiologic role. The cause in most instances, however, is unknown.

The less common hereditary form of the disease is inherited as an autosomal dominant trait. This hereditary form, first described by Sir William Osler in 1888, has been reviewed in detail by Donaldson and Rosen. They have also emphasized the biochemical abnormality in patients with the disease: the absence from the serum of a normally naturally occurring inhibitor of $C'1$ esterase which is a specific α-2 globulin in the complement system. This deficiency causes increased consumption of $C'2$ and $C'4$, with formation of a kininlike substance that causes an increase in vascular permeability and edema. Patients with nonhereditary angioneurotic edema have normal quantities of the inhibitor.

Clinical Features. Angioneurotic edema of

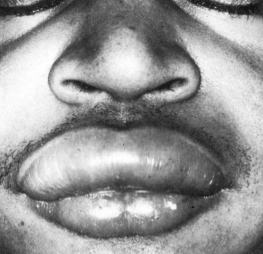

Figure 10–48. *Angioneurotic edema.*
The patient exhibits diffuse swelling of the cheeks and lips.

either type manifests itself as a smooth, diffuse edematous swelling particularly involving the face around the lips, chin and eyes, the tongue, and sometimes the hands and feet (Fig. 10–48). The swelling may involve any area, however, and the parotid gland has been reported to be affected in a number of cases. The eyes may be swollen shut and the lips extremely puffy. The symptoms appear rapidly, sometimes being present when the patient awakens in the morning. A feeling of tenseness or an itching or prickly sensation sometimes precedes the urticarial swelling. The skin is of normal color or slightly pink.

The condition usually lasts for only 24 to 36 hours, although some cases persist for several days. The frequency of the attacks cannot be predicted; sometimes they appear daily, other times at intervals of months or even years. The disease affects both sexes about equally, but is infrequent in children. Some cases seem to originate at puberty.

The hereditary form may be more dangerous because there is sometimes visceral involvement. Vomiting and abdominal pain may occur, and, especially dangerous, edema of the glottis which can result in death through suffocation.

The mechanism of development of the swelling in angioneurotic edema appears to be a vasodilatation, brought about by the release of histamine or a histamine-like substance, with subsequent transudation of plasma.

Treatment and Prognosis. When the etiologic agent, such as food, can be discovered, its elimination from the diet will prevent recurrent attacks. The causative agent can seldom be detected, however. Once developed, the edema can be treated by antihistamine drugs with usually prompt relief.

The disease is annoying, but in itself is seldom dangerous unless edema of the glottis or respiratory tract occurs. In such instances an emergency tracheotomy may be necessary.

Albright and Taylor have emphasized that local traumatic injury, which may occur in even such minor oral surgery as tooth extraction, is the most consistent precipitating event in an acute attack of hereditary angioneurotic edema. Heft and Flynn have pointed out that this form of the disease carries a high morbidity and cited examples of cases treated successfully with ε-aminocaproic acid and also by androgens. ε-aminocaproic acid is an antifibrinolytic agent which blocks the activation of plasmin, which in turn activates the complement cascade.

Drug Allergy

(Drug Idiosyncrasy; Drug Sensitivity; Stomatitis or Dermatitis Medicamentosa)

Drug allergy includes a variety of sensitivity reactions following exposure to any one of a great many drugs and chemicals but is not related to any pharmacologic activity or toxicity of these materials. Practically every known drug has been recognized at one time or another as capable of producing an allergic reaction in a sensitive person. Certain drugs, however, have a far greater tendency to produce reactions than others. Furthermore, some patients have a greater susceptibility to drugs and manifest reactions more readily than others. This is particularly true in patients who have other allergic diseases, such as asthma or hay fever.

It is impossible to list even a small portion of the drugs which have been known to produce an allergic reaction. Certain drugs, however, invoke reactions in such a high percentage of cases that this fact is of considerable clinical importance and warrants special note. These drugs include the following:

Aminopyrine	Gold
Arsphenamine	Iodides
Aspirin	Penicillin
Barbiturates	Phenolphthalein
Bromides	Quinine
Chloramphenicol	Streptomycin
Chlortetracycline	Sulfonamides
Dilantin	Thiouracil

Clinical Features. One of the most common allergic reactions to a drug is a manifestation that is similar to serum sickness and includes skin lesions, arthralgia, fever and lymphadenopathy. Agranulocytosis (q.v.) also sometimes occurs as a drug reaction. The skin lesions are of an erythematous type, as in erythema multiforme (q.v.), or they may be urticarial in nature. Sometimes an exfoliative dermatitis occurs. A "fixed" drug eruption may occur in patients who are administered on repeated occasions a drug to which they are sensitive. This "fixed" eruption consists in the appearance of a skin reaction at the same sites each time and is apparently due to local sensitization of the tissues. Nevertheless *the skin "patch" test is negative*. The various reactions are seldom anaphylactic in suddenness of appearance, but instead occur several hours to several days or longer after the beginning of the drug administration. Occasionally an immediate severe reaction occurs.

Oral Manifestations. Oral reactions to the administration of various drugs are considerably less common than are analogous cutaneous reactions. The reason for this is not clear. The oral lesions, sometimes referred to as stomatitis medicamentosa, are usually diffuse in distribution and vary in appearance from multiple areas of erythema to extensive areas of erosion or ulceration. In the early stages of the reaction, vesicles or even bullae may be found on the mucosa. Occasionally, purpuric spots appear, and angioneurotic edema is sometimes seen.

Involvement of the gingiva, palate, lips and tongue is particularly common (Fig. 10–49). The ulceration and necrosis of the gingiva often resemble acute necrotizing gingivitis or Vincent's infection. Hairy tongue, either black, brown or yellow, has been reported as a complication of antibiotic therapy, particularly with penicillin. In this condition there are elongation and staining of the filiform papillae, producing a heavy coating of the tongue. It has been suggested that this reaction is due not to the direct effect of the antibiotic on the tongue, but to the alteration of oral bacterial flora, with an overgrowth of fungal elements and subsequent overgrowth of papillae. Alteration of intestinal flora with disturbances in elaboration of vitamins or vitamin components may also play some role, since vitamin deficiencies are readily mirrored in the tongue. The lingual papillae will sometimes be desquamated after antibiotic therapy, leaving a smooth, painful, inflamed tongue which may become eroded.

The mercury in both silver and copper amalgam restorations has been suspected for many

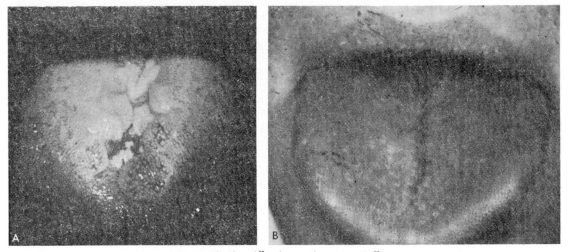

Figure 10–49. *Allergic reactions to penicillin.*
The tongue may become ulcerated (A) or denuded of papillae (B) in a penicillin reaction. (Courtesy of Dr. Boynton H. Booth.)

years of being potentially hazardous. The recent studies of Frykholm indicate that true mercury poisoning is unlikely, but that a mercury allergy due to exposure to dental amalgam is entirely possible. Such occurrences are extremely rare, however, considering the number of persons whose teeth contain amalgam restorations.

Treatment and Prognosis. The signs and symptoms of drug allergy usually regress with discontinuance of the causative agent. The acute signs may be relieved by the administration of antihistaminic drugs or cortisone. Recurrence can be prevented only by complete abstinence from use of the particular drug involved.

Contact Stomatitis and Dermatitis

(Stomatitis and Dermatitis Venenata)

A contact allergy is a type of reaction in which a lesion of the skin or mucous membrane occurs at a localized site after repeated contact with the causative agent. This form of allergy appears to result from a combination of the contactant with proteins of the epidermal cells, thus forming an antigen. This antigen in turn induces the formation of antibodies, which are not usually circulating, but which produce the usual antigen-antibody reaction.

There have been literally thousands of contactants identified as causing an allergic dermatitis. These vary from simple chemical elements to exceedingly complex organic substances. Many of these materials have come to represent hazards of occupation because of the wide use of organic compounds in industry. Certain initiating agents produce lesions upon contact because of their inherent irritating nature rather than as a result of an allergic phenomenon. In general, the reaction to the true contactant does not appear immediately as do reactions to simply irritating substances such as inorganic acids or other escharotics.

It would be inappropriate to attempt to list even the more common contactants which are recognized as causing dermatitis, because of the overwhelming numbers. But there is a well-recognized group of materials which frequently cause oral lesions, stomatitis venenata, and which for this reason are of special interest to the dentist. These may be classified as follows:

1. Dental or cosmetic preparations
   a. Dentifrices
   b. Mouthwashes
   c. Denture powders
   d. Lipstick, candy, cough drops, chewing gum
2. Dental materials
   a. Vulcanite
   b. Acrylic
   c. Metal alloy bases
3. Dental therapeutic agents
   a. Alcohol
   b. Antibiotics
   c. Chloroform
   d. Iodides
   e. Phenol
   f. Procaine
   g. Volatile oils

Clinical Features. Contact dermatitis is manifested by the occurrence of an itching or burning sensation at the site of contact, followed shortly by the appearance of an erythema and then vesicle formation. After rupture of the vesicles, erosion may become extensive, and if secondary infection occurs, the lesions may be serious. In chronic contact the skin may become thickened and dry.

Oral Manifestations. Contact stomatitis, or stomatitis venenata, demonstrates a variety of manifestations analogous to dermatitis venenata. After contact with some material to which the patient is sensitive, the mucosa becomes remarkably inflamed and edematous, the reaction imparting a smooth, shiny appearance to the surface. These symptoms are usually accompanied by a rather severe burning sensation, but pruritus occurs in some instances. Small vesicles may form, but these are transient and soon rupture to form small areas of erosion and ulceration which may become extensive in some cases (Fig. 10–50). Secondary infection is particularly common.

The reaction to various dental or cosmetic preparations is not especially common. Nearly every brand of dentifrice, however, has been reported to produce a contact stomatitis in certain persons. In most instances the flavoring agent is responsible. The same holds true for mouthwashes, denture powders, candy and chewing gum. Lipstick will sometimes incite a particularly violent reaction of the lips in a sensitized woman, producing severe edema and ulceration.

Certain dental materials have been implicated in causing a contact stomatitis. Vulcanite frequently produces burning of the mucosa in patients with dentures constructed from this material. This is of little clinical significance today because of its infrequent use. Acrylic has been reported occasionally to induce a contact allergy when used either as a denture base or as a filling material. The sensitivity may develop shortly after insertion of the denture or filling or not for a considerable period of time, even many months. The tissues in contact with the material become highly inflamed and are painful. In most cases the patient has been found by means of the patch test to be sensitive to the monomer, and such sensitivity is most common in cases of incomplete polymerization of the acrylic. It is important to realize that the majority of cases of inflamed mucosa that appear to arise from contact with an acrylic denture are not due to an acrylic sensitivity, but to the fact that the denture does not fit properly and is physically irritating. True acrylic sensitivity is extremely uncommon. Allergy to metal base alloys is also rare.

A report by Lea and his co-workers has emphasized the irritating and sensitizing capacities of the epoxy resins, some of which are now in use in dental practice. They studied numerous compounds and found that at least one uncured resin, one uncured resin modifier and several amine curing agents were both irritating and sensitizing to skin and thus, presumably, to oral mucous membrane.

It is of interest to point out here that the subcutaneous implantation of methyl methac-

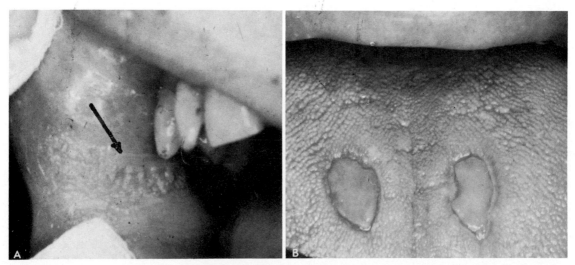

Figure 10–50. *Contact stomatitis.*
The vesicular eruption of the buccal mucosa in *A* was due to chewing leaves of the poison ivy plant, while the ulcers of the tongue in *B* were caused by application of "headache powder." (*A*, Courtesy of Dr. Henry M. Swenson and *B*, of Dr. Stephen F. Dachi.)

Table 10–4. Oral Manifestations of Occupational Disease According to the Etiologic Agent*

PHYSICAL STATE	PRINCIPAL ACTION	ETIOLOGIC AGENT — SPECIFIC FACTOR	OCCUPATION	POSSIBLE ORAL MANIFESTATIONS
Solid	Physical	Instruments for prehension	Cobblers, carpenters, glass blowers, musicians (wind instruments), seamstresses	Localized abrasion
	Chemical	Tar	Fishermen, asphalt and coal tar workers, pavers, pitch roofers, wood preservers	Stomatitis, carcinoma of lip and mucosa
Dust	Physical	Inorganic Copper, iron, nickel, chromium, coal, etc.	Bronzers, cement workers, electrotypers, grinders (metal), miners, stone cutters	Staining of teeth, pigmentation of gingiva, generalized abrasion, calculus, gingivostomatitis, hemorrhage
	Physical	Organic Bone, celluloid, sawdust, flour, tobacco	Bone, celluloid, flour, sawmill, textile, and tobacco workers	Staining of teeth, pigmentation of gingiva, generalized abrasion, calculus, gingivostomatitis, hemorrhage
	Chemical	Inorganic Arsenic	Chemical workers, electroplaters, metal refiners, rubber mixers, lead smelters, insecticide makers	Necrosis of bone
	Chemical	Bismuth	Bismuth handlers, dusting powder makers	Blue pigmentation of gingiva, oral mucosa, gingivostomatitis
	Chemical	Chromium	Aniline compound, chrome, photographic and steel workers, blue printers, rubber mixers	Necrosis of bone, ulceration of oral tissue
	Chemical	Fluorine	Cryolite workers	Osteosclerosis
	Chemical	Lead	Electrotypers, insecticide and storage battery makers, lead refiners, printers, rubber compounders	Blue-black pigmentation of gingiva, gingivostomatitis
	Chemical	Mercury	Bronzers (gun barrels), battery and paint makers, dentists, detonators, explosives and mercury salts workers	Gingivostomatitis, osteomyelitis, ptyalism
	Chemical	Phosphorus (white, yellow)	Brass founders, match factory, phosphor bronze workers, fertilizer and fireworks makers	Gingivostomatitis, ulceration of oral tissues, osteomyelitis
	Chemical	Organic Sugar	Refiners, bakers, candy makers	Caries
Liquid	Physical	Hot food (coffee, tea, soup)	Tasters	Stomatitis, leukoplakia
	Physical	Aniline	Aniline, coal tar, explosives workers, painters, tannery workers, vulcanizers	Blue coloration of lips and gingiva
	Chemical	Benzene	Coke oven and lacquer workers, dry cleaners, vulcanizers, smokeless powder makers	Hemorrhage from gingiva, stomatitis, blue coloration of lips
	Chemical	Cresol	Coal tar, rubber, tar, distillery and surgical dressing workers, disinfectant makers	Stomatitis
	Chemical	Wine and liquor	Tasters	Anesthesia and paresthesia of tongue
Gas	Physical	Atmosphere Increased pressure	Divers, caisson workers	Bleeding from gingiva
	Physical	Decreased pressure	Aviators	Bleeding from gingiva
	Physical	Acids: H_2SO_4, HNO_3, HCl, HF	Acid and cartridge dippers, petroleum refiners, explosives and gun cotton workers, galvanizers	Bleeding from gingiva, stomatitis, decalcification of enamel and dentin
	Physical	Amyl acetate	Alcohol, distillery, explosives, shellac, smokeless powder and shoe factory workers	Stomatitis
	Chemical	Acrolein	Bone grinders, lard, soap, linoleum makers, varnish boilers	Stomatitis
	Chemical	SO_2, NH_3, BR, Cl_2	Acetylene, dye, photographic film, phosgene makers, sugar refiners, refrigerating plant, disinfectant, laundry workers	Stomatitis
	Chemical	CO, CO_2	Miners, smelters, gasoline motor workers	Coloration of lips (cherry red, blue)
Ray	Physico-chemical	Radium, x-ray	Technicians, watch dial painters, research men	Gingivitis, periodontitis, osteomyelitis and necrosis, xerostomia, osteosclerosis
	Physico-chemical	Actinic	Sailors, fishermen	Carcinoma of lip

* From I. Schour and B. G. Sarnat: Oral manifestations of occupational origin: J.A.M.A. *120*:1197, 1942. (Courtesy of Dr. Isaac Schour.)

rylate in mice was reported by Laskin and his co-workers to result in a 25 per cent incidence of fibrosarcoma. Tumor formation in human beings after implantation of acrylic has not been reported.

A variety of therapeutic agents used topically in the oral cavity may produce bothersome or even serious allergic reactions. These include such common materials as antibiotics, alcohol, chloroform, phenol or the volatile oils. In the case of antibiotic lozenges or troches, it is frequently the flavoring agent rather than the antibiotic itself which causes the reaction. Of particular significance to the dentist is the fairly common allergy to procaine. This danger is of greater importance to the dentist than to patients, since the most common site of eruption is on the hands of the dentist. Considering the necessarily constant use of this local anesthetic agent, this can be professionally very serious. It may be necessary to discontinue all contact with and use of the solution, or to use rubber gloves when administering the anesthetic.

Treatment and Prognosis. The only treatment for contact dermatitis or stomatitis consists in discontinuing all contact with the offending material. When this is done, there is usually prompt remission of all lesions.

OCCUPATIONAL INJURIES OF THE ORAL CAVITY

Injuries of the oral cavity which occur as a direct result of the occupation of the patient are of rather common occurrence. In recent years industrial health programs have recognized the necessity of maintaining oral health and have emphasized the need for special precautions to prevent oral injuries.

Comprehensive studies of the oral manifestations of occupational injuries were made by Schour and Sarnat and by Walters and his co-workers. In many occupations the inherent dangers have been recognized and precautionary steps have been taken to prevent injuries. Such remarkable advances have been made in the application of organic chemicals in industrial techniques that health officers, including the dentist, must constantly be alert against new hazards. Examples of occupational injuries are listed in Table 10–4.

The examination of the oral cavity in the study of occupational disease is of generally accepted importance, since local effects are recorded both in the teeth themselves and in the soft tissues. Damage to the enamel and dentin is usually permanent and is an indicator of past occupation. The systemic effects may be transmitted to the oral cavity through the blood stream and the saliva and are frequently characteristic. Although early recognition and treatment of oral occupational diseases are important, the prevention of these diseases must be the goal of our public health authorities.

REFERENCES

Adrian, R. M., Hood, A. F., and Skarin, A. T.: Mucocutaneous reactions to antineoplastic agents. CA, 30:143, 1980.

Akers, L. H.: Ulcerative stomatitis following therapeutic use of mercury and bismuth. J. Am. Dent. Assoc., 23:781, 1936.

Albright, B. W., and Taylor, C. G.: Hereditary angioneurotic edema: report of a case. J. Oral Surg., 37:888, 1979.

Altshuller, L. F., Halak, D. B., Landing, B. H., and Kehoe, R. A.: Deciduous teeth as an index of body burden of lead. J. Pediatr., 60:224, 1962.

Anderson, G. M.: Practical Orthodontics. 9th ed. St. Louis, C. V. Mosby Company, 1960.

Andreasen, J. O.: Etiology and pathogenesis of traumatic dental injuries: A clinical study of 1,298 cases. Scand.J. Dent. Res., 78:329, 1970.

Idem: Fractures of the alveolar process of the jaw: a clinical and radiographic follow-up study. Scand. J. Dent. Res., 78:263, 1970.

Idem: Luxation of permanent teeth due to trauma: a clinical and radiographic follow-up study of 189 injured teeth. Scand. J. Dent. Res., 78:273, 1970.

Andreasen, J. O., and Hjørting-Hansen, E.: Intraalveolar root fractures: radiographic and histologic study of 50 cases. J. Oral Surg., 25:414, 1967.

Armstrong, W. D., and Simon, W. J.: Penetration of radiocalcium at the margins of filling materials. J. Am. Dent. Assoc., 43:684, 1951.

Ball, J. S., and Ferguson, A. W.: Permanent discoloration of primary dentition by nitrofurantoin. Br. Med. J., 2:1103, 1962.

Barker, B. F., Jensen, J. L., and Howell, F. V.: Focal osteoporotic bone marrow defects of the jaws. Oral Surg., 38:404, 1974.

Barker, J. N.: The sterilization of dentin. Aust. J. Dent., 39:156, 1935.

Bartels, H. A.: Significance of yeastlike organisms in denture sore mouths. Am. J. Orthod., 23:90, 1937.

Baum, H. B.: Occupational diseases of the mouth. Dent. Cosmos. 76:247, 1934.

Beasley, J. D., III: Traumatic cyst of the jaws: report of 30 cases. J. Am. Dent. Assoc., 92:145, 1976.

Bergendal, T., and Isacsson, G.: Effect of nystatin in the treatment of denture stomatitis. Scand. J. Dent. Res., 88:446, 1980.

Bernier, J. L., and Knapp, M. J.: New pulpal response to high-speed dental instruments. Oral Surg., 11:167, 1958.

Besic, F. C.: Fate of bacteria sealed in dental cavities. J. Dent. Res., 22:349, 1943.

Bhaskar, S. N., Beasley, J. D., III, and Cutright, D. E.:

Inflammatory papillary hyperplasia of the oral mucosa: report of 341 cases. J. Am. Dent. Assoc., 81:949, 1970.

Bhaskar, S. N., Bolden, T. E., and Weinmann, J. P.: Experimental obstructive adenitis in the mouse. J. Dent. Res., 35:852, 1956.

Idem: Pathogenesis of mucoceles. J. Dent. Res., 35:863, 1956.

Blaschke, D. D., and Brady, F. A.: The maxillary antrolith. Oral Surg., 48:187, 1979.

Bourgoyne, J. R.: Sialolithiasis. Oral Surg., 1:719, 1948.

Box, H. K; Red bone-marrow in human jaws. Bull. No. 20. Can. Dent. Res. Fndn., 1933.

Idem: Bone resorption in red marrow hyperplasias in human jaws. Bull. No. 21. Can. Dent. Res. Fndn., 1936.

Boyce, F. F.: Human bites. South. Med. J., 35:631, 1942.

Brännström, M.: Reaction of the pulp to amalgam fillings. Odontol. Revy, 14:244, 1963.

Brännström, M., and Söremark, R.: The penetration of ²²Na ions around amalgam restorations with and without cavity varnish. Odontol. Revy, 13:331, 1962.

Breitner, C., and Tischler, M.: Über die Beeinflussung der Zahnkeime durch orthodontische Bewegung der Milchzähne, Z. Stomatol., 32:1383, 1934.

Brown, L. R., Dreizen, S., Handler, S., and Johnston, D. A.: Effect of radiation-induced xerostomia on human oral microflora. J. Dent. Res., 54:740, 1975.

Brunner, H.: Pathology of ranula. Oral Surg., 2:1591, 1949.

Buchner, A., and Hansen, L. S.: Amalgam pigmentation (amalgam tattoo) of the oral mucosa. Oral Surg., 49:139, 1980.

Budtz-Jørgensen, E.: Denture stomatitis. III. Histopathology of trauma- and candida-induced inflammatory lesions of the palatal mucosa. Acta Odontol. Scand., 28:551, 1970.

Budtz-Jørgensen, E., and Bertram, U.: Denture stomatitis. I. The etiology in relation to trauma and infection. Acta Odontol. Scand., 28:71, 1970.

Idem: Denture stomatitis. II. The effect of antifungal and prosthetic treatment. Acta Odontol. Scand., 28:283, 1970.

Burstone, M. S.: The effect of x-ray irradiation on the teeth and supporting structures of the mouse. J. Dent. Res., 29:220, 1950.

Idem: Radiobiology of the oral tissues. J. Am. Dent. Assoc., 47:630, 1953.

Butt, B. G., Harris, N. O., Shannon, I., and Zander, H. A.: Ultrasonic removal of tooth structure. I. A histopathologic evaluation of pulpal response in monkeys after ultrasonic cavity preparation. J. Am. Dent. Assoc., 55:32, 1957.

Cahn, L. R.: The denture sore mouth. Ann. Dent., 3:33, 1936.

Canizares, O.: Contact dermatitis due to the acrylic materials used in artificial nails. Arch. Dermatol., 74:141, 1956.

Carl, W., Schaaf, N. G., and Chen, T. Y.: Oral care of patients irradiated for cancer of the head and neck. Cancer, 30:448, 1972.

Carl, W., and Wood, R.: Effects of radiation on the developing dentition and supporting bone. J. Am. Dent. Assoc., 101:646, 1980.

Casamassimo, P. S., and Lilly, G. E.: Mucosal cysts of the maxillary sinus: a clinical and radiographic study. Oral Surg., 50:282, 1980.

Cawson, R. A.: Denture sore mouth and angular cheilitis. Br. Dent. J., 115:441, 1963.

Claus, E. C., and Orban, B: Fractured vital teeth. Oral Surg., 6:605, 1953.

Colby, R. A.: Radiation effects on structures of the oral cavity: a review. J. Am. Dent. Assoc., 29:1446, 1942.

Coy, H. D., Bear, D. M., and Kreshover, S. J.: Autopolymerizing resin fillings. J. Am. Dent. Assoc., 44:251, 1952.

Crawford, B. E., and Weathers, D R.: Osteoporotic marrow defects of the jaws. J. Oral Surg., 28:600, 1970.

Criep, L.: Allergy and Clinical Immunology. New York, Grune & Stratton, 1976.

Cruikshank, L. C.: Dental disease and its relation to antisyphilitic treatment. Br. J. Vener. Dis., 14:280, 1938.

Curtis, A. C., and Taylor, H., Jr.: Allergic dermatoses of importance to the dentist. Am. J. Orthod. Oral Surg., 33:201, 1947.

Cutright, D. E.: The histopathologic findings in 583 cases of epulis fissuratum. Oral Surg., 37:401, 1974.

Cutright, D. E.: Morphogenesis of inflammatory papillary hyperplasia. J. Prosthet. Dent., 33:380, 1975.

Dachi, S. F., Ross, A., and Stigers, R. W.: Effects of prednisolone on the thermal sensitivity and pulpal reactions of amalgam-restored teeth. J. Am. Dent. Assoc., 69:565, 1964.

Daly, T. E., and Drane, J. B.: Management of dental problems in irradiated patients. Refresher course. Radiological Society of North America, Chicago, 1972.

Idem: Effects of prednisolone on the thermal sensitivity and pulpal reactions of silicate-restored teeth. J. Prosthet. Dent. 14:1124, 1964.

del Regato, J. A.: Dental lesions observed after roentgen therapy in cancer of buccal cavity, pharynx and larynx. Am. J. Roentgenol., 42:404, 1939.

Diamond, R. D., Stanley, H. R., and Swerdlow, H.: Reparative dentin formation resulting from cavity preparation. J. Prosthet. Dent., 16:1127, 1966.

Donaldson, V. H., and Rosen, F. S.: Hereditary angioneurotic edema: a clinical survey. Pediatrics, 37:1017, 1966.

Dreizen, S., Daly, T. E., Drane, J. B., and Brown, L. R.: Oral complications of cancer radiotherapy. Postgrad. Med., 61:85, 1977.

Dreizen, S., McCredie, K. B., Dicke, K. A., Zander, A. R., and Peters, L.: Oral complications of bone marrow transplantation in adults with acute leukemia. Postgrad. Med., 66:187, 1979.

Ellis, R. G., and Davey, K. W.: The Classification and Treatment of Injuries to the Teeth of Children. 5th ed. Chicago, Year Book Publishers, Inc., 1970.

English, J. A., Schlack, C. A., and Ellinger, F.: Oral manifestations of ionizing radiation. II. Effect of 200 KV. X-ray on rat incisor teeth when administered locally to the head in the 1,500 R dose range. J. Dent. Res., 33:377, 1954.

Ennis, L. M., Berry, H. M., and Phillips, J. E.: Dental Roentgenology. Philadelphia, Lea & Febiger, 1967.

Esterberg, H. L., and White, P. H.: Sodium Dilantin gingival hyperplasia. J. Am. Dent. Assoc., 32:16, 1945.

Ettinger, R. L.: The etiology of inflammatory papillary hyperplasia. J. Prosthet. Dent., 34:254, 1975.

Evelyn, K. A.: Medical applications of artificial radioactive isotopes. Can. Med. Assoc. J., 56:547, 1947.

Fajardo, L. F., and Berthrong, M.: Radiation injury in surgical pathology. Part III. Salivary glands, pancreas and skin. Am. J. Surg. Pathol., 5:279, 1981.

Fasoli, G.: Silikatcement und pulpa Veranderungen. Z. Stomatol., 22:222, 1924.

Fernström, A. I. B., Frykholm, K. O., and Huldt, S.: Mercury allergy with eczematous dermatitis due to silver-amalgam fillings. Br. Dent. J., 113:204, 1962.

Finnerud, C. W.: Perlèche; its nosologic status. J.A.M.A, *126*:737, 1944.

Fish, E. W.: Reaction of the dental pulp to peripheral injury of the dentin. Proc. R. Soc. Med., Sect. Odontol., *108*:196, 1931.

Idem: The reaction of dental pulp to peripheral injury of the dentine. Br. Dent. J., *52*:338, 1931.

Fisher, A. A.: Allergic sensitization of the skin and oral mucosa to acrylic denture materials. J.A.M.A., *156*:238, 1954.

Fisher, A. K., and Rashid, P. J.: Inflammatory papillary hyperplasia of the palatal mucosa. Oral Surg., *5*:191, 1952.

Frandsen, A. M.: Effects of roentgen irradiation of the jaws on socket healing in young rats. Acta Odontol. Scand., *20*:307, 1962.

Frankel, M. A.: Tetracycline antibiotics and tooth discoloration. J. Dent. Child., *37*:117, 1970.

Frykholm, K. O.: On mercury from dental amalgam: its toxic and allergic effects and some comments on occupational hygiene. Acta Odontol. Scand., *15*(Suppl. 22): 1957.

Gardner, A. F., Stoller, S. M., and Steig, J. M.: A study of the traumatic bone cyst of the jaw. Can. Dent. Assoc., J., *28*:151, 1962.

Gelbke, H.: The influence of pressure and tension on growing bone in experiments with animals. J. Bone Joint Surg., *33A*:947, 1951.

Giansanti, J. S., Cramer, J. R., and Weathers, D. R.: Palatal erythema: another etiologic factor. Oral Surg., *40*:379, 1975.

Glaros, A. G., and Rao, S. M.: Effects of bruxism: a review of the literature. J. Prosthet. Dent., *38*:149, 1977.

Glickman, I., and Bibby, B. G.: Effect of sodium perborate upon the gingival mucosa: a controlled experiment. J. Am. Dent. Assoc., *31*:1201, 1944.

Glickman, I., and Lewitus, M. P.: Hyperplasia of the gingivae associated with Dilantin (sodium diphenylhydantoinate) therapy. J. Am. Dent. Assoc., *28*:199, 1941.

Going, R. E.: Status report on cement bases, cavity liners, varnishes, primers, and cleansers. J. Am. Dent. Assoc., *85*:654, 1972.

Goldman, L., Gray, J. A., Goldman, J., Goldman, B., and Meyer, R.: Effect of laser beam impacts on teeth. J. Am. Dent. Assoc., *70*:601, 1965.

Gordon, N. C., Brown, S., Khosla, V. M., and Hansen, L. S.: Lead poisoning. Oral Surg., *47*:500, 1979.

Gormley, M. B., Marshall, J., Jarrett, W., and Bromberg, B.: Thermal trauma: a review of 22 electrical burns of the lip. J. Oral Surg., *30*:531, 1972.

Gottlieb, B.: Some orthodontic problems in histologic illumination. Am. J. Orthod., *32*:113, 1946.

Gregory, G. T., and Shafer, W. G.: Surgical ciliated cysts of the maxilla: report of cases. J. Oral Surg., *16*:251, 1958.

Grossman, E. R., Walchek, A., and Freedman, H.: Tetracyclines and permanent teeth: the relation between dose and tooth color. Pediatrics, *47*:567, 1971.

Grossman, L. I.: Pulp reactions to the insertion of self-curing acrylic resin filling materials. J. Am. Dent. Assoc., *46*:265, 1952.

Grubrich, W.: Veründergungen an orthodontisch bewegten Zähnen. Korr. Zahnärtze, *54*:153, 1930.

Gubler, W.: Zur Frage der orthodontisch verursachten Wurzelresorption. Schweiz. Mschr. Zahnheilk., *41*:1011, 1931.

Guernsey, L. H.: Reactive inflammatory papillary hyperplasia of the palate. Oral Surg., *26*:814, 1965.

Gurley, W. D., and Van Huysen, G.: Histologic response of teeth of dogs to operative procedures. J. Dent. Res., *19*:179, 1940.

Idem: Histologic changes in teeth due to plastic filling materials. J. Am. Dent. Assoc., *24*:1807, 1937.

Halstead, C. L.: Mucosal cysts of the maxillary sinus: report of 75 cases. J. Am. Dent. Assoc., *87*:1435, 1973.

Hansen, L. S., Sapone, J., and Sproat, R. C.: Traumatic bone cysts of jaws. Oral Surg., *37*:899, 1974.

Hardwick, J. L.: Sterilisation of carious dentin. Proc. R. Soc. Med., *42*:815, 1949.

Harrison, J. D.: Salivary mucoceles. Oral Surg., *39*:268, 1975.

Harrison, J. D., and Garrett, J. R.: Histological effects of ductal ligation of salivary glands of the cat. J. Path., *118*:245, 1976.

Harrison, J. D., Rowley, P. S. A., and Peters, P. D.: Amalgam tattoos: light and electron microscopy and electron-probe micro-analysis. J. Pathol., *121*:83, 1977.

Healey, H. G., Patterson, S. S., and Van Huysen, G.: Pulp reaction to ultrasonic cavity preparation. U.S. Armed Forces Med. J., *7*:1956.

Heft, M. W. and Flynn, P. M.: Hereditary angioedema: review of literature and dental treatment. J. Am. Dent. Assoc., *95*:986, 1977.

Henschel, C. J.: The friction of revolving steel burrs. J. Am. Dent. Assoc., *31*:895, 1944.

Idem: Heat impact of revolving instruments on vital dentin tubules. J. Dent. Res., *22*:323, 1943.

Herzberg, B. L.: Bone changes incident to orthodontic tooth movement in man. J. Am. Dent. Assoc., *19*:1777, 1932.

Hjørting-Hansen, E., and Holst, E.: Morsicatio mucosae oris and suctio mucosae oris. Scand. J. Dent. Res., *78*:492, 1970.

Howe, G. L.: Haemorrhagic cysts of the mandible–I, II. Br. J. Oral Surg., *3*:55, 77, 1965.

Hurt, W. C.: Mucous cysts. Oral Surg., *3*:425, 1950.

Ivy, R. H.: Hemorrhagic or traumatic cysts of the mandible. Surg., Gynecol. Obstet., *65*:640, 1937.

James, V. E., and Diefenbach, G. B.: Prevention of histopathologic changes in young dogs' teeth by use of zinc oxide and eugenol. J. Am. Dent. Assoc., *29*:583, 1942.

James, V. E., Schour, I., and Spence, J. M.: Response of human pulp to gutta-percha and cavity preparation. J. Am. Dent. Assoc., *49*:639, 1954.

Jensen, J. L., Howell, F. V., Rick, G. M., and Correll, R. W.: Minor salivary gland calculi. Oral Surg., *47*:44, 1979.

Johnson, A. L., Appleton, J. L., Jr., and Rittershofer, L. S.: Tissue changes involved in tooth movement. Int. J. Orthod. *12*:889, 1926.

Kaneshiro, S., Nakajima, T., Yoshikawa, Y., Iwasaki, H., and Tokiwa, N.: The postoperative maxillary cyst: report of 71 cases. J. Oral Surg., *39*:191, 1981.

Karges, M. A., Eversole, L. R., and Poindexter, B. J., Jr.: Antrolith: report of case and review of literature. J. Oral Surg., *29*:812, 1971.

Kashima, H. K., Kirkham, W. R., and Andrews, J. R.: Postirradiation sialadenitis: a study of the clinical features, histopathologic changes and serum enzyme variations following irradiation of human salivary glands. Am. J. Roentgenol., Radium Ther. Nucl. Med., *94*:271, 1965.

Kinerly, T., Jarabak, J. P., Phatak, N. M., and Dement, J.: Laser effect on tissue and material related to dentistry. J. Am. Dent. Assoc., *70*:593, 1965.

King, J. D.: Experimental investigations of parodontal disease in the ferret and related lesions in man. (2)

Gingival hyperplasia due to epanutin therapy. Br. Dent. J., *83*:148, 1947.

Knapp, M. J., and Bernier, J. L.: The response of oral tissues to ultrasound. J. Am. Dent. Assoc., *58*:50, 1959.

Kramer, J., and McLean, L.: The response of the human pulp to self polymerising acrylic restorations. Br. Dent. J., *92*:255, 1952.

Kraus, A.: Kann von dem unter einer Fuellung unbehandeltem Zurueckgelassenem Cariosem Dentin die Karies weiterschreiten? Zahn. Rundsch., *42*:1093, 1943.

Kronfeld, R.: The process of repair following tooth fracture. J. Dent. Res., *11*:247, 1931.

Kutscher, A. H., Zegarelli, E. V., Tovell, H. M. M., and Hochberg, B.: Discoloration of teeth induced by tetracycline. J.A.M.A., *184*:586, 1963.

Langeland, K.: Tissue changes in the dental pulp. Odontol. Tidskr., *65*:239, 1957.

Lantz, B.: Cervicofacial emphysema. A report of three cases with periodontal etiology. Odontol. Revy, *15*:279, 1964.

Laskin, D. M., and Donohue, W. B.: Treatment of human bites of the lip. J. Oral Surg., *16*:236, 1958.

Laskin, D. M., Robinson, I. B., and Weinmann, J. P.: Experimental production of sarcomas by methyl methacrylate implants. Proc. Soc. Exp. Biol. Med., *87*:329, 1954.

Lawrence, E. A.: Osteoradionecrosis of the mandible. Am. J. Roentgenol. Radium Ther., *55*:733, 1946.

Lea, W. A., Jr., Block, W. D., and Cornish, H. H.: The irritating and sensitizing capacity of epoxy resins. A.M.A. Arch. Dermatol., *78*:304, 1958.

Lefkowitz, W., Seelig, A., and Zachinsky, L.: Pulp response to a self-curing acrylic filling material. N. Y. Dent. J., *15*:376, 1949.

Lehner, T.: Oral candidosis. Dent. Practit., *17*:209, 1967.

Leist, M.: Über die Einwirkung der Roentgenstrahlen und des Radiums auf Zahne ünd Kiefer. Strahlentherapie, *24*:268, 1927.

Levy, B. M., ReMine, W. H., and Devine, K. D.: Salivary gland calculi: pain, swelling associated with eating. J.A.M.A., *181*:1115, 1962.

Levy, B. M., Rugh, R., Lunin, L., Chilton, N., and Moss M.: The effect of a single subacute x-ray exposure to the fetus on skeletal growth; a quantitative study. J. Morphol., *93*:561, 1953.

Lisanti, V. F., and Zander, H. A.: Thermal injury to normal dog teeth: in vivo measurements of pulp temperature increases and their effect on the pulp tissue. J. Dent. Res., *31*:548, 1952.

Lobene, R. R., and Fine, S.: Interaction of laser radiation with oral hard tissues. J. Prosthet. Dent., *16*:589, 1966.

Loeb, L.: Effects of roentgen rays and radioactive substances on living cells and tissues. J. Cancer Res., *7*:229, 1922.

Longenecker, C. G.: Venous air embolism during operations on the head and neck: report of a case. Plast. Reconstr. Surg., *36*:619, 1965.

Low-Beer, B. V. A.: Radiation therapy and dental medicine. Oral Surg., *4*:739, 1951.

Lura, H. E.: Tissue reactions of bone upon mechanical stresses. Am. J. Orthod., *38*:453, 1952.

Lynch, M. (ed.): Burket's Oral Medicine. 7th ed. Philadelphia, J. B. Lippincott Company, 1977.

Manley, E. B.: Effect of filling materials on the human tooth pulp. Proc. R. Soc. Med., Sect. Odontol., *34*:693, 1941.

Idem: Preliminary investigations into reaction of pulp to various filling materials. Br. Dent. J., *60*:321, 1936.

Idem: A review of pulp reactions to chemical irritations. Int. Dent. J., *1*:36, 1950.

Marshall, J. A.: Root absorption of permanent teeth– a study of bone and tooth movement. J. Am. Dent. Assoc., *17*:1221, 1930.

Idem: A study of bone and tooth changes incident to experimental tooth movement and its application to orthodontic practice. Int. J. Orthod., *19*:1, 1933.

Medak, H., Schour, I., and Klauber, W. A.: The effect of single doses of irradiation upon the eruption of the upper rat incisor. J. Dent. Res., *29*:839, 1950.

Meklas, J. F.: Bruxism: diagnosis and treatment. J. Acad. Gen. Dent., *19*:31, 1971.

Meyer, I.: Osteoradionecrosis of the Jaws. Chicago, Year Book Publishers, Inc., 1958.

Meyer, I, Shklar, G., and Turner, J.: Tissue healing and infection in experimental animals irradiated with cobalt-60 and orthovoltage. Oral Surg., *21*:333, 1966.

Miller, G.: Fat embolism: a comprehensive review. J. Oral Surg., *33*:91, 1975.

Mitchell, D. F., and Jensen, J. R.: Preliminary report on the reaction of the dental pulp to cavity preparation using an ultrasonic device. J. Am. Dent. Assoc., *55*:57, 1957.

Moffitt, J. M., Cooley, R. O., Olsen, N. H., and Hefferren, J. J.: Prediction of tetracycline-induced tooth discoloration. J. Am. Dent. Assoc., *88*:547, 1974.

Morris, C. R., Steed, D. L., and Jacoby, J. J.: Traumatic bone cysts. J. Oral Surg., *28*:188, 1970.

Morrish, R. B., Jr., Chan, E. , Silverman, S., Jr., Meyer, J., Fu, K. K., and Greenspan, D.: Osteonecrosis in patients irradiated for head and neck carcinoma. Cancer, *47*:1980, 1981.

Moyers, R. E.: The periodontal membrane in orthodontia. J. Am. Dent. Assoc., *40*:22, 1950.

Myall, R. W. T., Eastep, P. B., and Silver, J. G.: Mucous retention cysts of the maxillary antrum. J. Am. Dent. Assoc., *89*:1338, 1974.

Nadler, S. C.: Bruxism, a classification: critical review. J. Am. Dent. Assoc., *54*:615, 1957.

Nathanson, N. R., and Quinn, T. W.: Ranula: a review of the literature and report of three cases. Oral Surg., *5*:250, 1952.

Needleman, H. L., and Berkowitz, R. J.: Electric trauma to the oral tissues of children. ASDC J. Dent. Child., *41*:19, 1974.

Newton, A. V.: Denture sore mouth: a possible aetiology. Br. Dent. J., *112*:357, 1962.

Noble, W. H.: Mediastinal emphysema resulting from extraction of an impacted mandibular third molar. J. Am. Dent. Assoc., *84*:368, 1972.

Nuki, K., and Cooper, S. H.: The role of inflammation in the pathogenesis of gingival enlargement during the administration of diphenylhydantoin sodium in cats. J. Periodont. Res., *7*:102, 1972.

Nygaard-Østby, B.: Pulp reactions to direct filling resins. J. Am. Dent. Assoc., *50*:7, 1955.

Idem: Clinical and experimental experience with Borden Airotor. Nor. Tannlaegeforen. Tidskr. *68*:124, 1958.

Ohba, T., Yang, R. -C., Chen, C. -Y., and Uneoka, M.: Postoperative maxillary cyst. Int. J. Oral Surg., *9*:480, 1980.

Olech, E., Sicher, H., and Weinmann, J. P.: Traumatic mandibular bone cysts. Oral Surg., *4*:1160, 1951.

Oman, C. R.: Further report on use of ultrasonics in dentistry. Ann. Dent., *14*:1, 1955.

Oppenheim, A.: Bone changes during tooth movement. Int. J. Orthod., *16*:535, 1930.

Idem: Human tissue response to orthodontic intervention

of short and long duration. Am. J. Orthod. Oral Surg., 28:263, 1942.

Idem: Tissue changes, particularly of the bone incident to tooth movement. Am. J. Orthod., 3:57, 113, 1911–1912.

Palazzi, S.: Über die anatomischen Veränderungen der Zahnpulpa im Gefolge von Silikatzementfüllungen. Z. Stomatol., 21:279, 1923.

Peck, S., and Peck, H.: Laser radiation: some specific dental effects and an evaluation of its potential in dentistry. J. Prosthet. Dent., 17:195, 1967.

Peyton, F. A., and Vaughn, R. C.: Thermal changes developed during the cutting of tooth tissue. Fortn. Rev., 20:9, 1950.

Phillips, R. W.: Skinner's Science of Dental Materials. 8th ed. Philadelphia, W. B. Saunders Company, 1982.

Pindborg, J. J.: Clinical radiographic and histological aspects of intra-alveolar fractures of upper central incisors. Acta Odontol. Scand., 13:41, 1955–56.

Poyton, H. G.: The effects of radiation on teeth. Oral Surg., 26:639, 1968.

Pullon, P. A., and Miller, A. S.: Sialolithiasis of accessory salivary glands: review of 55 cases. J. Oral Surg., 30:832, 1972.

Quincke, H.: Über akutes umschriebenes Hautödem. Monatschr. Prak. Dermat., 1:129, 1882.

Ramanathan, K., Ganesan, T. J., and Raghavan, K. V.: Salivary mucoceles—racial and histological variations. Med. J. Malaysia, 4:302, 1977.

Reitan, K.: The initial tissue reactions incident to orthodontic tooth movement. Acta Odontol. Scand. (Suppl. 6): 1951.

Idem: Tissue changes following experimental tooth movement as related to the time factor. Dent. Record, 73:559, 1953.

Renner, R. P., Lee, M., Andors, L., and McNamara, T. F.: The role of C. albicans in denture stomatitis. Oral Surg., 47:323, 1979.

Rhymes, R., Jr: Postextraction subcutaneous emphysema. Oral Surg., 17:271, 1964.

Rickles, N. H.: Procaine allergy in dental patients: diagnosis and management; a preliminary report. Oral Surg., 6:375, 1953.

Robinson, H. B. G.: Pulpal effects of operative dentistry. J. Prosthet. Dent., 7:282, 1957.

Robinson, L., and Hjørting-Hansen, E.: Pathologic changes associated with mucous retention cysts of minor salivary glands. Oral Surg., 18:191, 1964.

Rovelstad, G. H., and St. John, W. E.: Condition of the young dental pulp after the application of sodium fluoride to freshly cut dentin. J. Am. Dent. Assoc., 39:670, 1949.

Rycroft, R. J. G.: Contact dermatitis from acrylic compounds. Br. J. Dermatol., 96:685, 1977.

Samuels, H. S.: Contact glossitis from autopolymerizing resin splint. U.S. Armed Forces Med. J., 11:1501, 1960.

Sandstedt, C.: Einige Beiträge zur Theorie der Zahnregulierung. Nord. Tandläkare Tidskr., 1904, 1905.

Schlesinger, S. L., Borbotsina, J., and O'Neill, L.: Petechial hemorrhages of the soft palate secondary to fellatio. Oral Surg., 40:376, 1975.

Schour, I., and Sarnat, B. G.: Oral manifestations of occupational origin. J.A.M.A., 120:1197, 1942.

Schützmannsky, G.: Unfallverletzungen an jugendlichen Zähnen, Dtsch. Stomatol., 13:919, 1963.

Schwartz, A. M.: Tissue changes incidental to orthodontic tooth movement. Int. J. Orthod., 18:331, 1932.

Schwartz, H. C.: Rhinolithiasis: a disorder not to be approached transorally. J. Am. Dent. Assoc., 98:228, 1979.

Seelig, A.: The effect of direct filling resins on the tooth pulp. J. Am. Dent. Assoc., 44:261, 1952.

Seelig, A., and Lefkowitz, W.: Pulp response to filling materials. N. Y. Dent. J., 16:540, 1950.

Segreto, V. A., Jerman, A. C., and Shannon, I. L.: Absorption and excretion of mercury in dental personnel: preliminary study. USAF School of Aerospace Medicine, Aerospace Medical Division (AFSC). Brooks Air Force Base, Texas, June, 1968.

Sewerin, I.: A clinical and epidemiologic study of morsicatio buccarum/labiorum. Scand. J. Dent. Res., 79:73, 1971.

Shafer, W. G.: The effect of single and fractionated doses of selectively applied x-ray irradiation on the histologic structure of the major salivary glands of the rat. J. Dent. Res., 32:796, 1953.

Idem: Effect of Dilantin sodium on various cell lines in tissue culture. Proc. Soc. Exp. Biol. Med., 108:694, 1961.

Shafer, W. G., Beatty, R. E., and Davis, W. B.: Effect of Dilantin sodium on tensile strength of healing wounds. Proc. Soc. Exp. Biol. Med., 98:348, 1958.

Shroff, F. R.: Effects of filling materials on the dental pulp. N. Z. Dent. J., 42:99, 145, 1946; 43:35, 1947.

Sieverink, N. P. J. B.: The simple bone cyst. Drukkerij Schippers, Nijmegen, 1974.

Silverman, F. N., and Cassady, H. A.: Acrodynia following ingestion of mercurial ointment; late dental sequelae. N. Eng. J. Med., 247:343, 1952.

Skillen, W. G., and Reitan, K.: Tissue changes following rotation of teeth in the dog. Angle Orthod., 10:140, 1940.

Smith, R. A.: The effect of roentgen rays on the developing teeth of rats. J. Am. Dent. Assoc., 18:111, 1931.

Southby, R.: Pink disease with clinical approach to possible etiology. Med. J. Aust., 2:801, 1949.

Spiegel, L.: Discoloration of skin and mucous membrane resembling argyria following use of bismuth and silver arsphenamine. Arch. Dermatol. Syph., 23:266, 1931.

Standish, S. M., and Shafer, W. G.: Serial histologic effects of rat submaxillary and sublingual salivary gland duct and blood vessel ligation. J. Dent. Res., 36:866, 1957.

Idem: Focal osteoporotic bone marrow defects of the jaws. J. Oral Surg., 20:123, 1962.

Idem: The mucous retention phenomenon. J. Oral Surg., 17:15, 1959.

Stanley, H. R., Jr.: Methods and criteria in evaluation of dentin and pulp response. Int. Dent. J., 20:507, 1970.

Idem: The protective effect of reparative dentin and how it compares to man-made liners. J. Am. Acad. Gold Foil Oper., 14:29, 1971.

Idem: Traumatic capacity of high-speed and ultrasonic dental instrumentation. J. Am. Dent. Assoc., 63:749, 1961.

Stanley, H. R., and Swerdlow, H.: An approach to biologic variation in human pulpal studies. J. Prosthet. Dent., 14:365, 1964.

Idem: Accelerated handpiece speeds: the potential abuse of high speed techniques. Dent. Clin. North Am., 4:621, 1960.

Idem: Reaction of the human pulp to cavity preparation: results produced by eight different operative grinding technics. J. Am. Dent. Assoc., 58:49, 1959.

Stein, M., Brady, L. W., and Raventos, A.: The effects of radiation on extraction-wound healing in the rat. Cancer, 10:1167, 1957.

Stern, R. H.: The laser in dentistry: a review of the literature. J. Dent. Assoc. S. Afr., 29:173, 1974.

Stern, R. H., and Sognnaes, R. F.: Laser beam effect on dental hard tissues. J. Dent. Res., 43:873, 1964.

Stuteville, O. H.: A summary review of tissue changes incident to tooth movement. Angle Orthod., 8:1, 1938.

Swerdlow, H., and Stanley, H. R., Jr.: Reaction of the human dental pulp to cavity preparation. I. Effect of water spray at 20,000 rpm. J. Am. Dent. Assoc., 56:317, 1958.

Idem: Reaction of the human dental pulp to cavity preparation. II. At 150,000 rpm with an air-water spray. J. Prosthet. Dent., 9:121, 1959.

Idem: Response of the human dental pulp to amalgam restorations. Oral Surg., 15:499, 1962.

Taylor, R. G., Shklar, G., and Roeber, F.: The effect of laser radiation on teeth, dental pulp, and oral mucosa of experimental animals. Oral Surg., 19:786, 1965.

Thoma, K. H.: Papillomatosis of the palate. Oral Surg., 5:214, 1952.

Thomas, B. O. A.: Penetration of phenol in tooth structure. J. Dent. Res., 20:435, 1941.

Toller, P. A.: Radioactive isotope and other investigations in a case of haemorrhagic cyst of the mandible. Br. J. Oral Surg., 2:86, 1964.

Toto, P. D.: Mucopolysaccharide keratin dystrophy of the oral epithelium. Oral Surg., 22:47, 1966.

Tribondeau, L., and Recamier, D.: Alterations des yeux et du séquelette facial d'un chat nouveau-né par roentgenisation. C. R. Soc. Biol. (Paris), 58:1031, 1905.

Tsuzuki, M.: Experimental studies on the biological action of hard roentgen rays. Am. J. Roentgenol. 16:134, 1926.

Turrell, A. J. W.: Allergy to denture-base materials: fallacy or reality. Br. Dent. J., 120:415, 1966.

Ultrasonic Dental Research Group of Chicago: Using the ultrasonic dental unit in restorative technics. Ill. Dent. J., 25:770, 1956.

Urist, M. R., and Ibsen, K. H.: Chemical reactivity of mineralized tissue with oxytetracycline. Arch. Pathol., 76:484, 1963.

van den Akker, H. P., Bays, R. A., and Becker, A. E.: Plunging or cervical ranula. J. Maxillofac. Surg., 6:286, 1978.

Van Huysen, G., and Fly, W.: Artificial dentures and the oral mucosa. J. Prosthet. Dent., 4:446, 1954.

Van Huysen, G., and Gurley, W. D.: Histologic changes in teeth of dogs following preparation of cavities of various depths and their exposure to oral fluids. J. Am. Dent. Assoc., 26:87, 1939.

Wakely, C.: The surgery of the salivary glands. Ann. R. Coll. Surg., 3:289, 1948.

Waldo, C. M., and Rothblatt, J. M.: Histologic response to tooth movement in the laboratory rat. J. Dent. Res., 33:481, 1954.

Waldron, C. A.: Solitary (hemorrhagic) cyst of the mandible. Oral Surg., 7:88, 1954.

Wallman, I. S., and Hilton, H. B.: Teeth pigmented by tetracycline. Lancet, 1:827, 1962.

Walters, F. J., Fridl, J. W., Nelson, R. L., and Trost, J. W.: Oral Manifestations of Occupational Origin: An Annotated Bibliography. Washington, D.C., Federal Security Agency, Public Health Service, 1952.

Warkany, J., and Hubbard, D. M.: Acrodynia and mercury. J. Pediat., 42:365, 1953.

Warren, S.: Effects of radiation of normal tissues. Arch. Pathol., 34:443, 562, 749, 917, 1070, 1942, 35:121, 304, 1943.

Watson, W. L., and Scarborough, J. E.: Osteoradionecrosis in intraoral cancer. Am. J. Roentgenol. Radium Ther., 40:524, 1938.

Weinstein, R. A., Stephen, R. J., Morof, A., and Choukas, N. C.: Human bites: review of the literature and report of case. J. Oral Surg., 31:792, 1973.

Whinery, J. G.: Progressive bone cavities of the mandible. Oral Surg., 8:903, 1955.

Witkop, C. J., Jr., and Wolf, R. O.: Hypoplasia and intrinsic staining of enamel following tetracycline therapy. J.A.M.A., 185:1008, 1963.

Wolcott, R. B., Paffenbarger, G. C., and Schoonover, J. C.: Direct resinous filling materials: temperature rise during polymerization. J. Am. Dent. Assoc., 42:253, 1951.

Wood, J. F. L.: Mucosal reaction to cobalt-chromium alloy. Brit. Dent. J., 136:423, 1974.

Wright, R. W.: Round shadows in the maxillary sinuses, Laryngoscope, 56:455, 1946.

Yamamoto, H., Okabe, H., Ooya, K., Hanaoka, S., Ohta, S., and Kataoka, K.: Laser effect on vital oral tissues: A preliminary investigation. J. Oral Path., 1:256, 1973.

Zach, L., and Brown, G. N.: Pulpal effect of ultrasonic cavity preparation: preliminary report. N. Y. Dent. J., 22:9, 1956.

Zander, H. A.: The effect of self-curing resins on the dental pulp. Oral Surg., 4:1563, 1951.

Idem: The reaction of dental pulps to silicate cement. J. Am. Dent. Assoc., 33:1233, 1946.

Zander, H. A., and Burrill, D. Y.: Penetration of silver nitrate solution in dentin. J. Dent. Res., 22:85, 1943.

Zander, H. A., and Pejko, I.: Protection of pulp under silicate cements with cavity varnishes and cement linings. J. Am. Dent. Assoc., 34:811, 1947.

Zander, H. A., and Smith, H. W.: Penetration of silver nitrate into dentin. J. Dent. Res., 24:121, 1945.

Ziskin, D. E., Stowe, L. R., and Zegarelli, E. V.: Dilantin hyperplastic gingivitis. Am. J. Orthod., 27:350, 1941.

Zussman, W. V.: Tetracycline-induced fluorescence in dentin and enamel matrix. Lab. Invest., 15:589, 1966.

CHAPTER 11

Healing of Oral Wounds

The healing of wounds is one of the most interesting of the many phenomena which characterize the living organism. The ability of damaged tissue to repair itself is a response of life itself, and within this very process may lie the final understanding of nature. It is said that an unhealed wound will eventually result in the death of the organism. Therefore, wound healing must be considered one of the primary survival mechanisms from birth onward. It should be clearly understood that the healing of a wound is not an isolated, solitary phenomenon but actually a very complex series of biologic events. Classic reviews of this dynamic process are those of Arey in 1936 and of Schilling in 1968.

Repair of tissue is generally considered to be a phase of the inflammatory reaction, since it cannot be separated from the preceding vascular and cellular phenomena occurring in response to an injury. Healing of all tissues after injury has an essentially identical pattern, but this healing may be modified considerably, depending upon numerous intrinsic and extrinsic factors.

Oral wounds are common, some being sustained accidentally (e.g., jaw fractures) and others being inflicted by the dentist for a specific purpose (e.g., extraction wounds, biopsy wounds). The unusual anatomic situation of the oral cavity—the teeth protruding from the bone, the constant inflammation present in the gingival tissues, the presence of countless microorganisms in a warm, moist medium of saliva—all contribute to modify the healing reaction of the various wounds. It is these reparative phenomena and their alterations from the basic pattern which will be discussed in this section.

GENERAL FACTORS AFFECTING THE HEALING OF ORAL WOUNDS

There are a number of general factors which may influence the rate of healing of wounds of the oral cavity. Although interference with the normal healing phenomena is not a common occurrence, the possible causes must be recognized by the dentist.

Location of Wound. The particular location of a wound is important and may modify the rate of healing. Wounds in an area in which there is a good vascular bed heal considerably more rapidly than wounds in an area which is relatively avascular.

Immobilization of the wound is also important in the healing reaction. If the wound is in an area subjected to constant movement so that formation of the new connective tissue is continuously disrupted (e.g., in the corner of the mouth), delayed healing will result. Immobilization is particularly important in the healing of fractures, for without it bony union may be delayed or even completely inhibited.

Physical Factors. *Severe trauma* to tissue is obviously a deterrent to rapid wound healing. Under certain situations, however, mild traumatic injury may actually favor the healing process. For example, it is well recognized that a second wound inflicted in the site of a healing initial wound heals more rapidly than the initial or single wound.

The *local temperature* in the area of a wound influences the rate of healing, probably through the effect on local circulation and cell multiplication. Thus, in environmental hyperthermia, wound healing is accelerated, while in hypothermia healing is delayed.

594

The effect of *x-ray radiation* on the healing of wounds has been rather extensively studied, and the data indicate generally that low doses of radiation tend to stimulate healing, while large focal doses of radiation or total body radiation tend to suppress healing.

Circulatory Factors. *Anemia* has been reported to delay wound healing, although not all studies have confirmed this observation. Similarly, *dehydration* has been found to affect adversely a healing wound.

Nutritional Factors. It has been shown that delay in healing of wounds may occur in a person who is deficient in any of a vast variety of essential foods.

Protein is one of the most important substances which may influence the speed of wound healing. Numerous clinical studies have indicated that poorly nourished patients whose low protein intake results in a protein deficiency manifested by a hypoproteinemia exhibit a delay in the appearance of new fibroblasts as well as a decreased rate of multiplication of fibroblasts in wounds. Conversely, it has been shown that feeding high protein diets to animals will increase the rate of fibroblastic proliferation and cause wounds to heal more rapidly. The exact manner in which protein influences the wound is not known, although there is considerable evidence that this effect is related to dietary compounds containing free sulfhydryl groups. Of all the essential amino acids, only methionine furnishes such a group, and studies have shown that administration of methionine to hypoproteinemic animals restores the rate of wound healing to a normal level.

Vitamins are another group of nutritional factors related to wound healing. One of these which has been known for many years to influence the rate of wound healing is vitamin C, or ascorbic acid. It has been shown that the mechanism by which it acts is through regulation of collagen formation and formation of normal intercellular ground substance of the connective tissue. It appears that, in scurvy or ascorbic acid deficiency, this inhibitory effect on wound healing is specifically related to interference with the production of mucopolysaccharides which make up the cement substance. Microscopically, it is recognized that fibroblastic proliferation in a wound of a scorbutic animal continues longer than in control animals. This is interpreted to mean that there is prolonged need for formation of connective tissue, and this is borne out by the fact that scorbutic animals exhibit a decreased tensile strength of the healing wounds.

There have been no extensive studies of the possible role of vitamins A and D in wound healing, but the available reports indicate that a vitamin A deficiency retards healing and that vitamins A and D, as in cod liver oil, may be factors in promoting tissue repair.

There have been surprisingly few investigations on the relation of the vitamin B complex to wound healing. The available studies indicate that riboflavin and pyridoxine deficiencies result in a delay in the healing process.

Age of Patient. Wounds in younger persons heal considerably more rapidly than wounds in elderly persons, and the rate of healing appears to be in inverse proportion to the age of the patient. The cause for this is unknown, but probably relates to the general reduction in the rate of tissue metabolism as the person ages, which itself may be a manifestation of decreased circulatory efficiency.

The classic tissue culture studies of Carrel and Ebeling in 1921 disclosed that serum from young animals did not contain any *stimulating* factor for fibroblastic proliferation; instead, it was found, serum from old animals contained a *restraining* factor against cell multiplication.

Infection. It has been demonstrated that wounds which are completely protected from bacterial irritation heal considerably more slowly than wounds which are exposed to bacteria or other mild physical irritation. Furthermore, Lattes and his co-workers showed that bacterial infection of wounds suppressed the cortisone-inhibitory effect on fibroplasia in the experimental animal. Some studies on germ-free animals with experimental wounds, primarily incised and closed, have shown a reduction in tensile strength, as compared to control animals, thus indicating that the germ-free state is a deterrent to wound healing.

It is obvious, however, that severe bacterial infection slows the healing of wounds. In view of the vast bacterial flora of the oral cavity, one might question whether all wounds of the oral cavity are not heavily infected. Since the antibody titer of a person against his own microorganisms is usually extremely high, there is seldom cause to worry about infection from autoinoculation. Occasionally, however, the resistance of the tissue is decreased, either locally or on a systemic basis, and an oral wound becomes massively infected and heals slowly, if at all.

Hormonal Factors. Adrenocorticotropic hormone (ACTH) and cortisone are substances that have been repeatedly shown to interfere with the healing of wounds. Not long after ACTH and cortisone were first used clinically, it was noted that wounds in recipients of these compounds exhibited delayed healing. Since this observation, a number of careful experimental studies were carried out in which it was shown that in patients receiving ACTH or cortisone the growth of granulation tissue was inhibited, apparently because of inhibition of proliferation of new fibroblasts and new endothelial sprouts and because of a depression of the inflammatory reaction. There is apparently not an actual suppression of mesenchymal activity, but rather a delay in the mesenchymal reaction. An experimental study by Shafer on the healing of extraction wounds in rats receiving cortisone showed that the healing of such wounds is delayed. This would suggest that patients receiving cortisone should be carefully evaluated by the dentist before he carries out oral surgical procedures.

Numerous investigators also have studied the effects of administration of pituitary growth hormone and thyroid hormone (thyroxin) and concluded that these had no significant role in wound healing. The opposite situations, obtained by surgical ablation of the pituitary gland and thyroid gland, have also been reported as having no significant effects on wound repair. There is one interesting experimental study in the literature which showed that wound healing was delayed during pregnancy, but this has not been confirmed clinically.

Diabetes mellitus (insulin deficiency) is one of the most widely recognized diseases in which there is significant, clinically evident retardation in repair of wounds after surgical procedures, including oral operations such as tooth extraction. Wounds in diabetic patients are notoriously slow to heal and frequently show complications in the repair process. The exact mechanism of this phenomenon is not known, but is probably related to the disturbance in carbohydrate metabolism at the cellular level in the local area of the wound. Because of this recognized relation of insulin deficiency to wound healing, a number of investigators have studied the effect of administration of insulin to normal animals (hyperinsulinism), but the reports are indecisive as to influence on wound healing. Nevertheless tissue culture studies have almost invariably shown stimulation of fibroblastic proliferation when insulin was added to the growth medium.

Miscellaneous Factors. A vast variety of other factors have also been studied in relation to wound healing, and these have been reviewed in an extensive discussion by El-Kha-shab. These factors include enzymes, such as trypsin, streptokinase, alkaline phosphatase, and coenzyme adenosine 5-monophosphate; growth-promoting factors such as cartilage and mucopolysaccharide, N-acetyl-D-glucosamine, tissue extracts and pantothenyl alcohol; hydroxyproline; hydrogen-ion concentration; electrolyte balance; therapeutic agents such as Dilantin sodium, sulfonamides and antibiotics; anticoagulants such as heparin and Dicumarol; emollients; sclerosing agents; cancericidal alkylating agents; carcinogenic agents; metals, particularly trace elements such as zinc and copper; deuterium oxide; antigen-antibody reactions; and lathyrism.

The effects of suture materials on healing skin wounds also have been studied by many investigators. A large comparative study in dogs was reported by Van Winkle and his co-workers, who concluded that there were no differences in healing among wounds closed with different suture materials up to a postoperative period of about one month. However, on a more long-term basis, they found that wounds sutured with nonabsorbable sutures were weaker than those sutured with absorbable ones and that, in general, there was a lower incidence of wound infection with monofilament sutures than with multifilament sutures. However, in some findings these investigators noted that when compared with other similar studies there were species differences, and they cautioned against direct application of such observations to the human patient.

In addition, chemical tissue adhesives have been widely utilized in surgical procedures involving numerous organs. Recently, use of certain of these adhesives, chiefly butyl and isobutyl cyanoacrylate, has been applied to a variety of procedures in the oral cavity performed in dental practice. Their chief attributes are (1) their ability to act as a surface tissue adhesive in the presence of moisture, and (2) their hemostatic and bacteriostatic effects. Bhaskar and Frisch have reviewed the use of cyanoacrylate adhesives in dentistry, concluding that butyl cyanoacrylate not only is well tolerated by tissues and permits uncomplicated healing but also generally hastens the healing process. While still in the investigative phase, it has been successfully tested as a surface dressing after gingivectomy on mucoperiosteal flaps, biopsy sites, extraction wounds, aphthous ulcers, leukemic ulcerations, pulp capping and in the grafting of mucosal tissues from one region of the mouth to another.

It may be concluded that the repair of damaged tissue is a vital, dynamic process which may be influenced by a multitude of exogenous and endogenous factors. That alteration in this process does not occur more frequently than it does is proof of the inherent resistance of the living organism to those factors which could interfere with perpetuation of life. In certain instances this resistance is diminished, and pathologic alterations in the repair phenomenon occur. The factors which may be responsible for this unfortunate occurrence must be recognized and understood so that, in such an eventuality, proper measures may be taken to correct the problem.

BIOPSY AND HEALING OF THE BIOPSY WOUND

Biopsy is the removal of tissue from the living organism for the purposes of microscopic examination and diagnosis. Although the diagnosis of many lesions can be made clinically by the dentist with experience, such a diagnosis is generally only a provisional one contingent upon the final report on the tissue specimen by the pathologist. The use of the biopsy is not restricted to the diagnosis of tumors, but is invaluable in determining the nature of any unusual lesion. Unfortunately, many lesions do not present a specific microscopic appearance, and for this reason a definitive diagnosis cannot always be rendered. Although the microscope in the hands of a qualified pathologist is an irreplaceable diagnostic tool, its limitations must always be kept in mind. Fortunately, with the rapid advances now occurring in scientific techniques adaptable to microscopic diagnosis, such as histochemical techniques, fluorescent microscopy, microradiography, histoautoradiography, transmission and scanning electron microscopy, and so forth, this sphere of diagnostic limitation is gradually shrinking.

Types of Biopsy. Total excision of a small lesion for microscopic study is called *excisional biopsy*. The pathologist will usually be able to tell the operator whether the lesion was removed in entirety by observing the appearance of the tissue along the line of excision. The excisional biopsy is preferred if the size of the lesion is such that it may be removed along with a margin of normal tissue and the wound can be closed primarily.

Some lesions are too large to excise initially without having established a diagnosis, or are of such a nature that excision would be inadvisable. In such instances, a small section is removed for examination; this is termed an *incisional or diagnostic biopsy* (Fig. 11–1). It is most useful in dealing with large lesions, lesions which the operator suspects may be treated by some means other than surgery once the diagnosis is made, or lesions in which the diagnosis will determine whether the treatment should be conservative or radical.

There are several methods by which material may be obtained from a lesion for microscopic study: (1) surgical excision by scalpel; (2) surgical removal by cautery or a high-frequency cutting knife; (3) removal by biopsy forceps or biopsy punch; (4) aspiration through a needle with a large lumen; (5) the exfoliative cytology

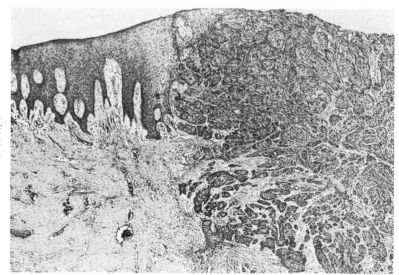

Figure 11–1. *Epidermoid carcinoma, diagnostic biopsy.* An adequate border of normal mucosa was obtained with the biopsy of the neoplastic mass, and no attempt was made initially to excise the lesion completely.

technique, whereby the surface of a lesion is either wiped with some form of sponge material which is then sectioned, or scraped and smeared on a microscope slide and studied by the pathologist for the presence of atypical or diagnostic cells.

The needle biopsy has little value in the diagnosis of oral lesions. The scalpel is the instrument of choice, since it cleanly removes the tissue and does not dehydrate it as cautery or the high-frequency cutting knife may. This latter instrument is of great value, however, in dealing with vascular lesions, where it controls bleeding at the biopsy site.

Exfoliative Cytology. Considerable interest has developed in the use of exfoliative oral cytology for the diagnosis of oral carcinoma, similar to its widespread use in the diagnosis of carcinoma of the uterine cervix (Fig. 11–2). In a review of the historic background of oral cytology, Von Haam cited numerous series of cases of patients with oral cancer in which the diagnostic accuracy of cytologic smears was compared with that of the surgical biopsy and was found to be almost identical. He concluded that: (1) cytology is not a substitute for, but an adjunct to, the surgical biopsy; (2) it is a quick, simple, painless and bloodless procedure; (3) it helps as a check against false-negative biopsies;

(4) it is especially helpful in follow-up detection of recurrent carcinoma in previously treated cases; and (5) it is valuable for screening lesions whose gross appearance is such that biopsy is not warranted. Obviously, the use of the cytologic smear is predicated upon the proper preparation of the smear by the clinician and sufficient experience in its evaluation by the cytologist.

The preferred technique is a relatively simple one. It consists essentially of cleansing the surface of the oral lesion of debris and mucin, and then vigorously scraping the entire surface of the lesion several times with a metal cement spatula or a moistened tongue blade. The collected material is then quickly spread evenly over a microscopic slide and fixed immediately before the smear dries. The fixative may be either a commercial preparation such as Spraycyte, 95 per cent alcohol, or equal parts of alcohol and ether. After the slide is flooded with the fixative, it should be allowed to stand for 30 minutes to air-dry. Slides are *never* flame-fixed in the same manner as bacteriologic smears. It is essential that the procedure be repeated and a second smear be prepared for submission to the cytologist. In preparing the duplicate slide, a separate scraping should be utilized. Two smears are always submitted from

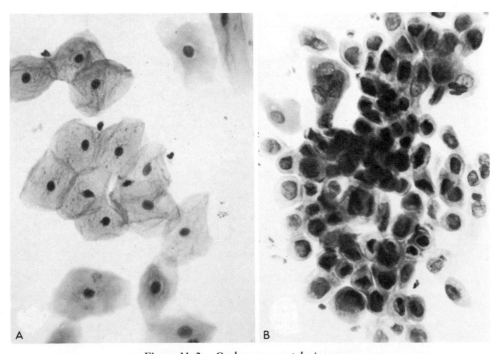

Figure 11–2. *Oral mucosa, cytologic smears.*
Normal epithelial cells are shown *(A)*, contrasted with malignant cells from a patient with epidermoid carcinoma *(B)*.

each lesion, since additional staining techniques are frequently employed.

The cytologic smear will usually be reported by the cytologist as falling into one of five classes:

Class I: (Normal.) Indicates that only normal cells were observed.
Class II: (Atypical.) Indicates the presence of minor atypia but no evidence of malignant changes.
Class III: (Indeterminate.) This is an in-between cytology that separates cancer from noncancer diagnosis. The cells display wider atypia that may be suggestive of cancer, but they are not clear-cut and may represent precancerous lesions or carcinoma in situ. Biopsy is *recommended*.
Class IV: (Suggestive of cancer.) A few cells with malignant characteristics or many cells with borderline characteristics. Biopsy is *mandatory*.
Class V: (Positive for cancer.) Cells that are obviously malignant. Biopsy is *mandatory*.

It should be remembered that the majority of benign lesions that occur in the oral cavity do not lend themselves to cytologic smear. For example, lesions which have a normal-appearing and intact surface, such as a fibroma, should be excised and never smeared. In addition, most authorities agree that leukoplakia does not lend itself to cytologic diagnosis because of the scarcity of viable surface cells in the smears taken from such lesions. Finally, it should be remembered that a negative cytology report does not rule out cancer and that a repeat smear or biopsy is indicated in all clinically suspicious lesions.

It has been recognized that the exfoliative oral cytologic smear is also of value in the diagnosis of diseases other than carcinoma. This is the case in diseases which are characterized by the presence of certain specific cells. Thus, cytologic smears have been useful in the diagnosis of lesions of herpes simplex infection, herpes zoster, pemphigus vulgaris, benign familial pemphigus, keratosis follicularis, hereditary benign intraepithelial dyskeratosis, white sponge nevus, and pernicious and sickle cell anemia.

Biopsy Technique. Biopsy technique is a simple procedure and may be carried out by any dentist as a routine office procedure if certain precautions are taken and certain rules are followed. The advantages of a biopsy so far outweigh its disadvantages or potential dangers that the biopsy is seldom, if ever, contraindicated in case of a lesion in which the diagnosis has not been established. To ensure obtaining a proper specimen for the pathologist, the following points must be considered:

1. Do not paint the surface of the area to be biopsied with iodine or a highly colored antiseptic.

2. If using infiltration anesthesia, do not inject anesthetic solution directly into the lesion. Inject around the periphery of the lesion instead.

3. Use a sharp scalpel to avoid tearing tissue.

4. Remove a border of normal tissue with the specimen if at all possible.

5. Use care not to mutilate the specimen when grasping it with forceps.

6. Fix the tissue immediately upon removal in 10 per cent formalin or 70 per cent alcohol. If the specimen is thin, place it upon a piece of glazed paper and drop into fixative; this prevents curling of tissue.

The Biopsy Report. The report of the biopsy is usually returned to the operator by the pathologist within a few days unless some special procedures, such as decalcification of tooth or bone substance or application of special stains, are necessary.

A negative biopsy report or a diagnosis not in conformity with the expected diagnosis should never be considered final. It means only that there are no features to suggest the expected diagnosis in that *particular piece* of tissue which was removed at that *particular time*. A repeat biopsy should *always* be performed when there is any doubt about the adequacy or representative nature of the original specimen.

Healing of the Biopsy Wound. The healing of a biopsy wound of the oral cavity is identical with the healing of a similar wound in any other part of the body and thus may be classified as either primary healing or secondary healing. The nature of the healing process depends upon whether the edges of the wound can be brought into apposition, often by suturing, or whether the lesion must fill in gradually with granulation tissue.

PRIMARY HEALING. Primary healing, healing by primary intention or healing by first intention is that type of healing which occurs after the excision of a piece of tissue with the close apposition of the edges of the wound. This is the form of healing one might expect after the excision of a lesion in an area of the oral cavity where the pliability of the tissues is such that the wound may be drawn together and sutured.

When the edges of the wound are brought into contact and held in place by sutures, the blood clots, and in a matter of hours numerous leukocytes are mobilized to the area. Connective tissue cells in the immediate vicinity undergo transformation into fibroblasts which in turn undergo mitotic division, and the new fibroblasts begin to migrate into and across the line of incision. In time, these cells form thin, delicate collagen fibrils which intertwine and coalesce in a general direction parallel to the surface of the wound. At the same time, endothelial cells of the capillaries begin to proliferate, and small capillary buds grow out and across the wound. These buds eventually form new capillaries which fill with blood, and a rich network of young capillaries and capillary loops is formed.

When there is a close apposition of the edges of the wound, the surface epithelium proliferates rapidly across the line of incision and re-establishes the integrity of the surface. The delicate connective tissue fibrils eventually coalesce into denser bundles and usually contract, so that in time all that is left to indicate the biopsy area is a small linear scar which may be depressed below the surface. Because there is no defect which must be filled with new tissue, this type of wound heals rapidly (Fig. 11–3).

SECONDARY HEALING. Secondary healing, healing by second intention, healing by granulation or healing of an open wound occurs when there is loss of tissue and the edges of the wound cannot be approximated. Healing of this type is often spoken of as a process in which the wound "granulates in," since the material which fills the defect during the healing process is called granulation tissue. This type of wound is a result of biopsy of a lesion in an area of the oral cavity in which the tissues are not pliable and in which the edges cannot be approximated. For example, removal of a lesion of the palate or a large lesion of the alveolar ridge is usually followed by healing by second intention, since the edges of the wound cannot be coapted.

After the removal of the lesion, the blood filling the defect clots and the repair process begins. It is basically identical with healing by primary intention except that the fibroblasts and capillaries have a greater distance to migrate; more granulation tissue must form, and of necessity the healing is slower. Cellular proliferation begins around the periphery of the wound, and the fibroblasts and endothelial cells grow into the clot along fibrin strands. In addition, polymorphonuclear leukocytes and, later, lymphocytes, and mononuclear phagocytes migrate into the granulation tissue from the adjacent vessels and tissues. Large numbers of leukocytes also accumulate on the surface of the wound. As the granulation tissue matures, it becomes more fibrous through condensation of collagen bundles, and the surface of the granulation tissue becomes epithelized. As in healing by primary intention, the collagen fibrils coalesce; the lesion becomes somewhat less vascular, and eventually the only evidence

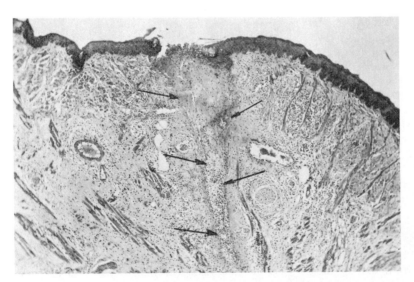

Figure 11–3. *Primary healing of a wound.*

The thin linear incision shows re-establishment of continuity of the tissue after only 48 hours.

of the wound may be a small depressed area of the mucosa.

HEALING OF THE GINGIVECTOMY WOUND

The elimination of the periodontal pocket by gingivectomy has become a routine clinical procedure principally because of the excellent results which are generally attained. Numerous techniques are in use for the removal of the tissue, and different types of postoperative packing material are applied to control bleeding, maintain tissue position, relieve pain and keep the fresh wounds free of debris. Despite these variations, the general features of the healing process are similar and must be understood before attempting to carry out such a surgical procedure.

Orban and Archer studied the wound healing following gingivectomy without the application of a surgical packing or dressing, while Bernier and Kaplan carried out a similar investigation, but used a zinc oxide-eugenol packing.

An interesting finding of acceleration of gingival wound healing in nonepileptic patients receiving Dilantin sodium was reported by Shapiro. He pointed out, however, that this accelerated healing may not be important in gingivectomy in which recession of tissue is the primary objective.

Early Healing Phase. Healing of the gingivectomy wound takes place rapidly regardless of whether a postoperative pack is used. There is some evidence, however, that healing may be slightly facilitated by the dressing.

Two days after the gingivectomy the surface of the tissue is covered by a grayish blood clot, and beneath this clot there is histologic evidence of delicate connective tissue proliferation. Even at this early stage there is also considerable activity of the epithelial cells bordering the wound preparatory to beginning of actual epithelization. Four days after the operation the deeper portion of the blood clot demonstrates considerable organization, while the more superficial portion exhibits dense numbers of polymorphonuclear leukocytes entrapped in the fibrinous meshwork. There is proliferation of young capillaries and young connective tissue cells into the base of the blood clot. Infiltration of polymorphonuclear leukocytes in the deeper connective tissue is present in varying degrees. The epithelium has extended over a portion of the wound below the

necrotic surface layer of the clot, but above the proliferating and organizing connective tissue.

Late Healing Phase. Continuation of the healing process is manifested by a condensation of the young connective tissue with nearly complete organization of the clot after eight to ten days. Clinically, at this period, the wound has a red, granular appearance and bleeds readily. Epithelization is usually complete within ten to fourteen days after gingivectomy. The epithelium remains thin, however, and begins to mature and form rete pegs only after the two-week interval. At this time the inflammatory cells have largely disappeared, except for those in the subepithelial zone.

Healing of the interproximal tissue appears to lag behind that adjacent to the labial or buccal surfaces. This may be partly because the epithelium which covers the interproximal tissue must grow in from the labial and lingual areas, a relatively great distance.

The surface epithelium grows downward along the surface of the cementum within a month after gingivectomy. This is a rather shallow proliferation which, nevertheless, is in close physical apposition to the tooth.

Healing of the gingivectomy wound is basically similar to the healing of wounds elsewhere in the body, but is somewhat modified by the special anatomy of the involved region. The chronic inflammation present in the diseased gingiva does not adversely affect the healing process and actually may provide some stimulus for healing.

HEALING OF THE EXTRACTION WOUND

A thorough understanding of the phenomenon of healing of extraction wounds is imperative to the dentist, since vast numbers of teeth are extracted because of pulp and periapical infection as well as various forms of periodontal disease, and there is an ever-present possibility of complications in the healing process.

A number of careful scientific studies have been carried out, both on the experimental animal and in the human being, dealing with undisturbed as well as complicated extraction wound healing. The investigations of Schram on dogs, of Claflin on both dogs and humans, of Mangos on humans, of Simpson on monkeys and of Amler and his associates on humans all may be cited as representative of such work, and all are in general agreement on the sequence of events in this particular reaction. The healing of an extraction wound does not differ from the healing of other wounds of the body except as it is modified by the peculiar anatomic situation which exists after the removal of a tooth. The healing process to be described here is a composite of the various studies reported in the literature and, while minor variations in the time sequence have been described, the uncomplicated healing of an extraction wound in the human may be expected to parallel that described later. Normal human biologic variation precludes the establishment of a day-to-day timetable for such healing wounds; the healing process can only be described as an "average" sequence of events.

Immediate Reaction Following Extraction. After the removal of a tooth, the blood which fills the socket coagulates, red blood cells being entrapped in the fibrin meshwork, and the ends of the torn blood vessels in the periodontal ligament become sealed off. The hours after tooth extraction are critical, for if the blood clot is dislodged, healing may be greatly delayed and may be extremely painful.

Within the first 24 to 48 hours after extraction, a variety of phenomena occur which consist principally of alterations in the vascular bed. There are vasodilatation and engorgement of the blood vessels in the remnants of the periodontal ligament and the mobilization of leukocytes to the immediate area around the clot. The surface of the blood clot is covered by a thick layer of fibrin, but at this early period visible evidence of reactivity on the part of the body in the form of a layering of leukocytes here is not particularly prominent. The clot itself shows areas of contraction. It is important to recognize that the collapse of the unsupported gingival tissue into the opening of a fresh extraction wound is of great aid in maintaining the clot in position.

First-Week Wound. Within the first week after tooth extraction, proliferation of fibroblasts from connective tissue cells in the remnants of the periodontal ligament is evident, and these fibroblasts have begun to grow into the clot around the entire periphery (Figs. 11–4, 11–5). This clot forms an actual scaffold upon which cells associated with the healing process may migrate. It is only a temporary structure, however, and is gradually replaced by granulation tissue. The epithelium at the periphery of the wound exhibits evidence of proliferation in the form of mild mitotic activity even at this time. The crest of the alveolar bone which makes up

the margin or neck of the socket exhibits beginning osteoclastic activity. Endothelial cell proliferation signaling the beginning of capillary ingrowth may be seen in the periodontal ligament area.

During this period, the blood clot begins to undergo organization by the ingrowth around the periphery of fibroblasts and occasional small capillaries from the residual periodontal ligament. Remnants of this periodontal ligament are still visible, but as yet there is no evidence of significant new osteoid formation, although in some cases it may have just commenced. An extremely thick layer of leukocytes has gathered over the surface of the clot, and the edge of the wound continues to exhibit epithelial proliferation.

Second-Week Wound. During the second week after extraction of the tooth, the blood clot is becoming organized by fibroblasts growing into the clot on the fibrinous meshwork (Figs. 11–4, 11–5). At this stage, new delicate capillaries have penetrated to the center of the clot. The remnants of the periodontal ligament have been gradually undergoing degeneration and are no longer recognizable as such. Instead, the wall of the bony socket now appears slightly frayed. In some instances, trabeculae of osteoid can be seen extending outward from the wall of the alveolus. Epithelial proliferation over the surface of the wound has been extensive, although the wound is usually not covered, particularly in the case of large posterior teeth. In smaller sockets, epithelization may be complete. The margin of the alveolar socket exhibits prominent osteoclastic resorption. Fragments of necrotic bone which may have been fractured from the rim of the socket during the extraction are seen in the process of resorption or sequestration.

Third-Week Wound. As the healing process continues into the third week, the original clot appears almost completely organized by maturing granulation tissue (Figs. 11–4, 11–5). Very young trabeculae of osteoid or uncalcified bone are forming around the entire periphery of the wound from the socket wall. This early bone is formed by osteoblasts derived from pluripotential cells of the original periodontal ligament which assume an osteogenic function. The original cortical bone of the alveolar socket undergoes remodeling so that it no longer consists of such a dense layer. The crest of the alveolar bone has been rounded off by osteoclastic resorption. By this time the surface of the wound may have become completely epithelized.

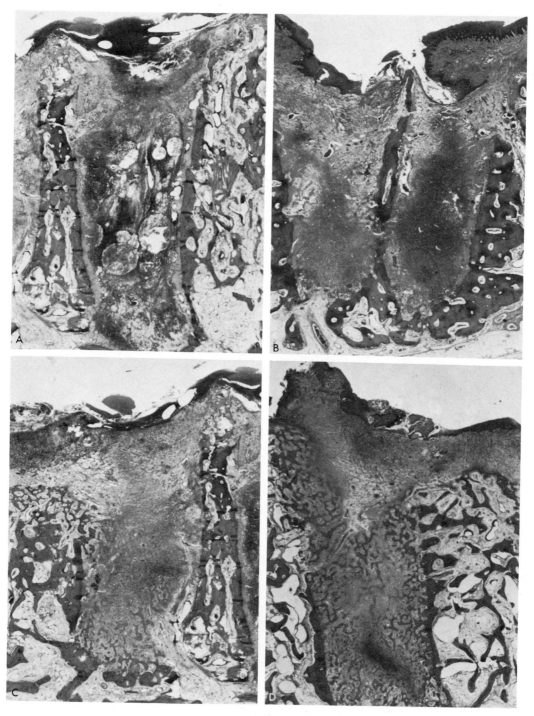

Figure 11–4. *Healing extraction wounds.*
The 4-day postextraction wound *(A)*, 7-day postextraction wound *(B)*, 14-day postextraction wound *(C)*, and 21-day postextraction wound *(D)* in the dog illustrate the progressive nature of the healing process. Extraction wounds in dogs heal at a somewhat more rapid rate than those in humans.

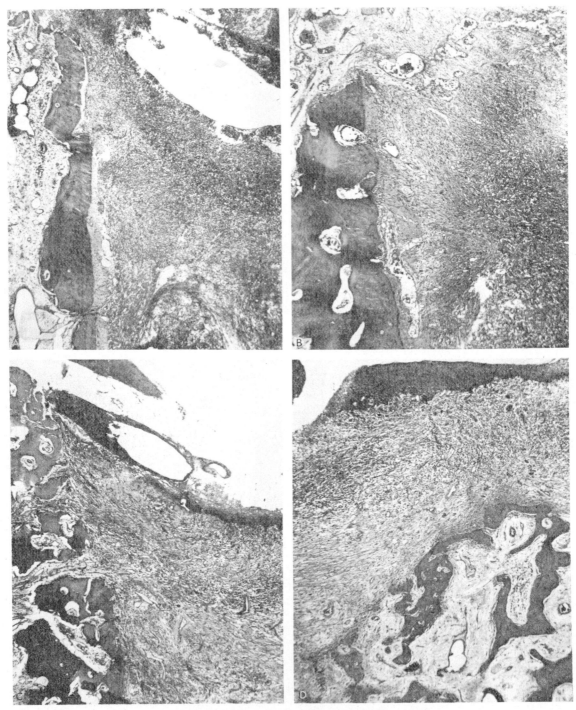

Figure 11–5. *Healing extraction wounds.*
The 4-day postextraction wound (*A*), 7-day postextraction wound (*B*), 14-day postextraction wound (*C*), and 21-day postextraction wound (*D*) in the dog under high magnification illustrate the progressive changes in the alveolar crest, periodontal ligament and superficial portion of the wound.

Fourth-Week Wound. During the fourth week after the extraction, the wound begins the final stage of healing, in which there is continued deposition and remodeling resorption of the bone filling the alveolar socket (Figs. 11–4, 11–5). However, this maturative remodeling will continue for several more weeks. Much of this early bone is poorly calcified, as is evident from its general radiolucency on the roentgenogram. Roentgenographic evidence of bone formation does not become prominent until the sixth or eighth week after tooth extraction. There is still roentgenographic evidence of differences in the new bone of the alveolar socket and the adjacent bone for as long as four to six months after extraction in some cases (Fig. 11–6). Because the crest of alveolar bone undergoes a considerable amount of osteoclastic resorption during the healing process and because the bone filling the socket does not extend above the alveolar crest, it is obvious that the crest of the healed socket is below that of the adjacent teeth. Surgical removal of teeth, during which the outer plate of bone is removed, nearly always results in loss of bone from the crest and buccal aspects, producing in turn a smaller alveolar ridge than that after simple forceps removal of teeth. This may be of considerable significance in the preparation of a prosthetic appliance.

COMPLICATIONS IN THE HEALING OF EXTRACTION WOUNDS

"Dry Socket"

(Alveolitis Sicca Dolorosa; Alveolalgia; Postoperative Osteitis; Localized Acute Alveolar Osteomyelitis; Alveolar Osteitis)

The most common complication in the healing of human extraction wounds is that condition known as a "dry socket." The "dry socket" is basically a focal osteomyelitis in which the blood clot has disintegrated or been lost, with the production of a foul odor and severe pain, but no suppuration. The condition derives its name from the fact that after the clot is lost the socket has a dry appearance because of the exposed bone.

The condition is most frequently associated with difficult or traumatic extractions and thus most commonly follows removal of an impacted mandibular third molar. In a series of 138 "dry sockets" among 6403 teeth extracted in human patients, Krogh reported that 95 per cent were in lower bicuspid and molar sockets, and this is confirmed by most other large series of cases. The reported frequency of occurrence of "dry socket" in most series is between 1 per cent and 3.2 per cent of all extractions. Sometimes the "dry socket" is a sequela of normal extraction of an erupted tooth resulting from a dislodgment or a disintegration of the clot and the subsequent infection of the exposed bone. This complication usually arises within the first few days after extraction, but has been known to occur even a week or longer after extraction. It has been reported by Macgregor that teeth which fracture during extraction more frequently develop "dry socket" than teeth removed in toto. He also noted that there does not appear to be any significant relationship between the general health of an individual and the occurrence of "dry socket."

The "dry socket" is extremely painful and is usually treated by the insertion of a packing material containing an obtundent. The exposed bone is necrotic, and sequestration of fragments is common. The healing of such infected wounds is extremely slow, and little can be done for the patient other than to relieve the subjective symptoms.

Some investigators have suggested that complications in the healing of extraction wound sockets can conceivably be eliminated or at least decreased in incidence and degree of severity by the insertion of one agent or another in the tooth socket at the time of extraction. Some of the agents which have been used have been thought to hasten formation of the blood clot, to protect the socket against bacterial infection and to promote healing. Drug therapy for "dry socket" has been reviewed by Rothenberg and Landman.

A variety of agents used in recent years in both experimental studies on animals and in clinical studies on human beings have generally been antibacterial substances such as certain of the sulfonamides or the antibiotics.

Versnel reported that a sulfanilamide-sulfathiazole cone placed in the fresh tooth socket of a dog remained as a well-tolerated foreign material. But this agent retarded blood clot formation and even caused some breakdown of the clot. Furthermore, it caused a remarkable delay in epithelization of the surface of the wound. Oxidized cellulose inserted into a socket for its hemostatic properties produced retardation of healing similar to that of the combined sulfonamides.

Sulfathiazole was evaluated by use in human

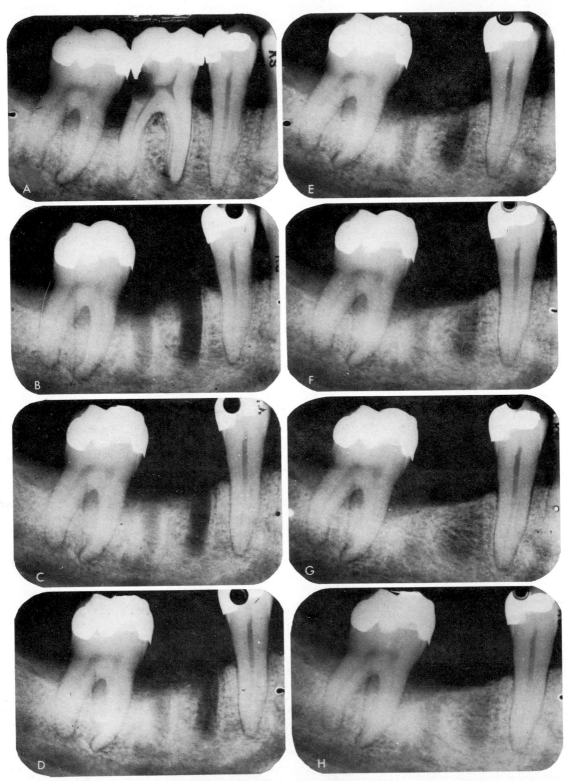

Figure 11–6. *Healing extraction wound.*

The roentgenographic features of the healing wound are shown serially: *(A)* tooth just before extraction; *(B)* after two weeks; *(C)* after one month; *(D)* after two months; *(E)* after four months; *(F)* after six months; *(G)* after eight months; *(H)* after fourteen months.

impacted third molar extraction wounds by Olech, who reported that though it was a clinical impression that the sulfonamide promoted healing and lessened the incidence of postoperative complications, this could not be supported by statistical analysis.

Millhon and his associates reported that sulfathiazole, 60 per cent in a glycerin base, when placed in the extraction socket, reduced the frequency of "dry socket" in a series of human patients with impacted lower third molars. However, these authors astutely observed that the use of sulfonamides cannot prevent the disagreeable results expected to follow careless surgical technique. They also pointed out that sulfathiazole is of no value in treatment of "dry sockets" once the symptoms have developed. Davis and his associates also found a 38 per cent reduction in the frequency of complicated healing after the use of sulfanilamide and sulfathiazole cones, while Rud reported a reduction in postoperative pain after removal of impacted lower third molars following use of sulfanilamide and sulfathiazole cones.

Olech also tested the effect of the insertion of penicillin into the sockets of human patients, but came to the same general conclusions that healing was not significantly promoted and that postoperative complications were not decreased. On this basis he concluded that the local implantation of these chemotherapeutic agents into sockets of impacted teeth was not justified. Similar studies of Versnel, using penicillin in dog extraction wounds, confirm the fact that this antibiotic does not promote healing.

A clinical study of the healing of human extraction wounds implanted with pure crystalline penicillin G tablets was reported by Holland and Tam. They found that there were no observable clinical differences during the postoperative period between the experimental group and a control group whose sockets were implanted locally with a lactose placebo tablet. Fewer cases of local osteitis occurred with the use of penicillin, but the difference was not statistically significant.

The local implantation of Aureomycin in extraction wound sockets of human mandibular bicuspid and molar teeth was studied by Verbic. In these cases it was found that the antibiotic resulted in a significant reduction in the incidence of decomposition of blood clots in addition to a decreased incidence of postoperative pain and swelling after one week. There was no evidence of a foreign body reaction or a toxicity reaction.

Quinley reported a reduction in the incidence of "dry sockets" to 0.78 per cent with the use of tetracycline hydrochloride tablets placed in the extraction sockets, while Stickel and Clark reported a 50 per cent decrease in the incidence of "dry sockets" when the tetracycline hydrochloride was administered systemically. In the study of Quinley, the local use of antibiotics occasionally resulted in a foreign body reaction. *Myospherulosis* is a complication of healing of an extraction wound or soft tissue wound into which there has been placed antibiotic ointment with a petrolatum base. This treatment results in the formation of clear spaces within the area of healing and the presence of altered erythrocytes which assume the appearance of solitary or clusters of spherules that have been mistaken for large microorganisms. This condition has been reviewed by Dunlap and Barker, who also presented two characteristic cases.

Hansen has reported encouraging results in the use of trypsin in cases of "dry socket" to relieve pain and promote healing. Trypsin itself is not bacteriostatic but by digesting necrotic tissue and debris, it appears to restrain bacterial growth. However, Gustafson and Wallenius have found that the use of trypsin statistically decreased the duration of pain by only about two days, but that there were no significant differences in the frequency of "dry socket" between trypsin applied locally and placebos. In addition, they noted a high percentage of side effects as the result of use of trypsin; these include erosions of the tongue, lips and buccal mucosa and burning sensations of the mouth.

Lilly and his associates studied the use of a phenolated antiseptic mouthrinse prior to extraction of mandibular third molars and reported a decrease in the incidence of "dry sockets" following such oral lavage as compared to the incidence in a group of patients not treated in this fashion.

Probably the oldest and most widely used method of treatment for "dry socket" is simply palliative medication and permitting nature to heal the wound. There are many palliative medicaments that have been used, such as iodoform gauze with a variety of incorporated dressing materials, zinc oxide and eugenol, and a large number of commercial compounds.

The various studies dealing with the prevention of extraction wound healing complications indicate that the routine use of agents inserted into the sockets is of only questionable value. There may be some benefit derived in cases of difficult extractions, but since the actual incidence of complications in even these cases is

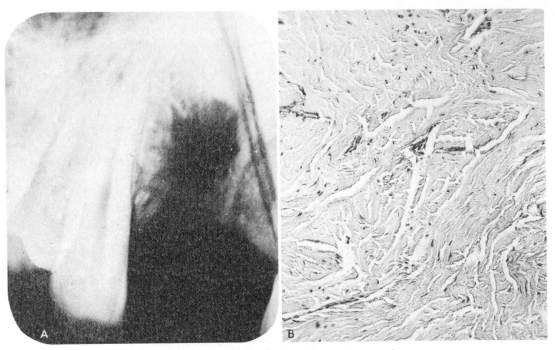

Figure 11–7. *Fibrous healing of extraction wound.*

low, chemotherapeutic adjuncts cannot be routinely recommended.

Probably the most important single factor in the prevention of extraction complications is gentleness in handling living tissues. One should strive to produce as little trauma as is possible, consistent with the successful completion of the operation.

Fibrous Healing of Extraction Wound

Fibrous healing of an extraction wound is an uncommon complication, usually following a difficult, complicated or surgical extraction of a tooth. It occurs most frequently when the tooth extraction is accompanied by loss of both the lingual and labial or buccal plates of bones with accompanying loss of periosteum.

The exact mechanism of development of this condition is not known, but is apparently related to the necessity of the labial and lingual periosteum for normal healing. The lesion is generally asymptomatic and is discovered only during roentgenographic examination.

Roentgenographic Features. The lesion appears as a rather well-circumscribed radiolucent area in the site of a previous extraction wound and may be mistaken for residual infection, e.g., a residual cyst or granuloma (Fig. 11–7,

A). There is no certain way of differentiating fibrous healing from residual infection without surgical exploration. At the time of surgery, simply a dense mass of fibrous connective tissue or scar tissue will be found.

Histologic Features. The area of fibrous healing consists of dense bundles of collagen fibers with only occasional fibrocytes and few blood vessels (Fig. 11–7, *B*). The lesion is essentially fibrous scar tissue with little or no evidence of ossification. Inflammatory cell infiltration is minimal or absent.

Treatment and Prognosis. Excision of the lesion for the purpose of establishing a diagnosis will sometimes, but not always, result in normal healing and subsequent bony repair of the fibrous defect.

HEALING OF THE FRACTURE

Fractures of the jaws are common injuries, and their manner of healing must be appreciated. Although it would seem that the sequence of events is a well-understood and thoroughly described phenomenon, there are surprisingly many controversial points about the general features of bone repair. There is at present great emphasis on the investigation of bone physiology and physiopathology, and certainly many of the challenging and perplexing unanswered problems will soon be clarified.

Immediate Effects of Fracture. When fracture of a bone occurs, the haversian vessels of the bone are torn at the fracture site, as are the vessels of the periosteum and the marrow cavity that happen to cross the fracture line. Because of the disruption of vessels, there is considerable extravasation of blood in this general area, but at the same time there is loss of circulation and lack of local blood supply. Circulation actually stops as far proximal to the fracture site as there is an anastomosis of undamaged vessels.

The haversian canals of bone contain only a single vessel. When the flow of blood in this vessel is interrupted by tearing at the fracture site, the bone cells or osteocytes of the haversian system supplied by this vessel die. The dead bone extends away from the fracture area to the site of the anastomosing circulation, and the distance may measure several millimeters or more. Because of the overlapping pattern of the blood supply of bone, seldom can a definite line of demarcation between living bone and dead bone be discerned. Concomitant with the disruption of the blood supply, there is death of the bone marrow adjacent to the fracture line. The tearing of the blood vessels in the periosteum also contributes to the local death of bone, since branches of the periosteal vessels supply the haversian vessels.

The blood clot which forms was once thought to play an important role in healing of the fracture through the replacement by granulation tissue and its subsequent replacement by bone. Most authorities now feel that the role of the blood clot in the healing process is only a passive one and that the newly forming bone, the callus, forms outside the granulation tissue replacement. Actually, the presence of the clot is not necessary for invasion of osteogenic cells, although frank necrosis of the clot may cause some retardation in the healing process.

Callus Formation. The callus is the structure which unites the fractured ends of bone, and it is composed of varying amounts of fibrous tissue, cartilage and bone. The external callus consists of the new tissue which forms around the outside of the two fragments of bone (Fig. 11–8). The internal callus is the new tissue arising from the marrow cavity.

The periosteum is an important structure in callus formation and ultimate healing of the fracture, and for this reason its preservation is essential. The cells of the periosteum immediately adjacent to the periosteum torn at the fracture line usually die. Peripheral to this area, however, may be found a flurry of cellular activity within a matter of hours after the injury. The outer or fibrous layer of periosteum is relatively inert and is actually lifted away from the surface of bone by the proliferation of cells in the osteogenic or inner layer of the periosteum. These cells assume the features of osteoblasts and, within a few days after the fracture, begin formation of a small amount of new bone at some distance from the fracture. The continued proliferation of these osteogenic cells forms a collar of callus around or over the surface of the fracture.

The new bone which begins to form in the

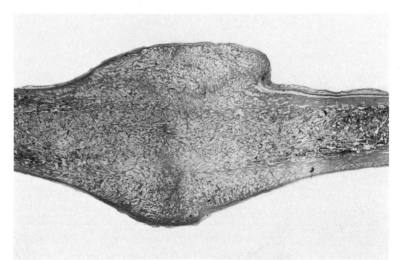

Figure 11–8. *Healing fracture.* The external callus is particularly prominent.

external callus usually consists of irregular trabeculae often laid down at right angles to the surface. This differentiation of cells into osteoblasts and subsequent formation of bone occur in the deepest part of the callus collar. Away from the fracture line in the rapidly growing area of the collar, varying numbers of cells of the osteogenic layer differentiate into chondroblasts rather than osteoblasts, and actually form cartilage. This cartilage fuses with the bone, although there is no sharp line of demarcation. The fact that the cells of the osteogenic layer may differentiate into chondroblasts rather than osteoblasts indicates their pluripotentiality and emphasizes that, in bones preformed in cartilage, the periosteum was once a perichondrium (Fig. 11–9).

The amount of cartilage formed in a callus may vary remarkably in different cases, and is determined by several factors. One factor of importance is the vascularity of the local environment. In a well-vascularized area the tendency is to form bone, but in a poorly vascularized environment cartilage develops. It will be noted that in the callus, bone forms adjacent to the blood vessels, while the cartilage forms from cells which have proliferated so rapidly that the

blood vessels have not kept pace and are outdistanced. The speed of healing, then, is another factor determining how much cartilage forms. In slow healing, cartilage formation is minimal. Finally, movement of the fragments is often associated with formation of considerable amounts of cartilage. In completely immobilized fractures little cartilage is laid down.

As callus formation progresses, the cartilage cells begin to mature, and the cartilage begins to calcify in a fashion similar to normal endochondral bone formation. This calcification is prominent adjacent to blood vessels developing in the immediate vicinity. The calcified cartilage is gradually resorbed and replaced by bone.

The internal callus forms from the endosteum of the haversian canals and undifferentiated cells of the bone marrow. Shortly after the fracture has occurred, the endosteum begins to proliferate and within a week or two begins formation of new bone and cartilage. The new bone formed at the end of each fragment gradually unites and establishes continuity of the bone.

Remodeling of the Callus. The external and internal calluses which unite the two fragments of bone must be remodeled because there is always an overabundance of new bone produced to strengthen the healing site. In addition, the new bone is frequently joined with fragments of the original dead bone. These fragments are slowly resorbed and replaced by a mature type of bone which follows normal stress patterns. The external callus is also remodeled so that in time the excess bone is removed. Ultimately, the bone in a fracture site is nearly indistinguishable from that existing before the fracture was sustained.

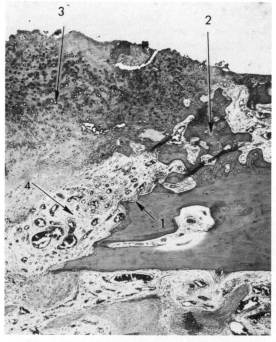

Figure 11–9. *Healing fracture of a long bone.*
The external callus above the fracture line *(1)* is composed of new bone *(2)*, cartilage *(3)* and vascular connective tissue *(4)*.

COMPLICATIONS OF FRACTURE HEALING

Nonunion of the fragments of bone is an occasional complication of the healing process. This results when the calluses of osteogenic tissue over each of the two fragments fail to meet and fuse or when endosteal formation of bone is inadequate. The causes of nonunion are not always clear, although in general it may be said that anything which delays growth and fusion of the collars is a factor. Nonunion is relatively common in elderly persons, in whom it is apparently related to a lack of osteogenic potential of cells.

Fibrous union in fractures is another complication of healing which arises usually as a result of lack of immobilization of the damaged bone. The fractured ends or fragments are united by fibrous tissue, but there is failure of ossification. In certain circumstances this may produce a pseudoarthrosis.

Lack of calcification of newly formed bone in the callus may occur, but only in unusual circumstances of dietary deficiency or mineral imbalance, which is seldom seen clinically. This may be produced in the experimental animal. Key and Odell reported that the opposite situation—an excess of minerals in the diet of normal rats—failed to accelerate the healing of experimental fractures of the femur.

REPLANTATION AND TRANSPLANTATION OF TEETH

Both replantation and transplantation of teeth have been recognized clinical procedures for many years. Because of the generally poor success of these particular techniques, they gradually fell into disuse. In recent years, however, there has been a remarkable revival of interest in replantation and transplantation of teeth, due in part to the availability of antibiotics which readily control infection and in part to a greater knowledge of tissue reactions.

The literature now contains over 2000 reported cases of replanted teeth, over 250 reported cases of autogenous transplanted teeth and over 375 reported cases of homogenous transplanted teeth, all in humans. An exceedingly thorough review of this topic, including all of these reported cases, has been published by Natiella and his associates.

REPLANTATION OF TEETH

Replantation refers to the insertion of a vital or nonvital tooth into the same alveolar socket from which it was removed or otherwise lost. This procedure finds its greatest use after traumatic injuries resulting in avulsion or other accidental loss of a tooth. However, it has been used in other unique situations as well. For example, unerupted teeth involved by dentigerous cysts have been replanted after removal of the cyst.

Many investigators believe that a tooth may be replanted without root canal therapy if root formation has not been completed and the apex is open. In some cases, the pulp tissue will undergo necrosis within a short period. In other instances, there is apparently revascularization and reinnervation, with the establishment of vital pulp responses. The majority of investigators believe that mature teeth with complete root formation must have the root canals filled before replantation or else pulp necrosis will result. In at least some of these cases, if the root canal is not filled, there is gradual obliteration of the pulp chamber and canal by bonelike material.

There has been some question of whether the preservation of the periodontal ligament on the root surface is of importance in the successful retention of a replanted tooth. Most investigations reveal that preservation of the periodontal ligament is an important factor in successful replantation. Partially formed teeth often have the ability to complete root formation as well as to re-establish a normal periodontal ligament space. Mature teeth may also develop a reasonably normal periodontal ligament, although the more common finding is varying degrees of resorption of cementum and dentin followed by subsequent replacement by bone resulting in a certain degree of ankylosis. There is some evidence to indicate that injury to the periodontal ligament or alterations in the cementum are important factors favoring root resorption and subsequent ankylosis. It also has been suggested by some investigators that whenever the extraoral period for the tooth exceeds 60 minutes, the chance for successful replantation with repair is significantly reduced, particularly if the storage of the tooth is in a dry rather than moist environment. There are a number of other factors which have also been considered of importance in determining whether a replanted tooth will be retained. For example, many investigators have stressed the necessity for handling the tooth to be replanted with great care so that there is no stripping or tearing of periodontal ligament fibers or of cementum. The matter of sterilization of the tooth has been argued, some investigators cautioning against sterilization but others recommending one of a large variety of sterilizing solutions in which the tooth should be placed for varying periods of time. Finally, fixation of the replanted tooth has also been the source of some disagreement. Some investigators believe that no splinting should be done, while others have used a variety of appliances including stainless steel wires, acrylic splints, orthodontic banding, arch wires with wire ligatures and even surgical cement with gauze, with recom-

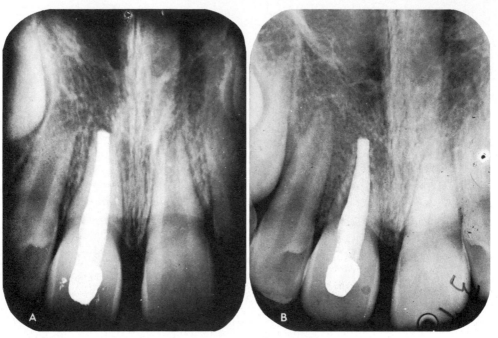

Figure 11–10. *Replanted tooth.*

A, Tooth immediately after replantation; *B,* tooth several months later, showing root resorption. (Courtesy of Dr. Samuel S. Patterson.)

mendations that these splints remain in place for a few days to several months. There is still no general agreement on many of these fine details.

Unfortunately, root resorption is totally unpredictable in its degree and time of onset. In some cases, root resorption may begin within a matter of weeks to a few months after replantation, while in other cases, gross resorption may take as long as 10 years. It appears likely that the roots of many replanted teeth are constantly being resorbed, but the rate at which this occurs varies remarkably between different cases. If the process is extremely slow, so that it takes place over a period of years, the operative procedure may be considered a clinical success. If root resorption is rapid, the tooth will be quickly exfoliated. Many cases are considered successful clinical results if the tooth is maintained beyond the period of two years (Fig. 11–10).

Unfortunately, there are many unknown factors which influence root resorption and ultimately determine the prognosis of a replanted tooth. In some cases, even after the most meticulous root canal therapy and sterilization, the tooth is either quickly resorbed or quickly exfoliated. Further investigation of this procedure is needed.

TRANSPLANTATION OF TEETH

The transplantation of teeth finds its greatest use in the replacement of teeth damaged beyond repair by caries. Generally, it is the mandibular first molar which is replaced by a developing third molar. Although the best results are obtained from autogenous transplants, investigations also have been carried out dealing with homologous transplants. The proceedings of a symposium on transplantation in dentistry were published in the *International Dental Journal* in June 1972.

The criteria of a satisfactory transplantation, as listed by Agnew and Fong, are that the transplant (1) has become organically integrated with its new environment; (2) is free of discernible periapical or lateral lesions; (3) is capable of effective masticatory function; (4) shares adequately in the maintenance of physiologic maxillomandibular and muscular relations; (5) displays, clinically and roentgenographically, such status of gingiva, periodontal ligament and bone (lamina dura and supporting bone) and such measure of the root length and over-all stability as seems compatible with indefinite maintenance; and (6) is esthetically acceptable.

These same investigators carried out on monkeys a critical experimental study dealing with histologic observation of developing teeth transplanted into prepared sockets of freshly extracted teeth. Their report indicated that no generalized pulpal necrosis necessarily occurs after the transplantation. Actually, the pulp becomes revascularized, and there is continued growth of the root dentin, although the shape of the root may be distorted. A functional, viable, highly cellular periodontal ligament develops, the tooth reattaching in the bony socket, and the gingival epithelium and epithelial attachment closely resemble those of normal teeth. The normal color and luster of the tooth are usually maintained. These findings appear similar to those few histologic studies reported in humans.

Most failures of autogenous transplants have been teeth that simply dropped out, had to be extracted or underwent severe resorption of the roots. Interestingly, these transplanted teeth may become carious, just as do normal teeth, and may even develop pulpitis and periapical infection.

Homologous transplants of preserved frozen teeth have also been successfully carried out. The establishment of "tooth banks" has even been proposed to simplify the procedure. There are several techniques available for the preservation of teeth, and these have been discussed by Pafford. They include (1) regular freezing, (2) freeze-drying, or lyophilization, (3) vitrification, and (4) chemical coagulation, as by thimerosal (Merthiolate). Teeth may apparently be used even after storage for months.

Teeth that have been preserved frozen and have been transplanted may be retained by the patient in some cases indefinitely. The gingival tissues heal promptly, and reattachment occurs within a few weeks, although readaptation of bone may take several months. The dentin of the transplanted tooth may be maintained in its normal state. Revascularization of the pulp is necessary if the tooth is to be retained indefinitely. New cementum may be laid down on the root surface after transplantation, and there is re-formation of the connective tissue fibers of the periodontal ligament. Unsuccessful transplants are usually lost because of root resorption or local infection.

It must be recognized that replantation and transplantation of teeth are sufficiently established as procedures that can be utilized in the routine dental practice. Care must be exercised in selecting the proper cases and in following certain principles of treatment, but favorable long-term results should be expected as the rule rather than the exception.

REFERENCES

Agnew, R. G., and Fong, C. C.: Histologic studies on experimental transplantation of teeth, Oral Surg., 9:18, 1956.

Amler, M. H.: The time sequence of tissue regeneration in human extraction wounds. Oral Surg., 27:309, 1969.

Idem: Pathogenesis of disturbed extraction wounds. J. Oral Surg., 31:666, 1973.

Idem: The age factor in human extraction wound healing. J. Oral Surg., 35:193, 1977.

Amler, M. H., Johnson, P. L., and Salman, I.: Histological and histochemical investigation of human alveolar socket healing in undisturbed extraction wounds. J. Am. Dent. Assoc., 61:32, 1960.

Amler, M. H., Salman, I., and Bungener, H.: Reticular and collagen fiber characteristics in human bone healing. Oral Surg., 17:785, 1964.

Andreasen, J. O., and Hjørting-Hansen, E.: Intraalveolar root fractures: radiographic and histologic study of 50 cases. J. Oral Surg., 25:414, 1967.

Arey, L. B.: Wound healing. Physiol. Rev., 16:327, 1936.

Bernier, J. L., and Kaplan, H.: The repair of gingival tissue after surgical intervention. J. Am. Dent. Assoc., 35:697, 1947.

Bhaskar, S. N., and Frisch, J.: Use of cyanoacrylate adhesives in dentistry. J. Am. Dent. Assoc., 77:831, 1968.

Borea, G.: Tooth germ transplantation. Int. Dent. J., 22:301, 1972.

Bourne, G. H. (ed.): The Biochemistry and Physiology of Bone. New York, Academic Press, 1956.

Carrel, A., and Ebeling, A. H.: Age and multiplication of fibroblasts. J. Exp. Med., 34:599, 1921.

Idem: The fundamental properties of the fibroblast and the macrophage. J. Exp. Med., 44:261, 285, 1926.

Claflin, R. S.: Healing of disturbed and undisturbed extraction wounds. J. Am. Dent. Assoc., 23:945, 1936.

Cook, R. M.: The current status of autogenous transplantation as applied to the maxillary canine. Int. Dent. J. 22:286, 1972.

Costich, E. R., Haley, E., and Hoek, R.: Plantation of teeth; a review of the literature. N.Y. State Dent. J., 29:3, 1963.

Crandon, J. H., Lund, C. C., and Dill, D. B.: Experimental human scurvy. N. Eng. J. Med., 223:353, 1940.

Davis, W. H., Hubbell, A. O., Bogart, W. E., and Graves, V. M.: Extraction wound healing: clinical observations. J. Oral Surg., 13:244, 1955.

Dunlap, C. L., and Barker, B. F.: Myospherulosis of the jaws. Oral Surg., 50:238, 1980.

El-Khashab, M.: The effects of a sclerosing solution on connective tissue and experimental wound healing in the rat. M.S.D. Thesis, Indiana University, 1961.

Frandsen, A. M.: Effects of roentgen irradiation of the jaws on socket healing in young rats. Acta Odontol. Scand., 20:307, 1962.

Gustafson, G., and Wallenius, K.: Effect of local application of trypsin on postextraction alveolar osteitis. Oral Surg., 14:280, 1961.

Ham, A. W.: Some histophysiological problems peculiar to calcified tissues. J. Bone Joint Surg., 34A:701, 1952.

Hansen, E. H.: Alveolitis sicca dolorosa (dry socket): frequency of occurrence and treatment with trypsin. J. Oral Surg., 18:409, 1960.

Hansen, J. and Fiboek, B.: Clinical experience of auto- and allotransplantation of teeth. Int. Dent. J., 22:270, 1972.

Harvey, S. C.: The healing of the wound as a biologic phenomenon. Surgery, 25:655, 1949.

Harvey, S. C., and Howes, E. L.: The effect of high protein

diet on the velocity of growth of fibroblasts in the healing wound. Ann. Surg., *91*:641, 1930.

Holland, M. R., and Tam, J. C.: The use of pure crystalline penicillin G tablets in extraction wounds. Oral Surg., 7:145, 1954.

Kay, L. W.: Investigations into the nature of pericoronitis. Br. J. Oral Surg., 3:188, 1966; *4*:52, 1966.

Key, J. A., and Odell, R. T.: Failure of excess minerals in the diet to accelerate the healing of experimental fractures. J. Bone Joint Surg., *37A*:37, 1955.

Krogh, H. W.: Incidence of dry socket. J. Am. Dent. Assoc., *24*:1829, 1937.

Lattes, R., Martin, J. R., and Ragan, C.: Suppression of cortisone effect on repair in the presence of local bacterial infection. Am. J. Pathol., *30*:901, 1954.

Lilly, G. E., Osbon, D. B., Rael, E. M., Samuels, H. S., and Jones J. C.: Alveolar osteitis associated with mandibular third molar extractions. J. Am. Dent. Assoc., *88*:802, 1974.

Macgregor, A. J.: Etiology of dry socket. Br. J. Oral Surg., 6:49, 1968.

Mangos, J. F.: The healing of extraction wounds. N. Z. Dent. J., *37*:4, 1941.

Marchand, F.: Der Process der Wundheilung, Stuttgart, Ferdinand Enke, 1901.

McLean, F. C., and Urist, M. R.: Bone: An Introduction to the Physiology of Skeletal Tissue. 2nd ed. Chicago, University of Chicago Press, 1961.

Medak, H., McGrew, E. A., Burlakow, P., and Tiecke, R. W.: Atlas of Oral Cytology. U.S. Public Health Service Publication No. 1949, 1970.

Menkin, V.: Biochemical Mechanisms in Inflammation, 2nd ed. Springfield, Ill., Charles C Thomas, 1956.

Idem: Dynamics of Inflammation. New York, Macmillan Company, 1940.

Millhon, J. A., Austin, L. T., Stafne, E. C., and Gardner, B. S.: An evaluation of the sulfa drug and other dressings in "dry socket" in lower third molars. J. Am. Dent. Assoc., *30*:1839, 1943.

Natiella, J. R., Armitage, J. E., and Greene, G. W.: The replantation and transplantation of teeth. A review. Oral Surg., 29:397, 1970.

Olech, E.: Value of implantation of certain chemotherapeutic agents in sockets of impacted lower third molars. J. Am. Dent. Assoc., *46*:154, 1953.

Orban, B., and Archer, E. A.: Dynamics of wound healing following elimination of gingival pockets. Am. J. Orthod. Oral Surg., *31*:40, 1945.

Pafford, E. M.: Homogeneous transplants of preserved frozen teeth. Oral Surg., 9:55, 1956.

Patterson, W. B. (ed.): Wound Healing and Tissue Repair. Chicago, University of Chicago Press, 1959.

Quinley, J. F.: "Dry socket" after mandibular odontectomy and use of soluble tetracycline hydrochloride. Oral Surg., *13*:38, 1960.

Rothenberg, F., and Landman, R.: A review of drug therapy for dry socket. J. Oral Ther., 2:229, 1965.

Rud, J., Baggesen, H., and Møller, J. F.: Effect of the sulfa cones and suturing on the incidence of pain after removal of impacted lower third molars. J. Oral Surg., Anesthet. Hosp. Dent. Serv., *21*:219, 1963.

Schilling, J. A.: Wound healing. Physiol. Rev., *48*:374, 1968.

Schram, W. R.: A histologic study of repair in the maxillary bones following surgery. J. Am. Dent. Assoc., *16*:1987, 1929.

Shafer, W. G.: The effect of cortisone on the healing of extraction wounds in the rat. J. Dent. Res., *33*:4, 1954.

Shapiro, M.: Acceleration of gingival wound healing in non-epileptic patients receiving diphenylhydantoin sodium (Dilantin, Epanutin). Exp. Med. Surg., *16*:41, 1958.

Simpson, H. E.: Effects of suturing extraction wounds in macacus rhesus monkeys. J. Oral Surg., Anesthet. Hosp. Dent. Serv., *18*:461, 1960.

Idem: Experimental investigation into the healing of extraction wounds in macacus rhesus monkeys. J. Oral Surg., Anesthet. Hosp. Dent. Serv., *18*:391, 1960.

Idem: The healing of extraction wounds. Br. Dent. J., *126*:550, 1969.

Idem: Healing of surgical extraction wounds in macacus rhesus monkeys. I. The effect of burs. J. Oral Surg., Anesthet. Hosp. Dent. Serv., *19*:3, 1961.

Idem: Healing of surgical extraction wounds in macacus rhesus monkeys. II. The effect of chisels. J. Oral Surg., Anesthet. Hosp. Dent. Serv., *19*:126, 1961.

Idem: Healing of surgical extraction wounds in macacus rhesus monkeys. III. Effect of removal of alveolar crests after extraction of teeth by means of forceps. J. Oral Surg., Anesthet. Hosp. Dent. Serv., *19*:227, 1961.

Söder, P-Ö.: Autotransplantation of teeth with use of cell cultivation technique. Int. Dent. J., *22*:327, 1972.

Stickel, F. R., and Clark, H. B.: Prophylactic use of tetracycline after removal of impacted teeth. J. Oral Surg., Anesthet. Hosp. Dent. Serv., *19*:149, 1961.

Swanson, A E.: Reducing the incidence of dry socket; a clinical appraisal. J. Can. Dent. Assoc., *32*:25, 1966.

Thoma, K. H. (ed.): Symposium on transplantation, replantation, and surgical positioning of teeth. Oral Surg., 9:1, 1956.

Van Winkle, W., Jr., Hastings, J. C., Hines D., and Nichols, W.: Effect of suture materials on healing skin wounds. Surg. Gynecol. Obstet., *140*:1, 1975.

Verbic, R. L.: Local implantation of Aureomycin in extraction wounds: a preliminary study. J. Am. Dent. Assoc., *46*:160, 1953.

Versnel, J. C.: Healing of extraction wounds after introduction of hemostatics and antibiotics. J. Am. Dent. Assoc., *46*:146, 1953.

Von Haam, E.: The historical background of oral cytology. Acta Cytol., 9:270, 1965.

SECTION IV

DISTURBANCES OF METABOLISM

CHAPTER 12

Oral Aspects of Metabolic Disease

Man is a complex biologic unit in a complex environment. If we isolate him from his social environment, we may conceive of him as an individual. The concept of individuality, which applies not only to man, but also to other biologic as well as inanimate objects, is one of wholeness, of complete integration. The term "individual" comes from the Latin *individuus*, meaning indivisible. In a literal sense, therefore, the term signifies that an organism cannot be divided without losing its identity. Loeb described individual man as a "mosaic of many tissues and organs," each one functioning and *metabolizing* in its own peculiar way. Each tissue or organ has properties not restricted to it, but common to all parts of the organism, and it is these common properties which bind the tissues and organs well together into a unit.

We cannot, however, isolate man from his social environment. Each individual is dependent on society for the needs of his daily life, and society is dependent for its well-being on the health of its individual members. Health is largely determined by man's reaction to his environment, both social and physical, but different individuals behave differently in the same environment and under apparently identical conditions. On this basis we recognize the variations of the substratum upon which environmental factors act. Individual variations in response to the internal and external environment are dependent upon constitution. Each response represents a complex interplay between the genetic and environmental factors acting on the individual.

Certain characteristics of an organism are fixed in the germ cells and give rise to definite metabolic, structural and functional conditions in the individual. These inherited features represent the core of his constitution, the unchangeable part of it. In actual life, however, it is often difficult to separate this core from effects produced by the environment.

It might be well to visualize man—the organism—as a universe: a universe of cells living together within a restricted framework. Some of the individuals (the cells) of this universe form rather tightly knit communities (the organs) which perform highly specialized tasks. Each individual within the community responds to his inner as well as his outer environment, and each is influenced by his neighbor. The outer environment in this instance is fluid—mostly water. Each individual cell influences the tissue fluid in some manner by removing and/or adding metabolic products. Each cell or organ system reacts to its changing environment within the limits of its inherent capabilities. If an analogy is drawn between the cell as an individual within the organism and the organism as an individual within the cosmos, the complexity of the interrelations becomes apparent, even though the nature of the interrelations is nebulous.

Duncan defined metabolism as "the sum total of tissue activity as considered in terms of physicochemical changes associated with and regulated by the availability, utilization and disposal of protein, fat, carbohydrate, vitamins, minerals, water and the influences which the endocrines exert on these processes." Alterations from these normal metabolic processes constitute the *disturbances of metabolism.* One recognizes immediately that this definition embodies a concept of cellular change as influenced not only by intrinsic factors, but also by such extrinsic factors as food supply, temperature, altitude, society; in other words, by environment.

The volume of literature pertaining to metabolism is rapidly surpassing the ability of investigators to keep pace with it. Obviously it is

616

the structure and function of cells. Phosphates are utilized in the formation of phosphoproteins, such as milk casein, and in the formation of the nerve phosphatides and the nucleoproteins of cells. They provide the energy-rich bonds in such compounds as adenosine triphosphate, which is important in muscle contraction, and they form part of such coenzymes as pyridoxal phosphate, which is necessary in decarboxylation and transamination of certain amino acids, such as tyrosine, tryptophan and arginine.

The normal inorganic phosphate level of blood in adults ranges from 2 to 4 mg./dl., while in children its range is from 3 to 5 mg./dl. These blood levels are maintained by a balance of various factors, such as parathyroid hormone, phosphatase activity, and vitamin D.

REQUIREMENTS AND ABSORPTION. The suggested daily dietary intake of phosphorus ranges from 240 mg. for infants to 800 mg. for adults. As with calcium, adolescents and pregnant and lactating women are advised to increase their daily dietary phosphorus intake by 50 per cent to 1200 mg.

Absorption of phosphorus takes place in the small intestine in the form of soluble inorganic phosphate. Approximately 70 per cent of food phosphorus is absorbed in the form of orthophosphate after intestinal phosphatase releases the food-bound phosphorus during the digestive process. An excess of calcium, iron or aluminum may interfere with the absorption of phosphorus because of a tendency to form insoluble phosphates in the intestinal tract.

When young rats are placed on a low phosphorus diet, there is some retardation in growth. The only specific gross or microscopic alterations are found in the skeletal system, where severe rickets is present (Fig. 12–1). This finding appears after the rats have been on the experimental phosphorus-deficient diet for only one week.

Phosphate depletion in man is nonexistent under most dietary regimens. Long-term antacid use, however, will render phosphate unabsorbable. Lotz and co-workers have described such a condition, which is characterized by weakness, malaise, anorexia and bone pain. Increased calciuria results in a negative calcium balance with bone demineralization.

EXCRETION. Excretion of phosphorus occurs primarily in the urine. Almost two-thirds of the total phosphorus excreted is found in the urine as phosphates of various cations. Fecal phosphorus, which is usually composed of unab-

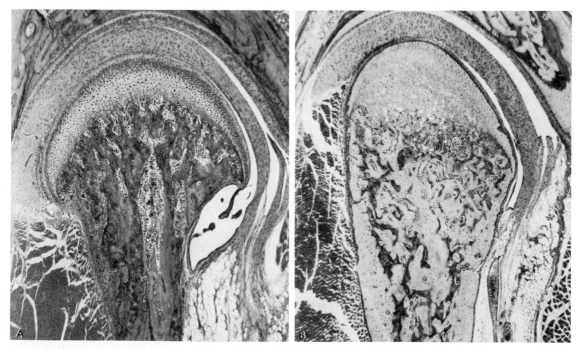

Figure 12–1. *Phosphorus deficiency.*
A, Sagittal section of mandibular joint of a normal rat 70 days of age. *B,* Sagittal section of mandibular joint of rat 70 days old, which received a phosphorus-deficiency diet since weaning at 21 days of age. (Courtesy of Dr. Herman Becks.)

sorbed as well as re-excreted phosphate, is usually excreted as calcium phosphate.

Magnesium. Magnesium appears to participate in practically every phosphorylating mechanism. In addition, this ion is necessary for the activity of certain enzymes, such as phosphatase and cocarboxylase. Although the concentration of magnesium in the intracellular fluids is not as great as the concentration of potassium, magnesium is widely distributed in the tissues of the animal body. The body of a 70 kg. man contains approximately 25 mg. of magnesium. Over half of this amount is found in the bones, and one quarter in the muscles. The remainder is distributed between liver, pancreas, erythrocytes, serum and cerebrospinal fluid. Hypermagnesemia is rare because of the renal capacity to excrete excess ion. The administration of magnesium-containing antacids to patients with renal insufficiency has resulted in central nervous system depression. Somjen and co-workers have also reported severe voluntary muscle paralysis with hypermagnesemia. Controlled human hypomagnesemia was studied by Shils, who noted a concurrent hypocalcemia and hypokalemia despite normal dietary calcium and phosphorus intake. Clinically the patients exhibited personality change, anorexia, nausea and vomiting, and carpopedal spasms.

REQUIREMENTS. The recommended daily dietary allowance for magnesium ranges from 50 mg. for infants to 400 mg. for teenage males. A daily increase of 150 mg. is suggested during pregnancy and lactation. Like calcium, magnesium is ingested in inorganic and organic forms. It is also absorbed and excreted in the same manner as calcium. Almost 60 per cent of the excreted magnesium is fecal, the rest being urinary. High calcium diets raise the requirement for magnesium.

High magnesium intake will produce rickets in growing animals, especially if the phosphorus and calcium intake is relatively low. The normal serum magnesium level is 1 to 3 mg./dl. When the level reaches 5 mg./dl., mild sedative or hypnotic effects may occur. Profound coma and even death may result when the serum level reaches 18 to 21 mg. A distinct but not fully understood relationship exists between magnesium, calcium, parathyroid hormone and bone metabolism. Buckle and co-workers have shown that hypomagnesemia and hypocalcemia have identical effects on the parathyroid glands, i.e., increased parathyroid hormone production. An apparent contradiction exists in that despite elevated hormone levels, many affected individuals exhibit hypocalcemia. Recent studies have indicated that the parathyroid hormone produced is defective, but some investigators have described hypomagnesemic patients who were refractory to exogenous parathyroid extract, which indicates a bone defect rather than a glandular abnormality.

DEFICIENCY. Magnesium deficiency in experimental animals leads to disturbances in the neuromuscular and vascular systems as well as to changes in the teeth, liver and kidneys. The effects of magnesium-deficient diets on the teeth and their supporting structures have been thoroughly described by Becks and Furuta and by Klein and his associates. Diets containing only 13 ppm of magnesium caused the ameloblasts from the labial side near the apex of the growing incisor tooth in rats to show various stages of localized degeneration with subsequent formation of enamel hypoplasia. The hypoplastic areas increased in size and number with the duration of the experiment, although the changes were noted in all animals after 41 days.

The syndrome of human magnesium-deficiency tetany was first described by Vallee and his associates in 1960. The condition is virtually identical with that of hypocalcemic tetany from which it can be differentiated only by chemical means. Clinically, patients with this deficiency exhibit a semicoma; severe neuromuscular hyperirritability, including carpopedal spasm and a positive Chvostek's sign; athetoid movements; marked susceptibility to auditory, visual and mechanical stimuli; a decreased serum magnesium; and a normal serum calcium concentration. Precipitating factors are a severe dietary inadequacy of magnesium or excessive losses of this ion due to vomiting, intestinal malabsorption and the administration of large amounts of magnesium-free parenteral fluids which induce a large urine volume. The tetany appears when the serum magnesium level is depressed below 1.30 mEq. per liter. Treatment by the intramuscular injection of magnesium sulfate is followed by a prompt rise in serum magnesium and a concomitant disappearance of the tetany and the convulsions. Discontinuance of the therapy in the presence of the precipitating factors results in a rapid reappearance of the tetany.

Pathologic Calcification. Pathologic calcification is commonly classified as (1) dystrophic calcification, (2) metastatic calcification, and (3) calcinosis. It is not always possible to make a clear distinction between these various forms.

DYSTROPHIC CALCIFICATION. In the dystrophic form of calcification, calcium salts are deposited in dead or degenerating tissues. This is the most frequent type of pathologic calcification and is found in a wide variety of tissues. Areas of tuberculous necrosis, blood vessels in arteriosclerosis, scars and areas of fatty degeneration are commonly recognized as sites of dystrophic calcification by the general pathologist. This type of calcification is not dependent upon an increase in the amount of circulating blood calcium, but appears to be related to a change in the local condition of the tissues. A local alkalinity in comparison with adjacent undamaged tissues appears to be an important factor in initiating the precipitation of calcium in degenerating or nonvital tissues.

In the mouth, areas of dystrophic calcification may frequently be found in the gingiva, tongue or cheek. Such areas are also found in the benign fibromas of the mouth and adjacent structures (Fig. 12–2). One of the most common intraoral dystrophic calcifications is found in the pulp of teeth, and this has been discussed in Chapter 5. Boyle described the pulp calcifications as calcific degeneration of the pulp tissue. They are usually found in the teeth of older persons, although they also may be seen in young people. They may occur in the wall of blood vessels or in the perineural connective tissue of the pulp, or they may be rather diffusely scattered both in the pulp chamber and in the root canal. They appear as fine fibrillar calcifications which may coalesce to form large masses of calcific material.

Hill classified calcific degenerations of the pulp into two types. The first, a nodular type, is a result of calcification of hyalinized connective tissue. Such calcification is usually perivascular or perineural and is often associated with increased fibrosis. The calcium deposits are most frequently found in the coronal portion of the pulp chamber and increase in size by accretion and deposition of calcium along the collagenous fibrils. The second type of calcification of the pulp is that found in and around necrotic cells and corpora amylacea. It occurs in a multicentric manner and is most frequently found in the radicular portion of the pulp canal. This type of calcification always shows a nidus in the center and increases in size by concrescence which is obvious on histologic examination.

Many of the deposits of calcareous material are found in degenerative processes of the pulp as well as in pulps which are the seat of inflammatory processes. In these cases the calcifications probably have the same relation to body health as calcifications within arterial walls in arteriosclerosis. This type of calcification probably does not cause pulpal inflammation, and there is no justification for considering it a source of dental infection. The other types of pulp stones or pulp nodules (denticles) are discussed in Chapter 5.

METASTATIC CALCIFICATION. In metastatic calcification, calcium salts are precipitated in previously undamaged tissues. This precipitation is due to an excess of blood calcium and occurs particularly in such diseases as hyperparathyroidism, which depletes the bone of

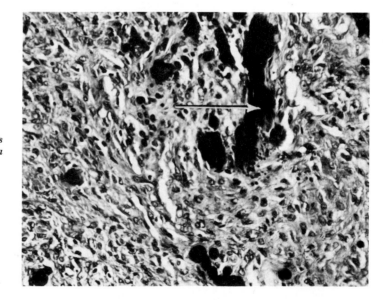

Figure 12–2. *Focal calcification is illustrated in the photomicrograph of a fibroma of the gingiva.*

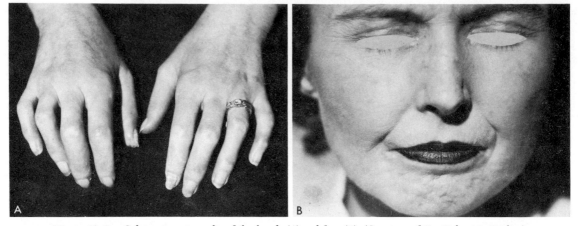

Figure 12–3.   Calcinosis universalis of the hands (A) and face (B). (Courtesy of Dr. Robert J. Gorlin.)

calcium and causes a high level of blood calcium. Metastatic calcifications also occur in hypervitaminosis D. In this type of calcification the deposits of calcium occur mainly in the kidneys, lungs, gastric mucosa and media of blood vessels. Since any degenerating or necrotic tissue will also be calcified when there is an increase in blood calcium levels, the differentiation between metastatic calcification and dystrophic calcification becomes extremely difficult.

CALCINOSIS. Calcinosis is the presence of calcifications in or under the skin. There are two forms of calcinosis: calcinosis circumscripta, which, as the name suggests, is a circumscribed form, and calcinosis universalis, which is a generalized form. Calcinosis universalis is often associated with scleroderma and sometimes dermatomyositis. These different forms of calcinosis have been discussed by Johnson (Fig. 12–3).

SODIUM AND POTASSIUM

Sodium.   The sodium ion content of the normal (70 kg.) adult male ranges from 83 to 97 gm. Over one-third of this amount is in the skeleton, of which 65 to 75 per cent is unexchangeable. Most of the remaining sodium is extracellular and accounts for 90 per cent of the basic ions of both extracellular fluid and plasma. Enamel ash contains about 0.3 per cent. The question of whether the sodium of the dental tissues is associated with the inorganic or organic fractions or with small quantities of tissue fluid present in the teeth remains unanswered.

Sodium ions play an important role in the maintenance of the acid-base equilibrium as well as of osmotic pressure, which depends largely on total base. In fact, the bulk of basic metabolic energy expenditure is concerned exclusively with the maintenance of proper intracellular sodium concentration, i.e., the sodium pump. When tissues are depleted of potassium, sodium may substitute for it, regulating the contraction of the heart. Little else is known of the functions of this element in the animal organism.

REQUIREMENTS AND EXCRETION. The minimal requirement of salt is thought to be about 0.5 gm. The lower limit of salt intake is not really known. The estimate of 0.5 gm. was reached based on the salt intake of breast-fed infants. Breast milk contains 0.4 gm. NaCl per liter. Interestingly, cow's milk contains 1.7 gm. NaCl per liter. The maximal intake without accumulating edema fluid is 35 to 40 gm. per day. In the United States, the average dietary intake of sodium is 10 to 15 gm. per day. The normal blood level is 160 mg./dl. of whole blood, or 340 mg./dl. of plasma (147.8 mEq./liter of plasma).

Under conditions of profuse sweating, 1 gm. of salt should be ingested for each liter of water in excess of 4 liters. Sweat may contain 2 to 3 gm. of salt per liter in hot environments if the person has not been acclimatized; after acclimatization, 0.5 gm. of salt per liter is found.

The kidney is the principal organ for the excretion of water and salt. Abnormal losses of either sodium or chloride must be balanced by the kidney. When the diet is low in salt, or when there is profuse sweating, practically no sodium or chloride is found in the urine. The regulatory mechanism controlling the reabsorption of sodium and chloride by the renal tubules is controlled in part by the adrenal glands. An inadequate intake or excessive loss of sodium stimulates the adrenal cortex to secrete aldosterone, a steroid hormone which acts directly on the renal tubules to increase reabsorption and to conserve sodium. The adrenal glands also control, to a smaller degree, the salt content of sweat.

Desoxycorticosterone, cortisone and hydrocortisone act to increase the tubular reabsorption of glomerular filtrate sodium and to decrease tubular reabsorption of filtrate potassium. It should be realized, therefore, that care must be taken in using these drugs to avoid edema resulting from excess sodium retention. Potassium loss must also be anticipated and provided for by increased potassium ingestion.

Many of the features of Addison's disease are referable to salt depletion. In this disease extracellular water and sodium are rapidly excreted by the kidneys, resulting in a fall of plasma sodium concentration and an increase in the serum potassium level. Water migrates intercellularly, and the result is a deprivation of both sodium and water.

Studies with radioactive sodium (Na^{22}) have shown that the sodium of bone, which constitutes about 30 per cent of the body sodium, is located on the surface of the apatite crystal lattice.

DEFICIENCY. Sodium deficiency in man probably never occurs in an uncomplicated form, but it may be present as a sodium and chloride deficiency. When diets very low in salt are used for long periods of time, gradual weakness, excessive fatigue, lassitude, apathy, anorexia, a sense of exhaustion, nausea, muscle cramps and peripheral vascular collapse may ensue.

Potassium. Most of the potassium of the body is intracellular. It is the predominant base in the cells. Radioactive potassium (K^{42}) studies have indicated that there is a constant exchange of potassium between its intracellular and extracellular phases, although it is clear from the studies of Peters and Van Slyke that potassium is prevented from diffusing freely out of cells by a membrane or by some other restraining factor or factors in the cellular or extracellular fluids.

REQUIREMENTS AND EXCRETION. The average American diet contains 2 to 4 gm. of potassium daily, although normal function can be maintained by a normal person on smaller intakes. The requirement for potassium is greatest during periods of rapid growth. About 90 per cent of the excreted potassium is eliminated in the urine. This urinary excretion is influenced by aldosterone which controls the active tubular secretion of potassium. The normal blood plasma level is about 4 mEq./liter of plasma.

DEFICIENCY. Primary dietary deficiency of potassium has not been observed, but depletion secondary to some pathologic condition has been encountered. It may occur in gastrointestinal disorders, in which there may be a loss of potassium through diarrhea and vomiting. It may also occur in general malnutritional states. It develops as a result of the administration of diuretics or ion-exchange resins. Excessive doses of cortisone or hydrocortisone may result in potassium depletion, and potassium deficiency is common in diabetic acidosis during insulin therapy.

Death in potassium deficiency may result from cardiac or respiratory failure or from paralytic ileus. The signs of potassium deficiency are primarily those of decreased muscular irritability, muscular weakness, reduced or absent reflexes, mental confusion, paralysis, disturbances in conductivity and contractility of heart muscle and alterations in the gastrointestinal tract.

HYPERKALEMIA. Hyperkalemia, which may result from extensive tissue breakdown, adrenal insufficiency, advanced dehydration or administration of excessive amounts of potassium, will produce such signs and symptoms as mental confusion, numbness and tingling of the extremities, pallor, cold skin, weakness, disturbances in cardiac rhythm, and peripheral collapse, as noted by Darrow.

The effects of potassium deficiency or of excess potassium on the oral structures per se have not been reported.

CHLORINE

The metabolism of chlorine, together with that of sodium and potassium, is closely related to the water balance and the acid-base equilibrium of the body. The average intake is 6 to 9 gm. per day. Quantitatively, chlorine and sodium are the most important mineral constituents of the extracellular fluids. Chlorine is excreted primarily through the kidney. It is one of the so-called threshold substances which are reabsorbed into the circulation after passing through the glomeruli to maintain normal body fluid concentrations. The normal blood plasma concentration of chlorine is 550 to 650 mg./dl. as sodium chloride.

Chloride activates salivary amylase. Little else is known of the function of chlorine in the animal organism. Rats placed on a synthetic diet low in chlorides failed to grow normally. The only histologic lesions reported were in the kidney.

The role of chloride per se in sodium deficiency in man is not clear. Large quantities of chloride ions may be lost in pyloric obstruction with gastric tetany, leading to signs of hyperexcitability and convulsions. These may be prevented by the administration of chloride ions. No oral manifestations of chloride deficiency have been reported.

TRACE ELEMENTS

A large number of elements have been shown to occur in a wide range of animal tissues and fluids in such minute quantities that they are usually described as "traces." Demonstration of a physiologic role for many of these elements has lagged far behind their mere detection in the living organism. It has been shown that both barium and strontium are essential for growth and especially for calcification of the bones and teeth of rats and guinea pigs. Mertz has reported silicon, vanadium, nickel and arsenic to be essential in various animal species. However, no imbalances in humans have been reported.

Iodine. Iodine is essential for the formation of thyroid hormone. No other function for iodine in the nutrition of higher animals is known. Iodine deficiency in man results in goiter. Iodine deficiency in experimental animals does not lead to colloid goiter. On the other hand, addition of iodine to the salt or water supply of endemic goiter areas has been successful in acting as a prophylactic in colloid goiter. About one third of the total body iodine is found in the thyroid. The precise mechanism of conversion of thyroid-concentrated iodine to colloid is unclear. However, thyroxin formation is intimately related to tyrosine metabolism.

The ovaries also contain a high concentration of iodine. Normal whole blood contains an average of 8 to 12 mcg./dl. (range, 3 to 30 mcg.); protein-bound iodine varies from 3 to 8 mcg./dl. The level of protein-bound iodine is increased during pregnancy and in hyperthyroidism and decreased in hypothyroidism.

The effects of the thyroid gland on oral structures will be considered in the section dealing with the endocrine glands.

Copper. Copper deficiency in experimental animals leads to anemia. Minimum copper requirements for man are not known, but are thought to be approximately 1 to 2 mg. per day. Acute copper deficiency in human beings has not been demonstrated.

The value of copper supplements, with and without iron, in the treatment of anemias of infancy and childhood and of secondary anemias of adults has been extensively studied. Copper is necessary for normal erythropoiesis as well as for iron absorption. Iron absorption is mediated by ceruloplasmin, which acts as a ferroxidase. Other metalloenzymes which require copper are cytochrome c oxidase, superoxide dismutase, tyrosinase and lysyl oxidase. Human copper deficiency diseases of importance are hepatolenticular degeneration (Wilson's disease) and Menkes' syndrome (steely- or kinky-hair syndrome).

Iron. Iron is absorbed in the upper portion of the duodenum, either as ferrous or as ferric salts, depending on the species studied. Absorption depends on the amount of the element that the organism has stored. If the tissues are depleted, iron is absorbed rapidly; if sufficient quantities are present, absorption is slight. Since little excretion of iron takes place either by the alimentary canal or by the kidneys, this element has been called a "one-way substance."

Few studies have been reported on the histopathologic changes occurring in the tissues of human beings or experimental animals with iron deficiency anemias. Iron deficiency in the human being, particularly in women and children, however, is more common than has been realized. Changes in the resulting anemia include formation of an esophageal web in the Plummer-Vinson syndrome, spooning of the nails (koilonychia), normoblastic arrest in the bone marrow and microcytosis, anisocytosis and hypochromia of the erythrocytes in the peripheral blood. For the oral findings in iron deficiency anemias, see Chapter 14. We should emphasize here, however, that sore tongue, similar to that found in nicotinic acid and riboflavin deficiencies, has been described in the iron deficiency anemias. These anemias respond well to iron therapy.

Iron overload can occur in a number of conditions. Idiopathic hemochromatosis results in excessive iron absorption. Hemoglobinopathies such as sideroblastic anemia and thalassemia can also cause iron overload. Bantu siderosis, a form of iron overload resulting from ingestion of homemade beer fermented in iron pots, has been extensively described.

Zinc. The concentration of zinc in enamel and dentin is about 0.02 per cent, which is higher than in any other tissue of the body. Bone, nails and hair have slightly lower concentrations. A strange and unexplained observation is that the teeth of tuberculous patients apparently have a higher zinc concentration than the teeth of normal people.

In 1961, Prasad and his associates reported a symptom complex of dwarfism and hypogonadism in male Iranians which stemmed from a deficiency of zinc in the diet. This deficiency was thought to occur from zinc binding with phytates present in bread. Subsequent studies in Egypt by Prasad and his co-workers confirmed this impression. The zinc-deficient subjects appeared much younger than their stated age, lacked facial, axillary and pubic hair, had atrophic testes and small external genitalia and were retarded in bone age. The zinc content of the plasma, red blood cells and hair was consistently lower than in normal ethnically identical controls. Radioisotope studies demonstrated a significantly increased plasma zinc turnover and a decreased excretion of Zn^{65} in the urine and stools of the dwarfs, indicative of zinc retention and conservation. A low plasma level of alkaline phosphatase, a zinc-containing enzyme, was also found in these patients.

Zinc deficiency in humans results in a number of disorders involving taste, keratogenesis, bone growth, wound healing, and reproduction. Acrodermatitis enteropathica, a specific multiorgan disorder resulting from zinc deficiency, has been described. Its symptoms include diarrhea and a wide range of mucocutaneous problems including vesicles, eczematoid and hyperkeratotic plaques, alopecia, stomatitis, and glossitis.

Manganese. Manganese is another indispensable trace element. Although it is especially abundant in the liver, it is distributed throughout all the organs. It is necessary for the activation of phosphatase and forms a part of the enzyme arginase.

There is no evidence of manganese deficiency in man.

Cobalt. In the naturally occurring cobalt-deficiency areas of North America, Europe, Australia, New Zealand and Africa, only sheep, cattle and goats show the effects of the deficiency on blood formation; horses and pigs develop normally. This element does not seem to have a storage depot in the animal organism.

Vitamin B_{12} contains about 4.5 per cent cobalt. If this is the only cobalt required by man, the amount must be infinitesimal, since 1 to 2 micrograms of vitamin B_{12} by injection each day will adequately treat pernicious anemia.

Chromium. Chromium deficiency has been described in cases of malnutrition and total parenteral alimentation. The total body content of chromium is less than 6 mg. It appears to have a role in carbohydrate and lipid metabolism. Mertz has suggested that chromium may facilitate insulin binding to cell membranes via a "chromium bridge." While it may potentiate insulin action, chromium is not thought to be a hypoglycemic agent per se.

Selenium. Burk and co-workers have described selenium deficiency in humans with protein-energy malnutrition. Rotruck and co-workers have reported that glutathione peroxidase is a selenoenzyme that is responsible for eliminating potentially harmful peroxides and free radicals. Selenium concentration in the blood is about 0.22 mcg./ml.

Fluoride. Using Mertz's definition of essentiality—that an element is essential if a deficiency of that element results in suboptimal physiologic function—fluoride is essential in human nutrition. Reports of the effect on animals of diets low in fluoride have been conflicting. With the exception of McClendon's work, there have been no published findings which indicate that fluoride is essential to animal growth, development, and reproduction. McClendon, using hydroponic techniques for preparing fluoride-free foods, showed that a few rats raised on such foods evidenced such severe caries that they were unable to eat and eventually starved.

The effects of fluoride as a prophylactic in dental caries are reviewed elsewhere. We should mention here, however, some of the work done on toxic fluorosis. It has been estimated that the average American diet contains about 0.2 to 0.3 mg. of fluoride per day. If 1 ppm of fluoride is added to the drinking water, about 1 to 2 mg. of fluoride will be added to the diet daily. Balance studies in man have shown that when the quantities of fluoride ingested do not exceed 4 to 5 mg. daily, little is retained by the body. This finding indicates the safety of the preventive dentistry programs based on the addition of fluoride to drinking water in concentrations of approximately 1 ppm.

Although fluoride normally accumulates slowly in bones as the person ages, it accumulates rapidly if ingested in abnormally high quantities. One must remember, however, that the rates of absorption and excretion as well as the rate of retention are related to the nature of the diet; e.g., intakes of calcium above certain minimal levels will reduce the absorption of dietary fluoride.

Chronic fluoride intoxication, such as that found in cryolite workers in Denmark, is characterized by widespread calcification of tendons and muscle sheaths, by extensive arthritic changes in the spine, producing rigidity, and by osteosclerosis of the bones.

DISTURBANCES IN PROTEIN METABOLISM

All living tissues, whether plant or animal, contain proteins. The fundamental difference between the protein metabolism of plants and that of animals is the ability of plants to synthesize proteins from the nitrogen and sulfur of the soil and from the carbon, oxygen and hydrogen of the air. Animals must ingest, break down, absorb and rearrange dietary proteins to form tissue proteins. The chemical process of digestion, which is essentially hydrolytic, is common to all heterotrophic organisms. Substances of high molecular weight—proteins, nucleic acids, and carbohydrates—are hydrolyzed to yield smaller molecules which are absorbed and assimilated.

Proteins constitute the most important group of foodstuffs. In addition to contributing to cells and intercellular materials, proteins and their constituent amino acids are of importance in the formation of hormones, enzymes, plasma proteins, antibodies and numerous other physiologically active substances.

Comparatively little is known of the processes by which digested protein is recombined to form body proteins. Build-up of body protein is particularly active during growth, late pregnancy and lactation. There is apparently a constant flux of tissue breakdown and tissue formation, producing a dynamic equilibrium.

Protein deficiency (marasmus) is usually associated with energy deficiency and occurs in many pathologic states besides simple starvation. Protein deficiency is common in prolonged febrile illness, in massive burns and large chronic ulcers, in "stress," hyperthyroidism and other hypermetabolic states, in conditions interfering with digestion and absorption and in metabolic diseases which interfere with utilization.

The clinical findings in protein deficiency include loss of weight and of subcutaneous fat, wasting of muscles, pigment changes in the skin with hair loss, hypotension, weakness and edema. Anemia is common. A decrease in serum proteins, hemoconcentration and a decrease in blood volume are other frequent findings.

In *kwashiorkor*, a combined protein-energy deficiency in children in many parts of the world, the oral lesions, when apparent, include a bright reddening of the tongue with a loss of papillae, bilateral angular cheilosis, fissuring of the lips and a loss of circumoral pigmentation. In addition, the mouths of kwashiorkor patients have been described by Van Wyk as being dry, dirty, caries-free and easily traumatized, with the epithelium readily becoming detached from the underlying tissues, leaving a raw, bleeding surface. In oral cytologic smears from his patients, he described a perinuclear vacuolization or halo around the nucleus in a remarkable number of the epithelial cells present and interpreted this as a sign of epithelial atrophy.

King has pointed out that about half of the world's population live in areas where the lack of milk, meat, poultry, fish, eggs, and so on, leads to early retardation of growth. Typically, children so retarded have edema, episodes of diarrhea, skin pigmentation, liver enlargement, alopecia, and poor resistance to infection, especially of the lungs and intestinal tract. The death rate may reach 25 times that considered normal for the age group. Those that survive show permanent physical stunting. This stunted condition is so general that it is often mistaken for a genetic phenomenon. In some areas 50 per cent of the children die before school age. It is significant that most of the children exhibit a normal growth rate up to weaning time.

Frandsen and his co-workers, Chawla and Glickman, Di Orio and co-workers, Navia, Aponte-Merced and Navia, Menaker and Navia and Navia and co-workers have studied the effects of protein and protein-energy deprivation on salivary glands and teeth and their supporting structures in experimental animals. Overall growth and growth of the jaws were decreased. Eruption was delayed, and incisor and molar growth was retarded. Radicular osteocementum was decreased. The enamel of affected incisors exhibited increased acid solubility. Increased dental caries was also reported. The gingiva and periodontal membranes exhibited varying degrees of degeneration. Salivary volume was decreased as were the DNA, RNA and protein concentrations of affected animals.

The severity of these changes was dependent on the degree of protein deprivation.

Protein Requirements. The accepted figure of 1 gm. of protein for each kilogram of body weight is designed to give a factor of safety to cover individual differences in requirement. Protein is required in increased quantity in the last half of pregnancy and during lactation and in even greater amounts in infancy, childhood and adolescence.

INDIVIDUAL AMINO ACIDS

The inadequacy of zein as a sole source of protein in rat nutrition brought out the importance of the variations in amino acid content of different proteins and led to the work of Rose and his collaborators and others on the essential and nonessential amino acids. The essential amino acids are histidine, isoleucine, leucine, lysine, methionine, phenylalanine, threonine, tryptophan and valine. This list of nine essential amino acids must not be accepted as final, however; more may have to be added, and some may eventually be dropped. The original concepts of "essential" and "nonessential" must be modified, since the determination of essentiality depends not only on the species studied, but also on the experimental criteria used (e.g., nitrogen balance, growth), the age of the animal used and the presence or absence of vitamins in the diet. For example, arginine is nonessen-

tial in the adult. However, infants are incapable of producing sufficient amounts of arginine for normal physiologic functions. Therefore arginine is considered essential in infants. It is unlikely, however, that a deficiency of a single essential amino acid occurs in humans.

AMYLOIDOSIS

Amyloid is a complex material with at least two distinct forms. Type A (secondary) amyloid is a fibrillar protein of unknown origin that is seen in prolonged inflammatory diseases, genetic diseases, and syndromes such as familial Mediterranean fever. Type B (primary) amyloid is thought to be of immune origin because of its sequence homology with the NH_2 terminal end of immunoglobulin light chains. Type B amyloid is commonly seen in patients with multiple myeloma and macroglobulinemia. Clinically asymptomatic patients found to have type B amyloid have serum and urine immunoglobulin abnormalities. A third type of amyloid (type C) includes amyloid of aging, localized nonspecific amyloid, and amyloid adjacent to APUD (*A*mine *P*recursor *U*ptake and *D*ecarboxylase) tumors, i.e., pheochromocytoma (Fig. 12–4). A review of the association of amyloid with a variety of diseases in man and animals has been published by Rigdon. The most common diseases predisposing to amyloidosis are the collagen diseases, particularly rheumatoid

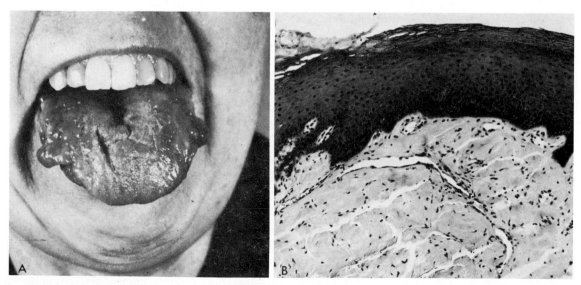

Figure 12–4. *Amyloidosis.*
Amyloid tumors of the tongue (*A*). The photomicrograph (*B*) illustrates a section through such a nodule. (Courtesy of Dr. Boynton H. Booth.)

arthritis, chronic infections such as tuberculosis and osteomyelitis, regional enteritis, ulcerative colitis, and certain malignant diseases, particularly multiple myeloma, Hodgkin's disease and renal cell carcinoma. Since modern surgery and medicine have largely eliminated chronic suppurative disease, rheumatoid arthritis and myeloma are now the chief predisposing causes for amyloidosis. Excellent reviews of amyloidosis were written by Franklin and by Kyle and Bayrd.

While any organ may be involved, those most commonly affected are the kidneys, heart, gastrointestinal tract, liver and spleen. Amyloidosis is also seen with considerable frequency in the respiratory tract, skin, eye, adrenals and nerves, and may involve bone. A primary localized cutaneous amyloidosis is also recognized. Amyloidosis itself is generally considered to be an irreversible disease.

Amyloid deposition in the tongue, resulting in macroglossia, and gingiva is also reported to be commonly seen. Because of the reported frequency of amyloid in gingival tissues, it has often been suggested that the gingival biopsy may be used conveniently for the diagnosis of amyloidosis. However, the results have been quite varied, some investigators reporting a high incidence of positive biopsies, while others have found so few positive results that the technique has been considered of little value. This subject has been reviewed by Lovett and his associates. Ulmansky, and Stanback and Peagler have discussed the oral manifestations of primary amyloidosis, and van der Waal and co-workers have reported on the significance of amyloidosis in oral surgery.

The amyloid in the microscopic sections of involved tissue appears as a hyaline, homogeneous material, often perivascular in distribution. It is best demonstrated by special stains such as Congo red and crystal violet or by the thioflavin-T fluorescent technique.

PORPHYRIA

Porphyria is a term which has been generally used to connote one of the inborn errors of porphyrin metabolism, characterized by overproduction of uroporphyrin and related substances. Not all cases of porphyria, however, represent a constitutional disturbance, since porphyria may appear as a sequel to some infections or intoxications. The classification of the porphyrias remains unsettled, although the newest and most basic classification defines two types: (1) Erythropoietic porphyria, characterized by early photosensitivity, splenomegaly, and excessive abnormal porphyrin formation in developing erythrocytes. Two subclasses, uroporphyria (congenital porphyria) and protoporphyria, have been described based on their respective porphyrin precursor type. (2) Hepatic porphyria, also a multisystem disorder, which has four subclasses; acute intermittent porphyria, porphyria variegata, porphyria cutanea tarda and hereditary coproporphyria. Heritable enzymatic effects have been identified in uroporphyria, acute intermittent porphyria and porphyria cutanea tarda. An excellent review of the porphyrias has been published by Elder and co-workers.

Erythropoietic Uroporphyria (Congenital Porphyria). This disease, the most important of the group, is transmitted as a nonsex-linked recessive character, both sexes being equally affected. The first sign of erythropoietic porphyria is usually the excretion of red urine containing much uroporphyrin. This may be noted at birth or only during the first years of life. Photosensitivity is frequently absent in the neonatal period, but may become apparent during the first years of life as exposure to sunlight increases. A vesicular or bullous eruption appears on the face, back of the hands and other exposed parts of the body (Fig. 12–5). The vesicles contain a serous fluid which usually exhibits red fluorescence. Ruptured vesicles heal slowly and leave depressed, pigmented scars. Occasionally the cutaneous manifestations may be relatively mild, resulting in little scarring. There is an interesting oral finding. The deciduous and permanent teeth may show a red or brownish discoloration, although this is not invariably present. Under ultraviolet light, however, the teeth always exhibit red fluorescence. Deposition of porphyrin in the developing teeth and bones is believed to be due to its physical affinity for calcium phosphate. The presence of porphyrin in the deciduous teeth indicates that the metabolic disorder may have been present during fetal life.

DISTURBANCES IN CARBOHYDRATE METABOLISM

Almost nothing is known of the effects of carbohydrate-deficient diets on the oral structures. Since carbohydrates form such a large

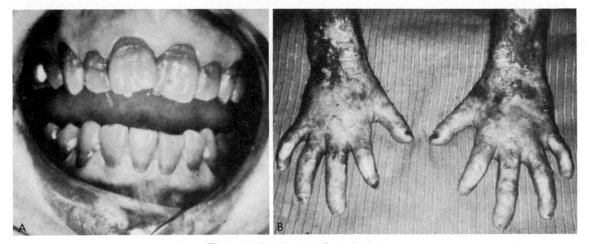

Figure 12–5. *Congenital porphyria.*
The intrinsic brown pigmentation of the teeth is seen in A, while the active skin lesions as well as scarring are shown in B. (Courtesy of Dr. Sidney B. Finn.)

part of our diet, however, and since they are of great importance to general health, they will be considered briefly here.

About half of the average American diet is made up of carbohydrates. The proportion of carbohydrates in the diet is even higher in many countries where proteinaceous foods and fats are expensive and not readily available. There are no requirements for carbohydrates in the sense implied by the phrase "essential amino acid requirements," because carbohydrates may be derived from noncarbohydrate sources. The digestion products of fats, proteins and carbohydrates follow metabolic pathways, some of which lead to "metabolic pools" where the molecules lose their identity as to original source. Here many of the organic moieties undergo a random distribution as they leave the pool for redistribution and recombination for storage or fuel.

MUCOPOLYSACCHARIDOSES

Among the more important carbohydrates in the body are the mucopolysaccharides, hexosamine-containing polysaccharides which are components of connective tissue ground substance and also of epithelial mucins. In the connective tissue, the acid mucopolysaccharides are most important because of their many functions, including their capacity for binding cations and basic groups in an ion-exchange type of reaction. In addition, they may be important in detoxification mechanisms and may function

in the distribution of water and electrolytes between the cells and circulating fluids.

There is an important group of diseases which represent a primary genetically determined disturbance of mucopolysaccharide metabolism. These are collectively known as the mucopolysaccharidoses, and they have been discussed in detail by McKusick and his associates and by Neufeld and Fratantoni. The specific diseases constituting this group are shown in Table 12–1 with certain of their clinical, genetic and biochemical features. The Hurler syndrome is the prototype of this group and is probably the most common component. For this reason, and because of the chemical similarities of the other mucopolysaccharidoses to it, only the Hurler syndrome will be discussed here. The dental manifestations of a number of the mucopolysaccharidoses have been described in the literature, including studies by Gardner, Galili and co-workers and Webman and associates.

Hurler Syndrome

(Mucopolysaccharidosis I: MPS IH; Gargoylism)

Hurler syndrome is a disturbance of mucopolysaccharide metabolism exhibiting a variety of classic clinical features. It is characterized by an elevated mucopolysaccharide excretion level in the urine. The disease, in which there is an excessive intracellular accumulation of both chondroitin sulfate B and heparitin sulfate in those tissues and organs where they are normally found, is inherited as an autosomal recessive trait.

Table 12–1. The Genetic Mucopolysaccharidoses*

	DESIGNATION	CLINICAL FEATURES	GENETICS	EXCESSIVE URINARY MPS	SUBSTANCE DEFICIENT
MPS I H	Hurler syndrome	Early clouding of cornea, grave manifestations, death usually before age 10	Homozygous for MPS I H gene	Dermatan sulfate Heparan sulfate	α-L-iduronidase (formerly called Hurler corrective factor)
MPS I S	Scheie syndrome	Stiff joints, cloudy cornea, aortic regurgitation, normal intelligence, ?normal life-span	Homozygosity for MPS I S gene	Dermatan sulfate Heparan sulfate	α-L-iduronidase
MPS I H/S	Hurler-Scheie compound	Phenotype intermediate between Hurler and Scheie	Genetic compound of MPS I H and I S genes	Dermatan sulfate Heparan sulfate	α-L-iduronidase
MPS II A	Hunter syndrome, severe	No clouding of cornea, milder course than in MPS I H but death usually before age 15 years	Hemizygous for X-linked gene	Dermatan sulfate Heparan sulfate	Hunter corrective factor
MPS II B	Hunter syndrome, mild	Survival to 30's to 50's, fair intelligence	Hemizygous for X-linked allele for mild form	Dermatan sulfate Heparan sulfate	Hunter corrective factor
MPS III A	Sanfilippo syndrome A	Identical phenotype:	Homozygous for Sanfilippo A gene	Heparan sulfate	Heparan sulfate sulfatase
MPS III B	Sanfilippo syndrome B	Mild somatic, severe central nervous system effects	Homozygous for Sanfilippo B (at different locus)	Heparan sulfate	N-acetyl-α-D-glucosaminidase
MPS IV	Morquio syndrome (probably more than one allelic form)	Severe bone changes of distinctive type, cloudy cornea, aortic regurgitation	Homozygous for Morquio gene	Keratan sulfate	Unknown
MPS V	Vacant				
MPS VI A	Maroteaux-Lamy syndrome, classic form	Severe osseous and corneal change, normal intellect	Homozygous for M-L gene	Dermatan sulfate	Maroteaux-Lamy corrective factor
MPS VI B	Maroteaux-Lamy syndrome, mild form	Severe osseous and corneal change, normal intellect	Homozygous for allele at M-L locus	Dermatan sulfate	Maroteaux-Lamy corrective factor
MPS VII	β-glucuronidase deficiency (more than one allelic form?)	Hepatosplenomegaly, dysostosis multiplex, white cell inclusions, mental retardation	Homozygous for mutant gene at beta-glucuronidase locus	Dermatan sulfate	β-glucuronidase

*By permission of Dr. Victor A. McKusick. From McKusick, V. A.: Heritable Disorders of Connective Tissue. 4th ed. St. Louis, C. V. Mosby Co, 1972.

Clinical Features. The disease usually becomes apparent within the first two years of life, progresses during early childhood and adolescence and terminates in death usually before puberty. The head appears large and the facial characteristics are quite typical, consisting of a prominent forehead, broad saddle nose and wide nostrils, hypertelorism, puffy eyelids with coarse bushy eyebrows, thick lips, large tongue, open mouth and nasal congestion with noisy breathing. Progressive corneal clouding is a classic manifestation of the disease as is hepatosplenomegaly, resulting in a protuberant abdomen. A short neck and spinal abnormalities are typical, while flexion contractures result in the "claw hand." These dwarfed individuals are mentally retarded.

Oral Manifestations. The oral manifestations of the Hurler syndrome have been reviewed by Gardner. These consist of a shortening and broadening of the mandible with prominent gonions, a wide intergonial distance and a greater than normal distance around the arch from ramus to ramus accounting, at least in part, for the typical spacing of the teeth. Localized areas of bone destruction in the jaws may be found which appear to represent hyperplastic dental follicles with large pools of metachromatic material, probably mucopolysaccharide. The teeth themselves are frequently described as being small, widely spaced and misshapen. However, many investigators have been unable to demonstrate abnormalities of the teeth, except for some delay in the time of eruption.

Gingival hyperplasia has been repeatedly described in patients with Hurler syndrome, although it is not a constant feature of the disease. In some patients the gingiva appears normal, while in others the gingiva appears enlarged as a result of local factors such as poor oral hygiene or mouth breathing. In occasional patients, the gingival tissues appear to be involved in a manner similar to fibromatosis gingivae. Finally, the tongue is also characteristically enlarged.

Histologic Features. There is excessive accumulation of intracellular mucopolysaccharide in many tissues and organs throughout the body including the liver, spleen, reticuloendothelial system, nervous system, cartilage, bone, and heart. Abnormal deposits are also found in many sites, with involved fibroblasts assuming the appearance of "clear" or "gargoyle" cells.

Gardner has reported the demonstration of these "Hurler cells" or "gargoyle cells" in the gingival tissues of affected patients. The Hurler cells are relatively large, with metachromatically staining cytoplasm which is either agranular or finely granular, often with crescent-shaped nuclei. These cells are not identified with hematoxylin and eosin but become evident with toluidine blue or with Alcian blue/aldehyde fuchsin stains. Some difficulty may be encountered in differentiating these from mast cells.

Laboratory Findings. There is an elevated level of mucopolysaccharides in the urine. In addition, metachromatic granules or Reilly bodies can often be demonstrated in the cytoplasm of circulating lymphocytes.

Treatment. There is no treatment for the disease.

Lipoid Proteinosis

(Hyalinosis Cutis et Mucosae)

Lipoid proteinosis is a disease thought to represent either a disturbance in mucopolysaccharide metabolism, possibly being related to the mucopolysaccharidoses, or an alteration involving lipoprotein material. It is transmitted as an autosomal recessive characteristic.

Clinical Features. These patients develop solitary or clustered yellowish-white, waxy nodules, varying in size from a millimeter to 0.5 cm. in diameter, on the skin of the face, neck, hands, axillae, scrotum, perineal areas and intergluteal cleft. Similar lesions occur on the margins of the eyelids as well as keratotic, verrucous clusters of papules on the elbows and knees. In addition, there is often intracranial calcification above the pituitary fossa in the hippocampus, falx cerebri or temporal lobes.

One of the characteristic features of the disease is the inability of infants to cry at birth and the hoarseness of the voice also present from birth, all a result of similar yellowish-white plaques in the epiglottis, aryepiglottic folds and interarytenoid region. On laryngoscopic examination, the cords are seen to be thickened and nodular. On rare occasion, dyspnea may be so severe as to necessitate stripping the nodules from the cords or laryngectomy.

Oral Manifestations. The oral cavity is usually severely affected in this disease with much of the oral mucous membrane developing the characteristic yellowish-white papular plaques which become increasingly more prevalent and prominent from childhood into adult life. The lips become thickened and nodular while the

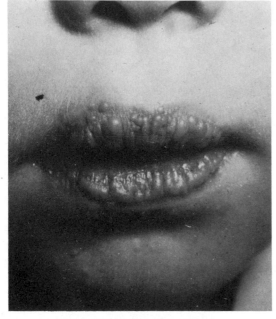

Figure 12–6. *Lipoid proteinosis.*
(Courtesy of Dr. Robert J. Gorlin.)

tongue becomes thickened, enlarged, very firm to palpation and sometimes bound to the floor of the mouth (Fig. 12–6). Recurrent painful parotitis may occur as a result of involvement of the buccal mucosa, with stenosis of the parotid duct opening. Congenital absence of teeth and severe enamel hypoplasia have also been reported. The oral manifestations of the disease have been discussed by Gorlin, Williams, and Hofer and Bergenholtz.

Histologic Features. The plaques microscopically exhibit hyalinosis of the connective tissue beginning around the subepithelial capillaries. This hyalin material stains intensely with the periodic acid–Schiff stain.

Treatment. There is no treatment for the disease.

HEREDITARY FRUCTOSE INTOLERANCE

Over 25 years ago Chambers and Pratt reported an unusual case of a young woman who repeatedly became nauseated and vomited after the ingestion of fruit or cane sugar. Numerous reports have since appeared in the literature, and over two dozen families have been diagnosed as having hereditary fructose intolerance.

Clinical Features. The disease is transmitted as an autosomal recessive trait and is manifested by hypoglycemia and vomiting after the inges-

tion of fructose-containing foods. It results from a deficiency in fructose 1-phosphate aldolase. Affected individuals rapidly acquire an intense aversion to all sweets and fruits.

Oral Manifestations. Newbrun and co-workers recently reported on the dietary habits and dental health of 17 affected individuals. Subjects with hereditary fructose intolerance had a total sucrose intake of less than 5 per cent of that of controls. Caries scores (DMFS) were less than 10 per cent of those of controls. This study confirms the previous observations of Cornblath and co-workers, Levin and colleagues and Marthaler and Froesch.

DISTURBANCES IN LIPID METABOLISM

Lipid metabolism is concerned with the assimilation, utilization, replacement and synthesis of the various fatty acids of the cell. All living cells contain fatty acids, largely in the form of esters with glycerol, cholesterol or other alcohols, or combined with phosphoric acids, nitrogenous bases or carbohydrates.

There seems to be some evidence of the existence of "essential fatty acids." Hansen studied a group of children with eczema and found a significant lowering of the iodine number of their serum fatty acids. Their skin lesions improved when large doses of high-iodine-number oils were administered.

Disturbances of lipid metabolism are rare, but they do occur. These disturbances have been classified as "lipoid storage diseases," xanthomatoses, lipid granulomas, and so on. Several disease entities have been identified on the basis of the particular lipid involved. Letterer-Siwe disease, Hand-Schüller-Christian disease, and eosinophilic granuloma have historically been classified as nonlipid reticuloendothelioses or histiocytosis X. Letterer-Siwe disease is currently considered to be a lymphomatous proliferation of poorly differentiated histiocytes, whereas Hand-Schüller-Christian disease and eosinophilic granuloma are thought to be non-neoplastic reactions of well-differentiated histiocytes to an unknown stimulus. The only distinction between the two is that eosinophilic granuloma is a solitary or unifocal lesion.

The lipid reticuloendothelioses include a variety of lipid storage diseases classified on the basis of the specific lysosomal enzymes and the lipid substrate accumulated by the cell. Two of these diseases, Gaucher's disease and Niemann-Pick disease, are of particular importance in dentistry and will be discussed in detail.

NONLIPID RETICULOENDOTHELIOSES

(Histiocytosis X Disease)

Hand-Schüller-Christian disease, Letterer-Siwe disease, and eosinophilic granuloma of bone have traditionally been grouped under the generic term histiocytosis X. It should be noted, however, that a number of investigators, including Liebermann and colleagues, Cline and co-workers and Otani, have presented data that Letterer-Siwe disease is not a severe fulminant form of Hand-Schüller-Christian disease but a separate nosologic entity. However, other recent reports in the literature, most recently that of Rapidis and co-workers, contest these findings. Other published reviews include those by Avioli and co-workers, Enriquez and associates, Lucaya, Cheyne, and Daneshbod and Kissane. Excellent articles on the head and neck manifestations of histiocytosis X have been published by Lovestedt, Chase and his co-workers and Hartman.

The etiology and pathogenesis of the diseases remain elusive; however, the fact that they stem from a proliferative reticuloendothelial disturbance rather than an enzymatic deficiency involving lipid catabolism necessitates their separation from the true lipid storage diseases (lipid reticuloendotheliosis).

Hand-Schüller-Christian Disease

(Multifocal Eosinophilic Granuloma)

Hand-Schüller-Christian disease is characterized by widespread skeletal and extraskeletal lesions and a chronic clinical course. It occurs primarily in early life, usually before the age of five, but it has been reported in adolescents and even in young adults. It is more common in boys than in girls, with a sex ratio of approximately two to one.

Hand-Schüller-Christian disease has certain features in common with Letterer-Siwe disease and eosinophilic granuloma, and some features which serve to distinguish it from the others. In all three diseases the proliferative cell is the histiocyte. In Hand-Schüller-Christian disease both the skeletal system and soft tissues may be involved, while in eosinophilic granuloma, only the bone is affected, although soft-tissue extension is often observed. Letterer-Siwe disease is an acute, fulminating disease with widespread lesions of both skeletal and extraskeletal tissues, including the skin.

Clinical Features. Hand-Schüller-Christian disease is characterized by the classic triad of single or multiple areas of "punched-out" bone destruction in the skull, unilateral or bilateral exophthalmos, and diabetes insipidus with or without other manifestations of dyspituitarism such as polyuria, dwarfism or infantilism. The complete triad occurs in only about 25 per cent of affected patients. Involvement of the facial bones, which is frequently associated with soft-tissue swelling and tenderness, causes facial asymmetry. Otitis media is also common. Other bones are frequently involved, particularly the femur, ribs, vertebrae, pelvis, humerus and scapula. Any of the visceral organs also may be involved, and the skin sometimes exhibits papular or nodular lesions, as discussed by Winkelmann.

Oral Manifestations. Oral manifestations may be one of the earliest signs of the presence of the disease. In reported series, the frequency of oral involvement varies widely, ranging from 5 per cent to over 75 per cent of patients.

These oral manifestations are often nonspecific and include sore mouth, with or without ulcerative lesions; halitosis, gingivitis and suppuration; an unpleasant taste; loose and sore teeth with precocious exfoliation of teeth; and failure of healing of tooth sockets following extraction (Fig. 12–7). Loss of supporting alveolar bone mimicking advanced periodontal disease is characteristic, and this finding in a child should always be viewed with suspicion. The oral findings have been discussed by Sedano and his associates and by Jones and his co-workers.

Roentgenographic Features. The individual lesions, particularly in the skull, are usually sharply outlined, although the lesions in the jaws may be more diffuse. The lesions in the jaws are usually manifested simply as destruction of alveolar bone with tooth displacement (Fig. 12–7).

Histologic Features. Hand-Schüller-Christian disease is usually considered as manifesting four stages during the progression of the characteristic lesion. These are (1) a proliferative histiocytic phase with accumulation of collections of eosinophilic leukocytes scattered throughout the sheets of histiocytes; (2) a vascular-granulomatous phase with persistence of histiocytes and eosinophils, sometimes with aggregation of lipid-laden (cholesterol) macrophages; (3) a diffuse xanthomatous phase with abundance of these "foam cells"; and (4) a fibrous or healing phase (Fig. 12–7).

Laboratory Features. Anemia and, less frequently, leukopenia and thrombocytopenia are occasionally found. The serum cholesterol level

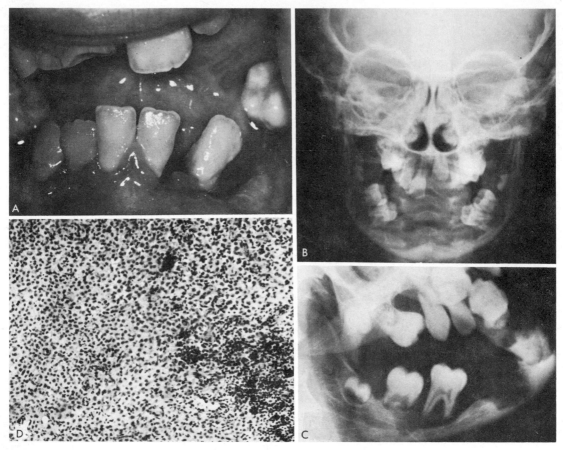

Figure 12–7. Hand-Schüller-Christian disease.
Clinically (A) the teeth are loose and have migrated. The gingiva is red, tender, swollen and hyperplastic. The roentgenograms (B, C) show lesions in the maxilla and mandible with severe loss of supporting bone. The microscopic appearance (D) is characteristic, showing sheets of proliferating histiocytes.

is nearly always normal, although the tissue cholesterol content may be elevated remarkably.

Treatment and Prognosis. The prognosis in Hand-Schüller-Christian disease is good. Approximately half of the patients undergo spontaneous remission over a period of years. The treatment of choice is curettage or excision of lesions. Inaccessible lesions may be irradiated. Some patients benefit from chemotherapeutic drugs, including prednisone, vinblastine and cyclophosphamide. One of the most significant factors influencing the morbidity and mortality of the disease is the extent of the disease at the time of initial diagnosis and the number of organ systems involved.

Eosinophilic Granuloma

(Unifocal Eosinophilic Granuloma)

The term "eosinophilic granuloma of bone" was introduced by Lichtenstein and Jaffe in

1940, although the lesion to which it referred had been described by others before them. The term is used to describe a lesion of bone which is primarily a histiocytic proliferation, with an abundance of eosinophilic leukocytes but no intracellular lipid accumulation. This disease occurs primarily in older children and young adults, and the proportion of males to females is about two to one.

Clinical Features. Clinically, the lesion may present no physical signs or symptoms and may be found only upon an incidental roentgenographic examination of the bones of the head or other areas. On the other hand, there may be local pain, swelling and tenderness. The lesion may occur in the jaw and overlying soft tissues of the mouth, so that the differential diagnosis between eosinophilic granuloma and some form of dental disease becomes imperative. Although the skull and mandible are common sites of involvement, the femur, humerus, ribs, and other bones may also be affected. General malaise and fever occasionally accom-

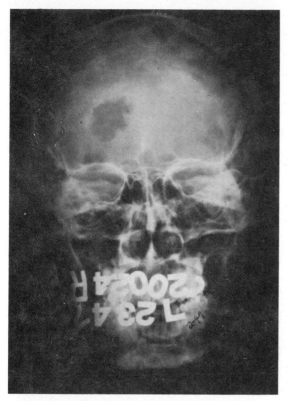

Figure 12–8. *Eosinophilic granuloma.*
The roentgenogram shows the typical irregular radiolucent areas of the skull. (Courtesy of Dr. M. Pleasure, Bronx Veterans Administration Hospital.)

pany the eosinophilic granuloma of bone. The lesions are destructive and are well demarcated, roughly round or oval in shape. The area destroyed is replaced by a soft tissue, the composition of which varies, depending upon the stage at which the lesion is examined. The tissue of the early lesion is soft and brown and, since there is no necrosis, is not friable. Later the lesion becomes fibrous and grayish.

Roentgenographic Features. The lesions appear as irregular radiolucent areas usually involving superficial alveolar bone (Fig. 12–8). The cortex is often destroyed, and pathologic fractures may occur. If the lesions are in the jaw, they usually appear as single or multiple areas of rarefaction which may be so well circumscribed as to resemble cysts of the jaw, periapical granulomas or even periodontal disease (Fig. 12–9).

Histologic Features. Microscopically (Fig. 12–10), the primary cell is the histiocyte, which grows in sheets or sheetlike collections. The histiocytes may coalesce and form multinucleated giant cells, but this is quite uncommon. The early lesions also contain large numbers of focal collections of eosinophils. When the lesion matures, fibrosis occurs. In these older lesions the eosinophils become less numerous, and they may even disappear so that the lesion approximates the histologic picture of Hand-Schüller-Christian disease.

Treatment and Prognosis. The prognosis in the majority of cases is excellent, since curettage and/or x-ray therapy are curative, symptoms usually subsiding within two weeks after treatment.

Letterer-Siwe Disease

Letterer-Siwe disease is an acute, often fulminating histiocytic disorder which invariably occurs in infants, usually before the age of three years.

Clinical Features. The initial manifestation of this disease is often a skin rash involving the trunk, scalp and extremities. This rash may be erythematous, purpuric or ecchymotic, sometimes with ulceration. The patients will also commonly have a persistent, low-grade spiking fever with malaise and irritability. Splenomegaly, hepatomegaly, and lymphadenopathy are early manifestations as well as nodular or diffuse involvement of visceral organs, particularly the lungs and gastrointestinal tract, later in the course of the disease. Diffuse involvement of the skeletal system also usually occurs later in the disease.

Oral Manifestations. The oral lesions may consist of ulcerative lesions, although gingival hyperplasia has also been described. Furthermore, diffuse destruction of bone of the maxilla and mandible may occur, causing loosening and premature loss of teeth. In some cases the disease has such a rapid course that significant oral involvement does not occur.

Histologic Features. The microscopic appearance of the lesions is very similar to that seen in Hand-Schüller-Christian disease where there is basically a histiocytic proliferation with or without eosinophils. However, these histiocytes do not contain significant amounts of cholesterol so that foam cells are not a feature of the disease, nor is fibrosis encountered. In some cases cytologically altered histiocytes are present in sufficient numbers to resemble a histiocytic lymphoma.

Laboratory Features. Progressive anemia is often present as well as leukopenia or thrombocytopenia.

Treatment and Prognosis. The prognosis in Letterer-Siwe disease is extremely poor. In the majority of cases, the course of the disease is rapid and terminates fatally in a short time.

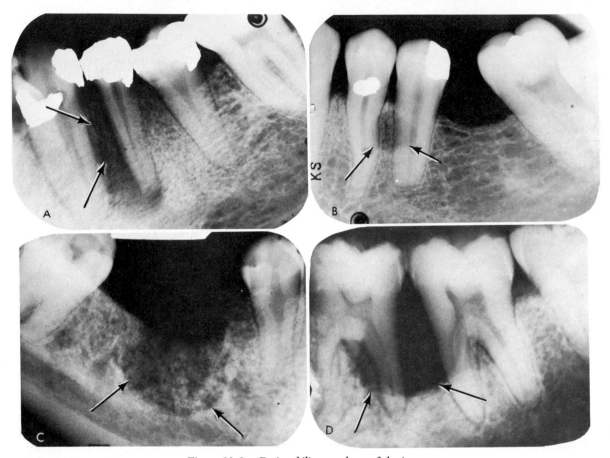

Figure 12–9.   *Eosinophilic granuloma of the jaws.*
These four cases exemplify the variable roentgenographic appearance of the disease in the jaws. (*D*, Courtesy of Dr. Charles A. Waldron.)

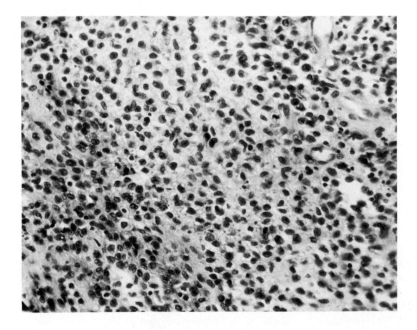

Figure 12–10.   *Eosinophilic granuloma.*
The photomicrograph shows sheets of histiocytes and many eosinophils.

However, some patients show response to chemotherapy and are sometimes maintained in
remission for years.

LIPID RETICULOENDOTHELIOSES

Disturbances in sphingomyelin and glucosyl
ceramide metabolism are characteristic of
Gaucher's disease and Niemann-Pick disease,
respectively. Both are inborn errors of lipid
metabolism and are inherited in an autosomal
recessive pattern. Although each disease is pan-
ethnic, both are much more common in Jews
of Ashkenazic origin. The gene frequency
among Ashkenazic Jews ranges from an estimated 1:100 in Niemann-Pick disease to 1:20 in
Gaucher's disease.

There are a variety of other inborn errors of
lipid metabolism that occur, including Tay-
Sachs disease (amaurotic familial idiocy), Fa-
bry's disease (angiokeratoma corporis diffusum
universale), generalized gangliosidosis, and
metachromatic leukodystrophy. It is of interest
that biopsy of the dental pulp has been reported
by Gardner and Zeman to be reliable in establishing a positive diagnosis of metachromatic
leukodystrophy and has been considered by
them to be the simplest method for the pro-
curement of tissue. These latter sphingolipidoses have been discussed by Knudson and by
Brady but, because of their general lack of oral
involvement or significant oral manifestations,
will not be discussed here.

Gaucher's Disease

Gaucher's disease is an autosomal recessive
defect of lipid metabolism in which kerasin is
deposited throughout the entire reticuloendothelial system as a result of a deficiency in
glucocerebrosidase, an enzyme necessary for
the degradation of the glucocerebroside. This
disease is the most common sphingolipid storage disease, with an incidence of one in every
2500 births in Ashkenazic Jews. The lipid-filled
histiocytes are known as "Gaucher's cells" and
are pathognomonic of this disease. These cells
are commonly seen in the spleen, lymph nodes,
liver and bone marrow.

Clinical Features. Gaucher's disease has
been divided into three clinical forms (types I,
II, and III). Type I (chronic non-neuronopathic)
is the most common and by definition has no
cerebral involvement. While the disease may
be apparent in infancy, most individuals remain
asymptomatic until adolescence, when they
present with hepatosplenomegaly. Osteolytic
disease ensues along with pulmonary dysfunction. Pneumonia is frequently the cause of
death. Type II (acute neuronopathic) is characterized by hepatosplenomegaly and developmental central nervous system disorders. The
signs and symptoms are apparent within the
first few months after birth, and the average
survival time is about nine months. The principal cause of death is anoxia and infection
secondary to pulmonary involvement. Type III
(subacute neuronopathic) resembles type II but
has a later onset and a more protracted clinical
course. In all three types of Gaucher's disease
sternal puncture or examination of the biopsies
of the spleen or liver will reveal the typical
Gaucher's cell. This is a round pale cell, measuring between 20 and 80 microns in diameter,
containing a small eccentric nucleus and a wrinkled or "crumpled silk" cytoplasm.

When bone is involved, the bone marrow
shows diffuse changes. Numerous large, foamy,
slightly granular cells with small, round pyknotic nuclei, which are the Gaucher's cells,
group together and replace the normal marrow
structure. These skeletal manifestations have
been discussed by Amstutz and Carey. Gaucher's cell accumulations are also found in the
spleen, the lymph nodes and the liver. An
excellent review of both the infantile and adult
forms of Gaucher's disease was published by
Levin.

Treatment and Prognosis. The prognosis of
the malignant infantile form is very poor, the
disease resulting in death usually within the
first year. The less virulent form may persist
until the sixth decade of life, when the patients
usually die of some intercurrent infection.

Brady and co-workers have reported that the
administration of purified glucocerebrosidase to
affected patients results in a dramatic decrease
in hepatic accumulations of glucocerebroside.
Although this therapeutic regime is experimental and fraught with potential side effects, it
nevertheless holds promise for future treatment
of the disease.

Niemann-Pick Disease

Niemann-Pick disease is the least common of
the genetic disturbances of lipid metabolism. It
is inherited as an autosomal recessive trait. In
this disease there is an abnormal storage of
phospholipids, mostly sphingomyelin, due to a
lack of sphingomyelinase. Currently the disease

is divided into five clinical types based on onset, central nervous system involvement, and variations in ancestry and enzyme activity. Like Gaucher's disease, it is more common in Ashkenazic Jews and has a pathognomonic cell, the Niemann-Pick cell. Niemann-Pick cells are foamy, lipid-laden cells distributed throughout the reticuloendothelial system. Unlike Gaucher cells, they are positive for cholesterol and only weakly positive for alkaline phosphatase. They are most easily distinguished from Gaucher cells by phase or electron microscopy. Epstein and co-workers have developed a procedure for detecting Niemann-Pick disease in utero by measuring sphingomyelinase activity in cultured amniotic cells. The clinical findings in this disease have been discussed by Gildenhorn and Amromin as well as by Knudson.

Enzyme replacement therapy in Niemann-Pick disease is currently being explored. Current treatment is symptomatic and consists mainly of antibiotic therapy for infections resulting from pulmonary involvement. Organ transplantation, e.g., the liver, has been proposed. To date the prognosis is poor, and the vast majority of patients die of the disease.

THE AVITAMINOSES

A vitamin is usually defined as an organic substance not made by the body, which is soluble in either fat or water and ordinarily is needed in only minute quantities to act as a cofactor in a variety of metabolic reactions. The word "vitamin" has reference to the fact that the substance it designates is essential to life. The term, therefore, is functional and not chemically descriptive.

It is useful to consider the vitamins together, for they share certain features. They are present and active in amounts that are minute in contrast to the considerable quantities of the ordinary nutrients. They differ from other nutrients in that many of them are inactivated by heat and oxidation. Some of the vitamins occur in natural sources in a physiologically inactive form. These are called provitamins. They become active only after conversion within the animal. For example, vitamin A exists in plants as carotene, which is activated in the liver. As will be seen with vitamin D and to a certain extent with vitamin A, recent evidence points to a hormonal rather than a coenzyme role for certain vitamins. Because of historical convention and the lack of conclusive evidence that

vitamins have a hormonal activity, these compounds will be discussed with the remainder of the vitamins.

Although the avitaminoses are an assorted group of diseases, and as unrelated to each other as the chemical constituents of the various vitamins, they too share enough common characteristics to justify their inclusion as a single group of diseases. The avitaminoses are due to the *absence* of minute amounts of biologically important materials rather than to the *presence* of minute amounts of biologically active materials (infectious agents). They cause disease not in a positive but in a negative way. The deficiency is the disease. Another characteristic of the deficiency diseases is that they may be present in varying degrees. There may be latent infection, but not a partial infection. A malignant growth is present or it is not. Deficiency diseases, however, may occur in partial form; i.e., they may occur to a mild degree, and in their incipient forms the lesions and symptoms might be difficult to recognize. They may also occur in more severe forms, but they are seldom so serious as to be the immediate cause of death.

THE FAT-SOLUBLE VITAMINS

Vitamin A

The therapeutic usefulness of vitamin A has been known since the time of the Egyptian pharaohs. The Ebers papyrus (circa 1500 B.C.) recommends liver as a cure for night blindness. However, the isolation, synthesis and recognition of the metabolic functions of vitamin A were not discovered until the twentieth century. The classic works of McCollum and Davis, Drummond, and Steenbock and co-workers provided a foundation upon which more recent vitamin A research is based. An excellent treatise on vitamin A was published by Moore in 1957.

The best known and most intensively studied role for vitamin A is that in vision. George Wald was awarded the Nobel Prize for medicine in 1967 for his discovery of the role of vitamin A in vision, and he has published an excellent review of the subject. Briefly, rhodopsin (visual purple) is formed by the union of vitamin A (11-*cis* retinal) and a protein, opsin, in the rods of the retina. When stimulated by light, the 11-*cis* retinal is isomerized to the all-*trans* retinal form and split from the protein moiety. The electrical potential generated during this process is transmitted to the brain via the optic nerve, resulting in visual sensation. In the dark, the all-*trans* form is enzymatically isomerized back to the 11-*cis* form and subsequently binds to opsin, thus completing the cycle. A continuous supply of vitamin A is therefore necessary for rod (low-light) vision, and the first manifestation of vitamin A deficiency is an impaired, low-light vision, i.e., night blindness.

Current research indicates that in addition to its role in vision and lysosomal stability, vitamin A may have a hormonal function in the regulation of epithelial differentiation. Intracellular receptors have been identified and may transport vitamin A molecules to the cell nucleus, where they interact with DNA to direct cellular differentiation.

The classic work of Wolbach and Howe on the dental changes in vitamin A deficiency of the rat and guinea pig was confirmed and elaborated by Schour and his co-workers. Excellent reviews have been written by Frandsen and Jolly. Most of our knowledge of the dental effects of vitamin A deficiency is based on findings in the continuously developing and erupting incisor tooth of the rat.

It is well established that vitamin A is concerned primarily with the process of differentiation of epithelial cells. In vitamin A deficiency the epithelial cells fail to differentiate. This means that the cells in the basal layer lose their specificity and tend to form a stratified squa-

mous epithelium with keratin production, independent of the type of cell previously formed by the basal cells. Thus one of the basic changes is a keratinizing metaplasia of epithelial cells. This occurs throughout the body, including the mucous membranes of the trachea, conjunctiva, and ureter, and the salivary and other glands (Fig. 12–11).

In the developing tooth of the rat that is deficient in vitamin A, the odontogenic epithelium fails to undergo normal histodifferentiation and morphodifferentiation, and the result is an increased rate of cell proliferation. Therefore epithelial invasion of pulpal tissue is characteristic in vitamin A deficiency.

In young rats whose mothers are maintained on a diet deficient in vitamin A for five months preceding their birth, changes are more severe, resulting in a distortion of the shape of both the incisors and the molars. Since the enamel-forming cells are disturbed, enamel matrix is arrested and/or poorly defined so that calcification is disturbed and enamel hypoplasia results. The dentin, too, is atypical in structure, lacking the normal tubular arrangement and containing cellular and vascular inclusions. Harris and Navia recently reported an increase in caries susceptibility of the rat molars of pups nursed by vitamin A-deficient dams, indicating a pre-eruptive role for vitamin A in tooth development. Posteruptive vitamin A deficiency has been reported to result in higher caries scores. However, Salley and co-workers posited that this

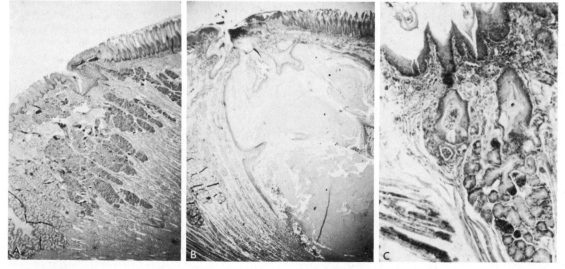

Figure 12–11. *Vitamin A deficiency.*
Photomicrographs of the tongue of a normal rat (*A*) and of vitamin A-deficient rats (*B, C*). There is squamous metaplasia in the mucous glands of the tongue and a large cyst filled with keratinaceous material (*B*).

increase in caries may be due to changes in salivary gland function rather than to dental changes per se.

The teeth of animals on a vitamin A deficient diet contain less total ash than the teeth of normal animals. Eruption rate is retarded, and in prolonged deficiencies eruption ceases completely. The alveolar bone is retarded in its rate of formation. The gingival epithelium becomes hyperplastic and in prolonged deficiencies shows keratinization. This tissue is easily invaded by bacteria that may cause periodontal disease and microabscess formation. The major and minor salivary glands undergo the typical keratinizing metaplasia. This is characteristic, of course, of all the epithelial cells in vitamin A deficiency. Most of the changes described are reversible with the feeding of vitamin A to deficient animals.

REQUIREMENTS. The recommended daily dietary allowance for vitamin A ranges from 420 mcg. to 800 to 1000 mcg. of retinol equivalents (R.E.) for adolescent and adult females and males. (1 R.E. = 1 mcg. retinal or 6 mcg. β-carotene.) Pregnant and lactating females should increase their daily intake by 200 and 400 mcg. R.E., respectively.

Clinical Features of Vitamin A Deficiency. The prominent manifestations of vitamin A deficiency in man are night blindness, xerophthalmia and keratomalacia. Hyperkeratotic changes in the oral epithelium of adults have also been noted. Follicular keratotic changes have been described in naturally occurring vitamin A deficiency by Frazier and Hu and by Sweet and K'ang. Hume and Krebs, and Steffens and co-workers studied controlled vitamin A deficiency in humans and were able to produce cutaneous manifestations in only one patient.

In the human infant, keratinizing metaplasia appears in the trachea and bronchi, kidney, pelvis, conjunctiva, cornea, salivary glands and genitourinary tract. Documented autopsy studies have been published by Wilson and DuBois and by Blackfan and Wolbach. If vitamin A deficiency were to cause changes in the human tooth bud, the deficiency state would have to occur before the sixth year of life, since by that time the crowns of all the teeth except the third molars are completely formed. The only cases of changes in human tooth buds attributable to vitamin A deficiency are those described by Boyle and by Dinnerman. Their findings were similar to those described in the rat incisor tooth in vitamin A deficiency. An excellent

symposium on vitamin A deficiency and its clinical implications may be found in the Federation Proceedings for 1958.

Hypervitaminosis A. Cases of hypervitaminosis A in children are reported with increasing frequency. The syndrome in children is characterized by anorexia, low-grade fever, hepatomegaly, sparse hair and increased vitamin A serum levels. Roentgenograms of the long bones show fragmentation of the distal fibular epiphyses and pronounced periosteal thickening. A case of adult hypervitaminosis A has been reported by Furman.

Vitamin D

Vitamin D (1,25-dihydroxycholecalciferol) is one of a number of compounds that are grouped together as the hydroxylated cholecalciferols. Vitamin D is commonly referred to as the antirachitic vitamin, although a variety of biochemical analogs have similar activity, e.g., vitamin D_2 (ergocalciferol) and vitamin D_3 (cholecalciferol). Mellanby demonstrated in 1919 that rickets could be produced experimentally and prevented by cod-liver oil administration. Shortly thereafter, McCollum and co-workers distinguished the antirachitic factor from the previously discovered vitamin A in cod-liver oil. Finally Steenbock reported in 1924 that antirachitic activity could be produced in food and animals by exposing them to ultraviolet radiation.

The metabolism and action of vitamin D have been widely described and will not be repeated in detail here. A schematic representation is provided in Figure 12–12. An excellent review of this subject has been published by Haussler and McCain.

Vitamin D has always been classified as a vitamin; however, it is probably best thought of as a hormone. Unlike a true vitamin, the hydroxylated cholecalciferols are not essential nutrients. Vitamin D_3 is formed from 7-dehydrocholesterol, which is an intermediate compound in the synthesis of cholesterol. 7-dehydrocholesterol is ultimately formed from acetyl-CoA, which is never in short supply. The hydroxylated cholecalciferols have the same basic biochemical structure as the steroid hormones, and they control calcium ion concentration in a manner similar to sodium and potassium ion concentration regulation by the mineralocorticoids. Also, vitamin D is not required in many cell cultures. Finally, vitamin D exerts its major influence by combining with nonhistone pro-

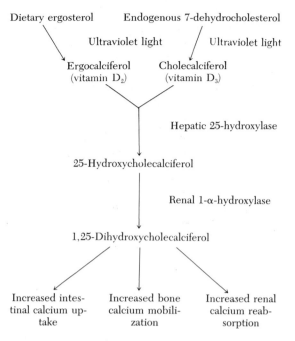

Dietary ergosterol   Endogenous 7-dehydrocholesterol

Ultraviolet light   Ultraviolet light

Ergocalciferol   Cholecalciferol
(vitamin D₂)   (vitamin D₃)

Hepatic 25-hydroxylase

25-Hydroxycholecalciferol

Renal 1-α-hydroxylase

1,25-Dihydroxycholecalciferol

Increased intes-   Increased bone   Increased renal
tinal calcium up-   calcium mobili-   calcium reab-
take   zation   sorption

Figure 12–12. Schematic representation of the metabolism and action of vitamin D.

teins in the nuclei of intestinal epithelial cells. This combination, in turn, exposes a portion of the genetic material for transcription of a specific protein, calcium-binding protein.

Relationship to Calcium and Phosphorus Homeostasis. A discussion of vitamin D is incomplete without mentioning its relationship to calcium and phosphorus homeostasis. In its role as an activator of calcium-binding protein, vitamin D has protean manifestations in parathyroid function, which subsequently affect calcium and phosphorus levels in the body. Hypervitaminosis D, as seen in over-zealous food faddists, results in hypercalcemia with irreversible renal and vascular damage. Hypovitaminosis D, although now uncommon because of dietary fortification, can and does result in secondary hyperparathyroidism. Parathyroid hormone levels are elevated, and serum calcium levels are maintained at the expense of bone calcium. Serum phosphate levels are decreased as a result of the effect of parathyroid hormone on renal excretion of phosphate. Serum alkaline phosphatase levels are increased due to the bones' attempt at re-formation. Dietary calcium forms insoluble calcium phosphates in the intestines because of its increased concentration.

REQUIREMENTS. The recommended daily dietary allowance of vitamin D from infancy through puberty is 10 mcg. of cholecalciferol (400 I.U. of vitamin D). Rickets can be pre-

vented and growth will proceed at a normal rate with significantly less vitamin D (2 to 5 mcg. of cholecalciferol), provided adequate amounts of calcium and phosphorus are present in the diet. Calcium uptake will be reduced slightly (25 to 30 per cent compared with 35 to 40 per cent) with decreased vitamin D intake. The recommended daily dietary intake tapers off to 7.5 mcg. in young adulthood and should be maintained at 5 mcg. after the age of twenty-five. Pregnant and lactating females should increase their daily intake by 5 mcg.

Vitamin D-Deficient Rickets

In common parlance, rickets refers to any disorder in the vitamin D–calcium-phosphorus axis which results in hypomineralized bone matrix, i.e., a failure of endochondral calcification. It should be realized that such a defect may result from a number of etiologies; thus there are a variety of forms of "rickets." A comprehensive review of rickets has been published by Pitt and Haussler.

Historically, vitamin D-deficient rickets developed in urban areas that were deprived of adequate sunlight. When air pollution filters out the ultraviolet portion of the spectrum, cholecalciferol formation is blocked. Infants rapidly develop the characteristic bony deformities. Identical lesions are seen in sun-rich areas where the diet is high in phytate, which binds the available dietary calcium. Social customs, e.g., the use of the purdah, may also result in rickets. The age of onset of the deficiency is important in the eventual morbidity, with premature infants being at highest risk. Although the incidence of rickets in Western societies has been drastically decreased because of food fortification with irradiated ergosterol, e.g., ergocalciferol in milk, Richards and co-workers have reported an incidence of radiographic changes consistent with rickets in 9 per cent of young children in Glasgow, Scotland.

Clinical Features. The rat is the laboratory animal commonly used for the experimental investigation of rickets. The effects of rickets are reflected only in the bones and teeth of the afflicted animal. The changes in the bones are found in the epiphyseal plate, the metaphysis and the shaft. Since the degree of change encountered depends on the rate of growth of the bones at the time of the deficiency, young animals are more seriously affected than older animals.

In young rats placed on rachitogenic diets, the first change seen is the cessation of calcification of their epiphyseal disks. Since the intercellular ground substance does not become calcified, the cartilage cells are not denied nutrition. Therefore they do not die, and their continued growth and multiplication lead to an increase in the width of the disk. The disk thickens irregularly because some focal areas usually calcify. The osteoblasts continue to lay down osteoid around the bone and cartilage spicules in the metaphysis, as well as beneath the periosteum in the region of the metaphysis and other areas of the shaft. The changes in the ribs and long bones of children with rickets are essentially the same as those described for the rat. Since undermineralized bone is not as capable of supporting weight as normal bone, children with rickets show bowing of the legs.

Oral Manifestations. Mellanby was the first to report the effects of rickets on the teeth, which included developmental abnormalities of dentin and enamel, delayed eruption, and misalignment of the teeth in the jaws. Her later work showed that affected teeth had a higher caries index than those of controls. In human rachitic teeth there is an abnormally wide predentin zone and much interglobular dentin. Although many reports are found in the literature linking rickets with enamel hypoplasia, infantile rickets does not always result in hypoplastic enamel. The eruption rate of the deciduous and permanent teeth, however, is retarded in rickets.

Osteomalacia

(Adult Rickets)

Osteomalacia is the adult equivalent of juvenile (vitamin D-deficient) rickets. Unlike juvenile rickets, only the flat bones and the diaphyses of the long bones are affected. The disease is most commonly seen in postmenopausal females with a history of low dietary calcium intake and little exposure to ultraviolet light. This disorder is endemic in certain areas of India, Japan, and China. Malabsorption is also a commonly reported etiology.

Clinical Features. Essentially there is a remodeling of bone in the absence of adequate calcium, which results in a softening and distortion of the skeleton and an increased tendency towards fracture. Pelvic deformities are commonly seen in affected multiparous females.

Oral Manifestations. Taylor and Day have reported a 50 per cent incidence of severe periodontitis in a series of 22 Indian women with osteomalacia. These data are questionable in view of the prevalence of endemic periodontal disease in this population group.

Roentgenographic Features. Radiologically there are severe asymmetric deformities of all stress-bearing bones e.g., the pelvis, spine and long bones of the legs. Longitudinal hairline fractures are seen in the long bones.

Histologic Features. The histologic findings in osteomalacia, like those in rickets, are nonspecific. There is an attempt at bone remodeling with inadequate calcification of bone matrix. The cortical bone is thin, and osteoid borders are found on the trabeculae.

Treatment and Prognosis. The treatment (and for that matter prevention) of osteomalacia consists of dietary enrichment of Vitamin D, usually in the form of milk, and the certainty of adequate dietary calcium. Hormonal therapy and fluoride administration have also been reported to be useful in the treatment of the disease. If the osteomalacia is secondary to malabsorption, the daily dietary fat intake must be severely restricted. While the mortality associated with osteomalacia is negligible, the morbidity is prominent and related to the extent of the disease at the time of initial diagnosis. Complications may arise from long bone fractures and compression of the spinal vertebrae.

Vitamin D-Resistant Rickets

(Familial Hypophosphatemia; Refractory Rickets; Phosphate Diabetes)

In recent years a number of isolated renal tubular defects, associated with an inability to reabsorb certain metabolites such as water, phosphate, calcium, and potassium, have been recognized. Some defects in reabsorption may lead to rickets or osteomalacia. Albright and co-workers first described a case of vitamin D-resistant rickets in 1937. Shortly thereafter, Christensen described a familial pattern of occurrence. Twenty years after its initial description, Winters and colleagues and Graham and co-workers proposed that the disorder was an X-linked dominant defect in renal phosphate metabolism. A large series of cases has been investigated by Stickler and associates.

The disease is now recognized as a specific disorder characterized by (1) hypophosphatemia and hyperphosphaturia associated with decreased renal tubular reabsorption of inorganic phosphates, (2) familial occurrence, being inherited as an X-linked dominant trait, (3) rickets or osteomalacia which does not respond to the usual doses of vitamin D, (4) normocalcemia with high-normal parathyroid hormone levels, (5) diminished intestinal calcium and phosphate absorption, (6) decreased growth with short stature, (7) normal vitamin D metabolism, and (8) the absence of other related abnormalities. This definition excludes conditions such as sporadic, nonfamilial vitamin D-resistant rickets and familial vitamin D-resistant rickets associated with normal or high serum concentration of inorganic phosphate.

Clinical Features. The mildest form of this disease is a simple hypophosphatemia without clinical manifestations other than a slight decrease in the height of the patient as compared with a normophosphatemic sibling. In hypophosphatemic adults the varying degrees of deformities due to rickets in childhood constitute more serious disturbances, such as bowing of the legs, shortening of stature, continuing osteomalacia and the presence of pseudofractures.

In children affected with this form of resistant rickets the disease is usually first recognized when the child begins to walk. The history or x-ray examination, however, might reveal abnormalities such as skull deformities, retardation of eruption of teeth and "sitting" deformities of the legs. Such children usually have received prophylactic doses of vitamin D but have failed to respond. Permanent deformities and short stature are often present.

Among family members with hypophosphatemia, females show considerably less bone disease than males. Few patients have the muscular weakness and atony which are so prominent and frequent in vitamin D-deficient rickets.

Oral Manifestations. Vitamin D-resistant rickets has marked effects on the teeth and supporting structures. These have been discussed in detail by many workers including Marks and his associates, Archard and Witkop, Tracy and his associates, Vasilakis and co-workers, Ainley, and Cohen and Becker.

Characteristically, there is histologic evidence of widespread formation of globular, hypocalcified dentin, with clefts and tubular defects occurring in the region of the pulp horns. In addition, these pulp horns are elongated and extend high, often reaching nearly to the dentinoenamel junction. This may even be evident on the roentgenogram (Fig. 12–13). Because of these defects, there is commonly invasion of the pulp by microorganisms without demonstrable destruction of the tubular matrix. Following this, there is often periapical involvement of grossly normal-appearing deciduous or permanent teeth, followed by the development of multiple gingival fistulas. In addition to abnormal cementum, the lamina dura around the teeth is also reported to be frequently absent or poorly defined on the roentgenogram, and the alveolar bone pattern is often abnormal.

Histologic Features. Alterations are found primarily in the cartilage plate and shaft of the long bones and are characterized by a failure of bone salts to be deposited in the cartilage matrix between the rows of hypertrophic cells, so that these cells are not invaded and destroyed by capillaries. The histologic picture is characterized by a broad zone between the multiplying cartilage cells and the shaft, the so-called rachitic metaphysis. This is composed of tongues of cartilage which extend down toward the shaft and are separated from one another by collections of capillaries. This zone contains trabeculae made up of uncalcified cartilage matrix upon which osteoid has been deposited. Since osteoblastic activity is not affected, osteoid is found deposited on preexisting bony trabeculae. The calcification is interfered with, so the osteoid does not calcify and is not remodeled.

Treatment and Prognosis. The treatment of vitamin D-resistant rickets is highly individualized. Massive doses of vitamin D frequently result in repair, but the risk of hypervitaminosis D in such cases is considerable. Success has been reported using 25-hydroxycholecalciferol in lower dosages than conventional vitamin D (10,000 to 25,000 I.U. per day of 25-hydroxycholecalciferol, as opposed to 50,000 to 100,000 I.U. per day of vitamin D). Healing of the rickets can be initiated by measures other than prescribing massive doses of vitamin D. Such methods include immobilization and administration of large amounts of phosphate. Decreased dosages of vitamin D (15,000 to 50,000 I.U. per day) combined with supplemental oral phosphate have been used successfully.

Renal Rickets

(Renal Osteodystrophy)

Painful, crippling bone disease is a common finding in patients with chronic renal disease. Renal rickets results from the inability of diseased kidneys to synthesize 1-α-hydoxylase and convert 25-hydroxycholecalciferol to the active form of vitamin D. Calcium absorption in the intestines is impaired, with a dramatic increase in fecal calcium excretion and negative calcium

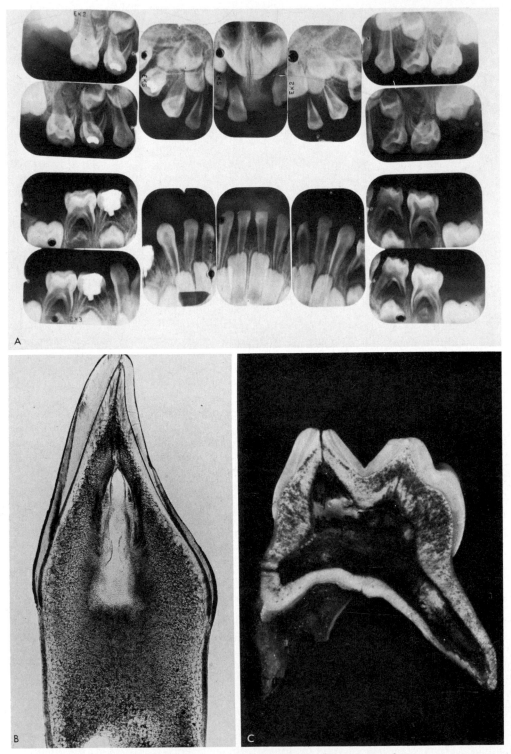

Figure 12–13. *Vitamin D-resistant rickets in a boy six years of age.*

The full mouth roentgenograms (*A*) show the wide root canals and pulp chambers. A ground section of an incisor tooth (*B*) shows the interglobular nature of the dentin. The deciduous molar (*C*) when split shows the relatively small quantity of dentin as well as the poor quality of the dentin. Note the connection between the pulp chamber and the occlusal surface of the tooth, a common finding in this disease, accounting for the frequent pulp infection and periapical involvement without the presence of a carious lesion. (Courtesy of Dr. S. S. Arnim.)

balance. Secondary hyperparathyroidism may lead to a superimposed osteitis fibrosis cystica.

Treatment and Prognosis. Renal osteodystrophy is refractory to physiologic doses of vitamin D. Kaye and Sagar have reported success in treating renal rickets with dihydrotachysterol, a vitamin D analog. Catto and co-workers have administered 1-α-hydroxycholecalciferol and reported good treatment success. The prognosis for the bone disease is guarded because of the inability to cure the underlying renal disease. Renal transplant patients function adequately after an initial post-transplantation hypercalcemia.

Hypophosphatasia

(Hypophosphatasemia)

Hypophosphatasia, a hereditary disease first recognized as an entity by Rathbun in 1948, is transmitted as a recessive autosomal characteristic. Since then many cases have been reported and several reviews of the disease presented. One such excellent review, that of Bruckner and his associates, stressed the dental findings in this condition as observed in a series of cases. Ritchie, Haupt and associates, Kjellmann and co-workers, Beumer and colleagues, Brittain and co-workers, and Witkop and Rao have discussed in detail the oral manifestations of hypophosphatasia.

The basic disorder is a deficiency of the enzyme alkaline phosphatase in serum or tissues and excretion of phosphoethanolamine in the urine. The severity of the disease is not directly related to serum alkaline phosphatase levels. There is an interesting similarity of many aspects of this disease to the condition known as "vitamin D-resistant rickets with familial hypophosphatemia."

Clinical Features. On the basis of clinical manifestations and chronology of the appearance of bone disease, hypophosphatasia is divided into three clinical forms: (1) infantile, (2) childhood, and (3) adult. The infantile form is manifested by severe rickets, hypercalcemia, bone abnormalities, and failure to thrive. Most of these cases are lethal. Hypophosphatasia of childhood is characterized by premature exfoliation of deciduous teeth, increased infection, growth retardation and rachitic-like deformities, including deformed extremities, costochondral junction enlargement (rachitic rosary) and failure of the calvarium to calcify. Pulmonary, gastrointestinal and renal disorders are also present. The adult form includes spontaneous fractures, prior history of rickets and osseous radiolucencies.

Oral Manifestations. The earliest manifestation of the disease may be loosening and premature loss of deciduous teeth, chiefly the incisors. There are varying reports of gingivitis; however it does not appear to be a consistent feature of the disease.

Roentgenographic Features. The metaphyses of long bones have been described as showing "spotty," "streaky," or irregular ossification.

Dental roentgenograms generally reveal hypocalcification of teeth and the presence of large pulp chambers, as well as alveolar bone loss; however, these findings have not been consistently reported.

Histologic Features. The long bones characteristically exhibit an increased width of proliferating cartilage with widening of the hypertrophic cell zone, irregularity of cell columns, irregular penetration of the cartilage by marrow with persistence of numerous cartilage islands in the marrow, and formation of large amounts of osteoid which is inadequately calcified. These findings are indistinguishable from those in true rickets.

The teeth present a unique appearance characterized by the absence of cementum, presumably as a result of failure of cementogenesis, so that there is no sound functional attachment of the tooth to bone by periodontal ligament (Fig. 12–14). This lack of attachment is thought to account for the early spontaneous exfoliation of the deciduous teeth. Occasional foci of poorly formed cementum may be found on some teeth.

Treatment. Therapeutic measures are generally unsuccessful. Vitamin D in high doses has resulted in partial improvement in some cases, but this may lead to deposition of calcium in many tissues, including the kidney. Bongiovanni and co-workers have reported that administration of high oral doses of phosphate results in moderate improvement in bone calcification as judged radiologically.

Pseudohypophosphatasia

A disease resembling classic hypophosphatasia but with a normal serum alkaline phosphatase level has been reported by Scriver and Cameron. Patients afflicted by pseudohypophosphatasia exhibit osteopathy of the long bones and skull, premature loss of deciduous teeth, hypotonia, hypercalcemia and phosphoethanolaminuria. Only the alkaline phosphatase

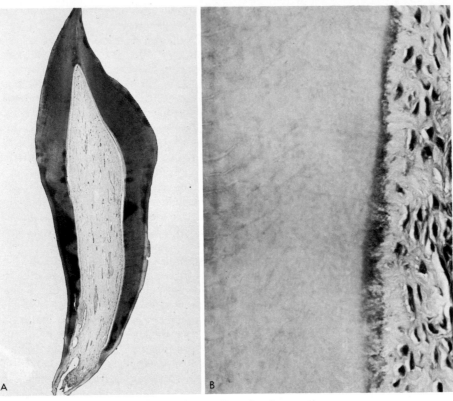

Figure 12–14. *Hypophosphatasia.*
A maxillary deciduous incisor of a patient with hypophosphatasia which was exfoliated at 15 months of age (*A*). The tooth root showed only a poor attempt at cementogenesis indicated by the granular, basophilic material between the dentin on the left and the periodontal fibers on the right (*B*). (Courtesy of Dr. Robert J. Bruckner.)

level remains normal. This disease also appears to be hereditary. Méhes and co-workers have reported the appearance of hypophosphatasia and pseudohypophosphatasia in the same kindred. This suggests that the two diseases may represent variations of a basic metabolic effect.

Vitamin E

Sixty years ago Evans and Bishop noted that a fat-soluble factor prevented fetal resorption in animals. This factor was named vitamin E and given the generic name of tocopherol, which means "the alcohol which brings forth offspring." Olcott and Emerson soon recognized the antioxidant properties of vitamin E. The main function of vitamin E is to prevent peroxidation of polyunsaturated fatty acids.

Vitamin E deficiency in experimental animals results in multisystem disorders, including decreased male fertility, impaired fetal-maternal vascular relationships, nutritional muscular dys-

trophy and encephalomalacia, increased vascular disruption, and hemolysis. All of these disorders can be attributed in part to the increased peroxidation of unsaturated fatty acids in vitamin E-deficient animals. Irving has described a loss of pigment and atrophic, degenerative changes in the enamel organ of vitamin E-deficient rats.

Infants are born with low levels of vitamin E and are particularly susceptible to vitamin E deficiency, especially if they are fed diets high in polyunsaturated fatty acids. Hassan and co-workers have described this syndrome, which consists of edema, desquamating erythematous papular dermatitis, thrombocytosis and anemia. Chronic steatorrhea, for example, as it occurs with cystic fibrosis, results in hypovitaminosis E and is manifested by muscular dystrophy–type symptoms, with elevated serum creatinine phosphokinase activity and creatinuria. This secondary vitamin E deficiency has been discussed by Nitowsky and co-workers.

REQUIREMENTS. The recommended daily dietary allowance for vitamin E ranges from 3 mg. of d-α-tocopherol for infants to 10 mg. for adult males. Increased intake in pregnant and lactating women is suggested, especially in view of the low perinatal levels of vitamin E in the infant. The average intake of vitamin E in the United States is 15 mg. per day; therefore, deficiency states are rare in the absence of underlying steatorrhea and malabsorption.

Vitamin E has gained a great deal of public and scientific attention in the past decade because of its role as a polyunsaturated fatty acid antioxidant. One of the prevailing theories of aging states that aging is, in part, a progressive accumulation of cellular damage resulting from free radicals. As an antioxidant, vitamin E may play a role in the prevention of free radical damage. This subject has been reviewed by Pryor. There are interesting but inconclusive animal studies to support this particular aging hypothesis. Unfortunately, publication of these results prompted megadose consumption of vitamin E by ill-advised members of the lay public. Based on the lack of toxic symptoms in nutrition faddists, vitamin E is thought by Farrel and Bieri to be one of the least toxic of the vitamins.

THE WATER-SOLUBLE VITAMINS

Vitamin K

In 1929, Dam noticed a peculiar hemorrhagic diathesis in chicks fed a fat-extracted diet. This clotting defect was not due to a deficiency of vitamins A, D, or E, which had previously been discovered. The new substance was named vitamin K or "koagulation vitamin." Like other fat-soluble vitamins, vitamin K is absorbed from the gut and is transported to the liver via lymph chylomicrons.

Dam and his co-workers later provided evidence that vitamin K was intimately involved in both the extrinsic and intrinsic systems of coagulation, particularly with prothrombin (Factor II) synthesis. Other investigators have since shown a role for vitamin K in the regulation of levels of Factors VII, IX, and X (proconvertin, Christmas factor and Stuart-Prower factor, respectively). Prior to Dam's discovery of vitamin K, Schofield had described a hemorrhagic disease in cattle which had consumed spoiled clover. Campbell and co-workers later described this vitamin K antagonist and identified it as Dicumarol. A coumarin analog, warfarin is commonly used as an anticoagulant in both humans and animals.

Primary vitamin K deficiency is rare in humans; however, newborns are particularly susceptible to vitamin K deficiency, and hypoprothrombinemia due to poor placental lipid transmission and a lack of vitamin K-synthesizing gastrointestinal flora may ensue. Secondary hypovitaminosis K may occur in adults with impaired fat absorption, which may accompany obstructive jaundice, sprue, ulcerative colitis and surgical bowel resection. Iatrogenic deficiency of vitamin K may occur secondary to antibiotic sterilization of the gut.

The most common oral manifestation of vitamin K deficiency is gingival bleeding. Prothrombin levels below 35 per cent will result in bleeding after toothbrushing; however, when prothrombin levels fall below 20 per cent, spontaneous gingival hemorrhages will occur.

REQUIREMENTS. The minimum daily dietary requirement of vitamin K is estimated to be between 1 to 2 mcg./kg., depending on the amount of gut bacterial production of the vitamin. The "normal mixed diet" in the United States is estimated to contain 300 to 500 mcg. of vitamin K, which is more than enough to meet minimum daily requirements.

Vitamin C

Vitamin C has been the object of intensive research for many years. Scurvy, which results from vitamin C deficiency, has been known since the time of the Ebers papyrus in Egypt (1500 B.C.). The effect on history, through the occurrence of scurvy in military troops, is notable. British sailors in the nineteenth century were referred to as "limeys" because of their consumption of citrus fruits to prevent scurvy while on long voyages. Hodges and co-workers have described the changes seen in experimental scurvy in man, and an excellent review has been written by Lloyd and Sinclair.

Svirbely and Szent-Györgyi isolated hexuronic acid (ascorbic acid) in 1928 and reported the results in 1932. A similar isolation procedure was reported by King and Waugh in 1932. Within two years the structure of vitamin C was determined and synthesized. Interestingly, most animals are capable of synthesizing their own vitamin C. Burns has postulated that humans, monkeys and guinea pigs are incapable of endogenous vitamin C production owing to an inability to convert L-gulonolactone (a glucose metabolite) to L-ascorbic acid. Because of this inherent defect, guinea pigs are the animal model of choice in studying scurvy.

Vitamin C is necessary for a number of metabolic processes, including hydrogen ion transfers and maintenance of intracellular oxidation-reduction potentials. It also acts as an antioxidant, facilitates iron uptake in the intestinal tract, and is involved in the formation of folinic acid (the active form of folic acid). Standinger and associates and Goldberg have reported that ascorbic acid is critical in hydroxylation reactions which require reduced iron or copper. Its role in the hydroxylation of proline in collagen synthesis has been described by Peterkovsky and Udenfriend. Tryptophan, norepinephrine, and tyrosine metabolism all require vitamin C.

In general, the action of vitamin C appears to be to further the normal development of intercellular ground substances in bone, dentin and other connective tissues, since all signs of the deficiency of ascorbic acid are associated with disturbances in these tissues.

The dental changes in scorbutic guinea pigs are so consistent and characteristic that Hojer and Crampton devised biologic assay methods for vitamin C by grading the histologic changes in the mandibular incisor. The characteristic change in the teeth of scorbutic guinea pigs is the atrophy and disorganization of the odontoblasts, resulting early in the deficiency state in the production of irregularly laid down dentin with few, irregularly arranged tubules. Eventually dentin formation ceases, and the predentin becomes hypercalcified, producing a heavy, basophilic staining line between dentin and pulp. The odontoblasts finally become indistinguishable from other pulpal cells (Fig. 12–15).

In scorbutic monkeys, hypertrophy of the gingiva covering the entire crowns of the teeth was reported by Goldman. In some cases subperiosteal hemorrhages lifted the gingiva from the underlying bone. Focal areas of necrosis of the free margin of the gingiva also occurred. The alveolar bone showed atrophic changes, and the marrow spaces were replaced by fibroblasts growing in an edematous space.

REQUIREMENTS. The recommended dietary intake for vitamin C ranges from 35 mg. in infants to 60 mg. in adults. Pregnant and lactating women should increase their daily intake by 20 mg. and 40 mg., respectively.

Clinical Features of Scurvy. The oral effects of vitamin C deficiency in humans occur chiefly in the gingival and periodontal tissues. The interdental and marginal gingiva is bright red with a swollen, smooth, shiny surface. In fully developed scurvy the gingiva becomes boggy, ulcerates and bleeds. The color changes to a violaceous red. In infants the enlarged tissue may cover the clinical crowns of the teeth (Fig. 12–16). In almost all cases of acute or chronic scurvy the gingival ulcers show the typical organisms, and the patients have the typical foul breath of persons with fusospirochetal stomatitis. In the severe chronic cases of scurvy, hemorrhages into and swelling of the periodontal membranes occur, followed by loss of bone and loosening of the teeth, which eventually exfoliate.

Boyle studied the deciduous and permanent

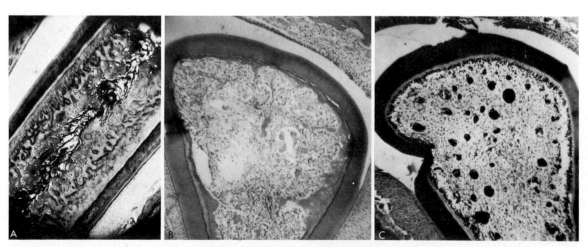

Figure 12–15. *Vitamin C deficiency.*
Photomicrographs of incisor teeth of guinea pigs with incomplete or early vitamin C deficiency showing the abnormal irregular dentin, (A) longitudinal and (B) cross section. The odontoblasts eventually fail to lay down dentin (C).

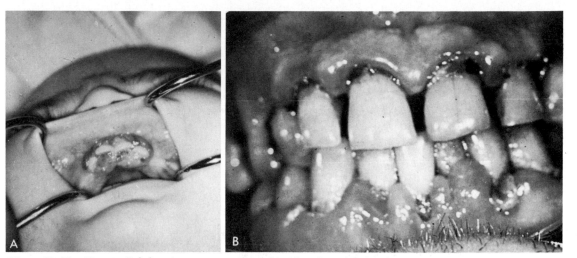

Figure 12–16. Vitamin C deficiency or scurvy in an infant (A) and an adult (B). (A, Courtesy of Dr. E. V. Zegarelli; B, Courtesy of Dr. E. R. Costich.)

tooth germs of scorbutic infants and found only small cysts and minute hemorrhages in some specimens.

Vitamin C is a threshold substance and is excreted primarily through the kidney. The degree of tissue saturation is the factor which determines the amount excreted. If intake has been normal, a slight increase in intake above normal will be excreted. If, on the other hand, the tissues are under-saturated through low intake or through excess metabolism of vitamin C, even high doses may be largely retained.

The role of ascorbic acid in collagen formation has been extensively studied from many aspects. It has been found that wounds produced in scorbutic guinea pigs fail to heal properly. Although there is fibroblastic proliferation in the wound area, the fibroblasts appear immature and fail to produce collagen. They do form a fluid-like material around themselves, representing an ineffectual attempt at collagen formation.

Histologic Features. The bone changes in scurvy were well reviewed by Follis in his book on the pathology of nutritional disease. He pointed out that in scurvy the osteoblasts fail to form osteoid. The cartilage cells of the epiphyseal plate continue to proliferate in normal fashion, and salts are deposited in the matrix between the columns of cartilage cells. But the osteoblasts fail to lay down osteoid on the spicules of calcified cartilage matrix. In addition, the calcified matrix material is not destroyed, so that a wide zone of calcified but nonossified matrix, called the scorbutic lattice,

develops in the metaphysis. The spicules are nonresistant to weight-bearing and motion stresses, and they are therefore liable to fracture. The changes which accompany the fractures lead to the characteristic lesions of the skeleton in scurvy.

As the "lattice" increases in width, a more and more fragile zone develops, so that eventually complete fracture of the spicules occurs with separation and deformity of the cartilage-shaft junction. This fracturing of the calcified matrix material leads to the classic picture of scurvy, the so-called *Trümmerfeldzone* or region of complete disintegration. About the fractures and clefts there are pink-staining hyaline material, immature-looking fibroblasts and macrophages containing hemosiderin. The area beneath the *Trümmerfeldzone* is free of hematopoietic cells and is made up of connective tissue cells, the so-called *Gerüstmark*. The reason for the migration of marrow cells out of the area, leaving only connective tissue elements, is not clear. In addition, subperiosteal hemorrhages are frequent in scorbutic animals.

Vitamin B Complex

Unlike the oral manifestations of vitamin A deficiency and the other vitamin deficiencies heretofore described, the oral signs of deficiencies of the B vitamins occur primarily in the oral soft tissues: the tongue, mucous membranes, gingiva and lips. Since much of our knowledge of the avitaminoses B is derived from clinical observation, the mechanism of action and the histologic details of the oral lesions associated with the various vitamin B deficiencies still remain to be elucidated.

At present the vitamin B group contains 11 well-characterized vitamins: thiamin, riboflavin, niacin, pyridoxine, pantothenic acid, biotin, folic acid, vitamin B_{12}, inositol, para-aminobenzoic acid and choline. Nearly every one of these vitamins forms part of a coenzyme essential for the metabolism of proteins, carbohydrates or fats.

The B-complex vitamins are needed by all living cells, but with the exception of nicotinic acid and choline, animal tissues are incapable of synthesizing them. The B vitamins must therefore be absorbed from the intestinal tract either from ingested food or from the products of the intestinal flora, or from both.

Most B-complex vitamins occur in nature in bound form within the cells of vegetable or animal tissues. These cellular structures must therefore be broken down by the digestion for the liberation of the vitamin and its eventual absorption from the gut. With the possible exception of vitamin B_{12}, the vitamins of the B complex are not stored in any appreciable amount in the tissues of the body, so if the intake exceeds the requirement, the excess is excreted in the urine.

Although the functions of individual vitamins, whether fat- or water-soluble, vary greatly, vitamins tend to occur together in nature to some extent. It should be remembered, therefore, that though a lesion induced by the elimination of a single vitamin from an experimental diet may occur in experimental animals and may even be induced in human subjects, lesions occurring naturally are probably associated with a deficiency of many of the essential nutrients. We are seeing only the most prominent clinical symptom and not the entire patient when we observe an angular cheilosis and assume that it is due to riboflavin deficiency. We must also remember that, though the most frequent cause of a nutritional deficiency is decreased intake of the essential nutrient, impaired absorption from the alimentary canal, failure of utilization by the tissues, inadequate storage, increased metabolism due to rapid growth, fever, pregnancy and other factors all contribute to clinical deficiency states.

Pathologic conditions other than deficiency states may impose special demands for vitamins. Adequate nutrition is obviously important in the treatment of disease, but the diet must be governed by the nature of the disturbance. The indiscriminate use of the B vitamins is of no value in the treatment of general ill health.

Thiamin. Thiamin (vitamin B_1) is a colorless basic organic compound composed of a sulfated pyrimidine ring. It is readily absorbed from both the small and large intestines. It is phosphorylated mainly by the liver and to a lesser extent by the kidney. In tissues, thiamin is found as thiamin pyrophosphate (cocarboxylase), rarely as free thiamin.

Clinical Features of Thiamin Deficiency. In man, thiamin deficiency leads to beriberi. This disease is characterized by multiple neuritis, often associated with congestive heart failure, generalized edema and sudden death. The disease is generally insidious in onset and chronic in course.

REQUIREMENTS. The recommended daily dietary allowance for thiamin ranges from 0.3 mg. for infants to 1.5 mg. for young adult males. Pregnant and lactating women should increase their daily intake by 0.4 mg. and 0.5 mg., respectively.

There is no convincing evidence that thiamin exerts an influence on oral tissues. There are reported cases of oral manifestations of thiamin deficiency, but they are not supported by the experience of volunteer human subjects who lived on diets containing very low levels of thiamin for six months and showed no oral lesions.

Riboflavin. Riboflavin (vitamin B_2) is a fully dialyzable, intensely yellow water-soluble pigment which is decomposed by light. It fluoresces green under ultraviolet illumination, is readily absorbed from the intestinal tract and is phosphorylated in the walls of the intestine as well as in other tissues of the body.

Riboflavin is a constituent of two different groups of coenzymes, riboflavin 5'-phosphate (flavin mononucleotide or FMN) and flavin adenine dinucleotide (FAD). These coenzymes are essential to the oxidative enzyme systems utilizing the electron transport system.

REQUIREMENTS. The recommended daily dietary allowance for riboflavin ranges from 0.4 mg. for infants to 1.7 mg. for young adult males. Pregnant and lactating women should increase their daily dietary intake by 0.3 mg. and 0.5 mg., respectively.

Clinical Features of Riboflavin Deficiency. Riboflavin deficiency is particularly common among children who do not drink milk. In endemic areas, the incidence is greater during the spring and summer months than in other seasons.

A long period of vague, nondescript symptoms usually precedes the appearance of diagnostic lesions. The diagnostic lesions of ariboflavinosis are usually limited to the mouth and perioral regions. The oral manifestations of the disease are well recognized, since they have been experimentally produced by Sebrell and Butler in 18 healthy women placed on a riboflavin-deficient diet. Although the exact mechanism involved in the production of the oral lesion is not understood, the clinical stages have been clearly defined.

In the mild deficiency state there is a glossitis which begins with soreness of the tip and/or the lateral margins of the tongue (Fig. 12–17). The filiform papillae become atrophic, while the fungiform papillae remain normal or become engorged and mushroom shaped, giving the tongue surface a reddened, coarsely granular appearance. The lesions extend backward over the dorsum of the tongue. In severe cases the tongue may become glazed and smooth, owing to complete atrophy of all papillae. In many cases the tongue has a magenta color which can be easily distinguished from cyanosis.

Paleness of the lips, especially at the angles of the mouth, but not involving the moist areas of the buccal mucosa, is the earliest sign of the deficiency disease. The pallor, which usually continues for days, is followed by cheilosis, which is evidenced by a maceration and fissuring at the angles of the mouth. The fissures may be single or multiple. Later the macerated lesions develop a dry yellow crust which can be removed without causing bleeding. The lips become unusually red and shiny because of a desquamation of the epithelium. As the disease progresses, the angular cheilosis spreads to the cheek. The fissures become deeper, bleed easily and are painful when secondarily infected with oral and/or skin microorganisms. Deep lesions leave scars on healing. The gingival tissues are not involved.

Riboflavin deficiency also affects the nasolabial folds and the alae nasi, which exhibit a scaly, greasy dermatitis. A fine scaly dermatitis may also occur on the hands, vulva, anus and perineum. Ocular changes, consisting of corneal vascularization, photophobia and a superficial and interstitial keratitis, have also been described. Considering that flavoproteins are widely distributed throughout the body, it is surprising that the lesions are so well localized.

In the differential diagnosis of ariboflavinosis, it is important to remember that bilateral angular cheilosis is a nonspecific lesion. Older people with greatly decreased vertical dimension, either through faulty dentures or through attrition of the natural dentition, frequently show the nonspecific angular cheilosis.

Niacin. In the living organism, ingested niacin is transformed into nicotinic acid amide, which is utilized to form coenzyme I (nicotinamide-adenine dinucleotide, or NAD) and coenzyme II (nicotinamide-adenine dinucleotide phosphate, or NADP). A deficiency of this vitamin leads to the classic symptoms of pellagra in human beings and to black tongue in dogs.

Pellagra as a widespread problem in the southeastern United States has largely disappeared. Spies and Butt formulated a working hypothesis of the pathogenesis of the disease as follows:

When the available nicotinic acid amide or compounds with similar functions are not adequate to supply the needs of the body for reasons of decreased supply, inadequate assimilation, increased demand, or increased loss, a disorder in respiratory enzyme systems occurs. As a result a state of generalized reduction in normal cellular respiration supervenes. When this biochemical lesion is severe enough, or has existed long enough, it is translated into functional disturbances in various organ systems of the body. Vasomotor instability in the skin, functional disorders of the alimentary canal, the nervous system, and the circulatory system may occur. It is probable that the most readily affected systems are those weakened by hereditary predisposition or trauma in the wear and tear of everyday life. This may explain the infinite variety of the clinical picture. Finally severe or persisting alterations in physiology lead to structural changes in various tissues which ultimately present the diagnostic lesions of pellagra.

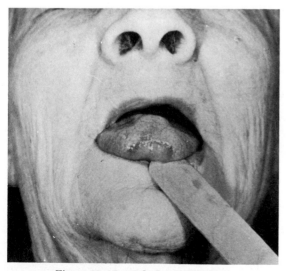

Figure 12–17. *Riboflavin deficiency.*
The atrophy of the filiform papillae gives the tip of the tongue a smooth, almost ulcerated appearance.

A metabolic interrelationship between the amino acid tryptophan and nicotinic acid has been demonstrated in a number of mammalian species including man. Pyridoxal-5-phosphate is required for the conversion of tryptophan into nicotinic acid in the tissues. The accepted conversion ratio (Niacin Equivalents) is 60 mg. tryptophan to 1 mg. nicotinic acid.

Clinical Features of Pellagra. The mucous membrane lesions affecting the tongue, oral cavity and vagina are usually the earliest lesions diagnostic of the disease. Other lesions common in pellagra are the typical dermal lesions of bilaterally symmetric, sharply outlined, roughened, keratotic areas (Fig. 12–18). (The word "pellagra" means rough skin.) Mental symptoms and weight loss also occur.

In the prodromal stage of nicotinic acid deficiency, the patient may complain of loss of appetite and vague gastrointestinal symptoms. General weakness, lassitude, mental confusion, forgetfulness and other ill defined symptoms develop. The patient then usually complains of a burning sensation in the tongue, which becomes swollen and presses against the teeth, causing indentations. The tip and lateral margins of the tongue become red.

In the acute stages of pellagra the entire oral mucosa becomes fiery red and painful. The mouth feels as though it had been scalded. Salivation is profuse. The epithelium of the entire tongue desquamates. Tenderness, pain,

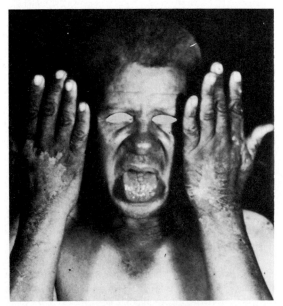

Figure 12–18. *Pellagra.*
(Courtesy of Dr. Boynton H. Booth.)

redness and ulcerations begin at the interdental gingival papillae and spread rapidly. Superimposed acute necrotizing ulcerative gingivostomatitis or Vincent's infection involving the gingiva, tongue and oral mucosa is a common sequel.

REQUIREMENTS. The recommended daily dietary allowance for niacin ranges from 6 mg. of Niacin Equivalents (N.E.) in infants to 10 mg. N.E. in young adult males. Pregnant and lactating women should increase their daily intakes by 2 mg. and 5 mg. N.E., respectively.

Pantothenic Acid. The role of pantothenic acid in metabolic processes is not at all clear. It is a constituent of coenzyme A and is widely distributed in foods. Since no evidence of human pantothenic acid deficiency has been recorded, the human requirement for this vitamin is unknown. Five to 10 mg. per day is considered adequate for children and adults. The average daily American diet contains between 5 and 20 mg. of pantothenic acid.

Pyridoxine. Pyridoxine (vitamin B_6) is actually a complex of three related substances: pyridoxine, pyridoxal and pyridoxamine. Pyridoxine is the most active compound when ingested.

Pyridoxine plays an important role in protein metabolism, since pyridoxine-deficient animals placed on a high protein diet exhibit the characteristic lesions sooner and die more quickly than animals whose pyridoxine-deficient diets contain smaller amounts of protein. This vitamin has also been shown to be involved in tryptophan metabolism. If young dogs deficient in pyridoxine are fed tryptophan, both kynurenin and xanthurenic acid are excreted in the urine. If pyridoxine is fed to the animals, xanthurenic acid is not excreted, but kynurenin and kynurenic acid are found in the urine. Thus, pyridoxine apparently determines whether xanthurenic acid or kynurenic acid will be excreted after tryptophan feeding. The finding of xanthurenic acid in the urine has been suggested as a biologic test for vitamin B_6 deficiency.

Hawkins and Barsky reported that mental depression, mental confusion, albuminuria and leukopenia occurred in normal people placed on a pyridoxine-deficient diet. The oral lesions of experimentally induced pyridoxine deficiency bear a striking resemblance to pellagrous stomatitis.

In some people with angular cheilosis, pyridoxine administration will effect a cure when riboflavin and nicotinic acid will not.

The minimum daily dietary allowance for

pyridoxine is 2.0 mg. for adults. Pregnant and lactating women should increase their daily intake by 2.5 mg.

Choline. Choline is an important constituent of lecithin, certain sphingomyelins, and acetylcholine. Little is known of choline requirements, since the need for choline is dependent on their sources of methyl groups in the diet, especially methionine.

Choline deficiency per se probably does not occur. It is possible, however, in cases in which general dietary protein is low to postulate a deficiency of choline and its precursor, methionine. Diets high in choline, methionine, and proteins are used in the treatment of fatty liver and cirrhosis, especially in chronic alcoholics; however, the results have not been promising.

No oral lesions have been ascribed to choline deficiency in man.

Biotin. It is unlikely that biotin deficiency ever develops spontaneously in man. In animals, biotin deficiency is characterized by a scaly, greasy dermatitis and eventual alopecia. No dental changes are described in biotin-deficient animals.

Inositol. Although inositol has been shown to be necessary for growth in experimental animals, no histologic studies have been reported on animals depleted of inositol. Little is known of its role in animal or human nutrition.

Folic Acid. Various macrocytic anemias, sprue, addisonian (pernicious) anemia and macrocytic anemia of infancy respond well to folic acid. Folic acid is essential for the growth of many animal species and is also essential in man. The primary function of folic acid is the transfer of one-carbon moieties in a number of metabolic reactions. Folic acid is also necessary for purine synthesis, the conversion of homocysteine to methionine, and the conversion of uridylate to thymidylate. The synthesis of DNA is impossible in the absence of folic acid.

Clinical Features of Folic Acid Deficiency. Folic acid deficiency in man is characterized by glossitis, diarrhea and macrocytic anemia. The glossitis appears initially as a swelling and redness of the tip and lateral margins of the dorsum. The filiform papillae are the first to disappear, the fungiform papillae remaining as prominent spots. In advanced cases, the fungiform papillae are lost and the tongue becomes slick, smooth and either pallid or fiery red in color. These are the toxic symptoms following aminopterin therapy for leukemia. Aminopterin interferes with the conversion of folic acid to folinic acid. Administration of folic acid in aminopterin toxicity quickly alleviates the glossitis and reverses the symptoms of gastrointestinal disturbances.

The minimum daily dietary allowance for folic acid ranges from 30 mcg. in infants to 400 mcg. in adults. Pregnant women should double their daily intake, while nursing mothers should increase their intake by 25 per cent.

Vitamin B$_{12}$. This vitamin includes a group of closely related compounds, the most common form being cyanocobalamin. It is the antipernicious anemia factor, and it has also been used in trigeminal neuralgia with some success. The oral manifestations of pernicious anemia are detailed in Chapter 14. Massive doses, 1000 mcg. daily, must be used for the treatment of trigeminal neuralgia.

The minimum daily dietary allowance for vitamin B$_{12}$ ranges from 0.5 mcg. in infants to 3.0 mcg. in adults. Pregnant and lactating women should increase their intake by 30 per cent.

DISTURBANCES IN HORMONE METABOLISM

No tissue in the mammalian body is exempt from some sort of hormonal influence, either in the course of its development and growth or in its functional activities. Yet the chemical structures of most hormonal substances are either unknown or only partially defined. Physiologic investigations of the hormones have been centered on their more specific actions, but it is becoming evident that the spheres of action of the hormones are extremely broad and reach far beyond the limits implied by the tissue of origin and its known interrelations with other organs and tissues. As Pincus points out, the expected action of ovarian estrogen as a promoter of female reproductive tract growth and of estrous behavior is accompanied by many activities outside of the reproductive sphere. Estrogens are hair- and bone-growth regulators; they are thymolytic, mitogenetic in the epidermis, enzyme-inhibitory in the adrenal cortex, phagocyte-stimulating, alkalosis-inducing, tumorigenic, antigoitrogenic and antihyperglycemic. Similar multiplicities of action may be listed for most of the known hormones.

We can readily note that the hormones vary tremendously in chemical composition and in biologic activity. They are united only by their definition as internal secretions.

Over fifty biologically active substances circulate continuously in the blood of mammals as hormones; yet, with few exceptions, these substances are not essential for life. In the rat, for example, neither thyroidectomy, gonadectomy nor hypophysectomy is fatal. Yet after such operations the rates of certain processes are reduced to a minimum and cannot be speeded up if the need arises. Although animals with inadequate hormone balance may live, their mental and physical vigor, their adaptability and drive, are gone or reduced. The mental dullness of the hypothyroid person is a good example of the influence of hormonal defect on the optimal rate of living.

Much experimental work has been done on the symptom-complex production as a result of the removal of one or more endocrine glands. Studies after the injection of the active principle of one or more of the endocrine glands, either into an intact animal or into an animal from which an endocrine gland or glands had previously been removed, have added tremendously to the literature on the mode of action of the hormones. In addition, the treatment of human symptoms indicating a deficiency of a particular hormone with the hormone preparation has added much to our knowledge of endocrinology.

With the accelerating increase of literature on the physiology and biochemistry of the hormones, any attempt to review the field would be overwhelming for both the writer and the reader. We will, therefore, restrict our observations to the oral pathology of the disturbances in hormone metabolism.

THE PITUITARY GROUP OF HORMONES

The pituitary is considered the master gland of the body. Harvey Cushing's admirable words adequately describe its function. He stated, "Here in this well-concealed spot, almost to be covered by a thumb nail, lies the very mainspring of primitive existence, vegetative, emotional and reproductive."

The pituitary consists of an anterior lobe and a posterior lobe. The anterior lobe is derived from Rathke's pouch and is therefore epithelial in origin. The posterior lobe develops from the floor of the third ventricle and is composed of nervous tissue. The anterior lobe is glandular in structure and is the active part of the organ. To date, at least six hormones have been identified as coming from the anterior pituitary: the somatotropic, the thyrotropic, the adrenocorticotropic, two gonadotropic and the lactogenic

hormones. In addition, the anterior lobe is said to have ketogenic, anti-insulin, diabetogenic, parathyrogenic and pancreatotropic activity. Removal of the pituitary gland brings the entire internal secretory system into discordance because of a progressive atrophy of all the endocrine glands except, possibly, the parathyroids.

Although the physiologic activity of the posterior lobe has never been proved, extracts of this lobe have a remarkably high pharmacologic potency. Three types of activity, vasoconstrictive, oxytocic and antidiuretic, have been reported.

Experiments in which the pituitary is removed or in which crude extracts of the gland are injected can give little information about which particular hormone is responsible for the effects observed. Precise information can be obtained only by studying the response of an animal to purified hormones. As yet, this approach has not been thoroughly carried out for dental effects. The evidence indicates that the growth hormone is mainly responsible for the effects of pituitary extracts on teeth, but that the thyrotropic hormone also plays a role. The entire spectrum of human growth hormone has been reviewed by Root.

A few workers have studied the relation of the pituitary gland to dental development, notably Schour and Van Dyke and Baume, Becks and associates. Working with rats, they found that after hypophysectomy there was a progressive retardation of eruption of the incisor tooth, which eventually ceased to erupt. The tooth attained only about two-thirds normal size and showed a distortion of form, especially at the basal end. When an extract of the anterior lobe of the pituitary was injected into the hypophysectomized rats, the eruption rate of the incisor tooth returned to normal.

Becks and his associates pointed out that the only constant pathognomonic sign of hypophysectomy in the rat was a thickening of the dentinal walls at the expense of the pulp chamber (Fig. 12–19). Baume and his associates reported that amelogenesis, and particularly the activities of the odontogenic epithelium, depended directly on the secretion of the anterior pituitary, whereas dentinogenesis and cementogenesis were able to proceed at a depressed rate without the pituitary hormones. They also pointed out some interesting interrelations. They suggested that the histologic changes in the enamel organ of the incisors of hypophysectomized rats were comparable to those of thyroidectomized animals of an equal postoperative interval. They also called attention to the simi-

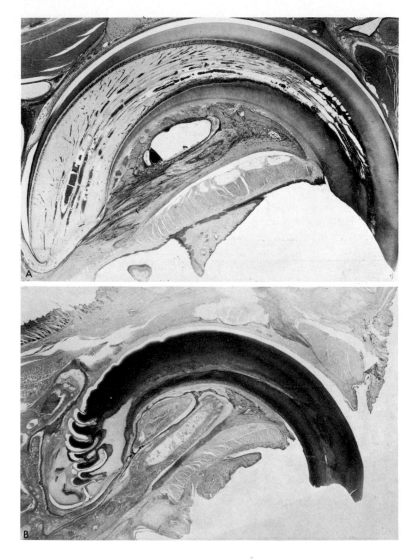

Figure 12–19. *Hypophysectomy.* Photomicrographs of a maxillary incisor tooth of a normal rat (*A*) and of a hypophysectomized rat (*B*). (Courtesy of Dr. Herman Becks.)

larity of the folding of the apical third of the incisor tooth of hypophysectomized animals to the changes in the teeth of magnesium-deficient animals, and they suggested that the changes in hypophysectomy may be related to salt and mineral metabolism, thus implicating the adrenal gland and its mineralocorticoids.

Collins and co-workers showed that the chronic administration of pure growth hormone to hypophysectomized animals allowed the incisors to erupt, but at only half the normal rate. The ameloblasts showed evidence of atrophy, but the dentin formed at a rate of 10 microns instead of the normal 16 microns per day. Baume and his associates injected thyroxin into hypophysectomized animals, either alone or with purified growth hormone. Their findings led them to the following explanation. The pituitary gland influences eruption not only with its thyrotropin, but also with its growth hormone. The effects of thyroxin on dental growth and development are quantitatively and qualitatively different from those of the pituitary growth hormone. Quantitatively, thyroxin is the factor which stimulates eruptive movement and tooth size, but it has little influence on alveolar growth. Growth hormone, on the other hand, spurs dental as well as alveolar growth, but has little effect on eruption rate. It is also possible that other endocrine organs, by virtue of their effects on metabolic interrelations, also affect tooth development and eruption.

Hypopituitarism

In man, some indication of the role played by the pituitary in the development of the oral tissues can be gained from studies of hypopituitarism as well as hyperpituitarism.

Clinical Features. The typical evidences of hypopituitarism resulting in pituitary dwarfism are a diminutive but well-proportioned body, fine, silky, sparse hair on the head and other hairy regions, wrinkled atrophic skin and, often, hypogonadism. The deficiency may be congenital, or it may be due to a destructive disease of the pituitary, such as an infarct occurring before puberty. There is no distinctive pattern to the basal metabolism in this disease.

In pituitary dwarfs the eruption rate and the shedding time of the teeth are delayed, as is the growth of the body in general. The clinical crowns appear smaller than normal because, even though eruption does occur, it is not complete. The dental arch is smaller than normal and therefore cannot accommodate all the teeth, so that a malocclusion develops. The anatomic crowns of the teeth in pituitary dwarfism are not noticeably smaller than normal, contrary to what might be expected in light of the animal experiments. Still, there are no reports of a careful statistical study of crown size in dwarfism. The roots of the teeth are shorter than normal in dwarfism, and the supporting structures are retarded in growth. The osseous development of the maxilla is not as retarded as that of the mandible.

Hypopituitarism in the adult is usually due to an infarction of the pituitary called Simmonds' disease. It is characterized by loss of weight and diminished sexual function. The basal metabolic rate is markedly lowered, and since Simmonds' disease represents a panhypopituitarism, there is a decrease in the activity of the many hormones of the pituitary gland and of those glands that are under pituitary regulation. In this disease the skin shows atrophic alterations. Changes in the head include thin eyebrows, loss of eyelashes, sharp features, thin lips and an immobile expression. No specific dental changes have been described in Simmonds' disease.

Hyperpituitarism

An increase in the number of granules in the acidophilic cells or an adenoma of the anterior lobe of the pituitary is associated with gigantism or acromegaly. If the increase occurs before the epiphyses of the long bones are closed, gigantism results; if the increase occurs later in life, i.e., after epiphyseal closure, acromegaly develops.

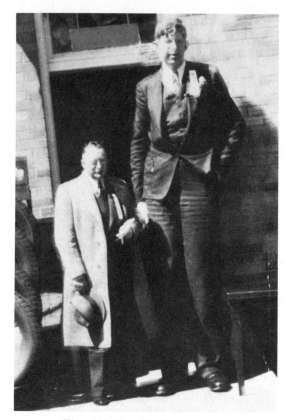

Figure 12–20. *Pituitary gigantism.*
This patient was 8 feet 6 inches tall and weighed over 425 pounds.

Clinical Features. Gigantism is characterized by a general symmetric overgrowth of the body, some persons with this disturbance attaining a height of over 8 feet (Fig. 12–20). Later in life such people usually show genital underdevelopment and excessive perspiration, and they complain of headache, lassitude, fatigue, muscle and joint pains and hot flashes.

The teeth in gigantism are proportional to the size of the jaws and the rest of the body. The roots may be longer than normal.

Acromegaly is a relatively rare disease in which there is hypersecretion by the anterior lobe, the influence being effected after ossification is complete. The following symptoms occur in acromegaly: temporal headaches, photophobia and reduction in vision. The terminal phalanges of the hands and feet become large. The ribs also increase in size.

The lips become thick and Negroid. The tongue also becomes enlarged and shows indentations on the sides from pressure against the teeth. Microscopically, the surface epithelium and the connective tissues are hyperplastic.

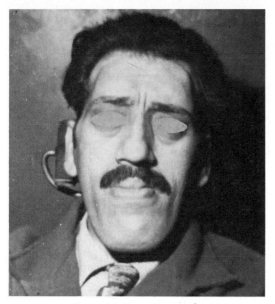

Figure 12–21. *Acromegaly.*
The patient shows the typical facies of the acromegalic. (Courtesy of Dr. E. V. Zegarelli.)

The mandible, because of accelerated condylar growth, becomes large. The resulting prognathism may be extreme, giving the head a typical acromegalic appearance (Fig. 12–21). The teeth in the mandible are usually tipped to the buccal or labial side, owing to the enlargement of the tongue.

THYROID HORMONE

Administration of thyroid gland or its derivatives, including thyroxin, causes an increased uptake of oxygen by the body as a whole. The precise cellular and enzymatic mechanism for its effect is not known. It is probably not due to increased glycolysis. In addition to increasing oxygenation, the thyroid hormone influences a variety of other actions which affect almost every other function and tissue of the mammalian body. It therefore plays an essential role in differentiation, growth, maturation, water balance, electrolyte balance, protein storage, carbohydrate and lipid metabolism, and other physiologic functions.

Calcitonin, a hypoglycemic polypeptide secreted by the "C" cells of the ultimobranchial elements of the thyroid gland, has gained increasing attention in recent years. It has been isolated, identified, sequenced and, more recently, synthesized. Calcitonin is responsive to hypercalcemia and acts to lower the plasma calcium level. Another of its actions is to inhibit resorption of bone mineral. Its use in human disease is still under active investigation. Excellent reviews of this hormone have been published by Foster, by Hirsch and Munson and by Rasmussen and Pechet.

Hypothyroidism

A failure of thyrotropic function on the part of the pituitary gland or an atrophy or destruction of the thyroid gland per se leads to an inability of the thyroid to produce sufficient hormone to meet the requirements of the body. If this failure occurs in infancy, cretinism results. If it occurs in the child, juvenile myxedema occurs; if in the adult, myxedema results. Myxedema is not a rare disease. Hospital records show that 4 to 8 of every 10,000 admissions enter with myxedema.

Clinical Features. Congenital hypothyroidism, or cretinism, leads to mental defects, retarded somatic growth, generalized edema and other changes, depending on the severity of the deficiency of thyroid hormone. The dentofacial changes in cretinism are also related to the degree of thyroid deficiency. Usually the base of the skull is shortened, leading to a retraction of the bridge of the nose with flaring. The face is wide and fails to develop in a longitudinal direction. The mandible is underdeveloped, and the maxilla is overdeveloped. The hair is sparse and brittle; the fingernails are brittle, and the sweat glands are atrophic.

The dental changes in juvenile hypothyroidism have been reviewed by Hinrichs, who also presented 36 cases. He indicated that the longer the time between the onset of the disease and the institution of treatment, the greater is the likelihood that the developing dentition will be affected. However, with a few exceptions, he found no striking morphologic changes in the teeth of the patients in his series.

Characteristically, the tongue is enlarged by edema fluid. It may protrude continuously, and such protrusion may lead to malocclusion. The eruption rate of the teeth is delayed, and the deciduous teeth are retained beyond the normal shedding time. Myxedema, the disease produced by thyroid deficiency in adults or children, is usually caused by atrophy of the thyroid gland of unknown etiology. The metabolic rate is lowered, although this finding should not be used as a diagnostic test for myxedema. Concentration of serum protein-bound iodine and radioactive iodine uptake or excretion studies are the diagnostic tests of value.

The myxedematous swelling is probably an extravascular, extracellular accumulation of water and protein in the tissues. The protein has a greater osmotic effect than the serum proteins, accounting for the increased blood protein concentration and decreased plasma volume which are found in myxedema.

The clinical orofacial findings in myxedematous patients are apparently limited to the soft tissues of the face and mouth. The lips, nose, eyelids and suborbital tissues are edematous and swollen. The tongue is large and edematous, frequently interfering with speech.

Hyperthyroidism

There is apparently some debate as to whether hyperthyroidism should be considered a single disease entity or should be subdivided into several types. Boothby and Plummer described two fundamentally different types of hyperthyroidism: (1) exophthalmic goiter, characterized by diffuse hyperplasia of the thyroid and by eye signs, and (2) toxic adenoma, in which hyperfunction originates in a benign tumor of the thyroid gland. In either case, we are concerned with the manifestations of excess circulating thyroid hormone.

Most of the symptoms of hyperthyroidism are due to an increased metabolic activity of the tissues of the body. This is usually manifested as an increased basal metabolic rate. The serum protein-bound iodine concentration is elevated. The urinary iodine excretion is reduced because of the increased iodine uptake by the thyroid gland.

Clinical Features. Alveolar atrophy occurs in advanced cases. In children, shedding of the deciduous teeth occurs earlier than normal, and eruption of the permanent teeth is greatly accelerated.

Patients suffering from hyperthyroidism usually present a facial expression of surprise or excitement, with wide-eyed staring. Such patients are nervous and highly emotional; they have increased sensitivity to epinephrine and are usually hypertensive. Thoma warns that they make very poor dental patients.

GONADAL HORMONES

Little is known of the relation of disturbances of metabolism of the sex hormones to oral pathology. Some evidence suggests that certain imbalances of estrogenic hormones might be reflected in the oral mucosa. In some women a gingivitis occurs periodically with abnormal or difficult menstruation. During the menopause the oral epithelium is said to become thinner than normal. In some patients a burning sensation of the tongue occurs during or after the menopause, while in other patients a "dry feeling" of the mouth is observed with or without an actual diminution of saliva.

Shafer and Muhler demonstrated a diminution in size and in number of granular tubules in the submaxillary glands of rats after either gonadectomy or the administering of estrogenic substances. Much further work is necessary to clarify the effects of the sex hormones on the oral and dental tissues.

PARATHYROID HORMONE

Two well-defined clinical entities are associated with the parathyroid glands: hyperparathyroidism, which manifests its symptoms primarily in the bones and the kidneys, and hypoparathyroid tetany.

Primary Hyperparathyroidism

Primary hyperparathyroidism is a disease in which the parathyroid glands elaborate an excessive quantity of parathyroid hormone. This increased activity is usually due to an adenoma of one or more of the four parathyroid glands, to a hyperplasia of the parathyroid tissue or, rarely, to a functional carcinoma of the parathyroid. The role of the parathyroid tumor in primary hyperparathyroidism has been discussed by Lloyd.

Parathyroid hormone is known to be a protein with a molecular weight of approximately 9500. It consists of a single polypeptide chain and contains no cysteine. It can be partially hydrolyzed without losing biologic activity so that there may be an active "core." The hormone has been crystallized but, as yet, not synthesized.

The bone disturbances in hyperparathyroidism vary from vague to roentgenographically characteristic lesions and even gross clinical evidence of bone lesions. Hypercalcemia may be manifested by poor muscle tone and decreased neuromuscular excitability.

Clinical Features. Hyperparathyroidism is a relatively rare disease which is said to be three times as common in women as in men. It usually affects people of middle age, but it may occur in childhood or in later life. In contrast to these statistics, Silverman and his co-workers, who reviewed 42 consecutive dentulous patients with hyperparathyroidism, found no correlation between sex and age and any aspect of the disease. Pathologic fracture may be the first symptom of the disease, although bone pain and joint stiffness are frequently early symptoms. In Silverman's group the most common significant early clinical finding was urinary tract stone, which occurred in 33 of the 42 patients. Occasionally the first sign of the disease may be a giant cell tumor or a "cyst" of the jaw. The effects of the disease on bone are of special interest to dentists. Almost all patients with hyperparathyroidism have skeletal lesions, some of which may occur in the skull or jaws. The loss of phosphorus and calcium in this disturbance results in a generalized osteoporosis with abortive attempts at bone repair and new bone formation. The new bone may be resorbed, and the resorption may lead eventually to pseudocyst formation, the extent of which depends on the duration and intensity of the disease. According to Schour and Massler, malocclusion caused by a sudden drifting with definite spacing of the teeth may be one of the first signs of the disease. An extensive review and discussion of this disease was published by Teng and Nathan.

Roentgenographic Features. The roentgenographic findings in this disease are of particular importance. The bones of affected persons show a general radiolucency as compared with those of normal people. Later, sharply defined round or oval radiolucent areas develop, which may be lobulated (Fig. 12–22). If such a lobulated

lesion develops in the mandible, it must be carefully differentiated from ameloblastoma, which frequently has the same appearance.

Small cystic areas may be seen in the calvarium, and large and/or small sharply defined radiolucencies may be present in the maxilla and/or mandible (Fig. 12–23). These small cystic areas must be differentiated from the lesions of multiple myeloma and eosinophilic granuloma. In the jaws, the bone roentgenogram in hyperparathyroidism has been described as having a "ground-glass" appearance. The lamina dura around the teeth may be partially lost (Fig. 12–24). Twenty of Silverman's 42 patients had normal dental radiograms, and 17 showed intact lamina dura but abnormal appearing alveolar bone. None showed complete loss of lamina dura, and only five showed partial loss.

Histologic Features. Histologic findings in the bone lesions of hyperparathyroidism are not pathognomonic of the disease, but are of considerable assistance in making the diagnosis. The most characteristic change in the bone is an osteoclastic resorption of the trabeculae of the spongiosa and along the blood vessels in the haversian system of the cortex. In the areas of resorption one also finds many plump osteoblasts lining islands of osteoid. Fibrosis, especially of the marrow spaces, is marked. The fibroblasts replace resorbed trabeculae, and in the fibrotic islands there is recent and old hemorrhage, with much hemosiderin in evidence. As the disease progresses, "osteoclastomas" develop, characterized by masses of fibroblasts growing in a loose syncytium, among which are numerous capillaries and endothelium-lined blood spaces, red blood cells, many areas of yellow or brown hemosiderin and innumerable multinucleated giant cells. These

Figure 12–22. *Primary hyperparathyroidism.*
The circumscribed radiolucent defect in the proximal end of the tibia was accompanied by multiple lesions of other bones, including the jaws.

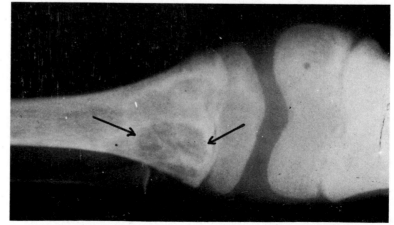

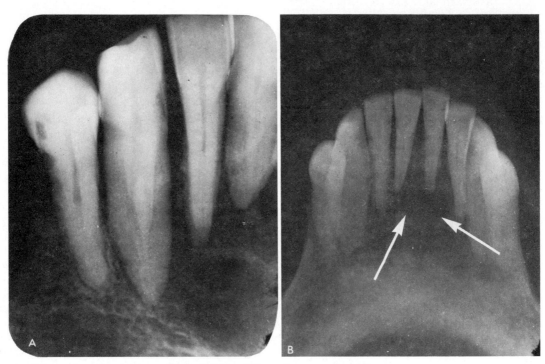

Figure 12–23. *Primary hyperparathyroidism.*
The periapical radiolucencies could be mistaken for apical infection. (Courtesy of Dr. Charles A. Waldron.)

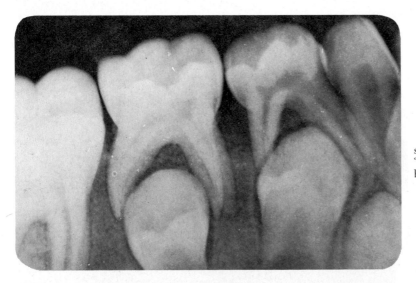

Figure 12–24.
Hyperparathyroidism.
The roentgenogram shows absence of the lamina dura and "ground-glass" appearance of the bone.

latter lesions are indistinguishable microscopically from the central giant cell granuloma of bone. Therefore, any patient who has a lesion diagnosed as a central giant cell lesion should be evaluated medically to rule out the possibility of hyperparathyroidism. This is most easily accomplished by a serum calcium level determination. If hyperparathyroidism is present, the serum calcium will be elevated above the normal level of 9 to 12 mg./dl.

Treatment and Prognosis. Excision of the parathyroid tumor will cure the patient. Careful examination of all parathyroid glands at the time of surgery should be carried out since multiple tumors occur with some frequency. Furthermore, since multiple tumors may develop over an extended period of time, patients who have had one parathyroid tumor should be followed for life.

Secondary Hyperparathyroidism

Hyperparathyroidism can also occur secondary to other disorders, the most common being end-stage renal disease. Massry and co-workers reported an incidence of hyperparathyroidism in patients with chronic renal failure ranging from 18 per cent after one year on dialysis to 92 per cent after more than two years. Giant cell lesions were not reported until 1963, however, by Fordham and Williams. Thirty patients undergoing chronic hemodialysis were studied by Spolnik and his associates, and 22 (73 per cent) of these were found to have roentgenographic evidence of bone disease involving the jaws, including 7 "brown tumors" (four in one patient) with loss of lamina dura also a prominent finding.

Hypoparathyroidism

Elimination of the parathyroid glands—by surgical removal, by destruction due to thrombosis of the blood vessels or disease of the glands, or in rare cases by congenital absence—leads to hypoparathyroidism. The disease is characterized metabolically by a decreased excretion of calcium. The blood chemistry shows a low concentration of serum calcium and a high concentration of serum phosphorus. If the calcium level of the serum falls to 7 to 8 mg./dl., there is increased neuromuscular excitability, which must be elicited, since it is not manifest. When the serum calcium level falls to 5 to 6 mg./dl., tetany and the characteristic carpopedal spasms are apparent.

Albright and Strock observed aplasia or hypoplasia of the teeth when hypoparathyroidism developed before the teeth were entirely formed. Similar changes are reported by Frensilli and his associates (Fig. 12–25).

Chronic candidosis, which is refractory to antifungal therapy such as nystatin, is sometimes seen in cases of idiopathic hypoparathyroidism. Such a case has been reported and discussed by Greenberg and his associates. The candidosis usually develops very early in life and precedes the hypocalcemia. The exact relationship between these two occurrences is not clear but it has been suggested that the *Candida* infection may cause the hypoparathyroidism by inducing an "immune response." Enamel hy-

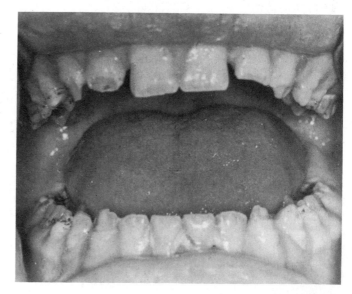

Figure 12–25. *Hypoparathyroidism.* The patient, demonstrating enamel hypoplasia, suffered from hypoparathyroidism in infancy. (Courtesy of Dr. E. V. Zegarelli.)

poplasia frequently accompanies this "syndrome."

Pseudohypoparathyroidism is a condition resembling idiopathic hypoparathyroidism in all respects, including the hypocalcemia and hyperphosphatemia, the drug-refractory candidosis and the enamel hypoplasia, except that parathyroid extract has little or no effect in correcting the hypocalcemia. This disease has been discussed by Croft and his co-workers.

ADRENAL HORMONES

A little over one hundred years ago (1855), Addison published his classic report on chronic adrenal cortical insufficiency, which is still called Addison's disease. Only in the last twenty-five years has it been recognized that the adrenal cortex, as such, plays the essential role in maintaining life. In that period, however, many substances have been isolated from the adrenal cortex, and intensive studies of the physiologic activity of adrenal cortical steroids are still being made. Much has been learned about the adrenal cortex, but much is still unknown. When the final story is written, we shall probably find that most of the metabolic interrelations in human physiology are mediated through the adrenals.

The action of the medullary portion of the adrenal gland is ascribed to epinephrine and norepinephrine. Norepinephrine may be a precursor of epinephrine, and for practical purposes one may consider the action of the hormones of the adrenal medulla to be that of epinephrine. Its effect on the various tissues of the body is similar to that of sympathetic nervous system stimulation. Increased amounts of epinephrine in the body lead to an elevated basal metabolism, mediated through its effect on liver and on carbohydrate metabolism rather than on the thyroid gland.

The effects of epinephrine and norepinephrine on the circulatory system have been extensively studied. Epinephrine in physiologic doses (1 mcg./kg.) causes a constriction of the arterioles and capillaries of the skin, mucous membranes and abdominal viscera, but a dilatation of the vessels of skeletal and heart muscle. The net result is a rise in blood pressure due to a sufficient vasoconstriction of the end capillaries and small arterioles of the skin and other organs. Epinephrine also relaxes the smooth muscles of the stomach, intestine, bronchioles and wall of the urinary bladder, while

it excites the muscles of the gallbladder, ureter and sphincters of the intestine. Recent studies have shown that under controlled conditions epinephrine acts as an over-all vasodilator drug and a powerful cardiac stimulant, while norepinephrine in comparable doses acts as an over-all vasoconstrictor substance.

The formation and liberation of the adrenal cortical steroids appear to be dependent upon the action of the pituitary adrenocorticotropic hormone (ACTH). At least six adrenal cortical steroids have been identified, and several unknown factors have been observed. Those identified are corticosterone, 17-hydroxycorticosterone, 17-hydroxyprogesterone, 11-dehydrocorticosterone, 11-desoxycorticosterone and 17-hydroxy-11-dehydrocorticosterone (cortisone). These steroids are intimately concerned with carbohydrate metabolism, mineral metabolism, protein and fat metabolism and fluid and electrolyte balance.

So much work is being done at this time on the metabolic influences of the adrenal cortex that almost anything written now will soon be obsolete. What little we know about the cortical hormones of the adrenal gland as they relate to oral pathology is summarized below.

Acute Insufficiency of the Adrenal Cortex

Acute adrenal cortical insufficiency is relatively rare. It usually occurs in connection with an acute septicemia and is called Waterhouse-Friderichsen syndrome. This disease occurs primarily in children, but it also occurs in adults. It is characterized by a rapidly fulminating septic course, a pronounced purpura and death within 48 to 72 hours. Meningococci, streptococci and pneumococci are the organisms most often responsible for the disease. At autopsy the conspicuous change seen is bilateral adrenal hemorrhage (Fig. 12–26).

The use of antibiotics and cortisone has changed the course of the disease from its usual fatal termination to recovery in some cases.

Chronic Insufficiency of the Adrenal Cortex: Addison's Disease

Modern medicine can add little to the description of the disease reported by Addison in 1855. Clinically, the disease is characterized by a bronzing of the skin, a pigmentation of the mucous membranes (Fig. 12–27), feeble heart action, general debility, vomiting, diarrhea and severe anemia. The pale brown to deep choco-

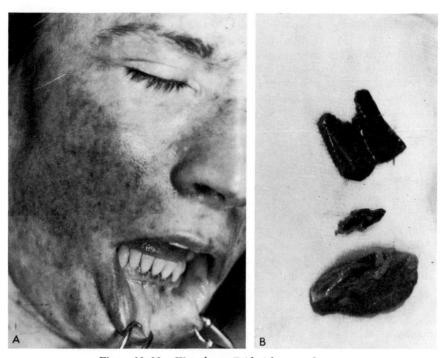

Figure 12–26. *Waterhouse-Friderichsen syndrome.*
There are petechial hemorrhages and purpura in the skin and oral mucosa (A). The adrenal glands are hemorrhagic (B).

Figure 12–27. *Addison's disease.*
There is pigmentation of the lips and oral mucosa. (Courtesy of Dr. Stephen F. Dachi.)

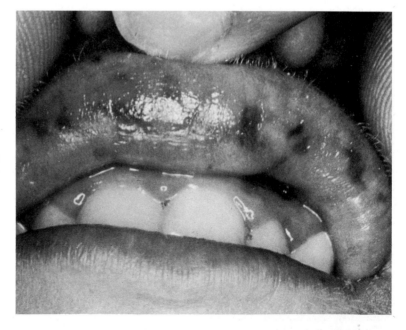

late pigmentation of the oral mucosa, spreading over the buccal mucosa from the angles of the mouth and/or developing on the gingiva, tongue and lips, may be the first evidence of the disease.

The diagnosis of Addison's disease is based on the clinical signs as well as on characteristic changes in the blood sodium and chloride levels. Biopsy of the oral lesions shows acanthosis with silver-positive granules in the cells of the stratum germinativum.

Hyperfunction of the Adrenal Gland

Adrenogenital Syndrome. A condition known as the adrenogenital syndrome results when hyperplasia or tumors of the adrenal cortex occur. Depending on the age at onset and the sex of the person affected, the clinical signs are pseudohermaphroditism, sexual precocity and virilism in women or feminization in men. If the disease begins early, premature eruption of the teeth may occur.

Cushing's Syndrome. This syndrome is a result of hormonal excess resulting from any of the following: (1) hyperplastic adrenal cortices without any other clinically evident endocrine lesion; (2) adrenal cortical adenoma or carcinoma; (3) ectopically located adrenal-like tumor, for example, of an ovary; (4) ACTH-secreting tumor of the anterior pituitary associated with adrenal cortical hyperplasia; or (5) nonpituitary carcinoma, for example, of a lung or the pancreas, with secretion of an ACTH-like material that induces adrenal cortical hyperplasia. When the syndrome is associated with spontaneous bilateral adrenal hyperplasia, it is referred to as Cushing's disease. In adults, it is recognized that Cushing's disease represents approximately 75 per cent of the cases of Cushing's syndrome. While Cushing's disease is uncommon in children, McArthur and his associates have reported a series of 13 cases in patients under the age of 15 years. The pathogenesis of this disease has been reviewed by Hunder.

It is characterized by a rapidly acquired adiposity about the upper portion of the body, mooning of the face, a tendency to become round-shouldered and develop a "buffalo hump" at the base of the neck, alteration in hair distribution, a dusky plethoric appearance with formation of purple striae, muscular weakness, vascular hypertension, glycosuria not controlled by insulin, and albuminuria.

The oral pathologist's primary concern with this peculiar disease state lies in the bone changes. In children there may be osteoporosis and premature cessation of epiphyseal growth, while in adults there is a severe osteoporosis.

The mechanism for the bone changes is not well understood. Apparently, 11-desoxycorticosterone is relatively unimportant in the pathogenesis of Cushing's syndrome. Albright's explanation for the pathogenesis of the disease is based on the S-F-N (sugar-fat-nitrogen) hormone group of steroids in which the "N" hormone is considered an anabolic one, stimulating osteogenesis and causing closure of the epiphysis, and the "S" hormone is considered an antianabolic one. The mechanism of osteoporosis is then explained on the basis of an excess of "S" hormone, leading to a retardation of osteoblastic activity and reduction in matrix formation.

We appreciate the fact that a number of complex interrelations are concerned in the normal and abnormal control of bone growth and maturation. Considerable interest is now centering on these interrelations and on the precise metabolic or endocrine pathways by which particular hormones influence skeletal growth. Little definite evidence on these topics exists as yet, but some information is available on the effects of cortisone on bone growth. For example, Follis showed that cortisone injections in rats produced retardation and arrest of and interference with resorption of bone. In other species, only retardation of bone growth was found.

Fraser and Fainstat demonstrated that in certain strains of mice the injection of cortisone into pregnant females produced a high percentage of cleft palates in the offspring. This effect was not due primarily to the inhibition of growth, since cleft palate was produced even when the cortisone was administered after the palate had already closed. Doig and Coltman reported several cases of cleft palate in children born of mothers who conceived while receiving injections of cortisone or who received injections of cortisone during the first three months of pregnancy. Obviously, more work is needed in this field before definite conclusions can be drawn.

Stress and the "Adaptation Syndrome"

The extensive studies of Hans Selye have done much to stimulate thinking and research in the area of "stress" and the adrenal gland. He formulated a theory of response to prolonged stress as a part of the individual's adaptative mechanism which may lead to clinical signs and symptoms called the "general adaptation syndrome." At present the theory is a controversial one, and much research is being done to clarify the points of controversy.

Any wasting disease produces atrophy of the adrenal cortex and loss of adrenal lipid. The mechanism for this finding is not known. Selye states that the adrenal changes are due to prolonged stress, with mobilization of lipids and ultimate exhaustion atrophy of the cortical cells. Apparently the hormones of the adrenal cortex are necessary for cellular enzymes to catalyze the energy-producing processes of cells. All "stressor" agents, such as cold, heat and trauma, increase the metabolic demands of the organism and stimulate adrenocortical function through

stimulation of the pituitary to secrete ACTH. If the stress is continued, the pituitary and the adrenal cortex produce excessive amounts of hormones to increase resistance. Eventually pathologic changes occur in those tissues which respond to the hormonal stimulation, and the diseases of adaptation (hypertension, periarteritis nodosa, and others) result.

Since there is a considerable amount of evidence against Selye's theory, and since the entire field of adrenal mechanisms in pathologic processes is in a state of flux, only a brief résumé of Selye's theory will be presented. The reader is directed to Selye's original papers (1946, 1948) and to the excellent critical review by Sayers (1950) for a more comprehensive coverage of the subject.

Selye states that the "stressed" person passes through a succession of stages. The first is the "alarm reaction," which consists of a shock phase and then a countershock phase. The next is the "adaptation stage," in which his resistance to the original stressor is greater, but his resistance to other stressor agents is lowered. If the stressor is continued, he eventually enters a stage of exhaustion and dies. If the stressor is removed, he enters a stage of convalescence and recovers. Figure 12–28 shows diagrammatically the control of adrenocortical activity.

Many people are receiving large doses of cortisone for the treatment of various diseases. We must remember that cortisone interferes with formation of granulation tissue, proliferation of fibroblasts and production of ground substance. Since these tissues and cellular products are essential to wound healing, it is important to recognize that surgery is hazardous in hyperadrenocorticism.

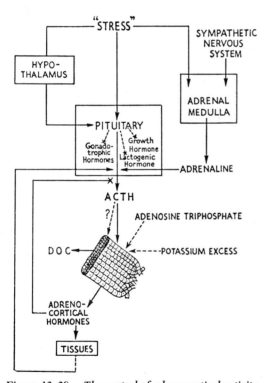

Figure 12–28. *The control of adrenocortical activity.*
Stress may act on the pituitary or through the hypothalamus to stimulate the secretion of ACTH at the expense of other pituitary hormones. ACTH stimulates the zona fasciculata and zona reticularis, though possibly not the zona glomerulosa, which may secrete DOC independently. The level of adrenocortical hormones in the blood controls the rate of production of ACTH. Rapid utilization of cortical hormones by the tissues lowers the blood level of cortical hormones and thus stimulates ACTH production. Adrenaline (epinephrine) may also stimulate ACTH production, and adenosine triphosphate or potassium excess may stimulate the adrenal cortex. (From P. M. F. Bishop: Cameron's Recent Advances in Endocrinology. 7th ed. London, J. & A. Churchill, Ltd., 1954.)

PANCREATIC HORMONE: INSULIN

Diabetes Mellitus

Diabetes is a biochemical lesion, and though no complete correlation exists between the occurrence of the disease and histologically demonstrable changes in the pancreas, the role of insulin in the control of the disease and historical considerations make it legitimate to discuss diabetes in the section on the pancreas. Because recent investigations have shown that other endocrine organs play a role in its production, many writers consider diabetes mellitus more generally a disease of metabolism.

Diabetes is a disorder of carbohydrate metabolism characterized by hyperglycemia and glycosuria, reflecting a distortion in the equilibrium between utilization of glucose by the tissues, liberation of glucose by the liver and production-liberation of pancreatic, anterior pituitary and adrenocortical hormones. This metabolic disorder lowers tissue resistance to infection.

Because of the lowered tissue resistance, patients with untreated or inadequately controlled diabetes sometimes exhibit a fulminating periodontitis with periodontal abscess formation and inflamed, painful and even hermorrhagic gingival papillae. Bernick and co-workers studied a series of 50 diabetic children and found that gingivitis was increased; however, the rate of caries formation was not related to the duration of the disease. Lin and colleagues noted a significant thickening of the basement membranes of gingival vessels and proposed that gingival biopsies may be useful as an adjunct in the diagnosis of diabetes. Because of excessive fluid loss, diabetic patients commonly complain of dry mouth. Even minor oral surgery is contraindicated in uncontrolled diabetic patients. Vascular changes in the dental pulp, gingiva and periodontal ligament have been reported in diabetic patients by Russell.

Controlled diabetic patients should undergo dental operations only after consultation with the physician who is treating the patient. There are no oral manifestations of controlled diabetes mellitus.

Progeria

(Hutchinson-Gilford Syndrome)

Progeria is a very rare disease originally described by Hutchinson in 1886. It is of unknown etiology and is characterized by dwarfism and premature senility. It is thought to be transmitted as an autosomal recessive trait. The term itself means prematurely old. Progeria has been discussed in an article by DeBusk.

Clinical Features. Affected infants appear normal at birth, but the typical clinical features become manifest within the first few years. The patients all have an amazing resemblance to each other, exhibiting alopecia, pigmented areas of the trunk, atrophic skin, prominent veins and loss of subcutaneous fat. The individuals have a high-pitched, squeaky voice, a beaklike nose and a hypoplastic mandible. Coxa valga is also a constant feature, as is severe atherosclerosis. Exophthalmos may be present, as may muscular atrophy and joint deformities.

The intelligence of individuals with this disease is generally either normal or above normal. Even at a very early age, the patient resembles a wizened little old person.

Oral Manifestations. The oral findings in progeria have been described by Gardner and Majka. These basically consist of the accelerated formation of irregular secondary dentin, apparently a manifestation of the premature aging process. Delayed eruption of teeth has also been reported by Wesley and colleagues.

Treatment and Prognosis. There is no treatment for this disease, and no patient with progeria has been reported living beyond the age of 27 years.

REFERENCES

Ainley, J. E.: Manifestations of familial hypophosphatemia. J. Endodont., 4:26, 1978.

Albright, F.: Cushing's syndrome: its pathological physiology, its relationship to the adrenogenital syndrome and its connection with the problem of the reaction of the body to injurious agents ("alarm reaction of Selye"). Harvey Lect. Series, 38:123, 1942–1943.

Albright, F., and Strock, M. S.: Association of a calcification of dentin with hypoparathyroidism in rats and cure of same with parathormone, with some correlated observations in man. J. Clin. Invest., 12:974, 1933.

Albright, F., Butler, A. M., and Bloomberg, E.: Rickets resistant to vitamin D therapy. Am. J. Dis. Child., 54:529, 1937.

Alfin-Slater, R., and Kritchevsky, D.: Human Nutrition: A Comprehensive Treatise. New York, Plenum Press, 1979.

Amstutz, H. C., and Carey, E. J.: Skeletal manifestations and treatment of Gaucher's disease. Review of twenty cases. J. Bone Joint Surg., 48-A:670, 1966.

Aponte-Merced, L., and Navia, J. M.: Pre-eruptive protein-energy malnutrition and acid solubility of rat molar enamel surfaces. Arch. Oral Biol., 25:701, 1980.

Archard, H. O., and Witkop, C. J., Jr.: Hereditary hypophosphatemia (vitamin D-resistant rickets) presenting primary dental manifestations. Oral Surg., 22:184, 1966.

Arcomano, J. P., Barnett, J. C., and Wunderlich, H. O.: Histiocytosis X. Am. J. Roentgenol., Radium Ther. Nucl. Med., 85:663, 1961.

Avioli, L. V., Lasersohn, J. T., and Lopresti, J. M.: Histiocytosis X (Schüller-Christian disease): a clinico-pathological survey, review of ten patients and the results of prednisone therapy. Medicine, 42:119, 1963.

Baratieri, A., Miani, C., and Sacchi, A.: A histochemical study of gingival hyperplasia in atypical mucopolysaccharidosis. Parodont. Acad. Rev., 4:163, 1968.

Batson, R., Shapiro, J., Christie, A., and Riley, H. D., Jr.: Acute nonlipid disseminated reticuloendotheliosis. Am. J. Dis. Child., 90:323, 1955.

Baume, L. J., Becks, H., and Evans, H. M.: Hormonal control of tooth eruption. III. The response of the incisors of hypophysectomized rats to growth hormone, thyroxin or the combination of both. J. Dent. Res., 33:104, 1954.

Baume, L. J., Becks, H., Ray, J. D., and Evans, H. M.: Hormonal control of tooth eruption. II. The effects of hypophysectomy on the upper rat incisor following progressively longer intervals. J. Dent. Res., 33:91, 1954.

Bavetta, L. A., and Bernick, S.: Lysine deficiency and dental structures. J. Am. Dent. Assoc., 50:427, 1955.

Bavetta, L. A., Bernick, S., Geiger, D., and Bergren, W.: The effect of tryptophane deficiency on the jaws of rats. J. Dent. Res., 33:309, 1954.

Becks, H., and Furuta, W. J.: Effects of magnesium deficient diets on oral and dental structures. I. Changes in the enamel epithelium. J. Am. Dent. Assoc., 26:883, 1939. II. Changes in the enamel structure. J. Am. Dent. Assoc., 28:1083, 1941. III. Changes in dentine and pulp tissue. Am. J. Orthod. Oral Surg., 28:1, 1942. IV. Changes in paradental bone structure. J. Dent. Res., 22:215, 1943.

Becks, H., Collins, D. A., Simpson, M. E., and Evans, H. M.: Changes in the central incisors of hypophysectomized female rats after different postoperative periods. Arch. Pathol., 41:457, 1946.

Bender, I. B.: Dental observations in Gaucher's disease. J. Dent. Res., 17:359, 1938.

Bernick, S., Bavetta, L. A., and Baker, R.: Histochemical and electron microscopy studies on tryptophane deficient dentin. J. Dent. Res., 34:671, 1955.

Bernick, S. M., Cohen, D. W., Baker, L., and Laster, L.: Dental disease in children with diabetes mellitus. J. Periodontol., 46:241, 1975.

Beumer, J., Trowbridge, H. O., Silverman, S., and Eisenberg, E.: Childhood hypophosphatasia and the premature loss of teeth. Oral Surg., 35:631, 1973.

Blackfan, K. D., and Wolbach, S. B.: Vitamin A deficiency in infants. A clinical and pathological study. J. Pediatr., 3:679, 1933.

Bodansky, M., and Bodansky, O.: Biochemistry of Disease. 2nd ed. New York, Macmillan Company, 1952.

Bondy, P. K., and Rosenberg, L. E.: Diseases of Metabolism. 8th ed. Philadelphia, W. B. Saunders Company, 1980.

Bongiovanni, A. M., Album, M. M., Root, A. W., Hope, J. W., Marino, J., and Spencer, D.: Studies on hypophosphatasia and response to high phosphate intake. Am. J. Med. Sci., 255:163, 1968.

Boothby, W. M., and Plummer, W. A.: Diseases of the thyroid gland. Oxford Med., 3:389, 1936.

Bourne, G. H., and Kidder, G. W.: Biochemistry and Physiology of Nutrition. New York, Academic Press, Inc., 1953.

Boyle, P. E.: Manifestations of vitamin A deficiency in a human tooth germ. J. Dent. Res., 13:39, 1933.

Idem: Kronfeld's Histopathology of the Teeth and Their Surrounding Structures. 3rd ed. Philadelphia, Lea & Febiger, 1949.

Boyle, P. E., Bessey, O. A., and Wolbach, S. B.: Experimental alveolar bone atrophy produced by ascorbic acid deficiency and its relation to pyorrhea alveolaris. Proc. Soc. Exp. Biol. Med., 36:733, 1937.

Boyle, P. E., Wolbach, S. B., and Bessey, O. A.: Histopathology of teeth of guinea pigs in acute and chronic vitamin C deficiency. J. Dent. Res., 15:331, 1936.

Brady, R. O.: The sphingolipidoses. N. Engl. J. Med., 275:312, 1966.

Brady, R. O., Pentchev, P. G., Gal, A. E., Hibbert, S. R., and Dekeban, A. S.: Replacement therapy for inherited enzyme deficiency: use of purified glucocerebrosidase in Gaucher's disease. N. Engl. J. Med., 291:989, 1974.

Brittain, J. M., Oldenberg, T. R., and Burkes, E. J.: Odontohypophosphatasia: report of two cases. J. Dent. Child., 43:38, 1976.

Brownstein, M. H., and Helwig, E. B.: The cutaneous amyloidoses. I. Localized forms. Arch. Dermatol., 102:8, 1970.

Bruckner, R. J., Rickles, N. H., and Porter, D. R.: Hypophosphatasia with premature shedding of teeth and aplasia of cementum. Oral Surg., 15:1351, 1962.

Brunner, H.: Eosinophilic granuloma of mouth, pharynx, and nasal passages. Oral Surg., 4:623, 1951.

Buckle, R. M., Care, A. D., Cooper, C. W., and Gitelman, H. J.: The influence of plasma magnesium concentration on parathyroid hormone secretion. J. Endocrinol., 42:529, 1968.

Burk, R. F., Jr., Pearson, W. N., Wood, R. P., and Viteri, F.: Blood selenium levels and in vitro red blood cell uptake of 75-Se in kwashiorkor. Am. J. Clin. Nutr., 20:723, 1967.

Burns, J. J.: Biosynthesis of L-ascorbic acid; basic defect in scurvy. Am. J. Med., 26:740, 1959.

Campbell, H. A., Smith, W. K., Roberts, W. L., and Link, K. P.: Studies on the hemorrhagic sweet clover disease. II. The bioassay of hemorrhagic concentrates by following the prothrombin level in the plasma of rabbit blood. J. Biol. Chem., 138:1, 1941.

Catto, G. R. D., MacLeod, M., Pelc, B., and Kodicek, E.: 1-α-Hydroxycholecalciferol: a treatment for renal bone disease. Br. Med. J., 1:12, 1975.

Chambers, R. A., and Pratt, R. T. C.: Idiosyncrasy to fructose. Lancet, 2:340, 1956.

Chase, D. C., Eversole, L. R., and Hale, H. D.: Histiocytosis-X with jaw involvement. J. Oral Surg., 32:494, 1974.

Chawla, T. N., and Glickman, I.: Protein deprivation and the periodontal structures of the albino rat. Oral Surg., 4:578, 1951.

Cheyne, C.: Histiocytosis X. J. Bone Joint Surg., 53-B:366, 1971.

Christensen, J. F.: Three familial cases of atypical late rickets. Acta Paediatr. Scand., 28:247, 1940–41.

Cline, M. J., and Golde, D. W.: A review and reevaluation of the histiocytic disorders. Am. J. Med., 55:49, 1973.

Cohen, S., and Becker, G. L.: Origin, diagnosis and treatment of the dental manifestations of vitamin-D resistant rickets: review of the literature and report of case. J. Am. Dent. Assoc., 92:120, 1976.

Collins, D. A., Becks, H., Asling, C. W., Simpson, M. E., and Evans, H. M.: The growth of hypophysectomized female rats following chronic treatment with pure pituitary growth hormone. V. Skeletal changes: skull and dentition. Growth, 13:207, 1949.

Comar, C. L., and Bronner, F.: Mineral Metabolism. New York, Academic Press, Inc., 1960.

Cornblath, M., Rosenthal, I. M., Reisner, S. H., Wybregt, S. H., and Crone, R. K.: Hereditary fructose intolerance. New Engl. J. Med., 269:1271, 1963.

Crampton, E. W.: The growth of the odontoblasts of the incisor teeth as a criterion of the vitamin C intake of the guinea pig. J. Nutr., 33:491, 1947.

Croft, L. K., Witkop, C. J., Jr., and Glas, J. E.: Pseudohypoparathyroidism. Oral Surg., 20:758, 1965.

Cushing, H.: The Pituitary Body and Its Disorders. Philadelphia, J. B. Lippincott Company, 1912.

Dam, H.: Cholesterinstoffwechsel in Hühnereiern und Hühnehen. Biochem. Z., 215:475, 1929.

Dam, H., Schønheyder, F., and Tage-Hansen, E.: Studies on the mode of action of vitamin K. Biochem. J., 30:1075, 1936.

Daneshbod, K., and Kissane, J. M.: Idiopathic differentiated histiocytosis. Am. J. Clin. Pathol., 7:381, 1978.

Darrow, D. C.: Body-fluid physiology: the role of potassium in clinical disturbances of body water and electrolyte. N. Eng. J. Med., 242:978, 1014, 1950.

DeBusk, F. L.: The Hutchinson-Gilford Progeria syndrome. J. Pediatr., *80*:697, 1972.

Dinnerman, M.: Vitamin A deficiency in unerupted teeth of infants. Oral Surg., *4*:1024, 1951.

Di Orio, L. P., Miller, S. A., and Navia, J. M.: The separate effects of protein and calorie malnutrition on the development and growth of rat bones and teeth. J. Nutr., *103*:856, 1973.

Doig, R. K., and Coltman, O. M.: Cleft palate following cortisone therapy in early pregnancy. Lancet, *2*:730, 1956.

Drummond, J. C.: LIX: The nomenclature of the so-called accessory food factors (vitamins). Biochem. J., *14*:660, 1920.

Duncan, G. G.: Diseases of Metabolism. 4th ed. Philadelphia, W. B. Saunders Company, 1959.

Elder, G. H., Gray, C. H., and Nicholson, D. C.: The porphyrias: a review. J. Clin. Pathol., *25*:1013, 1972.

Enriquez, P., Dahlin, D. C., Hayles, A. B., and Henderson, E. D.: Histiocytosis X: a clinical study. Mayo Clin. Proc., *42*:88, 1967.

Epstein, C. J., Brady, R. O., Schneider, E. L., Bradley, R. M., and Shapiro, D.: In utero diagnosis of Niemann-Pick disease. Am. J. Hum. Genet., *23*:533, 1971.

Evans, H. M., and Bishop, K. S.: On the existence of a hitherto unrecognized dietary factory essential for reproduction. Science, *56*:650, 1922.

Farrell, P. M., and Bieri, J. G.: Megavitamin E. Supplementation in man. Am. J. Clin. Nutr., *28*:1381, 1975.

Federation Proceedings Conference: Hypovitaminosis A. Fed. Proc., *17*:103, 1958.

Fish, E. W., and Harris, L. J.: The effects of vitamin C deficiency on tooth structure in guinea pigs. Br. Dent. J., *58*:31, 1935.

Fletcher, P. D., Scopp, I. W., and Hersh, R. A.: Oral manifestations of secondary hyperparathyroidism related to long-term hemodialysis therapy. Oral Surg., *43*:218, 1977.

Follis, R. H., Jr.: The Pathology of Nutritional Disease. Springfield, Ill., Charles C Thomas, 1948.

Idem: Effect of cortisone on growing bones of the rat. Proc. Soc. Exp. Biol. Med., *76*:722, 1951.

Idem: Non-effect of cortisone on growing bones of mice, guinea pigs and rabbits. Proc. Soc. Exp. Biol. Med., *78*:723, 1951.

Idem: Deficiency Disease. Springfield, Ill., Charles C Thomas, 1958.

Food and Nutrition Board, National Academy of Sciences, National Research Council: Recommended Dietary Allowances, 9th rev. ed., Washington, D.C., 1980.

Fordham, C. C., and Williams, T. F.: Brown tumor and secondary hyperparathyroidism. N. Engl. J. Med., *269*:129, 1963.

Foster, G. V.: Calcitonin (thyrocalcitonin). N. Engl. J. Med., *279*:349, 1968.

Frandsen, A. M.: Experimental investigations of socket healing and periodontal disease in rats. Acta Odont. Scand., *21*(Suppl. 37):53, 1963.

Frandsen, A. M., Becks, H., Nelson, M. M., and Evans, H.: The effects of various levels of dietary protein on the periodontal tissues of young rats. J. Periodontol., *24*:135, 1953.

Franklin, E. C.: Amyloidosis. Bull. Rheum. Dis., *26*:832, 1975.

Fraser, F. C., and Fainstat, T. D.: Production of congenital defects in the offspring of pregnant mice treated with cortisone. Pediatrics, *8*:527, 1951.

Frazier, C. N., and Hu, C. K.: Cutaneous lesions associated with deficiency in vitamin A in man. Arch. Int. Med., *48*:507, 1931.

Frazier, C. N., and Hu, C. K.: Nature and distribution according to age of cutaneous manifestations of vitamin A deficiency: study of 207 cases. Arch. Derm. Syph., *33*:825, 1936.

Frensilli, J. A., and Hinrichs, E. H.: Dental changes of idiopathic hypoparathyroidism: report of three cases. J. Oral Surg., *29*:727, 1971.

Furman, K. I.: Acute hypervitaminosis A in an adult. Am. J. Clin. Nutr., *26*:575, 1973.

Galili, D., Yatziv, S., and Russell, A.: Massive gingival hyperplasia preceding dental eruption in I-cell disease. Oral Surg., *37*:533, 1974.

Gardner, D. G.: Metachromatic cells in the gingiva in Hurler's syndrome. Oral Surg., *26*:782, 1968.

Idem: The oral manifestations of Hurler's syndrome. Oral Surg., *32*:46, 1971.

Idem: The dental manifestations of the Morquio syndrome (Mucopolysaccharidosis Type IV). Am. J. Dis. Child., *129*:1445, 1975.

Gardner, D. G., and Majka, M.: The early formation of irregular secondary dentine in progeria. Oral Surg., *28*:877, 1969.

Gardner, D. G., and Zeman, W.: Biopsy of the dental pulp in the diagnosis of metachromatic leucodystrophy. Dev. Med. Child Neurol., *7*:620, 1965.

Gildenhorn, H. L., and Amromin, G. D.: Report of a case with Niemann-Pick disease: correlation of roentgenographic and autopsy findings. Am. J. Roentgenol., Radium Ther. Nucl. Med., *85*:680, 1961.

Glickman, I.: Acute vitamin C deficiency and the periodontal tissues. II. The effect of acute vitamin C deficiency upon the response of the periodontal tissues of the guinea pig to artificially induced inflammation. J. Dent. Res., *27*:201, 1948.

Goldberg, A.: The enzymatic formation of haem by the incorporation of iron in protoporphyrin; importance of ascorbic acid, ergothioneine and glutathione. Br. J. Haematol., *5*:150, 1959.

Goldman, H.: Experimental hyperthyroidism in guinea pigs. Am. J. Orthod. Oral Surg., *29*:665, 1943.

Idem: Report of histopathologic study of jaws of diet-deficiency in monkeys, and its relation to Vincent's infection. Am. J. Orthod. Oral Surg., *29*:480, 1943.

Goodhart, R. S., and Shils, M. E.: Modern Nutrition in Health and Disease. 6th ed. Philadelphia, Lea and Febiger, 1980.

Goodman, D. S.: Vitamin A and retinoids: Recent advances. Fed. Proc., *38*:2501, 1979.

Idem: Vitamin A metabolism. Fed. Proc., *39*:2716, 1980.

Gorlin, R. J.: Genetic disorders affecting mucous membranes. Oral Surg., *28*:512, 1969.

Graham, J. B., McFalls, V. W., and Winters, R. W.: Familial hypophosphatemia with vitamin D resistant rickets II. Three additional kindreds of sex-linked dominant type with a genetic analysis of four such families. Am. J. Hum. Genet., *11*:311, 1959.

Green, D. E.: Currents of Biochemical Research, New York, Interscience Publishers, Inc., 1956.

Greenberg, D. M. (ed.): Metabolic Pathways. Vol. I—Carbohydrates, Lipids, and Related Compounds. 3rd ed. New York, Academic Press, Inc., 1967.

Idem: Metabolic Pathways. Vol. II—Amino Acids, Nucleic Acids, Porphyrins, Vitamins, and Coenzymes. 3rd ed. New York, Academic Press, Inc., 1968.

Idem: Metabolic Pathways. Vol. III—Amino Acids and Tetrapyrroles. 3rd ed. New York, Academic Press, Inc., 1969.

Idem: Metabolic Pathways. Vol. IV—Nucleic Acids, Protein Synthesis and Coenzymes. 3rd ed. New York, Academic Press, Inc., 1970.

Greenberg, M. S., Brightman, V. J., Lynch, M. A., and Ship, I. I.: Idiopathic hypoparathyroidism, chronic candidiasis, and dental hypoplasia. Oral Surg., 28:42, 1969.

Gÿorgy, P., and Pearson, W. N.: The Vitamins: Chemistry, Physiology, Pathology, Methods. 2nd ed. New York, Academic Press, Inc., 1967.

Hansen, A. E.: Serum lipids in eczema and in other pathologic conditions. Am. J. Dis. Child., 53:933, 1937.

Harris, S. S., and Navia, J. M.: Vitamin A deficiency and caries susceptibility of rat molars. Arch. Oral Biol., 25:415, 1980.

Hartman, K. S.: Histiocytosis-X: a review of 114 cases with oral involvement. Oral Surg., 49:38, 1980.

Hassan, H., Hashim, S. A., Van Itallie, T. B., and Sebrell, W. H.: Syndrome in premature infants associated with low plasma vitamin E levels and high polyunsaturated fatty acid diet. Am. J. Clin. Nutr., 19:147, 1966.

Haussler, M. R., and McCain, T. A.: Basic and clinical concepts related to vitamin D metabolism and action I. New Engl. J. Med., 297:974, 1977.

Idem: Basic and clinical concepts related to vitamin D metabolism and action II. New Engl. J. Med., 297:1041, 1977.

Hawkins, W. W., and Barsky, J.: An experiment on human vitamin B_6 deprivation. Science, 108:284, 1948.

Hill, T. J.: A Textbook of Oral Pathology. 4th ed. Philadelphia, Lea & Febiger, 1949.

Hinrichs, E. H.: Dental changes in juvenile hypothyroidism. J. Dent. Child., 23:167, 1966.

Hirsch, P. F., and Munson, P. L.: Thyrocalcitonin. Physiol. Rev., 49:548, 1969.

Hodges, R. E., Baker, E. M., Hood, J., Sauberlich, H. E., and March, S. C.: Experimental scurvy in man. Am. J. Clin. Nutr., 22:535, 1969.

Hofer, P. A., and Bergenholtz, A.: Oral manifestations in Urbach-Wiethe disease (lipoglycoproteinosis; lipoid proteinosis; hyalinosis cutis et mucosae). Odont. Revy., 26:39, 1975.

Hojer, A.: Method for determining the antiscorbutic value of a food stuff by means of histological examination of the teeth of young guinea pigs. Br. J. Exp. Pathol., 7:356, 1926.

Hokin, L. E.: Metabolic Pathways: Metabolic Transport. Vol. VI. 3rd ed. New York, Academic Press, Inc., 1972.

Houpt, M. I., Kenny, F. M., and Listgarten, M.: Hypophosphatasia: case reports. J. Dent. Child., 37:126, 1970.

Hume, E. M., and Krebs, H. A.: Vitamin A requirement of human adults: an experimental study of vitamin A deprivation in man. A report of the Vitamin A Subcommittee of the Accessory Food Factors Committee. Med. Res. Coun. Spec. Rep., Ser. no. 264, London, HMSO, 1949.

Hunder, G. G.: Pathogenesis of Cushing's disease. Mayo Clin. Proc., 41:29, 1966.

Irving, J. T.: Enamel organ of the rat's incisor tooth in vitamin E deficiency. Nature, 150:122, 1942.

Idem: The effects of avitaminosis and hypervitaminosis A upon the incisor teeth and incisal alveolar bone of rats. J. Physiol., 108:92, 1949.

Jaffe, H. L., and Lichtenstein, L.: Eosinophilic granuloma of bone. Arch. Pathol., 37:99, 1944.

Jardon, O. M., Burney, D. W., and Fink, R. L.: Hypophosphatasia in an adult. J. Bone Joint Surg., 52-A: 1477, 1970.

Johnson, R. H.: A unique case of pathologic calcification? Oral Surg., 32:66, 1971.

Jolly, M.: Vitamin A deficiency: a review I. J. Oral Therapeut. Pharmacol., 3:364, 1967.

Idem: Vitamin A deficiency: a review II. J. Oral Therapeut. Pharmacol., 3:439, 1967.

Jones, J. C., Lilly, G. E., and Marlette, R. H.: Histiocytosis X. J. Oral Surg., 28:461, 1970.

Kaye, M., and Sagar, S.: Effect of dihydrotachysterol on calcium absorption in uremia. Metabolism, 21:815, 1972.

King, C. G.: Protein malnutrition: a major international problem. News Report. Natl. Acad. Sci., Natl. Res. Council, 12:37, 1962.

King, C. G., and Waugh, W. A.: The chemical nature of vitamin C. Science, 75:357, 1932.

Kjellman, M., Oldfelt, V., Nordenram, A., and Olow-Nordenram, M.: Five cases of hypophosphatasia with dental findings. Int. J. Oral Surg., 2:152, 1973.

Klein, H., Orent, E., and McCollum, E. V.: The effects of magnesium deficiency on the teeth and their supporting structures in rats. Am. J. Physiol., 112:256, 1935.

Knudson, A. G., Jr.: Inborn errors of sphingolipid metabolism. Am. J. Clin. Nutr., 9:55, 1961.

Kosowicz, J., and Rzymski, K.: Abnormalities of tooth development in pituitary dwarfism. Oral Surg., 44:853, 1977.

Kruger, G. O., Prickman, L. E., and Pugh, D. G.: So-called eosinophilic granuloma of ribs and jaws associated with visceral (pulmonary) involvement characteristic of xanthomatosis. Oral Surg., 2:770, 1949.

Kyle, R. A., and Bayrd, E. D.: Amyloidosis: review of 236 cases. Medicine, 54:271, 1975.

Lahey, M. E.: Prognosis in reticuloendotheliosis in children. J. Pediatr., 60:664, 1962.

Levin, B.: Gaucher's disease. Clinical and roentgenologic manifestations. Am. J. Roentgenol., Radium Ther. Nucl. Med., 85:685, 1961.

Levin, B., Oberholzer, V. G., Snodgrass, G. J. A. I., Stimmler, L., and Wilmers, M. J.: Fructosemia: an inborn error of fructose metabolism. Arch. Dis. Child., 38:220, 1963.

Levin, B., Snodgrass, G. J. A. I., Oberholzer, V. G., Burgess, E. A., and Dobbs, R. A.: Fructosemia: observation on seven cases. Am. J. Med., 45:826, 1968.

Levin, L. S., Jorgenson, R. J., and Salinas, C. F.: Oral findings in the Morquio syndrome (mucopolysaccharidosis IV). Oral Surg., 39:390, 1975.

Levy, B. M.: Effects of pantothenic acid deficiency on the mandibular joints and periodontal structures of mice. J. Am. Dent. Assoc., 38:215, 1949.

Idem: The effect of pyridoxine deficiency on the jaws of mice. J. Dent. Res., 29:349, 1950.

Idem: The effect of riboflavin deficiency on the growth of the mandibular condyle of mice. Oral Surg., 2:89, 1949.

Levy, B. M., and Silberberg, R.: Effect of riboflavin deficiency on endochondral ossification of mice. Proc. Soc. Exp. Biol. Med., 63:355, 1946.

Lichtenstein, L.: Histiocytosis X. Integration of eosinophilic granuloma of bone, "Letterer-Siwe disease," and "Schüller-Christian disease" as related manifestations of a single nosologic entity. Arch. Pathol., 56:84, 1953.

Lichtenstein, L., and Jaffe, H. L.: Eosinophilic granuloma of bone. Am. J. Pathol., 16:595, 1940.

Lieberman, P. H., Jones, C. R., Dargeon, H. W. K., and Begg, C. F.: A reappraisal of eosinophilic granuloma of bone, Hand-Schüller-Christian syndrome and Letterer-Siwe syndrome. Medicine, 48:375, 1969.

Lin, J. H., Duffy, J. L., and Roginsky, M. S.: Microcirculation in diabetes mellitus. Hum. Pathol., 6:77, 1975.

Lloyd, B. B., and Sinclair, H. M.: In Bourne and Kidder, Chap. 11.

Lloyd, H. M.: Primary hyperparathyroidism: an analysis of the role of the parathyroid tumor. Medicine, 47:53, 1968.

Loeb, L.: The Biological Basis of Individuality. Springfield, Ill., Charles C Thomas, 1945.

Lotz, M., Zisman, E., and Bartter, F. C.: Evidence for a phosphorus-depletion syndrome in man. New Engl. J. Med., 278:409, 1968.

Lovestedt, S. A.: Oral manifestations of histiocytosis-X. Dent. Radiog. Photog., 50:21, 1977.

Lovett, D. W., Cross, K. R., and Van Allen, M.: The prevalence of amyloids in gingival tissues. Oral Surg., 20:444, 1965.

Lucaya, J.: Histiocytosis X. Am. J. Dis. Child., 121:289, 1971.

Margolin, F. R., and Steinbach, H. L.: Progeria. Hutchinson-Gilford syndrome. Am. J. Roentgenol., Radium Ther. Nucl. Med., 103:173, 1968.

Marks, S. C., Lindahl, R. L., and Bawden, J. W.: Dental and cephalometric findings in vitamin D resistant rickets. J. Dent. Child., 32:259, 1965.

Marthaler, T. M., and Froesch, E. R.: Hereditary fructose intolerance. Dental status of eight patients. Br. Dent. J., 123:597, 1967.

Massry, S. G., Coburn, J. W., Popovtzer, M. M., Shenaberger, J. H., Maxwell, M. H., and Kleeman, C. R.: Secondary hyperparathyroidism in chronic renal failure. Arch. Intern. Med., 124:431, 1969.

McArthur, R. G., Cloutier, M. D., Hayles, A. B., and Sprague, R. G.: Cushing's disease in children. Findings in 13 cases. Mayo Clin. Proc., 47:318, 1972.

McClendon, J. F.: Fluorine is necessary in the diet of the rat. Fed. Proc., 3:94, 1944.

McCollum, E. V., and Davis, M.: The nature of the dietary deficiencies of rice. J. Biol. Chem., 23:181, 1915.

McCollum, E. V., Simonds, N., Becker, J. E., and Shipley, P. G.: Studies on experimental rickets XXI. An experimental demonstration of the existence of a vitamin which promotes calcium deposition. J. Biol. Chem., 53:293, 1922.

McGavran, M. H., and Spady, H. A.: Eosinophilic granuloma of bone: a study of twenty-eight cases. J. Bone Joint Surg., 42-A:979, 1960.

McKusick, V. A.: Heritable Diseases of Connective Tissue. 4th ed. St. Louis, C. V. Mosby Company, 1972.

McKusick, V. A., Kaplan, D., Wise, D., Hanley, W. B., Suddarth, S. B., Sevick, M. E., and Maumanee, A. E.: The genetic mucopolysaccharidoses. Medicine, 44:445, 1965.

Méhes, K., Klujber, L., Lassu, G., and Kajtár, P.: Hypophosphatasia: screening and family investigators in an endogamous Hungarian village. Clin. Genet., 3:60, 1972.

Mellanby, E.: A further demonstration of the part played by accessory food factors in the aetiology of rickets. J. Physiol., 52:53, 1919.

Mellanby, E.: An experimental investigation on rickets. Lancet, 1:407, 1919.

Mellanby, M.: The influence of diet on teeth formation. Lancet, 2:767, 1918.

Mellanby, M. T.: Diet and the teeth; an experimental study. Med. Res. Coun. Spec. Rep. Ser. no. 191, London, HMSO, 1934.

Menaker, L., and Navia, J. M.: Effect of undernutrition during the perinatal period on caries development in the rat: II. Caries susceptibility in underfed rats supplemented with protein or calorie additions during the suckling period. J. Dent. Res., 52:680, 1973.

Idem: Effect of undernutrition during the perinatal period on caries development in the rat: III. Effects of undernutrition on biochemical parameters in the developing submandibular salivary gland. J. Dent. Res., 52:688, 1973.

Idem: Effect of undernutrition during the perinatal period on caries development in the rat: IV. Effects of differential tooth eruption and exposure to a cariogenic diet on subsequent dental caries incidence. J. Dent. Res., 52:692, 1973.

Idem: Effect of undernutrition during the perinatal period on caries development in the rat: V. Changes in whole saliva volume and protein content. J. Dent. Res., 53:592, 1974.

Mertz, W.: The essential trace elements. Science, 213:1332, 1981.

Moch, W. S.: Gaucher's disease with mandibular bone lesions. Oral Surg., 6:1250, 1953.

Moore, T.: Vitamin A. Elsevier, Amsterdam, 1957.

Navia, J. M.: Evaluation of nutritional and dietary factors that modify animal caries. J. Dent. Res., 49:1213, 1970.

Navia, J. M., Di Orio, L. P., Menaker, L., and Miller, S.: Effect of undernutrition during the perinatal period on caries development in the rat. J. Dent. Res., 49:1091, 1970.

Neufeld, E. F., and Fratantoni, J. C.: Inborn errors of mucopolysaccharide metabolism. Faulty degradative mechanisms are implicated in this group of human diseases. Science, 169:141, 1970.

Newbrun, E., Hoover, C., Mettraux, G., and Graf, H.: Comparison of dietary habits and dental health of subjects with hereditary fructose intolerance and control subjects. J. Am. Dent. Assoc., 101:619, 1980.

Nitowsky, H. M., Cornblath, M., and Gordon, H. H.: Studies of tocopherol deficiency in infants and children. II. Plasma tocopherol and erythrocyte hemolysis in hydrogen peroxide. Am. J. Dis. Child., 92:164, 1956.

Nitowsky, H. M., Tildon, J. T., Levin, S., and Gordon, H. H.: Studies of tocopherol deficiency in infants and children. VII. The effect of tocopherol in urinary, plasma and muscle creatinine. Am. J. Clin. Nutr., 10:368, 1962.

Nordin, B. E. C.: Pathogenesis of osteoporosis. Lancet, 1:1011, 1961.

Olcott, H. S., and Emerson, O. H.: Antioxidants and the autoxidation of fats IX. The antioxidant properties of the tocopherols. J. Am. Chem. Soc., 59:1008, 1937.

Otani, S.: A discussion of eosinophilic granuloma of bone, Letterer-Siwe disease and Schüller-Christian disease. Mt. Sinai J. Med., 24:1079, 1957.

Otani, S., and Ehrlich, J. C.: Solitary granuloma of bone simulating primary neoplasm. Am. J. Pathol., 16:479, 1940.

Peterkofsky, B., and Udenfriend, S.: Enzymatic hydroxylation of proline in microsomal polypeptide leading to formation of collagen. Proc. Natl. Acad. Sci. U.S.A., 53:335, 1965.

Peters, S. P., and Van Slyke, D. D.: Quantitative Clinical Chemistry. Vol. 1. Baltimore, Williams & Wilkins Company, 1931.

Pincus, G.: In Green, Chap. 7.

Pitt, M. J., and Haussler, M. R.: Vitamin D: Biochemistry and clinical applications. Skeletal Radiol., 1:198, 1977.

Prasad, A. S., Halsted, J. A., and Nadimi, M.: Syndrome of iron deficiency anemia, hepatosplenomegaly, hypogonadism, dwarfism and geophagia. Am. J. Med., 31:532, 1961.

Prasad, A. S., Miale, A., Jr., Farid, Z., Sandstead, H. H., Schulert, A. R., and Darby, W. J.: Biochemical studies on dwarfism, hypogonadism and anemia. Arch. Intern. Med., 111:65, 1963.

Prasad, A. S., Schulert, A. R., Miale, A., Jr., Farid, Z., and Sandstead, H. H.: Zinc and iron deficiency in male subjects with dwarfism and hypogonadism but without ancylostomiasis, schistosomiasis, or severe anemia. Am. J. Clin. Nutr., 12:437, 1963.

Pryor, W. A.: Free radical pathology. Chem. Eng. News, 49:34, 1971.

Rapidis, A. D., Longdon, J. D., Harvey, P. W., and Patel, M. F.: Histiocytosis-X. An analysis of 50 cases. Int. J. Oral Surg., 7:76, 1978.

Rasmussen, H., and Pechet, M. M.: Calcitonin. Sci. Am., 223:42, October, 1970.

Rathbun, J. C.: Hypophosphatasia. Am. J. Dis. Child., 75:822, 1948.

Reich, C., Seife, M., and Kessler, B. J.: Gaucher's disease: a review and discussion of twenty cases. Medicine, 30:1, 1951.

Richards, I. D. G., Sweet, E. M., and Arneil, G. C.: Infantile rickets persists in Glasgow. Lancet, 1:803, 1968.

Rigdon, R. H.: Occurrence and association of amyloid with diseases in birds and mammals including man: a review. Tex. Rep. Biol. Med., 32:665, 1974.

Ritchie, G. MacL.: Hypophosphatasia. A metabolic disease with important dental manifestations. Arch. Dis. Child., 39:584, 1964.

Rogers, D. R.: Screening for amyloid with the thioflavin-T fluorescent method. Am. J. Clin. Pathol., 44:59, 1965.

Root, A.: Growth hormone, Pediatrics, 36:940, 1965.

Rose, W. C., Haines, W. J., and Johnson, J. E.: The role of the amino acids in human nutrition. J. Biol. Chem., 146:683, 1942.

Rotruck, J. T., Pope, A. L., Ganther, H. E., Swanson, A. B., Hafeman, D. G., and Hoekstra, W. G.: Selenium: biochemical role as a component of glutathione peroxidase. Science, 179:588, 1973.

Russell, B. G.: Gingival changes in diabetes mellitus. Acta Pathol. Microbiol. Scand., 68:161, 1966.

Idem: The dental pulp in diabetes mellitus. Acta Pathol. Microbiol. Scand., 70:319, 1967.

Idem: The periodontal membrane in diabetes mellitus. Acta Pathol. Microbiol. Scand., 70:318, 1967.

Salley, J. J., Bryson, W. F., and Eshleman, J. R.: The effect of chronic vitamin A deficiency on dental caries in the Syrian hamster. J. Dent. Res., 38:1038, 1959.

Sayers, G.: The adrenal cortex and homeostasis. Physiol. Rev., 30:241, 1950.

Sbarbaro, J. L., and Francis, K. C.: Eosinophilic granuloma of bone. J.AM.A., 178:706, 1961.

Schofield, F. W.: A brief account of a disease of cattle simulating hemorrhagic septicemia due to feeding of sweet clover. Can. Vet. J., 3:74, 1922.

Schour, I., and Massler, M.: Endocrines and dentistry. J. Am. Dent. Assoc., 30:597, 763, 943, 1943.

Idem: The effects of dietary deficiencies upon the oral structures. Physiol. Rev., 25:442, 1945.

Schour, I., and Van Dyke, H. B.: Changes in the teeth following hypophysectomy. I. Changes in the incisor of the white rat. Am. J. Anat., 50:397, 1932.

Schour, I., Hoffman, M. M., and Smith, M. C.: Changes in the incisor teeth of albino rats with vitamin A deficiency and the effects of replacement therapy. Am. J. Pathol., 17:529, 1941.

Schroff, J.: Eosinophilic granuloma of bone. Oral Surg., 1:256, 1948.

Scriver, C. R., and Cameron, D.: Pseudohypophosphatasia. N. Engl. J. Med., 281:604, 1969.

Sebrell, W. H., and Butler, R. E.: Riboflavin deficiency in man (ariboflavinosis). Public Health Rep., 54:2121, 1939.

Sebrell, W. H., and Harris, R. S.: The Vitamins. New York, Academic Press, Inc., 1967.

Sedano, H. O., Cernea, P., Hosxe, G., and Gorlin, R. J.: Histiocytosis X. Clinical, radiologic, and histologic findings with special attention to oral manifestations. Oral Surg., 27:760, 1969.

Selye, H.: General adaptation syndrome and diseases of adaptation. J. Clin. Endocr., 6:117, 1946.

Idem: The alarm reaction and the diseases of adaptation. Ann. Intern. Med., 26:403, 1948.

Selye, H., et al.: Stress. Montreal, Acta Inc., 1950, 1951, 1952, 1953, 1954, 1955–56.

Shafer, W. G., and Muhler, J. C.: Effect of gonadectomy and sex hormones on the structure of the rat salivary glands. J. Dent. Res., 32:262, 1953.

Sherman, H. C.: Chemistry of Food and Nutrition. New York, Macmillan Company, 1947.

Shils, M. E.: Experimental human magnesium depletion. Medicine, 48:61, 1969.

Silverman, S., Gordon, G., Grant, T., Steinbach, H., Eisenberg, E., and Manson, R.: The dental structures in hyperparathyroidism. Oral Surg., 15:426, 1962.

Silverman, S., Jr., Ware, W. H., and Gillooly, C., Jr.: Dental aspects of hyperparathyroidism. Oral Surg., 26:184, 1968.

Sleeper, E. L.: Eosinophilic granuloma of bone: its relationship to Hand-Schüller-Christian and Letterer-Siwe's diseases, with emphasis upon oral symptoms and findings. Oral Surg., 4:896, 1951.

Somjen, G., Hilmy, M., and Stephens, C. R.: Failure to anesthetize human subjects by intravenous administration of magnesium sulfate. J. Pharmacol. Exp. Ther., 154:652, 1966.

Spies, T. D., and Butt, H. R.: In Duncan, Chap. 7.

Spolnik, K. J., Patterson, S. S., Maxwell, D. R., Kleit, S. A., and Cockerill, E. M.: Dental radiographic manifestations of end-stage renal disease. Dent. Radiogr. Photogr., 54:21, 1981.

Stahl, S. S., and Robertson, H. C.: Oral lesions in Hand-Schüller-Christian disease: report of case. Oral Surg., 8:319, 1955.

Stanback, J. S., and Peagler, F. D.: Primary amyloidosis. Review of the literature and report of a case. Oral Surg., 26:774, 1968.

Stanbury, J. B., Wyngaarden, J. B., and Fredrickson, D. S.: The Metabolic Basis of Inherited Disease. 4th ed. New York, McGraw-Hill Book Company, 1978.

Standinger, H. J., Krisch, K., and Leonhauser, S.: Role of ascorbic acid in microsomal electron transport and the possible relationship to hydroxylation reactions. Ann. N.Y. Acad. Sci., 92:195, 1961.

Steenbock, H.: The induction of growth promoting and calcifying properties in a ration by exposure to light. Science, 60:224, 1924.

Steenbock, H., and Black, A.: Fat soluble vitamins; the induction of growth promoting and calcifying properties in a ration by exposure to ultra-violet light. J. Biol. Chem., 61:405, 1924.

Steenbock, H., and Boutwell, P. W.: Fat soluble vitamine V. The stability of the fat soluble vitamine in plant materials. J. Biol. Chem., 41:163, 1920.

Steenbock, H., and Sell, M. T.: Fat soluble vitamine X. Further observations on the occurrence of the fat soluble vitamine with yellow plant pigments. J. Biol. Chem., 51:63, 1922.

Steenbock, H., Hart, E. B., and Jones, J. H.: Fat soluble vitamine XVIII. Sunlight in its relation to pork production on certain restricted rations. J. Biol. Chem., 61:405, 1924.

Steffens, L. F., Bair, H. L., and Sheard, C.: Dark adaptation and dietary deficiency in vitamin A. Am. J. Ophthalmol., 23:1325, 1940.

Stickler, G. B., Beabout, J. W., and Riggs, B. L.: Vitamin D-resistant rickets: clinical experience with 41 typical familial hypophosphatemic patients and 2 atypical non-familial cases. Mayo Clin. Proc., 45:197, 1970.

Svirbely, J. L., and Szent-Györgyi, A.: CV: the chemical nature of vitamin C. Biochem. J., 26:865, 1932.

Sweet, L. K., and K'ang, H. J.: Clinical and anatomic study of avitaminosis A among Chinese. Am. J. Dis. Child., 50:699, 1935.

Taylor, G. F., and Day, C. D. M.: Osteomalacia and dental caries. Br. Med. J., 2:221, 1940.

Teng, C. T., and Nathan, M. H.: Primary hyperparathyroidism. Am. J. Roentgenol., Radium Ther. Nucl. Med., 83:716, 1960.

Thoma, K. H.: Oral Pathology, 4th ed. St. Louis, C. V. Mosby Company, 1954.

Thompson, S. W., II, Gell, R. G., and Yamanaka, H. S.: A histochemical study of the protein nature of amyloid. Am. J. Pathol., 38:737, 1961.

Tracy, W. E., Steen, J. C., Steiner, J. E., and Buist, N. R. M.: Analysis of dentine pathogenesis in vitamin D-resistant rickets. Oral Surg., 32:38, 1971.

Ulmansky, M.: Primary amyloidosis of oral structures and pharynx. Report of a case. Oral Surg., 15:800, 1962.

Underwood, E. J.: Trace Elements in Human and Animal Nutrition. New York, Academic Press, Inc., 1977.

Vallee, B. L., Wacker, W. E. C., and Ulmer, D. D.: Magnesium deficiency tetany syndrome in man. N. Engl. J. Med., 262:155, 1960.

van der Waal, I., Fehmers, M. C. O., and Kraal, E. R.: Amyloidosis: its significance in oral surgery. Oral Surg., 36:469, 1973.

Van Wyk, C. W.: The oral mucosa in kwashiorkor: a clinico-cytological study. J. Dent. Assoc. S. Afr., 20:298, 1965.

Vasilakis, G. J., Nygaard, V. K., and DiPalma, D. M.: Vitamin D resistant rickets. A review and case report of an adolescent boy with a history of dental problems. J. Oral Med., 35:19, 1980.

Vogel, H. J.: Metabolic Pathways: Metabolic Regulation. Vol. V. 3rd Ed. New York, Academic Press, Inc., 1971.

Wald, G.: Molecular basis of visual excitation. Science, 162:230, 1968.

Warkany J., and Nelson, R. C.: Skeletal abnormalities induced in rats by maternal nutritional deficiency. Arch. Pathol., 34:375, 1942.

Webman, M. S., Hirsch, S. A., Webman, H., and Stanley, H. R.: Obliterated pulp cavities in the San Filippo syndrome (mucopolysaccharidosis III). Oral Surg., 43:734, 1977.

Weinfeld, A., Stern, M. H., and Marx, L. H.: Amyloid lesions of bone. Am. J. Roentgenol., Radium Ther. Nucl. Med., 108:799, 1970.

Wesley, R. K., Delaney, J. R., and Litt, R.: Progeria: clinical considerations for an isolated case. J. Dent. Child., 46:1, 1979.

Whedon, G. D.: Effects of high calcium intakes on bones, blood and tissue: relationship of calcium intake to balance in osteoporosis. Fed. Proc., 18:1112, 1959.

Williams, R. F.: Lipoid proteinosis. Report of a case. Oral Surg., 31:624, 1971.

Wilson, D. R., York, S. E., Jaworski, Z. F., and Yendt, E. R.: Studies in hypophosphatemic vitamin D-refractory osteomalacia in adults. Medicine, 44:99, 1965.

Wilson, J. R., and DuBois, R. O.: Report of a fatal case of keratomalacia in an infant with postmortem examination. Am. J. Dis. Child., 26:431, 1923.

Winkelmann, R. K.: The skin in histiocytosis X. Mayo Clin. Proc., 44:535, 1969.

Winters, R. W., Graham, J. B., Williams, T. F., McFalls, V. W., and Burnett, C. H.: A genetic study of familial hypophosphatemia and vitamin D resistant rickets. Trans. Assoc. Am. Physicians, 70:234, 1957.

Winters, R. W., Graham, J. B., Williams, T. F., McFalls, V. W., and Burnett, C. H.: A genetic study of familial hypophosphatemia and vitamin D resistant rickets with a review of the literature. Medicine, 37:97, 1958.

Witkop, C. J., and Rao, S.: Inherited defects in tooth structure. Birth Defects, 7:153, 1971.

Wolbach, S. B., and Bessey, O. A.: Tissue changes in vitamin deficiencies. Physiol. Rev., 22:233, 1942.

Wolbach, S. B., and Howe, P. R.: The incisor teeth of albino rats and guinea pigs in vitamin deficiency and repair. Am. J. Pathol., 9:275, 1933.

Ziskin, D. E., and Applebaum, E.: Effects of thyroidectomy and thyroid stimulation on growing permanent dentition of rhesus monkeys. J. Dent. Res., 20:21, 1941.

Ziskin, D. E., Applebaum, E., and Gorlin, R. J.: The effect of hypophysectomy upon the permanent dentition of rhesus monkeys. J. Dent. Res., 28:48, 1949.

Ziskin, D. E., Stein, G., Gross, P., and Runne, E.: Oral, gingival and periodontal pathology induced in rats on low pantothenic acid diet by toxic doses of zinc carbonate. Am. J. Orthod. Oral Surg., 33:407, 1947.

SECTION V

DISEASES OF SPECIFIC SYSTEMS

CHAPTER 13

Diseases of Bone and Joints

DISEASES OF BONE

Bone is a dense calcified tissue which is specifically affected by a variety of diseases that often cause it to react in a dynamic fashion. Some of these diseases involve the entire bony skeleton, while others affect only a single bone. It is characteristic for certain of these conditions to follow strict mendelian patterns of heredity, although sometimes a specific disease will be inherited in one case and apparently not in another. These diseases of bone, as a group, may arise at all ages; some characteristically are congenital and present at birth, while others develop in early childhood, young adulthood or even in later life.

The maxilla and mandible, like other bones, suffer from both the generalized and the localized forms of skeletal diseases. Although the basic reactions are the same, the peculiar anatomic arrangement of teeth embedded partially in bone, through which the bone may be subjected to an unusual variety of stresses, strains and infections, often produces a modified response of bone to the primary injury.

The diseases of bone to be considered in this chapter do not include specific infections, neoplasms or other recognized injuries restricted to the jaws, but constitute a group of generalized skeletal diseases which frequently manifest involvement of the maxilla or mandible.

Careful study of the various disease states affecting the skeleton has provided great insight into the many mysteries surrounding the normal physiology of bone. A false sense of understanding of bone metabolism arose within the past few decades, possibly because of an attempt to oversimplify one of the body's most complex tissues. Thorough investigative work on skeletal diseases coupled with intensive animal experimentation has only begun to lighten the darkness which frequently obscures scientific pursuits. The coming years will be extremely fruitful ones for clarification of the voids in our knowledge of bone physiopathology.

OSTEOGENESIS IMPERFECTA

("Brittle Bones"; Fragilitas Ossium; Osteopsathyrosis; Lobstein's Disease)

Osteogenesis imperfecta is a serious disease of unknown etiology which is closely related to dentinogenesis imperfecta, a milder condition affecting mesodermal tissues. Although osteogenesis imperfecta generally is recognized as representing a hereditary autosomal dominant characteristic, autosomal recessive and nonhereditary types also occur.

The disease in its usual form is present at birth (congenita or Vrolik's type), although some cases do not arise or are not recognized until later in childhood (tarda or Lobstein's type, gravis or levis). This latter variety of osteogenesis imperfecta has also been called osteopsathyrosis. Many infants afflicted with osteogenesis imperfecta are stillborn or die shortly after birth.

Clinical Features. The chief clinical characteristic of osteogenesis imperfecta is the extreme fragility and porosity of the bones, with an attendant proneness to fracture. The fractures heal readily, but the new bone is of a similar imperfect quality. It is common for fractures to occur while an infant is simply crawling or walking. If a person has suffered numerous fractures, particularly early in life, he may be seriously deformed by the time he reaches adulthood. Hyperplastic callus formation, which may or may not be related to actual fracture, occasionally occurs in some patients. This has been discussed by King and Bobechko in their review of the orthopedic problems associated with the disease. This callus may be so exuberant that it mimics osteosarcoma; in fact, several cases of true sarcoma arising in such calluses have been reported.

A second characteristic clinical feature of osteogenesis imperfecta is the occurrence of pale blue sclerae. The sclerae are abnormally thin, and for this reason the pigmented choroid shows through and produces the bluish color. However, the appearance of blue sclera is not confined to this disease since it may also be seen in osteopetrosis, fetal rickets, Marfan syndrome, and Ehlers-Danlos syndrome, as well as in normal infants. While the blue sclerae are a prominent sign in this disease, they are not invariably present. In a series of 42 patients reported by Bauze and his associates, 12 of the patients had white sclerae, and these were generally found in the older patients with the more severe disease and earlier onset of fractures.

In a thorough review of osteogenesis imperfecta and dentinogenesis imperfecta by Winter and Maiocco, the following additional signs and symptoms were described as being characteristic of osteogenesis imperfecta: deafness due to otosclerosis, abnormalities of the teeth (identical with those of dentinogenesis imperfecta, or "hereditary opalescent dentin"), laxity of the ligaments, a peculiar shape of the skull and an abnormal electrical reaction of the muscles.

Many patients with osteogenesis imperfecta also have a tendency for capillary bleeding although no specific blood dyscrasia or defect has been demonstrated.

Oral Manifestations. Osteogenesis imperfecta is basically a disturbance of mesodermal tissues, particularly the calcified tissues. When a widespread congenital disturbance in bone formation exists, it is only logical to expect a concomitant disturbance in dentin formation, and this is frequently the case. Osteogenesis imperfecta and dentinogenesis imperfecta are common companions, although many cases of dentinogenesis imperfecta do occur without the more generalized bone involvement.

The actual incidence of dentinogenesis imperfecta occurring in osteogenesis imperfecta has only been investigated in a few series of cases of significant size to warrant consideration. In the series of 90 patients with osteogenesis imperfecta reported by Falvo and his co-workers, 10 of 12 patients (83 per cent) with the congenita type had dentinogenesis imperfecta, as did 29 of 43 patients (67 per cent) with tarda

type and bowing of extremities and 20 of 35 patients (57 per cent) with tarda type but no bowing. Thus, a total of 65 per cent of the 90 patients with the bone disease had the dental disease as well. In a series of 42 patients reported by Bauze and his associates, 8 patients (19 per cent) had concomitant dental involvement, while in a group of 29 patients reported by Shoenfeld and his co-workers, 10 patients (34 per cent) were stated to have "teeth hypoplasia." Heys and her associates discussed the relation of these two diseases in a genealogical study of 18 families in which 167 individuals showed one or both conditions.

Histologic Features. The bones in patients with osteogenesis imperfecta exhibit thin cortices, sometimes being composed of immature spongy bone, while the trabeculae of the cancellous bone are delicate and often show microfractures (Fig. 13–1). Osteoblastic activity appears retarded and imperfect, and for this reason the thickness of the long bones is deficient. The basic defect appears to lie in the organic matrix with failure of fetal collagen to be transformed into mature collagen; calcification proceeds normally. There is some evidence that the progressive intermolecular cross-linkage of adjacent collagen molecules, which is an essential characteristic of normal collagen maturation, is defective in this disease. The length of the long bones is usually normal unless multiple fractures have caused undue shortening.

Treatment. There is no known treatment for osteogenesis imperfecta. Various substances have been administered in an attempt to induce osteosclerosis, but without success. Clinical improvement following the onset of puberty has been noted in some patients, especially in girls.

INFANTILE CORTICAL HYPEROSTOSIS

(Caffey's Disease; Caffey-Silverman Syndrome)

Infantile cortical hyperostosis was originally described independently by Caffey and Silverman and by Smyth and his co-workers as a syndrome of unknown etiology in which unusual cortical thickening occurred in certain bones of infants. It was soon discovered that none of a variety of diseases which may produce cortical thickening, such as scurvy, rickets, syphilis, bacterial osteitis, neoplastic disease and traumatic injury, are present in this condition.

Etiology. It has been suggested that infantile

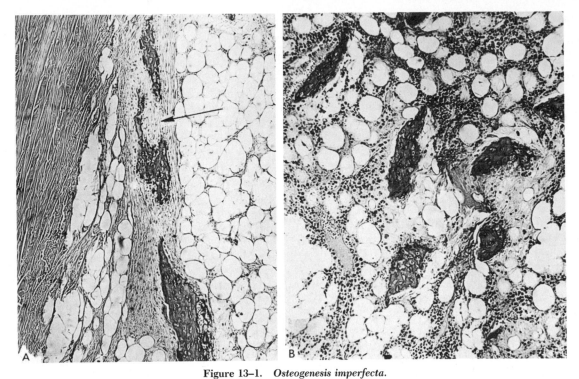

Figure 13–1. *Osteogenesis imperfecta.*
The cortex of bone is thin and replaced in some areas by fibrous tissue *(A)*. The cancellous bone is delicate and fragile *(B)*. (Courtesy of Dr. Frank Vellios.)

cortical hyperostosis may be an embryonal osteodysgenesis consequent to a local defect in the blood supply to the area. Another theory proposed is that an inherited defect of arterioles supplying the affected part results in hypoxia, producing focal necrosis of overlying soft tissues and periosteal proliferation. An allergic phenomenon has also been suggested as the basis of the disease, edema and inflammation producing periosteal elevation and subsequent deposition of calcium. There have been many reports of multiple cases in several generations of one family, thus lending strong support to the idea that, at least in some cases, it may follow a hereditary pattern, being transmitted as an autosomal dominant trait, probably with incomplete penetrance. For example, Newberg and Tampas have reported that in one family, a total of 21 members were afflicted with the disease. Saul and his associates have concluded that in the period from 1940 to 1960, sporadic cases of this disease occurred more commonly than familial cases and probably represented environmentally produced phenocopies but that such sporadic cases are rare today. At present, however, there is no general agreement on the etiology of infantile cortical hyperostosis.

It is of interest that some observations, such as those of Harris and Ramilo, have suggested a definite decrease in the number of patients being seen and diagnosed with this disease since 1968. However, this may be due to failure of identification or detection of the disease, especially if it is a mild form and the patient is relatively asymptomatic.

Clinical Features. Infantile cortical hyperostosis is characterized by the development of tender, deeply placed soft-tissue swellings and cortical thickening or hyperostosis involving various bones of the skeleton. It is significant that this disease usually arises during the first three months of life, but it may not appear before the second year. Interestingly, the disease has been demonstrated in the fetus in utero in a few cases as well as within the first few hours after birth. According to Saul and his associates, the familial type appears to have an earlier onset than the sporadic type, with 24 per cent of cases present at birth.

The mandible and the clavicles are the bones most frequently affected, the jaw involvement usually being manifested as a facial swelling. In fact, mandibular involvement is such a constant and striking feature of the disease that the question has been raised as to whether the diagnosis of the disease should ever be made in its absence. However, Saul and his co-workers reported that in the familial form of the disease mandibular involvement is less frequent and lower extremity involvement more frequent. Other bones which commonly demonstrate hyperostosis are the calvarium, scapula, ribs and tubular bones of the extremities, including the metatarsals. The soft-tissue swellings are associated with deep muscles and occur in general in the locations in which the hyperostoses subsequently arise. These swellings have been described in the scalp, face, neck, thorax and extremities.

Other signs and symptoms of this condition which have been described in some patients, but which are not inevitably present, include fever, hyperirritability, pseudoparalysis, dysphagia, pleurisy, anemia, leukocytosis, monocytosis, elevated sedimentation rate and increased serum alkaline phosphatase.

Oral Manifestations. The oral aspects of the disease have been studied by Burbank and his associates in a series of patients who had suffered from the condition during infancy. After careful follow-up examinations they found that some patients manifested a residual asymmetric deformity of the mandible, usually in the angle

and ramus area, even several years after the disease had subsided. A few patients with this deformity also had severe malocclusion. Despite the febrile component of the disease, no cases of enamel hypoplasia were observed.

Care must be taken not to confuse this disease with cherubism, in which bilateral enlargement of the mandible also occurs.

Roentgenographic Features. The roentgenographic appearance of the mandible in patients with infantile cortical hyperostosis is striking. The involvement may be unilateral or bilateral and is manifested as a gross thickening and sclerosis of the cortex due to an actively proliferating periosteum (Fig. 13–2). The hyperostosis usually lags behind the clinical appearance of the soft-tissue swellings so that inability to demonstrate roentgenographic evidence of the disease early in its course is not uncommon, and actually should be expected. Within a few weeks, however, the bony changes become obvious. Changes in other bones are similar to those occurring in the jaws.

Treatment and Prognosis. This disease appears to run a benign course, and active manifestations regress without treatment in several weeks to months. The course of the disease has not been altered by either sulfonamides or penicillin. On occasion, residual skeletal

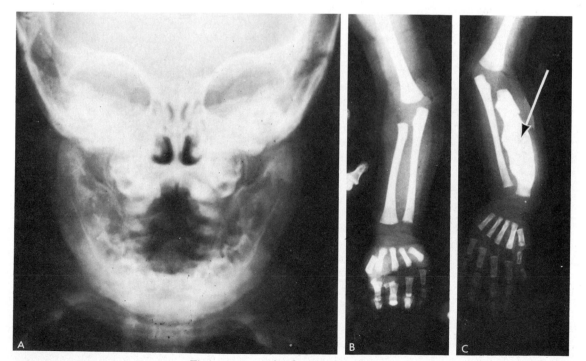

Figure 13–2. *Infantile cortical hyperostosis.*
There is thickening of the mandible *(A)* and of the radius in *C* as compared to the normal radius in *B (A,* Courtesy of Dr. F. Brooksaler: J. Pediatr., *48:*739, 1956.)

changes may persist into adult life. In addition, occasional cases of recurrence of pain and cortical thickening of bone in later childhood have been reported, such as that described by Blank.

CLEIDOCRANIAL DYSPLASIA

(Marie and Sainton's Disease; Scheuthauer-Marie-Sainton Syndrome; Mutational Dysostosis)

Cleidocranial dysplasia was referred to as cleidocranial dysostosis prior to the 1969 Paris conference on the nomenclature for constitutional disorders of bone, the proceedings of which were reprinted by McKusick and Scott. It is a disease of unknown etiology which is often but not always hereditary. When inherited, it appears as a dominant mendelian characteristic and may be transmitted by either sex. In those cases which appear to have developed sporadically, it has been suggested that they represent a recessively inherited disease or, more likely, either an incomplete penetrance in a genetic trait with variable gene expression or a true new dominant mutation. The disease affects men and women with equal frequency.

Clinical Features. Cleidocranial dysplasia is characterized by abnormalities of the skull, teeth, jaws and shoulder girdle as well as by occasional stunting of the long bones. In the skull the fontanels often remain open or at least exhibit delayed closing and for this reason tend to be rather large. The sutures also may remain open and wormian bones are common. The sagittal suture is characteristically sunken, giving the skull a flat appearance. Frontal, parietal, and occipital bones are prominent and the paranasal sinuses are underdeveloped and narrow. Based on the cephalic index, the head is brachycephalic, or wide and short, with the transverse diameter of the skull being increased. A variety of other skull abnormalities are sometimes present. An excellent review and discussion of the varied clinical findings in cleidocranial dysplasia has been published by Kalliala and Taskinen.

The defect of the shoulder girdle, from which the condition derives a portion of its name, ranges from complete absence of clavicles, in about 10 per cent of cases, to partial absence or even a simple thinning of one or both clavicles (Figs. 13–3, A; 13–4). Because of this clavicular disturbance, the patients have an unusual mobility of the shoulders and may be able to bring their shoulders forward until they meet in the midline (Fig. 13–3, A). Defects of the vertebral column, pelvis and long bones, as well as bones of the digits, are also relatively common. Thus cleidocranial dysplasia, once thought to be a disease involving only membranous bones, is now recognized as affecting the entire skeleton. In addition, changes outside the skeleton, such as anomalous muscles, have been reported, but these may be secondary to the bony involvement.

A disease known as *pycnodysostosis* or the Maroteaux-Lamy syndrome, which has most of

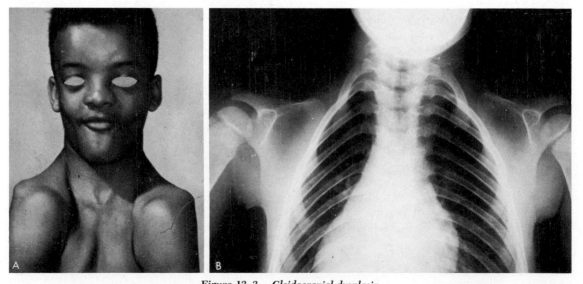

Figure 13–3.   *Cleidocranial dysplasia.*
The typical hypermobility of the shoulder *(A)* is made possible by the complete absence of the clavicles *(B)*. (Courtesy of Dr. Wilbur C. Moorman.)

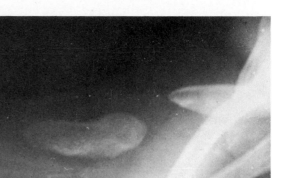

Figure 13–4. *Cleidocranial dysplasia.* There may be only hypoplasia of the clavicle rather than its complete absence.

the features of cleidocranial dysostosis, has also been described. However, patients with pycnodysostosis are also affected by dwarfism, their bones are dense and fragile, and they have partial agenesis of the terminal phalanges of the hands and feet. Neither of these latter two features are present in cleidocranial dysplasia, although the dense, fragile bones are similar to those seen in osteopetrosis or marble-bone disease. A thorough review of pycnodysostosis has been published by Elmore.

Oral Manifestations. Patients with cleidocranial dysplasia characteristically exhibit a high, narrow, arched palate, and actual cleft palate appears to be common. The maxilla is almost invariably reported to be underdeveloped and smaller than normal in relation to the mandible. However, Davis has reported that in a series of patients studied by cephalometric analysis all showed that the maxilla was of normal size and the position was either normal or anteriorly positioned in all cases. In addition, 70 per cent of the affected patients had larger mandibles than those of controls, which suggests that patients with cleidocranial dysplasia have enlarged mandibles rather than small maxillae, as reported in the literature. These findings remain to be confirmed. The lacrimal and zygomatic bones are also reported to be underdeveloped.

One of the outstanding oral findings is prolonged retention of the deciduous teeth and subsequent delay in eruption of the succedaneous teeth. Sometimes this delay in tooth eruption is permanent. The roots of the teeth are often somewhat short and thinner than usual and may be deformed.

In addition, Rushton reported that there is absence or paucity of cellular cementum on the roots of the permanent teeth, and this may be related to the failure of eruption so frequently seen. This has also been studied by Smith, who confirmed the absence of cellular cementum on both deciduous and permanent teeth. A surprising and unexplained feature was the absence of this cementum on the erupted teeth in both dentitions, with no increased thickening of the primary acellular cementum. The manner of anchorage of periodontal fibers and the maintenance of periodontal ligament width are also not understood in this disease. Furthermore, it is characteristic for numerous unerupted supernumerary teeth to be found by roentgenographic examination (Fig. 13–5). These are most prevalent in the mandibular premolar and incisor areas. Interestingly, partial anodontia has also been recorded in this condition but is rare.

Treatment and Prognosis. There is no specific treatment for cleidocranial dysplasia, although care of the oral conditions is important. The retained deciduous teeth should be restored if they become carious, since their extraction does not necessarily induce eruption of the permanent teeth. However, in recent years there has been increasing use of a multidisciplinary approach to treatment of these patients, utilizing the pedodontist, the orthodontist, and the oral surgeon. It has been found, as in the case reviewed by Hutton and his associates, that the permanent teeth do have the potential

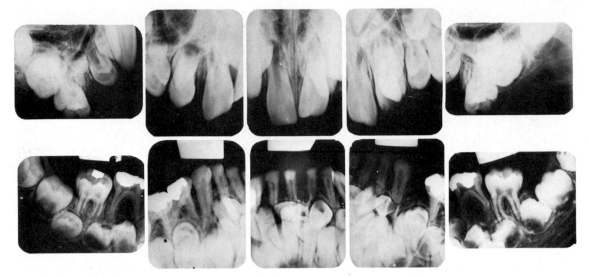

Figure 13–5. *Cleidocranial dysplasia.*
There are numerous unerupted and supernumerary teeth. (Courtesy of Dr. Wilbur C. Moorman.)

to erupt and that correct timing of surgical procedures for uncovering teeth and orthodontic repositioning can give excellent functional results.

CRANIOFACIAL DYSOSTOSIS

(Crouzon Disease or Syndrome)

The craniosynostosis syndromes constitute a group of conditions each characterized by premature craniosynostosis occurring in association with a variety of other abnormalities. These may or may not occur with syndactyly, anomalies of the hands and feet. The most common of the craniosynostotic syndromes occurring without syndactyly is craniofacial dysostosis, or Crouzon disease. The most common one occurring with syndactyly is the Apert syndrome, which is otherwise similar to Crouzon disease.

Craniofacial dysostosis is a genetic disease characterized by a variety of cranial deformities, facial malformations, eye changes and occasional other associated abnormalities. The majority of cases reported have followed a hereditary pattern, being transmitted as an autosomal dominant trait, but many cases with all apparent features of craniofacial dysostosis have shown no hereditary or familial history. Dunn, Kelln and his associates, and Gorlin and his co-workers have reviewed the history of this disease and discussed its differential diagnostic features.

Clinical Features. Although there is considerable individual variation in the appearance of patients with craniofacial dysostosis, the signs are all basically due to early synostosis of the sutures. The patients show a protuberant frontal region with an anteroposterior ridge overhanging the frontal eminence and often passing to the root of the nose (triangular frontal defect). The facial malformations consist of hypoplasia of the maxillae with mandibular prognathism and a high arched palate, cleft in some cases; the facial angle is exaggerated, and the patient's nose is described as resembling a parrot's beak. The eye changes often noted are hypertelorism, exophthalmos with divergent strabismus and optic neuritis and choked disks resulting frequently in blindness. Occasional other associated abnormalities are reported, such as spina bifida occulta. The mentality of the patient may or may not be retarded (Fig. 13–6).

It has been found that not all features are inevitably present in every case; e.g., the prognathic mandible may not be found, and there is often some overlap with other developmental syndromes.

Treatment and Prognosis. Craniectomy at a very early age to provide space for the rapidly developing brain has been used in treatment for some time. In the past few years, other very sophisticated surgical procedures have been developed by a limited number of skillful surgeons. These procedures were designed basically to improve the cosmetic appearance and vision of some patients with major craniofacial deformities such as those that accompany craniofacial dysostosis. These patients may ultimately come to lead a relatively normal life.

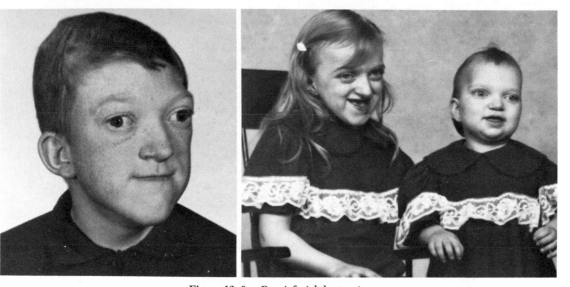

Figure 13–6. *Craniofacial dysostosis.*
A father (at an early age) and his two daughters are all affected by the condition. (Courtesy of Drs. David Bixler and Stephen G. Kaler.)

MANDIBULOFACIAL DYSOSTOSIS

(Treacher Collins Syndrome; Franceschetti Syndrome)

The term "branchial arch syndromes" has been used to describe a heterogeneous group of malformations of the head and neck characterized by anatomic alterations in the structures embryologically derived from the branchial arches. However, the term constitutes so large a group of syndromes that are individually recognizable as entities, albeit much overlap may exist between some, that it is of little use other than to indicate the part of the embryo involved by the disorders.

The mandibulofacial dysostosis syndrome encompasses a group of closely related defects of the head and face, often hereditary or familial in pattern, following an irregular form of dominant transmission. A historic review of the disease was made by Pavsek, who, in addition to reporting an additional case, summarized the embryologic faults of the conditions. There have been other excellent reviews by Rovin and his co-workers and by Fernandez and Ronis.

Clinical Features. Wide variations in the clinical expression of this syndrome are recognized, ranging from a complete, typical form manifesting all abnormalities listed below through incomplete, abortive, and atypical forms. The important clinical manifestations of the disease are (1) antimongoloid palpebral fissures with a coloboma of the outer portion of

the lower lids, and deficiency of the eyelashes (and sometimes the upper lids); (2) hypoplasia of the facial bones, especially of the malar bones and mandible; (3) malformation of the external ear, and occasionally of the middle and internal ears; (4) macrostomia, high palate (sometimes cleft) and abnormal position and malocclusion of the teeth; (5) blind fistulas between the angles of the ears and the angles of the mouth; (6) atypical hair growth in the form of a tongue-shaped process of the hairline extending towards the cheeks; and (7) other anomalies such as facial clefts and skeletal deformities (Fig. 13–7). The characteristic facies of the patients have often been described as being birdlike or fishlike in nature.

The syndrome is thought to result from a retardation or failure of differentiation of maxillary mesoderm at and after the 50-mm. stage of the embryo. The fact that the teeth of the upper jaw are usually unaffected, and ordinarily are present by the sixth week, is further evidence of retardation or arrest of differentiation at or after the second month of fetal life. The first visceral arch of the visceral mesoderm also advances secondarily to form the mandible, and again retardation occurs on the same basis.

A disease that has sometimes been confused with mandibulofacial dysostosis because of certain clinical features in common is *hemifacial microsomia* (also known as *oculoauriculovertebral dysplasia* or *Goldenhar syndrome*). However, hemifacial microsomia is sporadic in the

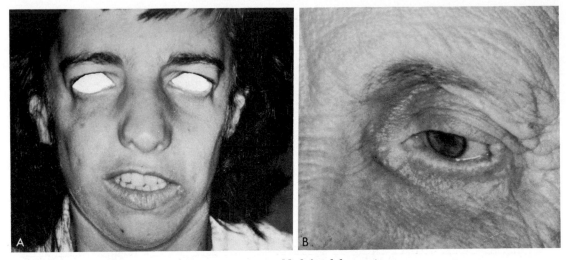

Figure 13–7. *Mandibulofacial dysostosis.*
(Courtesy of Dr. Stephen F. Dachi.)

vast majority of cases, although familial cases have been reported. In addition, as the name implies, this disease is unilateral and has been suggested to be related to an abnormality in the vascular supply of the head. It has been discussed in detail by Gorlin and his associates.

Roentgenographic Features. As Pavsek pointed out, the bodies of both malar bones tend to be grossly and symmetrically underdeveloped in mandibulofacial dysostosis. There may be agenesis of the malar bones with nonfusion of the zygomatic arches, as well as absence of the palatine bones. Cleft palate may be visible on the roentgenogram. There is usually hypogenesis, and sometimes agenesis, of the mandible. The paranasal sinuses are grossly underdeveloped, and the mastoids appear infantile and sclerotic. The auditory ossicles are often absent, and the cochlea and vestibular apparatus may be deficient. The cranial vault is normal in most instances.

Treatment and Prognosis. There is no treatment for this condition, but the prognosis is good, most patients living a normal life span.

PIERRE ROBIN SYNDROME

(Robin Anomalad)

This well-recognized disorder is considered to be a nonspecific anomalad which may occur either as an isolated defect or as a part of a broader group of malformations. The isolated defect is considered a sporadic or non-genetic condition with a very low recurrence risk in the

family. In contrast, the Pierre Robin syndrome in association with other genetic syndromes may carry a very high recurrence risk. The more commonly associated conditions have been listed by Gorlin and his associates and include the Stickler syndrome, the cerebrocostomandibular syndrome, the camptomelic syndrome and the persistent left superior vena cava syndrome.

The Pierre Robin syndrome or anomalad consists of cleft palate, micrognathia, and glossoptosis. An anomalad is a malformation together with its subsequently derived structural changes, the primary defect setting off a series of secondary or even tertiary events resulting in multiple anomalies. In the case of the Pierre Robin anomalad, the primary defect lies in arrested development and ensuing hypoplasia of the mandible, ultimately producing the characteristic "bird facies." This in turn prevents the normal descent of the tongue between the palatal shelves, resulting in cleft palate. Because of this "mechanism," cleft lip does not occur in association with the cleft palate.

The most important result of this jaw malformation is respiratory difficulty, although the exact explanation for its occurrence is uncertain. The usual suggestion is that failure of support of tongue musculature occurs because of the micrognathia, allowing the tongue to fall down and backward, partially obstructing the epiglottis. However, there is not full agreement on this point.

Other systemic findings may also be present in the Pierre Robin syndrome, including congenital heart defects, other skeletal anomalies and ocular lesions. In addition, mental retardation is present in a significant number of these patients.

MARFAN SYNDROME

(Marfan-Achard Syndrome; Arachnodactyly)

Marfan syndrome is a hereditary disease transmitted as an autosomal dominant trait. It is of interest that over 500 cases of this disease have been reported in the literature, one of the more famous instances being that of President Abraham Lincoln.

It is basically a disease of connective tissue related to a defective organization of collagen. It has been found that the collagen in this disease is abnormally soluble. Recent studies by Boucek and his associates have shown reduced amounts of chemically stable forms of intermolecular cross-links and suggested that an attenuation of probably nonenzymatic steps involved in the maturation of collagen causes the defective collagen organization in Marfan syndrome.

Clinical Features. The outstanding characteristic of Marfan syndrome is the excessive length of the tubular bones resulting in dolichostenomelia or disproportionately long thin extremities and arachnodactyly or spidery fingers. The shape of the skull and face is characteristically long and narrow, and commonly suggests the diagnosis of the disease. Other features of the disease include hyperextensibility of joints with habitual dislocations, kyphosis or scoliosis and flatfoot. Bilateral ectopia lentis, caused by weakening or rupture of the suspensory ligaments, is found in at least 50 per cent of patients, and myopia is usually present.

Cardiovascular complications are also a prominent feature of the disease and these include aortic aneurysm and aortic regurgitation, valvular defects, and enlargement of the heart.

Oral Manifestations. According to Baden and Spirgi, who have reviewed the oral manifestations of this disease, a high, arched palatal vault is very prevalent and may be a constant finding. Bifid uvula is also reported as well as malocclusion. In addition, multiple odontogenic cysts of the maxilla and mandible have occasionally been reported, most recently by Oatis and his co-workers. One additional finding sometimes present is temporomandibular dysarthrosis.

Treatment. There is no specific treatment and the prognosis is good.

DOWN SYNDROME

(Trisomy 21 Syndrome; Mongolism)

Down syndrome is a disease associated with subnormal mentality in which an extremely wide variety of anomalies and functional disorders may occur, two of the chief types being cranial and facial deformities.

Although many factors, such as advanced maternal age and uterine and placental abnormalities, have been regarded as causes of the disease, recent cytogenetic investigations now implicate a chromosomal aberration. This disease is, in fact, the most common chromosomal abnormality to occur in man.

It is now generally accepted that there are at least three forms of Down syndrome: one in which there is the typical trisomy 21 with 47 chromosomes (accounting for about 95 per cent of cases); another termed the translocation type, in which there appear to be only 46 chromosomes, although the extra chromosome material of number 21 is translocated to another chromosome of G or D group (about 3 per cent of cases); and another that is the result of chromosomal mosaicism (about 2 per cent). Children with the translocation type of Down syndrome are more commonly born to mothers under 30 years of age. The incidence of mongolism in subsequent siblings may be greatly increased in such instances. Mothers over 40 years rarely have translocation mongoloids. In contrast, the risk of having an affected child of the typical trisomy 21 type is approximately one in 2000 live births in women under 30 years of age but rises dramatically to one in 50 live births in women over 45 years of age.

It is of significant interest that individuals with Down syndrome, especially children, have an increased incidence of acute leukemia. Rowley presented data indicating that a gain of chromosome 21 occurs in the leukemic cells of constitutionally normal individuals with acute lymphocytic leukemia, particularly children, and postulated that the presence of an extra chromosome 21 in Down syndrome is the factor putting them at increased risk of acute leukemia.

Clinical Features. Patients with Down syndrome are characterized by a flat face, a large anterior fontanel, open sutures, small slanting eyes with epicanthal folds, open mouth, frequent prognathism, sexual underdevelopment, cardiac abnormalities and hypermobility of the joints. Actually, the defects are so varied in their occurrence that it is difficult to make a complete listing.

Oral Manifestations. The patients frequently exhibit macroglossia with protrusion of the tongue, as well as fissured tongue or pebbly tongue from enlargement of the papillae. They also commonly have a high arched palate. The teeth are sometimes malformed, enamel hypoplasia and microdontia being most common.

Cohen and his co-workers and Brown and Cunningham investigated the periodontal status of large groups of mongoloids and reported almost universal, severe, destructive periodontal disease that did not appear to be local in origin. Brown and Cunningham also commented on the surprising number of patients who had complete freedom from dental caries.

OSTEOPETROSIS

(Marble Bone Disease; Albers-Schönberg Disease; Osteosclerosis Fragilis Generalisata)

Osteopetrosis is an uncommon disease of unknown etiology. It may be subdivided into two main types: (1) a clinically benign dominantly inherited form, and (2) a clinically malignant recessively inherited form. Reported cases appear to be about equally divided between these two types.

It is of interest that a similar, but not identical, disease exists in certain strains of animals, including rats and mice. The *ia* strain of rat, for example, demonstrates the phenomenon of normal appositional bone growth, but failure of physiologic bone resorption. Osteoclasts are present in these animals in normal numbers, but appear afunctional. This finding may be related to the fact that the osteoclasts have been shown to be deficient in ribonucleic acid. The defective genes may also be associated with the parathyroid glands in these rats, since the injection of parathyroid hormone produces bone resorption. This suggests that it is necessary to have a certain level of parathyroid hormone in addition to the presence of osteoclasts if normal bone resorption is to occur. The grey-lethal strain of mouse exhibits a type of disturbance of bone metabolism similar to that of the *ia* rat.

Clinical Features. The clinical manifestations of the two forms of the disease are quite different and may be used to distinguish between them.

Malignant recessive osteopetrosis is the more severe form of the disease and either is present at birth (congenital or neonatal type), with some cases even being recognized in utero, or develops in very early life (infantile or childhood

type). In general, the earlier the disease appears, the more serious it is and many affected infants are stillborn or die very soon after birth.

Most bones of the skeleton are involved by the diffuse sclerotic process in both forms of the disease. However, in both forms, there may be less severe and less extensive involvement. In the malignant recessive disease, the most common clinical manifestation is optic atrophy (in over 75 per cent of cases), followed by hepatosplenomegaly, poor growth, frontal bossing, pathologic fractures, loss of hearing, facial palsy and genu valgum. Death in these patients is usually a result of anemia or secondary infection. No known patient with this form of osteopetrosis has survived past the age of 20 years.

Benign dominant osteopetrosis is a much less severe type of the disease which generally develops somewhat later in life; in fact, occasional cases are not diagnosed until middle age. These patients can be expected to survive into old age. This disease has been reviewed by Johnston and his associates.

Bone involvement, both extent and severity, is similar to that in the malignant recessive disease. However, nearly half of all patients with the benign form are totally asymptomatic. Pathologic fractures, often multiple, are the most common clinical manifestation (approximately 40 per cent of all cases), followed by bone pain, cranial nerve palsy (including optic and facial) and osteomyelitis. The cranial nerve involvement in both types of the disease is a result of narrowing of the cranial foramina by bone deposition with resulting impingement on the nerves.

Oral Manifestations. The jaws are involved in the same manner as the other bones in the body, and the oral manifestations have been reviewed by Kaslick and Brustein. However, a clear distinction has usually not been made as to the type of the disease present, benign or malignant.

The medullary spaces of the jaws are remarkably reduced in both dominant and recessive osteopetrosis so that there is a marked predilection for the development of osteomyelitis should infection gain entrance to the bone. This is a complication of dental extraction which has been reported frequently and discussed by Dyson. Similar findings were noted by Bjorvatn and his associates in four children with the malignant form of the disease. They stressed the necessity of administering large doses of antibiotics to control the recurring infection, which even then did not prevent the progressive osseous destruction. Fracture of the jaw during tooth extraction, even when the extraction is performed without undue force, may also occur because of the fragility of the bone.

It has been reported that the teeth are of defective quality, enamel hypoplasia, microscopic dentinal defects and arrested root development all having been described. However, this may not be true in the benign dominant form of the disease. It is also reported that the teeth are especially prone to dental caries. Since the dental findings have been recorded in so few cases, this observation is difficult to evaluate. An additional rather constant finding is retardation of tooth eruption due to the sclerosis of bone. This same phenomenon occurs in both the *ia* rat and the grey-lethal mouse, whose teeth become distorted in shape through eruptive pressure.

Roentgenographic Features. The roentgenographic picture of osteopetrosis, according to Johnston and his co-workers, remains the sine qua non of diagnosis. There is considerable variation in the severity of the disease, but the classic cases of osteopetrosis are characterized by a diffuse, homogeneous, symmetrically sclerotic appearance of all bones with clubbing and transverse striations of the ends of the long bones (Fig. 13–8). The medullary cavities are replaced by bone, and the cortex is thickened.

The jaws on occasion may be spared at least the severe involvement which the other bones suffer. When the jaws are affected, however, the density of the bone may be such that the roots of the teeth are nearly invisible on the dental roentgenograms.

Laboratory Findings. The patients manifest a myelophthisic anemia due to the displacement of hemopoietic marrow tissue by bone. The lymph nodes, liver, and spleen sometimes assume a hemopoietic function, and for this reason hepatomegaly may be present. Red blood cell counts below 1,000,000 cells per cubic millimeter may occur in cases of osteopetrosis. The serum calcium and phosphorus levels are usually within normal limits, as is the serum alkaline phosphatase level. An elevated serum acid phosphatase has been reported in patients with benign dominant osteopetrosis.

Histologic Features. Osteopetrosis is characterized by the endosteal production of bone with an apparent concomitant lack of physiologic bone resorption (Fig. 13–9). Osteoblasts are prominent, but osteoclasts are seldom found in significant numbers in tissue sections. The predominance of bone formation over resorption typically leads to the persistence of cartilaginous cores of bony trabeculae long after their replacement should have occurred in endochondral bones. The trabeculae themselves

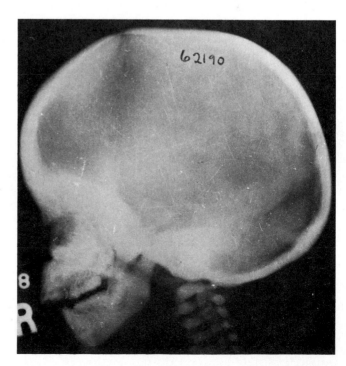

Figure 13–8. *Osteopetrosis.* The skull and jaws evidence dense diffuse radiopacity. (Courtesy of Dr. John A. Campbell.)

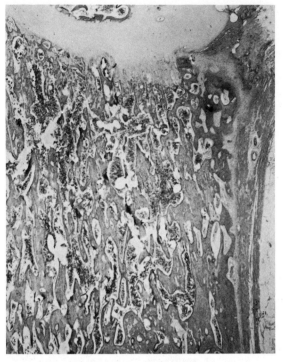

Figure 13–9. *Osteopetrosis.*
A photomicrograph of a long bone shows replacement of the marrow by endosteal bone. (Courtesy of Dr. Frank Vellios.)

are disorderly in arrangement, and the marrow tissue present is usually fibrous.

It has been reported by Johnston and his associates, however, that adult patients with benign osteopetrosis do not appear to have a deficiency in osteoclastic activity but rather an abnormality in the type and structure of bone. They found osteoblastic and osteoclastic activity with prominent remodeling of bone. However, by polarized light, the bone was found to be markedly deficient in collagen matrix fibrils and these seldom crossed from one osteone to another. This deficiency of fibrils could account for the tendency for fracture in these patients.

Treatment. No effective treatment has been discovered for osteopetrosis. Depletion of vitamin D or administration of vitamin A has failed to modify the course of the disease.

ACHONDROPLASIA

(Chondrodystrophia Fetalis)

Achondroplasia is a disturbance of endochondral bone formation which results in a characteristic form of dwarfism. It is a hereditary condition that is transmitted as an autosomal

dominant characteristic. This disease begins in utero and may actually be diagnosed before parturition, but it presents a high mortality rate. Eighty per cent of affected infants are either stillborn or die shortly after birth. Interestingly, twins are sometimes born of an affected parent, and occasionally only one of the pair is afflicted by the disease. These would obviously be fraternal twins.

Clinical Features. The achondroplastic dwarf is the most common type of dwarf and presents a characteristic physical appearance. He is quite short, usually under 1.4 meters, with short and thickened muscular extremities, a brachycephalic skull and bowed legs. The hands are usually small, and the fingers stubby. Lumbar lordosis with prominent buttocks and a protruding abdomen are often present, and many joints characteristically exhibit limitation of motion. Because of this, the arms do not hang freely at the sides, and the elbows often cannot be straightened (Fig. 13–10).

The incongruous appearance of the achondroplastic dwarf is in contrast to that of the pituitary dwarf, and the incongruity becomes more pronounced as he approaches adulthood and later life, chiefly because of the disproportionate size of the head in relation to the remainder of the body. Despite their misshapen appearance, achondroplastic dwarfs are of normal intelligence. Often they are also endowed with unusual strength and agility, characteristics which have led some to adopt the occupation of professional wrestler.

Oral Manifestations. The maxilla is often retruded because of restriction of growth of the base of the skull, and the retrusion may produce a relative mandibular prognathism (Fig. 13–11). The resultant disparity in size of the two jaws produces an obvious malocclusion. The dentition itself is usually normal, although congenitally missing teeth with disturbance in the shape of those present have been reported.

Roentgenographic Features. The long bones are shorter than normal, and there is thickening or mild clubbing of the ends. The epiphyses generally appear normal, but may close either early or late. The bones at the base of the skull fuse prematurely, producing shortening as well as a narrow foramen magnum. Except for the retrusion of the maxilla and the malocclusion between the two jaws, there are no changes in the jawbones.

Histologic Features. Achondroplasia is characterized by disturbances in the epiphyseal cartilage of long bones and ribs as well as in certain membrane bones of the base of the

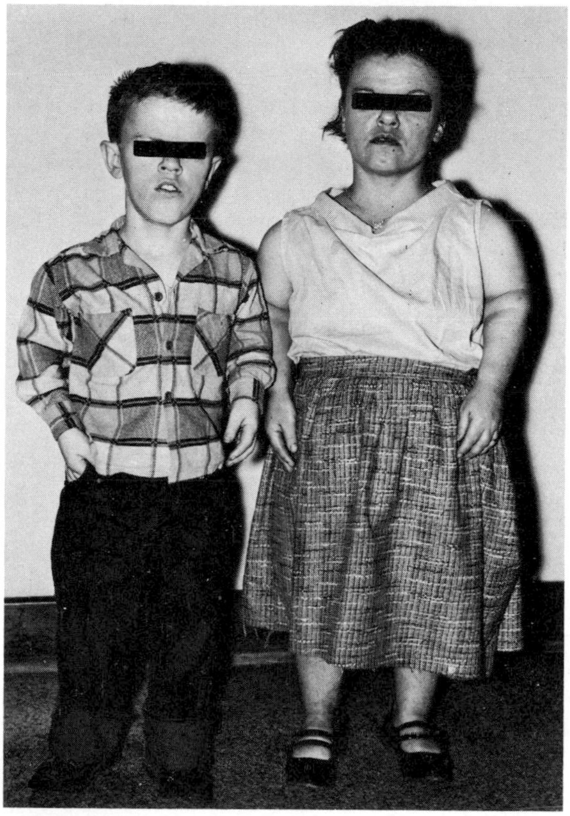

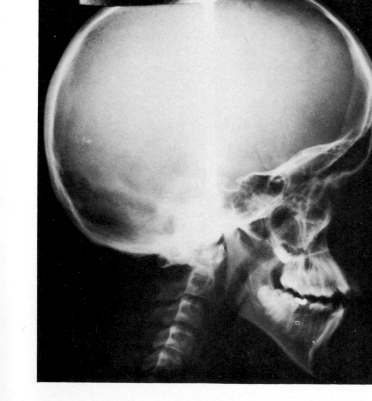

Figure 13–10. *Achondroplasia.*
The mother and son present the typical dwarfed appearance. (Courtesy of Dr. Ralph E. McDonald.)

Figure 13–11. *Achondroplasia.*
The lateral skull film illustrates the retruded maxilla which contributes to the characteristic facial appearance of the patient. (Courtesy of Dr. Ralph E. McDonald.)

skull. The basic defect appears as a retardation or even aplasia of the zone of provisional calcification of endochondral growth. The cartilage columns lack orderly arrangement, fail to calcify properly and are not resorbed and replaced by bone in the usual fashion. Since chondrocyte development is defective, the orderly longitudinal growth of bone is disrupted, resulting in stunting of the bone.

Treatment and Prognosis. There is no treatment for achondroplasia. If the patient survives past the first few years of life, the chances are excellent that he will have the life expectancy of a normal person.

OSTEITIS DEFORMANS

(Paget's Disease of Bone)

Osteitis deformans is a disease of bone which has been known for many years, at least since the original report of Paget in 1877, but which until recent years has been considered a rare occurrence. The widespread practice of routine skeletal roentgenographic examination of patients in hospitals as well as greater acceptance and use of postmortem examination has resulted in the discovery of relatively large numbers of cases which otherwise would have been overlooked and never recorded. Thus, although the incidence of the disease appears to be increasing, the apparent increase may be due only to the greater probability of discovery of the disease.

Etiology. The etiology of osteitis deformans is still unknown despite numerous theories that have been advanced over the years. Paget originally believed that the disease was an inflammatory one, and his view was supported by some later workers.

On the other hand, considerable evidence has been presented to confirm the hypothesis that a circulatory disturbance is the cause of the disease. It is well recognized that the bone in osteitis deformans is excessively vascular, and it has been suggested that the vessels are similar to arteriovenous aneurysms. There is a sizable group of other vascular alterations that occur concomitantly with the disease in a high proportion of the cases, and these include increased cardiac output, cardiac enlargement and arteriosclerosis among others.

Jaffe suggested some years ago that the cause of Paget's disease is a breakdown in the normal mechanism of creeping replacement to which bone is constantly subjected, and there are certain features of this disease which lend credence to this view.

Most recently, Rebel and his associates reported the presence of characteristic nuclear inclusions in the osteoclasts of four patients with Paget's disease; this was confirmed subsequently in numerous additional patients in other laboratories. Speculation has been advanced that these structures are viruses and that Paget's disease represents a condition caused by an infection by a "slow" virus. A "slow" virus is one which produces a disease with a prolonged incubation period (even years) prior to manifestation of the illness. One of the best known "slow" viral human diseases is subacute sclerosing panencephalitis, which is thought to be possibly related to measles. Interestingly, Rebel and his co-workers have recently reported viral antigens in the osteoclasts of patients with Paget's disease that were immunologically suggestive of measles or a measles-related virus. In his review of this theory of the etiology of the disease, Singer has pointed out that the protracted subclinical course, the absence of an acute inflammatory process, and geographic and familial clustering also favor a viral cause. Nevertheless, it still remains theory.

Clinical Features. Osteitis deformans occurs predominantly in patients over 40 years of age, the incidence increasing in the older age groups, but it has also been reported in young persons as early as the second decade of life. In the over-all series of 4164 autopsies of patients over 40 years of age reported by Schmorl, 138 cases of Paget's disease of bone were discovered, an incidence of 3 per cent. Some more recent studies have confirmed this incidence figure while others have reported a prevalence figure as low as 0.01 per cent. Both sexes are affected by the disease, but there is a slight predilection for men. Hereditary or familial tendencies have been reported in a number of instances. There is also a marked geographic predilection for occurrence, the disease being common in England, France and Germany but rare in certain other European countries, Africa, and the Middle and Far East. It occurs with moderate frequency in North America.

Osteitis deformans is a chronic disease, and symptoms develop slowly. Many times the disease is discovered only by accident, but eventually most patients complain of one or more of the following symptoms: bone pain, severe headache, deafness (due to involvement of the petrous portion of the temporal bone with compression of the cochlear nerve in its foramen), blindness or other visual disturbances (due to similar involvement of the optic nerve in its foramen), facial paralysis (due to pressure on the facial nerve), dizziness, weakness and mental disturbance.

The signs of the disease presented by the patients are not always obvious until it has become relatively far advanced, and this is true of jaw involvement also. These features include progressive enlargement of the skull, deformities of the spine, femur and tibia so that the patient actually becomes shorter, bowing of the legs, broadening and flattening of the chest and spinal curvature. With the waddling gait and the foregoing features, the patient often assumes a simian appearance, and his facial pattern may become grotesque. The involved bones become warm to the touch because of the increased vascularity, and they exhibit increased fragility with tendency for fracture. In fact, pathologic fracture is one of the most common complications of Paget's disease. It has variously been reported to occur in from 8 to over 30 per cent of all patients with the disease. Fracture healing is usually normal, although the callus may be abundant.

In the older literature, one of the classic initial complaints of patients with Paget's disease was their need to buy hats of increasingly larger size because of the skull enlargement. Interestingly, occasional cases are still seen today in which this is one of the initial clinical complaints or at least can be ascertained by questioning the patient. A thorough review of the clinical and metabolic features of Paget's disease has been published by de Deuxchaisnes and Krane.

Any bone in the skeleton may be involved, although there is a predilection for a certain distribution of lesions. The disease may be focal or localized in some patients and disseminated in others. In the series of autopsy cases reported by Schmorl, which undoubtedly did not include examination of the jaws, the following distribution of bone involvement was found:

Sacrum	56%	Left femur	15%
Spine	50%	Clavicle	13%
Right femur	31%	Tibia	8%
Skull	28%	Rib	7%
Sternum	23%	Humerus	4%
Pelvis	21%		

Involvement of the facial bones is occasionally seen also, and this entity was reviewed recently by Drury. It has sometimes been called *leontiasis ossea,* but, because this term is nonspe-

cific, Drury advocated discontinuing its use in referring to this disease.

Oral Manifestations. Involvement of the jaws in osteitis deformans is a rather common occurrence. Stafne and Austin reported 20 cases involving the maxilla and 3 cases involving the mandible in a series of 138 cases of generalized osteitis deformans, an incidence of 17 per cent jaw involvement. This predilection for the maxilla has also been noted in most other studies. A number of cases have been reported in which both jaws of a patient were involved. Cooke also provided an excellent study of 15 cases of Paget's disease of the jaws, while Tillman has reported 24 cases. Smith and Eveson also have recently reviewed this disease with particular reference to dentistry, analyzing 152 cases involving the jaws previously reported in the literature. Of these, 98 involved the maxilla, 28 the mandible and 26 both jaws. Thus, the ratio of involvement of maxilla to mandible was approximately 2.3:1.

The maxilla exhibits progressive enlargement, the alveolar ridge becomes widened and the palate is flattened (Fig. 13–12). If teeth are present, they may become loose and migrate, producing some spacing. When the mandible is involved, the findings are similar, but not usually as severe as in the maxilla. As the disease progresses, the mouth may remain open, exposing the teeth, because the lips are too small to cover the enlarged jaw.

Edentulous patients with dentures commonly complain of inability to wear their appliances because of increasing tightness due to expansion of the jaw. The dentures may be remade periodically to accommodate this increase in size of the jaws.

When the jaws are involved by Paget's disease, there is usually involvement of the skull as well. But there have been some cases reported in which the skull showed no evidence of the disease.

Roentgenographic Features. The roentgenographic features of osteitis deformans are varied and depend upon the stage of the disease encountered. Paget's disease has sometimes been described as a disorder characterized by an initial phase of deossification and softening, followed by a bizarre, dysplastic type of reossification not related to functional requirements, the two processes taking place simultaneously or alternately. With this in mind, the protean roentgenographic manifestations can be easily reconciled. Thus osteolytic areas of the skeleton are commonly associated with areas of osteoblastic activity. These destructive lesions may

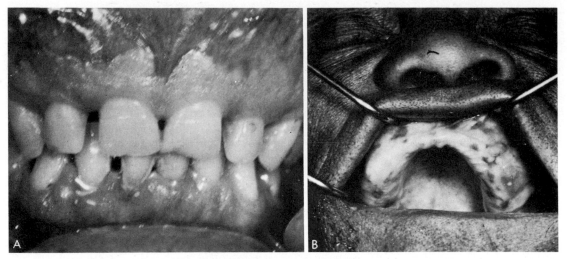

Figure 13–12.   *Osteitis deformans.*
There are diffuse enlargement of the maxilla and thickening of the dentulous *(A)* and edentulous *(B)* alveolar ridge. In addition, tipping of the teeth due to enlargement of the maxilla is obvious. *(B,* Courtesy of Dr. Robert J. Gorlin.)

be multiple and diffuse or isolated. The isolated lesion in the skull, when large, is sometimes referred to as "osteoporosis circumscripta."

The osteoblastic phase of osteitis deformans is the more commonly recognized one and inevitably occurs regardless of pre-existing osteolytic lesions. The osteoblastic areas, which appear as opacities in the roentgenogram, tend to be patchy in distribution, eventually becoming confluent, but often still showing minute areas of variation in radiodensity. This patchiness has been termed a "cotton-wool" appearance and is especially well demonstrated in the skull and jaws (Fig. 13–13).

Roentgenograms of the jaws may demonstrate even very early phases of the disease, although such phases may not be so specific as to be pathognomonic. An excellent description of the oral manifestations of early osteitis deformans has been provided by Spilka and Callahan. In such cases, poorly defined areas of osteoporosis may be noted, although of more diagnostic significance is the finding of loss of normal trabeculation and the appearance of irregular osteoblastic activity, again giving rise to the typical "cotton-wool" appearances of "Paget's bone" (Fig. 13–13, *B*). Although the disease is usually bilateral, it may show roentgenographic evidence of only unilateral involvement of the jaw, especially early in the course of the disease. This may closely simulate chronic, diffuse, sclerosing osteomyelitis.

The teeth themselves and adjacent bone present significant roentgenographic changes suggestive of osteitis deformans also. These consist characteristically of a rather pronounced hypercementosis and, often, loss of a well-defined lamina dura around the teeth. Root resorption has been reported in some cases, but this is unusual.

Laboratory Findings.   The serum calcium and serum phosphorus levels are usually within normal limits, even in cases of advanced osteitis deformans. The serum alkaline phosphatase level may be elevated, however, to extreme limits. Values as high as over 250 Bodansky units have been reported, particularly in patients in the osteoblastic phase of the disease, when there is rapid formation of new bone and when there is polyostotic involvement. In fact, there is no other disease of bone in which the serum alkaline phosphatase level may be as high as in Paget's disease. In the monostotic form of the disease, the alkaline phosphatase level seldom exceeds 50 Bodansky units. In the very early stage of the disease this phosphatase level may not be significantly elevated, although it is simply a matter of time before this does occur. The serum acid phosphatase level is not increased.

Histologic Features.   The microscopic appearance of the bone in cases of osteitis deformans varies remarkably, depending upon the stage of the disease encountered. Since the condition is characterized by both bone resorption and bone deposition, corresponding osteoclastic and osteoblastic activity may be expected to be evident. These concomitant processes occur in a haphazard fashion without regard to the patterns of stress. Since both processes may

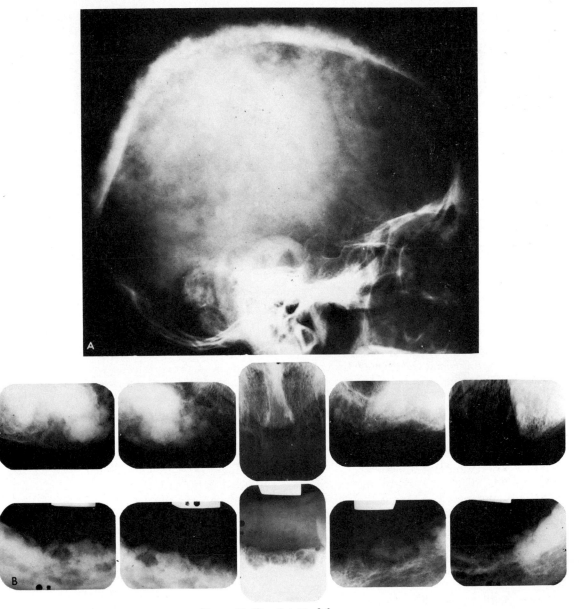

Figure 13–13. *Osteitis deformans.*
The roentgenograms of the skull (*A*) and the jaws (*B*) demonstrate the typical "cotton-wool" appearance. (*A*, Courtesy of Dr. John A. Campbell.)

occur in closely adjacent areas, the histologic picture is often a confusing one.

One of the most characteristic features of osteitis deformans is the formation of "mosaic" bone, a descriptive term used to indicate the appearance of bone which has been partially resorbed and then repaired, leaving deeply staining hematoxyphilic reversal lines (Fig. 13–14, *B*). These lines indicate the alternation between the resorptive and the formative phases, and when occurring over and over

again, eventuate in a "jigsaw-puzzle" appearance of the bone.

The bone may exhibit large numbers of osteoblasts or osteoclasts, or sometimes a combination of both, lining individual trabeculae, or the bone may be in a resting phase showing little cellular activity (Fig. 13–14, *C*). The marrow tends to be fibrous, although sometimes it is fatty. Inflammatory edema of the marrow is common, and focal collections of lymphocytes may be observed.

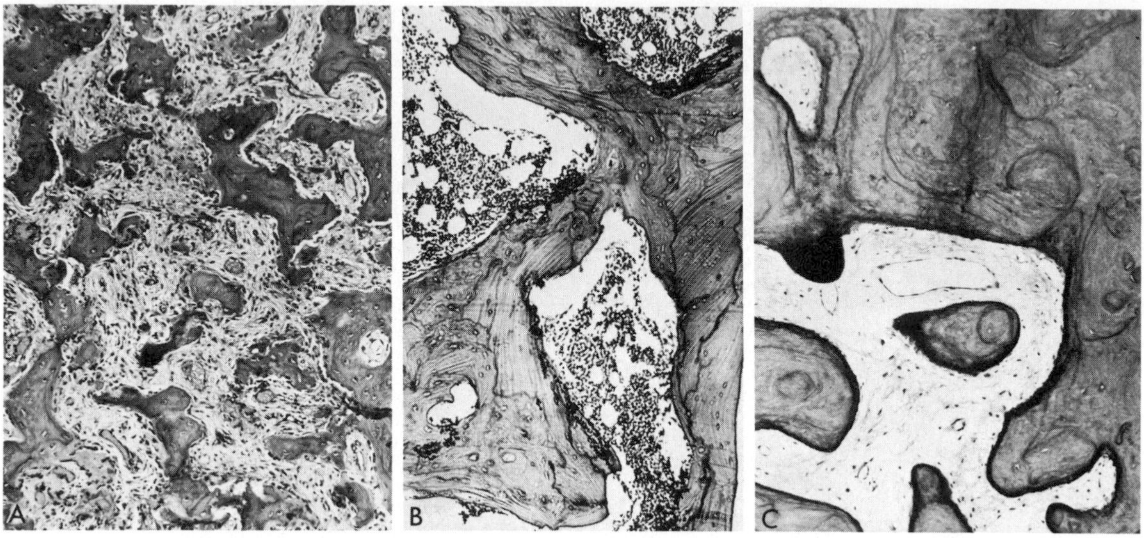

Figure 13–14. *Osteitis deformans.*
Photomicrographs of bone in different stages showing *(A)* reactive phase, *(B)* mosaic pattern, and *(C)* resting phase. Note the prominent resting and reversal lines in *B*.

The more rapidly bone is laid down, the more immature it is and the greater amounts of osteoid one may find. As bone formation lags and a resting phase is reached, the bone changes from a fibrillar type to a more mature lamellar variety (Fig. 13–14, *C*).

The proliferation of bone and concomitant hypercementosis sometimes result in obliteration of the periodontal ligament.

Treatment. There is no specific treatment for osteitis deformans. Vitamin, hormone and radiation therapy have all been utilized with sporadic reports of cures, but these have not been confirmed. Administration of fluoride has also been used but evidence is still lacking that it is of any significant benefit in controlling the disease.

Very promising results have recently been obtained in the treatment of this disease by the use of calcitonin, the parathormone antagonist produced by the thyroid gland which suppresses bone resorption. Diphosphonates have also been used with some success, since they also inhibit bone resorption as well as bone mineralization. Finally, one of the cytotoxic antibiotics, mithramycin, has been used therapeutically but has serious side effects. The use of these agents has been reviewed in detail by Smith and Eveson.

Prognosis. The disease is a chronic, slowly progressive one and seldom is a primary cause of death.

Complications may arise related to the bony alterations, including pathologic fractures, the skeletal deformities and the auditory and visual disturbances previously noted. The most serious complication of osteitis deformans is the development of osteosarcoma in a significant percentage of cases. The simultaneous occurrence of these two conditions is far too common to be due to chance, and it must be concluded that osteitis deformans predisposes to the development of the bone malignancy. It has been stated that the risk of osteosarcoma in Pagetic individuals over the age of 40 years is 30 times greater than in normal persons. Although the true frequency of malignant transformation is difficult to determine, Goldenberg reported an incidence of 15 per cent in one group of cases. Porretta and his associates reported 16 cases of osteosarcoma in 1753 cases of Paget's disease, an incidence of 0.9 per cent. In a review of the literature on this subject they found only one patient from a group of 128 with osteosarcoma developing in Paget's disease that survived for 5 years, and concluded that the prognosis for sarcoma in this situation is exceedingly poor. Interestingly, they also found that nearly 20 per cent of patients with sarcoma developing in Paget's disease had sustained a fracture of the bone at the site at which the sarcoma subsequently developed. The same workers have pointed out that if all cases of osteosarcoma are considered, between 2 and 5 per cent of these occur in patients with Paget's disease. Finally, in about 20 per cent of cases, the osteosarcoma is multicentric.

The cause of the development of the neoplasm is unknown, but Jaffe suggested that it is related to the remarkable proliferative capacities of the tissues in Paget's disease. In addition, Hutter and his group have drawn attention to the occurrence of giant cell tumors, both benign and malignant, as a complication of Paget's disease. Two such cases involving the jaws have been reported by Miller and his co-workers.

Differential Diagnosis. There are a number of bone diseases which, roentgenographically and/or microscopically, may resemble Paget's disease and must be differentiated. These include fibrous dysplasia of bone, hyperparathyroidism with bone involvement, subacute osteomyelitis, chronic sclerosing osteomyelitis, fibro-osteoma, osteosarcoma and other disseminated neoplasms such as metastatic carcinoma and multiple myeloma.

GENERALIZED CORTICAL HYPEROSTOSIS

(Van Buchem Disease or Syndrome; Endosteal Hyperostosis)

This disease of bone, described by Van Buchem and his associates in 1955, appears to represent an excessive deposition of endosteal bone throughout the skeleton in a pattern suggestive of a hereditary condition with an autosomal recessive characteristic.

Clinical Features. The disease is usually not discovered until adult life and, in nearly all reported cases, has been a chance finding. The facial appearance of these patients may be altered and this may be the reason that they seek professional advice. Such a case has been reported by Dyson. The face may appear swollen, particularly with widening at the angles of the mandible and at the bridge of the nose. Some patients also have loss of visual acuity, loss of facial sensation, some degree of facial paralysis and deafness, all due to cranial nerve involvement through closure of foramina. Intraorally, there is sometimes overgrowth of the alveolar process. Most patients, except for the facial appearance, appear normal and are free of symptoms, including bone tenderness.

Roentgenographic Features. A skeletal survey will reveal increased density of many bones of the body, although some bones, such as those of the hands and feet, may be unaffected. The skull also exhibits diffuse sclerosis, as may the jaws.

Histologic Features. The bone is normal dense bone but without evidence of remodeling.

Differential Diagnosis. Three other diseases must also be considered in the diagnosis inasmuch as they may also present widespread sclerosis: osteopetrosis (marble bone disease), osteitis deformans (Paget's disease of bone) and progressive diaphyseal dysplasia (Camurati-Engelmann disease).

Treatment and Prognosis. There is no treatment for the disease, although the patients usually lead a normal life.

MASSIVE OSTEOLYSIS

(Vanishing Bone; Disappearing Bone; Phantom Bone; Progressive Osteolysis; Gorham Syndrome)

Massive osteolysis is an unusual and uncommon disease characterized by spontaneous, progressive resorption of bone with ultimate total disappearance of the bone. It is of unknown etiology but appears to be related to an active hyperemia of bone. It must be differentiated from (1) osteolysis associated with an infection, such as osteomyelitis, or with rheumatoid arthritis, or (2) osteolysis associated with disease of the central nervous system, such as tabes dorsalis, syringomyelia, leprosy or myelodysplasia. The disease has been discussed in detail by Kery and Wouters.

Clinical Features. Massive osteolysis is most common in older children and young and middle-aged adults, affecting both sexes equally. Usually only one bone is affected in a given patient, although polyostotic cases have been reported. The most commonly affected bones are the clavicle, scapula, humerus, ribs, ilium, ischium, and sacrum.

The disease, which may or may not be painful, begins suddenly and advances rapidly until the involved bone is replaced by a thin layer of fibrous tissue surrounding a cavity. All laboratory values are usually normal.

Oral Manifestations. A number of cases have been reported involving the mandible and other facial bones, and these have been reviewed by Ellis and Adams and by Murphy and his co-workers. In only two of these cases was there destruction of the entire mandible. In at least three cases, there was concomitant involvement of the maxilla. The patient may present with pain or facial asymmetry or both. One of the consistent findings in the disease has been pathologic fracture following minor trauma.

Histologic Features. The typical histologic finding is replacement of bone by connective tissue containing many thin-walled blood vessels or anastomosing vascular spaces lined by endothelial cells. It does not represent a hemangioma of bone, which remains a localized lesion, although the term "hemangiomatosis" has been applied. Most authorities do not believe that the disease is due to increased osteoclastic activity, although osteoclasts may often be found in the tissues. On the other hand, their absence in areas of active resorption is often quite striking.

Treatment and Prognosis. There is no specific treatment. Radiation therapy has been of benefit in some cases, while surgical resection has stopped the progress of the disease in others. Left untreated, the disease commonly progresses to total destruction of the involved bone.

FIBROUS DYSPLASIA OF BONE

Fibrous dysplasia of bone is one of the most perplexing diseases of osseous tissue. It is a lesion of unknown etiology, uncertain pathogenesis and diverse histopathology. A wide variety of conditions, though differing remarkably in extent and presence of secondary involvement, have been included under the term "fibrous dysplasia." Central lesions of bone which exhibit general histologic features of fibrosis with varying degrees of simultaneous resorption and repair have been reported for many years under various uninformative terms. Since the original introduction of the term "fibrous dysplasia" by Lichtenstein in 1938, a gradual classification of the various forms of the disease has evolved. There is no universal acceptance of this classification, however, and, as our knowledge and experience increase, there undoubtedly will be modification if not actually a discarding of the entire scheme.

The terms "monostotic" and "polyostotic" have been applied to those forms of the disease in which, respectively, one or more than one bone is involved. Two apparently separate types of polyostotic fibrous dysplasia are described: (1) fibrous dysplasia involving a variable number of bones, although most of the skeleton is normal, accompanied by pigmented lesions of the skin or "café-au-lait" spots (Jaffe's type), and (2) an even more severe fibrous dysplasia involving nearly all bones in the skeleton and accompanied by pigmented lesions of the skin and, in addition, endocrine disturbances of varying types (Albright's syndrome).

Monostotic fibrous dysplasia, that form of the disease in which only a single bone is involved,

does not manifest extraskeletal lesions such as those seen in polyostotic fibrous dysplasia. Nevertheless this localized disease is fully as confusing because of its distribution, histologic variation, and clinical course.

Polyostotic Fibrous Dysplasia

The first recognized case of polyostotic fibrous dysplasia associated with skin lesions and endocrine disturbance was recorded by Weil in 1922. Since then a considerable number of cases have been reported, and the condition has been specifically described by Albright, from whom the apparent syndrome derives its eponym. Valuable series of cases have been discussed by Harris and his associates and by Van Horn and his associates.

Clinical Features. The disease usually manifests itself early in life with an evident deformity, bowing or thickening of long bones, often unilateral in distribution. Its onset is usually insidious although aching recurrent bone pain is the most common presenting skeletal symptom. The bones of the face and skull are frequently involved, and an obvious asymmetry may result; also involved may be the clavicles, pelvic bones, scapulae, long bones, and metacarpals and metatarsals. Because of the severe bone changes, spontaneous fractures are a common complication of the disease, and these may result in invalidism.

The skin lesions associated with the disease consist of irregularly pigmented melanotic spots, described as "café-au-lait" spots because of their light brown color. In addition, the female patients, but not males, may exhibit precocious puberty, sometimes beginning at the age of two or three years or even younger. Vaginal bleeding is a common manifestation. A variety of other disturbances of the endocrine system have been reported, including those relating to the pituitary, thyroid, parathyroid and ovary. In addition, the occasional occurrence of multiple intramuscular soft-tissue myxomas as an extraskeletal manifestation of polyostotic fibrous dysplasia has been discussed by Wirth and his associates.

Polyostotic fibrous dysplasia as severe as that in Albright's syndrome is a relatively uncommon disease. That form known as Jaffe's type is similar to Albright's syndrome except that the endocrine disturbances are absent and there is seldom extreme or diffuse involvement of bone. Thus it appears that this type of dysplasia is a mild or nonprogressive form of the disease.

Oral Manifestations. The oral manifestations of polyostotic fibrous dysplasia are related to the severe disturbance of the bony tissue. One-third of the polyostotic patients in the series of Van Horn and his associates had lesions in the mandible. The occurrence of maxillary lesions was not mentioned, although Harris and his group stated that maxillary and mandibular involvement was not rare.

There may be expansion and deformity of the jaws, and the eruption pattern of the teeth is disturbed because of the loss of normal support of the developing teeth. The endocrine disturbance also may alter the time of eruption of the teeth. A classic case with involvement of the maxilla has been reported by Church. In this instance there was no intraoral pigmentation, although it has been reported to occur.

Roentgenographic Features. The skeleton in polyostotic fibrous dysplasia may present an extremely variable roentgenographic appearance. In general, the medullary portions of bone are rarefied and present irregular trabeculations, often a multilocular cystic appearance. The cortical bone is usually thinned and often considerably expanded.

Laboratory Findings. There are no consistent significant changes in the serum calcium or phosphorus, although the serum alkaline phosphatase level is sometimes elevated. Premature secretion of pituitary follicle-stimulating hormone has been reported, as well as a moderately elevated basal metabolic rate.

Histologic Features. The lesions are composed of fibrillar connective tissue within which are numerous trabeculae of coarse, woven fiber bone, irregular in shape but evenly spaced, showing no relation to functional patterns. The osteocytes are quite large, and collagen fibers of these trabeculae can often be seen extending out into the fibrous tissue. Bone formation by stellate osteoblasts can be observed, although rows of cuboidal osteoblasts lined up on the surfaces of trabeculae are absent. These trabeculae typically have wide osteoid seams. Osteoclastic activity may be seen where the calcification of osteoid extends to the surface of the trabeculae.

Treatment and Prognosis. Mild cases of polyostotic fibrous dysplasia of bone may be treated surgically; the severe forms are impossible to treat in this manner, particularly since they tend to be progressive. For this reason, x-ray radiation has been used with some success. But this is hazardous because of the possibility of subsequent development of radiation-induced sarcomas, and these have been reported on numerous occasions. The prognosis depends upon the degree of involvement of the skeleton, but the uncomplicated disease is usually compatible with life. Occasional patients will die as a direct result of their fibrous dysplasia.

An additional complication is the malignant transformation of fibrous dysplasia, both polyostotic and monostotic, into osteosarcoma in patients who have not received radiotherapy. Sixteen such cases have been reviewed by Schwartz and Alpert, who noted that this was more common in the polyostotic form of the disease and that the most common site was the craniofacial region. Malignant transformation has also been discussed by Bell and Hinds.

Monostotic Fibrous Dysplasia of the Jaws

Monostotic fibrous dysplasia, though less serious than polyostotic fibrous dysplasia, is of greater concern to the dentist because of the frequency with which the jaws are affected. Nearly every bone has at one time or another been reported involved. In a series of 67 cases of monostotic fibrous dysplasia, Schlumberger found the following distribution:

Ribs	29 cases	Humerus	2 cases
Femur	9 cases	Ulna	2 cases
Tibia	8 cases	Vertebra	1 case
Maxilla	7 cases	Pelvis	1 case
Calvarium	5 cases	Fibula	1 case
Mandible	2 cases		

There is now evidence to indicate, however, that the incidence of jaw lesions is proportionately far greater than this study would indicate. It is now recognized that some cases of jaw lesions which in the past were diagnosed under a variety of other names are now embraced by the term "fibrous dysplasia." As an example, certain cases of so-called central giant cell tumors of the jaws have been found upon re-evaluation to be classifiable as fibrous dysplasia. This has been emphasized particularly by Jaffe, Lichtenstein and Portis and by Waldron. In past years the designation "ossifying fibroma" (q.v.) was a common one for a certain group of jaw lesions which occurred with considerable frequency. Many authorities now view at least some of these lesions as a type of monostotic fibrous dysplasia. Another lesion of bone, the nonosteogenic fibroma, also is considered by some investigators to be a form of fibrous dysplasia. The clinical term "leontiasis ossea" has often been applied to cases of fibrous dysplasia which affect the maxilla or facial bones and give the patient a leonine appearance. Thus it can be appreciated that fibrous dysplasia of bone has come to include a number of lesions once described by other terms. Although investigators differed as to the desirability of inclusion of certain bony lesions in this group, the trend in the past few years had been to recognize monostotic fibrous dysplasia as an entity with considerable clinical and histologic variation, probably dependent upon the stage or phase of the disease.

In contrast, however, it has been suggested that this trend to classify many fibro-osseous lesions of the jaws under the term "fibrous dysplasia" may be unfortunate, and many pathologists have now reverted again to the "purist" idea that fibrous dysplasia does represent a specific entity with well-defined microscopic and roentgenographic features. This would mean that there are certain fibro-osseous lesions of the jaws which would not be designated as fibrous dysplasia, and until more knowledge of the true nature of the lesions accumulates, some workers have simply classified them as "fibro-osseous lesions," after first being certain that they do not represent some specific entity.

Etiology. The etiology of monostotic fibrous dysplasia is unknown, and of the variety of possible factors which have been suggested, none has found general acceptance. Early investigators suggested that it was caused by aberrant activity in the bone-forming mesenchymal tissue. There is clinical evidence which indicates that local infections or trauma may eventuate in this disease under certain conditions as yet unrecognized. Some investigators insist that monostotic fibrous dysplasia is a peculiar reparative reaction on the part of bone to any one of a variety of injuries. However, some cases have been reported present at birth. Furthermore, most workers believe that, despite the similarity in nomenclature and histologic appearance, the monostotic form of the disease is not related to the polyostotic form and that the former does not progress to the latter.

Two cases of congenital monostotic fibrous dysplasia of the mandible have been reported by El Deeb and his associates, who have suggested that these may represent an autosomal recessive disorder.

Clinical Features. Monostotic fibrous dysplasia of the jaws occurs with apparently equal predilection for males and females, although some reports show a mild predominance of females. It is more common in children and young adults than in older persons. The mean age of occurrence in the 69 patients reported by Zimmerman and his associates was 27 years, while in 53 patients with craniofacial fibrous dysplasia reported by Gardner and Halpert, the mean age was 34 years.

The first clinical sign of the disease is a painless swelling or bulging of the jaw. The swelling usually involves the labial or buccal plate, seldom the lingual aspect, and when it involves the mandible it sometimes causes a protuberant excrescence of the inferior border. There may be some malalignment, tipping or displacement of the teeth due to the progressive expansile nature of the lesion, and tenderness may ultimately develop. The mucosa is almost invariably intact over the lesion.

Fibrous dysplasia of the maxilla is an especially serious form of the disease since it has a marked predilection for occurrence in children and is almost impossible to eradicate without radical, mutilating surgery (Fig. 13–15). These lesions are not well circumscribed, commonly extend locally to involve the maxillary sinus, the zygomatic process and the floor of the orbit, and even extend back toward the base of the skull. Severe malocclusion and bulging of the canine fossa or extreme prominence of the zygomatic process, producing a marked facial deformity, are typical sequelae of this disease in the maxilla. Thus, this form of the disease in this location need not be truly monostotic, but neither is it usually classified as a polyostotic type. It has sometimes been referred to as *craniofacial fibrous dysplasia*, since it does affect the craniofacial complex and is so characteristic in its clinical and roentgenographic features that it closely resembles a distinct entity. This form of the disease has been described in detail by Waldron and Giansanti and by Eversole and his associates.

Roentgenographic Features. The roentgenographic appearance of fibrous dysplasia of the jaw is extremely variable (Fig. 13–16). There are three basic patterns which may be seen. In one type, the lesion is generally a rather small unilocular radiolucency or a somewhat larger multilocular radiolucency, both with a rather well-circumscribed border and containing a network of fine bony trabeculae. In the second type, the pattern is similar except that increased trabeculation renders the lesion more opaque and typically mottled in appearance. The third type is quite opaque with many delicate trabeculae giving a "ground-glass" or "peau d'orange"

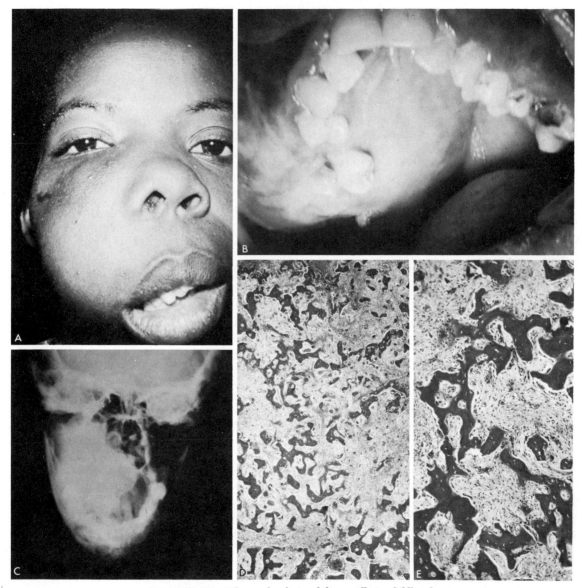

Figure 13–15. *Fibrous dysplasia of the maxilla in childhood.*
(Courtesy of Dr. Edward M. Pfafflin.)

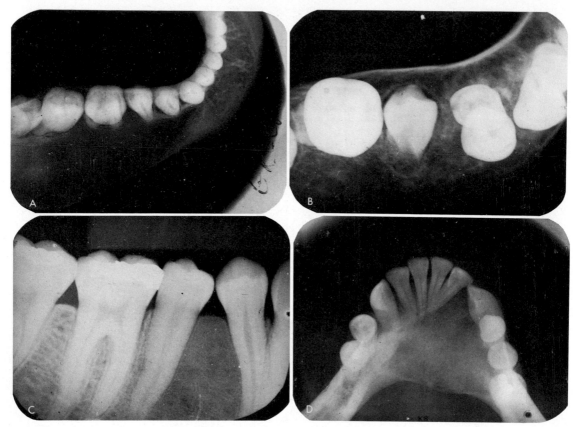

Figure 13–16. *Monostotic fibrous dysplasia of bone.*
The alteration and variation in trabecular pattern of bone are illustrated in four cases of fibrous dysplasia. (*A*, *D*, Courtesy of Dr. Wilbur C. Moorman and *C*, of Dr. Charles H. Redish.)

appearance to the lesion. This latter type characteristically is not well circumscribed but instead blends into the adjacent normal bone. Any of the three types may be found in either maxilla or mandible. In all types, generally the cortical bone becomes thinned because of the expansile nature of the growth, but seldom is this bony plate perforated, or is periosteal proliferation obvious. The roots of teeth in the involved areas may be separated or moved out of normal position but only occasionally exhibit severe resorption. In some cases, the bone appears so opaque that the roots of teeth may be indistinct or not visible.

It is of interest that, in craniofacial fibrous dysplasia, there is characteristic roentgenographic thickening of the base of the skull.

Histologic Features. There is considerable microscopic variation in cases of monostotic fibrous dysplasia of the jaws. The lesion is essentially a fibrous one made up of proliferating fibroblasts in a compact stroma of interlacing collagen fibers (Fig. 13–17, *A*, *B*). Irregular

trabeculae of bone are scattered throughout the lesion with no definite pattern of arrangement. Characteristically, some of these trabeculae are C-shaped or, as described by one author, Chinese character-shaped. These trabeculae are usually coarse woven bone but may be lamellar, although not as well organized as normal lamellar bone. The relationship of osteoblasts and osteoclasts to the trabecula is similar to that seen in the polyostotic form of the disease. Large lesions may show variation from area to area and sometimes present a greater bony reaction around the periphery of the lesion than in the central portion.

Some of the earlier literature dealing with this disease suggested that it represents a permanent maturation arrest in the woven bone stage and proposed that lesions demonstrating lamellar bone transformation should not be diagnosed as fibrous dysplasia. However, it is generally well accepted now, particularly on the basis of the work of Waldron and Giansanti, that lesions of fibrous dysplasia of the jaws,

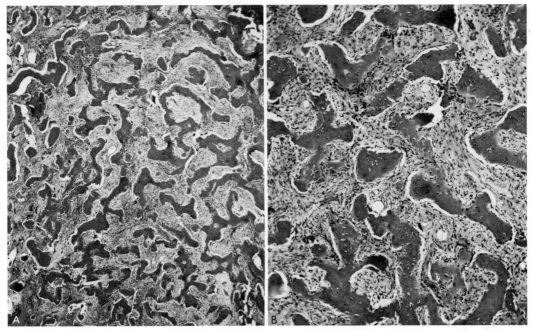

Figure 13–17.   Monostotic fibrous dysplasia of bone.

especially the craniofacial type, will mature over a period of time and the lesional tissue may show lamellar bone.

Treatment and Prognosis.   The treatment of monostotic fibrous dysplasia consists of surgical removal of the lesion. Unfortunately, the majority of lesions are too large at the time of original diagnosis to excise surgically without leaving a severe facial deformity or, in the case of the mandible, weakening the bone so as to invite pathologic fracture. In addition, many of the lesions, particularly those with the ground-glass or orange-peel roentgenographic appearance, are not circumscribed and would have to be block-resected. For these reasons, the majority of cases are simply treated by a conservative removal of that portion of the lesion contributing to the facial deformity. Periodic improvement of cosmetic appearance in this fashion seems more justifiable than the radical approach inasmuch as the lesion seldom jeopardizes the life of the patient. Because so few attempts at total removal of the lesion have been reported, any discussion of "recurrence rate" would be meaningless.

There are occasional cases reported in which monostotic fibrous dysplasia has undergone spontaneous malignant transformation into sarcoma, usually osteosarcoma, and these have been reviewed by Schwartz and Alpert.

In addition, Tanner and his associates re-ported four cases of sarcoma developing in the facial and jaw bone in patients whose lesions of fibrous dysplasia had all been treated by x-ray radiation between 3 and 25 years previously. Although it is difficult to prove a cause-and-effect relation, these four cases did fulfill the criteria for post-radiation sarcoma and once again emphasize the hazard of radiating benign lesions, especially those of bone.

CHERUBISM

(Familial Fibrous Dysplasia of the Jaws; Disseminated Juvenile Fibrous Dysplasia; Familial Multilocular Cystic Disease of the Jaws; Familial Fibrous Swelling of the Jaws; Hereditary Fibrous Dysplasia of the Jaws)

Cherubism is an uncommon disease involving the jaws which, despite several synonyms implying a relation to or a type of fibrous dysplasia, is not related to this latter condition. The first report of the disease was that of Jones in 1933, who also originated the descriptive term "cherubism" to indicate the unusual clinical appearance and facial deformity of patients with this disease.

Anderson and colleagues and McClendon and colleagues investigated the possible mode of inheritance of this condition in 65 patients representing 21 families. They concluded that the

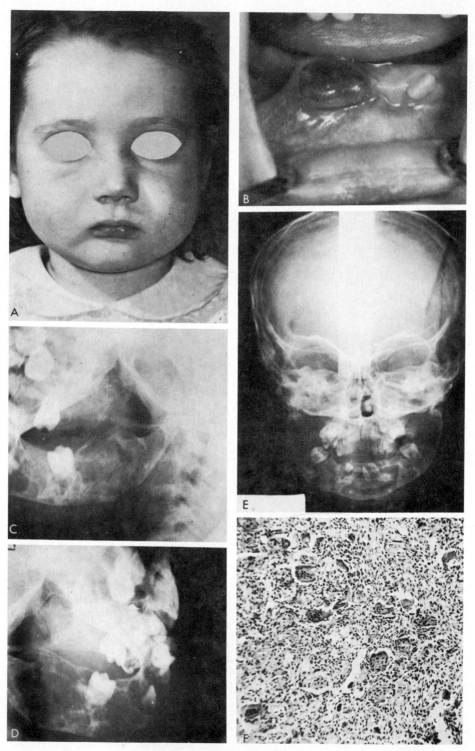

Figure 13–18.   Cherubism.
The patient has a cherubic appearance owing to the expansion of the jaws (A). Occasionally the mucosa will be perforated by the underlying bony lesion (B). The bilateral involvement of the mandible is seen in the lateral jaw and skull roentgenograms (C, D, E) where there has been serious destruction of bone. A biopsy of the bony lesion reveals a cellular fibrous mass with many interspersed multinucleated giant cells (F). (Courtesy of Dr. Ralph E. McDonald: Am. J. Dis. Child., 89:354, 1955.)

evidence supported the idea that cherubism is hereditary, the mode being an autosomal dominant gene with variable expressivity; penetrance of the dominant gene was approximately 100 per cent in males, but reduced in females to between 50 and 70 per cent. Nevertheless other genetic mechanisms are not precluded.

Clinical Features. Cherubism manifests itself in early childhood, often by the age of three or four years. The patients exhibit a progressive, painless, symmetric swelling of the jaws, mandible or maxilla, producing the typical chubby face suggestive of a cherub (Fig. 13–18, A). The vast majority of cases involve only the mandible. The jaws are firm and hard to palpation and reactive regional lymphadenopathy may be present. The palate may also be enlarged. There are no associated systemic manifestations, although in the excellent review and discussion by McClendon and his associates one patient was described as having pigmented skin lesions similar to those in polyostotic fibrous dysplasia.

The deciduous dentition may be spontaneously shed prematurely, beginning as early as three years of age. The permanent dentition is often defective, with absence of numerous teeth and displacement and lack of eruption of those present. The oral mucosa is usually intact and of normal color.

Roentgenographic Features. Roentgenograms reveal extensive bilateral destruction of bone of one or both jaws with expansion and severe thinning of the cortical plates. The body of the bone may present a multilocular appearance, and actual perforation of the cortex may occur (Fig. 13–18, C, D, E). The entire ramus may also be involved although the condyle is usually spared.

Numerous unerupted and displaced teeth are commonly seen, some of which may appear to be floating in cystlike spaces (Fig. 13–19). The other bones of the skull and the remainder of the skeleton usually present no abnormal findings, although accompanying lesions in other bones such as ribs and long bones are reported in a few cases.

Laboratory Findings. The values for the various formed elements of the blood as well as for serum calcium, phosphorus and alkaline phosphatase are usually within normal limits.

Histologic Features. The microscopic appearance of the tissue from the involved jaws is sometimes characterized by the presence of great numbers of large multinucleated giant cells in a loose, delicate fibrillar connective tissue stroma containing large numbers of fibroblasts and many small blood vessels (Fig. 13–18 F). A sprinkling of inflammatory cells may also be found in these lesions. The lesions are virtually indistinguishable from the central giant cell granuloma of the jaws (q.v.). Other times there are few multinucleated giant cells, and the lesion appears somewhat more fibrous. These appear to represent the somewhat older

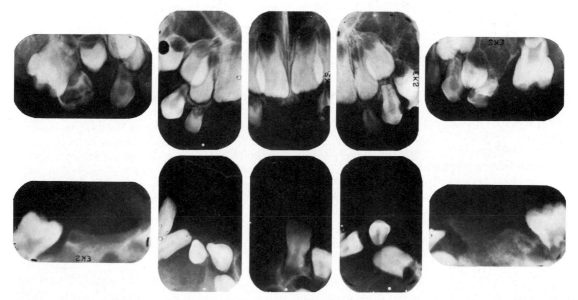

Figure 13–19. *Cherubism.*
The intraoral roentgenograms show the derangement of teeth and the many associated cystlike structures. (Courtesy of Dr. Ralph E. McDonald: Am. J. Dis. Child., 89:354, 1955.)

or regressing lesions. Epithelial remnants from the developing teeth are sometimes scattered throughout the lesions, and these may cloud the diagnosis of the primary disease by suggesting an odontogenic neoplasm. In addition, a peculiar perivascular, eosinophilic cuffing of the small capillaries in the lesions is sometimes found.

Treatment and Prognosis. There is general agreement that cherubism, although progressing rather rapidly during early childhood, tends to become static and may even show regression as the patient approaches puberty. In any event, the usually widespread involvement negates any possibility of surgical treatment aimed at curing the patient. When the patient becomes older, past puberty, surgical correction of the jaws for cosmetic reasons is sometimes advised. Radiation therapy for this benign bone disease is definitely contraindicated. By the age of 30 years, the patient's jaws may appear roentgenographically normal in bony structure.

DISEASES OF THE TEMPOROMANDIBULAR JOINT

The temporomandibular joint is one of the most important yet most poorly understood of the many joints in the body. Because of its unique anatomic position and association with other structures, the dentist in previous years often considered it outside his realm of responsibility. For this reason, the otolaryngologist contributed greatly to our knowledge of the anatomy and physiology of this joint and probably did much to stimulate the interest of the dental profession in this articulation. It is unfortunate that a great deal of misinformation about the temporomandibular joint has appeared in the medical and dental literature, arising chiefly through misinterpretation of anatomic and pathologic findings, and this has caused considerable confusion among investigators in their early phases of study.

It has been only within recent years that painstaking work dealing with the temporomandibular joint has been reported in any quantity, and the determined efforts of a number of workers have clarified much of the aura of mystery which surrounded this structure. As Schwartz pointed out, there have been more changes in concepts and methods of treatment in the past 25 years than in the previous 2500 years. Even today a great deal remains to be answered about the many osteopathoses that

occur here. Despite the many advances that have been made, most men experienced in the problems of the temporomandibular joint will agree that we are only at the threshold in our development of knowledge of its disturbances.

The diagnosis of these diseases has often been a perplexing problem because the clinician has been almost wholly dependent upon the description of the symptoms by the patient; seldom are definite clinical signs of temporomandibular joint disease manifested. Recent development of techniques for obtaining useful roentgenograms of this joint and the application of cinefluoroscopy and computerized axial tomography offer great promise of helping to solve the many unanswered questions pertaining to the temporomandibular joint in health and disease.

DEVELOPMENTAL DISTURBANCES OF THE TEMPOROMANDIBULAR JOINT

Aplasia of the Mandibular Condyle

Condylar aplasia, or failure of development of the mandibular condyle, may occur unilaterally or bilaterally, but in either event is a rare condition. Five cases have been reported by Kazanjian and isolated cases by other authors.

Clinical Features. This abnormality is frequently associated with other anatomically related defects such as a defective or absent external ear, an underdeveloped mandibular ramus or macrostomia. If the condylar aplasia is unilateral, there is obvious facial asymmetry, and both occlusion and mastication may be altered. A shift of the mandible toward the affected side occurs during opening. In bilateral cases this shift is not present.

Treatment. Treatment of condylar aplasia consists in osteoplasty, if the derangement is severe, and correction of the malocclusion by orthodontic appliances. If the patient exhibits little difficulty, surgical intervention is not warranted, although cosmetic surgery may aid in correcting facial deformity.

Hypoplasia of the Mandibular Condyle

Underdevelopment or defective formation of the mandibular condyle may be congenital or acquired. *Congenital* hypoplasia, which is of idiopathic origin, is characterized by unilateral or bilateral underdevelopment of the condyle beginning early in life.

The *acquired* form of hypoplasia may be due

to any agent which interferes with the normal development of the condyle. It has been suggested that this may occur in forceps deliveries that cause traumatic birth injury. External trauma to the condylar area in infants or younger children may also result in hypoplasia. Other cases have been observed in children following x-ray radiation over the temporomandibular joint area for local treatment of skin lesions such as the hemangioma, or "birthmark."

Infection spreading locally from the dental area or by the hematogenous route from a distant site may involve the joint, interfere with condylar growth and result in a hypoplastic condyle. Discussing arthritis in children, Kuhns and Swaim emphasized the fact that inflammation or a circulatory disorder in proximity to an epiphysis may result in a severe disturbance in growth.

A variety of endocrine and vitamin derangements in the experimental animal have been reported to cause disturbances in growth and development of the mandibular condyles. The possibility that such factors play any significant role in the development of human temporomandibular arthropathy has not been completely evaluated, but they are probably of minor clinical importance.

Clinical Features. The clinical deformity occasioned by condylar hypoplasia depends upon whether the disturbance has affected one or both condyles and upon the degree of the malformation. This in turn is directly related to the age of the patient at the time the involvement occurred, the duration of the injury and its severity. Unilateral involvement is the most common clinical type.

Severe unilateral arrest of growth will produce facial asymmetry, often accompanied by limitation of lateral excursion on one side and exaggeration of the antegonial notch of the mandible on the involved side. A mild disturbance presents only lesser degrees of these features, perhaps accompanied by a mandibular midline shift during opening and closing. The distortion of the mandible in this pathognomonic pattern results from lack of downward and forward growth of the body of the mandible due to the arrest of the chief growth center of the mandible, the condyle. Some growth continues at the outer posterior border of the angle of the mandible, resulting in thickening of the bone in this area. The older the patient at the time of the growth disturbance, the less severe will be the facial deformation. It should be remembered, however, that growth frequently

persists in this condyle until the age of 20 years and, even more important, that a growth potential is maintained indefinitely, unlike most other joints in the body.

Treatment and Prognosis. Treatment of condylar hypoplasia is a difficult problem since there are no available means of stimulating its growth locally or compensating for its failure. Although the condition itself is not necessarily a progressive one, the resulting disturbance may become more severe as the patient approaches puberty. Cartilage or bone transplants have been used to build up the underdeveloped parts, preceded in some cases by unilateral or bilateral sliding osteotomy, to improve the appearance of the patient with asymmetry and retrusion.

Hyperplasia of the Mandibular Condyle

Condylar hyperplasia is a rare unilateral enlargement of the condyle which should not be confused with a neoplasm of this structure, although it may superficially resemble an osteoma or chondroma.

The cause of this condition is obscure, but it has been suggested that mild chronic inflammation, resulting in a condition analogous to a proliferative osteomyelitis, stimulates the growth of the condyle or adjacent tissues. The unilateral occurrence strongly suggests a local phenomenon (Fig. 13–20).

Clinical Features. The patients usually exhibit a unilateral, slowly progressive elongation of the face with deviation of the chin away from the affected side. The enlarged condyle may be clinically evident or at least palpated and presents a striking roentgenographic appearance in both anteroposterior and lateral views as well as in specific condylar films. The affected joint may or may not be painful. A severe malocclusion is a usual sequela of the condition.

Treatment and Prognosis. The treatment of condylar hyperplasia usually involves resection of the condyle. This is generally sufficient to restore normal occlusion, although complete correction of the facial asymmetry may not be accomplished by this procedure.

TRAUMATIC DISTURBANCES OF THE TEMPOROMANDIBULAR JOINT

Luxation and Subluxation
(Complete and Incomplete Dislocation)

Dislocation of the temporomandibular joint occurs when the head of the condyle moves

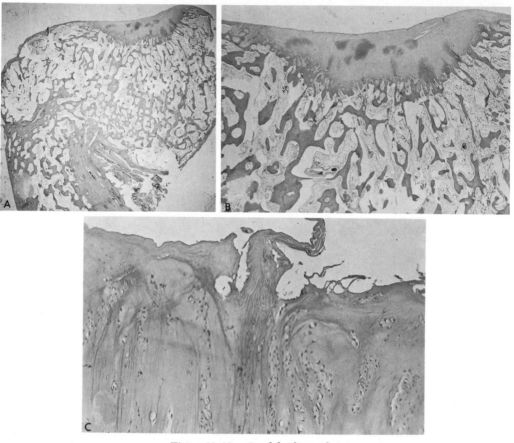

Figure 13–20. *Condylar hyperplasia.*

A, This demonstrates a low-power view of a condyle which shows hyperplasia as indicated by the increase in size of the condylar head. The articular surface of the condyle has been replaced by hyaline cartilage. B shows a higher magnification of the surface of the condyle which has been replaced by hyaline cartilage. C shows a high-power view of the cartilaginous surface with irregular formation of cartilage as indicated by the distribution of chondrocytes, small areas of tear, and the presence of abundant precipitated fibrin upon the cartilaginous surface and in the cartilaginous tears. Joints having such distribution of fibrin over the surface have a tendency to produce the so-called creak of leather sound which is due to the function of this surface against a similar change of the meniscus. (Courtesy of Dr. Donald A. Kerr.)

anteriorly over the articular eminence into such a position that it cannot be returned voluntarily to its normal position. Many workers believe that this inability to retrude the mandible is caused by spasm of the temporal muscle initiated by myotatic reflex. Thus, in movements of the mandible involving forward translation of the condyle, tension may be placed on the temporalis and lead to formation of the muscle spasm.

A great deal of confusion persists as to the use of the terms "luxation" and "subluxation." Luxation of the joint refers to complete dislocation, while subluxation is a partial or incomplete dislocation, actually a form of hypermobility. Despite wide acceptance of the term "subluxation," many investigators discourage its use, arguing that when the condyle is obviously

outside the limits of normal in its position, the joint is actually dislocated. It can be demonstrated that in cases of joint disturbances classified as subluxation, there is no abnormal joint relation visible on the temporomandibular roentgenogram. In such instances, though the condyle may lie well anterior to the articular eminence, such a position is normal for many persons.

Luxation may be acute, owing to a sudden traumatic injury resulting in fracture of the condyle or, more frequently, only in a stretching of the capsule, usually at the point of attachment for the external pterygoid muscle into the capsule. There is often some tearing of the tendon at this insertion point. Most commonly, however, luxation is a result of yawning or having the mouth opened too widely, as by a dentist extracting teeth or by a physician removing tonsils or through injudicious use of a mouth prop.

Clinical Features. The typical form of luxation is characterized by a sudden locking and immobilization of the jaws when the mouth is open, accompanied by prolonged spasmodic contraction of the temporal, internal pterygoid and masseter muscles, with protrusion of the jaw. All activities requiring motion of the mandible, such as eating or talking, are impossible; the mouth cannot be closed, and the patient frequently becomes panicky, especially if it is his first experience. In some instances the patient may be able to reduce the dislocation himself. This is particularly true in cases of chronic dislocation when the ligaments become stretched.

Superior and posterior dislocation of the condyle may occur in rare instances as the result of an acute traumatic impaction injury, and the head of the condyle may be forced through the glenoid fossa or tympanic plate into the middle cranial fossa.

Treatment. Reduction of a dislocated condyle is accomplished by inducing relaxation of the muscles and then guiding the head of the condyle under the articular eminence into its normal position by an inferior and posterior pressure of the thumbs in the mandibular molar area. The necessary relaxation can sometimes be brought about only by means of general anesthesia or by tiring the masticatory muscles by cupping the chin in the palm of the hand and applying a posterior and superior pressure for five to ten minutes.

Ankylosis

(Hypomobility)

Ankylosis of the temporomandibular joint is one of the most incapacitating of all diseases involving this structure.

Etiology. The most frequent causes of ankylosis of the temporomandibular joint are traumatic injuries and infections in and about the joint (Fig. 13–21). Straith and Lewis elaborated on the etiologic factors and enumerated them as follows: (1) abnormal intrauterine development, (2) birth injury (by forceps particularly), (3) trauma to the chin forcing the condyle against the glenoid fossa, particularly with bleeding into the joint space, (4) malunion of condylar fractures, (5) injuries associated with fractures of the malar-zygomatic compound, (6) loss of tissues with scarring, (7) congenital syph-

ilis, (8) primary inflammation of the joint (rheumatoid arthritis, infectious arthritis, Marie-Strümpell disease), (9) inflammation of the joint secondary to a local inflammatory process (e.g., otitis media, mastoiditis, osteomyelitis of the temporal bone or condyle), (10) inflammation of the joint secondary to a blood stream infection (e.g., septicemia, scarlet fever), (11) metastatic malignancies, and (12) inflammation secondary to radiation therapy.

Topazian has reviewed 229 cases of temporomandibular joint ankylosis and found that 49 per cent were a result of joint inflammation of one type or another, 31 per cent were related to trauma, and the remainder were idiopathic.

Clinical Features. This condition occurs at any age, but most cases occur before the age of ten years. Distribution is approximately equal between the sexes. The patient may or may not be able to open his mouth to any appreciable extent, depending on the type of ankylosis (Fig. 13–22). In complete ankylosis there is a bony fusion with absolute limitation of motion. There is usually somewhat greater motion in fibrous ankylosis than in bony ankylosis.

If the injury which brought about the ankylosis was sustained in infancy or childhood, at least before the age of 15 years, there is nearly always an associated facial deformity. The type of deformity is partially dependent upon whether the ankylosis is unilateral or bilateral. In unilateral ankylosis occurring at an early age, the chin is displaced laterally and backward on the affected side because of a failure of development of the mandible. When an attempt is made to open the mouth, the chin deviates toward the ankylosed side, if any motion is present. Bilateral ankylosis occurring in childhood results in underdevelopment of the lower portion of the face, a receding chin and micrognathia (Fig. 13–23). The maxillary incisors often manifest overjet due to failure of this mandibular growth.

Temporomandibular joint ankylosis has been divided into two types, depending upon the anatomic site of the ankylosis with respect to the joint itself: (1) intra-articular ankylosis and (2) extra-articular ankylosis. It is important that the distinction between the two types be made, but this is not usually difficult. In intra-articular ankylosis the joint undergoes progressive destruction of the meniscus with flattening of the mandibular fossa, thickening of the head of the condyle and narrowing of the joint space. The ankylosis is basically fibrous, although ossification in the scar may result in a bony union.

Extra-articular ankylosis results in a "splint-

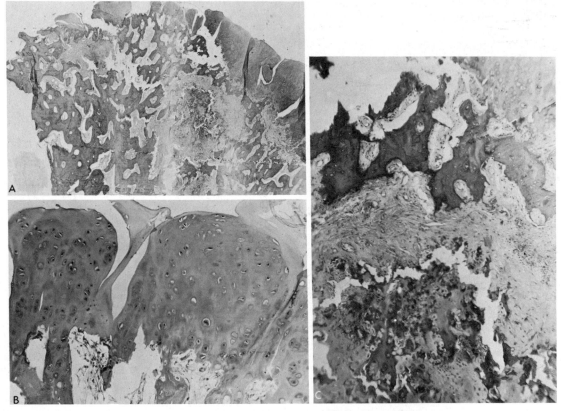

Figure 13–21. *Traumatic temporomandibular joint arthritis.*

A, There is replacement of much of the articular surface of the condylar head by hyaline cartilage. There has been complete destruction of the subarticular cortex, fibrosis, necrosis, and cartilage with ossification in areas of the condyle. *B* shows the residual bone and the area of degeneration with the formation of cartilage undergoing calcification and ossification. *C* shows a portion of the articular surface with the rents and tears which occur in the atypically formed cartilage covering the portion of the articular surface. The irregular distribution of the chondrocytes is evident. The irregularity of the condylar surface produced by the rents and tears in the cartilage plus the exposure of irregular projections of bone contributes to a grating sound and sensation in the joint as well as to its irregular movement. (Courtesy of Dr. Donald A. Kerr.)

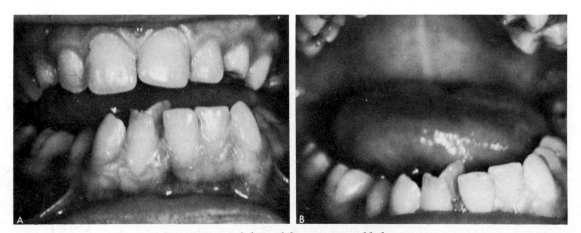

Figure 13–22. *Ankylosis of the temporomandibular joint.*

Furthest extent of opening possible before treatment *(A)* and after treatment *(B).* (Courtesy of Dr. Wilbur C. Moorman.)

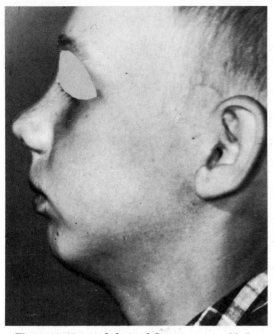

Figure 13–23. *Ankylosis of the temporomandibular joint.*
The receding chin is characteristic in these cases. (Courtesy of Dr. Wilbur C. Moorman.)

ing" of the temporomandibular joint by a fibrous or bony mass external to the joint proper, as in cases of infection in surrounding bone or extensive tissue destruction (Fig. 13–24). Kazanjian observed that movement is possible in extra-articular ankylosis when an attempt is made to thrust the chin forward, but that there is no movement in intra-articular ankylosis, especially of the bilateral type.

Roentgenographic Features. It is evident that every case of temporomandibular joint ankylosis must be carefully studied in every detail before a treatment plan is devised. One of the most important adjuncts to careful clinical examination is roentgenographic examination. It is usually but not always easy to demonstrate changes in the joint by this means. When such changes are obvious, they consist of an abnormal or irregular shape of the head of the condyle and a radiopacity indicative of the dense bone filling the joint space (Fig. 13–25).

Treatment. Treatment of temporomandibular bony ankylosis is surgical, usually complicated by the concomitant underdevelopment of the jaw. Basically, the operation consists of osteotomy or removal of a section of bone below the condyle. Fibrous ankylosis may be treated by functional methods.

Injuries of the Articular Disk

(Meniscus)

Complaints referable to injuries of the temporomandibular meniscus are relatively common in dental practice. Despite the frequency of occurrence, an aura of mystery too often surrounds these temporomandibular joint dysfunctions, and the tendency persists for patients to drift from one dentist to another, vainly seeking relief of their symptoms.

Etiology. One of the most common known causes of injury to the meniscus is malocclusion. This is usually a result of the bizarre pattern of mandibular excursions carried out during mastication. For example, in cases of excessive mandibular movement, the capsule is stretched in preventing too great an anterior condylar movement. Thus the adaptation of the disk to the condyle is lost, and the beginning of disk derangement is initiated (Fig. 13–26).

Some patients relate the beginning of their difficulties to a single episode of acute trauma directly to the jaw, such as a blow or a fall. In other cases patients will date their difficulties from one episode when the mouth was opened widely, as during yawning. Most authorities believe that such a single experience is not the actual cause of disk derangement, but merely a precipitating factor. Occasionally, inflammatory conditions such as rheumatoid arthritis have been suggested as the cause, but they are uncommon factors.

It is interesting and significant that Silver and his co-workers reported that 50 per cent of their patients with meniscus injuries were unable to offer any information about the cause of their problem.

Clinical Features. Meniscus injuries are far more common in females than in males, the percentage in the series of Silver and his associates and of Boman being 90 per cent and 86 per cent, respectively. Young adults are more frequently affected than children or persons past 40 years of age.

This form of disturbance is characterized by pain, snapping or clicking and crepitation in the joint area. The pain may be present only near completion of the opening motion. Joint noise in the form of snapping or clicking may be faint, audible only with a stethoscope, or so loud that it is obvious even to an observer standing near the patient. Transient or prolonged locking of the jaw may occur, almost invariably when the mouth is closed, unlike that seen in dislocation of the jaw, which occurs when the mouth is open.

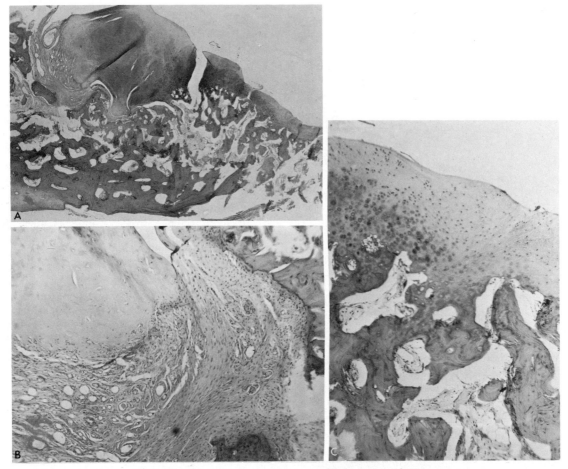

Figure 13–24.   *Traumatic temporomandibular joint arthritis.*

A, Low-power view of the surface and border of the articular surface of the condyle, showing extensive areas of alteration. In the center a large area of hyaline cartilage is present. To the right there is a replacement of the articular surface by hyaline cartilage. *B* shows a higher magnification of the boundary to the left of the large mass in which there is extensive fibrous proliferation with much angioblastic activity, and in the boundary, the formation of new bone. It is in this area that the so-called spurs of periarticular new bone formation occur, resulting in the process designated as lipping. *C*, High-power view of the articular surface showing the replacement of the condylar osseous cortex with hyaline cartilage and the intermingling of this cartilage with the trabecular bone of the body of the head of the condyle. Fibrosis of the marrow spaces is evident. (Courtesy of Dr. Donald A. Kerr.)

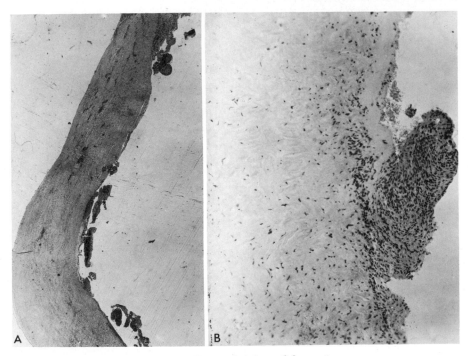

Figure 13–25. *Ankylosis of the temporomandibular joint.*
The irregular radiopacity represents an extra-articular anklyosis from splinting of the joint by excessive bone formation. (Courtesy of Dr. Wilbur C. Moorman.)

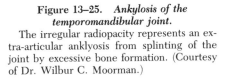

Figure 13–26. *Traumatic injury of the meniscus.*
A, In the central area of the disk the numerous small dark areas are areas of vascularization with accumulation of inflammatory cells. The material associated with the surface is attached fibrin, some of which is undergoing organization. The small round structures in the upper right area are organized fibrin, which in other sections show attachment to the surface of the meniscus. It is these bodies that become detached and free floating in the joint and are designated as "joint mice." B, A high-power view that shows the presence of fibrin on the surface of meniscus. This fibrin has undergone organization. These excrescences on the surface are responsible for some of the noise and irregular movement that occur in the traumatized temporomandibular joint. (Courtesy of Dr. Donald A. Kerr.)

Patients may complain also of dull pain in or around the ear or on the side of the jaw, with tinnitus and paresthesia of the tongue reported occasionally.

Roentgenographic studies of the temporomandibular joints in both closed and open positions are necessary for study of the condition, but unfortunately positive findings are absent in many cases.

Treatment. The treatment of meniscus disorders of the temporomandibular joint is varied and nonspecific. Immobilization of the jaws may be necessary in cases of severe pain. If an atypical masticatory pattern exists because of malocclusion, the malocclusion should be corrected if possible. Finally, meniscectomy or surgical removal of the disk has often proved beneficial. The treatment for each case depends upon careful individual evaluation, and no definite rules can be established.

Fractures of the Condyle

Condylar fracture results from an acute traumatic injury to the jaw and is accompanied by limitation of motion, pain and swelling over the involved condyle, deformity noted upon palpation and loss of normal condylar excursion.

The fractured condyle fragment is frequently displaced anteriorly and medially into the infratemporal region because of the forward pull of the external pterygoid muscle, and reduction of the fracture is often difficult because of this displacement. Many authorities believe that if reduction cannot be accomplished by conservative means, open reduction is usually not indicated even when the fracture is bilateral. Healing of such fractures without reduction seldom results in loss of function, limitation of motion or any other complication.

INFLAMMATORY DISTURBANCES OF THE TEMPOROMANDIBULAR JOINT

Arthritis, or inflammation of the joints, is one of the most prevalent diseases affecting the human race, and the temporomandibular joint does not escape this disease, although it is certainly not one of the joints most commonly involved. This particular joint may suffer from any form of arthritis, but there are three common types with which the dentist must be familiar: (1) arthritis due to a specific infection, (2) rheumatoid arthritis, and (3) osteoarthritis, or degenerative joint disease. These arthritides

of the temporomandibular joint have been reviewed and discussed by Mayne and Hatch.

Arthritis Due to a Specific Infection

The incidence of arthritis due to a specific infection is low when compared to the occurrence of rheumatoid arthritis and degenerative joint disease. There is a gamut of infections (such as those resulting from the gonococci, streptococci, staphylococci, pneumococci, and the tubercle bacillus) which may produce polyarticular involvement, either by blood stream or lymphatic metastasis or by direct extension from a focal infection. But the temporomandibular joint uniquely appears to escape such infection in most cases except in the event of gonococcal infection. Markowitz and Gerry indicated that only about 5 per cent of patients with gonorrhea suffer gonococcal arthritis, and of these, only about 3 per cent manifest temporomandibular joint involvement.

The most common form of infectious temporomandibular joint arthritis is that caused by direct extension of infection into the joint as a result of an adjacent cellulitis or osteomyelitis. Such an extension may follow dental infection, infection of the parotid gland, or even facial or ear infection.

Clinical Features. Patients suffering from acute infectious arthritis complain chiefly of severe pain in the joint, with extreme tenderness on palpation or manipulation over the joint area. The pain is of such intensity that motion is severely limited.

Healing of this form of arthritis often results in ankylosis, either osseous or fibrous. A fibrous ankylosis is more common, but in either event there is severe limitation of motion.

Histologic Features. Depending upon the severity of involvement, there is a variable amount of destruction of the articular cartilage and articular disk. Osteomyelitis with destruction of bone of the condyle may even be present. The joint spaces become obliterated in the healing phase by the development of granulation tissue and its subsequent transformation into dense scar tissue. In time, the disk may become completely replaced and the entire joint space may be filled with the cicatrix.

Treatment. The treatment of an infectious arthritis is chiefly the administration of antibiotics. If treatment is instituted in the acute phase, the sequelae will be less deforming or disabling than if the disease has been allowed to enter a chronic phase. In the advanced cases, meniscectomy or condylectomy has been advocated.

Rheumatoid Arthritis

Rheumatoid arthritis is a disease of unknown etiology which commonly begins in early adult life and affects women more frequently than men, in a ratio of at least 2 to 1. Although this disease is apparently not due to a specific bacterial infection, there is evidence to indicate that it may be a hypersensitivity reaction to bacterial toxins, specifically streptococci.

The distribution of joint involvement is nearly always polyarticular and frequently symmetrically bilateral. Patients usually manifest a long series of episodic exacerbations and remissions. Temporomandibular joint involvement in cases of rheumatoid arthritis is not particularly common despite the fact that this is a polyarticular disease. Comroe stated that this joint is involved in approximately 20 per cent of cases of rheumatoid arthritis.

Clinical Features. Rheumatoid arthritis, in its early stages, may be manifested by slight fever, loss of weight and fatigability. The joints affected are swollen, and the patient complains of pain and stiffness. Involvement of the temporomandibular joint may occur concomitantly with the other joint lesions or may arise at any subsequent time. The possibility of arthritic-like pain actually being caused by gout of the temporomandibular joint has been discussed by Kleinman and Ewbank.

Movement of the jaw, as during mastication or talking, causes pain and may be limited because of the stiffness. The stiffness is commonly at its height in the mornings and tends to diminish throughout the day with continued use of the jaw. Clicking and snapping of the joint are not common, but when they occur are due to alterations in the articular cartilage and meniscus. Over a period of years there may be ankylosis of the joint, but this is not inevitable.

In an investigation of 53 patients with rheumatoid arthritis by Crum and Loiselle, none were found to have any evidence of residual limitation of motion, swelling or tenderness in the temporomandibular joint. However, 43 per cent of these patients gave a history of temporomandibular joint symptoms at some time during the course of the disease, usually coinciding with acute systemic arthritic episodes.

It is of interest that the temporomandibular joint is frequently involved in the Marie-Strümpell type of rheumatoid arthritis. In this form of the disease there is usually sole involvement of the spine, sacroiliac and hip joint. The reason for the concomitant mandibular joint involvement is unknown, but has been recorded by Markowitz and Gerry.

Rheumatoid arthritis in children (Still's disease), when it involves the temporomandibular joint, may cause a malocclusion of the class II division 1 type with protrusion of maxillary incisors and an anterior open bite. Engel and his associates also found deformation of the mandible, characterized by shortening of the body and reduction in the height of the ramus due to failure of the growth center in the condylar area. The roentgenograms often revealed flattening and stunting of the condyles and a haziness about the joint indicative of periarticular fibrosis. These workers believe that this type of mandibular growth disturbance is characteristic of rheumatoid arthritis and that this disease should be considered when such a facial deformity occurs.

Histologic Features. There has been little opportunity for microscopic examination of the temporomandibular joint in cases of rheumatoid arthritis, and findings have been reported in but few cases. There is, however, no reason to expect the histologic features to be significantly different from those in other joints. Elsewhere, the disease is characterized by the ingrowth of granulation tissue to cover the articular surfaces, the invasion of cartilage and its replacement by granulation tissue, and the ultimate destruction of the articular cartilage. Eventually fibrous adhesions occur; the meniscus may become eroded, and fibrous ankylosis results. Occasionally the connective tissue becomes ossified and a true bony ankylosis occurs.

Treatment and Prognosis. There is no specific treatment for rheumatoid arthritis, although remarkable benefit may result from the administration of ACTH or cortisone. Once limitation of motion and deformity have occurred, surgical intervention in the form of condylectomy may be necessary to regain movement. There is, however, a great tendency for recurrence of the ankylosis.

Osteoarthritis

(Degenerative Joint Disease; Hypertrophic Arthritis)

Osteoarthritis is the most common type of arthritis and has been said to develop, at least to some degree, in all persons past 40 years of age. Although its etiology is unknown, it is a disease associated with the aging process. The joints first involved are those which bear the weight of the body and are thus subjected to continued stress and strain: the joints of the knees, hips and spine.

Clinical Features. Clinical signs and symptoms of osteoarthritis are often remarkably absent even in the face of severe histologic joint changes. Since the temporomandibular joint is not a weight-bearing joint, changes here are insignificant even though arthropathy may be present in other joints. Those changes that do occur may be a result of disturbed balance of the joint due to loss of all teeth or to external injury.

Patients with osteoarthritis of other joints may complain of clicking and snapping in the temporomandibular joint, but pain is not necessarily a feature. This joint noise is probably due to atypical disk motion resulting from discordant mandibular condyle-disk function on the basis of the changes in the articular cartilage. Limitation of motion or ankylosis rarely occurs.

Histologic Features. Changes occurring in the temporomandibular joint in osteoarthritis have been particularly described by Bauer, who also commented on the absence of subjective symptoms even when complete destruction of the disk was found.

The changes in the articular cartilage consist of loss of elasticity and surface erosions of varying degrees of severity, with the presence of vertical cracks extending often from the surface through the cartilaginous plate into the subchondral bone. Horizontal fissures may separate the cartilage from the underlying bone. The cartilage cells often exhibit degeneration, and there may be complete destruction of cartilage in localized areas. In other areas dystrophic calcification may occur in altered cartilage, and this can progress to actual ossification.

Bony protuberances or exostoses are common findings in osteoarthritis and develop both on the periphery of the cartilage and in the central portion of the articular plane, enlarging the condyle in its longitudinal axis. There may be bony lipping of the condyle and changes in its contour which may be visible in temporomandibular roentgenograms.

Alterations in the articular disk are similar to those occurring in the articular cartilage. The disk may exhibit cracks and fissures and may become hyalinized or even calcified in some cases. There may be necrosis or destruction of the disk, particularly opposite the exostoses; complete destruction of the disk has been known to occur.

Treatment. There is no treatment for this slowly progressive type of arthritis other than condylectomy.

Traumatic Arthritis

Traumatic arthritis of an acute or chronic nature is a common form of temporomandibular arthropathy and is described under Traumatic Disturbances of the Temporomandibular Joint.

NEOPLASTIC DISTURBANCES OF THE TEMPOROMANDIBULAR JOINT

Neoplasms and tumorlike growths, benign and malignant, may involve the temporomandibular joint, but such involvement is relatively uncommon. Such tumors may originate from the condyle, either the bone or the articular cartilage, or from the joint capsule. As might be expected, the connective tissue, cartilage and bone give rise to the majority of these tumors. Occasionally metastatic tumors have also been reported to involve the temporomandibular joint.

The rarity of these lesions precludes their discussion here, particularly since they exhibit no features significantly different from those of similar tumors occurring in other locations in and about the oral cavity which have already been described. A review of this subject was published by Thoma.

EXTRA-ARTICULAR DISTURBANCES OF THE TEMPOROMANDIBULAR JOINT

A variety of extra-articular disturbances may manifest themselves clinically as temporomandibular joint problems and, because of this masquerade, may prevent the examiner from arriving at a correct diagnosis. The most common presenting complaint is pain in the temporomandibular joint area, a symptom which justifiably implicates the joint as the possible source of difficulty.

Markowitz and Gerry reported that referred pain is a common source of arthralgia of this area. Impacted molar teeth on the same side as the temporomandibular joint pain were implicated, since removal of these teeth resulted in complete disappearance of the pain. These writers found also that sinusitis and middle ear disease often caused referral of pain to this joint. Still other conditions apparently causing referred pain were infratemporal cellulitis, impingement of the coronoid process on the tendon of the temporal muscle, neuritis of the third division of the fifth cranial nerve, including auriculotemporal neuritis; odontalgia; a foreign body in the infratemporal fossa; and overclosure of the mandible accompanied by severe dental attrition. Thus it must be remembered that since extra-articular disturbances may produce joint pain, the simple presence of pain in this area is not sufficient evidence to establish an incontrovertible diagnosis of primary joint disturbance.

One remaining condition must be discussed, since it has been described for a number of years as producing symptoms referable in part to the temporomandibular joint. This condition, which is the center of much controversy, is Costen's syndrome.

Costen's syndrome is a symptom complex originally described by Costen, an otolaryngologist, in 1934. Although Costen made an honest attempt to relate cases of impaired hearing, tinnitus, facial and temporal neuralgia, otalgia and glossodynia to a disturbance in temporomandibular joint function, it is unfortunate that the ascribed anatomic and physiologic basis for the syndrome is erroneous. More unfortunate is the fact that the misconceptions were fostered through ensuing years by many workers. Not until recently has a critical analysis of the anatomic descriptions of Costen and others revealed their misconceptions.

The symptoms constituting the syndrome originally defined by Costen consist of (1) impairment of hearing, either continuous or intermittent, (2) a "stuffy" sensation in the ears, especially at mealtime, (3) tinnitus, sometimes accompanied by a snapping noise when chewing, (4) otalgia, (5) dizziness, (6) headache about the vertex, occiput and behind the ears, sometimes increasing toward the end of the day, and (7) a burning sensation in the throat, tongue and side of the nose.

Temporomandibular joint dysfunction has usually been considered the basic disturbance leading to these symptoms. Since the arthropathy has been ascribed to malocclusion with an associated deep overbite, absence of molar teeth, poorly fitting dentures or an edentulous state, dentists became extremely interested in the condition. However, the consensus today, summarized by Zimmerman in the monograph

of Sarnat and Laskin, is that the concept of Costen's syndrome as a symptom-complex should be abandoned since the anatomic and physiologic foundation for the various symptoms, all predicated upon the idea of mandibular overclosure, cannot be substantiated.

MYOFASCIAL PAIN-DYSFUNCTION SYNDROME

(Temporomandibular Joint Pain-Dysfunction Syndrome; Masticatory Myalgesia Syndrome)

The concept of Costen's syndrome based on occlusal disharmony with resultant damage to the temporomandibular joint causing a wide variety of signs and symptoms based on anatomic and physiologic changes has now been almost totally discarded. In its place has arisen the concept delineated by Schwartz in 1955 under the term "temporomandibular joint pain-dysfunction syndrome" and subsequently designated by most workers as the "myofascial pain-dysfunction syndrome (MPD)." The studies of Schwartz resulted in discarding the mechanical concept of an occlusal etiology for TMJ problems and replacing it by the broader implications of a dysfunction of the entire masticatory apparatus, as well as recognition of certain psychologic characteristics of the patient, as being responsible for the syndrome.

Etiology. It is believed by many workers in this field today that the principal factor responsible for the manifestations of this syndrome is masticatory muscle spasm. This muscle spasm can be initiated as a result of muscular overextension, muscular overcontraction or muscle fatigue. Thus, muscular overextension may be produced by either dental restorations or prosthetic appliances which encroach on the intermaxillary space. In contrast, overcontraction may result from overclosure as a result of bilateral loss of posterior teeth or continued resorption of alveolar bone after construction of a prosthetic appliance. However, there is evidence that the most common cause of this syndrome is muscle fatigue caused by such chronic oral habits as grinding or clenching of the teeth. This in turn may result from irritating factors, such as an improperly occluding restoration or an overhanging margin on a restoration. These habits are believed to be an involuntary tension-relieving mechanism involving emotional as well as mechanical factors as etiologic agents. Thus, this explanation of the syndrome has been termed the "psycho-physiologic theory" by Laskin and his associates.

The development of masticatory muscle spasm as a result of any of the above mechanisms may lead to pain and limitation of motion as well as a minor shift in jaw rest position so that the teeth do not occlude properly. The teeth may gradually shift to accommodate this malocclusion, if it persists long enough, but then, when the spasm is relieved, the patients develop another occlusal imbalance when the relieved musculature permits return of the jaws to their original normal position.

In addition to the occlusal disharmony, masticatory muscle spasm is believed capable of producing at least two other organic changes— degenerative arthritis and muscle contracture. Any one or all of these conditions then become self-perpetuating because of the resultant altered chewing pattern, with continued insult and amplification of the original muscle spasm and pain.

Clinical Features. The vast majority of patients suffering from the myofascial pain-dysfunction syndrome, between 80 and 90 per cent, are female, usually below the age of 40 years.

There are four cardinal signs and symptoms of the syndrome: (1) pain, (2) muscle tenderness, (3) a clicking or popping noise in the temporomandibular joint, and (4) limitation of jaw motion, unilaterally or bilaterally in approximately an equal ratio, sometimes with deviation on opening. In addition to these four positive findings, these patients also have two typical negative disease characteristics: (1) an absence of clinical, roentgenographic or biochemical evidence of organic changes in the joint itself, and (2) lack of tenderness in the joint when it is palpated through the external auditory meatus. These classic manifestations of the disease have been discussed in detail by Greene and his associates.

The pain itself is usually unilateral and is described as a dull ache in the ear or preauricular area which may radiate to the angle of the mandible, temporal area or lateral cervical area. It frequently will vary in intensity between morning and the remainder of the day.

In a series of 277 patients with this syndrome reported by Greene and his associates, 81 per cent had tenderness in the masticatory and cervical musculature. The specific muscles affected were the lateral pterygoid (in 84 per cent of cases), masseter (in 70 per cent), temporalis (in 49 per cent), medial pterygoid (in 35 per cent) and the cervical, scalp and facial (in 43 per cent). Thus, the muscle tenderness is most common over the neck of the condyle, above the maxillary tuberosity, at the angle of the mandible and the temporal crest. A clicking or popping noise was present in 66 per cent of these patients, and limitation of motion in 63 per cent. Other less common symptoms included subluxation or dislocation in 17 per cent of cases, and miscellaneous features such as vertigo in 7 per cent.

Patients may occasionally relate the onset of their symptoms to some specific event such as a traumatic injury or the seating of a prosthetic appliance. However, in the majority of cases no such related incidents can be recalled by the patients. For example, in the series of Greene and his co-workers, 52 per cent of the patients could recall no incident related to the onset of the disease.

It also appears significant, since this disease is thought to have a psychologic or psychogenic component, that about 80 per cent of the patients in this study gave a history of other psychophysiologic diseases such as gastrointestinal ulcer, migraine headache or dermatitis. In addition, it was found that these patients had significantly higher urinary excretion levels of 17-OH steroids and catecholamines, which have been linked to the stress phenomenon, than a comparable group of control patients.

Treatment. The treatment for this syndrome is conservative. There is serious doubt that temporomandibular joint surgery, drug injection into the joint, or extensive occlusal equilibration or reconstruction is warranted. These are certainly contraindicated in the early phases of treatment. Relief of emotional factors, correction of any obvious faulty restorations and appliances, myotherapeutic exercises and physiotherapy and drug therapy (tranquilizers and muscle relaxants) are all a part of the armamentarium for use in the treatment of this disease.

REFERENCES

Albright, F., Butler, A. M., Hampton, A. D., and Smith, P.: Syndrome characterized by osteitis fibrosa disseminata, areas of pigmentation and endocrine dysfunction, with precocious puberty in females. N. Engl. J. Med., *216*:727, 1937.

Anderson, D. E., McClendon, J. L., and Cornelius, E. A.: Cherubism: hereditary fibrous dysplasia of the jaws. I. Genetic considerations. II. Pathologic considerations. Oral Surg., *15* (Suppl. 2):5, 17, 1962.

Baden, E., and Spirgi, M.: Oral manifestations of Marfan's syndrome. Oral Surg., *19*:757, 1965.

Bauer, W.: Osteo-arthritis deformans of the temporomandibular joint. Am. J. Pathol., *17*:129, 1940.

Bauze, R. J., Smith, R., and Francis, M. J. O.: A new look at osteogenesis imperfecta. J. Bone Joint Surg., 57B:1, 1975.

Bell, W. E.: Clinical diagnosis of the pain-dysfunction syndrome. J. Am. Dent. Assoc., 79:154, 1969.

Bell, W. H., and Hinds, E. C.: Fibrosarcoma complicating polyostotic fibrous dysplasia. Oral Surg., 23:299, 1967.

Bjorvatn, K., Gilhuus-Moe, O., and Aarskog, D.: Oral aspects of osteopetrosis. Scand. J. Dent. Res., 87:245, 1979.

Blank, E.: Recurrent Caffey's cortical hyperostosis and persistent deformity. Pediatrics, 55:856, 1975.

Boman, K.: Temporomandibular joint arthrosis and its treatment by extirpation of disk. Acta Chir. Scand., 95 (Suppl. 118): 1947.

Boucek, R. J., Noble, N. L., Gunja-Smith, Z., and Butler, W. T.: The Marfan syndrome: a deficiency in chemically stable collagen cross-links. N. Eng. J. Med., 305:988, 1981.

Brooke, R. I., Stenn, P. G., and Mothersill, K. J.: The diagnosis and conservative treatment of myofascial pain dysfunction syndrome. Oral Surg., 44:844, 1977.

Brooksaler, F., and Miller, J. E.: Infantile cortical hyperostosis. J. Pediatr., 48:739, 1956.

Brown, R. H., and Cunningham, W. M.: Some dental manifestations of mongolism. Oral Surg., 14:664, 1961.

Bruce, K. W., Bruwer, A., and Kennedy, R. L. J.: Familial intraosseous fibrous swellings of the jaws ("cherubism"). Oral Surg., 6:995, 1953.

Brussell, I. J.: Temporomandibular joint diseases: differential diagnosis and treatment. J. Am. Dent. Assoc., 39:532, 1949.

Burbank, P. M., Lovestedt, S. A., and Kennedy, R. L. J.: The dental aspects of infantile cortical hyperostosis. Oral Surg., 11:1126, 1958.

Burkhart, J. M., Burke, E. C., and Kelly, P. J.: The chondrodystrophies. Mayo Clin. Proc., 40:481, 1965.

Caffey, J., and Silverman, W. A.: Infantile cortical hyperostosis: preliminary report on new syndrome. Am. J. Roentgenol., 54:1, 1945.

Cahn, L. R.: Leontiasis ossea. Oral Surg., 6:201, 1953.

Carson, I. H.: Polyostotic fibrous dysplasia; report of case. Oral Surg., 7:524, 1954.

Cayler, G. G., and Peterson, C. A.: Infantile cortical hyperostosis. Am. J. Dis. Child., 91:119, 1956.

Chowers, I., Czackes, W., Ehrenfeld, E. N., and Landau, S.: Familial aminoaciduria in osteogenesis imperfecta. J.A.M.A., 181:771, 1962.

Church, L. E.: Polyostotic fibrous dysplasia of bone. Oral Surg., 11:184, 1958.

Cohen, B. H., Lilienfeld, A. M., and Sigler, A. T.: Some epidemiological aspects of mongolism: a review. Am. J. Public Health, 54:223, 1963.

Cohen, J.: Osteopetrosis. J. Bone Joint Surg., 33A:923, 1951.

Cohen, M. M., Jr.: The Robin anomalad—its nonspecificity and associated syndromes. J. Oral Surg., 34:587, 1976.

Cohen, M. M., Winer, R. A., Schwartz, S., and Shklar, G.: Oral aspects of mongolism. I. Periodontal disease in mongolism. Oral Surg., 14:92, 1961.

Comroe, B. I.: Arthritis and Allied Conditions. 3rd ed. Philadelphia, Lea & Febiger, 1948.

Cooke, B. E. D.: Paget's disease of the jaws: 15 cases. Ann. R. Coll. Surg. Engl., 19:223, 1956.

Cornelius, E. A., and McClendon, J. L.: Cherubism—hereditary fibrous dysplasia of the jaws: roentgenographic features. Am. J. Roentgenol., Radium Ther. Nucl. Med., 106:136, 1969.

Costen, J. B.: A syndrome of ear and sinus symptoms dependent upon disturbed function of the temporomandibular joint. Ann. Otol., Rhinol. Laryngol., 43:1, 1934.

Idem: Neuralgia and ear symptoms associated with disturbed function of the temporomandibular joint. J.A.M.A., 107:252, 1936.

Crum, R. J., and Loiselle, R. J.: Incidence of temporomandibular joint symptoms in male patients with rheumatoid arthritis. J. Am. Dent. Assoc., 81:129, 1970.

Davis, J. P.: A cephalometric investigation of cleidocranial dysplasia. Master's thesis, Indiana University School of Dentistry, 1974.

de Deuxchaisnes, C. N., and Krane, S. M.: Paget's disease of bone: clinical and metabolic observations. Medicine, 43:233, 1964.

Dingman, R. O.: Diagnosis and treatment of lesions of the temporomandibular joint. Am. J. Orthod. Oral Surg., 26:388, 1940.

Drury, B. J.: Paget's disease of the skull and facial bones. J. Bone Joint Surg., 44A:174, 1962.

Dunn, F. H.: Nonfamilial and nonhereditary craniofacial dysostosis: a variant of Crouzon's disease. Am. J. Roentgenol., Radium Ther. Nucl. Med., 84:472, 1960.

Duthie, R. B., and Townes, P. L.: The genetics of orthopaedic conditions. J. Bone Joint Surg., 49B:229, 1967.

Dyson, D. P.: Osteomyelitis of the jaws in Albers-Schonberg disease. Br. J. Oral Surg., 7:178, 1970.

Idem: Van Buchem's disease (hyperostosis corticalis generalisata familiaris). Br. J. Oral Surg., 9:237, 1972.

El Deeb, M., Waite, D. E., and Gorlin, R. J.: Congenital monostotic fibrous dysplasia—a new possibly autosomal recessive disorder. J. Oral Surg., 37:520, 1979.

El Deeb, M., Waite, D. E., and Jaspers, M. T.: Fibrous dysplasia of the jaws. Report of five cases. Oral Surg., 47:312, 1979.

Ellis, D. J., and Adams, T. O.: Massive osteolysis: report of a case. J. Oral Surg., 29:659, 1971.

Elmore, S. M.: Pycnodysostosis: a review. J. Bone Joint Surg., 49A:153, 1967.

Engel, M. B., and Brodie, A. G.: Condylar growth and mandibular deformities. Oral Surg., 1:790, 1948.

Engel, M. B., Richmond, J. B., and Brodie, A. G.: Mandibular growth disturbance in rheumatoid arthritis of childhood. Am. J. Dis. Child., 78:728, 1949.

Eversole, L. R., Sabes, W. R., and Rovin, S.: Fibrous dysplasia: a nosologic problem in the diagnosis of fibroosseous lesions of the jaws. J. Oral Path., 1:189, 1972.

Falvo, K. A., Root, L., and Bullough, P. G.: Osteogenesis imperfecta: clinical evaluation and management. J. Bone Joint Surg., 56A:783, 1974.

Fernandez, A. O., and Ronis, M. L.: The Treacher-Collins syndrome. Arch. Otolaryngol., 80:505, 1964.

Franceschetti, A., and Klein, D.: The mandibulo-facial dysostosis: a new hereditary syndrome. Acta Ophthalmol. (Kbh.), 27:143, 1949.

Gardner, A. F., and Halpert, L.: Fibrous dysplasia of the skull with special reference to the oral regions. Dent. Pract. Dent. Rec., 13:337, 1963.

Gerry, R. G.: Effects of trauma and hypermotility on the temporomandibular joint. Oral Surg., 7:876, 1954.

Glickman, I.: Fibrous dysplasia in alveolar bone. Oral Surg., 1:895, 1948.

Gold, L.: The classification and pathogenesis of fibrous dysplasia of the jaws. Oral Surg., 8:628, 725, 856, 1955.

Goldenberg, R. R.: The skull in Paget's disease. J. Bone Joint Surg., 33A:911, 1951.

Gorlin, R. J., Jue, K. L., Jacobsen, U., and Goldschmidt E.: Oculoauriculovertebral dysplasia. J. Pediatr., 63:991, 1963.

Gorlin, R. J., Pindborg, J. J., and Cohen, M. M., Jr.: Syndromes of the Head and Neck. 2nd ed. New York, McGraw-Hill Book Company, 1976.

Greene, C. S., and Laskin, D. M.: Long-term evaluation of conservative treatment for myofascial pain-dysfunction syndrome. J. Am. Dent. Assoc., 89:1365, 1974.

Greene, C. S., Lerman, M. D., Sutcher, H. D., and Laskin, D. M.: The TMJ pain-dysfunction syndrome: heterogeneity of the patient population. J. Am. Dent. Assoc., 79:1168, 1969.

Gutman, A. B., Tyson, T. L., and Gutman, E. B.: Serum calcium, inorganic phosphorus and phosphatase activity in hyperparathyroidism, Paget's disease, multiple myeloma and neoplastic diseases of the bone. Arch. Intern. Med., 57:379, 1936.

Hamner, J. E., III: The demonstration of perivascular collagen deposition in cherubism. Oral Surg., 27:129, 1969.

Harris, V. J., and Ramilo, J.: Caffey's disease: a case originating in the first metatarsal and review of a 12-year experience. A. J. R., 130:335, 1978.

Harris, W. H., Dudley, H., and Barry, R. J.: Natural history of fibrous dysplasia. An orthopedic, pathological, and roentgenographic study. J. Bone Joint Surg., 44A:207, 1962.

Hasenhuttl, K.: Osteopetrosis. J. Bone Joint Surg., 44A:359, 1962.

Heys, F. M., Blattner, R. J., and Robinson, H. B. G.: Osteogenesis imperfecta and odontogenesis imperfecta: clinical and genetic aspects in eighteen families, J. Pediatr., 56:234, 1960.

Horton, C. P.: Treatment of arthritic temporomandibular joints by intra-articular injection of hydrocortisone. Oral Surg., 6:826, 1953.

Hutter, R. V. P., Foote, F. W., Jr., Frazell, E. L., and Francis, K. C.: Giant cell tumors complicating Paget's disease of bone. Cancer, 16:1044, 1963.

Hutton, C. E., Bixler, D., and Garner, L. D.: Cleidocranial dysplasia—treatment of dental problems: report of case. J. Dent. Child., 48:456, 1981.

Jaffe, H. L.: Paget's disease of bone. Arch. Pathol., 15:83, 1933.

Idem: Giant cell reparative granuloma, traumatic bone cyst, and fibrous (fibro-osseous) dysplasia of the jawbones. Oral Surg., 6:159, 1953.

Jaffe, H. L., and Lichtenstein, L.: Non-osteogenic fibroma of bone. Am. J. Pathol., 18:205, 1942.

Jaffe, H. L., Lichtenstein, L., and Portis, R.: Giant cell tumor of bone, its pathologic appearance, grading, supposed variants and treatment. Arch. Pathol., 30:993, 1940.

Johnston, C. C., Jr., Lavy, N., Lord, T., Vellios, F., Merritt, A. D., and Deiss, W. P., Jr.: Osteopetrosis. A clinical, genetic, metabolic and morphologic study of the dominantly inherited, benign form. Medicine, 47:149, 1968.

Jones, W. A.: Familial multilocular cystic disease of the jaws. Am. J. Cancer, 17:946, 1933.

Jones, W. A., Gerrie, J., and Pritchard, J.: Cherubism: a familial fibrous dysplasia of the jaws. J. Bone Joint Surg., 32B:334, 1950.

Kalliala, E., and Taskinen, P. J.: Cleidocranial dysostosis. Oral Surg., 15:808, 1962.

Kazanjian, V. H.: Anklyosis of the temporomandibular joint. Surg., Gynecol. Obstet., 67:333, 1938.

Kaslick, R. S., and Brustein, H. C.: Clinical evaluation of osteopetrosis. Oral Surg., 15:71, 1962.

Kelln, E. E., Chaudhry, A. P., and Gorlin, R. J.: Oral manifestations of Crouzon's disease. Oral Surg., 13:1245, 1960.

Kery, L., and Wouters, H. W.: Massive osteolysis: report of two cases. J. Bone Joint Surg., 52B:452, 1970.

King, J. D., and Bobechko, W. P.: Osteogenesis imperfecta: an orthopaedic description and surgical review. J. Bone Joint Surg., 53B:72, 1971.

Kleinman, H. Z., and Ewbank, R. L.: Gout of the temporomandibular joint. Report of three cases. Oral Surg., 27:281, 1969.

Kneal, E., and Sante, L. R.: Osteopetrosis (marble bones). Am. J. Dis. Child., 81:693, 1951.

Kuhns, J. G., and Swaim, L. T.: Disturbances of growth in chronic arthritis in children. Am. J. Dis. Child., 43:1118, 1932.

Laskin, D. M.: Etiology of the pain-dysfunction syndrome. J. Am. Dent. Assoc., 79:147, 1969.

Lichtenstein, L.: Polyostotic fibrous dysplasia. Arch. Surg., 36:874, 1938.

Lichtenstein, L., and Jaffe, H. L.: Fibrous dysplasia of the bone. Arch. Pathol., 33:777, 1942.

Marbach, J. J.: Arthritis of the temporomandibular joints. Dent. Radiogr. Photogr., 42:51, 1969.

Markowitz, H. A., and Gerry, R. G.: Temporomandibular joint disease. Oral Surg., 2:1309, 1949; 3:75, 1950.

Mayne, J. G., and Hatch, G. S.: Arthritis of the temporomandibular joint. J. Am. Dent. Assoc., 79:125, 1969.

McClendon, J. L., Anderson, D. E., and Cornelius, E. A.: Cherubism: hereditary fibrous dysplasia of the jaws. II. Pathologic considerations. Oral Surg., 15 (Suppl. 2):17, 1962.

McDonald, R. E., and Shafer, W. G.: Disseminated juvenile fibrous dysplasia of the jaws. Am. J. Dis. Child., 89:354, 1955.

McKusick, V. A.: Heritable Disorders of Connective Tissue. 4th ed. St. Louis, C. V. Mosby Company, 1972.

McKusick, V. A., and Scott, C. I.: A nomenclature for constitutional disorders of bone. J. Bone Joint Surg., 53A:978, 1971.

Meijer, R., and Walker, J. C.: Waardenburg's syndrome. Plast. Reconstr. Surg., 34:363, 1964.

Miller, A. S., Cuttino, C. L., Elzay, R. P., Levy, W. M., and Harwick, R. D.: Giant cell tumor of the jaws associated with Paget's disease of bone. Report of two cases and review of the literature. Arch. Otolaryngol., 100:233, 1974.

Miller, C. W.: The temporomandibular joint. J. Am. Dent. Assoc., 44:386, 1952.

Montgomery, A. H.: Ossifying fibroma of the jaw. Arch. Surg., 15:30, 1927.

Moorman, W. C.: Diseases of the temporomandibular joint. Thesis, Indiana University, 1950.

Morgan, D. H.: Mandibular joint pathology. Importance of radiographs. Dent. Radiogr. Photogr., 43:3, 1970.

Murphy, J. B., Doku, H. C., and Carter, B. L.: Massive osteolysis: phantom bone disease. J. Oral Surg., 36:318, 1978.

Nagle, R. J.: Temporomandibular function. Oral Surg., 8:500, 1955.

Nelson, C. L., and Hutton, C. E.: Condylectomy for temporomandibular joint dysfunction. A survey of seventeen postoperative patients. Oral Surg., 51:351, 1981.

Newberg, A. H., and Tampas, J. P.: Familial infantile cortical hyperostosis: an update. A. J. R., 137:93, 1981.

Nicholas, J. A., Saville, P. D., and Bronner, F.: Osteoporosis, osteomalacia, and the skeletal system. J. Bone Joint Surg., 45A:391, 1963.

Novak, A. J., and Burket, L. W.: Oral aspects of Paget's disease, including case reports and necropsy findings. Am. J. Orthod. Oral Surg., 30:544, 1944.

Oatis, G. W., Jr., Burch, M. S., and Samuels, H. S.: Marfan's syndrome with multiple maxillary and mandibular cysts: report of case. J. Oral Surg., 29:515, 1971.

O'Riordan, M. L., Robinson, J. A., Buckton, K. E., and Evans, H. J.: Distinguishing between the chromosomes involved in Down's syndrome (trisomy 21) and chronic myeloid leukaemia (Ph¹) by fluorescence. Nature, 230:167, 1971.

Oshrain, H. I., and Sackler, A.: Involvement of the temporomandibular joint in a case of rheumatoid arthritis. Oral Surg., 8:1039, 1955.

Ozonoff, M. B., Steinbach, H. L., and Mamunes, P.: The trisomy 18 syndrome. Am. J. Roentgenol., Radium Ther. Nucl. Med., 91:618, 1964.

Pavsek, E. J.: Mandibulofacial dysostosis (Treacher-Collins syndrome). Am. J. Roentgenol., Radium Ther. Nucl. Med., 79:598, 1958.

Phemister, D. B., and Grimson, K. S.: Fibrous osteoma of the jaws. Ann. Surg., 105:564, 1937.

Pike, M. M.: Paget's disease with associated osteogenic sarcoma: report of three cases. Arch. Surg., 46:750, 1943.

Porretta, C. A., Dahlin, D. C., and Janes, J. M.: Sarcoma in Paget's disease of bone. J. Bone Joint Surg., 39A:1314, 1957.

Poswillo, D.: The pathogenesis of the first and second branchial arch syndrome. Oral Surg., 35:302, 1973.

Idem: The pathogenesis of the Treacher Collins syndrome (mandibulofacial dysostosis). Br. J. Oral Surg., 13:1, 1975.

Prowler, J. R., and Glassman, S.: Agenesis of the mandibular condyles. Oral Surg., 7:133, 1954.

Pugh, D. G.: Fibrous dysplasia of the skull; a probable explanation for leontiasis ossea. Radiology, 44:458, 1945.

Rebel, A., Malkani, K., Baslé, M., and Bregeon, Ch.: Is Paget's disease of bone a viral infection? Calcif. Tissue Res., 22: Suppl:283, 1977.

Rebel, A., Baslé, M., Pouplard, A., Kouyoumdjian, S., Filmon, R., and Lepatezour, A.: Viral antigens in osteoclasts from Paget's disease of bone. Lancet, 2:344, 1980.

Reed, R. J.: Fibrous dysplasia of bone. A review of 25 cases. Arch. Pathol., 75:480, 1963.

Robinson, H. B. G.: Osseous dysplasia; reaction of bone to injury. J. Oral Surg., 14:3, 1956.

Robinson, M.: Polyostotic fibrous dysplasia of bone. J. Am. Dent. Assoc., 42:47, 1951.

Rovin, S., Dachi, S. F., Borenstein, D. B., and Cotter, W. B.: Mandibulofacial dysostosis, a familial study of five generations. J. Pediatr., 64:215, 1964.

Rowley, J. D.: Down syndrome and acute leukaemia: Increased risk may be due to trisomy 21. Lancet, 2:1020, 1981.

Rushton, M. A.: An anomaly of cementum in cleidocranial dysostosis. Br. Dent. J., 100:81, 1956.

Sarnat, B. G., and Laskin, D. M.: Temporomandibular Joint: A Biological Basis for Clinical Practice. 3rd ed. Springfield, Ill., Charles C Thomas, 1980.

Saul, R. A., Lee, W. H., amd Stevenson, R. E.: Caffey's disease revisited. Am. J. Dis. Child., 136:56, 1982.

Schlumberger, H. G.: Fibrous dysplasia (ossifying fibroma) of the maxilla and mandible. Am. J. Orthod. Oral Surg., 32:579, 1946.

Idem: Fibrous dysplasia of single bones (monostotic fibrous dysplasia). Mil. Surgeon, 99:504, 1946.

Schmorl, G.: Über Osteitis deformans Paget. Virchows Arch. [Pathol. Anat.] 283:694, 1932.

Schreiber, H. R.: An anatomic and physiological approach to treatment of temporomandibular joint disturbances. J. Am. Dent. Assoc., 48:261, 1954.

Schwartz, D. T., and Alpert, M.: The malignant transformation of fibrous dysplasia. Am. J. Med. Sci., 247:1, 1964.

Schwartz, L.: Pain associated with the temporomandibular joint. J. Am. Dent. Assoc., 51:394, 1955.

Schwartz, L.: Disorders of the Temporomandibular Joint. Philadelphia, W. B. Saunders Company, 1959.

Schwarz, E.: The skull in skeletal dysplasias. Am. J. Roentgenol., Radium Ther. Nucl. Med., 89:928, 1963.

Sedano, H. O., Sauk, Jr., J. J., and Gorlin, R. J.: Oral Manifestations of Inherited Disorders. Woburn, Mass., Butterworth Publishers Inc., 1977.

Shapiro, H. H.: The anatomy of the temporomandibular joint. Oral Surg., 3:1521, 1950.

Shapiro, H. H., and Truex, R. C.: The temporomandibular joint and the auditory function. J. Am. Dent. Assoc., 30:1147, 1943.

Shoenfeld, Y., Fried, A., and Ehrenfeld, N. E.: Osteogenesis imperfecta. Am. J. Dis. Child., 129:679, 1975.

Silver, C. M., Simon, S. D., and Savastano, A. A.: Meniscus injuries of the temporomandibular joint. J. Bone Joint Surg., 38A:541, 1956.

Singer, F. R.: Paget's Disease of Bone. New York, Plenum Medical Book Company, 1977.

Singer, F. R.: Paget's disease of bone: a slow virus infection? Calcif. Tissue Int., 31:185, 1980.

Smith, B. J., and Eveson, J. W.: Paget's disease of bone with particular reference to dentistry. J. Oral Path., 10:233, 1981.

Smith, N. H. H.: A histologic study of cementum in a case of cleidocranial dysostosis. Oral Surg., 25:470, 1968.

Smyth, F. S., Potter, A., and Silverman, W.: Periosteal reaction, fever and irritability in young infants: new syndrome? Am. J. Dis. Child., 71:333, 1946.

Spilka, C. J., and Callahan, K. R.: A review of the differential diagnosis of oral manifestations in early osteitis deformans. Oral Surg., 11:809, 1958.

Spitzer, R.: A case of unilateral ankylosis of the temporomandibular joint with malposed unerupted mandibular molar. Oral Surg., 6:588, 1953.

Stafne, E. C., and Austin, L. T.: A study of dental roentgenograms in cases of Paget's disease (osteitis deformans), osteitis fibrosa cystica, and osteoma. J. Am. Dent. Assoc., 25:1202, 1938.

Stark, R. B., and Saunders, D. E.: The first branchial syndrome. The oral-mandibular-auricular syndrome. Plast. Reconstr. Surg., 29:229, 1962.

Stein, I., Stein, R. O., and Beller, M. L.: Living Bone in Health and Disease. Philadelphia, J. B. Lippincott Company, 1955.

Stout, A. P.: Fibrous and granulomatous lesions of the jaws. N. Y. Dent. J., 13:127, 1947.

Straith, C. L., and Lewis, J. R., Jr.: Ankylosis of the temporomandibular joint. Plast. Reconstr. Surg., 3:464, 1948.

Tampas, J. P., Van Buskirk, F. W., Peterson, O. S., Jr., and Soule, A. B.: Infantile cortical hyperostosis. J.A.M.A., 175:491, 1961.

Tanner, H. C., Jr., Dahlin, D. C., and Childs, D. S., Jr.: Sarcoma complicating fibrous dysplasia. Probable role of radiation therapy. Oral Surg., *14*:837, 1961.

Thoma, K. H.: Tumors of the condyle and temporomandibular joint. Oral Surg., 7:1091, 1954.

Tillman, H. H.: Paget's disease of bone. A clinical, radiographic, and histopathologic study of twenty-four cases involving the jaws. Oral Surg., *15*:1225, 1962.

Topazian, R. G.: Etiology of ankylosis of temporomandibular joint: analysis of 44 cases. J. Oral Surg., Anesth. Hosp. Dent. Serv., *22*:227, 1964.

Ulmansky, M., Hjørting-Hansen, E., and Andreasen, J. O.: Paget's disease of bone. Report of a case. Sart. Odontol. Tidskr., *72*:204, 1964.

Van Buchem, F. S. P., Hadders, H. N., and Ubbens, R.: An uncommon familial systemic disease of the skeleton: hyperostosis corticalis generalisata familialis. Acta Radiol., *44*:109, 1955.

Van Buskirk, F. W., Tampas, J. P., and Peterson, D. S., Jr.: Infantile cortical hyperostosis. An inquiry into its familial aspects. Am. J. Roentgenol. Radium Ther. Nucl. Med., *85*:613, 1961.

Van Horn, P. E., Jr., Dahlin, D. C., and Bickel, W. H.: Fibrous dysplasia: a clinical pathologic study of orthopedic surgical cases. Mayo Clin. Proc., *38*:175, 1963.

Von Wowern, N.: Cherubism. Int. J. Oral Surg., *1*:240, 1972.

Waldron, C. A.: Giant cell tumors of the jawbones. Oral Surg., 6:1055, 1953.

Waldron, C. A., and Giansanti, J. S.: Benign fibro-osseous lesions of the jaws: a clinical-radiologic-histologic review of sixty-five cases. Oral Surg., *35*:190, 340, 1973.

Wick, M. R., Siegal, G. P., Unni, K. K., McLeon, R. A., and Greditzer, H. G., III: Sarcomas of bone complicating osteitis deformans (Paget's disease). Fifty years' experience. Am. J. Surg. Pathol., *5*:47, 1981.

Wilner, D., and Sherman, R. S.: Roentgen diagnosis of Paget's disease (osteitis deformans). Dent. Radiogr. Photogr., *43*:47, 1970.

Winter, G. R., and Maiocco, P. D.: Osteogenesis imperfecta and odontogenesis imperfecta. Oral Surg., 2:782, 1949.

Wirth, W. A., Leavitt, D., and Enzinger, F. M.: Multiple intramuscular myxomas: another extraskeletal manifestation of fibrous dysplasia. Cancer, *27*:1167, 1971.

Woolf, R. M., Georgiade, N., and Pickrell, K.: Micrognathia and associated cleft palate (Pierre-Robin syndrome). Plast. Reconstr. Surg., *26*:199, 1960.

Yamane, G. M., and Fleuchaus, P. T.: Paget's disease (osteitis deformans). Oral Surg., 7:939, 1954.

Zimmerman, D. C., Dahlin, D. C., and Stafne, E. C.: Fibrous dysplasia of the maxilla and mandible. Oral Surg., *11*:55, 1958.

Zunin, C.: Two cases of Pierre-Robin's syndrome (micrognathia, cleft palate and glossoptosis). Pediatrics, *63*:95, 1955.

CHAPTER 14

Diseases of the Blood and Blood-Forming Organs

The formed elements of the blood, as well as its liquid portion, play extraordinary roles in many physiologic mechanisms and processes in the human body. When a disturbance of one of these constituents occurs, severe clinical manifestations result. In some cases the alteration of cells, serum, or other components is a result of a hereditary diathesis, nutritional deficiency, or exposure to certain chemicals. Other times, a focal or disseminated infection or a defect in one of the elements associated with the clotting mechanism causes the disturbance. A neoplastic overproduction of white cells is recognized as one of the most dreaded of blood dyscrasias.

The various blood diseases present polymorphic clinical expressions, one of which is the relatively constant involvement of oral structures. The dentist is often consulted by the patient suffering from one of the hematologic disorders who, unaware of his condition, only seeks relief of his harassing physical discomforts. Oral manifestations of many diseases of the blood are clinically similar to those lesions which occur in the oral cavity as a result of some local phenomenon, usually irritation or infection. For this reason a specific diagnosis of blood dyscrasia is difficult, if not impossible, to establish on the basis of the oral findings alone.

The hematologic disorders discussed in the following section are grouped, for ease of consideration, according to the cell type involved. No attempt is made to describe every known blood disease or even all the common ones. The sole criterion for inclusion in this section is the occurrence of oral manifestations and their obvious dental implications.

DISEASES INVOLVING THE RED BLOOD CELLS

ANEMIA

Anemia is defined as an abnormal reduction in the number of circulating red blood cells, the quantity of hemoglobin and the volume of packed red cells in a given unit of blood. The etiologies of the condition are extremely varied, and the classification presented in Table 14–1 based upon causes has been offered by Wintrobe.

In addition to this etiologic classification, a morphologic classification (Table 14–2) has been found of great value. It expresses the characteristic changes in the size and hemoglobin content of the red blood cell and thus acts as a guide to treatment.

A number of different types of anemia may exhibit oral manifestations. These may be unusually varied, but often are so characteristic that the dentist should at least strongly suspect, if not actually confirm, the diagnosis of the anemia. In the discussion to follow, only those forms of anemia which are known to exhibit specific oral signs and symptoms will be considered.

Pernicious Anemia

(Primary Anemia; Addison's Anemia; Biermer's Anemia)

Pernicious anemia is a relatively common chronic disease. Its long and interesting history

719

Table 14–1.   Etiologic Classification of the Anemias

I. Loss of blood
   A. Acute posthemorrhagic anemia
   B. Chronic posthemorrhagic anemia

II. Excessive destruction of red corpuscles
   A. Extracorpuscular causes
      1. Antibodies
      2. Infection (malaria, etc.)
      3. Splenic sequestration and destruction
      4. Associated disease states, e.g., lymphoma
      5. Drugs, chemicals, and physical agents
      6. Trauma to RBC
   B. Intracorpuscular hemolytic disease
      1. Hereditary
         a. Disorders of glycolysis
         b. Faulty synthesis or maintenance of reduced glutathione
         c. Qualitative or quantitative abnormalities in synthesis of globin
         d. Abnormalities of RBC membrane
         e. Erythropoietic porphyria
      2. Acquired
         a. Paroxysmal nocturnal hemoglobinuria
         b. Lead poisoning

III. Impaired blood production resulting from deficiency of substances essential for erythropoiesis
   A. Iron deficiency
      Experimentally; also copper and cobalt deficiencies
   B. Deficiency of various B vitamins
      Clinically, B_{12} and folic acid deficiencies (pernicious anemia and related macrocytic, megaloblastic anemias); pyridoxine-responsive anemia

      Experimentally, pyridoxine and niacine deficiencies; possibly also riboflavin, pantothenic acid and thiamine deficiencies
   C. Protein deficiency
   D. Possibly ascorbic acid deficiency

IV. Inadequate production of mature erythrocytes
   A. Deficiency of erythroblasts
      1. Atrophy of bone marrow: aplastic anemia
         a. Chemical or physical agents
         b. Hereditary
         c. Idiopathic
      2. Isolated erythroblastopenia ("pure red cell aplasia")
         a. Thymoma
         b. Chemical
         c. Antibodies
   B. Infiltration of bone marrow
      1. Leukemia, lymphomas
      2. Multiple myeloma
      3. Carcinoma, sarcoma
      4. Myelofibrosis
   C. Endocrine abnormality
      1. Myxedema
      2. Addisonian adrenal insufficiency
      3. Pituitary insufficiency
      4. Sometimes, hyperthyroidism
   D. Chronic renal disease
   E. Chronic inflammatory diseases
      1. Infections
      2. Noninfectious diseases, including granulomatous and collagen diseases
   F. Cirrhosis of liver

Modified from M. M. Wintrobe: Clinical Hematology. 8th ed. Philadelphia, Lea & Febiger, 1981.

culminated in the discovery by Whipple and by Minot and Murphy of the value of liver therapy. Although the exact nature of the disease is still unknown, it is generally recognized as being due to atrophy of gastric mucosa resulting in failure to secrete the still unidentified "intrinsic factor." Supposedly, this "intrinsic factor" is a substance present in normal gastric juice which is responsible for the intestinal absorption of the "extrinsic factor" (vitamin B_{12}), a substance now thought to be synonymous with the "erythrocyte-maturing factor" or "hemopoietic principle" and present in many foods, particularly liver, beef, milk and dairy products. Persons suffering from pernicious anemia have gastric juice which does not contain the "intrinsic fac-

Table 14–2.   Morphologic Classification of the Anemias

TYPE OF ANEMIA	DESCRIPTION	MOST COMMON CAUSES
1. Macrocytic	Increased MCV; increased MCH; normal MCH conc.	Lack of erythrocyte-maturing factors ("extrinsic" and "intrinsic" factors)
2. Normocytic	Reduction only in RBC number; normal MCV; normal MCH; normal MCH conc.	Hemorrhage; hemolysis; lack of blood formation; dilution of blood with fluid
3. Simple microcytic	Reduced MCV; reduced MCH; normal MCH conc.	Associated with infections and inflammatory diseases
4. Hypochromic microcytic	Reduced MCV; reduced MCH; reduced MCH conc.	Iron deficiency

MCV = mean corpuscular volume (Volume/RBC).
MCH = mean corpuscular hemoglobin (Hb./RBC).
MCH conc. = mean corpuscular hemoglobin concentration (Hb./Vol.).

tor" and, therefore, they are unable to absorb dietary vitamin B$_{12}$.

Clinical Features.   Pernicious anemia is rare before the age of 30 years and increases in frequency with advancing age. In the United States, males are affected more commonly than females; in other countries, notably Scandinavia, females are more commonly affected.

The disease is often characterized by the presence of a triad of symptoms: generalized weakness, a sore, painful tongue, and numbness or tingling of the extremities. In some cases the lingual manifestations are the first sign of the disease. Other typical complaints are easy fatigability, headache, dizziness, nausea, vomiting, diarrhea, loss of appetite, shortness of breath, loss of weight, pallor and abdominal pain.

Patients with severe anemia exhibit a yellowish tinge of the skin and sometimes of the sclerae. The skin is usually smooth and dry. Nervous system involvement is present in over 75 per cent of the cases of pernicious anemia, and this consists of sensory disturbances including the paresthetic sensations of the extremities described above, weakness, stiffness and difficulty in walking, general irritability, depression or drowsiness as well as incoordination and loss of vibratory sensation. These nervous aberrations are referable to the degeneration of posterior and lateral tracts of the spinal cord with loss of nerve fibers and degeneration of myelin sheaths. Degeneration of the peripheral nerves also occurs.

Oral Manifestations.   Glossitis is one of the more common symptoms of pernicious anemia. The patients complain of painful and burning lingual sensations which may be so annoying that the dentist is often consulted first for local relief.

The tongue is generally inflamed, often described as "beefy red" in color, either in entirety or in patches scattered over the dorsum and lateral borders (Fig. 14–1). In some cases small, shallow ulcers resembling aphthous ulcers occur on the tongue. Characteristically, with the glossitis, glossodynia and glossopyrosis, there is gradual atrophy of the papillae of the tongue that eventuates in a smooth or "bald" tongue which is often referred to as Hunter's glossitis or Moeller's glossitis and is similar to the "bald tongue of Sandwith" seen in pellagra. Loss or distortion of taste is sometimes reported accompanying these changes. The fiery red appearance of the tongue may undergo periods of remission, but recurrent attacks are common. On occasion the inflammation and burning sensation extend to involve the entire oral mucosa, but more frequently the rest of the oral mucosa exhibits only the pale yellowish tinge noted on the skin. Millard and Gobetti have emphasized that a nonspecific persistent or recurring stomatitis of unexplained local origin may be an

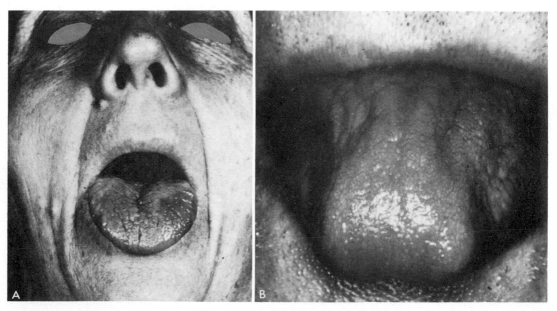

Figure 14–1. *Pernicious anemia.*
The tongue is inflamed and painful in each case, and there is beginning atrophy of the papillae in *A* and advanced atrophy in *B*. (Courtesy of Drs. Boynton H. Booth and Stephen F. Dachi.)

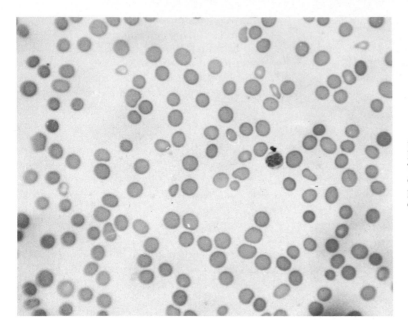

Figure 14–2. *Pernicious anemia.*
The peripheral blood smear from a typical case of pernicious anemia exhibits macrocytosis and poikilocytosis. The variation in size of erythrocytes is obvious. In addition, characteristic pear-shaped or "tear-drop" erythrocytes are also present.

early clinical manifestation of pernicious anemia. Not uncommonly the oral mucous membranes in patients with this disease become intolerant to dentures.

Farrant and Boen and Boddington have reported that cells from buccal scrapings of patients with pernicious anemia presented nuclear abnormalities consisting of enlargement, irregularity in shape and asymmetry. These were postulated to be due to a reduced rate of nucleic acid synthesis with a reduced rate of cell division. These epithelial cell alterations are rapidly reversible after administration of vitamin B_{12}.

Laboratory Findings. This chronic disease often exhibits periods of remission and exacerbation, and the blood changes generally parallel these clinical states. The red blood cell count is seriously decreased, often to 1,000,000 or less per cubic millimeter. Many of the cells exhibit macrocytosis; this, in fact, is one of the chief characteristics of the blood in this disease, although poikilocytosis, or variation in shape of cells, is also present (Fig. 14–2). The hemoglobin content of the red cells is increased, but this is only proportional to their increased size, since the mean corpuscular hemoglobin concentration is normal. A great many other red blood cell abnormalities have been described, particularly in advanced cases of anemia, including polychromatophilic cells, stippled cells, nucleated cells, Howell-Jolly bodies and Cabot's rings. Leukocytes are also often remarkably reduced in number, but are increased in average size and in number of lobes to the nucleus (becoming the so-called macropolycytes).

Bone marrow studies generally show great numbers of immature red cells or megaloblasts with few normoblasts, indicating maturation arrest at the more primitive megaloblast stage. Polymacrocytes ("macropolys") or large polymorphonuclear leukocytes with large polylobed nuclei are also typically found. The megakaryocytes appear normal.

Achlorhydria, or lack of gastric hydrochloric acid secretion, is a constant feature of the disease, and the pH of the gastric contents is usually high. This achlorhydria is probably associated with atrophy of the gastric mucosa, with a reduction in parietal cells, which commonly occurs in the presence of chronic inflammation. This atrophic gastritis may be related to the rather common occurrence of gastric carcinoma in patients with pernicious anemia. The incidence is between 5 and 10 per cent.

Treatment. The treatment of pernicious anemia consists in the administration of vitamin B_{12} and folic acid.

Sprue

(Idiopathic Steatorrhea; Celiac Disease)

Sprue is one disease of a large group which constitutes the "malabsorption syndrome." The disease, characterized by glossitis and diarrhea with large, pale, foul stools, was originally thought to occur only in tropical countries and has been termed "tropical sprue." It is found chiefly in persons subsisting on nutritionally inadequate diets, especially with a deficiency of vitamin B_{12} or folic acid. It is now recognized that a similar if not identical condition occurs in nontropical countries and is termed "nontropical sprue." This disease, also called "idiopathic steatorrhea" to distinguish it from steatorrhea resulting from fibrocystic disease of the pancreas with resultant decrease in pancreatic enzyme secretion, is generally accepted now as occurring as a result of susceptibility or intolerance to gluten wheat or rye flour. "Celiac disease" (or Gee-Herter disease) is the name applied to idiopathic steatorrhea when it occurs in children.

Sprue is not basically an anemic disorder. It is considered here, however, because it presents so many signs and symptoms in common with pernicious anemia that the differentiation is often difficult.

Clinical Features. Sprue occurs both in tropical countries and in temperate zones in persons of all ages, including infants.

The disease usually begins with intestinal disturbances, including diarrhea, constipation and flatulence. Excessive amounts of fat are passed in the stools, inducing a concomitant excessive loss of calcium, which in turn causes a calcium deficiency with ensuing low blood calcium levels and occasional tetany. This disturbance in calcium metabolism may result in osteoporosis as well as a great variety of skeletal abnormalities, especially if the disease occurs in children.

Nervous irritability as well as numbness and tingling of the extremities occurs, but seldom is there spinal cord involvement as in pernicious anemia. Malaise and generalized weakness are also common. The skin changes are often identical with those of pernicious anemia, but also include irregular brownish pigmentation, particularly on the face, neck, arms and legs, and drying of the skin with a scaly eruption.

Oral Manifestations. The oral changes in sprue are similar to those of pernicious anemia and have been described by Adlersberg from observation of 40 cases. There may be a severe glossitis with atrophy of the filiform papillae, although the fungiform papillae often persist for some time on the atrophic surface. Painful, burning sensations of the tongue and oral mucosa are common, and small, painful erosions may occur. These severe oral manifestations are seldom absent in cases of sprue (Fig. 14–3).

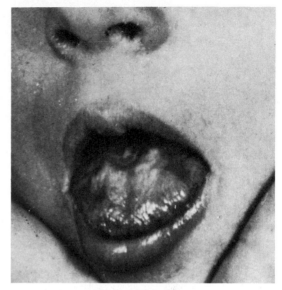

Figure 14–3. *Sprue.*
There is ulceration and inflammation of the tongue accompanied by a painful, burning sensation. (Courtesy of Dr. Boynton H. Booth.)

Tyldesley has reviewed this problem recently and concluded that there is an association between recurrent oral ulceration, or recurrent aphthous ulcers, and celiac disease and that proper dietary treatment leads to remission of the oral lesions.

Laboratory Findings. The blood and bone marrow changes are often identical with those of pernicious anemia and include a macrocytic anemia and leukopenia. Hypochromic microcytic anemia occasionally occurs. The patients do not usually exhibit achlorhydria, nor is the "intrinsic" factor absent.

Treatment. Sprue responds well in most cases to the administration of vitamin B_{12} and folic acid, although the diet must be carefully supervised and supplemented with vitamins and minerals. In cases of nontropical sprue, or gluten enteropathy, use of gluten wheat or rye flour should be discontinued.

Aplastic Anemia

Aplastic anemia is a disease characterized by a general lack of bone marrow activity; it may affect not only the red blood cells but also the white cells and platelets, resulting in a pancytopenia. The clinical manifestations of the disease vary according to the type of cell chiefly affected.

It is common to recognize two chief forms of aplastic anemia, primary and secondary. Primary aplastic anemia is a disease of unknown etiology which occurs most frequently in young adults, develops rapidly and usually terminates fatally. A disease known as *Fanconi's syndrome* consists of congenital, and sometimes familial, aplastic anemia associated with a variety of other congenital defects including bone abnormalities, microcephaly, hypogenitalism and a generalized olive-brown pigmentation of the skin.

Secondary aplastic anemia, on the other hand, is of known etiology, occurs at any age and presents a better prognosis, particularly if the cause is removed. The etiology of this secondary anemia is the exposure of the patient to various drugs or chemical substances or to radiant energy in the form of x-rays, radium or radioactive isotopes. In many cases the development of aplastic anemia after exposure to the drug or chemical seems to be an allergic phenomenon, since the amount of the substance absorbed is too small to result in an actual poisoning or intoxication. The chemicals which have been found most frequently to cause the development of this condition are acetophenetidin, amidopyrine, organic arsenicals, particularly sulfarsphenamine, benzol, chloramphenicol, quinacrine hydrochloride (Atabrine), trinitrotoluene, dinitrophenol, colloidal silver, bismuth, mercury, sulfonamides and penicillin, although many others have also produced the disease.

The effect of irradiation is usually more pronounced on the white blood cell series, although the development of aplastic anemia after exposure to x-ray radiation is well recognized.

Clinical Features. The clinical manifestations of aplastic anemia are referable not only to the anemia, but also to the leukopenia and thrombocytopenia which are variably present. There are few differences in the clinical features of the primary and secondary forms of the disease except in the ultimate prognosis.

The patients usually complain of severe weakness with dyspnea following even slight physical exertion and exhibit pallor of the skin. Numbness and tingling of the extremities and edema are also encountered. Petechiae in the skin and mucous membranes occur, owing to the platelet deficiency, while the neutropenia leads to a decreased resistance to infection.

Oral Manifestations. Petechiae, purpuric spots or frank hematomas of the oral mucosa may occur at any site, while hemorrhage into the oral cavity, especially spontaneous gingival hemorrhage, is present in some cases. Such findings are related to the blood platelet deficiency (Fig. 14–4). As a result of the neutropenia there is a generalized lack of resistance to infection, and this is manifested by the development of ulcerative lesions of the oral mucosa or pharynx. These may be extremely severe and may result in a condition resembling gangrene because of the lack of inflammatory cell response.

Laboratory Findings. The red blood cell count is remarkably diminished, often to as low as 1,000,000 cells per cubic millimeter, with a corresponding reduction in the hematocrit and hemoglobin levels. The reduced leukocyte count is at the expense of the granular series.

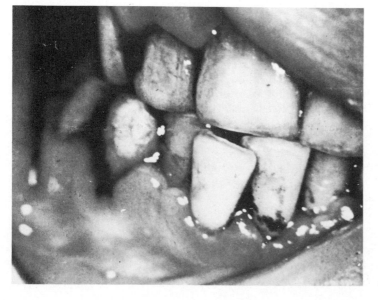

Figure 14–4. *Primary aplastic anemia.* The patient suffered from spontaneous hemorrhage from the gingiva.

The thrombocytopenia results in a prolonged bleeding time; the clotting time remains normal. Clot retraction is poor and the tourniquet test is positive.

Bone marrow smears exhibit variable findings depending on the extent of the anemia and/or pancytopenia. If only an anemia exists, there is erythropoietic depression. Occasionally, however, the marrow appears normal or even hyperplastic. In pancytopenia there is hypoplasia of all marrow elements, and only occasional cells of any type may be found. In cases of less severe damage, moderate numbers of primitive cells persist.

Treatment and Prognosis. There is no specific treatment for primary aplastic anemia, although the severity and rapid course of the disease can usually be attenuated by the administration of antibiotics and blood transfusions. The disease is fatal in an extremely high percentage of cases. In instances of secondary anemia the removal of the specific causative agent accompanied by the foregoing supportive treatment is usually sufficient. The prognosis is good.

Thalassemia

(Cooley's Anemia; Mediterranean Disease; Erythroblastic Anemia)

The thalassemia group of anemias is a heterogeneous group characterized by diminished synthesis of the α- or β-globin chain of hemoglobin A. The disease is inherited as an autosomal dominant trait and exhibits a racial pattern. Persons most commonly affected are those of Italian, Greek, Syrian, or Armenian nationalities, although a great many cases have been reported in persons from a variety of other countries in Europe or the Far East as well as in blacks in Africa and the United States.

The disease is termed α-thalassemia when there is deficient synthesis of the α chain and β-thalassemia when the β chain is deficient. Thus, in β-thalassemia there is an excess of α chains, producing "unstable hemoglobins" that damage the erythrocytes and increase their vulnerability to destruction. In heterozygotes, the disease is mild and is called *thalassemia minor* or *thalassemia trait*. It represents both α- and β-thalassemia. Homozygotes may exhibit a severe form of the disease that is called *thalassemia major* or *homozygous β-thalassemia*. Two other forms of thalassemia major that represent α-thalassemia also exist. These are (1)

hemoglobin H disease, which is a very mild form of the disease in which the patient may live a relatively normal life, and (2) hemoglobin Bart's disease, with hydrops fetalis, in which the infants are stillborn or die shortly after birth.

Clinical Features. The onset of the severe form of the disease (homozygous β-thalassemia) occurs within the first two years of life, often in the first few months. Siblings are commonly affected. The child has a yellowish pallor of the skin and exhibits fever, chills, malaise and a generalized weakness. Splenomegaly and hepatomegaly may cause protrusion of the abdomen. The face often develops mongoloid features due to prominence of the cheek bones, protrusion or flaring of the maxillary anterior teeth, and the depression of the bridge of the nose. The child does not appear acutely ill, but the disease follows an ingravescent course which is often aggravated by intercurrent infection. Some patients, however, die within a few months, especially when the disease is manifested at a very early age. Logothetis and his associates have shown that the degree of cephalofacial deformities in this disease (including prominent frontal and parietal bones, sunken nose bridge, protruding zygomas and mongoloid slanting eyes) is closely related to the severity of the disease and the time of institution of treatment.

Thalassemia minor (thalassemia trait) is generally without clinical manifestations.

Oral Manifestations. An unusual prominence of the premaxilla has been described in cases of erythroblastic anemia, such as that reported by Novak, and this results in an obvious malocclusion. The oral mucosa may exhibit the characteristic anemic pallor observed on the skin.

Laboratory Findings. The pronounced anemia is of a hypochromic microcytic type, the red cells exhibiting a poikilocytosis and anisocytosis. These cells are extremely pale, but in some instances appear as "target" cells with a condensation of coloring matter in the center of the cell. The presence of typical "safety-pin" cells and of normoblasts or nucleated red blood cells in the circulating blood is also a characteristic feature. The white blood cell count is frequently elevated, often as high as 10,000 to 25,000 or more per cubic millimeter.

Bone marrow smears show cellular hyperplasia with large numbers of immature, primitive and stem forms of red blood cells, all indicating maturation arrest. The serum bilirubin in these

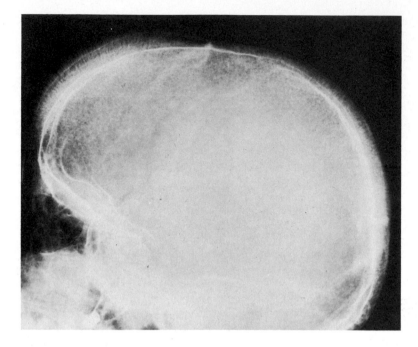

Figure 14–5. *Thalassemia.*
The "hair-on-end" effect is well
demonstrated in the roentgenogram.
(Courtesy of Dr. Robert J. Gorlin.)

patients is also elevated, indicative of the severe
hemosiderosis which is almost invariably present. This systemic hemosiderosis has suggested
a possible block in iron utilization with accumulation of iron pigment and subsequent inadequate formation of hemoglobin.

Roentgenographic Features. The skeletal
changes in thalassemia are most striking and
have been thoroughly described by Caffey. In
the skull there is extreme thickening of the
diploë; the inner and outer plates become
poorly defined, and the trabeculae between the
plates become elongated, producing a bristle-
like "crew-cut" or "hair-on-end" appearance of
the surface of the skull (Fig. 14–5).

Both the skull and long bones exhibit some
degree of osteoporosis, but spontaneous fracture of bones is not common. There is typically
a widening of the medulla with thinning of the
cortices of the long bones. The bony changes
may occur early in life and tend to persist,
particularly those in the skull.

Intraoral roentgenograms in some cases reveal a peculiar trabecular pattern of the maxilla
and mandible, characterized by an apparent
coarsening of some trabeculae and the blurring
and disappearance of others, resulting in a "salt
and pepper" effect. In general, the jaws exhibit
mild osteoporosis. According to Poyton and
Davey, who have reviewed the roentgenographic changes, thinning of the lamina dura

and circular radiolucencies in the alveolar bone
are also found.

Treatment. There is no treatment for this
form of anemia. The administration of liver
extract, iron or vitamin B_6 is fruitless. Blood
transfusions do provide temporary remissions.

The disease is usually fatal, although mild
forms which are compatible with life apparently
exist. Generally, the earlier in infancy the disease occurs, the more rapidly it proves fatal.
Death is generally due to intercurrent infection,
cardiac damage as a result of anoxia, or liver
failure.

Sickle Cell Anemia

Sickle cell anemia is a hereditary type of
chronic hemolytic anemia transmitted as a mendelian dominant, nonsex-linked characteristic,
which occurs almost exclusively in blacks, and
in whites of Mediterranean origin. The name is
derived from the peculiar microscopic appearance of sickle- or crescent-shaped erythrocytes
found in the circulating blood. Normal adult
hemoglobin (HbA) is genetically altered to produce sickle hemoglobin (HbS) by the substitution of valine for glutamine at the sixth position
of the β-globin chain. In the heterozygote, only
about 40 per cent of the hemoglobin is HbS, so
that the individual has only the sickle-cell trait
and manifests clinical evidence of sickling only

under conditions of severe hypoxia. About 8 per cent of American blacks are heterozygous for hemoglobin S. In the homozygote, nearly all hemoglobin is HbS, and the individual suffers from sickle cell anemia. This occurs in about one in 600 American blacks.

Clinical Features. Sickle cell anemia is more common in females and usually becomes clinically manifest before the age of 30 years. Patients manifest a variety of features related to the anemia per se. Thus the patient is weak, short of breath and easily fatigued. Pain in the joints, limbs and abdomen, as well as nausea and vomiting, is common. Systolic murmur and cardiomegaly also occur. One additional feature characteristically seen is packing of red blood cells in peripheral vessels with erythrostasis and subsequent local tissue anoxia. An infarct of the mandible on this basis has been reported by Walker and Schenck. Sickle cell crises may occur under a variety of situations, including the administration of a general anesthetic, probably as a result of decreased oxygenation of the blood. Other triggering causes of deoxygenation may include exercise or exertion, infections, pregnancy or even sleep.

Oral Manifestations. According to the studies of Robinson and Sarnat, a majority of patients with sickle cell anemia exhibit significant bone changes in the dental roentgenograms. These alterations consist of a mild to severe generalized osteoporosis and a loss of trabeculation of the jaw bones with the appearance of large, irregular marrow spaces. The trabecular change is prominent in the alveolar bone. There are no alterations in the lamina dura or periodontal ligament. Similar findings were reported by Morris and Stahl and by Prowler and Smith, not only in patients with sickle cell anemia but also in many with only the sickling trait. However, in a study of 80 patients with sickle cell anemia who were compared with an apparently normal group of patients, Mourshed and Tuckson stated that these two roentgenographic features of the jaws—increased radiolucency and coarse trabeculation—cannot be considered reliable diagnostic criteria for the disease.

Goldsby and Staats have reported morphologic alterations in the nuclei of epithelial cells in scrapings of the oral mucosa in 90 per cent of all studied cases of patients with homozygous sickle cell disease. These changes were chiefly nuclear enlargement, binucleation and an atypical chromatin distribution. These changes are similar to those that have been reported occurring in pernicious anemia and sprue (Fig. 14–6, A, B).

Roentgenographic Features. Roentgeno-

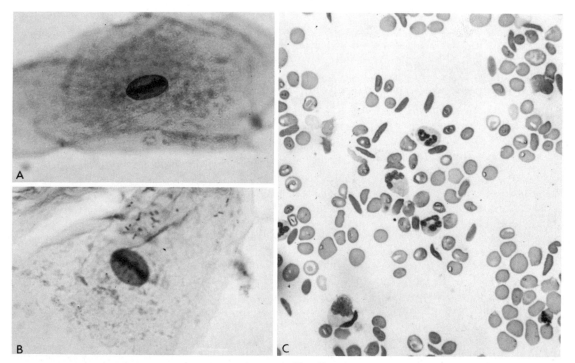

Figure 14–6. *Sickle cell anemia.*
Atypical chromatin bars are seen in cytologic smears from buccal mucosa (A, B), while numerous typical sickle-shaped erythrocytes are present in the peripheral blood smear (C).

grams of the skull exhibit an unusual appearance, with perpendicular trabeculations radiating outward from the inner table producing a "hair-on-end" pattern, identical to that seen in thalassemia, congenital hemolytic jaundice and sometimes in chronic iron deficiency anemia and secondary polycythemia of cyanotic congenital heart disease. The outer table of bone may appear absent and the diploë thickened. Generalized osteoporosis may be present. The long bones of children may exhibit enlarged medullary cavities with thin cortices, while the same bones in adults become sclerotic with cortical thickening due to fibrosis of the marrow.

Laboratory Findings. The red blood cell count may reach a level of 1,000,000 cells or less per cubic millimeter with a decreased hemoglobin level. On the blood smear, typical sickle-shaped red blood cells are commonly seen, although they are present also in cases of the sickle trait without clinical evidence of the disease (Fig. 14–6, C).

The sickle hemoglobin molecule undergoes gelation or crystallization when it is deoxygenated, and this physically distorts the erythrocyte, producing the sickle shape. These distorted cells then "logjam" and produce stasis within the microvasculature. Damage to erythrocyte membranes also occurs in sickled cells and leads to their fragmentation and intravascular hemolysis.

Treatment and Prognosis. There is no specific treatment for this disease except transfusion during a crisis. The prognosis is unpredictable. Many patients with the anemia die before the age of 30 years, but those patients with only the sickle cell trait have a better prognosis and may live a normal life span.

Erythroblastosis Fetalis

Congenital hemolytic anemia due to Rh incompatibility results from the destruction of fetal blood brought about by a reaction between maternal and fetal blood factors.

The Rh factor, named after the rhesus monkey, was discovered by Landsteiner and Wiener in 1940 as a factor in human red blood cells that would react with rabbit antiserum produced by administration of red blood cells from the rhesus monkey. The Rh factor, a dominant hereditary characteristic, is present in the red blood cells of approximately 85 per cent of the Caucasian population of the United States.

Pathogenesis. Erythroblastosis fetalis is essentially due to the inheritance by the fetus of a blood factor from the father that acts as a foreign antigen to the mother. The transplacental transfer of this antigen, actually transplacental leaks of red cells, from the fetus to the mother results in immunization of the mother and formation of antibodies which, when transferred back to the fetus by the same route, produce fetal hemolysis. Occasionally the ABO system may produce a similar type of immunization and hemolysis.

The basic inheritance of the Rh factor is relatively simple. If both parents are homozygously Rh-positive (have the Rh factor), the infant will be Rh-positive, but maternal immunization cannot occur, since both mother and fetus have the same antigen. If the mother is homozygously positive, but the father Rh-negative, the same situation actually exists, since both the mother and the fetus have the same antigen and no immunization can occur. If the father is Rh-positive and the mother Rh-negative, however, the fetus inherits the paternal factor, which may then act as an antigen to the mother and immunize her with resultant antibody formation.

The problem is complicated, however, by the occurrence of numerous immunologically distinct Rh antigens. The strongest of these antigens have been termed C, D and E, and the presence of any one of them constitutes an Rh-positive person. Each of these antigens is normally present in a specific gene, but, if absent, their place is taken by less potent Hr antigens, known as c, d and e. Thus, three Rh or Hr genes are inherited from each parent, constituting three pairs of factors. Any combination of C, D, E and c, d, e is therefore possible, but the only combination producing an Rh-negative person is cde-cde. The D antigen, by far the strongest, is most frequently responsible for the clinical manifestations of erythroblastosis fetalis, and the 85 per cent of the population generally considered Rh-positive actually have the D antigen homozygously (D-D) or heterozygously (D-d). The 15 per cent who are Rh-negative have the d antigen homozygously (d-d). Mathematically, according to the laws of random mating, there should be 10 cases of erythroblastosis fetalis in every 100 pregnancies. Clinically, it has been found that only one case in every 200 pregnancies occurs. There are several possible explanations for this discrepancy: (1) in some cases the mother may be unable to form antibodies even though immunized by the Rh-positive fetus; (2) even though the fetus is Rh-positive, transplacental transfer of the antigen does not occur, so that there is no maternal immunization; (3) immunization may occur, but its level is so low as to be clinically insignificant. Recent evidence has shown that, in general, women have a reduced immunologic responsiveness during pregnancy. Subsequent pregnancies might cause further immunization with increased antibody formation, so that in ensuing pregnancies clinical hemolysis does occur. This latter explanation is plausible since it explains adequately why the first pregnancy is often uneventful, while erythroblastosis frequently occurs in succeeding pregnancies.

It is of great interest to note that the frequency of erythroblastosis fetalis of Rh incompatibility has shown a dramatic decrease in the past few years and that the eventual elimination of the disease through immunization prevention techniques is a probability. At present, Rh-negative mothers are being given anti-D gamma globulin to prevent immunization, since it binds to antigenic receptor sites on fetal red cells, making them nonimmunogenic.

Clinical Features. The manifestations of the disease depend upon the severity of the hemolysis. Some infants are stillborn. Those that are born alive characteristically suffer from (1) anemia with pallor, (2) jaundice, (3) compensatory erythropoiesis, both medullary and extramedullary, and (4) edema resulting in fetal hydrops. It is of considerable interest that the severe anemia and jaundice do not begin to develop until at least several hours after birth and frequently not for several days. The most important aid in diagnosis of the disease is a positive direct Coombs test on cord blood.

Oral Manifestations. Erythroblastosis fetalis may be manifested in the teeth by the deposition of blood pigment in the enamel and dentin of the developing teeth, giving them a green, brown or blue hue (Fig. 14–7). Ground sections of these teeth give a positive test for bilirubin. The stain is intrinsic and does not involve teeth or portions of teeth developing after cessation of hemolysis shortly after birth.

Enamel hypoplasia is also reported occurring in some cases of erythroblastosis fetalis. This usually involves the incisal edges of the anterior teeth and the middle portion of the deciduous cuspid and first molar crown. Here a characteristic ringlike defect occurs which has been termed the "Rh hump" by Watson.

Many infants with this disease are stillborn, but an increasing number of those born alive have survived after a total replacement of their blood by transfusion at birth. Thus the dentist may expect to see more children with the peculiar pigmentation of teeth characteristic of the condition, and should be aware of its nature.

Laboratory Findings. The red blood count at birth may vary from less than 1,000,000 cells per cubic millimeter to near a normal level. There are characteristically large numbers of normoblasts, or nucleated red cells, in the circulating blood. Ultimately, severe anemia usually develops within a few days. The icterus index is invariably high and may reach a level of 100 units.

Treatment. No treatment for the tooth pigmentation is necessary, since it affects only the deciduous teeth and presents only a temporary cosmetic problem.

Iron-Deficiency Anemia and Plummer-Vinson Syndrome

Iron deficiency is an exceedingly prevalent form of anemia, particularly in females. It has

Figure 14–7. *Pigmentation of teeth in erythroblastosis fetalis.*
The teeth had a definite blue cast. The sharp line of separation between affected and unaffected tooth substance is seen near the cervical area of the mandibular cuspids and first molars. (Courtesy of Dr. Ralph E. McDonald.)

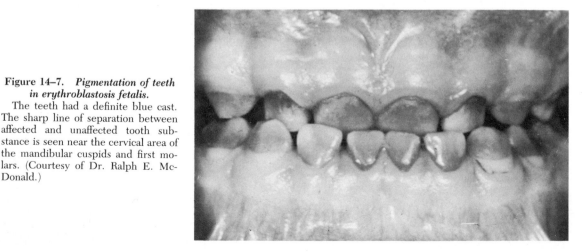

been estimated that between 5 and 30 per cent of women in the United States are iron deficient, while in some parts of the world, this may reach 50 per cent. Men are only rarely affected.

The iron deficiency leading to this anemia usually arises through (1) chronic blood loss (as in patients with a history of profuse menstruation, (2) inadequate dietary intake, (3) faulty iron absorption, or (4) increased requirements for iron, as during infancy, childhood and adolescence and during pregnancy.

The Plummer-Vinson syndrome is one manifestation of iron-deficiency anemia and was first described by Plummer in 1914 and by Vinson in 1922 under the term "hysterical dysphagia." Not until 1936, however, was the full clinical significance of the condition recognized. Ahlbom then defined it as a predisposition for the development of carcinoma in the upper alimentary tract. It is, in fact, one of the few known predisposing factors in oral cancer.

Clinical Features. While an iron-deficiency anemia may occur at any age, the Plummer-Vinson syndrome occurs chiefly in women in the fourth and fifth decades of life. Presenting symptoms of the anemia and the syndrome are cracks or fissures at the corners of the mouth, a lemon-tinted pallor of the skin, a smooth, red, painful tongue with atrophy of the filiform and later the fungiform papillae, and dysphagia resulting from an esophageal stricture or web. These oral findings are reminiscent of those seen in pernicious anemia. The mucous membranes of the oral cavity and esophagus are atrophic and show loss of normal keratinization. Koilonychia (spoon-shaped fingernails) or nails that are brittle and break easily have been reported in many patients; splenomegaly has also been reported in 20 to 30 per cent of the cases.

The depletion of iron stores in the body, manifested as iron-deficiency anemia, may be the direct cause of the mucous membrane atrophy, since the integrity of epithelium is dependent upon adequate serum iron levels. The atrophy of the mucous membranes of the upper alimentary tract predisposes to the development of carcinoma in these tissues. This relationship was first noted by Ahlbom, who reported that half of all women with carcinoma of the hypopharynx and upper part of the esophagus seen at Radiumhemmet in Stockholm suffered from Plummer-Vinson syndrome. Subsequently the predisposition to the development of oral carcinoma was also established.

Laboratory Findings. Blood examination reveals a hypochromic microcytic anemia of varying degree, while sternal marrow examination shows no megaloblasts typical of pernicious anemia. The red blood cell count is generally between 3,000,000 and 4,000,000 cells per cubic millimeter, and the hemoglobin is invariably low. That the anemia is of an iron-deficiency type can be confirmed by lack of a reticulocyte response following administration of vitamin B_{12}. Serum iron is low, and there is an absence of free hydrochloric acid in the stomach. The achlorhydria is generally the cause of the faulty absorption of iron, since the absence of hydrochloric acid prevents the conversion of unabsorbable dietary ferric iron to the absorbable ferrous state.

Unusual alterations in exfoliated squamous epithelial cells of the tongue in cases of severe iron-deficiency anemia have been reported by Monto and his associates. These changes consisted of a deficiency of keratinized cells, a reduced cytoplasmic diameter of cells with a paradoxical enlargement of the nucleus, and abnormal cellular maturation characterized by a disturbed nuclear pattern, an increase in nucleoli, presence of double nuclei and karyorrhexis.

Treatment and Prognosis. The anemia responds well to iron therapy and a high-protein diet. Because of the predisposition to the development of carcinoma of oral mucous membranes, it is essential that the diagnosis be established early so that treatment may be instituted as soon as possible.

POLYCYTHEMIA

Polycythemia is defined as an abnormal increase in the number of red blood cells in the peripheral blood, usually with an increased hemoglobin level. Three forms of the disease are recognized: (1) relative polycythemia, (2) primary polycythemia or erythremia (polycythemia rubra vera) of unknown etiology, and (3) secondary polycythemia or erythrocytosis, due to some known stimulus.

Relative polycythemia is an apparent increase in the number of circulating red blood cells that occurs as a result of loss of blood fluid with hemoconcentration of cells, and is seen in cases of excessive loss of body fluids such as chronic vomiting, diarrhea, or loss of electrolytes with accompanying loss of water. This increase in the number of red blood cells is only relative to the total blood volume and, therefore, is not a true polycythemia.

Primary polycythemia, or polycythemia rubra vera, is characterized by a true idiopathic increase in the number of circulating red blood cells and of the hemoglobin level.

Secondary polycythemia is similar to primary polycythemia except that the etiology is known. In general, the stimulus responsible for producing a secondary polycythemia is either (1) bone marrow anoxia or (2) production of an erythropoietic stimulator factor. Bone marrow anoxia may occur in numerous situations such as pulmonary dysfunction, heart disease, habitation at high altitudes or chronic carbon monoxide poisoning. Erythropoietic stimulatory factors include a variety of drugs and chemicals such as coal-tar derivatives, gum shellac, phosphorus, and various metals such as manganese, mercury, iron, bismuth, arsenic and cobalt. Some types of tumors such as certain brain tumors, liver and kidney carcinomas and the uterine myoma have also been reported associated with polycythemia. The mechanism for increased production of the red blood cells by these tumors is unknown, but has been postulated as due to elaboration of a specific factor which stimulates erythropoiesis.

Polycythemia Vera

(Polycythemia Rubra Vera; Erythremia; Vaquez's Disease; Osler's Disease)

Polycythemia vera is a chronic disease with an insidious onset characterized by an absolute increase in the number of circulating red blood cells and in the total blood volume. This abnormal finding is of unknown etiology, but in occasional cases has been reported as a familial disease. All manifestations of this disease are identical with those of secondary polycythemia, so the two conditions may be considered together here.

Clinical Features. Polycythemia vera often manifests itself primarily by headache or dizziness, weakness and lassitude, tinnitus, visual disturbances, mental confusion, slurring of the speech and inability to concentrate. The skin is flushed or diffusely reddened, as a result of capillary engorgement, as though the patient were continuously blushing. This condition is most obvious on the head, neck and extremities, although the digits may be cyanotic. The skin of the trunk is seldom involved.

Splenomegaly is one of the most constant features of polycythemia vera, and the spleen is sometimes painful. Gastric complaints such as gas pains, belching and peptic ulcers are common, and hemorrhage from varices in the gastrointestinal tract may occur.

The disease is more common in men and usually occurs in middle age or later.

Oral Manifestations. The oral mucous membranes appear deep purplish red, the gingiva and tongue being most prominently affected. The cyanosis is due to the presence of reduced hemoglobin in amounts exceeding 5 gm./dl. The gingivae are often engorged and swollen and bleed upon the slightest provocation. Submucosal petechiae are also common, as well as ecchymoses and hematomas. Intercurrent infection may occur, but this is not related directly to the disease.

Laboratory Findings. The red blood cell count is elevated and may even exceed 10,000,000 cells per cubic millimeter. The hemoglobin content of the blood is also increased, often as high as 20 gm./dl., although the color index is less than 1.0. Because of the great number of cells present, both the specific gravity and the viscosity of the blood are increased.

Leukocytosis is usual, as is a great increase in the number of platelets; in addition, the total blood volume is elevated through distention of even the smallest blood vessels of the body. There is usually hyperplasia of all elements of the bone marrow. Bleeding and clotting times are normal.

Treatment. No specific treatment for polycythemia is known, although several methods are used for relieving its symptoms. The patient may be periodically bled, or substances may be administered either to destroy blood (phenylhydrazine) or to interfere with its formation (nitrogen mustard or even x-ray radiation). In recent years the radioactive isotope of phosphorus, P^{32}, has been used. Any such treatment, however, produces only a remission of the disease; it does not effect a cure. The course of the disease may be protracted over many years.

DISEASES INVOLVING THE WHITE BLOOD CELLS

LEUKOPENIA

Leukopenia is an abnormal reduction in the number of white blood cells in the peripheral

Table 14–3.   Causes of Leukopenia

I. Infections
  A. Bacterial
    1. Typhoid fever
    2. Paratyphoid fever
    3. Brucellosis
    4. Tularemia (rarely)
  B. Viral and rickettsial
    1. Influenza
    2. Measles
    3. Rubella
    4. Chickenpox
    5. Infectious hepatitis
    6. Colorado tick fever
    7. Dengue
    8. Yellow fever
    9. Sandfly fever
  C. Protozoal
    1. Malaria
    2. Relapsing fever
    3. Kala-azar
  D. Any overwhelming infection
    1. Miliary tuberculosis
    2. Septicemia
II. Cachectic and debilitating states and inanition
III. Hemopoietic disorders, especially splenic
  A. Gaucher's disease
  B. Banti's disease
  C. Pernicious anemia (relapse)
  D. Aplastic anemia
  E. Chronic hypochromic anemia
  F. Myelophthisic anemia
  G. "Aleukemic" leukemia
  H. Agranulocytosis
IV. Chemical agents
  A. Agents commonly producing leukopenia in all patients if given in sufficient dose
    1. Mustards (sulfur and nitrogen mustards, triethylenemelamine [TEM], etc.)
    2. Urethane, busulfan, Demecolcin
    3. Benzene
    4. Antimetabolites (antifolic compounds, 6-mercaptopurine, etc.)
  B. Agents occasionally associated with leukopenia, apparently a result of individual sensitivity
    1. Analgesics, sedatives and anti-inflammatory agents (e.g., aminopyrine, dipyrone, phenacetin, phenylbutazone)
    2. Antithyroid drugs (e.g., the thiouracils)
    3. Anticonvulsants
    4. Sulfonamides
    5. Antihistamines
    6. Antimicrobial agents
    7. Tranquilizers (e.g., phenothiazines and others)
    8. Miscellaneous (e.g., dinitrophenol, phenindione, cimetidine, tolbutamide, chlorpropamide, carbutamide, gold salts, industrial chemicals)
    9. Many other drugs infrequently
V. Physical agents
  A. X-ray radiation and radioactive substances
VI. Anaphylactoid shock and early stages of reaction to foreign protein
VII. Certain diseases of unknown etiology, including hereditary and congenital
  A. Liver cirrhosis
  B. Felty's syndrome
  C. Disseminated lupus erythematosus
  D. Primary splenic neutropenia
  E. Cyclic neutropenia
  F. Chronic hypoplastic neutropenia

Modified from M. M. Wintrobe: Clinical Hematology. 8th ed. Philadelphia, Lea & Febiger, 1981.

blood stream. This decrease involves predominantly the granulocytes, although any of the cell types may be affected. The etiology of this particular sign of disease is extremely varied, but the classification shown in Table 14–3 has been devised by Wintrobe.

Oral lesions are present in certain diseases that are characterized by a reduction in the number of white cells. These lesions are related to the inability of the tissues to react in the usual manner to infection or trauma. Because of the dangerous sequelae which may result if the disease is not recognized, the dentist must be fully acquainted with each disorder and its serious consequences.

Agranulocytosis

(Granulocytopenia; Agranulocytic Angina; Malignant Leukopenia or Neutropenia)

Agranulocytosis is a serious disease involving the white blood cells. It is often classified with reference to etiology as primary or secondary in type, *primary agranulocytosis* being that form of the disease in which the etiology is unknown, and *secondary agranulocytosis* being that form in which the cause is recognized. Since the clinical and laboratory findings in both forms are identical, the disease will be discussed here as a single entity.

Etiology.   The most common known cause of agranulocytosis is the ingestion of any one of a considerable variety of drugs. Those compounds chiefly responsible for the disease are also those to which patients commonly manifest idiosyncrasy in the form of urticaria, cutaneous rashes and edema. For this reason and because often only small amounts of these drugs are necessary to produce the disease, it appears that the reaction may be an allergic phenomenon, although attempts to demonstrate antibodies in affected patients have not been successful. Moreover, in the case of some of the drugs, the disease occurs only after continued administration.

Kracke, in 1931, was one of the first to point out that a rapid increase in the number of cases of agranulocytosis occurred at the time of the introduction of certain coal-tar derivatives for use in therapy. The following drugs and compounds are some of those which have been reported to produce agranulocytosis in some persons:

Amidopyrine
Barbiturates
  (including amobarbital
  and phenobarbital)
Benzene
Bismuth
Chloramphenicol
Cinchophen
DDT
Dinitrophenol
Gold salts
Organic arsenicals
Phenacetin
Phenothiazines and
related compounds
  (including
  chlorpromazine,

promazine, mepazine,
prochlorperazine and
imipramine)
Phenylbutazone
Quinine
Sulfonamides
  (including
  sulfanilamide,
  sulfapyridine,
  sulfathiazole and
  sulfadiazine)
Thioglycolic acid
Thiouracil
Tolbutamide
Trimethadione
Tripelennamine

Most persons can be exposed to these drugs with near impunity; the hematologic reaction to the compounds is actually an uncommon one.

Clinical Features. Agranulocytosis occurs at any age, but is somewhat more common in adults, particularly women. The disease frequently affects workers in the health professions and in hospitals (e.g., physicians, dentists, nurses, hospital orderlies, and pharmacists), probably because they have easy access to the offending drugs and often use drug samples injudiciously.

The disease commences with a high fever, accompanied by chills and sore throat. The patient suffers malaise, weakness and prostration. The skin appears pale and anemic or, in some cases, jaundiced. The most characteristic feature of the disease is the presence of infection, particularly in the oral cavity, but also throughout the gastrointestinal tract, genitourinary tract, respiratory tract and skin. Regional lymphadenitis accompanies the infection in any of these locations.

The clinical signs and symptoms develop rapidly in the majority of cases, usually within a few days, and death may occur within a week.

Oral Manifestations. The oral lesions constitute an important phase of the clinical aspects of agranulocytosis. These appear as necrotizing ulcerations of the oral mucosa, tonsils and pharynx. Particularly involved are the gingiva and palate. The lesions appear as ragged necrotic ulcers covered by a gray or even black membrane (Fig. 14–8). Significantly, there is little or no apparent inflammatory cell infiltration around the periphery of the lesions, although hemorrhage does occur, especially from the gingiva. In addition, the patients often manifest excessive salivation.

It is obvious that all oral surgical procedures, particularly tooth extraction, are contraindicated in cases of agranulocytosis.

Histologic Features. The microscopic appearance of sections through the ulcerated oral lesions is a pathognomonic one and accounts for certain clinical features of the disease. Since

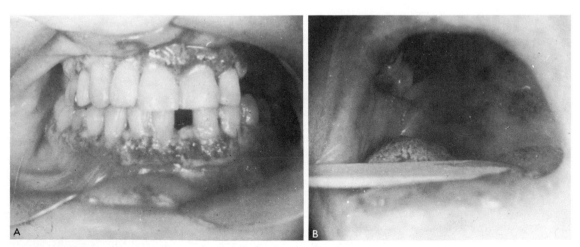

Figure 14–8. *Agranulocytosis.*
The necrotizing areas of ulceration on the gingivae (*A*) and palate (*B*) occurred after the use of a barbiturate. (Courtesy of Dr. Edward V. Zegarelli.)

the essential fault is the lack of development of normal granular leukocytes, the ulcerated areas exhibit no polymorphonuclear reaction to the bacteria in the tissues, and rampant necrosis ensues.

Bauer studied the microscopic appearance of the jaws in agranulocytosis and reported necrosis of the gingiva, beginning adjacent to the sulcus and spreading into the free gingiva, periodontal ligament and even alveolar bone. Rapid destruction of the supporting tissues of the teeth follows.

Laboratory Findings. The white blood cell count in agranulocytosis is often below 2000 cells per cubic millimeter with an almost complete absence of granulocytes or polymorphonuclear cells. The red blood cell count and platelet count are usually normal, although occasionally anemia is present.

The bone marrow is relatively normal except for the absence of granulocytes, metamyelocytes and myelocytes. Promyelocytes and myeloblasts are usually present in near normal numbers, however, and for this reason it appears that the basic defect is an arrest in cell maturation.

Treatment and Prognosis. The treatment of agranulocytosis is not specific, but should consist principally in recognition and withdrawal of the causative drug and in administration of antibiotic drugs to control the infection.

Death is usually related to massive infection, and for this reason the disease carried a high mortality before the advent of the antibiotics. In some series the mortality rate was 70 to 90 per cent. Today, although it is still a serious disease, agranulocytosis has a good prognosis if the responsible agent is discovered.

Cyclic Neutropenia

(Periodic Neutropenia; Cyclic Agranulocytic Angina; Periodic Agranulocytosis)

Cyclic neutropenia is an unusual form of agranulocytosis characterized by a periodic or cyclic diminution in circulating polymorphonuclear neutrophilic leukocytes as a result of bone marrow maturation arrest, accompanied by mild clinical manifestations, which spontaneously regresses only to recur subsequently in a rhythmic pattern. The etiology of this disease is unknown. Excellent reviews of cyclic neutropenia with its oral manifestations have been published by Page and Good, Becker and his co-workers, and Gorlin and Chaudhry. Although the role of hormonal and allergic factors in the etiology of

the disease has been suggested by some workers, there is no sound evidence to indicate that this is the case. There appear to exist at least two additional rare hereditary forms of the disease, one cyclic and the other noncyclic. In addition, a chronic idiopathic neutropenia, noncyclic and nonfamilial, associated with severe persistent gingivitis has been reported by Kyle and Linman.

Clinical Features. This type of agranulocytosis may occur at any age, although the majority of cases have been reported in infants or young children. The symptoms are similar to those of typical agranulocytosis except that they are usually milder. The patients manifest fever, malaise, sore throat, stomatitis and regional lymphadenopathy, as well as headache, arthritis, cutaneous infection and conjunctivitis. In contrast to other types of primary agranulocytosis, rampant bacterial infection is not a significant feature, presumably because the neutrophil count is low for such a short time.

Oral Manifestations. Patients with this disease typically exhibit a severe gingivitis, sometimes a stomatitis with ulceration, which corresponds to the period of the neutropenia and is due to bacterial invasion, chiefly from the gingival sulcus, in the absence of a defense mechanism (Fig. 14–9). With return of the neutrophil count to normal, the gingiva assumes a nearly normal clinical appearance. In children the repeated insult of infection often leads to considerable loss of supporting bone around the teeth (Fig. 14–10). The widespread severe ulceration usually seen in agranulocytosis does not often occur. However, isolated painful ulcers may occur which persist for 10 to 14 days and heal with scarring. On this basis, it has been suggested by Gorlin and Chaudhry that some cases diagnosed clinically as periadenitis mucosa necrotica recurrens may actually be cyclic neutropenia.

Roentgenographic Features. The intraoral roentgenograms typically exhibit mild to severe loss of superficial alveolar bone, even in children, as a result of the repeated cyclic gingivitis, advancing to periodontitis. In children this loss of bone around multiple teeth has sometimes been termed "prepubertal periodontitis," and it is frequently indicative of a serious systemic disease. Cohen and Morris have discussed the periodontal manifestations of cyclic neutropenia.

Laboratory Findings. Cyclic neutropenia is an unusual disease which manifests the clinical signs and symptoms and blood changes in a periodic fashion. The cycle commonly occurs

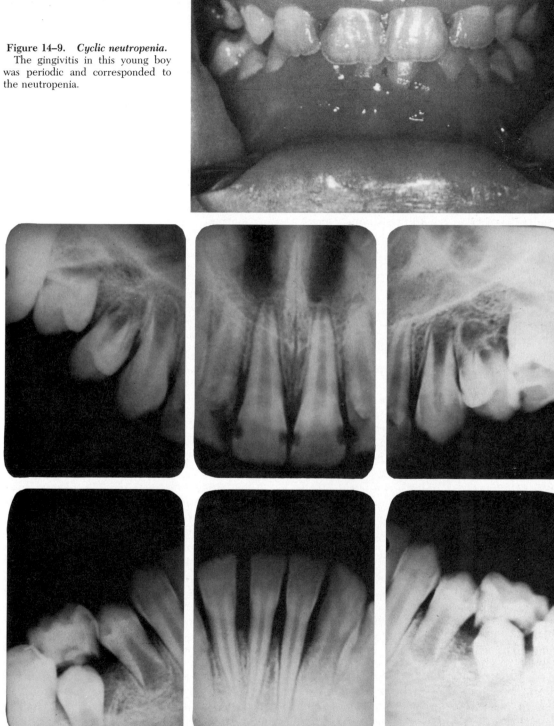

Figure 14–9. *Cyclic neutropenia.* The gingivitis in this young boy was periodic and corresponded to the neutropenia.

Figure 14–10. *Cyclic neutropenia.* The roentgenograms demonstrate beginning loss of alveolar bone even at an early age, due to the repeated episodes of gingival infection and inflammation.

every three weeks, although in some cases it may be several months or even longer in duration.

The patient may exhibit a normal blood count which, over a period of four to five days, begins to show a precipitous decline in the neutrophil count compensated by an increase in monocytes and lymphocytes. At the height of the disease, the neutrophils may completely disappear for a period of one or two days. Soon, however, the cells begin to reappear, and within four to five days the blood cell count and differential count are essentially normal.

Treatment and Prognosis. There is no specific treatment for the disease, although in some instances splenectomy has proved beneficial. Death occasionally results, usually from intercurrent infection, but the prognosis is generally far better than in typical agranulocytosis. The patients may suffer from their periodic disease for years.

Chédiak-Higashi Syndrome

Chédiak-Higashi syndrome is an uncommon genetic disease which is often fatal in early life as a result of a lymphoma-like terminal phase, hemorrhage, or infection. It is transmitted as an autosomal recessive trait.

Clinical Features. The characteristic clinical features of this disease consist of oculocutaneous albinism, photophobia, nystagmus, and recurrent infections. The degree of albinism and the structures involved are quite variable, as is pigmentary dilution of structures. Recurrent infections usually involve the respiratory tract and skin. Occasional other findings include neurologic problems, a variety of gastrointestinal disturbances, generalized lymphadenopathy and hepatosplenomegaly. The disease has sometimes been associated with the malignant lymphomas.

Oral Manifestations. Ulcerations of the oral mucosa, severe gingivitis, and glossitis are the commonly described oral lesions, as in the case-report of Gillig and Caldwell. Hamilton and Giansanti have pointed out that periodontal breakdown, probably related to defective leukocyte function, may also be a common oral feature.

Laboratory Findings. Hematologic studies show that the patients classically exhibit giant abnormal granules in the peripheral circulating leukocytes, in their marrow precursors, and in many other cells of the body as well. These granules are the hallmark of the syndrome and

are invariably present. They are thought to represent abnormal lysosomes and bear resemblance to toxic granulations and Döhle bodies. Pancytopenia is sometimes present.

Treatment. There is no specific treatment for the disease.

LEUKOCYTOSIS

Leukocytosis is defined as an abnormal increase in the number of circulating white blood cells. This condition is usually considered to be a manifestation of the reaction of the body to a pathologic situation. Any increase in the number of circulating white blood cells, particularly when involving only one type of cell, should prompt suspicion of and investigation for a particular disease, especially when the laboratory findings are correlated with the clinical findings in the patient. Care must be exercised in separating an absolute from a relative leukocytosis. but this should offer little difficulty.

A tabulation of the various conditions in which a pathologic increase in the number of each form of white blood cell is found has been compiled by Wintrobe. This classification is presented in (Table 14–4). In addition, a transient peripheral plasmacytosis, a cell not normally seen in circulating blood, may be found occasionally in a variety of pathologic situations or conditions listed in Table 14–5.

Infectious Mononucleosis

(Glandular Fever)

Infectious mononucleosis is a disease now known to be caused by the Epstein-Barr (EB) virus, a herpes-like virus, which is the same virus that has been implicated as the etiologic agent in Burkitt's African jaw lymphoma, nasopharyngeal carcinoma and lymphoblastic leukemia, all occurring in humans (q.v.).

The disease occurs chiefly in children and young adults. It has been transmitted experimentally to monkeys by the administration either of emulsified material from lymph nodes or of Seitz filtrate of the blood from affected human beings. The mechanism of human transmission is not entirely known, but one important means is thought to be through "deep kissing" or intimate oral exchange of saliva. For this reason, the condition has sometimes been called the "kissing disease." It is known that oral excretion of the EB virus may continue for

Table 14–4. Causes of Neutrophilia, Eosinophilia, Basophilia, Lymphocytosis and Monocytosis

NEUTROPHILIA

1. Acute infections, including localized infections, especially coccal, certain bacilli, fungi, spirochetes, viruses and parasites. Certain general infections, such as rheumatic fever, diphtheria and smallpox
2. Inflammatory conditions, such as coronary thrombosis, gout, collagen vascular disease, burns and hypersensitivity reactions
3. Intoxications
   a. Metabolic: uremia, diabetic acidosis, eclampsia
   b. Poisoning by chemicals and drugs: lead, mercury, digitalis; insect venoms: black widow spider; foreign proteins, after a preliminary leukopenia
4. Acute hemorrhage
5. Acute hemolysis
6. Malignant neoplasms when growing rapidly, especially in gastrointestinal tract, liver or bone marrow
7. Physiologic in the newborn, during labor, after strenuous exercise, after repeated vomiting, convulsions, paroxysmal tachycardia, after epinephrine injection
8. Myelocytic leukemia, polycythemia, myelofibrosis and myeloid metaplasia
9. Miscellaneous: chronic idiopathic neutropenia, hereditary neutrophilia, adrenocorticosteroids

EOSINOPHILIA

1. Allergic disorders: bronchial asthma, urticaria, angioneurotic edema, hay fever, some drug sensitivity
2. Skin diseases, especially pemphigus and dermatitis herpetiformis
3. Parasitic infestations, especially parasites which invade the tissues: e.g., trichinosis, echinococcus disease; less regularly in intestinal parasitism
4. Certain infections: e.g., scarlet fever, chorea, erythema multiforme
5. Certain diseases of the hemopoietic system: chronic myelocytic leukemia, polycythemia vera, Hodgkin's disease, after splenectomy, pernicious anemia
6. Malignant disease of any type, especially with metastasis or necrosis
7. Following irradiation
8. Loeffler's syndrome and pulmonary infiltration with eosinophilia
9. Tropical eosinophilia
10. Miscellaneous: periarteritis nodosa, rheumatoid arthritis, sarcoidosis, certain poisons, etc.
11. Inherited anomaly
12. Idiopathic

BASOPHILIA

1. Blood diseases: chronic myelocytic leukemia, erythremia, chronic anemia, chlorosis and Hodgkin's disease
2. Splenectomy
3. Infections: chronic inflammation of accessory sinuses, smallpox, chickenpox
4. After injection of foreign proteins
5. Myxedema
6. Some cases of nephrosis

LYMPHOCYTOSIS

1. Certain acute infections: pertussis, infectious mononucleosis, acute infectious lymphocytosis, infectious hepatitis
2. Chronic infections, such as tuberculosis, secondary and congenital syphilis and undulant fever
3. Lymphocytic leukemia, acute and chronic, some cases of lymphosarcoma, heavy chain disease
4. Hemopoietic disorders: relative lymphocytosis, in most conditions associated with neutropenia, exanthems, after the initial stage, especially in mumps and German measles, during convalescence from an acute infection, in thyrotoxicosis

MONOCYTOSIS

1. Certain bacterial infections: tuberculosis, subacute bacterial endocarditis, syphilis, brucellosis, rarely in typhoid
2. During subsidence of acute infections and recovery phase of agranulocytosis
3. Many protozoal and some rickettsial infections: malaria, Rocky Mountain spotted fever, typhus, kala-azar, trypanosomiasis, Oriental sore
4. Lymphoma, leukemia and other hematologic disorders: Hodgkin's disease and other lymphomas, monocytic leukemia, chronic myelocytic leukemia and "myeloproliferative" disorders, multiple myeloma
5. Lipid storage diseases, such as Gaucher's disease
6. Malignant neoplasms: carcinoma of ovary, stomach and breast
7. Collagen vascular disease: lupus erythematosus and rheumatoid arthritis
8. Granulomatous diseases: sarcoidosis, ulcerative colitis and regional arteritis
9. Tetrachlorethane poisoning
10. Chronic high-dose steroid therapy

Modified from M. M. Wintrobe: Clinical Hematology. 8th ed. Philadelphia, Lea & Febiger, 1981.

Table 14–5.   Causes of Peripheral Plasmacytosis

I. Infections
   A. Viral
      1. Rubella
      2. Rubeola
      3. Varicella
      4. Infectious mono-
         nucleosis
   B. Bacterial
      1. Streptococcal
      2. Diplococcal
      3. Syphilis
      4. Tuberculosis
   C. Protozoal
      1. Malaria
      2. Trichinosis
II. Serum sickness
   A. Drugs
      1. Penicillin

      2. Sulfisoxazole
   B. Antitoxins
      1. Equine tetanus
      2. Equine diphtheria
III. Neoplasia
   A. Hematologic
      1. Plasma-cell leukemia
      2. Chronic lymphocytic leukemia
   B. Nonhematologic
      1. Breast
      2. Prostate
IV. Miscellaneous
   A. Pokeweed mitogen
   B. Transfusion
   C. Hyperimmunization
   D. Trauma

From J. L. Moake, P. R. Landry, M. E. Oren, B. L. Sayer, and L. T. Heffner: Transient peripheral plasmacytosis. Am. J. Clin. Path., 62:8, 1974.

as long as 18 months following onset of the disease, although this excretion may be either constant or intermittent. The recent findings concerning the etiology of the disease have been reviewed in detail by Rapp and Hewetson.

Clinical Features. Frequently seen in epidemic form, infectious mononucleosis is char-

acterized by fever, sore throat, headache, chills, cough, nausea or vomiting and lymphadenopathy. Splenomegaly and hepatitis also occur with considerable frequency.

The cervical lymph nodes are usually the first to exhibit enlargement, followed by the nodes of the axilla and groin (Fig. 14–11,A). Pharyn-

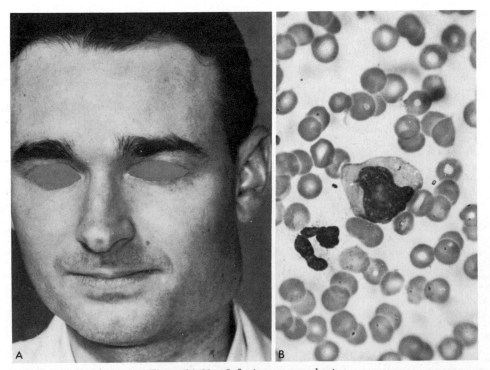

Figure 14–11. *Infectious mononucleosis.*
Severe cervical lymphadenopathy is present (A), while the peripheral blood smear exhibits numerous atypical lymphocytes with indented nuclei such as that illustrated (B).

Table 14–6. Manifestations of Infectious Mononucleosis

PHARYNGEAL LESIONS	% OF CASES	ORAL LESIONS	% OF CASES
Sore throat	56	Acute stomatitis and gingivitis	27
Pharyngitis and tonsillitis	35	Oral membrane, focal or extensive	9
Enlarged tonsils and pharyngeal lymphoid tissue	16	Oral palatal petechiae	5
Faucial and pharyngeal membrane	31	Oral ulceration	3

° Data compiled from series of 140 cases reported by W. Fraser-Moodie: Oral lesions in infectious mononucleosis. Oral Surg., *12*:685, 1959.

gitis and tonsillitis are common, but not invariably present, and skin rash has occasionally been reported.

The majority of cases in children appear to be asymptomatic. However, the peak incidence of the disease occurs in the 15- to 20-year-old age group. There does not appear to be a sex or seasonal predilection for occurrence.

Oral Manifestations. There are apparently no specific oral manifestations of infectious mononucleosis, although secondary lesions do occur. An excellent review of the literature and study of the oral lesions occurring in 140 patients with infectious mononucleosis was reported by Fraser-Moodie and is summarized in Table 14–6. The oral manifestations consisted chiefly of acute gingivitis and stomatitis, the appearance of a white or gray membrane in various areas, palatal petechiae and occasional oral ulcers. Of his entire series of 140 patients, 32 per cent exhibited oral manifestations, and,

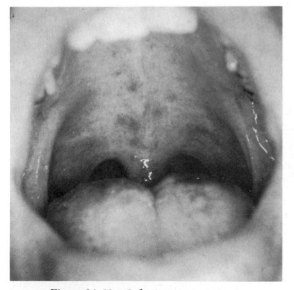

Figure 14–12. *Infectious mononucleosis.*
Palatal petechiae occurred as a prodromal manifestation of the disease.

interestingly, in 50 per cent of the patients with stomatitis the oral lesions were the first sign of the disease. Edema of the soft palate and uvula has also been reported in some cases.

Reports by Shiver and his co-workers and by Courant and Sobkov emphasized the finding of petechial hemorrhages of the soft palate near the junction with the hard palate as an early manifestation of infectious mononucleosis (Fig. 14–12). These have been described as pinpoint petechiae, numbering from a dozen to several hundred, which appeared a few days after other symptoms in 50 to 65 per cent of the patients in these series. The lesions persisted for 3 to 11 days and then gradually faded. They must be differentiated from areas of increased vascularity and pigmented areas. This occurrence of palatine petechiae as an early clinical diagnostic sign of infectious mononucleosis has also been confirmed by Schumacher and Barcay. They reported that approximately 7 per cent of a series of 452 patients with this disease had hemorrhagic manifestations, nearly half of these presenting with palatine petechiae. About one third of the patients with the hemorrhagic tendency exhibited oronasopharyngeal bleeding, including bleeding from the gingiva.

Laboratory Findings. The patient exhibits atypical lymphocytes in the circulating blood, as well as antibodies to the EB virus and an increased heterophil antibody titer (Fig. 14–11,*B*). However, the increased heterophil is present only in a small minority of children with the disease. The normal titer of agglutinins and hemolysins in human blood against sheep red blood cells does not exceed 1:8. In infectious mononucleosis, however, the titer may rise to 1:4096. This is referred to as a positive Paul-Bunnell test and is both characteristic and pathognomonic of the disease. An increase in the white blood cell count is also common, and this is almost invariably a lymphocytosis. In fact, infectious mononucleosis is defined partly on the basis that the patient has more than a 50 per cent lymphocytosis, of which 10 per cent or more are the "atypical" forms. These "atypical" forms consist of either oval, horseshoe-shaped or indented nuclei with dense, irregular nuclear chromatin and a basophilic, foamy or vacuolated cytoplasm. A thrombocytopenia is also present in some patients. It is an interesting finding that during the acute phase of infectious mononucleosis patients frequently have a normal sedimentation rate.

Treatment. There is no specific treatment for this disease. The various antibiotics have been used without great success. Bed rest and adequate diet are probably of as great a benefit as any other form of therapy. Short-term steroid therapy has occasionally been used, but the results have been somewhat inconsistent. The disease generally runs its course in two to four weeks, and there seldom are complications.

Leukemia

Leukemia is a disease characterized by the progressive overproduction of white blood cells which usually appear in the circulating blood in an immature form. This proliferation of white blood cells or their precursors occurs in such an uncoordinated and independent fashion that leukemia is generally considered a true malignant neoplasm, particularly since the disease is so often fatal. Any of the white blood cells may be involved by this disorder, and for this reason the disease is often classified according to the following types:

1. Myeloid (myelogenous, myelocytic) leukemia—involving the granulocyte series

2. Lymphoid (lymphogenous, lymphocytic, lymphatic) leukemia—involving the lymphocytic series

3. Monocytic leukemia—involving the monocyte series

This classification may be modified to indicate the course of the disease by application of the terms "acute," "subacute" and "chronic." An acute form of leukemia is one in which survival is less than six months; chronic leukemia implies a survival of over one year, and the subacute form lies between these two. In general, the course of the disease closely parallels the degree of anaplasia of the malignant cells; thus the more undifferentiated the cell, the more acute is the course. The relation of the leukemias to other malignant diseases of the lymphoid tissues is discussed under the section dealing with the malignant lymphomas.

Etiology. The etiology of leukemia is unknown. Certain aspects of the disease have suggested an infectious origin to some investigators, but a specific causative organism has never been isolated. Of these, viruses have been suspected for many years of being most closely related to this disease. It has been recognized for many years that a variety of animal leukemias were almost certainly of viral origin. It has been shown by Stewart and Eddy that the "polyoma" virus is capable of producing numerous different types of neoplasms in a variety of animals, one of these neoplasms being leukemia.

It is rather well accepted by most workers in the field of viral oncology today that avian, feline and murine leukemia are caused by leukemogenic viruses. However, the animals must be rendered immunologically vulnerable and it is possible that, in the human as well as in the experimental animal, radiation and a variety of chemicals, both of which have been closely associated with leukemia for many years, may be at least one key to this immunologic susceptibility. Not only is the incidence of leukemia among radiologists approximately ten times higher than among general practitioners of medicine, but also the data indicate a general rise in the incidence of this disease among the Japanese exposed to the atomic bomb blasts at Hiroshima and Nagasaki. In addition, chronic exposure to benzol, aniline dyes and related chemicals has been recognized for many years as being associated with the development of leukemia.

The Epstein-Barr (EB) virus, a herpes-like virus, has been implicated as being most likely a leukemogenic virus in humans because of the high antibody titer against this virus in leukemic patients, as well as the finding in leukemic cells of viruses with a morphologic similarity to the EB virus.

It is also recognized that chromosomal abnormalities commonly occur in leukemic patients, although the significance of this is not known. One such abnormality is the finding of the Philadelphia chromosome in between 85 and 95 per cent of patients with chronic myeloid leukemia. This Philadelphia chromosome, at one time thought to be a partial deletion of the long arm of chromosome 22, is now recognized as a translocation of chromosomal material from chromosome 22 to chromosome 9. In about 5 per cent of cases, the translocation occurs to other chromosomes. It is interesting to note that this chromosome disappears from the circulation during remission of the disease in many cases but will reappear when there is a relapse. In addition, a variety of other chromosomal abnormalities also have been recognized as occurring in over 50 per cent of patients with different forms of poorly differentiated leukemia.

It should be remembered that mongolism or Down syndrome is due to a defect or trisomy of chromosome 21. Interestingly, it has been found that the incidence of leukemia in mongoloids is between 3 and 15 to 20 times that of the general population. However, this type of leukemia in mongoloids is generally an acute form of leukemia in contrast to the chronic leukemia associated with the Philadelphia chromosome.

Intensive effort is now under way in attempting to prove the viral etiology of leukemia in humans. This effort has been discussed in detail by Rapp and Reed and by Gross. The importance of various cofactors or predisposing characteristics, such as genetics, age, hormones, immune competence and stress, must all be considered in determining the susceptibility to tumor development of an individual infected with an oncogenic virus. Only when this has been accomplished can there be any attempt at specific cure or even prevention of the disease.

Clinical Features. The age of the patients affected by leukemia varies remarkably, but generally may be correlated with the course of the disease. Thus acute leukemia is more common in children and young adults, while chronic leukemias are most frequently seen in adults of middle age or older. There are, however, many exceptions to this general rule. There is some difference in sex predilection, males being affected more often than females. No notable differences exist in the clinical manifestations of the morphologic forms of leukemia except that most cases of acute leukemia in adults are of the monocytic variety; thus all types of acute leukemia present a similar clinical picture and cannot be differentiated without recourse to laboratory studies. The same is true for chronic leukemia. For this reason the clinical features of leukemia can be discussed under the general categories of acute and chronic forms of the disease.

ACUTE LEUKEMIA. The development of acute leukemia is sudden, characterized by weakness, fever, headache, generalized swelling of lymph nodes, petechial or ecchymotic hemorrhages in the skin and mucous membranes and evidence of anemia. The lymphadenopathy is often the first sign of the disease, although many cases are recorded in which the oral lesions were the initial manifestation. In a survey of children with acute lymphoblastic leukemia, White has shown that in at least two-thirds of the cases, cervical lymph nodes are palpable before diagnosis and treatment of the disease have been established.

Numerous organs, such as the spleen, liver and kidney, become enlarged, owing to leukemic infiltration, especially in cases of long duration. In the fulminating variety of the disease there is not time for gross pathologic changes to develop. Hemorrhages are commonly due to the decrease in platelets incident to involvement of the bone marrow and decrease in megakaryocytes. Terminal infection is frequent and may be related to the crowding out of myeloid tissue which ordinarily produces granulocytes.

CHRONIC LEUKEMIA. In contrast to acute leukemia, chronic leukemia develops so insidiously that the disease may be present for months or even several years before the symptoms lead to discovery. It is not unusual for this form of leukemia to be found by a routine hematologic examination in which an unexplained leukocytosis is noted.

The patient may appear in excellent health or exhibit features such as an anemic pallor and emaciation suggestive of a chronic debilitating disease. Lymph node enlargement is common in chronic lymphatic leukemia, but uncommon in myeloid leukemia, as might be expected, particularly in the early stages of the disease. The protracted course of the disease allows sufficient time for full development of splenomegaly and hepatomegaly. Enlargement of the salivary glands and tonsils also may occur, owing to leukemic infiltration, and this results in xerostomia.

The skin is frequently involved in chronic leukemia and may manifest petechiae or ecchymoses. In other instances there may be leukemids: papules, pustules, bullae, areas of pigmentation, herpes zoster, itching and burning sensations or a variety of other disturbances. Finally, nodular lesions composed of leukemic cells may occur on the skin.

Destructive lesions of bone are reported in some cases of chronic leukemia, and these may result in pathologic fracture or osteomyelitis.

Laboratory Findings. Hematologic examination constitutes the basis for the final diagnosis of any type of leukemia. It is recognized, however, that "subleukemic" or "aleukemic" forms of the disease exist in which the white blood cell count of the peripheral blood is normal or even subnormal and in which there are or are not abnormal or immature leukocytes present.

ACUTE LEUKEMIA. Anemia and thrombocytopenia are both characteristic of acute leukemia. As a result, in some instances both bleeding time and coagulation time are prolonged. The tourniquet test is usually positive.

The leukocyte count may be subnormal, particularly in the early stages of the disease, but it usually rises in the terminal stages to 100,000 or more cells per cubic millimeter, and there is a corresponding increase in the proportion of the involved cell in the differential count. This increase in cells is due to a single cell type, usually very immature. In myeloid leukemia the predominant cell often resembles the myeloblast, or undifferentiated myelocyte. The cells of lymphoid leukemia may exhibit considerable variation in degree of differentiation. Monocytic leukemia also manifests poorly differentiated cells (Fig. 14–13).

In many instances it is difficult if not impossible for even an experienced hematologist to distinguish the exact type of acute leukemia. The term "stem cell leukemia" is sometimes applied to those types in which the leukemic cells are highly undifferentiated. Such cases are most difficult to diagnose.

CHRONIC LEUKEMIA. Anemia and thrombocytopenia are also common in the chronic form of leukemia. The leukocytosis may be great, and white blood cell counts of over 500,000 cells per cubic millimeter are not uncommon. On the other hand, very low white blood cell counts also occur. In all forms of the chronic dyscrasia the differential count is elevated in the cell type involved, and often over 95 per cent of the total number of cells are leukemic cells.

Oral Manifestations. Oral lesions occur in both acute and chronic forms of all types of leukemia: myeloid, lymphoid and monocytic. These manifestations are far more common, however, in the acute stage of the disease and, according to Burket, are most common in monocytic leukemia. In a series of cases he reported oral lesions in 87 per cent of patients with monocytic leukemia, in 40 per cent of patients with myeloid leukemia and in 23 per cent of those with lymphoid leukemia. Osgood found a similar high incidence of oral manifestations in monocytic leukemia, reporting that 80 per cent of affected patients exhibited gingival hyperplasia. An 80 per cent incidence of positive oral findings was reported in a series of 38 leukemic patients by Duffy and Driscoll. Interestingly, those patients not manifesting oral lesions were either very young children or edentulous persons. In a study of 292 children with leukemia of different types, Curtis found that only slightly less than 30 per cent had oral findings suggestive of leukemia. He pointed out that this infrequency of oral manifestations in childhood leukemia is due primarily to the high incidence of acute lymphocytic leukemia in this age group, since this type is least likely to produce oral lesions.

Often a patient with leukemia presents him-

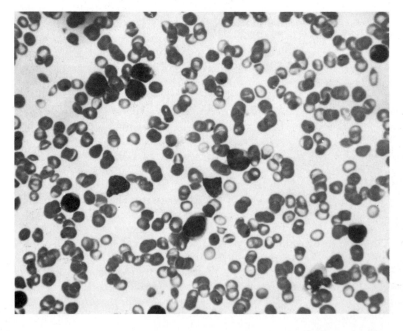

Figure 14–13. *Monocytic leukemia, acute.*

Vast numbers of atypical, pleomorphic monocytes are present in the peripheral blood smear.

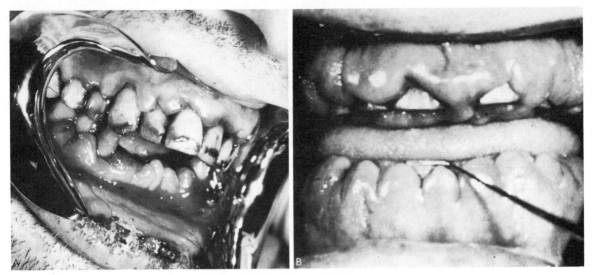

Figure 14–14. *Monocytic leukemia.*
The severe gingival hyperplasia may develop within a few weeks.

self to his dentist for treatment of oral lesions, not suspecting that they are more than local in nature. These primary clinical manifestations of the disease may consist of gingivitis, gingival hyperplasia, hemorrhage, petechiae and ulceration of the mucosa.

The gingival hyperplasia, which may be one of the most constant features of the disease except in edentulous patients, is usually generalized and varies in severity. In severe cases the teeth may be almost completely hidden (Fig. 14–14). The gingivae are boggy, edematous and deep red. They bleed easily. The gingival swelling is due to the leukemic infiltration in areas of mild chronic irritation (Fig. 14–15). Purpuric lesions of the oral mucosa analo-

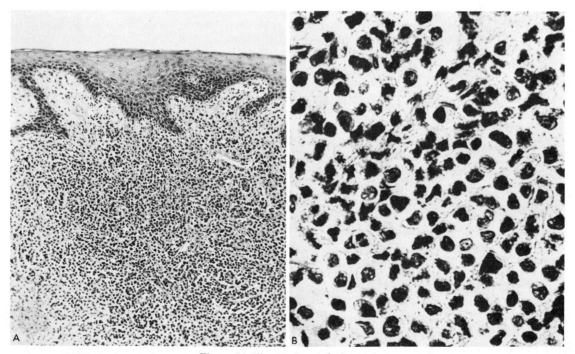

Figure 14–15. *Monocytic leukemia.*
The gingival tissue is densely infiltrated by atypical blood cells (A) with a mononuclear configuration (B).

gous to the cutaneous ecchymoses may also be seen.

The gingival hemorrhage which commmonly occurs is due to ulceration of the sulcus epithelium and necrosis of underlying tissue. Since the normal white blood cell distribution is greatly disturbed, a normal inflammatory response to even a mild infection is impossible. For this reason severe ulceration of the oral mucosa and even the development of a noma-like condition is not unusual. Thrombosis of gingival vessels appears to contribute to this phenomenon.

Rapid loosening of the teeth due to necrosis of the periodontal ligament has been reported, and destruction of alveolar bone also occurs in some cases. The use of panoramic radiographs in a study of 214 children with acute leukemia has been reported by Curtis to be useful in demonstrating previously overlooked changes in the jaws. Of this group, approximately 63 per cent exhibited osseous changes in the jaws, including alterations in developing tooth crypts, destruction of lamina dura, displacement of teeth and poor radiographic definition of bone, sometimes extending to the crest of alveolar bones, with destruction of the bone in this area.

It is imperative that the dentist maintain a high index of suspicion in cases of periodontal lesions with a somewhat unusual appearance. The complaint of a patient that he has experienced sudden gingival bleeding or gingival hyperplasia should suggest the possibility of leukemia. As Michaud and her co-workers have indicated in a study of 77 children with the disease, the oral manifestations of acute leukemia may be varied; they are not pathognomonic. Any disease that causes immunosuppression, bone marrow suppression, and disease of the blood-forming organs may have one or more of the oral findings of acute leukemia at the time of its initial diagnosis.

Treatment. Spectacular advances have been made in the treatment of the leukemias over the past few years. At one time, the prognosis for this disease was almost hopeless. Today, a wide array of chemotherapeutic drugs, radiation therapy and corticosteroids under certain circumstances offer prolonged remissions and apparent cures in at least some forms of the disease. For example, the most common form of leukemia in children, acute lymphocytic leukemia, once almost always fatal within a few months, now has a prolonged remission and a probable cure rate approaching 50 per cent. Because this area of treatment is changing so

rapidly with the introduction of new drugs and new techniques, to cite data on therapeutic responses would not be meaningful. It is sufficient to note that while leukemia is still a serious disease, the outlook for the leukemic patient today is far more promising than it was only a few decades ago and will probably continue to improve.

DISEASES INVOLVING THE BLOOD PLATELETS

The blood platelets have a variety of unique and very necessary functions which include: (1) adhesion to a variety of substances, primarily collagen fibrils in the damaged vessel wall, which initiates a secretory process in which there are extruded from the cell ("release reaction") granules including serotonin, adenosine triphosphate (ATP) and adenosine diphosphate (ADP). ADP can directly aggregate platelets, thus accounting for the primary and temporary arrest of bleeding after vascular wall disruption; and (2) participation in the blood-clotting mechanism by providing a lipid or lipoprotein surface that may catalyze one or more reactions in the conversion of prothrombin to thrombin. This thrombin, in addition to converting fibrinogen to fibrin, can also aggregate platelets. An additional function, recently discovered, is their synthesis of certain prostaglandins which act as potent inhibitors of platelet aggregation in normal blood flow.

There has been very extensive research within the past two decades to clarify our understanding of platelet function and, particularly, our understanding of the exact mechanisms involved in some of the bleeding disorders which may be encountered clinically. Thus, the finding of a prolonged bleeding time in a patient with a normal platelet count would suggest some disturbance in platelet function. This could be a result of (1) an inherent defect of the platelets, which is the usual case, or (2) a deficiency of a plasma factor necessary for some certain aspect of platelet function.

Platelet physiology and abnormalities in their function have been thoroughly reviewed by Weiss and by Zieve and Levin, and the reader is referred to these sources for a discussion of hemostasis. Only the more common and well-recognized diseases involving blood platelets can be discussed in this section, but it should be emphasized that new pathologic entities in this area are being reported frequently.

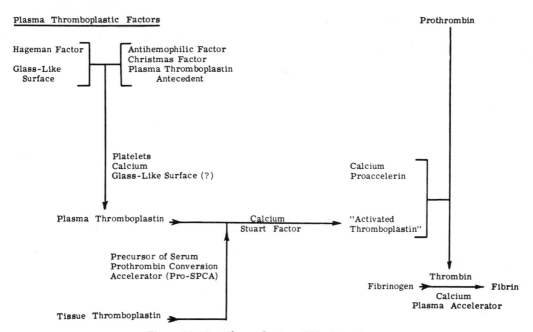

Figure 14–16. *The mechanism of blood clotting.*
(From O. D. Ratnoff: Bleeding Syndromes, A Clinical Manual. Springfield, Ill., Charles C Thomas, 1960.)

PURPURA

Purpura is defined as a purplish discoloration of the skin and mucous membranes due to the spontaneous extravasation of blood and, in itself, is a symptom rather than a disease entity. There are many causes of purpura, and the clinical manifestations of the condition are widely diversified.

Blood platelets play an obviously important role in the clotting mechanism, and if the platelets are defective or deficient, purpura may result (Fig. 14–16 and Table 14–7). On the other hand, many times purpura will occur even though there are adequate numbers of thrombocytes in the circulating blood; in such cases the purpura is due to an unexplained increase in capillary fragility. This variability in presence or absence of blood platelet deficiency in cases of purpura has formed the basis of the following classification:

1. Nonthrombocytopenic purpura
2. Thrombocytopenic purpura
   a. Primary or "essential" purpura
   b. Secondary or symptomatic purpura

Nonthrombocytopenic Purpura

Nonthrombocytopenic purpura constitutes a heterogeneous group of diseases which have in common only the fact that they may cause

Table 14–7. International Nomenclature of Blood Clotting Factors

FACTOR	PREFERRED SYNONYMS
I	Fibrinogen
II	Prothrombin
III	Tissue thromboplastin
IV	Ionized calcium
V	Accelerator globulin Proaccelerin Labile factor
(VI)	Term no longer used; Factor VI-activated Factor V
VII	Serum prothrombin conversion accelerator (SPCA) Convertin Stable factor
VIII	Antihemophilic globulin (AHG)
IX	Plasma thromboplastin component (PTC) Christmas factor
X	Stuart factor
XI	Plasma thromboplastin antecedent (PTA)
XII	Hageman factor
XIII	Fibrin stabilizing factor

purpura. As the name indicates, this type of purpura is not mediated through changes in the blood platelets, but rather through alterations in the capillaries themselves that result in many instances in increased permeability. The most common causes of nonthrombocytopenic purpura or conditions with which this form of purpura is associated are shown in Table 14–8.

The oral manifestations of this form of purpura vary considerably both in incidence of occurrence and in nature, and many of these will be discussed in other sections dealing with the specific etiologic agents. In general terms, the oral purpuric lesions resemble those to be described under Thrombocytopenic Purpura.

Table 14–8. Bleeding Disorders Due Mainly to Vascular Abnormalities (Nonthrombocytopenic Purpura)

I. Autoimmune
 1. Allergic purpuras
 2. Drug-induced vascular purpura
 3. Purpura fulminans
II. Infections
 1. Bacterial (meningococcemia and septicemia due to other organisms, typhoid fever, scarlet fever, diphtheria, tuberculosis, endocarditis, bacterial products, leptospirosis, others)
 2. Viral (smallpox, influenza, measles, others)
 3. Rickettsial (Rocky Mountain spotted fever, typhus, others)
 4. Protozoal (malaria, toxoplasmosis)
III. Structural Malformations
 1. Hereditary hemorrhagic telangiectasia
 2. Hereditary disorders of connective tissue (Ehlers-Danlos syndrome, osteogenesis imperfecta, pseudoxanthoma elasticum)
 3. Acquired disorders of connective tissues (scurvy, corticosteroid purpura, Cushing's disease, senile purpura, "cachectic" purpura)
IV. Miscellaneous
 1. Autoerythrocyte sensitization and related syndromes (DNA hypersensitivity, cutaneous hyperreactivity to hemoglobin, psychogenic purpura, vicarious bleeding)
 2. Paraproteinemias (hyperglobulinemic purpura, cryoglobulinemic purpura, Waldenström's macroglobulinemia, others)
 3. Purpura simplex and related disorders ("orthostatic" and "mechanical" purpura, factitial purpura)
 4. Purpura in association with certain skin diseases (annular telangiectatic purpura, angioma serpiginosum, Schamberg's disease, pigmented purpuric lichenoid dermatitis)
 5. Others (blood-borne tumor emboli, Kaposi's sarcoma, snake venoms, hemochromatosis, amyloidosis, other chronic diseases)

Modified from M. M. Wintrobe: Clinical Hematology. 8th ed. Philadelphia, Lea & Febiger, 1981.

Thrombocytopenic Purpura

Thrombocytopenia is a disease in which there is an abnormal reduction in the number of circulating blood platelets. When this occurs, the patient develops focal hemorrhages into various tissues and organs, including the skin and mucous membranes.

Two basic forms of thrombocytopenia are recognized: (1) primary, which is of unknown etiology; and (2) secondary, which may be due to a wide variety of situations listed in Table 14–9. One subtype, thrombotic thrombocytopenic purpura, will be discussed separately because of its unusual clinical and histologic features.

Primary thrombocytopenia (also called Werlhof's disease, purpura hemorrhagica and idiopathic purpura) is thought by some investigators to be an autoimmune disorder in which a person becomes immunized and develops antibodies against his own platelets. The discovery in the serum of thrombocytopenic patients of an antiplatelet globulin which results in a decrease in the number of circulating platelets when administered to normal patients has given credence to this theory. However, some cases appear due to the absence of a platelet-stimulating or megakaryocyte-ripening factor. The *acute* form of the primary type of disease commonly occurs in children, often following certain viral infections, while the *chronic* type occurs most frequently in adults, especially women of childbearing age.

The various manifestations of primary and secondary thrombocytopenic purpura are nearly identical and, for this reason, may be described together.

Clinical Features. Thrombocytopenic purpura is characterized by the spontaneous appearance of purpuric or hemorrhagic lesions of the skin which vary in size from tiny, red pinpoint petechiae to large purplish ecchymoses and even massive hematomas. The patient also exhibits a bruising tendency.

Epistaxis, or bleeding from the nose, is a common manifestation of the disease, as are bleeding in the urinary tract, resulting in hematuria, and bleeding in the gastrointestinal tract, producing melena or hematemesis. A possible complication is intracranial hemorrhage, which may result in hemiplegia. The spleen is usually not palpable. If it is palpable, leukemia should be suspected instead of thrombocytopenic purpura.

Table 14–9. Etiologic Classification of Secondary Thrombocytopenia

I. Conditions associated with a reduction of platelet production
   A. Hypoplasia or aplasia of megakaryocytes
      1. Ionizing radiation
      2. Drugs and chemicals (e.g., certain oncolytic compounds, organic solvents, chemo-
therapeutic agents, antibiotics, anticonvulsants, antihistamines, sedatives and tranquilizers, heavy metals, hair dyes and shoe polishes, insecticides, antithyroid drugs,
antidiabetic drugs and a variety of others)
      3. Congenital hypoplastic anemia
      4. Fanconi's familial anemia
      5. Congenital thrombocytopenia with absent radii
      6. Aplastic anemia with thymoma
      7. Agnogenic myeloid metaplasia
      8. "Idiopathic"
   B. Infiltration of marrow by abnormal cells
      1. Leukemia
      2. Metastatic tumors
      3. Multiple myeloma
      4. The histiocytoses
   C. Megaloblastic anemia
   D. Metabolic disorders
      1. Azotemia
      2. Hypothyroidism
   E. Infections (e.g., many bacterial diseases, including pneumococcal pneumonia, meningo-
coccal infection, erysipelas, scarlet fever, diphtheria, tuberculosis, bacterial endocarditis
and others; certain spirochetal infections, including syphilis; certain rickettsial infections; many viral infections, including measles, chickenpox, mumps, influenza, smallpox,
cat-scratch fever, infectious hepatitis and infectious mononucleosis; certain protozoan
and metazoan diseases)
II. Conditions associated with a reduction of platelet life-span
   A. Diseases related to immune mechanism
      1. Sensitivity to drugs (e.g., certain sedatives, antipyretics, chemotherapeutic agents,
cardiac therapeutic agents, antihistaminics, antidiabetic drugs and a variety of
others)
      2. Experimental anaphylaxis
      3. Infections (same as those listed in I, E above)
      4. Hemolytic anemias (e.g., acute idiopathic hemolytic anemia, toxemia of pregnancy,
incompatible transfusion reactions)
      5. Systemic lupus erythematosus
      6. Thrombotic thrombocytopenic purpura
      7. Idiopathic thrombocytopenic purpura
   B. Diseases resulting in platelet sequestration or utilization at an excessive rate
      1. Splenomegaly (e.g., congestive splenomegaly, Gaucher's disease, sarcoidosis, miliary
tuberculosis)
      2. Platelet sequestration (e.g., congenital hemangiomatosis, Kaposi's sarcoma, experi-
mental hypothermia)
      3. Intravascular coagulation: amniotic fluid embolism
III. Thrombocytopenia due to dilution of platelets by transfusion of platelet-poor blood
IV. Conditions in which thrombocytopenia is of idiopathic pathogenesis
   A. Infections (same as those listed in I, E above)
   B. Congenital thrombocytopenia with eczema and repeated infections
   C. Familial thrombocytopenia
   D. Onyalai
   E. Thermal burns
   F. Heat stroke
   G. Kwashiorkor
   H. Macroglobulinemia
   I. Hypofibrinogenemia with carcinoma, premature separation of placenta, etc.
   J. Paroxysmal nocturnal hemoglobinuria

Modified from O. D. Ratnoff: Bleeding Syndromes: a Clinical Manual. Springfield, Ill., Charles C
Thomas, 1960.

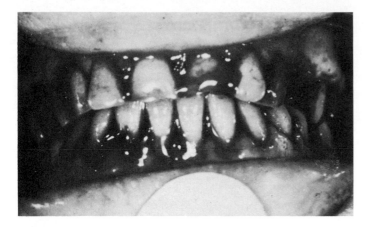

Figure 14–17. *Primary thrombocytopenic purpura.*
(Courtesy of Dr. Robert J. Gorlin.)

According to Wintrobe and his associates, over 80 per cent of cases of primary thrombocytopenic purpura occur before the age of 30 years, with the greatest incidence before 10 years. Many patients present a familial history of purpura. Secondary thrombocytopenia has no particular age predilection.

Oral Manifestations. One of the prominent manifestations of thrombocytopenic purpura is the severe and often profuse gingival hemorrhage which occurs in the majority of cases (Fig. 14–17). This hemorrhage may be spontaneous and often arises in the absence of skin lesions.

Petechiae also occur on the oral mucosa, commonly on the palate, and appear as numerous tiny, grouped clusters of reddish spots only a millimeter or less in diameter. Actual ecchymoses do occur here occasionally.

The tendency for excessive bleeding contraindicates any oral surgical procedure, particularly tooth extraction, until the deficiency has been compensated.

Laboratory Findings. The thrombocytopenia may be exceptionally severe, and the platelet count is usually below 60,000 platelets per cubic millimeter. As a consequence, the bleeding time is prolonged, often to one hour or more. The coagulation time is normal, although the clot does show failure of retraction. As might be expected from the clinical findings, the capillary fragility is increased and the tourniquet test is strongly positive. The red and white blood cell counts are normal unless secondarily disturbed by frequent episodes of hemorrhage or drug- or x-ray-induced pancytopenia.

It is important to understand the basic mechanisms underlying the determination of bleeding and clotting times. Cessation of bleeding,

as measured by the bleeding time, depends upon the physical blockade of severed capillaries by platelets; as long as the number of platelets present in the blood stream is normal and the platelets aggregate properly, there is no alteration in bleeding time. But if the number of circulating platelets is decreased, the normal platelet plugging of the capillaries occurs more slowly and the bleeding time is consequently prolonged. On the other hand, the role of the platelets in the blood clotting mechanism is through release of a thromboplastic factor from agglutinated platelets. This is present in sufficiently large quantities so that, even when there is a reduction in the number of circulating platelets, sufficient thromboplastic substance is released to maintain normal coagulation. Therefore, in thrombocytopenia, the coagulation time remains normal.

The blood platelets are probably also related to capillary fragility, although the exact mechanism is unknown. It has been suggested that all capillaries undergo "daily wear and tear" with minor injuries to their walls which are normally plugged by the platelets. If the platelets are diminished, however, there is failure of this maintenance of capillary integrity, resulting in an apparent increase in the capillary fragility.

Treatment and Prognosis. There is no specific treatment for this disease, although splenectomy probably has proved more beneficial than any other form of therapy aside from symptomatic relief such as transfusions and bed rest. Corticosteroids have been used in many cases with excellent results, although remissions may be temporary. The prognosis for patients with this disease is fairly good, since remissions are common. Unfortunately, exacerbations are also common. When death ensues, it is usually from sudden severe hemorrhage.

In secondary thrombocytopenia, correction or removal of the etiologic factor is essential.

Thrombotic Thrombocytopenic Purpura

This is an uncommon form of thrombocytopenic purpura which is of an obscure nature but may be immunologically mediated.

Clinical Features. The disease generally occurs in young adults and is more common in females than in males. It is characterized by thrombocytopenia, hemolytic anemia, fever, transitory neurologic dysfunction and renal failure.

Histologic Features. The major findings in this disease are the widespread microthrombi in the arterioles, venules, and capillaries in all tissues and organs throughout the body. These intravascular thrombi are composed of loose aggregates of platelets that become organized into amorphous plugs, which are then replaced by fibrin. All of the clinical features can be traced to the thrombosed microcirculation.

It has been reported by Goldenfarb and Finch that biopsy of gingival tissue in patients suspected of having this disease will frequently confirm the diagnosis. Although tissue from many other sites may be used, they believe that gingival tissue is preferable because of its accessibility, its highly vascular structure, and its amenability to rapid hemostasis. The characteristic microscopic gingival changes are described as occlusive subintimal deposits of PAS (periodic acid-Schiff)-positive material at arteriolocapillary junctions.

Treatment and Prognosis. At one time, this disease was almost uniformly fatal. However, many patients now survive with the help of modern therapeutic drugs and techniques, including corticosteroids, platelet aggregation inhibitors, splenectomy and exchange transfusions.

Aldrich Syndrome

(Wiskott-Aldrich Syndrome)

Aldrich syndrome is a rare, hereditary disease occurring in males and is transmitted as an X-linked recessive trait. Partial expression has been reported in females. The disease usually occurs in infancy or early childhood and is almost invariably fatal. It has been reviewed in detail by Perino and James, who have stressed the differential diagnosis of the disease.

Clinical Features. The disease is characterized by thrombocytopenic purpura, eczema, usually beginning on the face, and a markedly increased susceptibility to infection. Petechiae and a purpuric rash or ecchymoses of the skin may be early signs of the disease. The eczema has been thought to be allergic in nature. These patients commonly manifest boils, otitis media, bloody diarrhea, and respiratory infection. The increased susceptibility to infection appears related to an antibody deficiency—in particular, a poor antibody response to polysaccharide antigens despite a normal response to protein antigens. Serum IgM levels are low, but IgA and IgE levels may be normal or elevated. Thus, patients are unable to form antibody against polysaccharide-containing organisms such as pneumococci, *Hemophilus influenzae* and coliform bacilli. It is generally agreed that these patients have T- and B-cell abnormalities, although these cells may be relatively normal during early infancy.

One of the important features of the disease is the occurrence of a lymphoreticular malignant neoplasm, commonly a malignant lymphoma, which is often discovered incidentally at autopsy, although it is the specific cause of death in about 10 per cent of cases.

Oral Manifestations. Spontaneous bleeding of the gingiva is frequently seen as well as bleeding from the gastrointestinal tract and nose. Palatal petechiae may also be present.

Laboratory Findings. One of the basic defects appears to be both a qualitative and quantitative abnormality of the platelets. Because of the thrombocytopenia, generally between 18,000 and 80,000 per cubic millimeter, these patients have a prolonged bleeding time. In addition, there is considerable anisocytosis—alterations in the size and shape of platelets, with most platelets being smaller than normal. At the electron microscope level there are alterations in the cell membrane, while biochemically there is a deficiency of the adenosine diphosphate nucleotide storage pool, although platelets can aggregate. Quantitatively, there appears to be decreased production and defective maturation of platelets since normal megakaryocytes may be seen in the marrow, but little platelet formation. There also seems to be accelerated platelet clearance from peripheral blood.

Treatment and Prognosis. There is no specific treatment for the disease, and death usually occurs within the first five years of life as a result of secondary infection or hemorrhage. Some patients have been treated with antibiotics and platelet transfusions, bone marrow transplantation, and even transfer factor. The eventual prognosis, however, is poor.

THROMBOCYTASTHENIA

"Thrombocytasthenia" is the term used to designate a variety of diseases characterized by a *qualitative* defect in blood platelets. Some forms are congenital and/or familial, while others are acquired.

Familial Thrombasthenia

(Glanzmann Thrombasthenia or Disease)

Familial thrombasthenia is a hereditary, chronic hemorrhagic disease transmitted as an autosomal recessive trait. There appear to be at least several varieties or forms of Glanzmann disease, thus accounting for the heterogeneous nature of various descriptions of the condition and the bewildering array of biochemical alterations cited.

Clinical Features. Patients with this disease exhibit the usual characteristics of excessive bleeding, either spontaneous or following minor traumatic injury. Both sexes may be affected and, in females, the onset of menarche may be a critical event. Purpuric hemorrhages of skin are common, as are epistaxis and gastrointestinal bleeding. Hemarthrosis has also been reported.

Oral Manifestations. Spontaneous bleeding from the oral cavity, particularly gingival bleeding, is often seen in these patients as are palatal petechiae.

Laboratory Findings. The bleeding time is prolonged in familial thrombasthenia, while clot retraction characteristically is impaired. However, the platelet count is normal, as is the clotting time. The aggregation of platelets by epinephrine, ADP, and thrombin is defective. In addition, it is now recognized that there are reduced amounts of certain membrane glycoproteins on the surface of platelets in this disease. This membrane abnormality may be at least partly responsible for the hemostatic defect.

Treatment. There is no specific treatment. However, Perkin and his co-workers have discussed this disease and reported two cases of patients requiring oral surgery who were treated with a microfibrillar collagen preparation and with a fibrinolytic inhibitor, ϵ-aminocaproic acid, to control postoperative hemorrhage.

Thrombocytopathic Purpura

(Thrombocytopathia)

Thrombocytopathic purpura is a group of rare diseases of unknown etiology in which the patient manifests a bleeding tendency referable to qualitative defects in the blood platelets. It is not related to thrombocytopenic purpura, since the platelet count is usually normal, although the two diseases have been reported to occur simultaneously. It is clinically indistinguishable from thrombasthenia. An acquired form is also recognized associated with a variety of disease conditions such as uremia.

Clinical Features. Patients with thrombocytopathic purpura have a severe bleeding tendency and bruise easily after only minor trauma. Spontaneous ecchymoses are common, although petechial hemorrhages are rare. Epistaxis and bleeding into the gastrointestinal tract are frequent clinical findings. In some cases menstrual bleeding has been so severe as to require blood transfusions.

Oral Manifestations. The oral manifestations are those that might be expected in such a hemorrhagic disorder. Spontaneous gingival bleeding is common, while mucosal ecchymoses occasionally occur. Excessive and prolonged bleeding from dental extractions may be a serious management problem.

Laboratory Findings. The platelet count is nearly always normal, but the bleeding time is either normal or prolonged. This is generally due to defective platelet aggregation, even though there is normal release of ADP and ATP, so that normal capillary plugging is impaired. This failure of normal aggregation can often be seen in routine blood smears. Since there are a number of forms of this disease, a variety of different platelet defects seem to exist. For example, in one type called "storage pool disease," there is a deficiency in the nonmetabolic storage pool of platelet adenine nucleotides. Another form is the "Portsmouth syndrome," discussed by Roser and his associates, in which there is normal ADP-induced platelet aggregation but abnormal or absent collagen-induced aggregation. In the Bernard-

Soulier syndrome, there is normal platelet aggregation to collagen and ADP but an abnormal response to fibrinogen.

Treatment. There is no satisfactory treatment for this disease, although conventional hemostatic agents and blood transfusions aid in controlling the severe hemorrhage. Apparently, death due to prolonged bleeding is rare, but obviously could occur.

Thrombocythemia

(Thrombocytosis)

Thrombocythemia is a condition characterized by an increase in the number of circulating blood platelets. As in thrombocytopenia, two forms are recognized: primary (or "essential") and secondary. The etiology of primary thrombocythemia is unknown. Secondary thrombocythemia may occur after traumatic injury, surgical procedures or parturition. In addition, a number of cases have been reported to occur in association with polycythemia and myeloid leukemia, anemia, tuberculosis and sarcoidosis, hyperadrenalism, rheumatoid arthritis and bronchial carcinoma with osseous metastases.

Clinical Features. Patients with thrombocythemia almost invariably show a bleeding tendency in spite of the fact that their platelet count is elevated. Epistaxis and bleeding into the gastrointestinal tract as well as bleeding into the genitourinary tract and central nervous system are common. Hemorrhage into the skin is also found.

Oral Manifestations. Spontaneous gingival bleeding is one of the more commonly reported findings in cases of thrombocythemia, but petechiae are rare. Excessive and prolonged bleeding also frequently occurs after dental extractions. Pogrel has discussed this disease as a cause of oral hemorrhage.

Laboratory Findings. The platelet count in thrombocythemia is greatly increased, and it has been suggested that this high concentration interferes with the formation of thromboplastin. One case reported in the literature showed 14,000,000 platelets per cubic millimeter by a method whereby the normal value was approximately 250,000. In addition, there is abnormal platelet aggregation in response to several aggregating agents. The clotting time, prothrombin time, clot retraction and tourniquet test are all normal, although the bleeding time is frequently prolonged. In primary thrombocythemia, both the red and white blood cell counts are normal. But in secondary thrombocythemia there may be alterations in the red and white cell counts, depending upon the associated condition.

Treatment. The most common treatment has been the administration of radioactive phosphorus (P^{32}) and blood transfusions in cases of severe hemorrhage. Certain cytotoxic drugs, heparin during thrombotic episodes, corticosteroids and aspirin have also been used with some degree of success.

DISEASES INVOLVING SPECIFIC BLOOD FACTORS

HEMOPHILIA

(Bleeder's Disease; Disease of the Hapsburgs; The Disease of Kings)

Hemophilia is a blood disease with a long and interesting history. It is characterized by a prolonged coagulation time and hemorrhagic tendencies. The disease is hereditary, the defect being carried by the X chromosome, and is transmitted as a sex-linked mendelian recessive trait; thus hemophilia occurs only in males, but is transmitted through an unaffected daughter to a grandson. The sons of a hemophiliac are normal and are not carriers of the trait; the heterozygous daughters carry the defect to half their sons and as a recessive trait to half their daughters. The occurrence of hemophilia is theoretically possible in a homozygous female, and occasional rare cases have been recorded.

Etiology. There are a number of different types or varieties of hemophilia, and there has been extensive investigation and clarification of this disease in recent years. In light of our present knowledge, three chief forms of hemophilia may be described: hemophilia A (classic hemophilia), B, and C. Each of these differs from the others only in the particular deficiency of the blood clotting factor involved:

Type	Clotting Factor Deficiency
Hemophilia A	Plasma thromboplastinogen (antihemophilic globulin, AHG)
Hemophilia B	Plasma thromboplastin component (PTC)
Hemophilia C	Plasma thromboplastin antecedent (PTA)

A deficiency of AHG (Factor VIII) results in the occurrence of hemophilia A, which is the most common type of hemophilia. However, recent studies now show that Factor VIII is a glycoprotein which contains three distinct components: (1) a clot-promoting factor that corrects the coagulation defect in patients with classic hemophilia, (2) a Factor VIII antigen that is present in patients with classic hemophilia but deficient in those with von Willebrand's disease (q.v.), and (3) a component called the von Willebrand factor that is synthesized by endothelial cells that will correct the platelet adherence defect in von Willebrand's disease. Therefore, in hemophilia A (classic hemophilia), there is only an absence of the clot-promoting factor. Hemophilia B, due to a PTC deficiency, is also known as Christmas disease (named after the first patient in whom it was described). Apparently two forms of hemophilia B exist: one in which there are apparently normal levels of the inactive protein, another in which there are deficient levels of the coagulant factor. A PTA deficiency is the cause of hemophilia C. Despite the fact that different blood components are involved in each of these diseases, their clinical and oral manifestations are identical. They will

therefore be described together as a single disease. In addition, some of the characteristics of the various hemophilioid disorders are shown in Table 14–10.

Clinical Features. Patients with hemophilia exhibit persistent bleeding, either spontaneous or following even slight trauma that produces the mildest of abrasions or cuts. Hemorrhage into the subcutaneous tissues, internal organs, and joints is also a common feature and may result in massive hematomas. It is of interest, though still unexplained, that there is a wide range in the degree of severity of Factor VIII deficiencies, with some patients showing only rare and mild bleeding, and others frequent and severe bleeding.

The disease is usually present from birth, but may not become clinically apparent for several years. Spontaneous cyclic remissions and exacerbations of hemophilia are common.

Oral Manifestations. Hemorrhage from many sites in the oral cavity is a common finding in hemophilia, and gingival hemorrhage may be massive and prolonged. Even the physiologic

Table 14–10.   Characteristics of the Hemophilioid Disorders

DISORDER	MODE OF INHERITANCE	PROTHROMBIN TIME (PT)	PARTIAL THROMBOPLASTIN TIME (PTT)*	BLEEDING TIME
Hemophilia A	Sex-linked recessive	Normal	Prolonged	Normal
Hemophilia B	Sex-linked recessive	Normal	Prolonged	Normal
Vascular hemophilia	Autosomal dominant	Normal	Usually moderately prolonged	Prolonged
Factor II deficiency	?	Prolonged	Prolonged	Normal
Factor V deficiency	Autosomal recessive	Prolonged	Prolonged	Normal
Factor VII deficiency	Autosomal recessive	Prolonged	Normal	Normal
Factor X deficiency	Autosomal recessive	Prolonged	Prolonged	Normal
PTA deficiency	Incomplete recessive	Normal	Slightly prolonged	Normal
Fibrinogen deficiency	Autosomal recessive	Prolonged (or incoagulable)	Prolonged (or incoagulable)	Normal†
Factor XIII deficiency	Autosomal recessive	Normal	Normal	Normal

*Either original test or activated test (kaolin, etc.) may be used.
†May occasionally be prolonged.
   Courtesy of Dr. Harold R. Roberts. Modified from H. R. Roberts and K. M. Brinkhous: Blood coagulation and hemophilioid disorders. Postgrad. Med., 43:114, 1968.

processes of tooth eruption and exfoliation may be attended with severe prolonged hemorrhage. The oral manifestations of the various forms of hemophilia have been discussed by Spiegel and by Steg and his co-workers. In addition, mandibular "pseudotumor" of hemophilia has been reported by Stoneman and Beierl, a condition in which there is subperiosteal bleeding, with reactive new bone formation causing tumor-like expansion of the bone.

The problem of dental extractions is a difficult one in hemophiliacs. Without proper premedication, even a minor surgical procedure may result in death from exsanguination. Tooth extraction by means of rubber bands has often been used successfully, the rubber band being placed around the cervix of the tooth and allowed to migrate apically, causing exfoliation of the tooth through pressure necrosis of the periodontal ligament.

Laboratory Findings. The characteristic defect of hemophilia is a prolonged coagulation time. The bleeding time is normal, as is the prothrombin time and platelet aggregation. In vitro, the deficiency of the clot-promoting factor in the plasma of hemophiliacs impairs clotting because it appears to retard development of the substance responsible for conversion of prothrombin to thrombin. Separation of the various forms of hemophilia and proper diagnosis depends upon demonstration that the plasma of a patient with a known form of hemophilia does not correct the plasma clotting defect in the patient under observation.

Treatment and Prognosis. There is no known cure for hemophilia. The affected persons should be protected from traumatic injuries.

If a surgical procedure such as tooth extraction must be carried out, the operation should be considered a major one and performed only in a hospital.

The greatest number of fatalities in hemophiliacs have resulted from surgical procedures, including tooth extraction. Preoperative transfusion of whole blood and the administration of antihemophilic factor concentrate are recommended. Nevertheless, oral surgery is a dangerous procedure and should be avoided whenever possible. Unfortunately, a small percentage of hemophiliacs have circulating anticoagulant, probably an antibody, which specifically inactivates antihemophilic factor, negating the effects of transfusion.

The prognosis is variable, and many affected persons die during childhood.

VON WILLEBRAND'S DISEASE

(Pseudohemophilia; Vascular Hemophilia; Vascular Purpura)

Von Willebrand's disease, or pseudohemophilia, is a disease characterized by the tendency to excessive bleeding in patients who have a normal platelet count, normal clotting time, normal serum fibrinogen and normal prothrombin time. Only the bleeding time is prolonged. Therefore, other diseases characterized by an abnormal bleeding time must be ruled out before the diagnosis is established. In the past many diseases were included under this term, but separation became possible as our knowledge of blood factors broadened.

It is now accepted to be a hereditary disease, inherited as an autosomal dominant trait transmitted by and manifested in both males and females but detected more often in females. It might be best considered as a group of closely related diseases, or at least a disease with a number of known variants that is caused basically by qualitative and quantitative abnormalities in Factor VIII. Whereas classic hemophilia is caused by a deficiency of only one of the three components of Factor VIII (q.v.), classic von Willebrand's disease is caused by decreases in all three functional components of Factor VIII. However, proportional variabilities occur in decreases in these three components which accounts for the recognized variants of the disease. It is an exceedingly complex inherited coagulopathy which still is under active investigation. This disease is probably much more common than has been realized.

Clinical Features. Excessive bleeding, either spontaneously or following even minor trauma, is the chief feature of the disease. The most common sites of bleeding in a series of 64 cases reported by Estren and his co-workers were the nose, skin, and gingiva. Spontaneous nosebleeds occurred in 75 per cent of the cases in this series; spontaneous cutaneous ecchymoses occurred in 70 per cent of the cases. Bleeding into the gastrointestinal tract and severe menorrhagia are also common, although hemarthrosis is rare. This bleeding tendency is often cyclic or sporadic.

Oral Manifestations. Gingival bleeding occurred in this same series in 39 per cent of the patients. In some instances this was spontaneous bleeding; in other cases bleeding occurred only after brushing of the teeth.

The disease may be discovered after dental extractions because of the prolonged and excessive bleeding. The profuse bleeding may commence at the time of the extraction and continue indefinitely, or it may begin several hours subsequent to surgery and result in an almost unmanageable flow.

Laboratory Findings. The bleeding time of patients with this disease is increased to an extremely variable degree. Bleeding times of over 300 minutes have been recorded, but more often they range between several minutes and one hour. The bleeding time also shows wide variation in the same patient at different times. The clotting time of the blood is usually normal, but may be slightly prolonged, while capillary fragility is reportedly increased with a positive tourniquet test in about 50 per cent of cases. The clot retraction is normal. Characteristically, poor platelet adherence is also demonstrable.

Treatment. Bleeding episodes are best treated by transfusions of plasma and/or antihemophilic factor and by local control of hemostasis. Unfortunately, some patients become refractory to this treatment after repeated transfusions, and occasionally patients develop antibodies against antihemophilic factor.

Death from bleeding in pseudohemophilia is reportedly rare despite what appears to be excessive loss of blood. Nevertheless the inherent dangers of tooth extraction should be recognized by the dentist so that if such a procedure is absolutely necessary, he may be on guard to institute prompt measures to control bleeding, should it occur. In general, all surgical procedures of an unessential nature should be avoided.

PARAHEMOPHILIA

Parahemophilia is a rare hemorrhagic disorder, clinically similar to hemophilia, but caused by a deficiency of an unrelated blood factor, proaccelerin (Factor V), which is one of the substances responsible for the conversion of prothrombin to thrombin.

Clinical Features. Parahemophilia is generally thought to be inherited as an autosomal recessive trait. Both sexes are affected. Patients with parahemophilia exhibit severe bleeding tendency. Spontaneous epistaxis, bleeding into the gastrointestinal tract and menorrhagia are common. Cutaneous ecchymoses and hematomas are frequently seen, although petechiae are rare. Intraocular hemorrhage and hemorrhage into the central nervous system have been reported in some patients, but hemarthrosis is seldom seen.

Oral Manifestations. Spontaneous gingival bleeding occurs in some cases of parahemophilia. Petechiae of the oral mucosa are rare. Prolonged bleeding following dental extractions is common, and this may terminate fatally.

Laboratory Findings. The blood platelet level is normal in cases of parahemophilia. Both the clotting time and prothrombin time are prolonged, but the bleeding time is normal. The basic defect in the disease is the reduction of plasma proaccelerin.

Treatment. There is no effective treatment for parahemophilia. Transfusions, as well as freshly frozen plasma, are given to replace blood lost through hemorrhage or prior to a necessary surgical procedure. The prognosis is good, although a few deaths have been reported as a result of the hemorrhage.

AFIBRINOGENEMIA AND HYPOFIBRINOGENEMIA

(Hypofibrinogenopenia)

Afibrinogenemia is an uncommon disease in which the patient has little or no fibrinogen present in either his plasma or tissues. For this reason the blood cannot clot, even after the addition of thrombin.

A fibrinogen deficiency may be either congenital or acquired. *Congenital afibrinogenemia* is a rare hereditary disease, probably an autosomal recessive trait, occurring in both sexes, but with some predilection for males. It is present from the time of birth and appears to be due to an inability of the patient to synthesize fibrinogen rather than any excessive destruction of fibrinogen.

Acquired hypofibrinogenemia generally occurs secondary to defective fibrinogen formation, to an increase in fibrinogen consumption during intravascular clotting, or to destruction or digestion of fibrinogen by fibrinolytic or proteolytic enzymes circulating in the blood stream. It may also occur in extravascular sequestration of the protein, in loss of blood through hemorrhage, in a transfusion reaction and in association with other conditions, including amyloidosis, polycythemia, certain neoplasms, and pregnancy.

There is generally not a complete absence of fibrinogen in the acquired form of the disease as there is in the congenital type, and this accounts for the difference in use of the terms "afibrinogenemia" and "hypofibrinogenemia." But since the clinical features in both forms of the disease are almost identical, they will be described together.

Clinical Features. Patients with hypofibrinogenemia or afibrinogenemia exhibit severe bleeding episodes, throughout their lives in the congenital type, and the disease is clinically indistinguishable from hemophilia. However, characteristically in the congenital type, the patients may have long periods of freedom from bleeding. Epistaxis, bleeding into the gastrointestinal tract and central nervous system, and cutaneous ecchymoses and hematomas are all common. Hemarthrosis is not as prominent as in hemophilia. In affected females, menstrual bleeding is usually normal.

Oral Manifestations. The oral manifestations of congenital afibrinogenemia have been reviewed by Kranz and Ruff, and those of the acquired type by Rose. These consist of spontaneous gingival bleeding and prolonged and excessive bleeding following dental extractions. Petechiae of the oral mucosa are rare.

Laboratory Findings. Patients with congenital afibrinogenemia have normal red blood cell, white blood cell and platelet counts, although thrombocytopenia has been occasionally reported. The bleeding time may be normal or slightly prolonged. The most dramatic feature is that the clotting time and prothrombin time are infinite, although this is not necessarily the case in hypofibrinogenemia. The peripheral blood fails to clot even after the addition of thrombin. The tourniquet test in these patients is normal. Finally, the erythrocyte sedimentation rate is zero, the cells remaining suspended even after 24 hours.

Treatment. There is no specific treatment for the disease except for transfusions, particularly of concentrated fibrinogen, during bleeding episodes. Occasional patients develop antibodies against the administered fibrinogen, thus disrupting therapy. Unfortunately, the prognosis is poor, and many patients die of hemorrhage during infancy or early childhood. Some patients do reach adult life. The acquired form of the disease is less serious if recognized in time.

DYSFIBRINOGENEMIA

This is a congenital disease probably transmitted as an autosomal dominant characteristic which appears to represent a group of familial disorders rather than a single entity. For example, there may be impairment of the rate at which thrombin cleaves fibrinopeptides from fibrinogen. There may be replacement of one amino acid residue by another in the NH_2 terminal part of the Aα chain of fibrinogen, as

in fibrinogen Detroit, in which arginine replaces serine. In fibrinogen Philadelphia, the abnormal protein is catabolized at an accelerated rate.

The disease manifests itself clinically by a mild to severe bleeding tendency although, interestingly, paradoxical thrombosis has also been reported.

Fibrinogen is usually present in normal amounts in this disease, but is defective in its structure and coagulability so that the aggregation of fibrin monomers is impeded. In one variant, the abnormality of fibrinogen appears to be one manifesting defective cross-linking between fibrin strands after clotting has occurred.

FIBRIN-STABILIZING FACTOR DEFICIENCY

(Factor XIII Deficiency)

There have been sporadic cases reported of patients with a deficiency of the fibrin-stabilizing factor or Factor XIII. This congenital disease appears to be transmitted as an autosomal recessive trait with a high incidence of consanguinity. This condition has been reviewed by Rydell.

Biochemically, thrombin appears to activate Factor XIII from an inactive precursor form. This activated Factor XIII then cross-links fibrin or stabilizes it by transamidation. In the absence of this factor, there is failure of permanent peptide bonds between fibrin molecules so that the fibrinogen monomer aggregates (fibrins) break up under certain conditions.

Patients with this deficiency have severe postsurgical bleeding episodes which are typically delayed for 24 to 36 hours, hemarthrosis and defective wound healing. Bleeding and clotting times are both normal.

Treatment of the disease, prior to surgery, is the administration of Factor XIII in even small amounts.

MACROGLOBULINEMIA

(Macroglobulinemia of Waldenström)

Macroglobulinemia is not specifically a blood "factor" disease, but is included here because of the hemorrhagic tendency of the disease, thus mimicking the other hemorrhagic diatheses previously described. The condition was first described as an entity by Waldenström in 1948, and, by 1958, he found over 100 cases in the literature in his classic review of the disease. Since then many more cases have been discovered, and this disease should not be considered rare.

Etiology. The etiology of macroglobulinemia is unknown. It has been suggested to be related to (1) a variant of multiple myeloma, (2) the Bing-Neel syndrome (hyperglobulinemia with central nervous system involvement on a toxi-infectious basis), (3) a variety of plasmacytoma, or (4) an altered immunologic reaction.

It is now generally classified as a plasma cell dyscrasia so that the excessive proliferation of B-lymphocytes, the precursor of the plasma cell, results in the production of large amounts of electrophoretically homogeneous M-type IgM globulins which characterize the disease.

Clinical Features. Macroglobulinemia occurs most frequently in persons over the age of 50 years, seldom under 40 years. Males and females are about equally affected.

The chief clinical signs are pallor, weakness and weight loss, lymphadenopathy and hepatomegaly occurring commonly. Hemorrhages from the nasal and oral cavity are characteristic of the disease, and subarachnoid and ocular hemorrhages are also frequently seen, according to Voight and Frick. Bone lesions such as those that occur in myeloma are exceedingly rare.

Oral Manifestations. Oral lesions are common in macroglobulinemia, and these have been reviewed by Gamble and Driscoll. They consist of spontaneous gingival hemorrhage, often with continued oozing of blood; bleeding oral ulcers on the tongue, palate, buccal mucosa or gingiva; and focal areas of hyperemia which appear edematous and are painful. Severe and prolonged bleeding following dental extractions is common. Salivary gland involvement with xerostomia has also been reported.

These bleeding diatheses appear to be related to protein-protein interactions, with formation of complexes between IgM globulins and coagulation factors such as fibrinogen, thrombin and Factors V and VII, as well as interference with platelet agglutination and capillary damage.

Laboratory Findings. Waldenström was the first to demonstrate by ultracentrifugation technique that the serum of patients with this disease contained a fraction in the serum proteins, presumably globulins, with molecular weights near 1,000,000 as contrasted to the highest normal globulin molecular weight of 150,000. In addition to the macroglobulinemia and hyperglobulinemia, these patients generally manifested severe anemia with hemoglobin

levels near 4 to 6 gm./dl., an extremely elevated sedimentation rate, demonstrable euglobulins and frequent gelling of the serum upon cooling to room temperature or lower. The viscosity of the blood serum was usually extremely high.

The white blood cell and platelet counts, as well as the bleeding, clotting, and prothrombin times, are usually within normal limits, although lymphocytosis, neutropenia, and thrombocytopenia are occasionally observed.

Bone marrow smears are generally confusing, since they show an increase in mononuclear cells that have been interpreted variously as plasma cells, lymphoid cells, or lymphoid reticulosis.

Bence Jones proteinuria is present in a limited number of patients with macroglobulinemia.

Treatment. There is no specific treatment for the disease other than supportive therapy with whole blood replacement. Chlorambucil in relatively high doses has produced prolonged remissions in many patients. Repeated plasmapheresis has often been used for temporary treatment.

CRYOGLOBULINEMIA

Cryoglobulinemia is a disease characterized by the presence of cryoglobulins in varying amounts in the blood. These cryoglobulins are globulins which have the ability to precipitate on exposure to cold and redissolve upon return to body temperature. This condition has been discussed in detail by Brouet and his associates.

A mild cryoglobulinemia has been found to occur in a large variety of diseases including some of the collagen diseases such as rheumatoid arthritis, periarteritis nodosa and systemic lupus erythematosus, as well as in certain of the malignant lymphomas including lymphosarcoma, Hodgkin's disease and lymphatic leukemia. It is also sometimes found in polycythemia, heart disease and cirrhosis. In multiple myeloma, it has occasionally been found in large quantities. In some cases there is no apparent associated disease and, in these instances, it has been referred to as "essential cryoglobulinemia," or mixed IgG-IgM cryoglobulinemia.

Cryoglobulinemia does not usually produce clinical manifestations. On occasion, however, spontaneous bleeding from the nose and mouth with purpuric hemorrhages into the skin and retina may be found. Decubitus ulcers and gangrene of the lower extremities are also sometimes present.

REFERENCES

Adlersberg, D.: Newer advances in sprue. Oral Surg., *1*:1109, 1948.

Ahlbom, H. E.: Simple achlorhydric anemia, Plummer-Vinson syndrome, and carcinoma of the mouth, pharynx and oesophagus in women. Br. Med. J., *2*:231, 1936.

Banks, P.: Infectious mononucleosis; a problem of differential diagnosis to the oral surgeon. Br. J. Oral Surg., *4*:227, 1967.

Barnfield, W. F.: Leukemia and dental procedures. Am. J. Orthod. Oral Surg., *31*:329, 1945.

Barton, G. M. G.: Recurrent agranulocytosis. Lancet, *1*:103, 1948.

Bauer, W. H.: The supporting tissues of the tooth in acute secondary agranulocytosis (arsphenamine neutropenia). J. Dent. Res., *25*:501, 1946.

Becker, F. T., Coventry, W. D., and Tuura, J. L.: Recurrent oral and cutaneous infections associated with cyclic neutropenia. A.M.A. Arch. Dermatol., *80*:731, 1959.

Bender, I. B.: Bone changes in leucemia. Am. J. Orthod. oral Surg., *30*:556, 1944.

Berliner, D.: Spontaneous gingival bleeding in aplastic anemia. J. Maine Med. Assoc., *41*:200, 1950.

Bethell, F. H.: Leukemia: the relative incidence of its various forms, and their response to radiation therapy. Ann. Intern. Med., *18*:757, 1943.

Birch, C. L., and Snider, F. F.: Tooth extraction in hemophilia. J. Am. Dent. Assoc., *26*:1933, 1939.

Bizzozero, O. J., Jr., Johnson, K. G., and Ciocco, A.: Radiation-related leukemia in Hiroshima and Nagasaki, 1946–1964. I. Distribution, incidence and appearance time. N. Engl. J. Med., *274*:1095, 1966.

Boddington, M. M.: Changes in buccal cells in the anaemias. J. Clin. Pathol., *12*:222, 1959.

Boen, S. T.: Changes in the nuclei of squamous epithelial cells in pernicious anaemia. Acta Med. Scand., *159*:425, 1957.

Bowie, E. J. W., Thompson, J. H., Jr., and Owen, C. A., Jr.: The blood platelet (including a discussion of the qualitative platelet diseases). Mayo Clin. Proc., *40*:625, 1965.

Boyd, W. C.: Rh blood factors; an orientation review. Arch. Pathol., *40*:114, 1945.

Boyle, P. E., and Dinnerman, M.: Natural vital staining of the teeth of infants and children. Am. J. Orthod. Oral Surg., *27*:377, 1941.

Brinkhous, K. M. (ed.), and Denicola, P. (Assoc. Ed.): Hemophilia and Other Hemorrhagic States. Chapel Hill, N.C., University of North Carolina Press, 1959.

Brouet, J. C., Clauvel, J. P., Danon, F., Klein, M., and Seligmann, M.: Biologic and clinical significance of cryoglobulins. A report of 86 cases. Am. J. Med., *57*:775, 1974.

Brunning, R. D.: Philadelphia chromosome positive leukemia. Hum. Pathol., *11*:307, 1980.

Burket, L. W.: A histopathologic explanation for the oral lesions in the acute leucemias. Am. J. Orthod. Oral Surg., *30*:516, 1944.

Caffey, J.: Cooley's anemia: a review of the roentgenographic findings in the skeleton. Am. J. Roentgenol., Radium Ther., Nucl. Med., *78*:381, 1957.

Cahn, L.: A case of Plummer-Vinson syndrome. Oral Surg., *5*:325, 1952.

Cohen, D. W., and Morris, A. L.: Periodontal manifestations of cyclic neutropenia. J. Periodontol., *32*:159, 1961.

Cook, T. J.: Blood dyscrasias as related to periodontal disease: with special reference to leukemia. J. Periodontol., *18*:159, 1947.

Cooley, T. B., and Lee, O. P.: Erythroblastic anemia. Am. J. Dis. Child., *43*:705, 1932.

Courant, P., and Sobkov, T.: Oral manifestation of infectious mononucleosis. J. Periodontol., *40*:279, 1969.

Curtis, A. B.: Childhood leukemias: initial oral manifestations. J. Am. Dent. Assoc., *83*:159, 1971.

Idem: Childhood leukemias: osseous changes in jaws on panoramic dental radiographs. J. Am. Dent. Assoc., *83*:844, 1971.

Custer, R. P. (ed.): An Atlas of the Blood and Bone Marrow. 2nd ed. Philadelphia, W. B. Saunders Company, 1974.

Daniels, J. C., Ritzmann, S. E., and Levin, W. C.: Lymphocytes: morphological, developmental, and functional characteristics in health, disease, and experimental study—an analytical review. Tex. Rep. Biol. Med., *26*:5, 1968.

Duffy, J. H., and Driscoll, E. J.: Oral manifestations of leukemia. Oral Surg., *11*:484, 1958.

Dunnet, W. N.: Infectious mononucleosis. Br. Med. J., *1*:1187, 1963.

Erlandson, M. E., and Hilgartner, M.: Hemolytic disease in the neonatal period and early infancy. J. Pediatr., *54*:566, 1959.

Estren, S., Medal, L. S., and Dameshek, W.: Pseudohemophilia. Blood, *1*:504, 1946.

Farrant, P. C.: Nuclear changes in squamous cells from buccal mucosa in pernicious anaemia. B. Med. J., *1*:1694, 1960.

Fraser-Moodie, W.: Oral lesions in infectious mononucleosis. Oral Surg., *12*:685, 1959.

Friedman, L. L., Bowie, E. J. W., Thompson, J. H., Jr., Brown, A. L., Jr., and Owen, C. A., Jr.: Familial Glanzmann's thrombasthenia. Mayo Clin. Proc., *39*:908, 1964.

Gamble, J. W., and Driscoll, E. J.: Oral manifestations of macroglobulinemia of Waldenström. Oral Surg., *13*:104, 1960.

Gillig, J. L., and Caldwell, C. H.: The Chédiak-Higashi syndrome: case report. J. Dent. Child., *37*:527, 1970.

Goldenfarb, P. B., and Finch, S. C.: Thrombotic thrombocytopenic purpura. A ten-year survey. J.A.M.A., *226*:644, 1973.

Goldman, A. M.: Leukemia—importance of recognition by the dentist. N. Y. Dent. J., *15*:329, 1949.

Goldsby, J. W., and Staats, O. J.: Characteristic cellular changes in oral epithelial cells in sickle cell diseases. Cent. Afr. J. Med., *10*:336, 1964.

Idem: Nuclear changes of intraoral exfoliated cells of six patients with sickle-cell disease. Oral Surg., *16*:1042, 1963.

Goodheart, C. R.: Herpesviruses and cancer. J.A.M.A., *211*:91, 1970.

Gorlin, R. J., and Chaudhry, A. P.: The oral manifestations of cyclic (periodic) neutropenia. Arch. Dermatol., *82*:344, 1960.

Gross, L.: Mouse leukemia: an egg-borne virus disease (with a note on mouse salivary gland carcinoma). Acta Haematol. (Basel), *13*:13, 1955.

Gross, L.: Viral etiology of cancer and leukemia: A look into the past, present, and future—G.H.A. Clowes memorial lecture. Cancer Res., *38*:485, 1978.

Halliwell, H. L., and Brigham, L.: Pseudohemophilia. Ann. Intern. Med., *29*:803, 1948.

Hamilton, R. E., Jr., and Giansanti, J. S.: The Chédiak-Higashi syndrome. Oral Surg., *37*:754, 1974.

Hanzlik, P. J.: Agranulocytosis: a critical review of causes and treatment. J. Am. Dent. Assoc., 22:487, 1935.

Hastrup, J., and Grahl-Madsen, R.: Wiskott-Aldrich's syndrome; thrombocytopenia, eczema and recurrent infection. Danish Med. Bull., 12:99, 1965.

Hayward, J. R., and Capodanno, J. A.: Trigeminal neurologic signs in leukemia. J. Oral Surg., Anesth. Hosp. Dent. Serv., 21:499, 1963.

Henle, G., Henle, W., and Diehl, V.: Relation of Burkitt's tumor-associated herpes-type virus to infectious mononucleosis. Proc. Nat. Acad. Sci. U.S.A., 59:94, 1968.

Henle, W., Henle, G., Ho, H.-C., Burtin, P., Cachin, Y., Clifford, P., de Schryver, A., de-The, G., Diehl, V., and Klein, G.: Antibodies to Epstein-Barr virus in nasopharyngeal carcinoma, other head and neck neoplasms, and control groups. J. Natl. Cancer Inst., 44:225, 1970.

Henshaw, P. S., and Hawkins, J. W.: Incidence of leukemia in physicians. J. Natl. Cancer Inst., 4:339, 1944.

Hjørting-Hansen, E., Philipsen, H. P., and Drivsholm, A.: Oral manifestations of Waldenström's macroglobulinemia. Ugeskr. Laeger, 124:133, 1962.

Kanfer, J. N., Blume, R. S., Yankee, R. A., and Wolff, S. M.: Alteration of sphingolipid metabolism in leukocytes from patients with the Chédiak-Higashi syndrome. N. Engl. J. Med., 279:410, 1968.

Kauder, E., and Mauer, A. M.: Neutropenias of childhood. J. Pediatr., 69:147, 1966.

Kirschbaum, J. D., and Preuss, F. S.: Leukemia; a clinical and pathologic study of one hundred and twenty-three fatal cases in a series of 14,400 necropsies. Arch. Intern. Med., 71:777, 1943.

Kitchin, P. C.: Oral observations in the case of periodic agranulocytosis. J. Dent. Res., 14:315, 1934.

Kolmeier, K. H., and Bayrd, E. D.: Familial leukemia: report of instance and review of the literature. Proc. Mayo Clin., 38:523, 1963.

Kracke, R. R.: Recurrent agranulocytosis. Am. J. Clin. Pathol., 1:385, 1931.

Kranz, W. C., and Ruff, J. D.: Congenital absence of fibrinogen: a rare cause of oral bleeding. Oral Surg., 12:88, 1959.

Kyle, R. A., and Linman, J. W.: Gingivitis and chronic idiopathic neutropenia: report of two cases. Mayo Clin. Proc., 45:494, 1970.

Landsteiner, K., and Wiener, A. S.: Studies on an agglutinogen (Rh) in human blood reacting with anti-rhesus sera and with human isoantibodies. J. Exp. Med., 74:309, 1941.

Lange, R. D., Moloney, W. C., and Yamawaki, T.: Leukemia in atomic bomb survivors. I. General observations. Blood, 9:574, 1954.

Lawrence, J. S.: Irradiation leukemogenesis. J.A.M.A., 190:1049, 1964.

Lewis, E. B.: Leukemia and ionizing radiation. Science, 125:965, 1957.

Lewis, H. B.: Leukemia, multiple myeloma, and aplastic anemia in American radiologists. Science, 142:1492, 1963.

Lewis, J. H.: Coagulation defects. J.A.M.A., 178:1014, 1961.

Livingston, R. J., White, N. S., Catone, G. A., and Hartsock, R. J.: Diagnosis and treatment of von Willebrand's disease. J. Oral Surg., 32:65, 1974.

Logothetis, J., Economidou, J., Constantoulakis, M., Augoustaki, O., Loweenson, R. B., and Bilek, M.: Cephalofacial deformities in thalassemia major (Cooley's anemia). Am. J. Dis. Child., 121:300, 1971.

Marsland, E. A., and Gerrard, J. W.: Intrinsic staining of teeth following icterus gravis. Br. Dent. J., 94:305, 1953.

McCarthy, F. P., and Karcher, P. H.: The oral lesions of monocytic leukemia. N. Engl. J. Med., 234:787, 1946.

Michaud, M., Baehner, R. L., Bixler, D., and Kafrawy, A. H.: Oral manifestations of acute leukemia in children. J. Am. Dent. Assoc., 95:1145, 1977.

Millard, H. D., and Gobetti, J. P.: Nonspecific stomatitis—a presenting sign in pernicious anemia. Oral Surg., 39:562, 1975.

Miller, J.: Pigmentation of teeth due to rhesus factor. Br. Dent. J., 9:121, 1951.

Minot, G. R., and Murphy, E. J.: Treatment of pernicious anemia by a special diet. J.A.M.A., 87:470, 1926.

Moake, J. L., Landry, P. R., Oren, M. E., Sayer, B. L., and Heffner, L. T.: Transient peripheral plasmacytosis. Am. J. Clin. Pathol., 62:8, 1974.

Monto, R. W., Rizek, R. A., and Fine, G.: Observations on the exfoliative cytology and histology of the oral mucous membranes in iron deficiency. Oral Surg., 14:965, 1961.

Morris, A. L., and Stahl, S. S.: Intraoral roentgenographic changes in sickle-cell anemia. Oral Surg., 7:787, 1954.

Mourshed, F., and Tuckson, C. R.: A study of the radiographic features of the jaws in sickle cell anemia. Oral Surg., 37:812, 1974.

Niederman, J. C., Miller, G., Pearson, H. A., Pagano, J. S., and Dowaliby, J. M.: Infectious mononucleosis. Epstein-Barr-virus shedding in saliva and the oropharynx. N. Engl. J. Med., 294:1355, 1976.

Novak, A. J.: The oral manifestations of erythroblastic (Cooley's) anemia. Am. J. Orthod. Oral Surg., 30:539, 1944.

Osgood, E. E.: Monocytic leukemia. Arch. Int. Med., 59:931, 1931.

Page, A. R., and Good, R. A.: Studies on cyclic neutropenia. A.M.A. J. Dis. Child., 94:623, 1957.

Perino, K. E., and James, R. B.: Wiskott-Aldrich syndrome: review of literature and report of case. J. Oral Surg., 38:297, 1980.

Perkin, R. F., White, G. C., and Webster, W. P.: Glanzmann's thrombasthenia. Oral Surg., 47:36, 1979.

Pogrel, M. A.: Thrombocythemia as a cause of oral hemorrhage. Oral Surg., 44:535, 1977.

Porter, D. D., Wimberly, I., and Benyesh-Melnick, M.: Prevalence of antibodies to EB virus and other herpes viruses. J.A.M.A., 208:1675, 1969.

Powell, J. W., Weens, H. S., and Wenger, N. K.: The skull roentgenogram in iron deficiency anemia and in secondary polycythemia. Am. J. Roentgenol., Radium Ther. Nucl. Med., 95:143, 1965.

Poyton, H. G., and Davey, K. W.: Thalassemia. Changes visible in radiographs used in dentistry. Oral Surg., 25:564, 1968.

Prowler, J. R., and Smith, E. W.: Dental bone changes occurring in sickle-cell diseases and abnormal hemoglobin traits. Radiology, 65:762, 1955.

Quick, A. J., and Adlam, R. T.: Coexistence of von Willebrand's disease and hemophilia in a family. J.A.M.A., 185:635, 1963.

Ragab, A. H., and Vietti, T. J.: Infectious mononucleosis, lymphoblastic leukemia and the E. B. virus. Cancer, 24:261, 1969.

Rapaport, S. I.: Infectious mononucleosis. Ann. West. Med. Surg., 2:543, 1948.

Rapp, C. E., Jr., and Hewetson, J. F.: Infectious mononucleosis and the Epstein-Barr virus. Am. J. Dis. Child., 132:78, 1978.

Rapp, F., and Reed, C. L.: The viral etiology of cancer. A realistic approach. Cancer, 40:419, 1977.

Ratnoff, O. D.: Bleeding Syndromes: A Clinical Manual. Springfield, Ill., Charles C Thomas, 1960.

Ratnoff, O. D. (ed.): Treatment of Hemorrhagic Disorders. New York, Harper & Row, 1968.

Resch, C. A.: Oral manifestations of leucemia. Am. J. Orthod. Oral Surg., 26:901, 1940.

Rettberg, W. A. H.: Symptoms and signs referable to the oral cavity in blood dyscrasias. Oral Surg., 6:614, 1953.

Robbins, S. L., and Cotran, R. S.: Pathologic Basis of Disease. 2nd ed. Philadelphia, W. B. Saunders Company, 1979.

Robinson, I. B., and Sarnat, B. G.: Roentgen studies of the maxillae and mandible in sickle-cell anemia. Radiology, 58:517, 1952.

Rose, S. A.: Hypofibrinogenopenia. Oral Surg., 11:966, 1958.

Roser, S. M., Gracia, R., and Guralnick, W. C.: Portsmouth syndrome: review of the literature and clinicopathological correlation. J. Oral Surg., 33:668, 1975.

Rydell, R. O.: Blood factor XIII deficiency: review of literature and report of case. J. Oral Surg., 29:628, 1971.

Sandberg, A. A.: Chromosomes and leukemia. C. A., 15:2, 1965.

Schaar, F. E.: Familial idiopathic thrombocytopenic purpura. J. Pediatr., 62:546, 1963.

Schumacher, H. R., and Barcay, S. J.: Hemorrhagic phenomena in infectious mononucleosis. Am. J. Med. Sci., 234:175, 1962.

Segal, N. A.: Idiopathic thrombocytopenic purpura. Oral Surg., 6:631, 1953.

Shiver, C. B., Jr., Berg, P., and Frenkel, E. P.: Palatine petechiae, an early sign in infectious mononucleosis. J.A.M.A., 161:592, 1956.

Smith, H. W.: Oral manifestations and systemic blood diseases. W. V. Med. J., 43:236, 1947.

Sodeman, W. A., Jr., and Sodeman, T. M. (eds.): Sodeman's Pathologic Physiology: Mechanisms of Disease. 6th ed. Philadelphia, W. B. Saunders Company, 1979.

Southam, C. M., Craver, L. F., Dargeon, H. W., and Burchenal, J. H.: A study of the natural history of acute leukemia, with special reference to the duration of the disease and the occurrence of remissions. Cancer, 4:39, 1951.

Spiegel, L. H.: Christmas disease. Oral Surg., 11:376, 1958.

Stanbury, J. B., Wyngaarden, J. B., and Fredrickson, D. S. (eds.): The Metabolic Basis of Inherited Disease. 4th ed. New York, McGraw-Hill Book Company, 1978.

Steg, R. F., Gores, R. J., Thompson, J. H., Jr., and Owens, C. A., Jr.: Bleeding due to deficiency of plasma thromboplastin antecedent (PTA) and plasma thromboplastin component (PTC). Oral Surg., 13:671, 1960.

Stephens, D. J., and Lawrence, J. S.: Cyclical agranulocytic angina. Ann. Intern. Med., 9:31, 1935.

Stoneman, D. W., and Beierl, C. D.: Pseudotumor of hemophilia in the mandible. Oral Surg., 40:811, 1975.

Stoy, P. J.: Three cases of acute monocytic leukaemia, with special reference to their oral condition. Br. Dent. J., 92:144, 1952.

Tank, G.: Two cases of green pigmentation of the deciduous teeth associated with hemolytic disease of the newborn. J. Am. Dent. Assoc., 42:302, 1951.

Thoma, K. H., Cascario, N., Jr., and Bacevicz, F. J.: Erythroblastic anemia. Am. J. Orthod. Oral Surg., 30:643, 1944.

Tyldesley, W. R.: Recurrent oral ulceration and coeliac disease. A review. Br. Dent. J., 151:81, 1981.

Van Creveld, S.: Coagulation disorders in the newborn period. J. Pediatr., 54:633, 1959.

Vinson, P. P.: Hysterical dysphagia. Minn. Med., 5:107, 1922.

Voight, A. E., and Frick, P. G.: Macroglobulinemia of Waldenström: a review of the literature and presentation of a case. Ann. Intern. Med., 44:419, 1956.

Waldenström, J.: Two interesting syndromes with hyperglobulinemia. Schweiz. Med. Wochenschr., 78:927, 1948.

Waldenström, J.: Die Makroglobulinamie; in L. Heilmeyer (ed.): Ergebnisse der inneren Medizin und Kinderheilkunde. Berlin, Springer-Verlag, 1958.

Walker, R. D., and Schenck, K. L., Jr.: Infarct of the mandible in sickle cell anemia: report of a case. J. Am. Dent. Assoc., 87:661, 1973.

Watson, A. O.: Infantile cerebral palsy. A survey of dental conditions and treatment emphasizing the effect of parental Rh incompatibility on the deciduous teeth. Dent. J. Aust., 27:6, 72, 1955.

Weiss, H. J., Chervenick, P. A., Zalusky, R., and Factor, A.: A familial defect in platelet function associated with impaired release of adenosine diphosphate. N. Engl. J. Med., 281:1264, 1969.

Weiss, H. J.: Platelet physiology and abnormalities of platelet function. N. Engl. J. Med., 239:531, 1975.

Wentz, F. M., Anday, G., and Orban, B.: Histopathologic changes in the gingiva in leukemia. J. Periodontol., 20:119, 1949.

Whipple, G. H., and Robscheit-Robbins, F. S.: Blood regeneration in severe anemia. Am. J. Physiol., 72:395, 1925.

White, G. E.: Oral manifestations of leukemia in children. Oral Surg., 29:420, 1970.

Windhorst, D. B., Zelickson, A. S., and Good, R. A.: Chediak-Higashi syndrome: hereditary gigantism of cytoplasmic organelles. Science, 151:81, 1966.

Wintrobe, M. M.: Clinical Hematology. 8th ed. Philadelphia, Lea & Febiger, 1981.

Wintrobe, M. M., Hanrahan, E. M., Jr., and Thomas, C. B.: Purpura hemorrhagica, with special reference to course and treatment. J.A.M.A., 109:1170, 1937.

Wolff, J. A., and Ignatov, V. G.: Heterogeneity of thalassemia major. Am. J. Dis. Child., 105:234, 1963.

Wyngaarden, J. B., and Smith, L. H.: Cecil Textbook of Medicine. 16th ed. Philadelphia, W. B. Saunders Company, 1982.

Zieve, P. D. and Levin, J.: Disorders of Hemostasis. Vol. X in Major Problems in Internal Medicine. Philadelphia, W. B. Saunders Company, 1976.

CHAPTER 15

Diseases of the Periodontium

Diseases of the periodontal structures have been known since antiquity. Skulls of some ancient cave dwellers show evidence of chronic periodontal disease, while an acute form now known as acute necrotizing ulcerative gingivitis, or "Vincent's infection," was reported at least as early as 400 B.C. in soldiers in the Greek army of Xenophon. Man suffers to a greater extent from periodontal disturbances than lower animals; in fact, the lack of animal susceptibility to these afflictions has hampered research in this field.

Diseases of the periodontium are common and cause loss of more teeth in the adult than does any other disease. Classification of the various periodontal diseases is difficult because in nearly every case the condition begins as a minor localized disturbance which, unless adequately treated, may gradually progress until the alveolar bone is resorbed and the tooth is exfoliated. Also, a variety of local irritating factors and underlying systemic situations may alter the progress of the disease. The various resulting pathologic conditions are generally similar regardless of the etiologic factors involved. In other words, the reaction to injury that occurs in the gingiva and supporting tissues of the teeth is usually a chronic inflammatory response. Histologic studies of the periodontium seldom indicate the type of irritant causing the disease or suggest a specific method of therapy.

Periodontal diseases are classified into two general groups on the basis of the pathologic processes present: (1) *inflammation* (gingivitis and periodontitis), and (2) *dystrophy* (gingivosis and periodontosis, now usually termed "juvenile periodontitis"). The etiology of the inflammatory periodontal diseases is varied, but is usually divided into local factors and/or systemic factors which provoke or aggravate the inflam-

matory reaction. Dystrophic or regressive changes of the periodontium are caused by degenerative, circulatory or mechanical influences, or by other abnormalities which result in pathologic changes in the periodontium. The etiology of these different types of periodontal diseases is discussed in subsequent sections dealing with the specific conditions.

THE HEALTHY PERIODONTIUM

The healthy gingiva fits snugly around the teeth, filling each interproximal space between the teeth to the contact area (Fig. 15–1, A). The gingiva ends in a thin delicate edge called the "free gingiva," which is closely adherent to the tooth. A jet of air from a syringe will blow the free gingiva away from the tooth surface, but the gingiva settles back into place quickly. The color of the normal gingiva is a pale, "cool" coral pink, and in the adult the tissue is dense, firm to the touch and insensitive to moderate pressure; it does not bleed easily, and it has a stippled "orange peel" surface. The free and attached gingivae blend smoothly with the redder, glossy, unstippled alveolar mucosa of the vestibule and floor of the mouth. In children, the gingiva is not stippled and appears redder and more delicate. Roentgenograms show that the alveolar bone has a definite cribriform plate with uniform trabeculae and extends to a definite point between the teeth (Fig. 15–1, B).

Although the interdental tissues in a healthy young adult mouth are usually roughly pyramidal in shape, completely filling the space between the teeth almost to the contact area, Cohen has demonstrated that there is a small depression or concavity in the gingival interdental tissues just below the contact area. This concavity he labeled the "col," a term used by

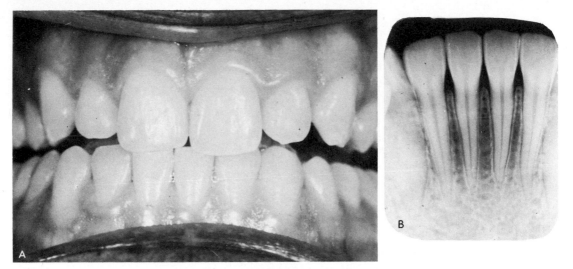

Figure 15–1. *Healthy gingivae (A) and healthy alveolar bone (B) in the young adult.*

mountaineers to describe a depression between two peaks. The "col" lies between the buccal and lingual papillae and is covered with a vestigial structure consisting of the epithelial remnants of the enamel organs of the two adjacent teeth. The buccal and lingual papillae are covered by keratinized, stratified squamous epithelium. The epithelium of the "col" is gradually replaced by stratified squamous epithelium unless interrupted by inflammation. Fish believes that a clinically healthy "col" covered with enamel epithelium is found only in adolescents or very young adults. If at this early age the "col" becomes inflamed or irritated from aggressive scaling, an infrabony pocket may develop, since the "col" is a vulnerable area of the periodontium.

After the adult tooth has passed through the pre-eruptive and prefunctional active phases of eruption and gained its normal position, it continues to maintain the vertical dimension of the jaws through the so-called functional phase, or continuous eruption. This latter process compensates for occlusal or incisal wear through a minute amount of eruption accomplished during the adult years. In cases of severe attrition, however, the small amount of continuous eruption may not maintain vertical dimension. Also during adulthood, the teeth are constantly subjected to the stresses of occlusion as well as to those of the tongue and facial musculature which may prompt that tooth movement called "mesial drift." Finally, there is a minor amount of tooth movement that results in slight shortening of the arch length due to lifetime attrition

of interproximal surfaces. Thus the tooth is not in a completely fixed state throughout life, but undergoes change in position in space because of function. Change in the position of teeth or in the forces which play on the teeth results in adaptations of the tooth attachment apparatus.

The most coronal portion of this attachment apparatus is called the "epithelial attachment" or "epithelial cuff." This is a band of modified stratified squamous epithelium, normally about 0.2 mm. in vertical dimension, wrapped around the neck of the erupted tooth in the adult (Fig. 15–2). This epithelium is continuous with the epithelium lining the gingival crevice (crevicular epithelium). The attachment epithelium, like all other surface epithelium throughout the body, is continuously replaced by multiplication of the basal cells to compensate for the desquamation of the surface cells. Whether or not this band is organically attached to the tooth is controversial, but the nature of its attachment does not seem to be as important as the fact that the epithelium is present at the site where the tooth extrudes into the oral cavity and that in health it covers the underlying living connective tissues and is in close adaptation to the tooth (Fig. 15–3). The epithelium in this area, whether attached firmly or lightly, is an external cover for the oral cavity which is resistant to the invasion of irritants and bacteria into the underlying connective tissues. It is a continuous, living, protective device around the neck of the tooth.

Immediately beneath the epithelial attachment there is usually a small number of lym-

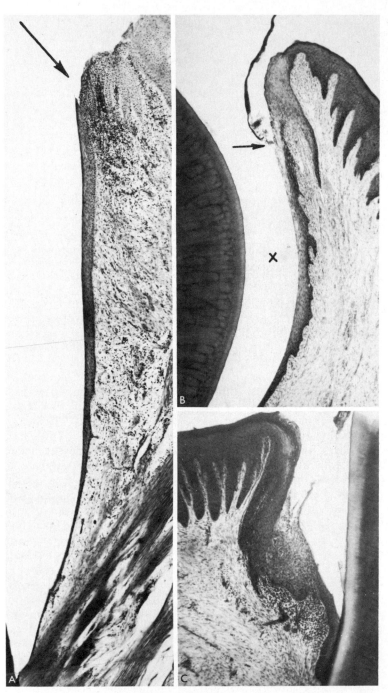

Figure 15–2. *Epithelial attachment.*

A, Epithelial attachment of erupting third molar. The attachment is long and narrow. Note also the mild inflammatory reaction at the base of the gingival crevice at the point indicated by the arrow. *B,* Epithelial attachment of lower first molar from a dog. The space *X* was filled with enamel before decalcification. The base of the gingival sulcus is indicated by the arrow. At this point the reduced enamel epithelium fuses with the crevicular epithelium. *C,* Epithelial attachment of erupted human tooth. (*A,* Photomicrograph by Dr. J. P. Weinmann; reproduced by courtesy of Dr. G. W. Burnett and the Williams & Wilkins Company. *B,* Courtesy of Dr. B. Orban and J. Periodontol.)

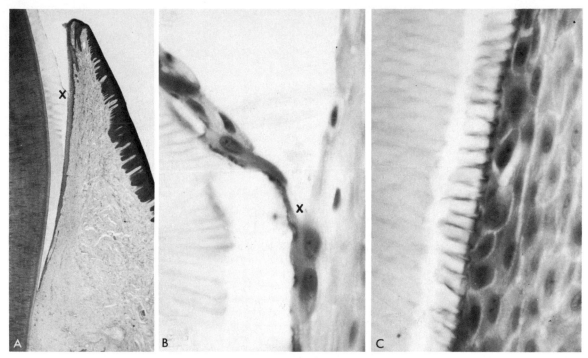

Figure 15–3. *Epithelial attachment on lower incisor of a dog.*
A, Bottom of the gingival sulcus is indicated at X. *B*, Higher magnification. The bottom of the gingival sulcus is indicated at X. *C*, The organic attachment of enamel epithelium to the enamel matrix is obvious. (Courtesy of Dr. B. Orban and J. Periodontol.)

phocytes. A few connective tissue fibers of the periodontal ligament, the free gingival group, project from the cementum of the tooth root out into the gingiva without attachment to bone. In this area there is a band of fibers situated horizontally around the necks of all the teeth.

The periodontal ligament is made up of collagen fibers, oxytalan fibers, fibroblasts, amorphous ground substance and interstitial tissue, cementoblasts, osteoblasts and osteoclasts, epithelial rests of Malassez, which are remnants of Hertwig's epithelial root sheath, thin-walled blood vessels, lymphatic vessels, and tactile sensory nerves (Figs. 15–4, 15–5).

The collagen fibers forming the periodontal ligament are attached to the cementum of the tooth and are inserted into the surrounding tissues. The fibers are arranged in poorly defined groups, usually described as follows: (1) The *gingival* group of fibers extend from cementum into the free and attached gingiva and hold the gingiva in apposition to the tooth. Careful study of marginal gingiva which is free of inflammation will reveal a small compact group of connective tissue fibers encircling the teeth. These "circular fibers" (ligamentum circulare), which help maintain the position of the free gingiva, are not found if inflammation is present and, according to Arnim and Hagerman, will be rebuilt if the inflammation subsides. (2) The *transseptal* fibers extend from the cementum of one tooth to the adjacent tooth in the interdental areas, coronal to the alveolar crest. (3) The *alveolar* group of fibers extend from the cementum toward the alveolar bone, and are usually divided into (a) *alveolar crest* fibers near the alveolar crest, (b) *horizontal* fibers in the coronal portion of the tooth, (c) *oblique* fibers which extend from the cementum coronally toward the alveolar bone and constitute the largest group, (d) *apical* fibers, consisting of fibers in the apical area, and (e) *interradicular* fibers, which extend from the interradicular cementum of multirooted teeth to the crest of the interradicular bone.

The collagen fibers hold the tooth in position, suspend it in the alveolus, and transform occlusal pressures to tensile forces on the alveolar bone. Although these fibers are not elastic fibers, they are wavy in arrangement, and under occlusal pressure they do straighten. Sicher has stated that although fiber bundles extend from cementum to bone, the individual fibers do not. The fibers from the cementum and the bone

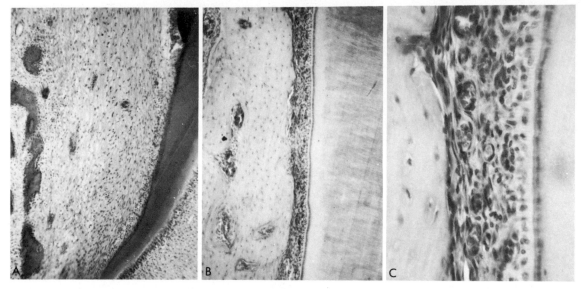

Figure 15–4. *Normal immature periodontium.*
The unoriented periodontal fibers of a developing tooth are illustrated in *A*. The periodontal ligament of an unerupted tooth is shown under low magnification in *B* and high magnification in *C*.

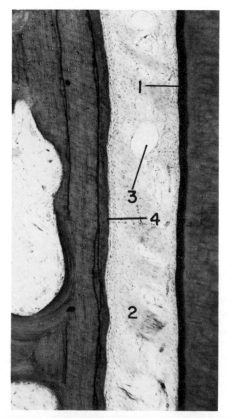

Figure 15–5. *Normal mature periodontium.*
Note the thin layer of cementum *(1)*, the periodontal fibers *(2)*, the large and empty capillaries *(3)*, and alveolar bone *(4)*.

are connected by an intermediate group of interlacing fibers in the middle of the periodontal ligament.

Oxytalan fibers are so named because they are acid-resistant, in contrast to collagen fibers. They are probably related to elastic fibers. An increase in the number of large oxytalan fibers in the transseptal region of periodontal ligaments supporting teeth which served as abutments for fixed bridges suggests that they may be related to stress. A concentration of these fibers is also frequently observed immediately inferior to the epithelial attachment, irrespective of its location on the tooth. Although oxytalan fibers may persist for a short time after the collagen fibers have been destroyed in periodontal disease, they ultimately disappear also, and there is no evidence that they deter the progress of a periodontal lesion.

The epithelial rests are found in all persons, but apparently their total number decreases with age. They vary in size from small resting types to larger proliferative masses of epithelial cells. Some are calcified and persist as cementicles. The majority of epithelial rests are located in the cervical area of the teeth at all ages except during the first and second decades, at which time the greatest number is found in the apical area. Reeve and Wentz have suggested that the greater persistence of epithelial rests in the cervical area may be correlated with and influenced by the constant inflammatory reaction present in the area of the gingival sulcus.

The width of the periodontal ligament of teeth in function (0.25 to 0.40 mm.) is much greater than the very thin periodontal ligament (0.10 to 0.15 mm.) of unerupted teeth. Similarly, alveolar bone is denser, with more trabeculae and thicker cribriform plates, while the cementum is also thicker as a result of increased function. The periodontium is a site of continuous readaptation due to its function. Periodontal ligament fibers are removed and replaced continuously throughout life, as are connective tissue fibers elsewhere in the body. The rate of this replacement process is unknown, but is probably variable and related, in part at least, to the physical forces applied to the periodontal ligament.

The cementum has no nerve supply of its own, but is rather a homogeneous matrix, comparable to bone, laid down on the tooth surface by cementoblasts which are active throughout

life. Thus cementum is continuously increasing in bulk around the tooth, unless it undergoes resorption in response to trauma, infection or altered function. Cementum often undergoes physiologic resorption and repair in microscopic areas (Fig. 15–6). At the other end of the periodontal ligament fibers, the alveolar bone also undergoes constant apposition by osteoblasts, in order that new periodontal fibers may be embedded into its substance.

The tooth is suspended in its position by the unique attachment (gomphosis) formed by strong connective tissue fibers. The functional arrangement of periodontal ligament fibers is such that physiologic force from any direction will result in tension on fiber groups and *not* in compression on bone or fiber groups. Tension on some groups and relaxation of others is the functional movement of periodontal ligament fibers. The tooth is continuously erupting to a slight degree and is always subject to movement, depending on physiologic or artificial stresses. Movement may be accomplished in the manner described above and hastened by resorption of alveolar bone. When alveolar bone is undergoing resorption, there is also an accompanying constant apposition elsewhere which maintains the tooth attachment, but allows movement at the same time.

Thus many vital, active functions of cell replacement and tissue apposition are occurring in the periodontium throughout life. Should irritants of any nature interfere with these processes, the delicate balance could be disturbed so that disease of the periodontal tissues might ensue.

DEPOSITS ON TEETH

The organic coverings of tooth enamel are divided into two types: (1) anatomic structures, and (2) acquired pellicle. The anatomic covering, formed during the developmental and eruptive stages, is known as Nasmyth's membrane or enamel cuticle, and remnants of this membrane may persist throughout the life of the tooth.

PELLICLE

The acquired pellicle is a thin deposit which may form shortly after eruption on the exposed surfaces of teeth. It is usually invisible grossly and is probably of no pathologic significance. It

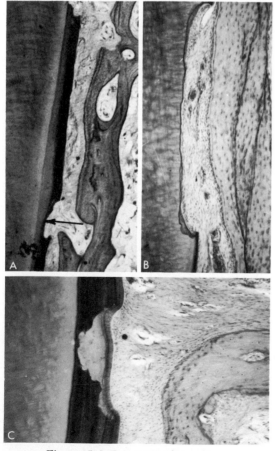

Figure 15–6. *Resorption of cementum.*
A and *B*, Focal microscopic resorption of cementum is common. *C*, Repair of an area of resorption is evident.

is re-formed within minutes after exposure of pumice-polished teeth to saliva in the mouth. It is fully formed in 30 minutes and reaches its mature thickness of 0.1 to 0.8 microns within 24 hours. It is free of bacteria and completely covers the tooth surface.

Pellicle has been thoroughly investigated by Meckle, by Leach and Saxton, and by Sönju and Rölla, utilizing electron microscopy, electron histochemistry, optical histochemistry, and chemistry. They found that the brownish-stained, smooth, structureless deposits, in contradistinction to plaque, did not stain with basic fuchsin. The brown pigment is due to the presence of tannins in the pellicle. The pellicle frequently penetrated some distance into the enamel, especially on the proximal surfaces of the teeth. The histochemistry and the electron histochemistry indicated that pellicles are of salivary origin. The histochemistry of the pellicle was found to be practically identical with that of dried salivary films on glass. In addition, similar structures formed in vitro by incubating enamel in saliva. The acquired pellicles were composed of mucoproteins or glycoproteins similar to those found in saliva and contained some lipid material. Primary amino acid groups and 1:2 glycol groups were also demonstrated by both electron histochemistry and chemical analysis. Bacterial enzymatic degradation of salivary glycoproteins apparently did not take place, either because the material was rapidly deposited before bacterial enzyme action could occur or because the stereo-chemical structure of the glycoproteins enabled them to resist enzymatic degradation. A persistent extraneous calcification was always observed in pellicle from the lingual surfaces of lower anterior teeth, but was of such small magnitude that it could not be resolved by light microscopy.

STAINS

The oral cavity is subjected to many types of exogenous and endogenous substances which can stain teeth, and since the oral flora in many cases contains chromogenic microorganisms, stained deposits are common on the teeth. Those stains which are incorporated into tooth structure (intrinsic stains, e.g., in porphyria, erythroblastosis fetalis and tetracycline therapy) are discussed elsewhere in this text.

Stain from Tobacco Smoking. On the teeth of persons who smoke there often occurs a yellowish-brown to black deposit as a result of the collection of tobacco tars and resins. (See Plate VI.) This stain will vary from a light brown, powdery deposit in the person who smokes an occasional cigarette to a dense black tarry deposit in the confirmed pipe smoker. The deposit is harmless to the teeth, although it should be removed because of its objectionable esthetic appearance and because it may be a nidus for calculus or have a mild irritant action on the gingiva. If dentin is exposed, as in older patients by attrition, the staining may be severe.

Brown Stain. A thin, brown, delicate pellicle-like structure may occur on teeth and is also thought to be composed of salivary mucin. Its occurrence on those surfaces of teeth most closely adjacent to the orifices of the salivary gland ducts tends to confirm its relation to saliva.

A delicate pigmented dental plaque, called by some the "mesenteric line," was described by Pickerill and appears to be a plaque of brown or black dots which may coalesce to form a thin, dark line on the enamel at the cervical margin of the tooth. Pickerill and Bibby and Shourie noted that the presence of this line is often associated with a relative freedom from dental caries.

Black Stain. In some patients, either children or adults, a thin, black deposit forms on the teeth, usually in a narrow line or band, just above the free gingiva. It is not associated with smoking. This black stain may be caused by chromogenic microorganisms, although none have been identified or cultured from adult stain. The black stain on primary teeth is associated with a low incidence of dental caries. Slots in 1974 demonstrated that the microflora of black stain was dominated by *Actinomyces* sp. and showed that they could produce black pigment in culture. The deposit is easily removed and often recurs slowly.

Green Stain. In some persons, most often children, there will frequently be a heavy gray-green stain especially prominent on the gingival third of the maxillary anterior teeth. This stain appears to be soft or "furry" and is difficult to remove, suggesting its association with the enamel cuticle. Sometimes a green stain of long standing covers a decalcified area of the enamel. No chromogenic microorganism has been identified which could cause green stain, although it has been assumed that such an organism is the cause. It has also been suggested that coloration of remnants of Nasmyth's membrane, possibly by blood pigment, may be responsible for the stain.

Orange Stain. Infrequently, a light, thin de-

PLATE VI

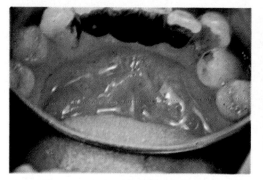

Tobacco stain

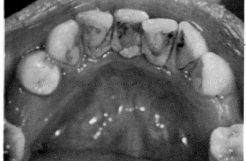

Calculus

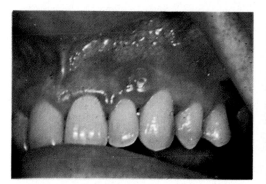

Lateral abscess

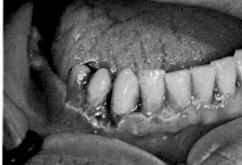

Acute necrotizing gingivitis

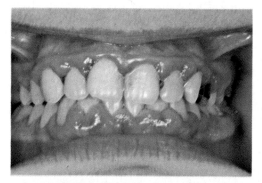

Inflammatory gingival hyperplasia

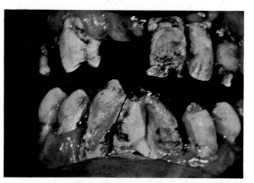

Advanced periodontitis

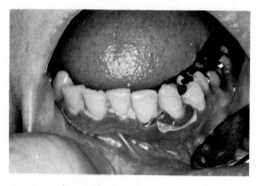

Chronic desquamative gingivitis

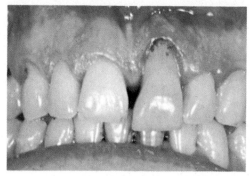

Gingival recession

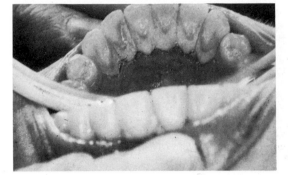

Figure 15–7. *Supragingival calculus on lingual surface of lower anterior teeth.*

posit of a material which has a brick-red to orange color is seen on teeth. The cause of this stain is not known, but it is also thought to be due to pigment-producing microorganisms. This stain is easily removed, is of no apparent significance and may or may not recur.

CALCULUS

In some children and most adults, varying amounts of a hard, stonelike concretion form on teeth or prosthetic appliances in the oral cavity (Figs. 15–7, 15–8). These deposits are called "calculus," "odontolithiasis," or "tartar." (See also Plate VI.) Calculus is attached dental plaque which has undergone mineralization.

Mandel considers calculus formation to be a triphasic process consisting of cuticle or pellicle deposition, bacterial colonization and plaque maturation, and mineralization, although all three steps may not always be essential. Frank and Brendel have indicated that bacteria can be attached directly to enamel without a cutic-

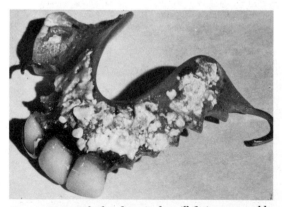

Figure 15–8. *Calculus deposited on ill-fitting removable partial denture.*

ular intermediary. Theilade and his co-workers have shown that calcareous deposits can occur in germ-free animals. Nevertheless, the usual process in man is probably a triphasic one.

Calculus is deposited as a soft, rather "greasy" material which gradually hardens by deposition of mineral salts in the organic interstices, until it may be at least as hard as cementum. It varies in color from yellow to dark brown or black, depending upon the amount of stain present on or within the deposit.

Distribution of Calculus. Calculus is classified or divided into two general types according to its location. Deposits above the gingiva on the exposed coronal surfaces of the teeth are spoken of as *supragingival calculus* (formerly called "salivary calculus"), while those covered by the free gingiva are spoken of as *subgingival calculus* (formerly called "serumal calculus"). The subgingival calculus is generally much harder, denser, less extensive, flatter, more brittle and darker in color than the supragingival calculus. Many investigators believe that both types of calculus result from a deposit of inorganic substances into bacterial plaque from saliva and that their physical differences are dependent only upon their environment. Many deposits include both types of calculus, one shading into the other, so that any actual division is indistinguishable. Other workers believe that saliva does not penetrate the gingival crevice and that the source of the inorganic salts in calculus is the blood or tissue fluid from the gingival tissues.

The greatest accumulations of calculus, both supragingival and subgingival, occur on those surfaces of the teeth that are closest to the orifices of the major salivary gland ducts. Thus the lingual surfaces of the mandibular anterior teeth opposite the submaxillary and sublingual gland openings and the buccal surfaces of the maxillary molars opposite the parotid duct opening are the common sites of deposition of calculus (Fig. 15–9). It may be localized in its distribution or generalized over many tooth surfaces.

Incidence of Calculus Deposition. Careful clinical observations have indicated that calculus is deposited at irregular intervals throughout life. Patients will sometimes demonstrate a rapid deposition for a short time and then no deposition of calculus for days or weeks.

Although there have been few epidemiologic studies on the incidence of calculus, several indices to evaluate the quantity of calculus have been developed. The Simplified Calculus Index

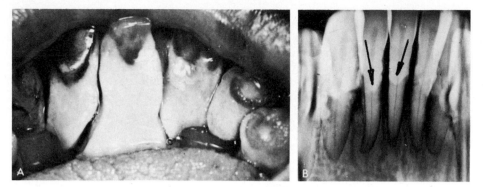

Figure 15–9. *Calculus.*

A, Massive amount of calculus in a patient who had not had a prophylaxis for many years. *B,* Roentgenographic appearance of teeth with a heavy calculus deposit.

of Greene and Vermillion and the Probe Method of Calculus Assessment of Volpe and co-workers were developed to measure the quantity of calculus formed in long-term longitudinal studies, whereas the Calculus Surface Index of Ennever and his co-workers was developed for short-term clinical trials of calculus inhibitory agents. In fact, the World Health Organization in 1978 proposed that since plaque and gingivitis were so closely correlated, it was unnecessary to assess plaque (and presumably calculus) in population studies and field trials.

Marshall-Day did report, however, that in a study of persons 13 to 60 years old, the 19- to 22-year age group showed an increase in calculus deposition over the younger age group and that there was a further sharp increase in the 31- to 34-year age group. The incidence of calculus reached a peak of 91 per cent of persons studied in the 56- to 59-year age group. Of the entire group, 71 per cent of men and 62 per cent of women manifested calculus formation. Twenty-six per cent exhibited supragingival calculus only, with no significant difference between men and women. Persons with subgingival calculus alone were comparatively rare, the incidence being 7 per cent for men and 8 per cent for women. After 30 years of age, by far the greater proportion of subjects studied exhibited both types of calculus.

Composition of Calculus. Calculus is composed of approximately 75 per cent calcium phosphate, 15 to 25 per cent water and organic material and the rest calcium carbonate and magnesium phosphate with traces of potassium, sodium, iron and other elements. When deposits of calculus are ashed and analyzed, their basic structure and composition are about the same, regardless of their location. As might be

expected, though, chemical analyses of calculus vary rather widely, depending upon the age of the calculus studied, the amount of food debris and bacterial elements present, and so forth. Calculus consists primarily of calcium phosphate arranged in a hydroxyapatite crystal lattice structure similar to that of bone, enamel and dentin. The similarity of chemical analyses and physical characteristics of dentin, enamel, cementum, bone and calculus indicates that removal of calculus from enamel, cementum or dentin must be done with care, or the dental tissues, especially the cementum, will be injured.

The organic stroma of the calculus in which the mineral salts are deposited consists of a tangled meshwork of microorganisms, especially gram-positive filamentous types, desquamated epithelial cells and other debris and white blood cells. Gram-negative filaments and cocci are also present in varying numbers. Mucin has been identified in calculus, as might be expected from its universal presence in saliva. Mandel and Levy have demonstrated a carbohydrate fraction, probably in combination with a protein, and lipid in calculus.

Attachment of Calculus. The manner of attachment of calculus to the tooth surface is an interesting problem, since it is well known that calculus may be scaled from the teeth very easily in some persons, but only with the greatest difficulty in others. This suggests that calculus may have more than one mode of attachment. Acquired pellicle formation has already been discussed. It is important to reiterate McDougall's findings that all plaques on enamel include an acquired cuticle or pellicle. Zander also investigated calculus attachment and observed four types of attachment of the organic calculus matrix to the tooth surface: (1) attachment to the secondary dental cuticle, (2) attachment to microscopic irregularities in the surface of the cementum corresponding to the previous location of Sharpey's fibers, (3) attachment by penetration of microorganisms of the calculus matrix into the cementum, and (4) attachment into areas of cementum resorption. He also found that one piece of calculus seldom attached by a single mode, but rather by some combination of modes.

Bacterial Colonization and Plaque Maturation. Many theories have been formulated to explain calculus deposition, but none of them is completely acceptable. No one yet knows exactly why calculus forms in some persons and not in others, or in the same person at some times but not at others.

Although the plaque associated with calculus and periodontal disease has not been as extensively studied as has carious plaque, there have been some important advances in our knowledge of the calculogenic plaque. Much of the work in this area has been stimulated by Mandel and his colleagues following the report of their mylar strip technique. The work of Mandel, of Howell, Rizzo and Paul, of Löe, Theilade, and Jensen, of Ritz and others all indicates that the early plaque is composed of a preponderance of coccal microbial forms. As the plaque ages, fusobacteria and filamentous organisms increase in number and, by the second or third week of plaque formation, about half of the organisms in the plaque are filamentous. Gram-positive cocci and rods make up the remainder of the plaque population. The population dynamics of plaque development indicates a progressive decline in aerobic organisms with a concomitant increase in anaerobic organisms.

There is increasing evidence that the various diseases included under the term "chronic periodontal disease" are in fact different diseases and may be associated with distinct microbial organisms. Reports from the laboratories of Socransky and his co-workers, of Slots and of Kornman and Loesche and others indicate that there is a certain specificity to the combination of bacteria in this subgingival plaque of such periodontal diseases as chronic gingivitis, acute necrotizing gingivitis, and juvenile periodontitis. The evidence for microbial specificity of individual periodontal diseases was well presented in a review by Löe in 1981.

There are several reports of microbial differences between clinical forms of periodontal disease. Studies by Tanner and co-workers showed that the predominant cultivable organisms from periodontitis lesions varied among patients. They pointed out that differences among the predominant cultivable microorganisms of individual forms of periodontitis were as large as differences between adult and juvenile periodontitis. Their studies were early attempts to distinguish "pathogens" associated with different clinical features of destructive periodontal disease. Studies of the plaque in various forms of periodontal disease indicate that there are indeed differences not only in clinical and microbial features but also in host responses to microbial complexes. For example, it is possible that *Peptococcus asaccharolyticus* and *Actinobacillus actinomycetem-comitans* play significant etiologic roles in distinctly different destructive forms of periodontal disease.

Plaque Mineralization. The investigations of Mandel and Levy, as well as Wasserman and his associates, on early, developing calculus utilizing histochemical as well as histologic techniques have added to our knowledge of calculus formation. They studied calculus formation by placing contoured strips around lower anterior teeth in patients known to form calculus rapidly. It was noted that the calcifying areas were frequently laminated by alternating dark- and light-staining bands, producing a concentric ringlike appearance similar to that of pulp stones and urinary calculi. This lamination had been noted by Black in human calculus 50 years earlier.

That bacteria may not be essential for calculus formation was demonstrated by the finding that calcareous deposits developed on the teeth of germ-free animals. Such calcified deposits may be laboratory curiosities and may or may not have relevance to human calculus formation. In any event, the human bacterial plaque does mineralize, but there is no evidence that viable microorganisms are essential for the process.

The major mineral present in calculus is a carbonate apatite similar to that formed in bones and teeth. It is not known why some dental plaques mineralize and others do not. The bulk of the calculus mass consists of mineralized bacteria, and the earliest visible mineral deposition is usually associated with them. Certain microorganisms, such as *Bacterionema matruchotii* and some strains of *Streptococcus mutans*, can be isolated from plaque and will form apatite intracellularly when cultured in a medium rich in calcium phosphate. In addition, dead microbial cells induce apatite formation when suspended in metastable calcium phosphate solutions. This finding suggested to Ennever and his co-workers that some component of the cell was functioning as a catalyst for apatite nucleation. They isolated such a catalyst from microbial cells and characterized it as a proteolipid, nonpolar protein-acidic phospholipid complex. Bacterial cells will not calcify if the proteolipid has been completely removed. Dental calculus matrix also contains proteolipid, which is essential for its remineralization in vitro after it has been decalcified. It is chemically similar to microbial proteolipid. Thus it appears that proteolipid derived from plaque microbial membranes provides the catalyst for calculus formation. Isolated proteolipid and synthetically prepared analogues have been used to determine the mechanism of calcification. An essential feature of the mechanism is the initial calcium binding by acidic phospholipids of the complex. The binding is followed by dehydration, which forms a microenvironment in which apatite nuclei are stabilized long enough for crystal growth.

Other *miscellaneous theories* of calculus formation have been advanced, but are generally not accepted because of lack of evidence. For example, it has been reported that animals on experimental diets deficient in certain vitamins acquire heavy deposits of calculus. The effects of other types of diet on calculus deposition have also received much attention. Baer and his co-workers found that a diet of fine physical consistency and a high caloric content resulted in calculus deposition in animals. A carbohydrate diet containing 66 per cent cornstarch produced more calculus than a similar diet containing 66 per cent sucrose or glucose. In at least one study conducted by the same investigators, a diet containing 62 per cent protein and 13 per cent sucrose did not produce any more calculus than one containing much less protein. These findings have not been confirmed in man.

Importance of Calculus. Calculus is so uniformly associated with periodontal diseases that some investigators have considered it a result rather than a cause of gingival inflammation. This seems most unlikely, however. Calculus is a hard, rough material that is adherent to the tooth surface, and therefore it moves with the tooth during function. For this reason, injury to the adjacent or overlying gingival tissues which do not move in unison with the teeth may result. Also, when pressure is placed on the gingiva during mastication, the underlying calculus may irritate the gingival tissues. Calculus, with its overlying mat of microorganisms, thus causes an inflammatory reaction in the gingiva (Fig. 15–10). Occasionally, however, supragingival calculus may collect in prodigious amounts with little more pathosis present than a superficial inflammation; this is probably due to high tissue resistance. Removal of calculus results in such rapid clinical improvement that it is difficult to believe that the calculus and associated microorganisms are not directly responsible for gingival inflammation.

Prevention of calculus formation is dependent

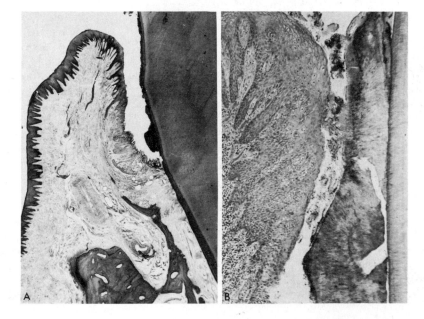

Figure 15–10. *Calculus.*
The gingival tissues opposite the rough deposits of calculus show inflammation and alterations in the epithelium. (*B*, Courtesy of Drs. J. P. Weinmann and G. W. Burnett and the Williams & Wilkins Company.)

primarily upon removal by the patient of the fresh, uncalcified deposits with toothbrush and dental floss.

CLASSIFICATION OF PERIODONTAL DISEASE

Many classifications of periodontal disease have been proposed. The report of the Committee on Classifications and Nomenclature of the American Academy of Periodontology in 1957 suggested that pathologic involvement of the periodontium may be grouped into the following four categories:

1. Inflammation (gingivitis, periodontitis)
2. Dystrophy (gingivosis, periodontosis, now termed juvenile periodontitis)
3. Neoplasia
4. Anomalies

Only the first two categories will be discussed in this chapter, since the others have been considered elsewhere.

GINGIVITIS

Gingivitis, inflammation of the gingival tissues, may occur in an acute, subacute or chronic form. The severity of the gingivitis depends upon the severity, duration and frequency of the local irritations, and the resistance of the oral tissues. Acute or even subacute gingivitis of any nature is not common and rarely occurs in persons who are in robust health. In contrast, chronic gingivitis is extremely common and, in older dentulous patients, is nearly universal in occurrence.

Etiology. The etiology of gingivitis is especially varied and has been divided into local and systemic factors. Those factors which have been most commonly cited are as follows:

LOCAL FACTORS
1. Microorganisms
2. Calculus
3. Food impaction
4. Faulty or irritating restorations or appliances
5. Mouth-breathing
6. Tooth malposition
7. Chemical or drug application, etc.

SYSTEMIC FACTORS
1. Nutritional disturbances
2. Drug action
3. Pregnancy, diabetes and other endocrine dysfunctions
4. Allergy
5. Heredity
6. Psychic phenomena
7. Specific granulomatous infections
8. Neutrophil dysfunction
9. Immunopathies

MICROORGANISMS. One must recognize the omnipresence of the many varieties of oral microorganisms growing as a film or plaque—for the most part on the nonself-cleansing areas of the teeth, particularly below the cervical convexity of the crown and in the cervical areas. Smears of the material taken from the normal gingival sulcus, from the gingival sulcus in a case of marginal periodontitis, or from the gingival pocket in advanced periodontal disease, all will reveal this myriad of microorganisms of many different types. Prominent among these will be cocci, various types of bacilli, fusiform organisms, spirochetes and, in advanced periodontitis, amoebas and trichomonads. The normal oral flora is so vast, however, and is made up of so many varieties of microorganisms that it has never been possible to prove conclusively that any one type is of greater importance than any other types of microorganisms as far as periodontal diseases are concerned. The plaque associated with gingivitis and early periodontitis is complex and heterogeneous. However, Slots and co-workers in 1978 demonstrated that in the early stages of gingivitis the *Actinomyces* group of organisms is the dominant genus in the supragingival plaque.

Plaque and plaque-derived endotoxins may act as irritants or antigens in both nonspecific acute inflammatory responses and immune mechanisms of defense. One of the prime functions of the immune response is to activate the inflammatory system. Both the nonspecific acute inflammatory reaction and the immune response are homeostatic mechanisms, each of which is usually successful in restoring and maintaining homeostasis. The growing weight of evidence suggests that the breakdown in host resistance dental plaque is a result of tissue injury brought about by the immune reaction. When both nonspecific and immunologically mediated inflammatory lesions of the gingiva occur, the lesion is no longer a self-limiting protective reaction and becomes progressively tissue destructive. There are many destructive enzymes released by polymorphonuclear leukocytes (PMNs) and numerous tissue destructive lymphokines and lymphotoxins elaborated by B- or T-lymphocytes. Thus, collagenase liberated by both PMNs and lymphocytes, other lysosomal enzyme secretions, lysosomal acid hydrolases (of macrophages), lymphotoxin-mediated cytotoxins and osteoclast-activating factor (OAF) are all tissue-destructive substances released as part of the inflammatory reaction to injury. The subject of host-parasite interactions in gingivitis and periodontitis was reviewed by MacPhee and Cowley in 1981.

Specific microorganisms sometimes cause an

inflammatory reaction of the gingiva, although the clinical appearance may be entirely nonspecific. For example, a monilial or a tuberculous infection may affect the gingiva. The herpes simplex virus and the fusospirochetal organisms of acute necrotizing gingivitis may also infect the gingiva. Furthermore, both a streptococcal and a staphylococcal gingivitis have been described as being due specifically to these organisms. Definite proof of a cause-and-effect relation here is difficult and questionable.

CALCULUS. Calculus, whether it is in a supragingival or a subgingival position, causes irritation of the contracting gingival tissue. This irritation is probably caused by the by-products of the microorganisms, although the mechanical friction resulting from the hard, rough surface of the calculus may play a role.

FOOD IMPACTION AND GENERAL ORAL NEGLECT. The impaction of food and the accumulation of debris on the teeth because of oral neglect result in gingivitis through irritation of the gingiva by toxins of microorganisms growing in this medium. The degradation products of the food debris may also prove irritating to the gingival tissues.

FAULTY OR IRRITATING RESTORATIONS OR APPLIANCES. Faulty restorations may act as irritants to gingival tissues and thereby induce gingivitis. Overhanging margins of proximal restorations may directly irritate the gingiva and in addition allow the collection of food debris and organisms which add further insult to these tissues. Improperly contoured restorations may also produce gingival irritation by causing food packing or abnormal excursions of food against the gingiva during mastication. Prosthetic or orthodontic appliances impinging on the gingival tissues produce gingivitis as a result of the pressure per se and of the trapping of food and microorganisms.

MOUTH-BREATHING. Drying of the oral mucous membrane because of breathing with the mouth open, because of an environment of excessive heat, or from excessive smoking, will result in gingival irritation, with accompanying inflammation or sometimes hyperplasia. Klingsburg and his co-workers reported that "exteriorizing" rodent oral mucous membranes, by removing part of the rat's lower lip, resulted in an increase in keratinization of the mucous membranes.

TOOTH MALPOSITION. Teeth which have erupted or which have been moved out of physiologic occlusion, where they are repeatedly subjected to abnormal forces during mastication, are apparently very susceptible to the development of periodontal disease. For example, a lower incisor may be "bucked" out of alignment in the second or third decade of life and suddenly, in its new position, receive much of the occlusal stress of one or two upper anterior teeth. Calculus may be deposited on the lingual surface of such a tooth; bacteria are at hand to attack the tissue around this tooth, and as a result of this combination of influences the gingival tissues may become inflamed and may recede. Teeth in labial positions have less osseous coverage over their radicular surface and hence are more susceptible to trauma from tooth brushing and other local irritations. Abnormally high frenal attachments also contribute to gingival recession.

CHEMICAL OR DRUG APPLICATION. Many drugs are at least potentially capable of inducing gingivitis, particularly an acute gingivitis, owing to a direct local or systemic irritating action. For example, phenol, silver nitrate, the volatile oils, or aspirin, if applied to the gingiva, will provoke an inflammatory reaction. Others, such as Dilantin sodium, produce gingival changes when administered systemically. These have been discussed specifically in the chapter on injuries caused by chemical agents.

An unusual type of gingivostomatitis first appeared in the United States about 1968. It had not been previously encountered, at least in the numbers found during the ensuing three- or four-year period. The clinical features of the disease were so characteristic that it could be readily recognized as a specific entity, probably with a common etiology. This disease was most prevalent in young females and often extended over a period of many months. There was intense hyperemia, edema and inflammation of the free and attached gingiva which, in severe cases, extended to involve the buccal and vestibular mucosa. Ordinarily, however, gingival involvement was restricted to the free and attached gingiva (alveolar mucosa) with a sharp line of demarcation from the normal-appearing vestibular mucosa. Filiform depapillation of the tongue occurred, as did atrophic, dry, scaly cheilitis with fissuring and maceration of the commissures. The tissues frequently burned and were quite sensitive to dentifrices and highly seasoned foods. Histologically, the gingiva characteristically exhibited mild epithelial hyperplasia with focal areas of liquefaction, forming microvesicles. A marked leukocytic infiltrate was invariably present throughout the entire thickness of epithelium. In the connective tissue, there was marked vascular dilatation with severe thinning of epithelium over the connective tissue pegs. Uniformly present was an intense plasma cell infiltrate, thus giving rise to the term *plasma cell gingivitis.* Although a number of etiologic factors such as hypersensitivity, allergy, endocrine disease, specific infection, etc. were proposed, it remained for Kerr and his associates in 1971 to identify the most probable causative agent. They found that the disease represented an allergic reaction to some component of chewing gum. If the patients eliminated the use of chewing gum, the tissues returned to normal. During the period of 1968 to 1972, some chewing gum manufacturers presumably used a new ingredient in their product but then discontinued its use and returned to their original formula. Since this period, the disease seems to have disappeared in the United States.

NUTRITIONAL DISTURBANCES. Nutritional imbalance is frequently manifested in changes in the gingiva and deeper underlying periodontium. The effects of nutritional deficiencies on these structures as well as on the oral cavity as a whole have been considered in detail in the chapter on oral aspects of metabolic disease and will not be reiterated here. It is sufficient to point out that adequate intake, absorption and utilization of the various vitamins, minerals and other foodstuffs are essential to the maintenance of a normal periodontium.

PREGNANCY. Many investigators have reported that the gingiva undergoes changes during pregnancy which have been termed "pregnancy gingivitis." Among studies of relatively large numbers of pregnant patients, the following may be cited as representative:

LOOBY (1946)—475 WOMEN	
Slight gingivitis	40%
"Hypertrophic" gingivitis	10
"Pregnancy tumor"	2

ZISKIN AND NESSE (1946)—416 WOMEN	
Pregnancy gingivitis	37.9%
Hypertrophic gingivitis	7.0
Raspberry-red gingiva	40.0
Combination	1.8

MAIER AND ORBAN (1949)—530 WOMEN	
No pathosis	44.6%
Mild inflammation	35.9
Moderate inflammation	17.5
Severe inflammation	1.5
"Pregnancy tumor"	0.5

The clinical appearance of the gingiva in the pregnant woman varies from no change to a smooth, shiny, deeply reddened marginal gingiva with frequent focal enlargement and intense hyperemia of the interdental papilla. Occasionally a single tumor-like mass will develop, the "pregnancy tumor," which is histologically identical with the pyogenic granuloma (q.v.). Pregnancy induces a hypersensitive response to a mild injury which otherwise would have been innocuous. This gingivitis, clinically nonspecific in appearance, may occur near the end of the first trimester and may regress or even completely disappear at the termination of the pregnancy.

DIABETES MELLITUS. Diabetes has been repeatedly reported in association with severe periodontal disease, especially in younger people. One is unable to prove that diabetes is a specific cause of severe periodontal disease, since many patients with diabetes have normal periodontal structures. However, in uncontrolled diabetes many metabolic processes are affected, including those which make up resistance to infection or trauma. For example, the uncontrolled diabetic may suffer from persistent chronic ulcers of the skin of the legs, presumably because resistance is lowered and any minor irritation such as trauma or bacterial infection of the skin will result in injury greater than that in the normal person. Also, the effectiveness of the healing process is decreased, probably as a result of a disturbance in cellular carbohydrate metabolism. Therefore, considering the periodontium, located in the oral cavity with its many factors predisposing to disease, including calculus, bacteria, and trauma, it is not surprising that this structure appears to break down more readily in persons with uncontrolled diabetes than in normal persons. Controlled experimental animal studies have been performed repeatedly in which the animals were made deficient in insulin production and yet no consistent special periodontal pathosis resulted. Perhaps the local factors were insufficient to overcome the inborn vitality of the periodontium in such cases.

It has been reported by Russell that nearly 40 per cent of a group of 37 diabetics exhibited gingival angiopathy in the form of PAS-positive, diastase-resistant thickening of vessel walls, of hyalinization of vessel walls and sometimes of luminal obliteration. Similar changes were also found in the periodontal ligament vessels of patients with diabetes mellitus.

OTHER ENDOCRINE DYSFUNCTIONS. Gingivitis is reported with some frequency to occur in association with *puberty*, the so-called puberty gingivitis. The gingiva appears hyperemic and edematous. The fact that many adolescents are chronic mouth-breathers as a result of lymphoid hyperplasia of the tonsils and adenoids has suggested to some workers that the endocrine basis is relatively unimportant, the local irritant (drying of the mucosa because of the mouth-breathing) being the actual cause of the condition.

Gingivitis associated with *menstruation* has been reported by many workers. In addition a nonspecific gingivitis with gingival bleeding—vicarious menstruation—may occur. This phenomenon is rare.

PSYCHIATRIC PHENOMENA. Psychiatric disturbances appear to have a definite influence upon the severity of periodontal disease. Belting and Gupta reported that the severity of periodontal disease was significantly greater in psychiatric patients than in a control group of patients; significant differences in severity were noted even when such variable factors as amounts of calculus, brushing frequency and bruxism were held constant in the two groups. The severity of periodontal disease increased significantly as the degree of anxiety increased. It was noted also that the severity of periodontal disease decreased significantly in both normal and psychiatric groups as the educational level of the patient increased.

Incidence. Numerous studies have been devoted to ascertaining the incidence or prevalence of gingival disease. It is a generally accepted fact that periodontal disease is worldwide in distribution and that there is no age group, except the very young infant, in which it does not occur. Although all races are affected, there is some difference in incidence between different races and different countries.

In the United States there have been only a few epidemiologic studies. Brucker, studying a group of children between the ages of 4 and 16 years, reported that the gingivae were normal in approximately 90 per cent of the individuals. Between 6 and 8 per cent of the children exhibited slight marginal gingivitis, while approximately 1.5 per cent demonstrated severe gingivitis. Massler and his associates found that only 9 per cent of a group of 5-year-old children in Chicago exhibited gingival disease, although the incidence increased sharply at age 7 years to 69 per cent, apparently in association with eruption of the permanent incisors and first molars. By the age of 11 years the incidence of gingival disease was approximately 80 per cent.

Marshall-Day and his associates studied the incidence of periodontal disease in a group of 1279 persons ranging in age from 13 to 65 years and residing in the Boston, Massachusetts, area. Their investigations revealed that the incidence of gingivitis was extremely high even in the early age groups, ranging from 80 per cent at ages 13 to 15 years to 95 per cent at age 60 years. An interestingly significant reduction in incidence of gingival disease to 62 per cent occurred in the late teens and early twenties. It was suggested that this reduction was associated with the end of puberty and/or social factors, the adolescents placing a greater emphasis on oral hygiene and esthetics than they had previously. In 10 of the 13 different age groups, males were affected more frequently than females, the overall average being 88 per cent for males and 80 per cent for females.

Other clinical studies on gingivitis have reported similar results.

Clinical Features. Specific forms of acute gingivitis will be discussed separately, and the present considerations will be limited to the most common form of gingival disease—chronic gingivitis.

The earliest manifestations of chronic gingivitis consist in slight alterations in the color of the free or marginal gingiva from a light pink to a deeper hue of pink, progressing to red or reddish blue as the hyperemia and inflammatory infiltrate become more intense. Bleeding from the gingival sulcus following even mild irritation such as tooth brushing is also an early feature of gingivitis. Edema, which invariably accompanies the inflammatory response and is an integral part of it, causes a slight swelling of the gingiva and loss of the characteristic normal stippling (Fig. 15–11). Inflammatory swelling of the interdental papillae often produces a somewhat bulbous appearance of these structures. This increase in the size of the gingiva favors the collection of more debris with increased bacterial accumulations, which in turn induce

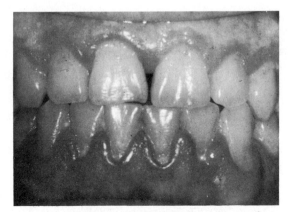

Figure 15–11. *Gingivitis.*
The inflammation of the gingiva results in swelling with reduction in and eventual loss of normal stippling.

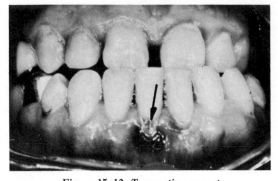

Figure 15–12. *Traumatic crescent.*
The recession and inflamed gingival tissue of the mandibular left central incisor resulted from local irritation and trauma.

more gingival irritation, thus bringing about a continuing cycle. When hyperemia and swelling of the marginal gingiva are confined to a localized area of the gingiva, the affected area sometimes assumes a crescent shape and has been termed a "traumatic crescent" (Figs. 15–12, 15–13).

Suppuration of the gingiva, manifested by the ability to express pus from the gingival sulcus by pressure, may occur in advanced chronic gingivitis.

Roentgenographic Features. Chronic gingivitis, in which the inflammation is limited strictly to the gingiva, does not manifest changes in the underlying bone. When bony changes become evident, the condition is termed "periodontitis."

Histologic Features. The gingiva in chronic gingivitis will reveal infiltration of the connective tissue by varying numbers of lymphocytes, monocytes and plasma cells. Polymorphonu-

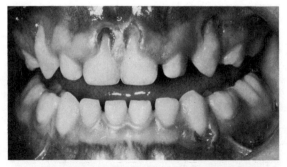

Figure 15–13. *Traumatic gingival recession.*
Gingival recession in a five-year-old girl caused by injury while sucking her finger. Stripping of the gingiva by a fingernail is a common manifestation of a habit that often has a psychogenic background. (Courtesy of Dr. Thompson M. Lewis: J. Periodontol., 33:353, 1962.)

clear leukocytes are occasionally noted, particularly beneath the crevicular epithelium. The crevicular epithelium is usually nonkeratinized and irregular. It is infiltrated by inflammatory cells and is frequently ulcerated (Fig. 15–14). The capillaries of the connective tissue are usually engorged and sometimes increased in number. Edema of the connective tissue may be prominent. The underlying periodontal ligament, except perhaps for those fibers of the free gingival group, is not involved, nor is the crest of the alveolar bone disturbed. The junction of the epithelial attachment to the tooth represents a weak point in the epithelial barrier to the oral environment, and at this point a collection of polymorphonuclear leukocytes and lymphocytes is nearly always found (Fig. 15–15).

Several investigators have applied histochemical techniques to studies of the normal and inflamed gingiva. Dewar and Turesky and his associates studied the glycogen content of the granular and spinous layers of the epithelium and found that it increases as the intensity of the underlying inflammation increases. Mast cells containing granules of sulfonated mucopolysaccharide are increased in the inflamed gingiva, but the significance of this finding is not clear. Alkaline phosphatase activity is somewhat increased in the inflamed gingiva, since it is present in the inflammatory and endothelial cells, and these are obviously present in larger numbers in chronic gingivitis. No remarkable differences were found in nucleic acid distribution between normal and inflamed gingiva, although the concentration of ribonucleic acid (RNA) was always lower in all cells of the crevicular epithelium and in the marginal epithelium where leukocytic infiltration had occurred. Histochemical studies of acid phosphatase in normal and inflamed human gingiva have shown that this enzyme is located almost exclusively in the epithelium. There is a greater reaction in the superficial layers (with the exception of the stratum corneum, which is acid phosphatase-free) and a gradual diminution toward the basal cell layer. The reaction is absent or very weak in the epithelial lining of the gingival sulci and periodontal pockets and in the epithelial attachment.

As in all infections, the immune response plays an important role in delineating the signs and symptoms of the process. Factors governing leukocyte migration and chemotactic activity obviously influence the host response. If the bacterial plaque does not evoke a positive

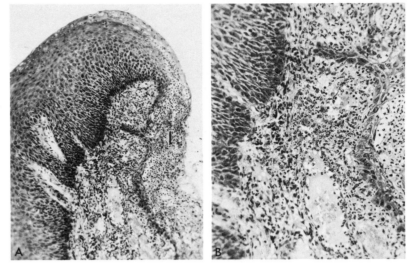

Figure 15–14. Gingivitis.
The gingiva is infiltrated by large numbers of lymphocytes, plasma cells and polymorphonuclear leukocytes. The crevicular epithelium (1) is invaded by these inflammatory cells and is degenerating. (A, Low-power, and B, high-power photomicrographs.)

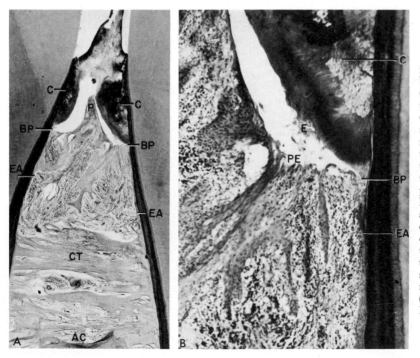

Figure 15–15. Gingivitis.
Photomicrograph of tissue from interproximal space between two bicuspids. AC marks alveolar crest; CT, transseptal fibers; P, interdental papilla; BP, bottom of pockets; C, calculus; EA, epithelial attachment. Photomicrograph on the right shows higher magnification of the bottom of the pocket BP with the calculus C in situ. In this case the calculus filled almost the entire pocket. PE, The pocket epithelium, which is broken in some areas; E, the epithelium which is clinging to the calculus; EA, the epithelial attachment alongside the tooth. Note the severe inflammatory reaction in the connective tissue and the elongated rete pegs resulting from this inflammation. (Courtesy of Dr. B. Orban and J. Periodontol.)

chemotactic response in the polymorphonuclear leukocytic cells, there will be few if any signs of inflammation. On the other hand, if the patient's leukocytes are unable to respond to the "call of the plaque," either because of a genetic defect or for some other reason, infection and tissue destruction may occur without the inflammatory reaction.

Treatment and Prognosis. Most cases of chronic gingivitis are due to local irritation. If the irritants are removed at this stage, the inflammation with its attendant swelling due to hyperemia, edema and leukocytic infiltration will disappear within a matter of hours or a few days, leaving no permanent damage. The fact that recovery usually follows the removal of irritants emphasizes the need for careful early treatment followed by proper toothbrushing and frequent prophylaxis. If there is poor response to good local therapy, a search should be made for systemic factors which might be complicating the case.

ACUTE NECROTIZING ULCERATIVE GINGIVITIS

(Vincent's Infection; Trench Mouth; Acute Ulceromembranous Gingivitis; Phagedenic Gingivitis; Fusospirochetal Gingivitis; Acute Ulcerative Gingivitis; etc.)

Acute necrotizing ulcerative gingivitis is a common specific type of gingivitis which has been recognized for centuries. The disease manifests both acute and recurrent (subacute) phases; a chronic stage also has been described, but most investigators believe that treating chronic necrotizing gingivitis as a separate entity cannot be justified, since it is neither clinically nor histologically specific. This inflammatory condition involves primarily the free gingival margin, the crest of the gingiva and the interdental papillae (Fig. 15–16). On rare occasions the lesions spread to the soft palate and tonsillar areas, and in such instances the term "Vincent's angina" has been applied.

Epidemiology. Acute necrotizing ulcerative gingivitis frequently occurs in an epidemic pattern, sweeping through groups of persons in close contact, especially those living under similar conditions. This was especially apparent during World War I, when the Allied troops suffered severely from the disease. It was at this time that the term "trench mouth" originated, since the disease was especially prevalent among the troops in the trenches. Similar sporadic outbreaks also occurred during World War II.

The pattern of spread of this disease in many instances indicated that it was a contagious infection, but this theory is not now accepted. Its occurrence in groups of persons can be explained on the basis of similar predisposing conditions among the members of the group which may cause gingivitis to develop in each, even though there is no actual contact between them. Nevertheless, acute necrotizing ulcerative gingivitis is still a disease deemed reportable by the boards of health in some states.

Clinical Features. Acute necrotizing ulcerative gingivitis may occur at any age, but is reportedly more common among young and middle-aged adults, 15 to 35 years old. It is an extremely rare finding in children, but a mistaken diagnosis is often made, particularly by physicians and school nurses, confusing this disease with primary herpetic gingivostomatitis.

The disease is characterized by the development of painful, hyperemic gingiva and sharply punched-out erosions of the interdental papillae (Fig. 15–16). The ulcerated remnants of the papillae and of the free gingiva bleed when touched and generally become covered by a gray, necrotic pseudomembrane (Fig. 15–17). The ulceration tends to spread and may eventually involve all gingival margins. It rather commonly begins at a single isolated focus, with a rapid onset. A typical fetid odor ultimately develops which may be extremely unpleasant. (See also Plate VI.)

The patient almost always complains of inability to eat because of the severe gingival pain or tenderness and the tendency for gingival

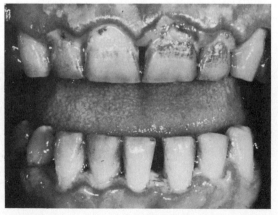

Figure 15–16. *Acute necrotizing ulcerative gingivitis.*
A typical, heavy, gray necrotic membrane covers the gingival tissues of the anterior teeth in this severe case. (Courtesy of Dr. Merrill Wheatcroft.)

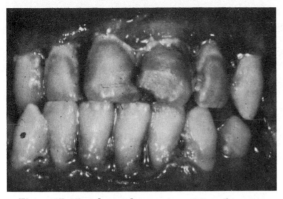

Figure 15–17. *Advanced acute necrotizing ulcerative gingivitis.*
Note the presence of a gray necrotic membrane and destruction of the interproximal tissues, particularly in the mandibular anterior region.

bleeding. The pain is of a superficial "pressure" type. The patient usually suffers from headache, malaise and a low-grade fever (99 to 102°F.). Excessive salivation with the presence of a metallic taste to the saliva is often noted, and regional lymphadenopathy is usually present.

In advanced and more serious cases there may be generalized or systemic manifestations, which may include leukocytosis, gastrointestinal disturbances and tachycardia.

After healing of acute necrotizing ulcerative gingivitis, the crests of the interdental papillae which have been destroyed, leaving a hollowed-out area, constitute an area which retains debris and microorganisms, and can serve as an "incubation zone." Such areas, along with gingival flaps of erupting third molars, are ideal locations for organisms to persist, and in many cases recurrence of acute necrotizing ulcerative gingivitis will begin here.

Etiology. Most investigators believe that acute necrotizing ulcerative gingivitis is a primary disease caused by a fusiform bacillus and *Borrelia vincentii*, a spirochete, coexisting in a symbiotic relationship. Both microorganisms are invariably present in profuse numbers in this "fusospirochetal" disease, although other spirochetes, fusiforms and filamentous organisms are also found. Some workers also include vibrio and coccal forms as important agents in the etiology of this disease. The fact that these two microorganisms, the fusiform bacillus and *Borrelia vincentii*, are found in moderate numbers in other oral diseases, including acute herpetic gingivostomatitis, as well as in many apparently healthy mouths, suggests that predisposing factors are essential to the develop-

ment of the acute necrotizing ulcerative gingivitis. This is particularly apparent in view of the fact that the disease has never been produced experimentally, in either human beings or animals, simply by oral inoculation of material from lesions in patients with the disease. Unsuccessful attempts were made by Schwartzman and Grossman to transmit the disease to 25 children by inoculation of infected material from gingival lesions in 7 cases of acute necrotizing ulcerative gingivitis. In 14 of the children the gingivae were traumatized by rubbing, but even this failed to induce the disease after local inoculation. King also attempted to produce the disease in his own mouth by inoculation of infected material, but he was unsuccessful even after traumatizing the gingiva, and the organisms promptly disappeared. He did show characteristic signs of acute necrotizing ulcerative gingivitis, however, after he became ill a short time later with several colds. Fusospirochetal abscesses can be produced in the experimental animal by the subcutaneous injection of gingival exudate or, as reported by Hampp and Mergenhagen, by subcutaneous injection of pure cultures of either *Borrelia vincentii* or *Borrelia buccale*. Rosebury suggested that the subcutaneous tissues are readily susceptible to infection by these microorganisms but that the gingival tissues are relatively resistant because previous contact of the oral tissues with the bacteria has resulted in a local immunity.

A decreased resistance to infection is one of the most important predisposing factors in the development of acute necrotizing ulcerative gingivitis. This was most apparent during World War I, when the Allied troops, living under poor sanitary conditions in the trenches and subsisting on inadequate diets, acquired this gingivitis in almost epidemic proportions, suggesting a contagious disease. According to Schluger, similar outbreaks occurred during and after World War II among soldiers in the field, when poor food, poor oral hygiene and fatigue prevailed. Undoubtedly, psychic phenomena can also be important predisposing factors.

Stones has reported that the incidence of acute necrotizing ulcerative gingivitis in Liverpool Dental Hospital (England) shows a significant seasonal variation, the highest incidence occurring between October and February, when respiratory infections and exanthemas are at their peak, and the lowest incidence occurring in July and August. Similar findings have been noted by Carter and Ball among the naval personnel at the Great Lakes Naval Training Center. Experimentally, fusospirochetal infection in dogs was produced by Swenson and Muhler after the administration of Scillaren-B, a mixture of glucosides which lower tissue resistance by inducing leukopenia.

Numerous investigators have reported that fusospirochetal infection may be produced more readily in animals deficient in various vitamins. Necrotizing lesions of the oral cavity have been produced in animals deficient in vitamin C and B complex, but it still remains to be proved that the lesions are due to fusospirochetal organisms. In some instances a relation between vitamin deficiency and acute necrotizing ulcerative gingivitis in humans has been suggested, but the data are conflicting, especially in view of the general inability to alter the course of the disease by administration of vitamins.

An excellent review of the etiology of this disease was published by Goldhaber and Giddon.

Bacteriologic Examination. Smears of material from the gingiva in cases of acute necrotizing ulcerative gingivitis show vast numbers of fusiform bacilli (genus Fusobacterium, or Fusiformis) and an oral spirochete (*Borrelia vincentii*), various other spirochetes, filamentous organisms, vibrios, cocci, desquamated epithelial cells and varying numbers of polymorphonuclear leukocytes (Figs. 15–18, 15–19). The relative numbers of microorganisms present vary with the stage of the disease, secondary invaders being more prominent in the later phases as well as in the subacute form of necrotizing gingivitis.

The fusiform bacillus associated with acute necrotizing ulcerative gingivitis is an elongated rod with tapered ends measuring 5 to 14 microns in length and 0.5 to 1.0 micron in diameter. This nonmotile organism is weakly gram-positive, occurs singly or in clusters and can be cultured under anaerobic conditions.

Borrelia vincentii is a gram-negative spirochete with three to six long, loose spirals. It measures approximately 10 to 15 microns in length, is actively motile and can be cultured anaerobically, although with some difficulty.

The diagnosis of acute necrotizing ulcerative gingivitis based upon a smear of gingival material is hazardous because of the nonspecific findings. Although the presence of the disease can often be confirmed when vast numbers of the spirochete and fusiform bacteria are found in the smear, somewhat lesser numbers are often seen in smears from "normal mouths," cases of acute herpetic gingivostomatitis, simple pericoronitis, marginal gingivitis and chronic gingivitis. Although the bacterial smear may be of value as an aid in diagnosis of atypical cases

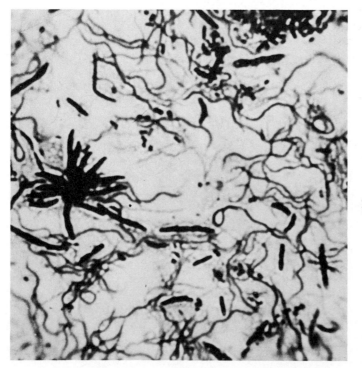

Figure 15–18. *Acute necrotizing ulcerative gingivitis.*
Photomicrograph of a smear from gingival exudate. Note the many spirochetes, fusiform bacteria, and other microorganisms.

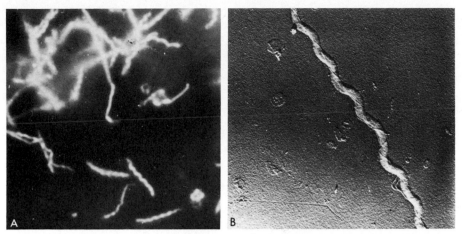

Figure 15–19. *Oral spirochetes.*
A, Darkfield examination. *B*, Electron photomicrograph, × 11,000 original magnification. (Courtesy of Dr. E. Hampp.)

of acute necrotizing ulcerative gingivitis, the final diagnosis is a clinical one.

Histologic Features. Microscopic examination of the gingiva in this disease reveals an acute gingivitis with extensive necrosis. The stratified squamous epithelium over the surface is ulcerated and replaced by a thick fibrinous exudate, or pseudomembrane, containing many polymorphonuclear leukocytes and microorganisms. Even in nonulcerated areas, a common feature noted by most investigators is the general lack of keratinization of the gingival tissues. The connective tissue is infiltrated by dense numbers of polymorphonuclear leukocytes and shows an intense hyperemia. The microscopic picture is an entirely nonspecific one (Fig. 15–20).

There is not complete agreement among investigators as to the penetration of the gingival tissues by the microorganisms associated with this disease. Vast numbers of both spirochetes and fusiform bacilli are found on the surface of the living tissue in and beneath the necrotic pseudomembrane. Both forms have also been reported as invading viable tissues to variable depths below the surface. The suggestion has been made that the presence of microorganisms in the tissues is due to surgical artefact. Schaffer, using light microscopy, failed to find bacteria penetrating vital tissues. Listgarten, on the other hand, utilizing electron microscopic techniques, was able to identify spirochetes between viable epithelial cells (Fig. 15–21).

Treatment and Prognosis. The treatment of acute necrotizing ulcerative gingivitis is extremely varied, depending upon the individual dentist's experience with the disease. Some prefer to treat this condition conservatively, instituting only superficial cleansing of the oral cavity in the early acute stage of the disease, followed by more thorough scaling and polishing as soon as the oral conditions permit. In many such cases prompt regression of the disease results even without medication. Other dentists prefer the use of oxygenating agents or antibiotics coupled with local treatment.

The usual case of acute necrotizing ulcerative gingivitis begins to subside in 48 hours with adequate treatment, and there may be little evidence ultimately of the presence of the disease. Sometimes there has been considerable destruction of tissue, the interdental papillae and marginal gingiva, and this may be evidenced after regression of the disease by the punched-out appearance of the interproximal gingiva and the apparent gingival recession (Fig. 15–22). Recontouring of gingival papillae is usually required; this can be accomplished by proper use of round tooth picks or by gingivoplasty. Treatment cannot be considered complete until the gingival tissue contours approximate the normal.

Acute gingivitis recurs with considerable frequency in patients who have been treated. Occasional serious sequelae have also been reported following this disease, such as gangrenous stomatitis or noma, septicemia and toxemia and even death.

GINGIVAL HYPERPLASIA

The gingival tissues in the healthy adult completely, though barely, fill the interproximal

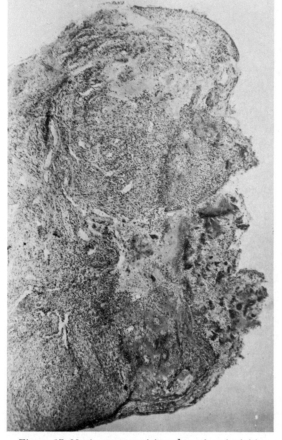

Figure 15–20. *Acute necrotizing ulcerative gingivitis.*
There is a nonspecific inflammatory reaction and ulceration of the gingival tissues. (Courtesy of Drs. E. Hampp and G. W. Burnett, and Williams & Wilkins Company.)

tissues which may result from a number of different conditions. Gingival enlargements are not to be confused with overgrowths of bone, or exostoses which are noted occasionally on the alveolar bone, usually at some distance from the gingiva.

There are many classifications of gingival hyperplasia, but the most practical one is as follows:

1. Inflammatory gingival hyperplasia
2. Noninflammatory (fibrous) gingival hyperplasia
3. Combination of inflammatory and fibrous hyperplasias

In inflammatory hyperplasia the enlarged gingivae are soft, edematous, hyperemic or cyanotic and sensitive to touch. They can easily be made to bleed, and they present a glossy, nonstippled surface. In noninflammatory or fibrous hyperplasia of the gingiva the enlarged tissue is firm, dense, resilient, normal in color or slightly paler than normal, sometimes well stippled, insensitive and not easily traumatized. Frequently there is a combination of the two types of enlargement. In most cases the enlargement results because of local irritations such as poor oral hygiene, accumulation of dental calculus or mouth breathing. The local irritation results in hyperemia, edema and lymphocytic infiltration. Many times the irritation results also in a proliferation of the fibrous elements of the gingival tissues. The proliferation on occasion may be increased by some predisposing systemic factor.

spaces between teeth, beginning near the contact area and extending apically and laterally in a smooth curve. Frequently, however, there is an increase in the size of the gingiva so that soft tissue overfills the interproximal spaces, balloons out over the teeth and protrudes into the oral cavity. The enlargement of the gingiva may be localized to one papilla or may involve several or all of the gingival papillae throughout the mouth (Fig. 15–23). The enlargement is usually more prominent on the labial and buccal surfaces, although it does occasionally develop in the lingual gingiva. It does not involve the vestibular mucosa.

An increase in the bulk of any tissue may be due to hypertrophy, i.e., an increase in the size of a structure due to an increase in the size of the individual cells involved, or to hyperplasia, i.e., to an increase in the number of cellular elements. "Gingival hyperplasia" is a general term for the gross increase in size of gingival

INFLAMMATORY GINGIVAL HYPERPLASIA

Inflammatory hyperplasia of the gingiva usually results from prolonged chronic inflammation of the gingival tissues (Fig. 15–24). Clinical examination often reveals the nature of the local irritation that causes the hyperplasia, but the histologic picture is usually nonspecific, showing merely inflammation of the gingiva. (See also Plate VI).

Inflammatory Hyperplasia Associated with Vitamin C Deficiency

The spongy, bleeding gums of scurvy, vitamin C deficiency (q.v.), have long been recognized as a specific entity. Although clinical scurvy is now rare, occasional cases are seen. Subclinical cases are probably common, since it has been reported that many patients do not

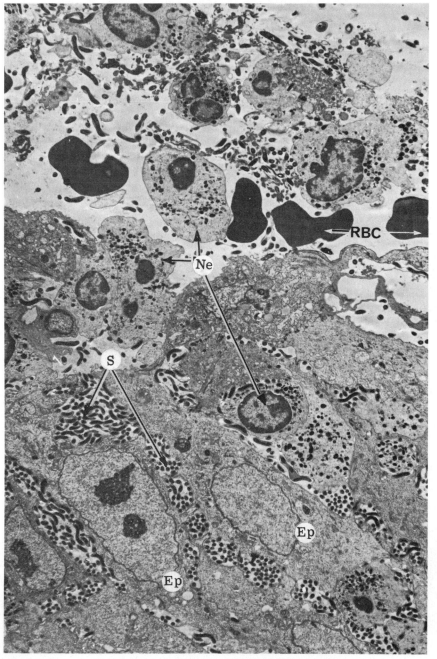

Figure 15–21. *Acute necrotizing ulcerative gingivitis.*
Electron microscope photomicrograph illustrates the epithelium adjacent to ulcerated lesion. Neutrophiles *(Ne)*, red blood cells *(RBC)*, microorganisms and cellular debris cover the epithelium. Dense masses of large and medium spirochetes *(S)* and some neutrophiles *(Ne)* distend the space between the epithelial cells *(Ep)*. Original magnification, × 3500. (Courtesy of Dr. Max A. Listgarten: J. Periodontol., *36:*328, 1965.)

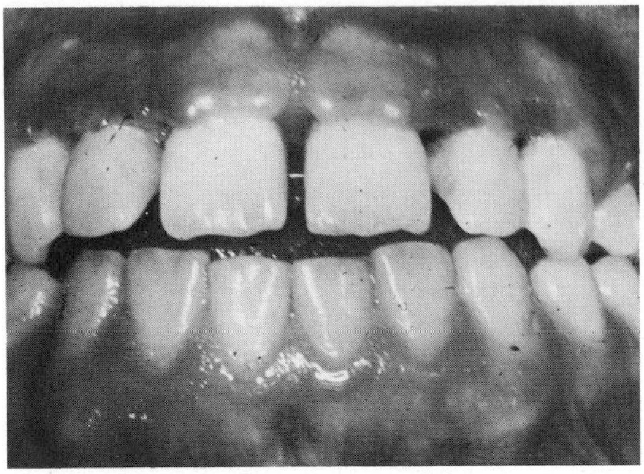

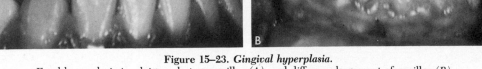

Figure 15–22. *Acute necrotizing ulcerative gingivitis after initial treatment.*

Note the persisting gray necrotic membrane on the free margin of the gingival tissue between the maxillary right central and lateral incisors. Note also the cupped-out gingival papillae between the maxillary anterior teeth which may become an incubation zone. Treatment must be continued until such areas are recontoured.

include adequate vitamin C in their diet. In such cases the gingivae become tender, swollen and edematous. They bleed upon the slightest provocation. Gingival sulci are often filled with partially clotted blood, and the crests of the interdental papillae are red or purple. There are sometimes ulceration and necrosis of the papillae as infection becomes superimposed upon the susceptible tissues. Hemorrhages following slight trauma to other parts of the body are also noted. Treatment includes improvement of oral hygiene and administration of vitamin C.

Inflammatory Hyperplasia Associated with Leukemia

Gingival hyperplasia is often an early finding in acute monocytic, lymphocytic or myelocytic

leukemia (q.v.). Gingival tissues are enlarged and are soft, edematous, easily compressed and tender. They show no signs of stippling. The color of the gingival tissue is sometimes bluish red, and the surface is glossy (Fig. 15–25). The gingivae are usually inflamed, owing to local infection, and occasionally an acute necrotizing gingivitis develops.

Histologic study of this type of gingival hyperplasia shows that the gingival tissues are packed with immature leukocytes, the specific type depending on the nature of the leukemia present. Capillaries are engorged, and the connective tissue is edematous and not well organized.

Inflammatory Hyperplasia Due to Endocrine Imbalance

Inflammatory gingival hyperplasia often occurs at puberty, particularly in girls. Some investigators think that this hyperplasia may result from an endocrine imbalance or readjustment in the endocrine balance at this particular stage of the patient's development. Others believe that at this age oral care is poor, perhaps because of local irritation associated with eruption of teeth. Also, nutrition may be inadequate, so that the inflammatory hyperplasia which occurs may be only indirectly associated with an endocrine disturbance.

During pregnancy one also notices a tendency for gingival hyperplasia of the inflammatory type. This proliferation may be due to disturbed nutrition, poor oral hygiene, or actually some systemic predisposition toward proliferation. The so-called pregnancy gingivitis, more properly spoken of as "gingivitis in pregnancy," is often associated with isolated gingival proliferation, sometimes so severe that it is

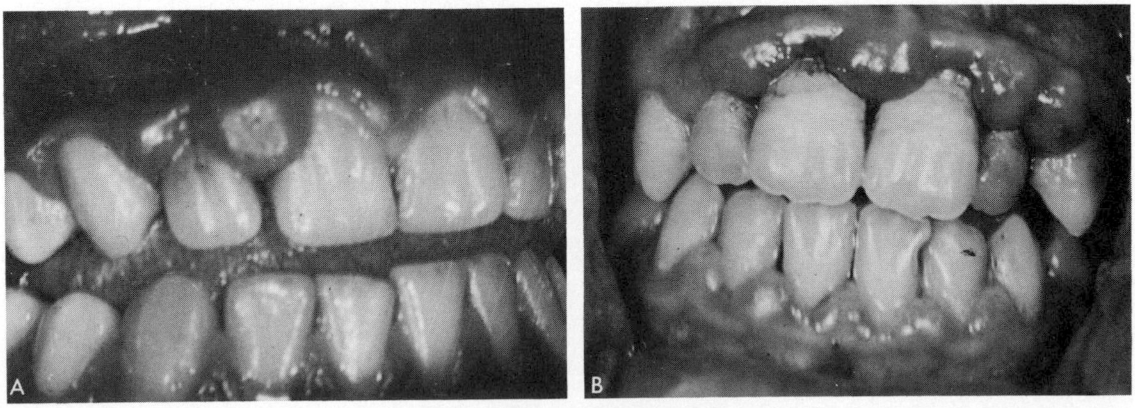

Figure 15–23. *Gingival hyperplasia.*
Focal hyperplasia involving only two papillae *(A)*, and diffuse enlargement of papillae *(B)*.

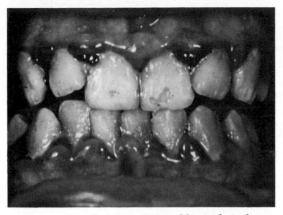

Figure 15–24. *Inflammatory gingival hyperplasia due to local irritation from collection of plaque.*

referred to as a "pregnancy tumor," which is basically a pyogenic granuloma (q.v.). These proliferations resemble those seen in some non-pregnant persons who have severe local irritations. Microscopic study of these gingival lesions reveals increased vascularity, multiplication of fibroblasts, edema and infiltration of leukocytes into the gingiva. *Diagnosis of the etiologic factors cannot be made by microscopic study.*

Inflammatory Hyperplasia Associated with Regional Enteritis (Crohn's Disease)

Regional enteritis is a slowly progressive disease of unknown etiology occurring in persons of all ages and both sexes. It is characterized by granulomatous, superficial ulcerations of the intestinal tract with frequent fistulae developing onto body surfaces or viscera, or between intestinal loops. This disease has been reported

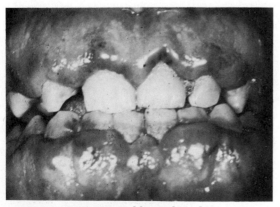

Figure 15–25. *Gingival hyperplasia due to acute monocytic leukemia.*

as having oral manifestations or oral extensions, and 24 such cases have been reviewed by Bernstein and McDonald. The most commonly involved areas are the buccal mucosa, where the lesions present a cobblestone appearance; the vestibule, where linear and hyperplastic folds and ulcers are found; the lips, which appear diffusely swollen and indurated; the gingiva and alveolar mucosa, which exhibit a granular erythematous swelling; and the palate, where multiple ulcers occur. The oral lesions may either precede or follow the appearance of the intestinal lesions and, like those lesions, commonly show periods of quiescence alternating with exacerbations of the process. The microscopic findings of the oral lesions are those of a chronic granulomatous disease, reminiscent of sarcoid. Typical cases also have been reported by Bottomley and his associates and by Eisenbud and his co-workers.

FIBROUS HYPERPLASIA OF THE GINGIVA

In contrast to the soft, edematous, hyperemic type of hyperplasia which is commonly seen in many patients is the fibrous type of hyperplasia. Often a single papilla or several papillae will be enlarged, and palpation will reveal that the enlargement is dense, insensitive and not easily irritated. It shows no tendency to bleed and presents a well-stippled surface which is normal in color. Microscopic study will show that the enlargement is due primarily to an increase in the bulk of mature fibrous connective tissue. Occasionally inflammatory changes are superimposed on the fibrous hyperplasia.

Chronic low-grade irritation of gingival tissues can cause localized hyperplasia of fibrous tissue. The treatment therefore is to remove the local irritation. If the fibrous hyperplasia is too extensive, surgical excision is desirable. The fibrous hyperplasia may gradually progress, although it is usually self-limiting.

Idiopathic Fibrous Hyperplasia

Patients are occasionally seen whose gingival tissues are so diffusely enlarged that the teeth are completely covered or, if the enlargement is present before tooth eruption, the dense fibrous tissue may interfere with or prevent eruption (Fig. 15–26). Other names for this condition are "fibromatosis" (q.v.), "fibromatosis gingivae," "elephantiasis gingivae" and "congenital macrogingiva." The cause of this devel-

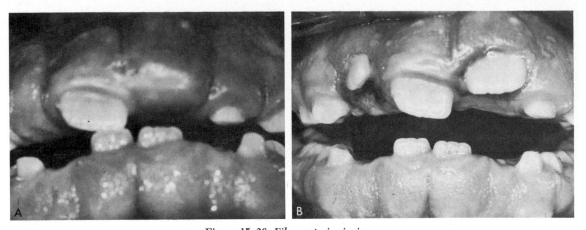

Figure 15–26. *Fibromatosis gingivae.*
Idiopathic fibrous hyperplasia (A) before and (B) after an incision had been made to allow eruption of the maxillary central incisor. Eventually these teeth assumed a relatively normal position.

opmental enlargement of gingival tissue is not known. It is probably genetic in some instances, since reports have been made of several cases occurring in the same family.

A typical case of idiopathic fibrous hyperplasia presents large masses of firm, dense, resilient, insensitive fibrous tissue that covers the alveolar ridges and extends over the teeth. It is normal in color, and the patient complains only of the deformity. Often the gingivae are so enlarged that the lips protrude, and the fibrous mat of tissue upon which the patient chews may be 25 mm. wide and as much as 15 mm. thick.

This hyperplasia may be noted at an early age and in a few cases even at birth. Teeth do not erupt normally because of the dense fibrous tissue.

Histologic sections of tissue from idiopathic fibrous hyperplasia of the gingiva show a moderate hyperplasia of the epithelium with mild hyperkeratosis and production of long rete pegs. The underlying stroma is made up almost entirely of dense bundles of mature fibrous tissue with few young fibroblasts present. Occasionally some chronic inflammation caused by local irritation may also be present.

Surgical removal of the excess fibrous tissue is the only treatment of value. Recurrence may follow.

Fibrous Hyperplasia Caused by Dilantin Sodium

It is now well established that fibrous hyperplasia of the gingiva sometimes occurs as a result of the use of the anticonvulsant drug, diphen-

ylhydantoin (Dilantin sodium) (q.v.). This drug is very effective in controlling epileptic seizures, but in some cases does have the side effect of causing fibrous hyperplasia of the gingiva.

The gingival hyperplasia may arise shortly after institution of Dilantin sodium therapy. It begins with the painless enlargement of one or two interdental papillae, which present an increased stippling and ultimately a roughened or pebbled surface with lobulations. The gingival tissues are dense, resilient, and insensitive; they show little or no tendency to bleed (Fig. 15–27).

The bulk of the enlargement is due primarily to proliferation of the fibrous connective tissue with numerous fibroblasts. There may be a superimposed chronic inflammation. The enlargement generally presents no difficulties, al-

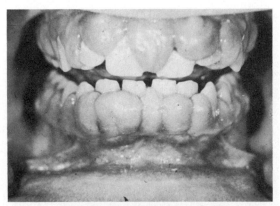

Figure 15–27. *Dilantin hyperplasia.*
Fibrous hyperplasia of the gingiva in an epileptic patient receiving Dilantin sodium. (Courtesy of Dr. B. Orban.)

though it is esthetically objectionable. It may be so severe as to interfere with function, and for this reason it may be surgically excised. Unfortunately, recurrence is common. It has been found that careful oral hygiene will result in slower development of the hyperplasia, and slower recurrence after surgical excision. Some regression of the hyperplasia may result if the use of the drug is discontinued.

There is no sharp line of demarcation between hyperplasia of connective tissue and benign neoplasia of fibroblasts; indeed, there are several conditions which resemble fibromas but which should not be so designated. Keloid is one such condition, and fibrous hyperplasia of the gingiva is another. Since these growths have never been reported to be precancerous, do not show unlimited growth and may involve one or many gingivae, it seems that they should not be classed as benign neoplasms.

PERIODONTITIS

(Periodontoclasia; Pyorrhea; Pyorrhea Alveolaris; Schmutz Pyorrhea)

The most common form of periodontal disease is that which is associated with local irritation. This begins as a marginal gingivitis which usually progresses, if untreated or treated improperly, to destructive chronic periodontitis. This type of periodontitis, sometimes referred to as marginal periodontitis, is most common in the adult, although it is found occasionally in children, especially when oral hygiene is lacking, or in certain cases of malocclusion. In the adult, periodontal disease of this type accounts for more than 90 per cent of the cases of periodontal disturbances and is responsible for greater tooth mortality than dental caries. In general, the treatment of this form of periodontal disease, as of all others, is dependent upon removal of etiologic factors, both local and systemic, the maintenance of good oral hygiene and the establishment of a stable, harmonious articulation free from traumatic interferences.

Etiology. Gingivitis may precede and develop into the more severe periodontitis which involves not only the gingiva, but also alveolar bone, cementum and periodontal ligament. Etiologic factors in general are the same as for gingivitis, but are usually more severe or of longer duration. Local factors, microbial plaque, calculus, food impactions and irritating margins of fillings appear to be most important in the development of this common form of

periodontal disease. The microflora in advanced periodontitis is characterized by the presence of large numbers of asaccharolytic microorganisms, including *Fusobacterium nucleatum, Bacteroides melaninogenicus, Eikenella corrodens, Bacteroides corrodens* and *Bacteroides capillosus.* Slots (1977) found that these organisms constituted up to 75 per cent of the isolates from periodontitis pockets.

Incidence. The incidence of periodontal disease is difficult to determine, and figures vary according to the criteria used by the individual investigators. This wide variation in the reported prevalence of periodontal disease is doubtless due to lack of uniformity in methods of assessment used and, of course, to inherent differences in the populations examined.

According to a study by Marshall-Day, chronic periodontal disease occurs rarely before 18 years of age, but increases in incidence so rapidly that after 45 years of age almost all subjects show evidence of localized or generalized bone loss. Incidence of bone loss in men is slightly higher than in women. The incidence of pocket formation increases constantly with age and reaches a peak of 94 per cent at ages 52 to 55 years. Abnormal tooth mobility is rarely encountered before 25 years of age, but increases sharply from 25 per cent at ages 35 to 39 to 49 per cent at ages 40 to 48, with a steady increase to 79 per cent at age 60. Localized or generalized clinically demonstrable suppuration occurs spontaneously or under digital pressure in almost 40 per cent of subjects at age 40 and approximately 50 per cent in the older age groups. There is also a rapid rise in tooth loss after 35 years of age, so that by 60 years of age, 60 per cent of the teeth have been lost and 26 per cent of patients are completely edentulous.

Clinical Features. Periodontitis usually begins as a simple marginal gingivitis as a reaction to plaque or calculus. An early, and perhaps the first, pathologic finding will be a tiny ulceration of the crevicular epithelium. Unless the irritants are removed, with the passage of time more plaque and calculus are deposited, and the marginal gingivitis becomes more severe. The gingiva becomes more inflamed and swollen, and with irritation the crevicular (pocket) epithelium suffers more frequent ulceration. It proliferates as a result of the inflammation so that at this stage there is a tendency for the epithelial attachment to extend or "migrate" apically on the tooth. As it does so, it is easily detached at its coronal portion. Through this process and because of the increased swelling of the marginal gingiva, the gingival crevice

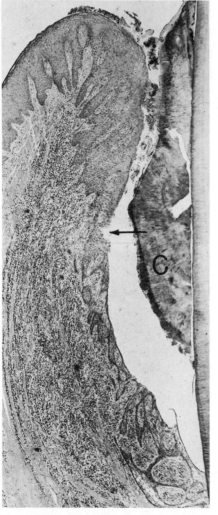

Figure 15–28. *Developing periodontal pocket.*
C labels a firmly attached deposit of subgingival calculus.
The arrow indicates a break in the integrity of the epithelial
lining of the pathologic pocket. Note the chronic inflammatory reaction in the soft tissue and the scarcity of gingival
fibers. (Courtesy of Drs. J. P. Weinmann and G. W.
Burnett, and Williams & Wilkins Company.)

gradually becomes deeper and is classified as
an early *periodontal pocket* (Fig. 15–28).

Clinically, the presence of calculus may be
detected at this stage. Subgingival calculus may
be more readily visualized if the free marginal
gingivae are blown back from the tooth by
compressed air. Besides the mild visible swelling and hyperemia of the gingivae there is also
a tendency for them to bleed readily; if the
gingivae are simply rubbed by the examiner,
minute "spontaneous" hemorrhages will often
appear in the region of the interdental papillae.
An unpleasant, almost foul type of halitosis may
also be present.

As periodontitis becomes more severe, the
teeth become mobile and give off a rather dull
sound when tapped with a metal instrument.
Suppurative material and other debris occasionally may be expressed from the pathologic
pocket adjacent to a tooth by slight pressure on
the gingiva. Compressed air and instrument
exploration will reveal that the tissue detach-
ment may be severe. The embrasures may be
open because the interdental papillae are deficient. The normal festooning is not apparent,
and the gingivae appear "boggy" because of
hyperemia and edema; no stippling is noted,
and the gingival tissues are smooth, shiny, and
perhaps redder or bluer than normal. The patient may have no subjective symptoms or may
complain of a bad taste, bleeding gums, and
hypersensitivity of the necks of the teeth due
to exposure of cementum as the soft tissues
recede. In other words, the patient has a severe
chronic gingivitis and an involvement of the
deeper portions of the periodontium. This is
the stage of severe periodontitis, or what Page
and Schroeder call the advanced lesion of periodontitis.

Gingival recession is a common phenomenon,
particularly in later years in life. In such cases
the gingival tissues recede toward the apex,
exposing cementum, sometimes to an alarming
degree. Since cementum is softer than enamel,
it is often worn away by a toothbrush and an
abrasive dentifrice. Gingival recession can occur
more rapidly if there has been rapid alveolar
bone loss, due to any cause, since gingival tissue
in health will maintain a uniform relation with
alveolar bone crest. Gingival recession often
begins as a thin break in the free gingiva
adjacent to the center of a tooth. This is called
a *Stillman's cleft* (Fig. 15–29). Abnormal frequency and direction of tooth brushing, occlusal
forces or a high muscle attachment will sometimes lead to gingival recession. Gingival recession is preceded by alveolar bone loss, but bone
loss is not necessarily accompanied by an equal
amount of recession.

Histologic Features. In marginal gingivitis
which is just beginning to undergo transition
into early periodontitis, the enlarged free marginal gingiva is densely infiltrated with lymphocytes and plasma cells, and the apical border of
the inflamed area approaches the crest of the
alveolar bone and the crestal fibers of the periodontal ligament (Figs. 15–30, 15–31). The
crevicular epithelium shows various degrees of
proliferation, and often tiny ulcerations. One of
the early microscopic signs of the encroachment
of the inflammatory process on the periodon-

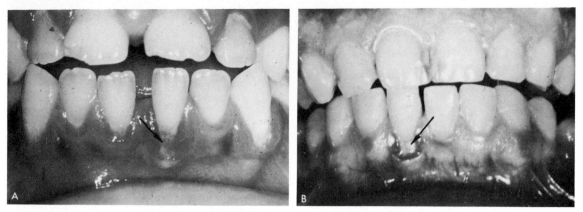

Figure 15–29. *Gingival recession (Stillman's cleft).*
The recession on the lower anterior teeth is due to poor oral hygiene and an abnormal amount of local irritation (*A* and *B*).

tium is the appearance of giant cells, osteoclasts, on the surface of the bone crest. They soon appear to lie in the little bays of bone resorption known as Howship's lacunae. The underlying tissues of the periodontium show no changes at this stage (Fig. 15–32). The pathologic process involves alveolar bone prior to involvement of the periodontal ligament.

The next stage of the progress of the disease is a continuation of the factors just described: (1) more plaque is deposited in an apical direction on the tooth; (2) more irritation of the free gingiva occurs; (3) the epithelial attachment proliferates apically down onto the cementum of the tooth and shows more ulceration; (4) the alveolar crest of bone is resorbed further api-

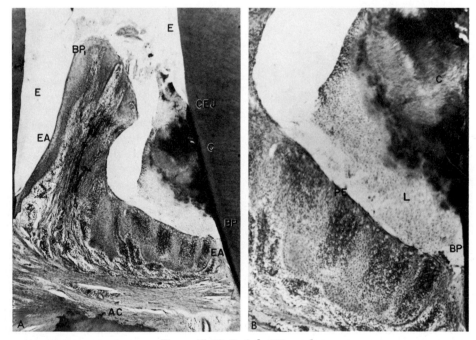

Figure 15–30. *Periodontitis, early.*
Photomicrographs of the interproximal space between a second and third molar. The bottom of the pocket on the third molar is on the enamel (*BP₁*), whereas it is on the cementum (*BP*) of the second molar. *E*, Enamel is lost in decalcification; *EA*, epithelial attachment; *CEJ*, cementoenamel junction; *C*, deposit of calculus; *AC*, alveolar crest showing resorption. The illustration on the right is a higher magnification of the bottom of the pocket, showing calculus (*C*) separated from the epithelium (*PE*), and leukocytes (*L*) which have migrated from the connective tissue. (Courtesy of Dr. B. Orban and J. Periodontol.)

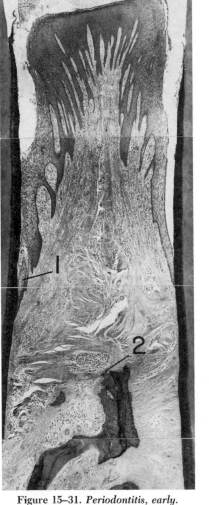

Figure 15–31. *Periodontitis, early.*
Composite photomicrograph of case of gingivitis gradually progressing toward a periodontitis. Note that the epithelium *(1)* is proliferating along the cementum and that there is a beginning resorption of alveolar bone *(2)*. (Courtesy of Drs. J. P. Weinmann and G. W. Burnett, and Williams & Wilkins Company.)

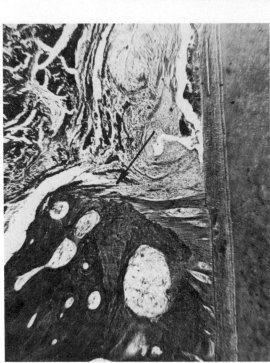
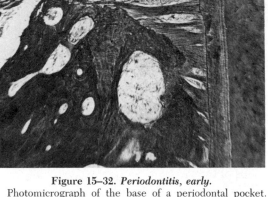

Figure 15–32. *Periodontitis, early.*
Photomicrograph of the base of a periodontal pocket. Note that the deeper periodontal ligament fibers are not involved, but there is a disturbance of some of the alveolar crest fibers. (Silver stain.)

cally; (5) principal periodontal ligament fibers become disorganized and detached from the tooth; and (6) a periodontal pocket exists between the free gingiva and the tooth, to depths of from 2 mm. down, until finally the apex of the tooth is approached. The deep pocket that then exists between the calculus- and plaque-covered tooth surface and the epithelial lining of the gingival tissues forms a protective trap for multiplying microorganisms and for leuko-cytic cellular exudate from the inflamed soft tissue of the pocket wall. The vicious cycle of irritant collection, inflammation and detach-ment continues, along with periodontal bone resorption in an apical direction (Fig. 15–33).

Immunologic Features. There is considera-ble evidence indicating that plaque-induced ef-fector mechanisms play a major role in the pathogenesis of inflammatory periodontal dis-ease. Both the cellular and humoral immuno-logic pathways have been implicated in the destruction of periodontal tissues. Correlations of varying magnitudes have been demonstrated between the clinical severity of periodontal disease and plaque antigen-induced peripheral blood lymphocyte blastogenesis by Ivanyi and Lehner (1971), by Horton and co-workers (1972), and by Mackler and associates (1974). The clinical severity of periodontal disease has also been correlated with salivary IgA concen-trations by Orstavik and Brandtzaeg (1975). Robertson and his co-workers (1980) studied the periodontal status of patients with primary immunodeficiencies and compared them with age-matched and plaque-matched individuals. Since most patients with immunodeficiency dis-eases have a short life span, most of the patients examined were younger than 15 years of age. There were, however, two patients, one 45

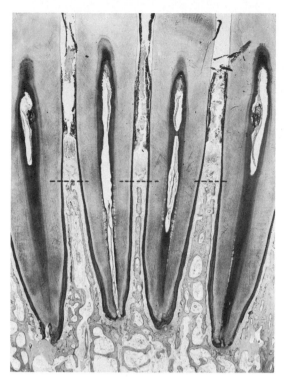

Figure 15–33. *Periodontitis.*
Note the collection of debris interproximally and the horizontal bone loss. (Courtesy of Dr. J. P. Weinmann.)

years old and the other 16 years old, with IgA deficiency, although low to undetectable levels of IgA were noted in all of the immunodeficient patients studied. Without exception, immunodeficient patients demonstrated less gingival inflammation than immunocompetent subjects matched in age and plaque index. These results are in accord with studies by Tollefsen and co-workers and by Kardachi and Newcomb of patients receiving immunosuppressant drugs. The diminished levels of gingival inflammation in immunodeficient patients can be explained if there was a qualitative difference in the oral microflora or if there was impairment in the host's ability to react to plaque. Brown and co-workers found very few differences in the microbial composition of dental plaque between the two patient groups reported on by Robertson and his co-workers (1980). However, significantly higher plaque levels of catalase-negative diphtheroids and Candida sp. were found in immunodeficient patients, whereas control groups had higher concentrations of Fusobacterium sp. They concluded that immunoglobulins have minimal influence on the microbial composition of dental plaque. Therefore, if den-

tal plaque is present and the reaction to it is absent or minimal, one would expect little periodontal disease. On the other hand, if the immunologic effector mechanisms are responsible for the signs or symptoms of periodontal disease, there would be inflammation and tissue destruction only in patients able to mount an immunologic response to the presence of dental plaque. Mackler and his co-workers reported in 1978 that the earlier mild gingivitis lesions contained predominantly thymus (T)-derived lymphocytes, whereas the more advanced lesions contained large numbers of B-lymphocytes and plasma cells. Thus, patients with humoral (B-lymphocyte) immunodeficiencies would be expected to have some gingival inflammation, since many such patients manifest normal T-cell mediated responses. In fact, some of the IgA-deficient patients in Robertson's study did show mild gingivitis, but it was less severe than in the age- and plaque-matched controls.

Evidence that the immune response is capable of destroying all periodontal tissues in experimental animals was provided by Levy and his colleagues (1976). When complete (CFA) and incomplete (IFA) Freund's adjuvant was injected into the periodontium of CFA-sensitized marmosets, capuchins, and rhesus monkeys, all animals developed a proliferative granulomatous reaction at the injection site. However, only in CFA-injected animals was there marked destructive periodontitis with considerable bone destruction. The injection of IFA into the periodontium of the same animals resulted in the formation of nondestructive proliferative granulation tissue.

It seems obvious then that the immune response, while often protective, can also be a highly destructive reaction to injury. The current state of knowledge of the histopathology and immunopathology of periodontitis has been summarized by Page and Schroeder.

CLASSIFICATION OF PERIODONTAL POCKETS. In a normal healthy periodontium the gingival tissues fit snugly around the teeth, and the gingival crevice approximates zero. In the presence of inflammation, however, the gingival tissues increase in bulk, causing an increase in the depth of the pocket around the teeth. If the pathologic changes are limited to the gingiva, this is called a *gingival* (or *pseudo-*) *pocket*. If, however, the base of the pocket has invaded further into the periodontium, it is called a *periodontal pocket*. The base of the periodontal pocket is on the tooth root, and the epithelial

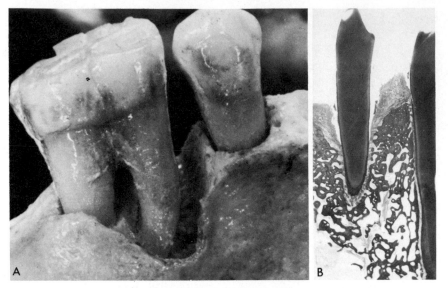

Figure 15–34. *Infra-bony pocket.*

A, Typical infra-bony pocket of the mandibular molar region. B, Photomicrograph of a similar pocket. (A, Courtesy of Dr. John Pritchard: J. Periodontol., *28*:202, 1957.)

attachment is on cementum. Although periodontal disease usually progresses apically and advances at the expense of the horizontal loss of the crest of the alveolar bone, sometimes the depth of the pocket extends apical to the crest of the alveolar bone. Such a pocket, which has bone on its lateral wall, is called an *infra-bony pocket,* and is the exception rather than the rule, since usually the bottom of the pathologic pocket is level with or coronal to the alveolar crest of bone (*supra-bony pocket*) (Fig. 15–34). The infra-bony pocket may result from food impaction and is frequently found along the tooth which has shifted considerably out of its usual position or has been subjected to severe occlusal trauma. Infra-bony pockets are classified according to their shape (narrow or broad) and the number of bony walls. According to Goldman and Cohen in a complete discussion of this condition, three-wall infra-bony pockets are commonly observed in the interdental areas where one finds an intact proximal wall as well as buccal and lingual walls of the alveolar process. Two-wall infra-bony pockets may be seen in the interdental areas, with the buccal and lingual walls intact, but the proximal wall destroyed. A "curtain" of soft tissue remains where the osseous wall has been destroyed. Infrabony pockets with one osseous wall are occasionally seen in the interdental area.

The type of periodontal pocket present can be determined by careful clinical examination and study of good roentgenograms. Consideration of the topography and type of infra-bony pocket is important in planning the treatment of periodontal disease. The most favorable type of pocket for reattachment to occur is, of course, the one with three osseous walls. A "slanting fill-in" of bone can occur in a pocket with two bony walls; but when only one wall is present, chances for formation of additional height of alveolar bone are poor.

Roentgenographic Features. The earliest change in the periodontal bone is a blunting of the alveolar crest due to beginning bone resorption (Fig. 15–35). As resorption progresses, there is horizontal loss of more bone, often with a tendency for a cupping out of the interdental alveolar bone. The periodontal ligament space retains its usual thickness, and generally no changes are noted except the superficial bone changes which actually may become extensive (Fig. 15–36). It is of interest that roentgenographic evidence of alveolar bone changes has been reported in about 12 per cent of cases in which pocket formation does not exist clinically.

Treatment and Prognosis. By careful complete periodontal treatment, teeth involved by periodontal disease can be saved if the bone loss has not been too extreme, if irritants are removed by scaling and curettage and if pockets are eliminated by gingival recession or by surgical removal of the gingiva (gingivectomy), if osseous deformities are eliminated and the

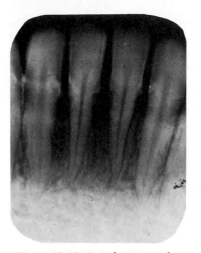

Figure 15–35. *Periodontitis, early.*
Note the blunting of the alveolar crest and loss of alveolar bone in the roentgenogram. (Courtesy of Dr. R. Gottsagen.)

tooth-supporting tissues recontoured to a normal physiologic architecture, if occlusal forces are balanced and systemic factors are corrected.

Clinicians for many years have demonstrated that after successful treatment for periodontitis, pathologic pockets are shallower, even though no tissue was removed. Obviously this loss of pocket depth can be caused either by gingival recession or by reattachment of periodontal ligament to the tooth surface next to the pocket. Actually, both recession and reattachment may occur in the same case. There is usually a

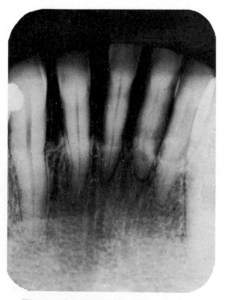

Figure 15–36. *Periodontitis, advanced.*

shrinkage or recession of the gingival tissues as inflammation and its associated edema and hyperemia are diminished, for as the gingival tissues return to a state of health the normal relation of gingiva to alveolar bone is gradually re-established just above the bone level. The distance from the crest of the gingiva to the base of the pocket is diminished by the reduction in the size of the gingiva.

The second possible explanation for the shallower pocket after therapy is that reattachment occurs. *Reattachment* may be defined as a re-establishment of fibrous connection of tooth to alveolar bone and gingiva by periodontal fibers in an area of cementum which was adjacent to a pathologic pocket. A typical epithelial attachment is described as re-forming. The cellular elements which would make reattachment possible are all present in the periodontium; resorption of bone and rebuilding of new bone with reattachment of new periodontal ligament fibers go on constantly.

Considering this problem from a purely theoretic point of view, if reattachment is to occur, it is necessary that connective tissues remain in contact with the tooth for an appreciable but as yet undetermined period of time. Since the cementum lining the pocket is necrotic, osteoclasts (cementoclasts) must resorb the cementum to a level at which it is viable. Next, cementoblasts must develop to deposit a new layer of cementum which traps ends of connective tissue fibers. Finally, new alveolar bone must be built opposite the newly attached periodontal fibers in response to the stimulus of the periodontal ligament.

Animal experiments have indicated that reattachment will not occur as long as inflammation persists in the tissues next to the tooth.

Factors interfering with reattachment include the following:

Crevicular Epithelium. For reattachment to occur, this epithelium must be destroyed or curetted away. Since cementum can be deposited only by connective tissue, the presence of epithelium interferes with reattachment. The fresh bleeding connective tissue surface will form a blood clot in contact with the tooth which can organize and contribute to reattachment. In certain cases, particularly those with infra-bony pockets, the blood clot is easily protected and healing occurs more easily.

Motion. During the period of reorganization the tooth must be at least relatively immobile, since motion would tend to disturb the healing process and allow any crevicular epithelium

remaining to proliferate and reline the pathologic pocket.

Inflammation itself apparently interferes
with reattachment, perhaps because cementoblasts cannot develop in areas of inflammation.

Necrotic cementum is also a barrier to reattachment, since new cementum apparently will
not be deposited upon cementum which has
been in contact with oral fluids and suppuration
for an appreciable time.

Other, as yet unknown, factors are also involved. Connective tissue can lie adjacent to
cementum for months without being lined by
epithelium or establishing a reattachment of
periodontal ligament to tooth.

There is now much experimental evidence to
prove that reattachment can occur in experimental animals, and many articles have been
published, some with histologic evidence, indicating that reattachment can occur in the
human patient.

Provided the condition is not too advanced
and therapy is adequate, periodontitis can be
arrested, and teeth can be maintained in function almost indefinitely. The inflammatory process gradually subsides; gingival tissues return
to normal size, color and contour; the teeth
become less mobile, and suppuration and
bleeding stop. The depth of the gingival crevice
approaches zero, owing to tissue shrinkage or
gingivectomy; stippling returns, and the case
appears normal, even though the gingival tissues and alveolar crest are apical to their original position. In other words, a new steady state
is reached, different from the original but compatible with the maintenance of good oral
health.

LATERAL PERIODONTAL ABSCESS
(Lateral Abscess)

Clinical Features. The lateral periodontal
abscess is related directly to a pre-existing periodontal pocket. When such a pocket reaches
sufficient depth, perhaps 5 to 8 mm., the soft
tissues around the neck of the tooth may approximate the tooth so tightly that the orifice of
the pocket is occluded. Bacteria multiply in the
depth of the pocket and cause sufficient irritation to form an acute abscess with exudation of
pus into this area. A foreign body, particularly
food debris, may also lead to abscess formation.
This may result in sufficient swelling to destroy
the cortical plate of bone, if it still exists, and
allow the abscess to balloon the overlying tissues, forming a "gum boil," or parulis (Fig. 15–
37, *A*). A direct incision perpendicular to the
long axis of the involved tooth will release pus,
while the introduction of a periodontal pocket
probe from the gingiva to the area will release
the pus around the neck of the tooth. If the
abscess does not drain spontaneously through
the gingival crevice, and if it is not treated, a
fistula may develop to release the pus spontaneously onto the mucosal surface (Fig. 15–37,
B). The acute periodontal abscess will cause the
afflicted tooth to be tender to percussion. (See
also Plate VI.)

The occurrence of periodontal abscesses of
both lateral and periapical types was reported
by Dinsdale and Holt in a group of 34 children
treated with cortisone for rheumatic fever. The
abscesses appeared within two weeks after therapy had been discontinued. The cortisone apparently actuated pre-existing periodontal le-

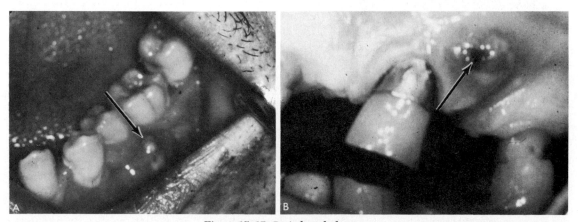

Figure 15–37. *Periodontal abscess.*
The abscess in *B* has perforated, forming a fistula.

sions, but the abscesses were unusual in that pain was very mild or even absent and there was no local swelling or cellulitis. Lymph node involvement was also rare. In some cases the only clinical manifestation of the abscess was the release of pus from the neck of a loose deciduous tooth upon pressure. It was particularly noted that the erythrocyte sedimentation rate, which is seldom elevated in normal children who have a periodontal abscess, was usually elevated in cortisone-treated children with rheumatic fever who had a periodontal abscess.

Histologic Features. Microscopically, the abscess resembles an abscess elsewhere. It consists of a central cavity filled with pus walled off on one side by the root of the tooth and on the other by connective tissue, because it is likely that in most instances the epithelial lining of the crevice will have been destroyed by the inflammatory process.

Treatment. Treatment of a periodontal abscess is similar to that of an abscess elsewhere. Careful insertion of a dull probe into the pocket along the tooth will usually produce drainage, and the acute symptoms will subside. The abscess will recur, however, unless the cause is removed and the depth of the pocket is reduced. Extraction of the tooth is indicated after the acute symptoms have subsided only in cases in which normal tissue contours cannot be developed and maintained.

CHRONIC DESQUAMATIVE GINGIVITIS

Chronic desquamative gingivitis is a term that has been used for many years to describe a unique condition of the gingiva characterized by intense redness and desquamation of the surface epithelium. At one time this was thought to be a specific degenerative disease of the gingival tissues, although of unknown etiology, and was sometimes also called "gingivosis." However, the term "gingivosis" was first used by Schour and Massler in 1947 to describe a probably unrelated disease of the gingiva which they found in a group of malnourished Italian children.

McCarthy and his co-workers studied 40 cases of chronic desquamative gingivitis and concluded in 1960 that it was not a specific disease entity but rather a clinical manifestation of several diseases and thus had several etiologies. The term "chronic desquamative gingivitis" is now used by most workers as a descriptive term for the oral manifestations of any one of a variety of diseases which, once identified, may permit a rational therapeutic approach of value for patient management.

Etiology. A classification of chronic desquamative gingivitis based on etiology was proposed by McCarthy and his co-workers. They suggested the causative factors to be: (1) certain dermatoses, (2) hormonal influences, (3) abnormal responses to irritation, (4) chronic infections, and (5) idiopathic. Subsequent studies such as those of Nisengard and Neiders and of Rogers and his associates have shown that the dermatoses are numerically the most important of the causative factors. For example, in the study of Nisengard and Neiders, 67 of the 100 patients exhibited immunofluorescent findings suggestive of or diagnostic of a dermatosis.

The most important dermatoses presenting oral findings categorized as a desquamative gingivitis are (1) cicatricial pemphigoid (benign mucous membrane pemphigoid), (2) pemphigus, and (3) lichen planus. These individual diseases along with their identification by immunofluorescence will be considered with other diseases of the skin in Chapter 16.

Clinical Features. Chronic desquamative gingivitis occurs in both sexes at any age from the teens to late adult life, but is predominant in women in the age group of 40 to 55 years.

In the patient with chronic desquamative gingivitis, the gingivae are red, swollen and glossy in appearance, occasionally with multiple vesicles and many superficial denuded areas which have an exposed bleeding connective tissue surface. The lesions, which may occur in edentulous mouths as well as in the mouths of patients with their natural dentition, exhibit a patchy distribution. If the nonulcerated gingivae are massaged, the epithelium readily strips or slides from the connective tissue to leave the raw, sensitive surface which bleeds readily (Fig. 15–38). This is termed "Nikolsky's sign" and consists in a slipping or peeling of the tissue at the dermal-epidermal junction under slight lateral pressure. Oral mucous membrane surfaces other than gingiva are sometimes involved also, particularly buccal mucosa (Plate VI).

Patients with chronic desquamative gingivitis complain of extremely sensitive gingival tissues. They often find it difficult to eat anything hot, cold or spicy, and tooth brushing is nearly impossible because of the ensuing pain and hemorrhage. A presumptive diagnosis is sometimes established when the patient reports that

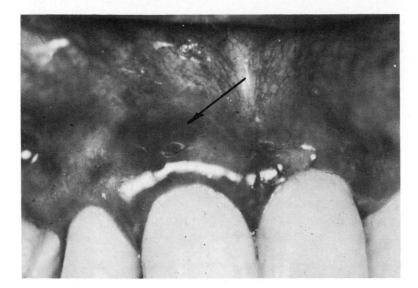

Figure 15–38. *Chronic desquamative gingivitis.* There are raw denuded areas on the gingival mucosa.

his mouth has been sensitive and extremely irritated for many months and no treatment has been successful. In fact, chronicity is one of the common features of the disease, some patients suffering for many years.

Histologic Features. The microscopic features of the lesion depend entirely upon the nature of the disease process involved and will be characteristic of that particular condition.

Treatment. The proper treatment of the condition will depend entirely upon the definitive diagnosis of the disease.

JUVENILE PERIODONTITIS

(Periodontosis)

Juvenile periodontitis, termed periodontosis until recent years, has been concisely defined by Baer as "a disease of the periodontium which can occur in an otherwise healthy adolescent, which is characterized by a rapid loss of alveolar bone about more than one tooth of the permanent dentition. There are two basic forms in which it occurs. In one form of the disease, the only teeth affected are the first molars and incisors. In the other, more generalized form, it may affect most of the dentition. The amount of destruction manifested is not commensurate with the amount of local irritants present."

Cases of juvenile periodontitis seldom exist per se for any great length of time, since most periodontal disturbances of noninflammatory origin become complicated by inflammation long before the affected tooth is lost.

Etiology. Becks reported the frequency of systemic disturbances in 80 cases of juvenile periodontitis. In 84 per cent of the cases endocrine disturbances were found; in 12 per cent other systemic disturbances were present; and in 4 per cent of the cases no disturbance could be identified. Goldman found lesions in the periodontal tissues of two spider monkeys that had died of amebic and bacillary dysentery. The appearance of the periodontal lesions in these monkeys resembled that seen in juvenile periodontitis.

Frandsen and co-workers found protein-free diets to be responsible for an increased rate of bone resorption and osteoporosis in the alveolar and supporting bone of the teeth of rats. The jaws of the protein-deficient rats were smaller than the jaws of rats to which normal protein was fed, and there was less osteocementum on the roots of their teeth. The interdental papillae and transseptal fibers were disturbed, and there was evidence of considerably more breaking down of tissue than of rebuilding.

Diets lacking in minerals, especially calcium and phosphorus, have been shown to produce in the supporting tissues of animals' teeth disturbances that resemble those found in the human patient with juvenile periodontitis.

Several investigators have shown a familial tendency for occurrence of the disease. For example, Baer has found it occurring in identical twins, parent-offsprings, siblings, first cousins, and uncles and nephews. He has also reported a tendency for the disease to follow the maternal side of the line.

More recent studies by Newman and Socransky (1977) have shown that the lesion of juvenile periodontitis is associated with the presence of subgingival plaque which is loosely attached to the root surfaces of involved teeth. Bacteriologic evaluation of the plaque revealed the presence of a sparse microbiota in which gram-negative capnophilic and anaerobic rods predominate. There is also evidence that the host defense seems to be impaired in individuals with juvenile periodontitis. Clark and colleagues demonstrated that patients with this disease frequently showed a defective neutrophil chemotactic response. In addition, serum from several patients examined contained a factor which markedly inhibited neutrophil chemotaxis. Similar findings have been reported by Cianciola and co-workers in 1977 and by Lavine and associates in 1979. A thorough general review of this disease, including the various theories on etiology, has been carried out by Kaslick and Chasens (1968), and by Liljenberg and Lindhe (1980).

Clinical Features. Juvenile periodontitis occurs in the adolescent period of life, during the years from 12 to 20, but is more prevalent clinically between the ages of 18 and 25 years. Females are consistently reported to be affected more frequently than males, by a ratio often as high as 3:1. It may appear in mouths in which the hygienic condition is faultless and in which no caries exists. It occurs entirely free from marginal inflammation, but usually is not discovered until marginal inflammation has become superimposed on the degenerative process.

The first indication to the patient of the presence of juvenile periodontitis is often a sudden symmetric pathologic drifting of teeth, usually the first permanent molars and then the anterior teeth. It is possible that these teeth are involved first because they erupt earlier than the other teeth.

Juvenile periodontitis in its early stages is not usually recognized clinically, although a roentgenogram would reveal alveolar bone loss in a local area. The first definite clinical evidence seen by the dentist is deep pocket formation, often on only one tooth, with the bone of the adjacent tooth roentgenographically normal. Actually, this is the beginning of the last stage in the development of the disease. At this point mouth fluids, microorganisms and debris enter the pocket, and the usual inflammatory symptoms follow.

As juvenile periodontitis progresses from its early stages, bone resorption may be observed before there is clinical evidence of pocket formation. Bone changes begin at or near the crest of the alveolar process. Rapid bone resorption widens the periodontal space, opening marrow spaces of the bone in which the disorganized periodontal ligament coalesces with the marrow tissue which has been changed from a fatty marrow to a fibrous tissue.

The degeneration and loss of the principal fibers of the periodontal ligament are soon followed by the proliferation of epithelium along the root surface.

Migration, or pathologic wandering of teeth, is often accompanied by extrusion of the affected tooth from its socket. Degenerative changes in the connective tissue of the periodontal ligament and the development of granulation tissue cause pressure upon the surface of the root, forcing the crown of the tooth from its normal position and often extruding it to a place where the occlusal force has a traumatic effect upon the supporting tissue. Trauma complicates the existing pathologic conditions and hastens the loosening of the tooth.

Pain is not usually present in juvenile periodontitis until late in the progress of the disease, when traumatic influences enter, or after pocket formation has occurred, when deep infection of the pocket tissue may take place. In this event lateral abscesses in the periodontal tissue frequently develop. It is not uncommon to observe the sudden development of an extremely deep pocket on the root of a tooth, extending almost to its apex.

JUVENILE (PRECOCIOUS) PERIODONTOSIS WITH PALMAR-PLANTAR HYPERKERATOSIS (PAPILLON-LEFÈVRE SYNDROME). Numerous cases of juvenile periodontosis occurring in association with certain skin lesions have been reported since the original case described in 1924 by Papillon and Lefèvre. An excellent discussion of this entity, with a review of the literature and presentation of additional cases, has been published by Gorlin and his co-workers.

The Papillon-Lefèvre syndrome is characterized by severe destruction of alveolar bone involving both the deciduous and permanent dentitions. Some reported cases have shown bone loss as early as two years of age with premature exfoliation of teeth. Inflammatory gingival enlargement, gingival ulceration, and formation of deep pockets are frequently present, although in other instances there is no inflammatory element and only the permanent dentition may be affected.

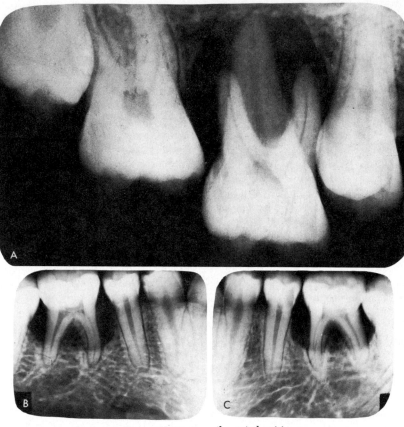

Figure 15–39. *Juvenile periodontitis.*

A, Enlarged roentgenogram of maxillary first permanent molar of a 16-year-old patient with juvenile periodontitis. Note almost complete absence of alveolar bone and thin, narrow roots. *B* and *C*, Roentgenograms of mandibular first permanent molars in the same case.

The characteristic skin lesions associated with the oral changes consist of keratotic lesions of the palmar and plantar surfaces (hyperkeratosis palmoplantaris). In addition, some patients manifest a generalized hyperhidrosis, very fine body hair, and a peculiar dirty-colored skin. These latter features are reminiscent of hereditary ectodermal dysplasia, and in some reported cases all aspects of this disease are present. Calcification of the falx cerebri or dura is also frequently reported.

The etiology of the Papillon-Lefèvre syndrome is unknown, but has been suggested to be related to a generalized epithelial dysplasia. The disease is thought to be familial, probably transmitted as an autosomal recessive characteristic.

Juvenile periodontosis without skin manifestations is also known to occur, and this substantiates the opinion of some workers that different types of periodontosis with different etiologies exist.

Roentgenographic Features. The roentgenograms in cases of junvenile periodontitis exhibit varying degrees of "vertical" pocket formation with localized alveolar bone loss and widening of the periodontal ligament space (Fig. 15–39). This "vertical" pocket formation, with the bone loss often more extensive on one tooth than on an adjacent tooth, differs from the "horizontal" type of bone loss in periodontitis. In periodontitis many teeth are involved to about the same degree, so that the bone loss appears to be "horizontal."

Histologic Features. The histopathology of juvenile periodontitis has been described by Orban and Weinmann as follows:

First stage: In the first stage degeneration of the principal fibers of the periodontal membrane occurs with a localized widening of the periodontal membrane due to resorption of the alveolar bone. During this process a proliferation of the capillaries can be observed with development of a loose connective tissue. There is no inflammation in this stage and no

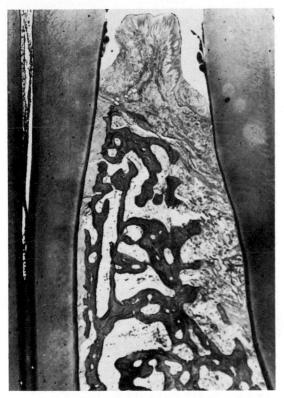

Figure 15–40. *Juvenile periodontitis.*
Photomicrograph of an early case. There is normal width of the periodontal membrane on the distal surface of the tooth on the left and degenerative connective tissue replacing the periodontal ligament on the mesial surface of the tooth on the right. Note also alveolar bone loss and lack of inflammation. (Courtesy of Dr. B. Orban and J. Periodontol.)

proliferation of the epithelial attachment. (Fig. 15–40.)

Second stage: The second stage is characterized by the proliferation of the epithelial attachment along the root surface. During this period there is a slight cellular infiltration in the connective tissue. These scattered cellular elements are of the plasma cell and polyblast type.

Third stage: In the third stage the epithelium of the proliferated attachment separates from the surface of the root, and deep gingival crevices develop. The inflammation increases due to irritation and infection from these deep crevices.

Treatment and Prognosis. The first step in the treatment of juvenile periodontitis should be the removal of those teeth that have a definitely hopeless prognosis because of looseness and loss of support or because they have moved so far out of alignment that they cannot be used. Teeth that have erupted so far that properly restored occlusion cannot be made should also be removed. Some teeth appear

hopeless when gingival inflammation is present, and the roentgenogram often reveals considerable loss of alveolar bone. Nevertheless such teeth frequently will be found favorable for further treatment after the usual routine procedure of scaling, polishing, and home care has been instituted.

The prognosis of juvenile periodontitis is less favorable than for other types of periodontal disease. The many factors that enter into the etiology of this disease make it exceedingly difficult to control, and at the same time the correction of systemic disturbances does not always result in an immediate response in the periodontal condition. Therefore the prognosis is not very encouraging. If a nutritional deficiency is corrected, the tooth affected by juvenile periodontitis may be repaired before pocket formation occurs. Sometimes a favorable change in the systemic condition may be brought about, resulting in repair in these areas; the teeth become firm in their new position, and no further progress of the disease is apparent.

PERIODONTAL TRAUMATISM

Excessive occlusal forces result in typical changes in the periodontal ligament and alveolar bone. If these abnormal occlusal forces are chronic and repeated over a long period of time, the periodontal ligament gradually becomes more dense, and the periodontal space widens. The alveolar bone becomes denser also and the teeth will show obvious "wear patterns," with definite facets on the crowns of teeth.

An acute traumatic force sufficient to produce traumatic injury to the periodontium also results in rather specific changes in the tooth attachment apparatus. For example, a force which tips a tooth sharply to the buccal results in a crushing of the periodontal ligament fibers and perhaps of the alveolar crest bone. The blood vessels in the involved area become thrombosed, and edema and extravasation of blood occur. On the opposite side of the tooth there is often a tearing of the periodontal ligament, and sometimes cementum or bone is torn loose. Since the tooth rotates around a fulcrum point slightly apical to the midroot, the same changes may occur near the apex on the opposite side. These changes result in tenderness of the tooth for a few days, but if the forces are not grossly excessive, eventually the damaged alveolar crest bone will be resorbed; new per-

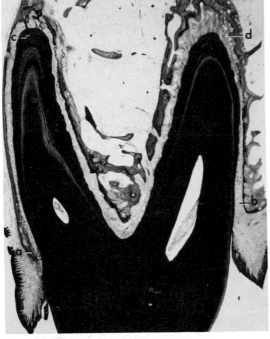

Figure 15–41. Periodontal traumatism.

A buccolingual section through the premolar of a rhesus monkey after excessive occlusal stresses had been applied for three days. Buccal alveolar margin (*a*), lingual alveolar margin (*b*), apex of mesiobuccal root (*c*), and apical area of lingual root (*d*). Note pressure necrosis at *a* and resorption of bone at *d*. (Courtesy of Dr. Frank M. Wentz: J. Periodontol., 29:117, 1958.)

iodontal fibers, cementum, and bone will be elaborated, and after a few weeks the tissues will return to normal, with the periodontal ligament space wider or the tooth reoriented in a new position.

When excessive forces occur in different and alternating directions, as may happen in cases of cusp interference, destruction of the supporting bone may occur around the entire periphery of the root, resulting in widening of the periodontal ligament space. This in turn, by interfering with mastication, favors collection of debris on teeth and predisposes to further periodontal disease.

Results of various types of trauma on the periodontium have been studied experimentally in laboratory animals. For example, Wentz and his co-workers subjected premolar teeth of rhesus monkeys to excessive occlusal stresses which tended to move the teeth buccally upon closure and lingually when the mouth was opened. Histologic studies after three days showed compression and pressure necrosis of the periodontal ligament, thrombosis of blood vessels, and beginning bone resorption at the buccal alveolar margin and lingual apical area (Figs. 15–41 and 15–42, A). Even though the excessive force was of but three days' duration, both areas also showed undermining resorption of alveolar bone, while on the opposite sides of

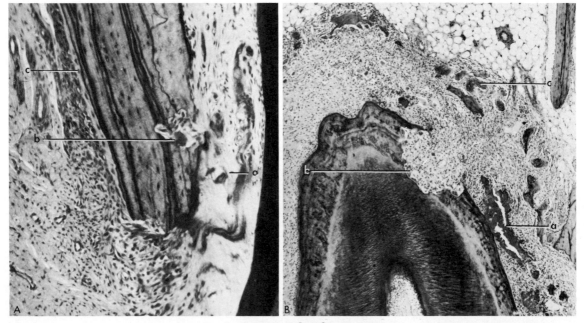

Figure 15–42. Periodontal traumatism.

A, Reaction of tissues after three days; high magnification of the pressure area (*a*) in Figure 15–41. Area of necrosis in the periodontal ligament (*a*), resorption of bone (*b*), and deposition of new bone (*c*). B, Reaction of tissues after 14 days; extensive necrosis near palatal root (*a*). Resorption has eliminated the area of compression (*b,c*). (Courtesy of Dr. Frank M. Wentz: J. Periodontol., 29:117, 1958.)

the root there was evidence of new bone formation on the endosteal surface of the alveolar bone. The characteristic cellular picture of inflammation was not present. After 14 days, the premolars used in the experiment were very loose. Histologic study revealed more extensive necrosis, undermining resorption of bone and adjoining root, and on the opposite side of the root, new bone formation (Fig. 15–42, *B*). After three and six months the involved teeth were still loose, but the traumatic tissue changes were no longer present. The periodontal ligament was lengthened, however, and the periodontal space was much wider (average 0.65 mm. as compared with 0.19 mm. in the control). New bone was noted on the buccal periosteal surface of the alveolar process. At no time was gingivitis or periodontitis noted. This experiment illustrates the damage to the periodontium that can occur from excessive occlusal stresses. If the damage is not enough to cause exfoliation of the tooth, the periodontium is gradually adapted to withstand the added stress.

In those cases in which the trauma is not immediately self-corrective it is imperative that correction of the occlusal relation, elimination of cuspal interference, and fixation or splinting of loose teeth be carried out to prevent further damage.

REFERENCES

Arnim, S. S., and Hagerman, D. A.: Connective tissue fibers of the marginal gingiva. J. Am. Dent. Assoc., 47:271, 1953.

Baer, P. N.: The case for periodontosis as a clinical entity. J. Periodontol., 42:516, 1971.

Idem: The relation of the physical character of the diet to the periodontium and periodontal disease. Oral Surg., 9:839, 1956.

Baer, P. N., and Newton, W. L.: The occurrence of periodontal disease in germfree mice. J. Dent. Res., 38:1238, 1959.

Baer, P. N., Stephan, R. M., and White, C. L.: Studies on experimental calculus formation in the rat. I. Effect of age, sex, strain, high carbohydrate, high protein diets. J. Periodontol., 32:190, 1961.

Becks, H.: Systemic background of paradentosis. J. Am. Dent. Assoc., 28:1447, 1941.

Belting, C. M.: A review of the epidemiology of periodontal diseases. J. Periodontol., 28:37, 1957.

Belting, C. M., and Gupta, O. P.: The influence of psychiatric disturbances on the severity of periodontal disease. J. Periodontol., 32:219, 1961.

Belting, C. M., Massler, M., and Schour, I.: Prevalence and incidence of alveolar bone disease in men. J. Am. Dent. Assoc., 47:190, 1953.

Bernstein, M. L., and McDonald, J. S.: Oral lesions in Crohn's disease: report of two cases and update of the literature. Oral Surg., 46:234, 1978.

Bibby, B. G.: A study of a pigmented dental plaque. J. Dent. Res., 11:855, 1931.

Bottomley, W. K., Giorgini, G. L., and Julienne, C. H.: Oral extension of regional enteritis (Crohn's disease). Oral Surg., 34:47, 1972.

Boyle, P. E., Bessey, O. A., and Wolbach, S. B.: Experimental production of the diffuse alveolar bone atrophy type of periodontal disease by diets deficient in ascorbic acid (vitamin C). J. Am. Dent. Assoc., 24:1768, 1937.

Brown, L. R., Mackler, B. F., Levy, B. M., Wright, T. E., Handler, S. F., Moylan, J. S., Perkins, D., and Keene, H. J.: Comparison of the plaque microflora in immunodeficient and immunocompetent dental patients. J. Dent. Res., 58:2344, 1979.

Brucker, M.: Studies on the incidence and cause of dental defects in children. III. Gingivitis. J. Dent. Res., 22:309, 1943.

Burnett, G. W., and Scherp, H. W.: Oral Microbiology and Infectious Disease. 3rd ed. Baltimore, Williams & Wilkins Company, 1968.

Cabrini, R. L., and Carranza, F. A., Jr.: Histochemical distribution of acid phosphates in human gingiva. J. Periodontol., 29:34, 1958.

Carranza, F. A., Jr., and Glickman, I.: Some observations on the microscopic features of infrabony pockets. J. Periodontol., 28:33, 1957.

Carter, W. J., and Ball, D. M.: Results of a three year study of Vincent's infection at the Great Lakes Naval Dental Department. J. Periodontol., 24:187, 1953.

Cianciola, L. J., Genco, R. J., Patters, M. R., McKenna, J., and Van Oss, C. J.: Defective polymorphonuclear leukocyte function in a human periodontal disease. Nature, 265:445, 1977.

Clark, R. A., Page, R. C., and Wilde, G.: Defective neutrophil chemotaxis in juvenile periodontitis. Infect. Immunol., 18:694, 1977.

Cohen, B.: Pathology of the interdental tissues. Dent. Pract., 9:167, 1959.

Cohen, B.: Morphological factors in the pathogenesis of periodontal disease. Br. Dent. J., 107:31,1959.

Idem: Studies of the interdental epithelial integument. (Abs.) J. Dent. Res., 38:219, 1959.

Coolidge, E., and Hine, M. K.: Periodontia. Philadelphia, Lea & Febiger, 1954.

Dewar, M. R.: Observations on the composition and metabolism of normal and inflamed gingivae. J. Periodontol., 26:29, 1955.

Idem: Mast cells in gingival tissue. J. Periodontol., 29:67, 1958.

Dinsdale, R. C. W., and Holt, K. S.: Activation of dental infection by cortisone. Studies in children with rheumatic fever. Ann. Rheum. Dis., 17:436, 1958.

Editorial : Scurvy and rickets are still with us. J.A.M.A., 137:465, 1948.

Eisenbud, L., Katzka, I., and Platt, J.: Oral manifestations in Crohn's disease. Oral Surg., 34:770, 1972.

Engel, M. B.: Water-soluble mucoproteins of the gingiva. J. Dent. Res., 32:779, 1953.

Engel, M. B., Ray, H. G., and Orban, B.: The pathogenesis of desquamative gingivitis: a disturbance of the connective tissue ground substance. J. Dent. Res., 29:410, 1950.

Ennever, J.: Intracellular calcification by oral filamentous microorganisms. J. Periodontol., 31:304, 1960.

Idem: Microbiologic mineralization: a calcifiable cellfree extract from a calcifiable microorganism. J. Dent. Res., 41:1381, 1962.

Ennever, J., Sturzenberger, O. P., and Radike, A. W.: Calculus surface index for scoring clinical calculus studies. J. Periodontol., 32:54, 1961.

Ennever, J., Vogel, J. J., Riggan, L. J., and Paoloski, S.
B.: Proteolipid and calculus matrix calcification in vitro.
J. Dent. Res., 56:140, 1977.

Ennever, J., Vogel, J. J., Boyan-Salyers, B., and Riggan,
L. J.: Characterization of calculus matrix calcification
nucleator. J. Dent. Res., 58:619, 1979.

Fish, W.: Etiology and prevention of periodontal breakdown,. Dent. Program, 1:234, 1961.

Fitzgerald, R. J., and McDaniel, E. G.: Dental calculus in
the germfree rat. Arch. Oral Biol., 2:239, 1960.

Forscher, B. K., Paulsen, A. G., and Hess, W. C.: The
pH of the periodontal pocket and the glycogen content
of the adjacent tissue. J. Dent. Res., 33:444, 1954.

Frandsen, A. M., Becks, H., Nelson, M. M., and Evans,
H. M.: The effects of various levels of dietary protein
on the periodontal tissue of young rats. J. Periodontol.,
24:135, 1953.

Frank, R. M., and Brendel, A.: Ultrastructure of the
approximal dental plaque and the underlying normal
and carious enamel. Arch. Oral Biol., 11:883, 1966.

Fullmer, H. M.: Observations on the development of
oxytalan fibers in the periodontium of man. J. Dent.
Res., 38:510, 1959.

Idem: Observations on the development of oxytalan fibers
in dental granulomas and radicular cysts. Arch. Pathol.,
70:59, 1960.

Idem: A histochemical study of periodontal disease in the
maxillary alveolar processes of 135 autopsies. J. Periodontol., 32:206, 1961.

Idem: A critique of normal connective tissues of the periodontium and some alterations with periodontal disease. J. Dent. Res., 41:223, 1962.

Gavin, J. B., and Collins, A. A.: The occurrence of bacteria
within the clinically healthy gingival crevice. J. Periodontol., 32:198, 1961.

Glickman, I.: Acute vitamin C deficiency and periodontal
disease. J. Dent. Res., 27:201, 1948.

Glickman, I., and Smulow, J. B.: Chronic desquamative
gingivitis—its nature and treatment. J. Periodontol.,
35:397, 1964.

Idem: Histopathology and histochemistry of chronic desquamative gingivitis. Oral Surg., 21:325, 1966.

Glickman, I., Morse, A., and Robinson, L.: The systemic
influence upon bone in periodontoclasia. J. Am. Dent.
Assoc., 31:1435, 1944.

Goldhaber, P., and Giddon, D. B.: Present concepts concerning the etiology and treatment of acute necrotizing
ulcerative gingivitis. Int. Dent. J., 14:468, 1964.

Goldman, H. M.: Periodontosis in the spider monkey. J.
Periodontol., 18:34, 1947.

Idem: The topography and role of the gingival fibers. J.
Dent. Res., 30:331, 1951.

Idem: Histologic topographic changes of inflammatory origin in the gingival fibers. J. Periodontol., 23:104, 1952.

Idem: The behavior of transseptal fibers. J. Dent. Res.,
36:249, 1957.

Idem: The extension of exudate into supporting structures
of teeth in marginal periodontitis. J Periodontol.,
28:175, 1957.

Goldman, H. M., and Cohen, D. W.: The infrabony pocket:
classification and treatment. J. Periodontol., 29:272,
1958.

Goldman, H. M., and Ruben, M. P.: Desquamative gingivitis and its response to topical triamcinolone therapy. Oral Surg., 21:579, 1966.

Gorlin, R. J., Sedano, H., and Anderson, V. E.: The
syndrome of palmar-plantar hyperkeratosis and premature periodontal destruction of the teeth. J. Pediatr., 65:895, 1964.

Gottlieb, B.: Etiology and therapy of alveolar pyorrhea.
Zeitschr. Stomatol., 18:59, 1920.

Idem: Diffuse atrophy of the alveolar bone. Zeitschr. Stomatol., 21:195, 1923.

Grant, D. A., and Orban, B.: Leukocytes in the epithelial
attachment. J. Periodontol., 31:87, 1960.

Greene, J. C., and Vermillion, J. R.: The simplified oral
hygiene index. J. Am. Dent. Assoc., 68:7, 1964.

Hampp, E. G., and Mergenhagen, S. E.: Experimental
infections with oral spirochetes. J. Infect. Dis., 109:43,
1961.

Hawes, R. R.: Report of three patients experiencing juvenile periodontosis and early loss of teeth. J. Dent.
Child., 27:169, 1960.

Henry, J. L., and Weinmann, J. P.: The pattern of resorption and repair of human cementum. J. Am. Dent.
Assoc., 42:270, 1951.

Hiatt, W. H., and Orban, B.: Hyperkeratosis of the oral
mucous membrane. J. Periodontol. 31:96, 1960.

Horton, J. E., Leikin, S., and Oppenheim, J. J.: Human
lympho-proliferative reaction to saliva and dental
plaque deposits: an in vitro correlation with periodontal
disease. J. Periodontol., 43:522, 1972.

Howell, A., Rizzo, A., and Paul, F.: Cultivable bacteria in
developing and mature human dental calculus. Arch.
Oral Biol., 10:307, 1965.

Ingle, J. I.: Papillon-Lefèvre syndrome: precocious periodontosis with associated epidermal lesions. J. Periodontol., 30:230, 1959.

Ivanyi, L., and Lehner, T.: Lymphocyte transformation by
sonicates of dental plaque in human periodontal disease. Arch. Oral Biol., 16:1117, 1971.

Kardachi, B. J., and Newcomb, G. M.: A clinical study of
gingival inflammation and renal transplant recipients
taking immunosuppressive drugs. J. Periodontol.,
49:307, 1978.

Kaslick, R. S., and Chasens, A. I.: Periodontosis with
periodontitis: a study involving young adult males. Part
I. Review of the literature and incidence in a military
population. Part II. Clinical, medical, and histopathologic studies. Oral Surg., 25:305, 327, 1968.

Katchburian, F.: Histochemical study of sulfhydryl (cysteine) and bisulfide (cystine) groups in human gingiva.
J. Periodontol., 31:154, 1960.

Kerr, D. A.: Stomatitis and gingivitis in the adolescent and
preadolescent. J. Am. Dent. Assoc., 44:27, 1952.

Kerr, D. A., McClatchey, K. D., and Regezi, J. A.: Allergic
gingivostomatitis (due to gum chewing). J. Periodontol., 42:709, 1971.

Idem: Idiopathic gingivostomatitis. Cheilitis, glossitis, gingivitis syndrome; atypical gingivostomatitis, plasma-
cell gingivitis, plasmacytosis of gingiva. Oral Surg.,
32:402, 1971.

King, J. D.: Nutritional and other factors in "trench mouth,"
with special reference to the nicotinic acid component
of the vitamin B_2 complex. Br. Dent. J., 74:113, 1943.

Klemperer, P.: The concept of collagen diseases. Am. J.
Pathol., 26:505, 1950.

Klingsburge, J., Cancellaro, L., and Butcher, E.: Effects
of aging on exteriorized rodent oral mucous membranes. I.A.D.R. Preprinted abst., 1960.

Kohl, J. T., and Zander, H. A.: Morphology of interdental
gingival tissues. Oral Surg., 14:287, 1961.

Kornman, K. S., and Loesche, W. J.: The subgingival
microbial flora during pregnancy. J. Periodont. Res.,
15:111, 1980.

Lavine, W. S., Maderazo, E. G., Stolman, J., Ward, P.
A., Cogen, R. B., Greenblatt, I., and Robertson, P.
B.: Impaired neutrophil chemotaxis in patients with

juvenile and rapidly progressing periodontitis. J. Periodont. Res., *14*:10, 1979.

Leach, S. A., and Saxton, C. A.: An electron microscopic study of the acquired pellicle and plaque formed on the enamel of human incisors. Arch. Oral Biol., *11*:1081, 1966.

Idem: The uneven distribution of calculus in the mouth. J. Periodontol., *22*:7, 1951.

Levy, B. M., Robertson, P. B., Dreizen, S., Mackler, B. F., and Bernick, S.: Adjuvant induced destructive periodontitis in nonhuman primates—a comparative study. J. Periodont. Res., *11*:54, 1976.

Lewis, T. M.: Gingival traumatization—a habit. J. Periodontol., *33*:353, 1962.

Liljenberg, B., and Lindhe, J.: Juvenile periodontitis. Some microbiological, histopathological and clinical characteristics. J. Clin. Periodontol., *70*:48, 1980.

Linghorne, W. J., and O'Connel, D. C.: Studies in the regeneration and reattachment of supporting structures of the teeth. I. Soft tissue reattachment. J. Dent. Res., *29*:419, 1950.

Listgarten, M. A.: Electron microscopic observations on the bacterial flora of acute necrotizing ulcerative gingivitis. J. Periodontol., *36*:328, 1965.

Listgarten, M. A., and Lewis, D. W.: The distribution of spirochetes in the lesion of acute necrotizing ulcerative gingivitis: an electron microscopic and statistical survey. J. Periodontol., *38*:379, 1967.

Löe, H.: The specific etiology of periodontal disease and its application to prevention; in F. A. Carranza and E. B. Kenney (eds.): Prevention of Periodontal Disease. Chicago, Quintessence Publishing Co., 1981.

Löe, H., Theilade, E., and Jensen, S. B.: Experimental gingivitis in man. J. Periodontol., *36*:177, 1965.

Looby, J. P.: in L. W. Burket (ed.): Oral Medicine. 6th ed. Philadelphia, J. B. Lippincott Company, 1971.

Macapanpan, L. C., Meyer, J., and Weinmann, J. P.: Mitotic activity of fibroblasts after damage to the periodontal membrane of rat molars. J. Periodontol., *25*:105, 1954.

MacDonald, J. B.: The Motile Non-Sporulating Anaerobic Rods of the Oral Cavity. Toronto, University of Toronto Press, 1953.

Mackler, B. F., Altman, L. C., Wahl, S., Rosenstreich, D. L., Oppenheim, J. J., and Mergenhagen, S. E.: Blastogenesis and lymphokine synthesis by T and B lymphocytes from patients with periodontal disease. Infect. Immunol., *10*:844, 1974.

Mackler, B. F., Faner, R. M., Schur, P., Wright, T. E., and Levy, B. M.: IgG subclasses in human periodontal disease. I. Distribution and incidence of IgG subclass bearing lymphocytes and plasma cells. J. Periodont. Res., *13*:109, 1978.

MacPhee, T., and Cowley, G.: Essentials of Periodontology and Periodontics. 3rd ed., Oxford, England, Blackwell Scientific Publications, 1981.

Maier, A. W., and Orban, B.: Gingivitis in pregnancy. Oral Surg., *2*:234, 1949.

Mandel, I., and Thompson, R. H.: The chemistry of parotid and submaxillary saliva in heavy calculus formers and non-formers. J Periodontol., *38*:310, 1967.

Mandel, I. D.: Plaque and calculus. Alabama J. Med. Sci., *5*:313, 1968.

Mandel, I. D., and Levy, B. M.: Studies on salivary calculus. I. Histochemical and chemical investigations of supra- and subgingival calculus. Oral Surg., *10*:874, 1957.

Mandel, I. D., Levy, B. M., and Wasserman, B. H.: Histochemistry of calculus formation. J. Periodontol., *28*:132, 1957.

Manson, J. D.: Juvenile periodontitis (periodontosis). Int. Dent. J., *27*:114, 1977.

Marshall-Day C. D.: The epidemiology of periodontal disease. J. Periodontol., *22*:13, 1951.

Marshall-Day, C. D., Stephens, R. G., and Quigley, L. F., Jr.: Periodontal disease; prevalence and incidence. J. Periodontol., *26*:185, 1955.

Massler, M., Schour, I., and Chopra, B.: Occurrence of gingivitis in suburban Chicago school children. J. Periodontol., *21*:146, 1950.

Massler, M., Rosenberg, H. M., Carter, W., and Schour, I.: Gingivitis in young adult males: lack of effectiveness of a permissive program of toothbrushing. J. Periodontol., *28*:111, ·1957.

McCarthy, F. P., McCarthy, P. L., and Shklar, G.: Chronic desquamative gingivitis: a reconsideration. Oral Surg., *13*:1300, 1960.

McCarthy, P. L., and Shklar, G.: Diseases of the Oral Mucosa. 2nd ed. Philadelphia, Lea & Febiger, 1980.

McDougall, W. F.: Studies on dental plaque. II. The histology of the developing interproximal plaque. Aust. Dent. J., *8*:398, 1963.

McHugh, W. D. (ed.): Dental Plaque. Edinburgh and London, E. & S. Livingston Ltd., 1970.

Meckel, A. H.: The formation and properties of organic films on teeth. Arch. Oral Biol., *10*:585, 1965.

Miller, S. C., and Firestone, J. M.: Psychosomatic factors in the etiology of periodontal disease. Am. J. Orthod. Oral Surg., *33*:675, 1947.

Muhlemann, H. R., and Schneider, V. K.: Early calculus formation. Helvetica Odont. Acta, *3*:22, 1959.

Newman, M. G., and Socransky, S. S.: Predominant cultivable microbiota in periodontosis. J. Periodont. Res. *12*:120, 1977.

Nisengard, R. J., and Neiders, M.: Desquamative lesions of the gingiva. J. Periodontol., *52*:500, 1981.

Nuckolls, J.: Development of the periodontal lesion. J. Periodontol., *23*:149, 191, 1952.

Orban, B.: Classification and nomenclature of periodontal diseases (based on pathology, etiology, and clinical picture). J. Periodontol., *13*:88, 1942.

Idem: Histopathology of periodontal diseases. Am. J. Orthod. Oral Surg., *33*:637, 1947.

Orban, B., and Weinmann, J. P.: Diffuse atrophy of the alveolar bone. J. Periodontol., *13*:31, 1942.

Orban, B., Bhatia, H., Kollar, J. A., and Wentz, F. M.: The epithelial attachment (the attached epithelial cuff). J. Periodontol., *27*:167, 1956.

Orstavik, D., and Brandtzaeg, P.: Secretion of parotid IgA in relation to gingival inflammation and dental caries experience in man. Arch. Oral Biol. *20*:701, 1975.

Page, R. C., and Schroeder, H. E.: Pathogenesis of inflammatory periodontal disease. A summary of current work. Lab. Invest., *33*:3235, 1976.

Papillon, M. M., and Lefèvre, P.: De cas de keratodermie palmaire et plantaire symetrique familiale (maladie de Meleda) chez le frère et la soeur. Coexistence dans les deux cas d'alterations dentaires graves. Bull. Soc. Fr. Dermatol. Syphilgr., *31*:82, 1924.

Pickerill, H. P.: A sign of immunity. Br. Dent. J., *44*:967, 1923.

Pierce, H. B., Newhall, C. A., Merrow, S. B., Lamden, M. P., Schweiker, C., and Laughlin, A.: Ascorbic acid supplementation. I. Response of gum tissue. Am. J. Clin. Nutri., *8*:353, 1960.

Pritchard, J.: The infrabony technic as a predictable procedure. J. Periodontol., *28*:202, 1957.

Ramfjord, S.: Experimental periodontal reattachment in rhesus monkeys. J. Periodontol., *22*:67, 1951.

Idem: The histopathology of inflammatory gingival enlargement. Oral Surg., 6:516, 1953.

Reeve, C. M., and Wentz, F.: Epithelial rests in human periodontal ligament. Oral Surg., 15:785, 1962.

Report of Committee on Classification and Nomenclature. J. Periodontol., 28:56, 1957.

Ritz, H. L.: Microbial population shifts in developing human dental plaque. Arch. Oral Biol., 12:1561, 1967.

Robertson, P. B., Mackler, B. F., Wright, T. E., and Levy, B. M.: Periodontal status of patients with abnormalities of the immune system. II. Observations over a 2-year period. J. Periodontol. 51:70, 1980.

Rogers, R. S., III, Sheridan, P. J., and Jordan, R. E.: Desquamative gingivitis. Clinical, histopathologic, and immunopathologic investigations. Oral Surg., 42:316, 1976.

Rosebury, T.: The nature and significance of infection in periodontal disease. Am. J. Orthod. Oral Surg., 33:658, 1947.

Idem: The role of infection in periodontal disease. Oral Surg., 5:363, 1952.

Rosebury, T., MacDonald, J. B., and Clark, A.: A bacteriologic survey of gingival scrapings from periodontal infections by direct examination, guinea pig inoculation and anaerobic cultivation. J. Dent. Res., 29:718, 1950.

Rosenthal, S. L., and Gootzeit, E.: Incidence of B. fusiformis and spirochetes in the edentulous mouth. J. Dent. Res., 21:373, 1942.

Russell, B. J.: Gingival changes in diabetes mellitus. I. Vascular changes. Acta Pathol. Microbiol. Scand., 68:161, 1966.

Saxén, L.: Juvenile periodontitis. J. Clin. Periodontol., 7:1, 1980.

Saxén, L.: Heredity of juvenile periodontitis. J. Clin. Periodontol., 7:276, 1980.

Schaffer, E. M.: Biopsy studies of necrotizing ulcerative gingivitis. J. Periodontol., 24:22, 1953.

Scherp, H. W.: Discussion of bacterial factors in periodontal disease. J. Dent. Res., 41:suppl. to No. 1:327, 1962.

Schluger, S.: Necrotizing ulcerative gingivitis in the army: incidence, communicability and treatment. J. Am. Dent. Assoc., 38:174, 1949.

Schour, I., and Massler, M.: Gingival disease (gingivosis) in hospitalized children in Naples (1945). Am. J. Orthod. Oral Surg., 33:757, 1947.

Schwartzman, J., and Grossman, L.: Vincent's ulceromembranous gingivostomatitis. Arch. Pediatr., 58:515, 1941.

Shourie, K. L.: Mesenteric line or pigmented plaque:a sign of comparative freedom from caries. J. Am. Dent. Assoc., 35:805, 1947.

Slots, J.: The microflora of black stain on human primary teeth. Scand. J. Dent. Res., 82:484, 1974.

Slots, J.: The predominant cultivable microflora of advanced periodontitis. Scand. J. Dent. Res., 85:114, 1977.

Slots, J., Moen, D. O., Langebaek, J., and Frandsen, A.: Microbiota of gingivitis in man. Scand. J. Dent. Res., 86:174, 1978.

Smith, D. T.: Oral Spirochetes and Related Organisms in Fuso-Spirochetal Disease. Baltimore, Williams & Wilkins Company, 1932.

Smith, G. H.: Factors affecting the deposition of dental calculus. Aust. J. Dent., 34:305, 1930.

Socransky, S. S.: Microbiology of periodontal disease—present status and future considerations. J. Periodontol., 48:497, 1977.

Sönju, T. and Rölla, G.: Chemical analysis of pellicle formed in two hours on cleaned human teeth in vivo. Rate of formation and amino acid analysis. Caries Res., 7:30, 1973.

Stammers, A. F.: Vincent's infection; observations and conclusions regarding the aetiology and treatment of 1,017, civilian cases. Br. Dent., J., 76:147, 1947.

Stones, H. H.: Oral and Dental Diseases. 5th ed. Baltimore, Williams & Wilkins Company, 1966.

Swenson, H. M., and Muhler, J. C.: Induced fusospirochetal infection in dogs. J. Dent. Res., 26:161, 1947.

Tanner, A.C.R., Haffergee, C., Bratthall, G. T., Visconti, R. A., and Socransky, S. S.: A study of the bacteria associated with advancing periodontal disease in man. J. Clin. Periodontol., 6:278, 1979.

Tenenbaum, B., and Karshan, M.: The composition and formation of salivary calculus. J. Periodontol., 15:72, 1944.

Theilade, J., Fitzgerald, R. J., Scott, D. B., and Nylen, M.: Electron microscopic observations of dental calculus in germfree and conventional rats. Arch. Oral Biol., 9:97, 1964.

Thoma, K. H.: Vincent's infection or fusospirochetosis. Am. J. Orthod. Oral Surg., 27:479, 1941.

Tollefsen, T., Soltvedt, E., and Koppang, H. S.: The effect of immunosuppressive agents on periodontal disease in man. J. Periodont. Res. 13:240, 1978.

Tollefsen, T., Koppang, H. S., and Messelt, E.: Immunosuppression and periodontal disease in man. Histological and ultrastructural observations. J. Periodont. Res. 17:329, 1982.

Turesky, S., Glickman, I., and Litwin, T.: A histochemical evaluation of normal and inflamed human gingivae. J. Dent. Res., 30:792, 1951.

van Palenstein Helderman, W. H.: Microbial etiology of periodontal disease. J. Clin. Periodontol., 8:261, 1981.

Vogel, R. I., and Deasy, M. J.: Juvenile periodontitis (periodontosis): current concepts. J. Am. Dent. Assoc., 97:843, 1978.

Volpe, A. R., Manhold, J. H., and Hazen, S. P.: In vivo calculus assessment: a method and its reproducibility. J. Periodontol., 36:292, 1965.

Waerhaug, J.: The gingival pocket. Odontol. Tidsk., 60:Suppl. 1, 1952.

Idem: Pathogenesis of pocket formation in traumatic occlusion. J. Periodontol., 26:107, 1955.

Wallman, I. S., and Hilton, H. B.: Teeth pigmented by tetracycline. Lancet, 1:827, 1962.

Wasserman, B. H., Mandel, I. D., and Levy, B. M.: In vitro calcification of dental calculus. J. Periodontol., 29:144, 1958.

Weinmann, J. P.: Progress of gingival inflammation into the supporting structures of the teeth. J. Periodontol., 12:71, 1941.

Weiss, M. D., Weinmann, J. P., and Meyer, J.: Degree of keratinization and glycogen content in the uninflamed and inflamed gingiva and alveolar mucosa. J. Periodontol., 30:208, 1959.

Wentz, F. M., Jarabak, J., and Orban, B.: Experimental occlusal trauma imitating cuspal interferences. J. Periodontol., 29:117, 1958.

Whitten, J. B., Jr.: The fine structure of desquamative stomatitis. J. Periodontol., 39:75, 1968.

World Health Organization: Epidemiology, etiology and prevention of periodontal diseases. Technical Report Series No. 621, Geneva, W.H.O., 1978.

Zander, H. A.: The attachment of calculus to root surfaces. J. Periodontol., 24:16, 1953.

Ziskin, D. E.: Effects of male sex hormone on gingivae and oral mucous membranes. J. Dent. Res., *20*:419, 1941.

Ziskin, D. E., and Blackberg, S. N.: The effect of castration and hypophysectomy on the gingival and oral mucous membranes of rhesus monkeys. J. Dent. Res., *19*:381, 1940.

Ziskin, D. E., and Moulton, R.: A comparison of oral and vaginal smears. J. Clin. Endocrinol., 8:2, 1948.

Ziskin, D. E., and Nesse, G. J.: Pregnancy gingivitis: history, classification, etiology, Am. J. Orthod. Oral Surg., *32*:390, 1946.

Ziskin, D. E., and Zegarelli, E. V.: Chronic desquamative gingivitis. Am. J. Orthod. Oral Surg., *31*:1, 1945.

Ziskin, D. E., Blackberg, S. N., and Slanetz, C. A.: Effects of subcutaneous injections of estrogenic and gonadotrophic hormones on gums and oral mucous membrane of normal and castrated rhesus monkeys. J. Dent. Res., *15*:407, 1936.

Ziskin, D. E., Zegarelli, E. V., and Slanetz, C.: Estrogen implants in dogs. Am. J. Orthod. Oral Surg., *33*:723, 1947.

CHAPTER 16

Diseases of the Skin

Dermatology, the specialized study of skin diseases, has become an important subdivision of the practice of medicine not only because of the many primary diseases that affect the skin, but also because of the common cutaneous manifestations of deeper visceral or systemic diseases. The dermatologist is well aware that many primary cutaneous diseases also involve the mucous membranes throughout the body, including the oral mucosa.

It is especially important for the dentist to recognize not only that some dermatoses exhibit concomitant lesions of the oral mucous membranes, but also that manifestation of some of the diseases may be preceded by oral lesions. Thus the dentist may be in a position to establish the diagnosis of a dermatologic disease before the cutaneous lesions become apparent.

There is no universally accepted classification of these dermatologic diseases. However, several broad groups of diseases may be separated out, all of which have significant interest to dentistry, on the basis of the nature of the disease process or the nature of the lesion itself.

One large group of specific lesions which has been recognized in recent years is that known as the *genodermatoses*. These basically represent hereditary skin disorders, many of which are also accompanied by various systemic manifestations of different altered enzyme functions. Some of these genodermatoses are characterized particularly by alterations in the normal keratinization process and these have been specifically referred to as *genokeratoses*. Unfortunately, there are numerous defects and considerable overlap in even such a simple scheme. There are, for example, numerous diseases characterized by alterations in the keratinization process which are not genetically transmitted and, therefore, are not genokeratoses. There is considerable value in classifying certain dermatologic diseases as vesiculobullous diseases because of the aid provided in the differential diagnosis of a given case in which vesicles and bullae are present. However, some of the vesiculobullous diseases are genetically transmitted and thus could also be classified as genodermatoses, while others have no hereditary pattern.

The dermatologic diseases with oral manifestations of one type or another that are discussed in this chapter are grouped for greatest ease of understanding because of certain similarities which exist.

HEREDITARY HYPOHIDROTIC (ANHIDROTIC) ECTODERMAL DYSPLASIA

Hereditary hypohidrotic (anhidrotic) ectodermal dysplasia is a specific syndrome characterized by a congenital dysplasia of one or more ectodermal structures and their accessory appendages, manifested primarily by hypohidrosis, hypotrichosis and hypodontia. It is the most common type of the various ectodermal dysplasias which, as a group, may present abnormalities of the skin, hair, nails, eyes, teeth, facies, sensorineural apparatus and adnexal glandular structures in various combinations and of varying severity. A listing of the more widely recognized main groups of ectodermal dysplasia has been reviewed by Giansanti and his associates but, because of their infrequent occurrence, they are not discussed here.

In the majority of cases of hereditary hypohidrotic (anhidrotic) ectodermal dysplasia it is an X-linked recessive mendelian character, males being affected much more frequently than females. However, in some forms the abnormality can also be transmitted as an autosomal dominant or recessive characteristic.

The term "congenital ectodermal defect," which has been applied to some cases of hereditary ectodermal dysplasia, is a less desirable term because it has often been used also to refer to a variety of other unrelated minor ectodermal aberrations.

Clinical Features. Patients with hereditary hypohidrotic (anhidrotic) ectodermal dysplasia usually exhibit a soft, smooth, thin, dry skin with partial or complete absence of sweat glands. Such persons cannot perspire, and they consequently suffer from hyperpyrexia and an inability to endure warm temperatures. Infants often exhibit this as their first symptom of the disease, developing unexplained fever with elevation of temperature. The sebaceous glands and hair follicles are often defective or absent.

The hair of the scalp and eyebrows tends to be fine, scanty and blond and resembles lanugo, which, in fact, is often absent. However, the mustache and beard are usually normal in appearance. The bridge of the nose is depressed; the supraorbital ridges and frontal bosses are pronounced and the lips protuberant (Fig. 16–1, A). It has been said that the facial appearance of these individuals is quite characteristic and that they resemble each other enough to be mistaken for siblings.

Koszewski and Hubbard reported a 25 per cent incidence of refractory chronic anemia in patients with hereditary ectodermal dysplasia.

Oral Manifestations. The oral findings are of particular interest, since patients with this abnormality invariably manifest anodontia or oli-

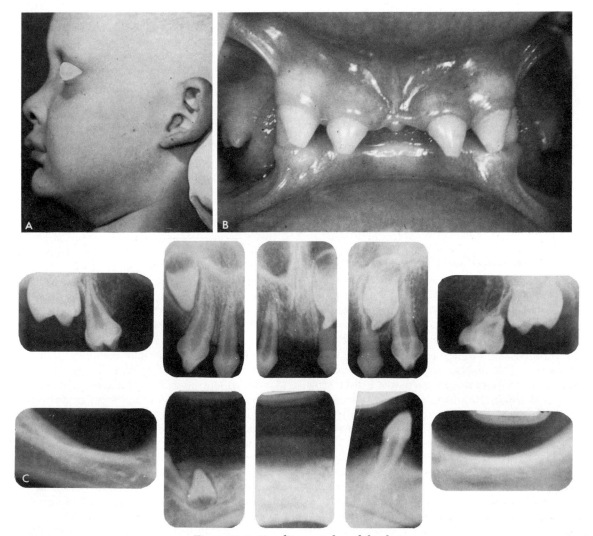

Figure 16–1. *Hereditary ectodermal dysplasia.*
A, The protuberant lips, the thin, scanty hair and the saddle-nose are characteristic of the disease. *B*, The teeth are cone-shaped. *C*, Roentgenogram shows congenitally missing teeth. (Courtesy of Dr. Ralph E. McDonald.)

godontia, complete or partial absence of teeth, with frequent malformation of any teeth present, both deciduous and permanent dentitions (Fig. 16–1, *B, C*). Where some teeth are present, they are commonly truncated or cone-shaped. It should be pointed out that even when complete anodontia exists, the growth of the jaw is not impaired. This would imply that the development of the jaws, except for the alveolar process, is not dependent upon the presence of teeth. However, since the alveolar process does not develop in the absence of teeth, there is a reduction from the normal vertical dimension resulting in the protuberant lips. In addition, the palatal arch is frequently high and a cleft palate may be present.

According to Bessermann-Nielsen, the salivary glands, including the intraoral accessory glands, are sometimes hypoplastic in this disease. This results in xerostomia, and the protuberant lips may be dry and cracked with pseudorhagades formation. As a related phenomenon, there may be hypoplasia of the nasal and pharyngeal mucous glands which leads to chronic rhinitis and/or pharyngitis, sometimes with associated dysphagia and hoarseness.

Treatment. There is no treatment for the condition, although, from a dental standpoint, partial or full dentures should be constructed for both functional and cosmetic purposes. Dentures may be used even in relatively young patients, but they must be reconstructed periodically as the jaws continue to grow.

CHONDROECTODERMAL DYSPLASIA

(Ellis-van Creveld Syndrome)

This uncommon disease is not classified as a dermatologic disease but is discussed here because of the similarity of certain of its features to those of hereditary anhidrotic ectodermal dysplasia. The disease appears to be inherited as an autosomal recessive characteristic with parental consanguinity in about 30 per cent of the cases. McKusick and his co-workers reported 52 cases of this condition among 30 families in an Amish isolate.

Clinical Features. Chondroectodermal dysplasia is characterized by a number of ectodermal disturbances, including involvement of the nails and teeth as well as chondrodysplasia, polydactyly and sometimes congenital heart disease.

The nails are generally hypoplastic with marked koilonychia. The sweat mechanism has been reported to be normal in contrast to that in hereditary anhidrotic ectodermal dysplasia. The arms and legs are shortened and thickened. The bilateral polydactyly affects the hands and occasionally the feet. Many additional malformations are often present, although cardiac abnormalities are present in only about half of all cases.

Oral Manifestations. A discussion of both the systemic and oral manifestations of the disease has been published by Gorlin and Pindborg, by McKusick and his associates and by Winter and Geddes.

The most constant oral finding is a fusion of the middle portion of the upper lip to the maxillary gingival margin eliminating the normal mucolateral sulcus. Thus, the middle portion of the upper lip appears hypoplastic.

Natal teeth, prematurely erupted deciduous teeth, frequently occur as well as congenital absence of teeth, particularly in the anterior mandibular segment. Tooth eruption is often delayed and those erupted are commonly defective, being small, cone-shaped, irregularly spaced and demonstrating enamel hypoplasia. Supernumerary teeth are also reported.

Treatment. There is no treatment for the disease. Some patients die in early childhood.

LICHEN PLANUS

(Lichen Ruber Planus)

Lichen planus is of particular interest to the dentist because involvement of the oral mucous membranes so frequently accompanies or precedes the appearance of lesions on the skin. It is one of the most common dermatologic diseases to manifest itself in the oral cavity and, therefore, should be completely familiar to the dentist, particularly since the diagnosis can often be established without a biopsy.

Clinical Features. The skin lesions of lichen planus appear as small, angular, flat-topped papules only a few millimeters in diameter. These may be discrete or gradually coalesce into larger plaques, each of which is covered by a fine, glistening scale. The papules are sharply demarcated from the surrounding skin. Early in the course of the disease the lesions appear red, but they soon take on a reddish-purple or violaceous hue. Later, a dirty brownish color develops. The center of the papule may be slightly umbilicated. Its surface is covered by characteristic, very fine grayish-white lines, called Wickham's striae. The lesions may

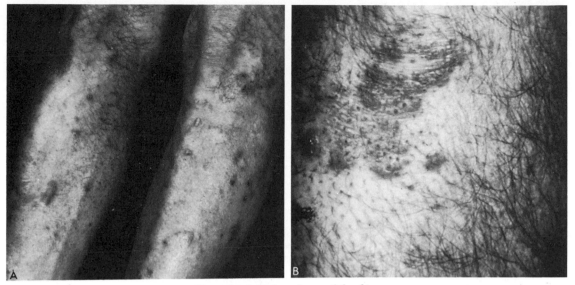

Figure 16–2. *Lichen planus of the skin.*

occur anywhere on the skin surface, but usually are distributed in a bilaterally symmetrical pattern, most often on the flexor surfaces of the wrist and forearms, the inner aspect of the knees and thighs, and the trunk, especially the sacral area (Fig. 16–2). The face frequently remains uninvolved. In chronic cases, hypertrophic plaques may develop, especially over the shins. The primary symptom of lichen planus is a severe pruritus that may be intolerable.

Lichen planus is a disease of adulthood, but occasionally children are affected. It is without a dramatic sex predilection in its occurrence, although females are affected somewhat more often than males in most reported series of cases.

The *etiology* of lichen planus is not known. It is interesting to note that the disease seldom is seen in carefree persons; the nervous, high-strung person is almost invariably the one in whom the condition develops. The course of the disease is long, from months to several years, frequently undergoing periods of remission followed by exacerbations which often correspond to periods of emotional upset, overwork, anxiety or some form of mental strain. Other causes suggested include traumatism (since outbreaks often develop along scratch lines), malnutrition and infection. The presence of immunoglobulins and complement has been reported at the epidermal-dermal junction of skin cases of lichen planus, thus suggesting a possible immune factor in the disease. However, this was far less conclusive in the oral lichen planus studies of Schiödt and his associates, of Daniels and Quadra-White and of Walker.

An interesting association of lichen planus, diabetes mellitus and vascular hypertension has been described by Grinspan, the triad being described as Grinspan's syndrome by Grupper. However, in a group of over 120 patients with oral lichen planus, Christensen and his co-workers could find neither a relationship to hypertension, as based on arterial pressure, nor any difference between the glucose tolerance of these patients and that of general population samples.

In addition, lichen planus has been reported in several members of one family, raising the question of a hereditary pattern. There is no sound evidence for this idea, however.

Oral Manifestations. The majority of patients with dermal lichen planus have associated oral lesions of the disease, according to the study of Shklar and McCarthy. Conversely, in a study of 115 patients with oral lichen planus by Andreasen, only 44 per cent had skin lesions as well.

In oral lichen planus, females are also affected more frequently than males. In the study of 326 such patients reported by Kovesi and Bánóczy, 63 per cent were women, while of 200 patients reported by Silverman and Griffith, 65 per cent were women. Similar to those with skin lichen planus, the majority of the patients were between 40 and 70 years of age.

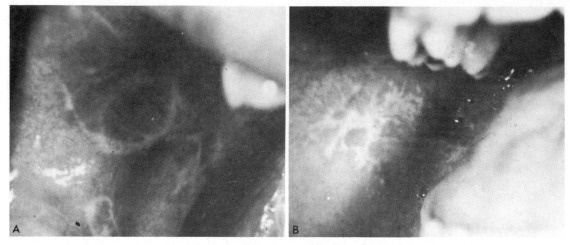

Figure 16–3. *Lichen planus of the buccal mucosa.*
These cases illustrate the typical patterns which the oral lesions assume.

In the oral cavity, the disease assumes a somewhat different clinical appearance than on the skin, and classically is characterized by lesions consisting of radiating white or gray, velvety, threadlike papules in a linear, annular or retiform arrangement forming typical lacy, reticular patches, rings and streaks over the buccal mucosa and to a lesser extent on the lips, tongue and palate. A tiny white elevated dot is frequently present at the intersection of the white lines, known here also as the striae of Wickham. When plaquelike lesions occur, radiating striae may often be seen on their periphery.

Shklar and McCarthy have reported the following distribution of oral lesions: buccal mu-

cosa, 80 per cent; tongue, 65 per cent; lips, 20 per cent; gingiva, floor of mouth and palate, less than 10 per cent (Figs. 16–3, 16–4). These oral lesions produce no significant symptoms, although occasionally patients will complain of a burning sensation in the involved areas. (See also Plate VII.)

Vesicle and bulla formation has been reported in oral lesions of lichen planus, but this is not a common finding, and the diagnosis of lichen planus from the clinical appearance of the lesions is extremely difficult. This *bullous* form of lichen planus has been discussed by Shklar and Andreasen. Still another type, the so-called *erosive* form of lichen planus, usually begins as such and not as a progressive process from

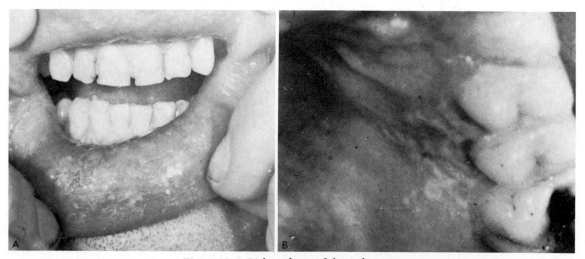

Figure 16–4. *Lichen planus of the oral mucosa.*
Lichen planus of the lips *(A)*, palate and gingiva *(B)*. *(A,* Courtesy of Dr. Edward V. Zegarelli.)

PLATE VII

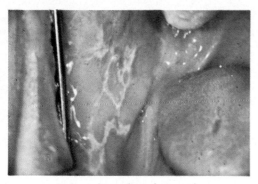

Lichen planus (buccal mucosa)

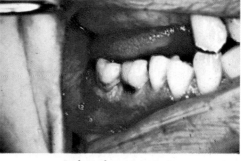

Lichen planus (gingiva)

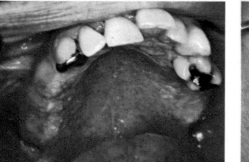

Lichen planus (palate)

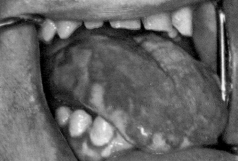

Stevens-Johnson syndrome

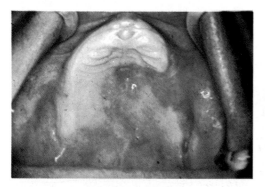

Pemphigus vulgaris

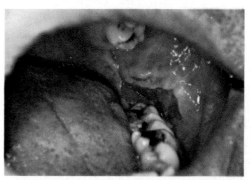

Pemphigus vulgaris

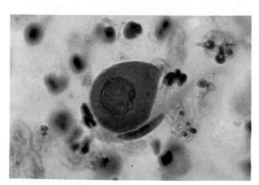

Pemphigus vulgaris, acantholytic
cell (cytologic smear)

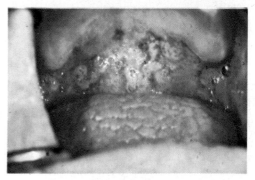

Pemphigoid

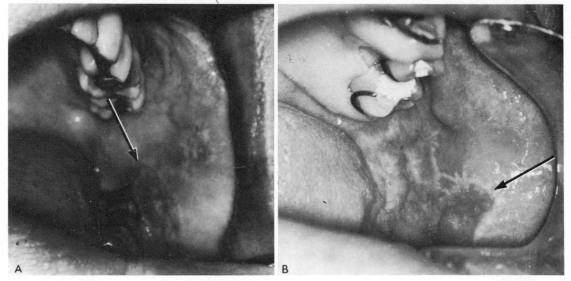

Figure 16–5. *Erosive lichen planus of the oral mucosa.*
(*B*, Courtesy of Dr. Edward V. Zegarelli.)

"nonerosive" lichen planus. Nevertheless the vesicular or bullous form of the disease may clinically resemble erosive lichen planus when the vesicles rupture. Eroded or frankly ulcerated lesions are irregular in size and shape and appear as raw, painful areas in the same general sites involved by the simple or reticular form of the disease (Fig. 16–5). Despite the erosion of the mucosa, the characteristic radiating striae may often be noted on the periphery of the individual lesions.

An *atrophic* form of lichen planus occurs with some frequency and appears clinically as smooth, red, poorly defined areas, often but not always with peripheral striae evident. As pointed out in Chapter 15, the term "chronic desquamative gingivitis" (q.v.) was at one time used to describe a red, diffuse, painful condition of the gingiva, usually found in postmenopausal women and generally quite refractory to therapy. It is now generally accepted that this is not an entity but represents a variety of conditions including the oral manifestations of several dermatologic diseases, one of which is lichen planus (usually the atrophic or erosive form), occurring on the gingiva.

A *hypertrophic* form of lichen planus may also occur on the oral mucosa, generally appearing as a well-circumscribed, elevated white lesion resembling leukoplakia. In such cases biopsy is usually necessary to establish the diagnosis.

The oral manifestations of lichen planus may occur weeks or months before the appearance of the skin lesions; in fact, in the clinical experience of most investigators, the great majority of patients exhibiting oral lichen planus do not have skin lesions present at the time of presentation of the oral lesions. Indeed, many patients with oral lichen planus never manifest the cutaneous form of the disease, although most patients are not followed up for a sufficiently long time to be absolutely certain of this.

Other mucous membranes may be affected also, such as those of the penis, vagina and epiglottis. Involvement of these locations may occur concomitant with or independent of oral lesions.

Histologic Features. The microscopic appearance of lichen planus is characteristic and pathognomonic. Typical findings include hyperparakeratosis or hyperorthokeratosis with thickening of the granular layer, acanthosis with intracellular edema of the spinous cells in some instances, the development of a "saw tooth" appearance of the rete pegs, necrosis or liquefaction degeneration of the basal layer of cells with the appearance of a thin band of eosinophilic coagulum in the place of this basal layer and, finally, infiltration of lymphocytes and only occasional plasma cells into the subepithelial layer of connective tissue (Fig. 16–6). True dyskeratosis does not occur. In some cases the hyperkeratosis and acanthosis are not prominent features, although they can usually be found in at least a few areas. Colloid bodies, also called Civatte bodies, hyaline bodies, or

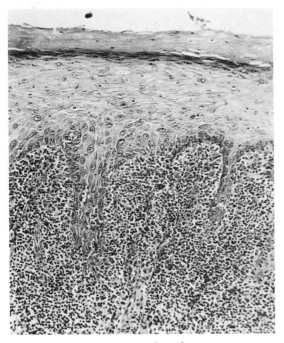

Figure 16–6. *Lichen planus.*
The photomicrograph illustrates the characteristic features of the disease.

cells appear to abut directly on the connective tissue, only a thin band of eosinophilic material separating the two. In a histochemical study of lichen planus, Abbey and Shklar reported that the basic pathosis appeared to be one of degeneration in the lower layers of the epithelium. In electron microscope studies, Pullon found two additional changes in the epithelium that are not apparent with the light microscope: (1) an irregularity of the nuclear membrane of the cells and (2) an increased thickening and granularity of epithelial tonofibrils. Ultrastructural studies of changes in the basal cell region have been reported by El-Labban and Kramer, who described a "dilution" of cytoplasmic contents of the basal epithelial cells without cell death and accumulation of fragments of lamina densa material, rather than liquefaction degeneration of the basal layer. The infiltration of lymphocytes characteristically is sharply limited to the papillary and most superficial portion of the reticular layers of connective tissue, the deeper connective tissue being almost free of inflammatory cells. Finally, an artifactual tearing is often seen between the connective tissue and epithelium, suggesting a weakness between these two structures. Although obviously a post-surgical, technical flaw, it is sometimes of aid in establishing the diagnosis of lichen planus.

Direct immunofluorescent studies of lichen planus by Daniels and Quadra-White have been most interesting. They have shown that nearly all specimens from oral lesions of this disease react with antifibrinogen and exhibit an intensely positive fluorescence that outlines the basement membrane zone with numerous irregular extensions into the superficial lamina propria (Fig. 16–7). This particular pattern is characteristic of both lichen planus and lupus

fibrillar bodies, are often present in the epithelium, mostly in the spinous and basal cell layers, appearing as round, eosinophilic globules probably representing degenerated epithelial cells or phagocytosed epithelial cell remnants within microphages according to the work of El-Labban and Kramer and of Griffin and his associates. These also appear to correspond to structures called "cytoid bodies" and despite the variation in terminology are known to occur in a variety of dermatoses. Owing to the degeneration of the basal layer of cells, the spinous

Figure 16–7. *Lichen planus.*
Oral specimen showing fluorescence in the superficial lamina propria and basement membrane zone with antifibrinogen. (Courtesy of Dr. Troy E. Daniels and C. V. Mosby Company. From Daniels, T. E., and Quadra-White, C.: Direct immunofluorescence in oral mucosal disease: a diagnostic analysis of 130 cases. Oral Surg., *51*:38, 1981).

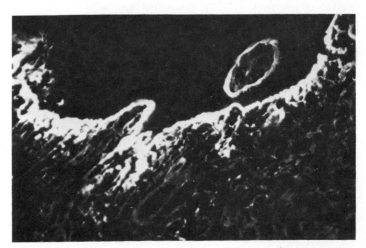

erythematosus. This is not present in pemphigoid or erythema multiforme, in both of which the fluorescence instead tends to form a patchy linear pattern, nor is it seen in pemphigus, in which the fluorescence has a granular pattern. These workers reported a general absence of immunoglobulins in lichen planus lesions while only a few specimens exhibited a fine granular fluorescence with anti-C3 (complement) at the basement membrane zone. They concluded that the pattern of fibrinogen deposition, in the absence of fluorescence by other reagents, is sufficiently unique to be used as a diagnostic criterion for oral mucosal lichen planus (see also p. 834).

Differential Diagnosis. It is important that lichen planus be differentiated from other lesions of the oral cavity which may present a similar clinical appearance, but which may have a different prognosis. Oral lesions which bear superficial resemblance to lichen planus include leukoplakia, candidiasis, pemphigus, cicatricial pemphigoid, erythema multiforme, syphilis, recurrent aphthae and lupus erythematosus (q.v.). Although microscopic examination of tissue may be necessary to establish a definitive diagnosis, the clinical characteristics of these various diseases are often sufficient to differentiate one from the other.

Treatment and Prognosis. There is no specific treatment for lichen planus. In the past, such compounds as arsenicals, mercurials and bismuth were used, but with only indifferent success. Although vitamin therapy has been advocated with some reported benefit, the value of such therapy is difficult to estimate. Corticosteroid therapy has been used in severe cases to relieve the inflammation and decrease the pruritus of skin lesions. The intraoral lesions also respond to corticosteroids, especially intralesional administration. This is particularly indicated in the erosive form or when there is significant pain. It is not uncommon for the disease to regress completely after stabilization of the emotional state of the patient.

Malignant Potential. Lichen planus, at one time, was thought to be a perfectly benign disease and was not considered a potentially premalignant condition. However, there has been a relatively large number of cases of epidermoid carcinoma developing in oral lesions of lichen planus reported in the literature. For example, Stillman and his associates reviewed 112 cases of oral cancer developing in lichen planus in 1973, while by 1978, Krutchkoff and his co-workers were able to tabulate 223

reported cases of malignant transformation in oral lichen planus. Of this latter group, over 90 per cent were considered unacceptable by Krutchkoff and his co-workers for various reasons, however. Inasmuch as both oral lichen planus and oral cancer are relatively common diseases, their simultaneous occurrence in the same patient at least in some cases may only be fortuitous. Nevertheless, the possibility of a true relationship between these two diseases, albeit quite a limited one, must be accepted pending clarification through further study. Interestingly and perhaps significantly, the majority of these reported cases of cancer have occurred in the erosive type of lichen planus. An analogous malignant transformation of dermal lichen planus has been reported but is very rare.

PSORIASIS

Psoriasis is one of the more common chronic inflammatory dermatologic diseases; the incidence among the population of the United States is estimated to be between 0.25 and 2 per cent. In rare instances it has been reported to manifest oral mucous membrane lesions.

Clinical Features. Psoriasis of the skin is characterized by the occurrence of small, sharply delineated, dry papules, each covered by a delicate silvery scale which has been described as resembling a thin layer of mica. If the deep scales are removed, one or more tiny bleeding points are disclosed, a characteristic feature termed *Auspitz's sign.* After removal of the scale the surface of the skin is red and dusky in appearance.

The cutaneous lesions, which are painless and seldom pruritic, may be few in number or extensive in distribution. The papules enlarge at the periphery and tend to become slightly infiltrating and elevated, smaller lesions coalescing to form large plaques of irregular outline. They are roughly symmetrical and are most frequently grouped on the extensor surfaces of the extremities, particularly the elbows and knees, the scalp, back and chest, face and abdomen. Involvement of the hands and feet, with the exception of the fingernail, is uncommon.

The disease commences with the appearance of a few small papules, which gradually increase in size. New lesions slowly arise over a period of weeks, months or even years. The disease may remain static for a long time, progress slowly to involve more and more skin area, or exhibit acute generalized exacerbations. The disease is more severe in the winter and less severe in the summer as a result of increased exposure to ultraviolet light; patients who move to a warm sunny climate usually undergo improvement in their condition. Mental anxiety or stress almost invariably appears to increase the severity of the disease or induce acute exacerbations. Arthritis is a complication in about 12 per cent of persons with psoriasis, according to Allen.

Psoriasis is uncommon in children, and seldom does a primary attack occur after the age of 45 years; it most frequently arises in the second and third decades of life. There is no sex predilection; neither do social conditions or occupation appear to play any part in the etiology of the disease.

The cause of psoriasis is unknown. It has been reported that heredity is a factor in some cases, and present evidence in these suggests a polygenic inheritance pattern, possibly transmitted as a simple dominant trait with a low penetrance based on known familial clustering and higher concordance rates in monozygotic versus dizygotic twins. Infection by various microorganisms, metabolic disturbance, endocrine dysfunction, neurogenic factors and trauma, as well as parturition, have been considered important precipitating factors in the onset of the disease by various workers, although most cases have no such known "trigger."

There is evidence also that psoriasis, as with many other human diseases, is associated with the human major histocompatibility (HLA) complex, implying that either the HLA antigen itself or a linked gene is directly involved in the disease process. It has also been shown by Guilhou and his associates that psoriatic patients have an increase in serum IgG and IgA, as well as salivary IgA, and an increase in IgE levels in some patients and the presence of anti-IgG activity in the serum of nearly one-half of psoriatic patients. These data, it was concluded, could be in favor of autoimmune processes in this disease. Finally, studies concerning the pathogenesis of the disease by Voorhees and his co-workers and Wright and his associates have suggested that the epidermal changes in this disease may be related to alterations in cellular levels of cyclic AMP and cyclic GMP.

Oral Manifestations. Most authorities consider psoriatic involvement of oral mucosa extremely rare and point out that many oral lesions occurring concomitant with psoriasis of the skin are actually other diseases such as leukoplakia or lichen planus. In fact some investigators deny the existence of oral psoriasis. For example, in a study of 100 patients with dermal psoriasis, Buchner and Begleiter found none with oral lesions of the disease. However, they did note in these patients an 11 per cent incidence of angular cheilosis, 6 per cent incidence of fissured tongue and 5 per cent incidence of benign migratory glossitis. Nevertheless it has been reported that in occasional cases

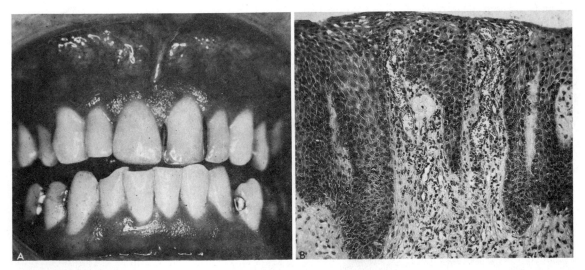

Figure 16–8. Psoriasis.
A, The patient manifested typical psoriasis of the skin and, in addition, presented granular gingival lesions which microscopically exhibited the characteristic psoriaform pattern. *B,* Photomicrograph of skin psoriasis exhibits the pathognomonic features of the disease. (Courtesy of Drs. Robert J. Gorlin and Frank Vellios.)

oral lesions have exhibited all histologic features of psoriasis and in some instances have been identical with the coexisting skin lesions.

Such lesions have been reported on the lips, buccal mucosa, palate, gingiva and floor of the mouth (Fig. 16–8,A). Clinically, they are described as gray or yellowish-white plaques; as silvery white, scaly lesions with an erythematous base; as multiple papular eruptions which may be ulcerated; or as small, papillary, elevated lesions with a scaly surface. Reports by Goldman and Bloom and by Levin emphasized the vagaries in the clinical appearance of oral psoriasis. Psoriasis of the gingiva was reported by Brayshaw and Orban and that of the alveolar ridge by Wooten and his associates in patients without skin lesions; however, cases of mucosal involvement without skin manifestations must be viewed with caution even though the histologic sections of the lesions do present a psoriaform pattern. White and his associates have reviewed the literature on intraoral psoriasis while reporting an additional case. Fischman and his co-workers studied an oral lesion in a patient with skin lesions of psoriasis utilizing light and electron microscopy, as well as immunologic methods, and noted in all instances that the findings in the oral lesion were similar to those in the skin lesions. They concluded that true oral lesions do occur in psoriasis.

The general problem of "psoriasiform" lesions of the oral mucosa has been reviewed by Weathers and his associates. These lesions included psoriasis, Reiter's syndrome, benign migratory glossitis and "ectopic geographic tongue," and the authors concluded that their exact interrelationship, if any, is still unknown.

Histologic Features. The microscopic appearance of psoriasis is characterized by uniform parakeratosis, absence of the stratum granulosum and elongation and clubbing of the rete pegs. The epithelium over the connective tissue papillae is thinned, and it is from these points that bleeding occurs when the scales are peeled off. Tortuous, dilated capillaries extending high in the papillae are prominent (Fig. 16–8, B). Intraepithelial microabscesses (Monro's abscesses) are a common but not invariable finding; they are reported by Pisanty and Ship to be absent in oral psoriasis. Mild lymphocytic and histiocytic infiltration of the connective tissue is also typical, particularly perivascular and periadnexal in location.

Related to the pathogenesis of psoriasis is the very rapid turnover rate of skin epithelial cells in psoriasis. Normal skin turnover time is approximately 28 days, while that of psoriatic skin is only 3 to 4 days. As would be expected, there is also a dramatic increase in the mitotic index of psoriatic skin which is said to even surpass that of epidermoid carcinoma.

Treatment. The lesions often disappear spontaneously for varying periods but will nearly always recur. There is no specific form of therapy for psoriasis. A variety of lotions and ointments have been classically prescribed, as well as ultraviolet light. The most commonly used topical medications are corticosteroids, tars and such drugs as iodochlorhydroxyquin, dihydroxyanthralin, and retinoic acid. In general, however, any relief obtained is only symptomatic and temporary. Although psoriasis is cosmetically disfiguring and sometimes restricts the patient's activities, the disease does not lead to serious consequences.

PITYRIASIS ROSEA

Pityriasis rosea is an acute skin eruption of unknown etiology. It seldom occurs in a true epidemic pattern, although occasional familial or household outbreaks are described. Still, there is little evidence to suggest that the disease is actually contagious.

Clinical Features. Pityriasis rosea is characterized by the appearance of superficial light red macules or papules, either generalized over most of the skin surface, with the usual exception of the face and hands, or localized to certain areas such as the trunk, thighs, axillae or groin. This generalized outbreak is frequently preceded by the appearance of a "primary lesion" or "herald spot" seven to ten days previously. This spot is brighter red and larger (3 to 4 cm. in diameter) than the multiple eruptions which follow its appearance. The individual exanthematous lesions are commonly ovoid, with the long axis parallel to the natural lines of cleavage of the skin, and are covered by a thin silvery scale.

The lesions often manifest mild itching, sometimes accompanied by headache and low-grade fever; cervical lymphadenopathy may also be present.

Pityriasis rosea usually runs its course in three to six weeks and seldom recurs. It is interesting that the disease occurs seasonally, being far more common in the spring and autumn than at other times. It involves young adults chiefly but shows no definite sex predilection, although in some studies there is a slight predominance in women.

The cause of pityriasis rosea is unknown. An

infectious etiology has been proposed and, though without conclusive evidence, a virus is most favored and seems to be a likely explanation. A relation to nervous strain or emotional disturbance has been noted, although this may be purely coincidental.

Oral Manifestations. It was pointed out by Guequierre and Wright, and confirmed by others, that involvement of the oral mucous membranes occurs with some frequency in pityriasis rosea. The oral lesions appear either concomitantly with or subsequent to the skin manifestations; they are not present throughout the clinical course of the disease, but are usually prominent during its most severe phase.

The oral lesions usually occur only on the buccal mucosa, although both tongue and palatal lesions have also been recorded. They appear as erythematous macules with or without a central area of grayish desquamation. The lesions may be single or multiple, are irregular in shape, occasionally show a raised border and vary in size from a few millimeters to 1 or 2 cm. in diameter. These lesions are asymptomatic and of no clinical significance. They clear simultaneously with the skin lesions.

Histologic Features. The microscopic changes in pityriasis rosea are not pathognomonic, but consist of slight acanthosis and focal parakeratosis with microvesiculation or simply sprinkling of leukocytes within the epithelium. In addition, edema, hyperemia and perivascular infiltration of lymphocytes, plasma cells and histiocytes are prominent in the superficial connective tissue. The histologic features suggest little more than a nonspecific dermatitis.

Treatment. Pityriasis rosea usually demands no treatment, since the disease is self-limiting and generally undergoes rapid, spontaneous regression.

ERYTHEMA MULTIFORME

(Erythema Multiforme Exudativum; Stevens-Johnson Syndrome; Ectodermosis Erosiva Pluriorificialis)

Erythema multiforme is a term applied to an acute dermatitis of unknown etiology and protean manifestations. Although the exact cause is obscure, a variety of different agents are known to precipitate an attack of the disease in about one-half of the cases. The remainder appear to be spontaneous, inasmuch as the patients are unable to relate any specific agent or event to the occurrence of the disease. The most common precipitating agent, discussed by Shelley, is herpes simplex infection, preceding the onset of erythema multiforme by one to three weeks. A number of other viral infections also may trigger the disease as well as bacterial and fungal infections, drug intake (e.g., barbiturates, phenylbutazone, digitalis, iodides, mercurials, penicillin, salicylates, sulfonamides and birth control pills), vaccination, radiation therapy and occasional other diseases (e.g., Crohn's disease, ulcerative colitis and infectious mononucleosis). These patients do not appear to have a related immunodeficiency. These various agents have been reviewed by Coursin and by Lozada and Silverman.

Clinical Features. Erythema multiforme occurs chiefly in young adults, although it may develop at any age, and affects males more frequently than females. This disease is characterized by the occurrence of asymptomatic, vividly erythematous discrete macules, papules or occasionally vesicles and bullae distributed in a rather symmetrical pattern most commonly over the hands and arms, feet and legs, face and neck. The individual lesions may vary considerably in size even in the same patient, but are generally only a few centimeters or less in diameter. A concentric ringlike appearance of

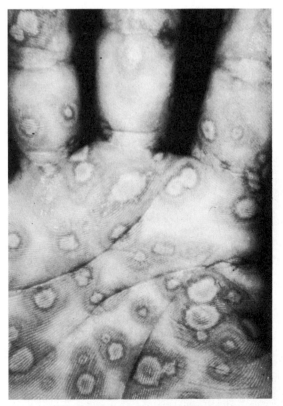

Figure 16–9. *Erythema multiforme.*
Typical "target" or "bull's eye" lesions of hand.

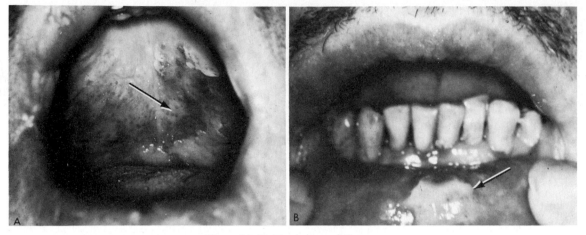

Figure 16–10. *Erythema multiforme.*
Lesions of the palate *(A)* and lip *(B)*.

the lesions, resulting from the varying shades of erythema, occurs in some cases and has given rise to the terms "target," "iris" or "bull's eye" in describing them (Fig. 16–9). They are most common on the hands, wrists and ankles. Mucous membrane involvement, including the oral cavity, is common. The lesions make their appearance rapidly, usually within a day or two, and persist for several days to a few weeks, gradually fading and eventually clearing. Recurrence of the disease over a period of years is common, however.

The *oral mucous membrane* lesions are not usually a significant feature of the disease except for the pain and discomfort they cause. The hyperemic macules, papules or vesicles may become eroded or ulcerated and bleed freely. The tongue, palate, buccal mucosa and gingiva are commonly diffusely involved (Fig. 16–10). Occasionally, mucous membrane lesions occur before the cutaneous manifestations, but oral involvement without dermal lesions has been questioned. Nevertheless, Lozada and Silverman have reported that 12 of 50 patients with erythema multiforme had oral lesions only.

STEVENS-JOHNSON SYNDROME. At one time considered to be a separate disease, Stevens-Johnson syndrome is now recognized as simply a very severe bullous form of erythema multiforme with widespread involvement typically including the skin, oral cavity, eyes and genitalia. It commences with the abrupt occurrence of fever, malaise, photophobia and eruptions of the oral mucosa, genitalia and skin. The cutaneous lesions in this mucocutaneous-ocular disease are similar to those of erythema multiforme, although they are commonly hemorhagic and are often vesicular or bullous.

Oral mucous membrane lesions may be extremely severe and so painful that mastication is impossible. Mucosal vesicles or bullae occur which rupture and leave surfaces covered with a thick white or yellow exudate. Erosions of the pharynx are also common. The lips may exhibit ulceration with bloody crusting and are painful (Fig. 16–11, *A*). The oral lesions may be the chief complaint of the patient and, understandably, have been mistaken for acute necrotizing ulcerative gingivostomatitis. Interestingly, however, it has been reported that the organisms of Vincent's infection are scarce in patients with this disease. (See also Plate VII.)

Eye lesions consist of photophobia, a characteristic of the disease referable to the conjunctivitis, corneal ulceration and panophthalmitis which may occur (Fig. 16–11, *B*). Keratoconjunctivitis sicca also has been described. Blindness may result chiefly from intercurrent bacterial infection.

Genital lesions are reported to consist of a nonspecific urethritis, balanitis and/or vaginal ulcers (Fig. 16–11, *C*).

Other reported complications are related to respiratory tract involvement such as tracheobronchial ulceration and pneumonia. The patients usually recover unless they succumb to a secondary infection.

Histologic Features. The microscopic appearance of erythema multiforme is not diagnostic. Although considerable variation occurs, corresponding to the variation in clinical appearance, the cutaneous or mucosal lesions generally exhibit intracellular edema of the spinous layer of epithelium and edema of the superficial connective tissue which may actually produce a subepidermal vesicle. In a study of oral lesions,

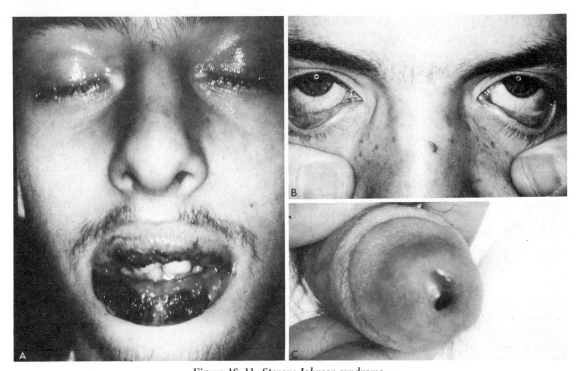

Figure 16–11. *Stevens-Johnson syndrome.*
Crusting ulcerated lesions of the oral cavity and lips *(A)*, conjunctivitis *(B)*, and urethritis *(C)* are characteristic of the disease.

Shklar has also described a zone of severe liquefaction degeneration in the upper layers of the epithelium, intraepithelial vesicle formation and thinning with frequent absence of the basement membrane. Dilatation of the superficial capillaries and lymphatic vessels in the uppermost layer of connective tissue is prominent, and a varying degree of inflammatory cell infiltration, chiefly lymphocytes, but often neutrophils and eosinophils, is also present. Similar findings were described by Buchner and his coworkers in a series of 25 cases. The findings have been confirmed in an electron microscope study by von Bülow and his co-workers.

Differential Diagnosis. The varied nature of the disease may present difficulty in diagnosis, particularly when the occurrence of cutaneous lesions is minimal. In the presence of oral lesions, aphthous stomatitis, contact dermatitis or stomatitis and acute necrotizing gingivitis must be considered, as well as pemphigus, dermatitis herpetiformis, bullous lichen planus, herpes zoster, chickenpox and toxic epidermal necrolysis (Lyell's disease).

Toxic epidermal necrolysis is a very serious, often fatal, bullous drug eruption, so severe that large sheets of skin peel off, giving the appearance of a widespread scalding burn. Oral erosions may also occur and have been de-

scribed by Giallorenzi and Goldstein. It is now considered to be a confluent form of Stevens-Johnson syndrome. Toxic epidermal necrolysis must be differentiated from the *staphylococcal scalded skin syndrome*, which appears clinically similar even though the latter is a milder disease with a better prognosis.

Treatment and Prognosis. There is no specific treatment for the disease, although in some cases ACTH, cortisone and chlortetracycline have shown promising results. Seldom is the patient's life endangered, but chronic episodic recurrences may be disconcerting.

MUCOCUTANEOUS LYMPH NODE SYNDROME

(Kawasaki Disease)

An acute self-limiting febrile illness in a large number of Japanese children was first described in 1967 by Kawasaki under the name mucocutaneous lymph node syndrome. It is now known to occur in other countries, with the first recognized case in the continental United States being seen in 1974. By the end of 1981, over 800 cases had been recorded in this country.

The etiology of the disease is still unknown

but has most frequently been suggested to be either a viral disease or a "collagen-vascular" disease. There does appear to be some genetic component.

Clinical Features. The vast majority of cases have occurred in children between 3 months and 12 years of age, although it has also been reported in adults. The most frequent symptoms of the disease, as determined by the Epidemiological Study Group of the Japanese MCLS Research Committee, are: (1) fever for five days or more, with no response to antibiotics (95 per cent of cases); (2) bilateral congestion of ocular conjunctiva (90 per cent); (3) changes in the extremities peripherally including indurative edema (75 per cent), erythema of palms and soles (90 per cent) and membranous desquamation of fingers and toes (95 per cent); (4) changes in lips and mouth including dryness, redness and fissuring of lips (90 per cent), strawberry-like reddening and swelling of tongue papillae (80 per cent) and diffuse reddening of oral and pharyngeal mucosa (90 per cent), sometimes with gingival ulceration; (5) polymorphous exanthema of torso without vesicles or crusts (90 per cent); and (6) acute, nonpurulent swelling of cervical lymph nodes of 1.5 cm. or more (75 per cent). Other less common findings include diarrhea, arthralgia, proteinuria, leukocytosis, increased sedimentation rate and positive C-reactive protein. One of the unfortunately common complications of the disease is cardiac abnormality. The United States Centers for Disease Control has reported that approximately 20 per cent of patients develop coronary-artery aneurysms in the second to fourth week of illness but that, at least in the Japanese cases, about half of these aneurysms disappear within two years.

While the vast majority of cases are self-limiting and nonfatal, occasional deaths do occur, almost invariably a result of the cardiac complications, usually a coronary thrombosis or vascular damage related to infantile periarteritis nodosa.

The implications of dental treatment in these patients have been reviewed by Taylor and Peterson.

Differential Diagnosis. Unfortunately, there are no laboratory tests available for confirmation of the diagnosis of the disease. Therefore, its diagnosis is based entirely on clinical manifestations. It must be carefully distinguished from scarlet fever, erythema multiforme or Stevens-Johnson syndrome.

PACHYONYCHIA CONGENITA

Pachyonychia congenita is an extremely uncommon disease, believed to be inherited as an autosomal dominant characteristic with incomplete penetrance, characterized by a variety of cutaneous and mucosal abnormalities.

Clinical Features. The skin lesions of pachyonychia congenita usually occur shortly after birth and consist of dystrophic changes in the fingernails and toenails, hyperkeratotic calluses of the palms and soles, follicular keratosis about the knees and elbows, and hyperhidrosis or excessive sweating of the hands and feet. The nail changes from which the disease derives its name consist of marked thickening, increasing toward the free border, with the nail bed becoming filled with yellowish keratotic debris, often causing the nail to project upward at the free edge. Associated sparse hair and corneal dyskeratosis producing corneal opacities have been reported also.

Oral Manifestations. Oral lesions are nearly always present, according to Gorlin and Chaudhry. They consist of either focal or generalized, white, opaque thickening of the mucosa involving the buccal mucosa, tongue or lips. These leukoplakic oral lesions should not be confused clinically with lichen planus. These have even been reported present at birth. Angular cheilosis is also reported to be commonly seen. Teeth present at birth, natal teeth, have been found on a number of occasions. Cases with typical oral lesions have been reported by Maser and by Young and Lenox.

Histologic Features. The mucous membrane exhibits acanthosis and intracellular edema or vacuolization of the spinous cells reminiscent of white sponge nevus. Parakeratosis is evident. There are no features pathognomonic of the disease, however.

Treatment. There is no treatment for the disease, which is not considered to be a serious condition.

KERATOSIS FOLLICULARIS

(Darier's Disease; Darier-White's Disease)

Keratosis follicularis is a genodermatosis transmitted as an autosomal dominant characteristic. However, many cases appear to occur as new mutations. There also is thought to be some relationship of the disease to vitamin A

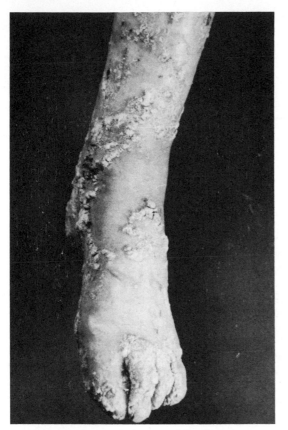

Figure 16–12. *Keratosis follicularis.*
(Courtesy of Dr. Dwight R. Weathers. Arch. Dermatol., *100*:50, 1969.)

metabolism, since some patients have low plasma levels of the vitamin.

Clinical Features. Keratosis follicularis usually is manifested during childhood or adolescence and has an equal sex distribution.

The cutaneous lesions appear as small, firm papules, which are red when they first appear, but characteristically become grayish brown or even purple, ulcerate and crust over (Fig. 16–12). Especially in the skin folds, the lesions tend to coalesce and produce verrucous or vegetating macerated, foul-smelling masses. They are generally distributed about the forehead, scalp, neck and over the shoulders, but often spread to the limbs, chest and genitalia. Palmar and plantar keratotic thickening may be so severe as to interfere with function. In severe cases, all the intertriginous areas are involved. Characteristic nail changes are also seen consisting of splintering, fissuring, longitudinal streaking and subungual keratosis.

Oral Manifestations. The oral mucosa is probably more commonly involved than is generally realized, according to Gorlin and Chaudhry, who found a number of reports of oral lesions in the literature. In addition, they pointed out that other mucosal surfaces such as vulva, pharynx and larynx have also been reported as sites of the disease. Mucosal lesions have been said to be apparent only when there is extensive skin involvement. However, Weathers and Driscoll have stated that severe skin involvement is not necessary for the occurrence of oral lesions, although the severity of oral involvement did tend to parallel that of the skin. Nevertheless, oral involvement has been reported in as high as 50 per cent of all cases.

The oral lesions appear as minute, whitish papules which feel rough upon palpation. Some cases have been described as rough, pebbly areas with verrucous white plaques or as having a cobblestone appearance as in the cases of Weather and his associates and Prindiville and Stern. These are most frequently found on the gingiva, tongue, hard and soft palates, buccal mucosa and even the pharynx (Fig. 16–13).

Histologic Features. The disease is misnamed, since the changes are not restricted to the hair follicles. The characteristic findings in skin lesions are hyperkeratosis, papillomatosis, acanthosis and a peculiar benign dyskeratosis. This benign dyskeratosis is characterized by rather typical cells called *corps ronds* and grains. The corps ronds are larger than normal squamous cells and have a round, homogeneous, basophilic nucleus with a dark eosinophilic cytoplasm and a distinct cell membrane. These are found usually in the granular layer and superficial spinous layer. The grains are small, elongated parakeratotic cells situated in the keratin layer. Both corps ronds and grains represent partially keratinized cells and are found also in the typical slitlike intradermal vesicles just above the basal layer of cells, the typical suprabasilar cleavage (Fig. 16–14). Acantholytic cells are commonly found floating in the lacunae produced by this intraepithelial separation. The microscopic features of the oral lesions are identical except that the hyperkeratotic changes are generally not pronounced.

In an excellent review of keratosis follicularis, Spouge and his associates have also described a peculiar hyperplasia of the epithelial rests of Malassez in the periodontal ligament with a maturation of these individual cells into prickle cells, some of which even exhibited individual cell keratinization.

The cytologic findings in scrapings taken from

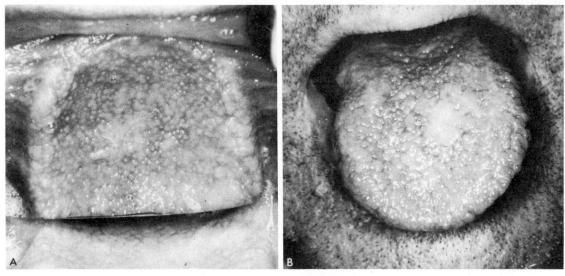

Figure 16–13. *Keratosis follicularis.*
(Courtesy of Dr. Dwight R. Weathers. Arch. Dermatol., *100*:50, 1969.)

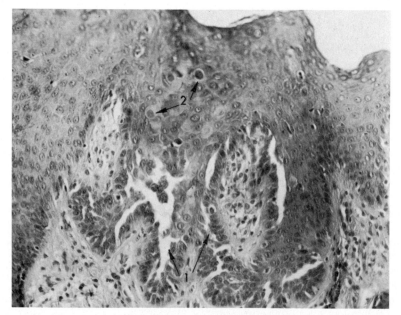

Figure 16–14. *Keratosis follicularis.*
Typical suprabasilar cleavage *(1)* and corps ronds *(2)* are evident. (Courtesy of Dr. William G. Sprague.)

the deeper portion of oral mucosal lesions have been described by Burlakow and his co-workers. They pointed out that, while some of the cells might be mistaken for malignant cells, the general cell population, the presence of grain cells and corps ronds and the "leafing-out" pattern of the parabasal cells should permit the correct diagnosis from such cytologic smears.

It has been demonstrated by the electron microscope that the basic defect in epidermal synthesis, turnover and resultant keratinization is related to a defect in the desmosome-tonofilament complex. It is also reported that there is a sevenfold decrease in turnover time of this epithelium.

Treatment. Treatment usually consists in the administration of large doses of vitamin A, but the results are variable. Corticosteroids are also used.

WARTY DYSKERATOMA

(Isolated Dyskeratosis Follicularis; Isolated Darier's Disease)

The warty dyskeratoma is a lesion which bears marked histologic similarity to keratosis follicularis but, in contrast to the latter, is usually a single isolated focus. The suggested origin of the lesion from the pilosebaceous apparatus would seem somewhat unlikely since oral lesions are known to occur.

Clinical Features. The skin lesions have occurred on the face, scalp or neck and upper chest in the majority of reported cases. They are almost invariably single lesions varying in size from only 1 to 10 mm. in diameter. They appear as elevated nodules, somewhat umbilicated, with a raised border and varying in color from yellow or brown to gray or black. Purulent drainage as well as bleeding frequently occurs.

There were 80 males and 32 females in a group of 112 cases of this lesion reviewed by Tanay and Mehregan and the majority occurred in middle-age or in older adults. In nearly every case, careful examination will reveal a hair passing through the lesion.

Oral Manifestations. Oral lesions are rare but do occur, three cases having been reported by Tomich and Burkes and several solitary cases reviewed by Patibanda and by Danforth and Green. These lesions were described as small whitish areas of the mucosa with a central depression and were situated on the alveolar ridge and palate. The patients were aware of the presence of these lesions and in at least two of these cases discomfort was present.

Histologic Features. The microscopic findings in the skin and mucosal lesions are identical except for the absence of a pilosebaceous structure in the oral lesions. The intraoral lesions exhibit a central orthokeratin or parakeratin core beneath which the epithelium shows a suprabasilar separation resulting in a cleftlike space containing acantholytic and benign dyskeratotic cells. The connective tissue papillae are covered usually by a single layer of basal cells while the underlying connective tissue shows a nonspecific chronic inflammatory cell infiltrate.

The term *focal acantholytic dyskeratosis* was suggested by Ackerman in 1972 for a clinically heterogeneous group of dermatologic conditions all characterized by certain histologic features which they share in unison but with no implied common etiology or pathogenesis. The warty dyskeratoma is one of the group fulfilling the criteria, and an intraoral case has been reported under the more inclusive generic term by Freedman and his associates.

Treatment and Prognosis. The lesions should be treated by surgical excision. There appears to be no malignant transformation in these lesions.

INCONTINENTIA PIGMENTI

(Bloch-Sulzberger Syndrome)

Incontinentia pigmenti is basically a genodermatosis, commonly presenting oral manifestations, and probably transmitted as a sex-linked dominant trait. Nearly all reported cases (over 600 in a world review by Carney) involve females, the disease being thought to be lethal for males. Morgan has reported an interesting cluster of four affected infants within a 6-month period in one city, whereas not a single case had been diagnosed in the previous 10 years in over 33,000 births.

Clinical Features. The disease generally appears shortly after birth and is characterized by the appearance of erythematous and vesiculobullous lesions on the trunk and extremities which frequently disappear, then reappear. This phase is often associated with a marked eosinophilia. These are gradually replaced by white keratotic, lichenoid, papillary or verrucous lesions which then persist for some months.

The third type of characteristic skin lesions in these infants are brownish-gray macules in a streaked, patchy distribution over the trunk and extremities, occurring subsequent to the verrucous, keratotic lesions. This pigmentation begins to fade within a few years. It is the heavy melanin pigmentation of the epithelium, dropping down into clusters of chromatophores in the upper dermis (incontinence), which gives the disease its name and is considered the hallmark of the syndrome.

A variety of associated defects are often seen in incontinentia pigmenti, including local or generalized baldness; ophthalmologic lesions including cataracts, optic atrophy, strabismus and retrolental fibroplasia; central nervous system involvement and lesions of the skeletal system.

Oral Manifestations. Oral changes in this disease have been recently described by Gorlin and Anderson and by Russell and Finn, among others, and appear limited to the teeth. Both the deciduous and permanent dentitions may be affected. These dental changes have been described as consisting of delayed tooth eruption, peg or cone-shaped tooth crowns, congenitally missing teeth, malformed teeth and additional cusps. The cone-shaped teeth are very similar to those seen in hereditary ectodermal dysplasia.

Treatment. No treatment is necessary.

POROKERATOSIS OF MIBELLI

Porokeratosis of Mibelli is an uncommon genokeratosis characterized by faulty keratinization of the skin followed by atrophy. It appears to be inherited as a simple dominant characteristic, although many sporadic cases are known. There is no adequate documentation that the lesions of porokeratosis, despite the name of the disease, have their origin in the epidermal pores of sweat glands.

Clinical Features. The majority of cases begin in early childhood but the progression of the lesions is generally exceedingly slow. It appears to occur in males with greater frequency than in females. The lesions themselves consist initially of crateriform keratotic papules which gradually enlarge to form elevated plaques ranging in size from a few millimeters to several centimeters. The lesions have a predilection for the extremities, particularly the hands and feet, as well as the shoulders, face and neck, and the genitalia. The nails commonly become thickened and ridged. The central portion of the lesions ultimately becomes atrophic, leaving permanent scarring. Epidermoid carcinoma has been reported developing in this atrophic skin. Lesions of the oral cavity are said to occur with considerable frequency in patients with this disease.

Histologic Features. The elevated horny margin of the lesion exhibits hyperkeratosis and acanthosis with a deep groove filled with parakeratin and a characteristic absence of the usual underlying granular layer. This constitutes the "cornoid lamella" which is characteristic of the lesion. The central portion of the lesion shows epithelial atrophy and occasionally dyskeratosis. The connective tissue beneath the cornoid lamella may exhibit a lymphocytic infiltrate.

Treatment. There is no treatment for the disease except for removal of individual lesions.

DYSKERATOSIS CONGENITA

Dyskeratosis congenita is a well-recognized but rare genokeratosis which is probably inherited as a recessive characteristic with nearly all reported cases occurring in males. The disease manifests three typical signs: oral leukoplakia, dystrophy of the nails and pigmentation of the skin. The importance of the syndrome lies in the high incidence of oral cancer which develops in the young affected adults.

Clinical Features. The nail changes are usually the first manifestation of the disease, becoming dystrophic and shedding some time after the age of 5 years. The grayish-brown skin pigmentation appears at the same time or a few years later and is distributed over the trunk, neck, and thighs. The skin may become atrophic and telangiectatic and the face appears red.

Occasional cases have also been reported with a wide spectrum of other minor manifestations including a frail skeleton, mental retardation, small sella turcica, dysphagia, transparent tympanic membranes, deafness, epiphora and eyelid infections, urethral anomalies, small testes, dental abnormalities and, commonly, hyperhidrosis of the palm and soles.

Oral Manifestations. The oral lesions in this disease appear to develop in a recognized sequence which has been outlined by Cannell. Thus, the oral lesions have their onset between the ages of 5 and 14 years and appear as diffusely distributed vesicles and ulcerations followed by the accumulation of white patches of necrotic epithelium and sometimes a superimposed monilial infection. Involvement of the tongue and buccal mucosa is particularly common. Between the approximate ages of 14 and 20 years, there are repeated, recurrent ulcerations and the development of erythroplasia or red mucosal lesions. Finally, between the ages of 20 and 30 years, there is development of erosive leukoplakia and carcinoma, frequently proving fatal between the ages of 30 and 50 years.

Other mucocutaneous areas may also be involved by similar lesions, including the rectum, vulva, vagina, urethra, upper gastrointestinal tract and respiratory tract.

Severe periodontal bone loss has been reported by Wald and Diner in a 15-year-old patient with dyskeratosis congenita. This might have been related to the pancytopenia present.

Histologic Features. The skin shows nothing specific except for increased numbers of melanin-containing chromatophores and increased vascularity. Oral lesions have not been thoroughly studied but the leukoplakic lesions appear to be nonspecific hyperparakeratosis or hyperorthokeratosis and acanthosis. Depending on the stage of the disease, the epithelium may show dysplasia. The exact nature of the preceding vesicles and ulcers has not been described.

Laboratory Findings. Many cases have been characterized also by hematologic changes including anemia, leukopenia, thrombocytopenia and pancytopenia. Some patients have developed Fanconi's anemia. In fact, the suggestion has been made that Fanconi's syndrome, or Fanconi's familial pancytopenia, is simply a varied expression of dyskeratosis congenita.

Treatment and Prognosis. There is no possible treatment for this disease. However, the high frequency of malignant transformation of oral lesions would necessitate careful periodic examination of the patient for such an occurrence.

WHITE SPONGE NEVUS

(Familial White Folded Dysplasia of Mucous Membrane; White Folded Gingivostomatitis; Oral Epithelial Nevus; Congenital Leukokeratosis; Cannon's Disease)

Familial white folded dysplasia is a relatively uncommon condition of the oral mucosa described by Cannon in 1935. The disease appears to follow a hereditary pattern as an autosomal dominant trait but with irregular penetrance and no definite sex predilection.

Clinical Features. This mucosal abnormality is congenital in many instances, children being born with the condition. In other cases it does not appear until infancy, childhood or even adolescence, by which time it has generally reached the full extent of its severity.

The oral lesions may be widespread, often involving the cheeks, palate, gingiva, floor of the mouth and portions of the tongue. The mucosa appears thickened and folded or corrugated with a soft or spongy texture and a peculiar white opalescent hue (Fig. 16–15, A).

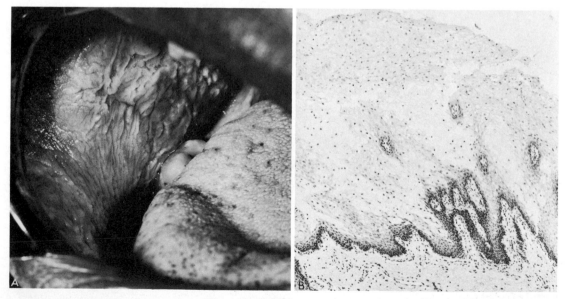

Figure 16–15. White sponge nevus.
The folded, spongy texture of the buccal mucosa is apparent in A. The typical intracellular edema and cellular pyknosis of the spinous cells are shown in B. (Courtesy of Dr. Carl J. Witkop.)

There is sometimes a minimal amount of folding present. Ragged white areas may also be present which can be removed sometimes by gentle rubbing without any ensuing bleeding. The lesions themselves are almost invariably asymptomatic. Bánóczy and her associates have provided a detailed review and discussion in their report of 45 cases of this disease.

In occasional cases reported in the literature, the oral lesions were accompanied by similar lesions of other mucosal surfaces, including the vagina and labia, anus, rectum and nasal cavity.

Histologic Features. The microscopic findings in familial white folded dysplasia are characteristic but not entirely pathognomonic of the disease. The epithelium is generally thickened, showing both hyperparakeratosis and acanthosis, and the basal layer is intact. The cells of the entire spinous layer, continuing to the very surface, exhibit intracellular edema (Fig. 16–15, *B*). These vacuolated cells may show pyknotic nuclei. In addition, parakeratin plugs running deep into the spinous layer are typically found. The submucosa may show a mild inflammatory cell infiltration, but this is not consistent.

Several electron microscope investigations of the white sponge nevus have been reported, the first being that of Whitten, and subsequent studies, those of McGinnis and Turner and of Frithiof and Bánóczy. There is some lack of agreement on interpretation of the ultrastructural findings in the various studies so that,

until these are resolved, their discussion in explanation of the light microscope findings should be deferred.

Treatment and Prognosis. There is no treatment for the condition, but since it is perfectly benign, the prognosis is excellent. There are no serious clinical complications.

HEREDITARY BENIGN INTRAEPITHELIAL DYSKERATOSIS

This unusual hereditary syndrome was discovered in 1954 in a racial isolate group of mixed Caucasian, Indian and Negro ancestry living in North Carolina. Since that time it has been thoroughly studied and described by Witkop and his co-workers. The disease appears superficially similar to familial white folded dysplasia or white sponge nevus in its hereditary pattern, although the clinical and microscopic features are different.

Clinical Features. The oral lesions of hereditary benign intraepithelial dyskeratosis appear generally as white, spongy, macerated lesions of the buccal mucosa, with or without folds (Fig. 16–16, *A*). They are also described on the floor of the mouth, ventral and lateral surfaces of the tongue, the gingiva and palate. These lesions vary from delicate, opalescent white membranous areas to a rough, shaggy mucosa. Lesions frequently involve the corners of the

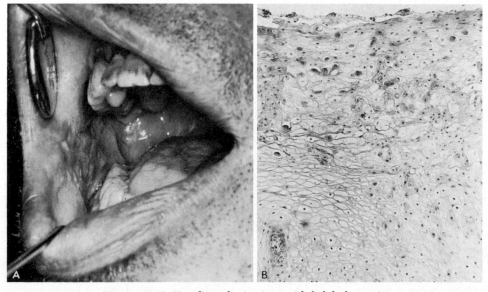

Figure 16–16. *Hereditary benign intraepithelial dyskeratosis.*
The white, macerated appearance of the lesions on the buccal mucosa is seen in *A.* The peculiar "dyskeratotic" cells are shown in *B.* (Courtesy of Dr. Carl J. Witkop.)

mouth and appear as soft plaques with pinpoint elevations when the mucosa is stretched.

Patients with this disease also manifest lesions of the eye characterized by superficial, foamy, gelatinous white plaques overlying the cornea, sometimes producing temporary blindness. In addition, the conjunctivae are usually intensely congested. Interestingly, these eye lesions in some cases show a seasonal variation, tending to appear or increase in severity in the spring and disappear, sometimes by spontaneous shedding of the pseudomembrane, in late summer or fall.

Histologic Features. Sections of the buccal mucosa exhibit thickening of the epithelium with pronounced hydropic degeneration. In addition, numerous round, waxy-appearing eosinophilic cells resembling minute epithelial pearls are evident, the "dyskeratotic" cells (Fig. 16–16, B). An excellent detailed description of the microscopic features of this disease has been provided by Witkop. Sadeghi and Witkop also have described ultrastructural differences between the mature dyskeratotic cells in this disease and in other dyskeratotic conditions of the mucous membranes.

Treatment and Prognosis. Witkop and his associates indicate that there is no increase in the death rate or in death from neoplastic disease in these patients, and therefore no treatment is indicated.

ACANTHOSIS NIGRICANS

Acanthosis nigricans is an unusual dermatosis which is usually classified into three main types: (1) benign, (2) malignant, and (3) pseudoacanthosis nigricans.

The *benign* form of the disease, which may be present at birth or occur later in childhood, particularly in puberty, appears to be a genetic disease inherited as a dominant characteristic and is exceedingly rare. It is never associated with internal malignancies.

The *malignant* form of the disease is invariably associated with internal malignancies (e.g., adenocarcinomas of various internal organs, particularly the stomach, or malignant lymphomas) which generally are highly malignant and metastasize early. In the majority of cases, the cutaneous lesions and the malignancies occur simultaneously. However, in a small number of cases, either may precede the other. This form of the disease usually develops after the age of 40 years but on rare occasion has been observed in childhood.

The *pseudoacanthosis nigricans* is that most common form of the disease which, at one time, was thought to be intimately associated with a variety of endocrinopathies. However, more recently it has been recognized as a disease that simulates true acanthosis nigricans in which lesions occur around body creases as a result of an underlying obesity, rather than as a true result of an endocrinologic problem. Interestingly, patients with this disease are invariably brunettes.

In recent years, it has been recognized that acanthosis nigricans may be associated with a variety of other diseases, including insulin-resistant diabetes, congenital lipodystrophy, lupoid hepatitis, hepatolenticular degeneration, hepatic cirrhosis, Bloom's syndrome, corticosteroid therapy and nicotinic acid therapy. This associated type has sometimes been considered a fourth form of the disease and termed *syndromal acanthosis nigricans*. Brown and Winkelmann have published an excellent review of this disease.

Clinical Features. The skin lesions in all forms of the disease are similar although the severity of the lesions and their distribution may vary from case to case. Generally, the skin lesions vary from a symmetric, mild hyperpigmentation and mild papillary hypertrophy of only small patchy areas to heavily pigmented, aggressively verrucous lesions involving much of the skin, especially the axillae, palms and soles, and face and neck (Fig. 16–17, A). The verrucous lesions are often pedunculated. Generalized pruritus is also a common finding.

Oral Manifestations. Oral mucous membrane involvement has been reported in between 25 and 50 per cent of all cases of acanthosis nigricans. The oral findings in the benign form have been described by Pindborg and Gorlin and, in the malignant form, by Bang. These oral findings in both forms appear essentially the same.

The tongue and lips appear to be most frequently involved, and to the greatest degree. There is hypertrophy of the filiform papillae producing a shaggy, papillomatous surface to the dorsal tongue. The lips may be enlarged and covered by papillomatous growths, particularly at the angles of the mouth. The buccal mucosa is less frequently involved, but generally shows a velvety white appearance with occasional papillary lesions. Similar findings may be seen in other areas, including the palate (Fig. 16–17, B, C, D). In addition, gingival enlargement has been reported, clinically resembling idiopathic fibromatosis.

Histologic Features. The histologic findings

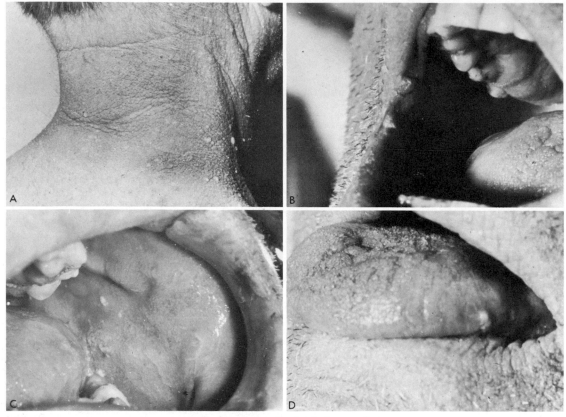

Figure 16–17. *Acanthosis nigricans maligna.*
Lesions of the skin *(A)*, and intraoral lesions of the commissure *(B)*, buccal mucosa *(C)*, and tongue *(D)* are illustrated. (Courtesy of Dr. Gisle Bang. Oral Surg., 29:370, 1970.)

are characteristic but not pathognomonic. There is generally a rather marked acanthosis, coupled with a peculiar incomplete parakeratosis. There is no increase in the number of melanophores in the oral mucosa in contrast to the skin lesions (Fig. 16–18).

Treatment. There is no treatment for the disease, although the essentiality of finding the associated malignant neoplasm in that form of the disease is obvious.

PEMPHIGUS

Pemphigus is a serious chronic skin disease characterized by the appearance of vesicles and bullae, small or large fluid-filled blisters, that develop in cycles. These are not pathognomonic, however, since vesicles and bullae may also develop in many other diseases. The etiology is still unknown despite numerous attempts in the past to implicate specific microorganisms. However, it is quite evident that an autoimmune mechanism is involved in the disease process inasmuch as intercellular antibodies may be demonstrated in the epithelium of the skin and oral mucosa of these patients and circulating intercellular antibodies are present in their serum.

Several types of pemphigus are recognized, but the basic lesion, the vesicle or bulla, is the same in each case. These types are:

1. Pemphigus vulgaris
2. Pemphigus vegetans
3. Pemphigus foliaceus
4. Pemphigus erythematosus

Allen pointed out that, despite the individual varieties of pemphigus described, there are several general features which most forms have in common. First, the initial lesion of any type of pemphigus is always the vesicle or bulla, even though the lesions in the later stages of the disease may be varied in nature—e.g., scaly, papillomatous. Secondly, the initial lesions occur most frequently on the trunk, although the oral mucosa is often the primary

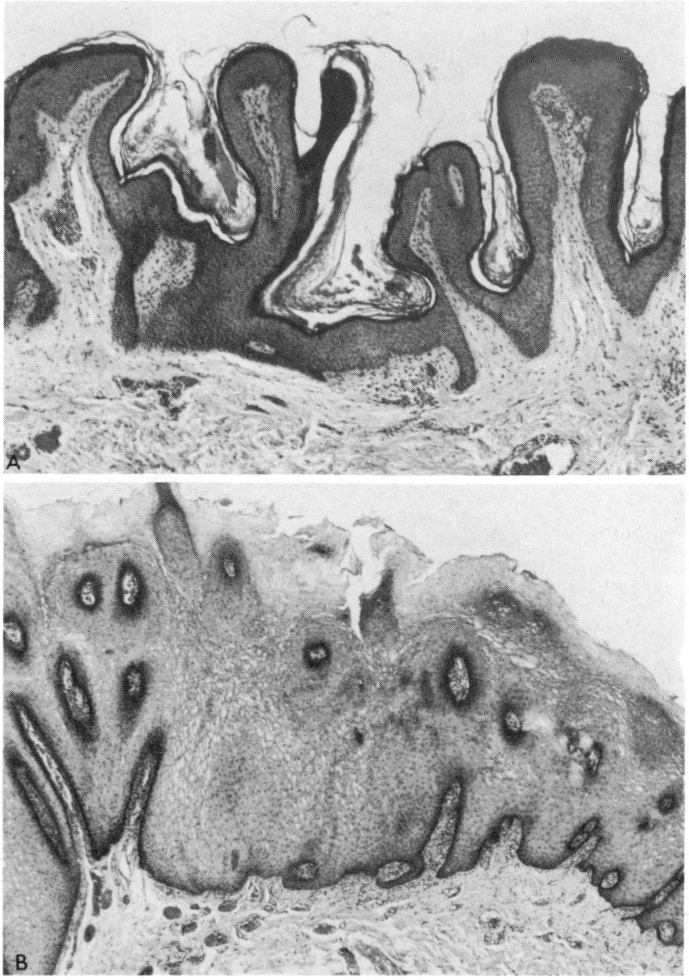

Figure 16–18. *Acanthosis nigricans maligna.*
Photomicrographs of lesions of the skin *(A)* and buccal mucosa *(B)* show the typical changes in each location. (Courtesy of Dr. Gisle Bang. Oral Surg., *29:*370, 1970.)

site of involvement in all forms except pemphigus foliaceus and pemphigus erythematosus. In fact, Allen stated: "It is the alert dentist who may make the original diagnosis which may be received skeptically because the skin may look completely normal at the time."

Clinical Features. Pemphigus of most types seldom occurs before the age of 30 years and is equally distributed in occurrence between males and females. Several cases have been described in childhood, however, and these have been reviewed by Bennett and his associates, who reported an additional case in an eight-year-old patient. It is also of interest that this disease is well recognized as occurring more frequently in Jewish persons, particularly the Ashkenazian group as reported by Pisanti and his co-workers.

Pemphigus vulgaris is characterized by the rapid appearance of vesicles and bullae, varying in diameter from a few millimeters to several centimeters, in such numbers that large areas of the skin surface may be covered (Fig. 16–19). These lesions contain a thin, watery fluid shortly after development, but this may soon become purulent or sanguineous. When the bullae rupture, they leave a raw eroded surface identical with that seen when focal areas of epithelium slide off either under oblique pressure or spontaneously without the prior formation of a vesicle or bulla. The loss of epithelium occasioned by rubbing apparently unaffected skin is termed *Nikolsky's sign.* It is a characteristic feature of pemphigus and is caused by prevesicular edema which disrupts the dermalepidermal junction. The course of pemphigus vulgaris is a variable one, the disease terminating in death or recovery within a few days or weeks, or being prolonged over a period of months or even years.

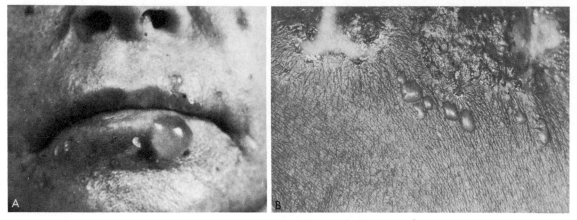

Figure 16–19. *Pemphigus vulgaris.*
Unruptured bullae and vesicles on the lips of *(A)* and skin *(B)*. *(A,* Courtesy of Dr. Boynton H. Booth.)

Pemphigus vegetans is now considered by most authorities to be a variant of pemphigus vulgaris. The flaccid bullae which develop then become eroded and form "vegetations" on some of the erosions (Fig. 16–20, *A, B*). These fungoid masses, which become covered by a purulent exudate and exhibit an inflamed border, frequently occur first on the nose and in the mouth, axillae and anogenital region and here bear close resemblance to condylomas. The disease usually terminates as pemphigus vulgaris, although long remissions are rather common in pemphigus vegetans.

Pemphigus foliaceus is manifested by characteristic early bullous lesions which rapidly rupture and dry to leave masses of flakes or scales suggestive of an exfoliative dermatitis or eczema. The disease may originate in this form or may develop from one of the other types of pemphigus. It is a relatively mild form of pem-

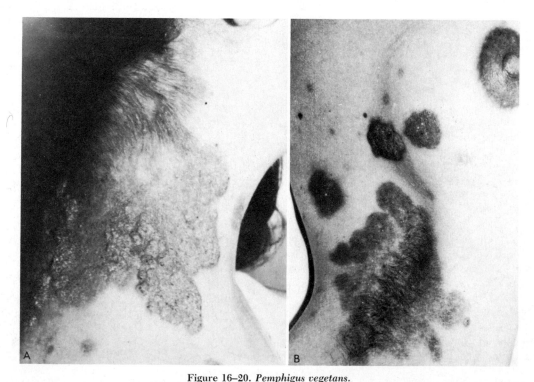

Figure 16–20. *Pemphigus vegetans.*
Vegetative lesions of the neck *(A)* and trunk *(B)*. (Courtesy of Dr. William C. Hurt. From Hurt, William C.: Oral Surg., *16*:1383, 1963.)

phigus, which is most common in older adults but may occur in young children as well.

Brazilian pemphigus (fogo selvagem or Brazilian wildfire) is a mild endemic form of pemphigus foliaceus found in tropical regions, particularly in Brazil, that often occurs in children and frequently in family groups. The course of the disease is similar to that of pemphigus foliaceus.

Pemphigus erythematosus (Senear-Usher syndrome) is a form of the disease which is characterized by the occurrence of bullae and vesicles concomitant with the appearance of crusted patches resembling seborrheic dermatitis or even lupus erythematosus. Periods of remission followed by exacerbation are common, but most cases ultimately terminate in pemphigus vulgaris or foliaceus.

The skin manifestations of any form of pemphigus may be accompanied by fever and malaise. Death may or may not rapidly ensue, depending upon the form of the disease. In the series of cases reported by Lever, wide variation occurred in the mortality rate.

Oral Manifestations. The oral lesions of the different types of pemphigus, which were specifically described by Lever, by Bernier and Tiecke, and by Zegarelli and Zegarelli, are stressed by most dermatologists because of their frequency of occurrence and because the mouth is often the site of the first manifestation of the disease.

The oral lesions are similar to those occurring on the skin, although intact bullae are rare, since they tend to rupture as soon as they form (Fig. 16–21). The oral mucosa also exhibits Nikolsky's phenomenon and may be denuded by the peripheral enlargement of the erosions. No intraoral site is immune to the development of the lesions, which bleed easily and are exquisitely tender. The pain may be so severe that the patient is unable to eat. The lesions tend to have a ragged border and be covered by a white or blood-tinged exudate. Extension onto the lips with the production of crusting may occur. In patients with this type of oral lesion, salivation is profuse, and the stench is overwhelming. (See also Plate VII.)

Pemphigus vulgaris, the most common form of pemphigus, typically shows oral lesions as either the initial or an early manifestation of the disease. In the series of 28 cases reported by Zegarelli and Zegarelli, the average duration between the onset of the oral lesions and the diagnosis of the disease was nearly seven months.

Oral lesions are reported to occur in over 50 per cent of cases of pemphigus vegetans. The proliferative vegetations seen in the cutaneous lesions of pemphigus vegetans are rare in the mouth, however. Instead, according to Hurt, who has reviewed this form of the disease, they form a serpiginous pattern in the mouth with the surface resembling pus. This can be wiped off, leaving a red, moist base that usually does not bleed and is not painful. This surface material often contains many eosinophils (Fig. 16–22, *A, B, C*).

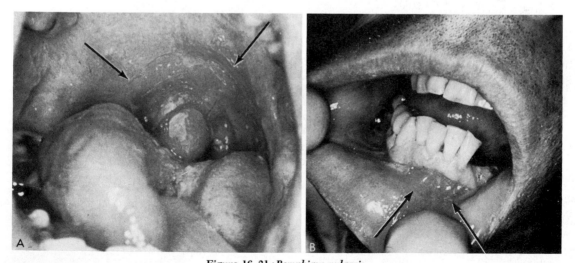

Figure 16–21.•*Pemphigus vulgaris.*
Rupture of bullae of the oral mucous membranes results in large, denuded, painful lesions. (Courtesy of Dr. Wilbur C. Moorman.)

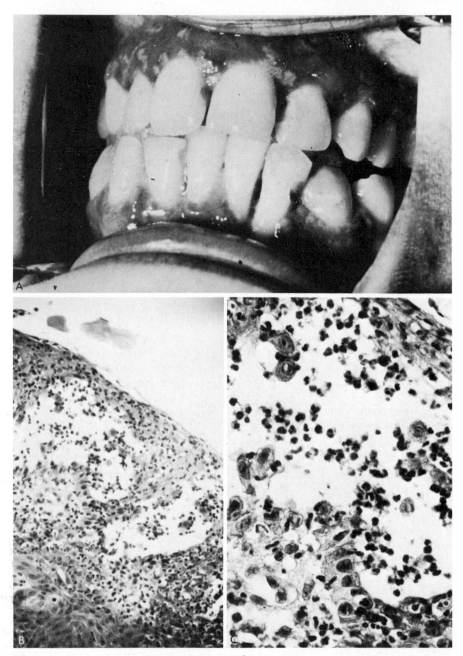

Figure 16–22. *Pemphigus vegetans.*
The oral lesions *(A)* were the initial manifestation of the disease. The low- and high-power photomicrographs *(B,C)* are from the gingival biopsy. (Courtesy of Dr. William C. Hurt. From Hurt, William C.: Oral Surg., *16*:1383, 1963.)

Oral lesions in pemphigus foliaceus are rare, according to Perry and Brunsting in their extensive study of this form of the disease.

Histologic Features. Pemphigus as an entity is characterized microscopically by the formation of a vesicle or bulla entirely intraepithelially, just above the basal layer producing the distinctive suprabasilar "split" (Fig. 16–23, *A*, *B*). Prevesicular edema appears to weaken this junction, and the intercellular bridges between the epithelial cells disappear. This results in loss of cohesiveness or acantholysis and, because of this, clumps of epithelial cells are often found lying free within the vesicular space (Fig. 16–23, *A*, *B*). These have been called "Tzanck cells" and are characterized particularly by degenerative changes which include swelling of the nuclei and hyperchromatic staining. These

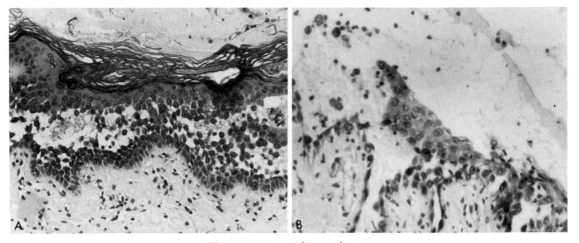

Figure 16–23. *Pemphigus vulgaris.*
A, Early stage of vesiculation with suprabasilar cleavage accompanied by prominent acantholysis and numerous Tzanck cells. B, In the bullous stage, acantholysis is still evident with occasional leukocytes in the bullous fluid. (Courtesy of Drs. Frank Vellios and Charles A. Waldron.)

changes are particularly obvious in cytologic smears taken from early, freshly opened vesicles (Fig. 16–24). Such smears form the basis for a rapid supplemental test for pemphigus, the

"Tzanck test," and these cytologic findings have been discussed in detail by Medak and his associates as well as by Shklar and Cataldo. Shklar has also reported that there is a marked

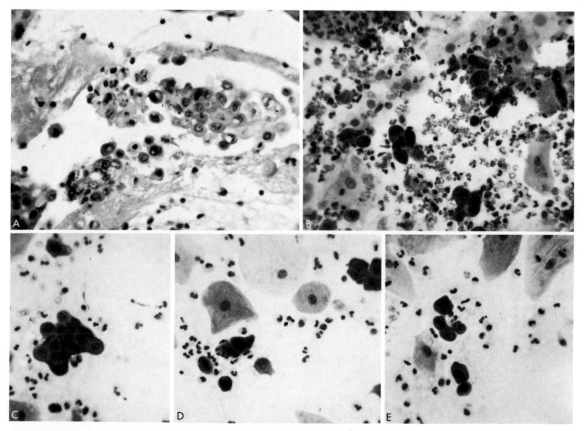

Figure 16–24. *Pemphigus vulgaris.*
The characteristic acantholytic cells are seen in the histologic section of the vesicle (A). These same cells are found on cytologic smear of the vesicle (B, C, D, E,).

increase in RNA in the cytoplasm of these acantholytic cells as well as in the epithelial cells at the floor of the vesicle.

The fluid in most vesicles, particularly those more than a day or two old, contains variable numbers of polymorphonuclear leukocytes and lymphocytes. The relative scarcity of inflammatory cell infiltration, however, in both the vesicular fluid and in the connective tissue at the base of the vesicle or bulla, is suggestive of pemphigus, since most other bullous diseases manifest marked inflammation. Once secondary infection occurs, this feature is masked.

Immunofluorescent testing has proven to be of great value in establishing the diagnosis of pemphigus, especially when the clinical or microscopic findings are inconclusive. In this test, *direct immunofluorescence* is used to demonstrate the presence of immunoglobulins, predominantly IgG but sometimes in combination with C3, IgA and IgM, in the intercellular spaces or intercellular substance in either the oral epithelium of the lesions or of clinically normal epithelium adjacent to the lesions. This test is carried out by incubating a biopsy specimen (either frozen section or one specially fixed in Michel solution) with a fluorescein-conjugated antiglobulin. *Indirect immunofluorescence* has also been used to substantiate the diagnosis of pemphigus. This is accomplished basically by incubating normal animal or human mucosa with serum from the patient suspected of having the disease and adding the fluorescein-conjugated human antiglobulin. A positive reaction in the tissue indicates the presence of circulating immunoglobulin antibodies. Daniels and Quadra-White have reported positive direct immunofluorescence for IgG in ten biopsies of ten patients (100 per cent) with pemphigus vulgaris (Fig. 16–25). Six of these ten also were positive for C3, while only one each was positive for IgA and IgM. Laskaris has also found, in testing a series of 58 patients with pemphigus vulgaris limited to the oral cavity, positive direct immunofluorescence in 57 (98 per cent), demonstrating intercellular substance deposition of IgG, either alone or in combination with C3, IgA, and IgM. By indirect immunofluorescence, Laskaris also reported that, when normal human oral mucosa was used as the substrate, circulating intercellular substance antibodies were present in 50 of the 58 patients (86 per cent).

Oral cytologic smears from patients with oral lesions of pemphigus vulgaris have also been tested for immunofluorescence and it has been

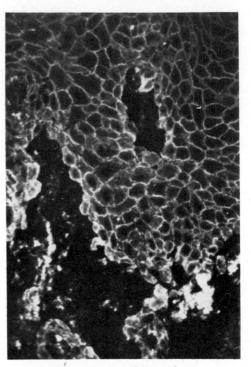

Figure 16–25. Pemphigus vulgaris.
Oral specimen showing intercellular space fluorescence throughout the epithelium with anti-IgG. At lower left there is an intraepithelial vesicle above the basal epithelial cells attached to the basement membrane zone. (Courtesy of Dr. Troy E. Daniels and C. V. Mosby Company. From Daniels, T. E., and Quadra-White, C.: Direct immunofluorescence in oral mucosal disease: a diagnostic analysis of 130 cases. Oral Surg., *51*:38, 1981.)

reported by Acosta and his associates that these smears were positive in all 13 patients tested by the direct technique for intercellular IgG deposition. It was concluded that the cytologic smear–direct immunofluorescence technique may be of value in the diagnosis of pemphigus.

Differential Diagnosis. Oral lesions constitute an important feature of pemphigus, and for this reason pemphigus must always be considered in the differential diagnosis of blister-like eruptions of oral mucous membranes. Some difficulty may be experienced in differentiating pemphigus from other bullous diseases such as dermatitis herpetiformis, erythema multiforme bullosum, bullous lichen planus, epidermolysis bullosa and other chronic bullous dermatoses such as bullous pemphigoid and cicatricial pemphigoid. Clinical experience, however, aided by the histologic appearance of the lesions, usually suffices to separate the diseases.

Treatment. Pemphigus is a serious disease. Prior to the advent of the corticosteroids, the mortality rate approximated 95 per cent, particularly for pemphigus vulgaris. Today, steroids and antibiotic therapy for secondary infection have reduced the mortality so that only 30 to 40 per cent of patients will die either of the disease or of the side effects of treatment. Some cases still run an acute course despite treatment and terminate in early death. Other cases, especially certain types such as pemphigus foliaceus, vegetans or erythematosus, may undergo prolonged remission in a varying percentage of instances.

It is important to realize that, while systemic therapy is important to the over-all treatment of the disease, topical therapy of both skin and oral lesions is especially necessary because of the pain and discomfort suffered by these patients.

FAMILIAL BENIGN CHRONIC PEMPHIGUS

(Hailey-Hailey Disease)

Familial benign chronic pemphigus is an uncommon dermatologic disease transmitted by an irregular dominant gene, although some patients do not manifest a familial history. Furthermore, in certain families, some generations may be symptom-free. The disease itself appears to represent an epidermal defect, either a fault in the synthesis or maturation of the tonofilament and desmosome complex.

Clinical Features. The disease first manifests itself during adolescence or young adult life, although there are occasional exceptions. There is no apparent predilection for occurrence in either sex.

The lesions themselves develop as small groups of vesicles appearing on normal or erythematous skin, which soon rupture to leave eroded, crusted areas. These lesions then appear to enlarge peripherally but heal in the center. Nikolsky's sign is present. It has been frequently noted that heat and sweating amplify the outbreak of the lesions while spontaneous remissions may occur in cold weather. The lesions themselves develop most commonly on those areas of skin which are exposed to friction—e.g., flexure surfaces of the axillae and groin, the neck and the genital area. Tender and enlarged regional lymph nodes may also be present.

It has been recognized that bacterial infection also appears to precipitate the appearance of lesions and, more recently, infection by *Candida albicans* has been implicated.

Oral Manifestations. Oral lesions occasionally occur in patients with familial benign chronic pemphigus, and these are similar to those occurring on the skin. The lesions develop as crops of vesicles which rapidly rupture leaving raw eroded areas.

Histologic Features. The histologic appearance of the epithelial lesions in familial benign chronic pemphigus bears remarkable similarity to that seen in pemphigus vulgaris and in keratosis follicularis or Darier's disease. However, in familial benign chronic pemphigus there is generally more extensive acantholysis than in pemphigus vulgaris and there is usually less damage to the acantholytic cells. One of the characteristic features of this disease is that occasional intercellular bridges persist so that adjacent epithelial cells still adhere to each other and are not entirely acantholytic. This appearance has been given the classic description of the "dilapidated brick wall" effect. Finally, benign dyskeratotic cells similar to the corps ronds of Darier's disease may be present.

Treatment and Prognosis. Antibiotic therapy is generally effective in controlling the lesions. Long remissions are common but seldom does the disease ever disappear spontaneously. It often becomes less severe as the patient ages.

CICATRICIAL PEMPHIGOID

(Benign Mucous Membrane Pemphigoid; Ocular Pemphigus)

Cicatricial pemphigoid is a vesiculobullous disease of unknown etiology but probably autoimmune in nature which is relatively uncommon, although it may occur more often than realized as a result of misdiagnosis. It has been discussed in detail by Shklar and McCarthy and more recently by Foster and Nally and by Mitchell and Smith.

Clinical Features. The disease occurs nearly twice as frequently in females as it does in males with the peak age of involvement being between 40 and 50 years. Typically, the vesiculobullous lesions occur on the oral mucous membranes and conjunctiva. Lesions also occur on the skin, particularly around the genitalia and near the body orifices in about 25 per cent of cases. Typically, these lesions heal by scar formation, particularly on the conjunctiva. Other mucous membrane surfaces may be involved such as the nose, larynx, pharynx, esophagus, vulva, vagina, penis and anus.

The ocular involvement is probably the most

serious complication of this disease. Following
the initial conjunctivitis, adhesions develop between the palpebral and bulbar conjunctivae
resulting in obliteration of the palpebral fissure,
with opacity of the cornea frequently leading to
complete blindness.

Oral Manifestations. The most consistent oral
lesions to occur are those involving the gingivae, although ultimately other sites in the oral
cavity become involved. The mucosal lesions
are also vesiculobullous in nature but appear to
be relatively thick-walled and, for this reason,
may persist for 24 to 48 hours before rupturing
and desquamating. Eventually their rupture
does occur leaving a raw, eroded, bleeding
surface. The gingivae frequently manifest a persistent erythema for weeks or even months after
the original erosions have healed (Fig. 16–26A).
These oral lesions rarely scar. In the past, this
disease has often been diagnosed as "chronic
desquamative gingivitis," a term now used only
in the descriptive sense and not as a specific
disease entity.

Histologic Features. The histologic findings in
cicatricial pemphigoid, in contrast to pemphigus
vulgaris, are nonspecific. The vesicles and bullae are subepidermal rather than suprabasilar
and there is no evidence of acantholysis (Fig.
16–26, *B*). The basement membrane structure
appears to detach with the epithelium from the
underlying connective tissue, as shown in the
electron microscope studies of Susi and Shklar.
There is a nonspecific chronic inflammatory
infiltrate in the connective tissue, chiefly lymphocytes, plasma cells and eosinophils.

Immunofluorescence studies have revealed
the presence of tissue-bound basement membrane zone antibodies in most patients with this
disease as well as circulating anti-basement
membrane zone antibodies in the serum of
some patients. Daniels and Quadra-White reported the results of direct immunofluoresence
examinations in 33 patients with cicatricial pemphigoid. Of these, they found that 17 (51 per
cent) showed a linear basement membrane zone
pattern of IgG, 10 (33 per cent) IgA, 12 (36 per
cent) IgM, and 32 (97 per cent) C3 (Fig. 16–
27). Laskaris and Angelopoulos also reported
both direct and indirect immunofluorescent
studies on 33 patients with cicatricial pemphigoid and found 32 of the 33 (97 per cent) had a
direct total positive basement membrane zone
pattern (IgG 32/33; IgA 9/33; IgM 4/33; C3 26/
33; fibrin 13/33), while only 12 of the 33 (36 per
cent) had an indirect positive using the patients'
serum and a substrate of normal human oral
mucosa (IgG only; all others negative). These
authors pointed out that the immunofluorescence pattern of cicatricial pemphigoid was indistinguishable from the pattern observed in
bullous pemphigoid and that this gave support
to the possibility that the two diseases may
represent variants of the same entity.

Differential Diagnosis. Because of the nonspecific microscopic findings on biopsy, a variety of other diseases must be considered in the
differential diagnosis. The chief of these are
pemphigus vulgaris, bullous pemphigoid, erosive lichen planus, and bullous erythema multiforme.

Treatment and Prognosis. In mild forms of
the disease, no treatment is necessary. However, if the bullous eruptions are severe or
there is conjunctival involvement, topical, intralesional or systemic corticosteroid therapy is
indicated. In very severe cases, immunosup-

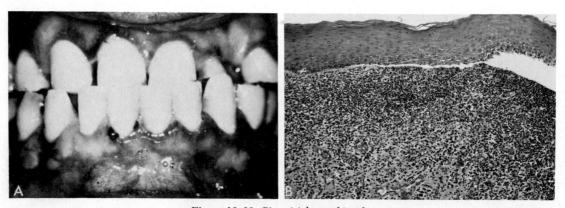

Figure 16–26. *Cicatricial pemphigoid.*
Erythematous and eroded areas are seen in *A*, while the typical subepidermal separation is apparent in *B*. (*A*, Courtesy
of Dr. Richard W. Henry.)

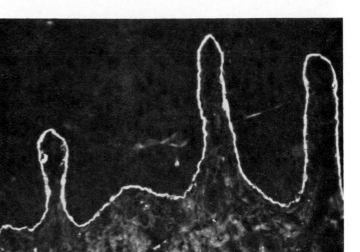

Figure 16–27. *Cicatricial pemphigoid.*
Oral specimen showing continuous linear fluorescence in the basement membrane zone with anti-C'3. (Courtesy of Dr. Troy E. Daniels and C. V. Mosby Company. From Daniels, T. E., and Quadra-White, C.: Direct immunofluorescence in oral mucosal disease: a diagnostic analysis of 130 cases. Oral Surg., *51*:38, 1981.)

pressive agents have been used. The disease characteristically has exacerbations and remissions but generally extends over a period of many years.

BULLOUS PEMPHIGOID

(Parapemphigus)

Bullous pemphigoid is a disease which differs markedly from pemphigus vulgaris but has many features in common with cicatricial pemphigoid. In fact, some investigators suggest that bullous pemphigoid and cicatricial pemphigoid are simply variants of a single entity. This has been discussed in detail by Person and Rogers. Still other dermatologists consider bullous pemphigoid to be a variant of dermatitis herpetiformis (q.v.).

Clinical Features. Bullous pemphigoid is basically a disease of elderly persons, approximately 80 per cent of patients being over 60 years of age. Nevertheless, it can occur earlier in life. There appears to be no sex predilection.

The cutaneous lesions begin as a generalized nonspecific rash, commonly on the limbs, which appears urticarial or eczematous and which may persist for several weeks to several months before the ultimate appearance of the vesiculobullous lesions. The vesicles and bullae arise in these prodromal skin lesions as well as in normal skin. In addition to the occurrence on the limbs, the abdomen is frequently affected. These vesicles and bullae are relatively thick-walled and may remain intact for some days. Rupture does not always occur, although when it does it leaves a raw, eroded area which heals rapidly.

Oral Manifestations. Oral lesions occur far less frequently in bullous pemphigoid than in cicatricial pemphigoid, varying from approximately 10 to 45 per cent in various reported series. These oral lesions of bullous pemphigoid have been reviewed by Shklar and his associates and are usually described as vesicles and areas of erosion and ulceration. An important feature of the oral involvement is the similarity of gingival lesions to those of cicatricial pemphigoid. This gingival involvement generally involves much, if not all, of the gingival mucosa and is exceedingly painful. The gingival tissues appear extremely erythematous and may desquamate as the result of even minor frictional trauma. The vesicles and ultimate erosions may develop not only on the gingival tissues but in any other area such as the buccal mucosa, palate, floor of the mouth and tongue.

Histologic Features. The vesicles and bullae in this disease are subepidermal and nonspecific. There is no evidence of acantholysis of epithelial cells; in fact, the epithelium appears relatively normal. The vesicles contain a fibrinous exudate admixed with occasional inflammatory cells.

Electron microscope studies have shown that, in contrast to cicatricial pemphigoid, the basement membrane remains attached to the connective tissue rather than to the overlying separated epithelium. In addition, these ultrastructural studies have shown that the primary changes in bullous pemphigoid appear to occur in the connective tissue where the blood vessels show alterations in their penetrability.

The basement membrane also shows thickening, with interruption of continuity.

Bullous pemphigoid is thought to be an autoimmune disease and circulating basement membrane zone antibodies have been found by the indirect immunofluorescence technique in about 80 per cent of patients with this disease, according to the study of 29 patients reported by Laskaris and Nicolis. Direct immunofluorescent studies of these same patients revealed tissue-bound anti-basement membrane zone antibodies of the IgG class in all oral mucosal biopsies (100 per cent) of patients who had both mucosal and skin lesions (14 patients), but in only 80 per cent of oral mucosal biopsies in the group of patients who had only skin lesions (15 patients).

Treatment and Prognosis. Treatment for the disease consists of systemic corticosteroid therapy. The mortality rate is not high and spontaneous remissions may occur.

EPIDERMOLYSIS BULLOSA

Epidermolysis bullosa is an uncommon group of dermatologic diseases in which bullae or vesicles occur on skin or mucous membrane surfaces spontaneously or after minor trauma. Several different forms of the condition are recognized and these may be classified as follows:

1. Epidermolysis bullosa simplex
   a. Generalized form
   b. Localized form (Weber-Cockayne syndrome, recurrent bullous eruption of hands and feet)
2. Epidermolysis bullosa dystrophic, dominant
3. Epidermolysis bullosa dystrophic, recessive
4. Junctional epidermolysis bullosa (epidermolysis bullosa letalis, junctional bullous epidermatosis, Herlitz's disease)
5. Epidermolysis bullosa acquisita (acquired)

There are distinct differences in the manifestations of these various types necessitating their individual consideration, and these have been reviewed in detail by Gorlin and by Crawford and his co-workers.

Epidermolysis Bullosa Simplex

Clinical Features. The *generalized* form of epidermolysis bullosa simplex is inherited as an autosomal dominant characteristic, manifests itself at birth or shortly thereafter and is characterized by the formation of vesicles and bullae, chiefly on the hands and feet at sites of friction or trauma. The knees, elbows and trunk are only rarely involved and the nails are only occasionally affected. When the blisters heal, usually within two to ten days, it is an important feature that there is no resultant scarring or permanent pigmentation. The disease appears to improve at puberty and prognosis is good for a normal life span.

The *localized* form of the disease (Weber-Cockayne syndrome), which is also familial may occur early in childhood or later in life and is commonly recurrent. The bullae only develop on the hands and feet, are related to frictional trauma and tend to exacerbate in hot weather. There is no scarring upon healing.

Oral Manifestations. Bullae of the oral cavity have been reported in occasional cases of generalized epidermolysis bullosa simplex, but it is doubtful that they actually occur. In addition, the teeth are not affected.

Histologic Features. In the generalized form of epidermolysis bullosa simplex, the vesicles and bullae develop as a result of destruction of basal and suprabasal cells so that some nuclei may persist on the floor of the blister, according to Lowe. The individual cells become edematous and show dissolution of organelles and tonofibrils with displacement of the nucleus to the upper end of the cell. The PAS (periodic acid-Schiff)-positive basement membrane remains on the dermal side of the separation. The elastic, pre-elastic and oxytalan fibers in the connective tissue are normal.

In the *localized* form of the disease, the bullae are intra-epidermal and suprabasal in location.

Epidermolysis Bullosa Dystrophic, Dominant

Clinical Features. This form of the disease may have its onset in infancy or it may be delayed until puberty. The blisters commonly develop on the ankles, knees, elbows, feet and head; healing results in scarring which is sometimes keloidal in type. In the majority of cases, the nails are thick and dystrophic, and milia are commonly present. However, the eye is never involved. Palmar-plantar keratoderma with hyperhidrosis also may occur as well as ichthyosis and sometimes hypertrichosis.

Oral Manifestations. Bullae of the oral cavity have been described as occurring in about 20 per cent of cases of this type, and Andreasen has described oral milia. The teeth are unaffected.

Histologic Features. The bullae in this form of the disease develop as a result of separation through the very thin, irregular PAS-positive basement membrane which becomes divided. The basal layer appears normal although flattened on the roof of the blister. The underlying connective tissue shows an absence of elastic and oxytalan fibers.

EPIDERMOLYSIS BULLOSA DYSTROPHIC, RECESSIVE

Clinical Features. This type of epidermolysis bullosa is the best known and classic form of the disease. It has its onset at birth or very shortly thereafter and is characterized by the formation of bullae spontaneously or at sites of trauma, friction or pressure (Fig. 16–28, A). The typical sites of involvement are the feet, buttocks, scapulae, elbows, fingers and occiput. The bullae contain a clear, bacteriologically sterile or sometimes blood-tinged fluid. When these bullae rupture or are peeled off under trauma or pressure, they leave a raw, painful surface. These patients frequently have a positive Nikolsky's sign. The bullae heal by scar, milia and pigmentation (Fig. 16–28, B). This scarring may result in afunctional club-like fists.

The hair may be sparse while the nails are usually dystrophic or absent.

Oral Manifestations. Oral bullae are common in this form of the disease. They may be preceded by the appearance of white spots or patches on the oral mucous membrane or the development of localized areas of inflammation. The bullae may be initiated by nursing or by any simple dental operative procedure in the oral cavity. Unless great caution is used, large areas of mucous membrane may be inadvertently denuded. These bullae are painful, especially when they rupture or when the epithelium desquamates (Fig. 16–28). Scar formation often results in obliteration of sulci and restriction of the tongue. Hoarseness and dysphagia may occur as a result of bullae of the larynx and pharynx. Esophageal involvement may produce serious stricture.

Dental defects have also been described, consisting of rudimentary teeth, congenitally absent teeth, hypoplastic teeth and crowns denuded of enamel. These have been discussed in detail by Arwill and his associates.

Histologic Features. The separation and bulla formation here occur immediately beneath the poorly defined PAS-positive basement membrane which remains attached to the roof of the blister. Fragments of the basement membrane may adhere to the dermis, however. The basal layer of cells is normal. The pre-elastic and oxytalan fibers in the connective tissue are increased in number. Elastic fibers are also increased but appear fragmented, according to Lowe.

JUNCTIONAL EPIDERMOLYSIS BULLOSA

It has been suggested by some workers that the junctional or lethal type is simply an ex-

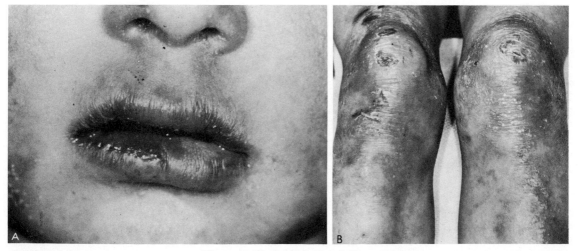

Figure 16–28. *Epidermolysis bullosa.*
A. The lower lip shows painful desquamation of the epithelium. *B,* The bullae and the typical scarring of the knees are indicative of the dystrophic recessive form of the disease. (Courtesy of Dr. John Mink.)

tremely severe form of the dystrophic recessive form which is incompatible with prolonged survival. However, some recent studies have suggested that the two may be distinctly different disorders. Clarification of this must await further study.

Clinical Features. Three criteria have been established for the diagnosis of this form of the disease. These are: (1) onset at birth, (2) absence of scarring, milia or pigmentation, and (3) death within three months of age. The bullae are similar to those seen in the dystrophic recessive type except that they commonly develop spontaneously, and sheets of skin may actually be shed.

Oral Manifestations. Oral bullae are frequently very extensive and, because of their extreme fragility, produce serious feeding problems. Similar lesions also occur in the upper respiratory tract, the bronchioles and the esophagus.

Severe disturbances in enamel and dentin formation of the deciduous teeth also occur but this is of only academic interest. These have been described by Arwill and his associates and by Gardner and Hudson in significant detail.

Histologic Features. The microscopic changes, including the location of the bullous cleavage, appear similar and probably identical to those occurring in the dystrophic recessive disease.

Epidermolysis Bullosa Acquisita

This is a rare form of epidermolysis bullosa in which there is no evidence of hereditary transmission. It is similar in many respects to the dystrophic form of the disease, including bullae developing at the sites of trauma, milia, mucous membrane involvement and dystrophy of the nails. However, the onset of the disease is in adult life. This condition has been discussed by Roenigk and his associates, who also reviewed the reported cases.

Treatment. This group of diseases cannot be cured so that therapy is chiefly symptomatic. The simplex form of the disease requires little treatment; the lethal form will terminate fatally in most cases regardless of management. In the dystrophic forms, prevention of trauma may reduce the incidence of bulla formation, but this is almost impossible to achieve. Antibiotics are useful in controlling secondary infection and corticosteroids have sometimes been found effective.

DERMATITIS HERPETIFORMIS
(Duhring-Brocq Disease)

Dermatitis herpetiformis is a rare, benign, chronic, recurrent dermatologic disease of unknown etiology. Patients with this disease have an interesting associated malabsorption enteropathy, similar in some respects to celiac disease. They commonly have a decrease in enzymatic disaccharidase and dipeptidase activities and villous atrophy of the small intestine. Whether the disease is a reaction pattern and whether the activity of the skin lesions can be correlated with the enteropathy is not yet known. However, the gluten-free diet found so useful in the control of celiac disease has been of less benefit in dermatitis herpetiformis.

Despite the name, it is totally unrelated to herpes simplex infection or the herpesvirus. Emotional disturbances and acute infections are both reported to precipitate an attack of the disease.

Clinical Features. The disease occurs chiefly between 20 and 55 yrs of age, although children occasionally are involved. Males are affected at least twice as frequently as females.

The first manifestations of the disease are usually pruritus and severe burning, followed by the development of erythematous papules, vesicles, bullae or pustules. These occur most frequently on the extremities, trunk and buttocks as well as on the face, scalp and sometimes oral cavity. The vesicle is the most common and characteristic lesion, usually occurring symmetrically and in groups. Pigmentation of involved areas of skin ultimately develops in most cases. Patients frequently show increased severity of the disease in summer months.

Oral Manifestations. Vesicles and bullae which rupture rapidly to leave areas of superficial ulceration at any intraoral site are the characteristic finding. These have been described by Russotto and Ship.

Histologic Features. The lesions begin by accumulation of neutrophils and eosinophils in the dermal papillae producing a microabscess. The connective tissue becomes necrotic and the overlying epithelium separates, usually forming a subepithelial vesicle with destruction of basement membrane. The presence of eosinophils is generally prominent and characteristic, aiding in the differential diagnosis by excluding epidermolysis bullosa, erythema multiforme and pemphigus.

Direct immunofluorescent staining of uninvolved paralesional skin has been shown by

Katz to be positive at the epidermal-dermal junction. Almost invariably, IgA alone or in combination with the immunoglobulins IgG or IgM will be found in the upper dermis. When IgA deposits occur at the dermal-epidermal junction in a linear pattern (about 14 per cent of cases) rather than as granules, the variant has been termed *linear IgA disease*. This has been discussed by Wiesenfeld and his colleagues, who also described the oral manifestations as being similar to those in the usual form of dermatitis herpetiformis.

Laboratory Findings. Some patients develop a blood eosinophilia of over 10 per cent. Interestingly, these patients also show a sensitivity to the halogens (chlorine, bromine, iodine and fluorine) both by patch test and after ingestion.

Treatment and Prognosis. Sulfapyridine is the treatment of choice; the disease usually does not respond to corticosteroid therapy. The disease runs a very prolonged course, often over 10 years. Prolonged remissions followed by recurrence are often seen, although some remissions are permanent. The longer the disease persists, the less severe are its manifestations in most cases.

ACRODERMATITIS ENTEROPATHICA

This is an uncommon genodermatosis, probably inherited as an autosomal recessive characteristic with about two-thirds of patients having a familial history. The basic defect appears to be related to a malabsorption of zinc through a genetic absence or deficiency in an intestinal zinc-binding ligand, possibly involving the zinc-rich Paneth cells concerned with some phase of zinc transport. Low serum zinc levels are confirmatory of this.

Clinical Features. The disease begins in the first few weeks or months of life with a localized eruption of the skin, particularly near the body orifices. Shortly, there is loss of hair and gastrointestinal disturbance accompanied by diarrhea. The skin lesions are vesiculobullous in nature and tend to occur in crops. These lesions rupture and become crusted and ultimately erythematous, scaling with a psoriasiform pattern. The skin lesions, and oral lesions as well, are prone to secondary infection, especially by *Candida albicans*. This is probably related to the deficiency in cell-mediated immunity reportedly manifested by the children.

Oral Manifestations. The oral mucosa, chiefly the buccal mucosa, becomes erythematous and edematous with erosive desquamative lesions.

These oral lesions have been described in the cases of Danbolt.

Treatment. This disease was considered fatal at one time, but the recent recognition of the true nature of the disease and its treatment by zinc supplement commonly results in excellent long-term survival. This treatment is so dramatic that all clinical manifestations may be reversed within just a few days.

LUPUS ERYTHEMATOSUS

Lupus erythematosus is a rather common disease of unknown etiology which has been described for many years. It exists in two basic forms: systemic lupus erythematosus and discoid lupus erythematosus. Some investigators believe that, despite the nomenclature, the discoid form of the disease is not related to systemic lupus erythematosus and represents solely a mucocutaneous disease. Other workers believe that discoid lupus erythematosus is but one manifestation of the generalized disease of systemic lupus erythematosus, even though it may take a long period of time for the other manifestations of systemic lupus to make their appearance. It should be noted that certain laboratory findings are common to both diseases, e.g., the presence of antinuclear antibodies, abnormal serum globulins, positive rheumatoid factor, elevated sedimentation rate and false-positive serologic test for syphilis.

Etiology. Regardless of whether these have been considered to be two separate disease entities or two forms of the same disease, the same etiologic factors have been considered for both systemic and discoid lupus erythematosus. These etiologic factors include a genetic predisposition to the disease and an immunologic abnormality, possibly mediated by a viral infection. The disease is characteristically classified as an autoimmune disease, since these patients develop antibodies to many of their own cells and cell components and tissues. In fact, some of the manifestations of the disease appear to result from the deposition of antigen-antibody complexes in the tissues.

Clinical Features. *Systemic lupus erythematosus* is a serious cutaneous-systemic disorder which characteristically manifests repeated remissions and exacerbations. This disease has its peak age of onset at about 30 years in females but about 40 years in males. The disease may occur in childhood as reported by Jacobs. There is a marked predilection for occurrence in females by a ratio of at least 8:1.

The cutaneous lesions consist of erythematous patches on the face which coalesce to form a roughly symmetrical pattern over the cheeks and across the bridge of the nose in a so-called butterfly distribution. Also involved are the neck, upper arms, shoulders and fingers. These lesions may present itching or burning sensations as well as areas of hyperpigmentation. The acute erythematous patches either arise on previously uninvolved skin or develop in old chronic lesions. Their severity is intensified by exposure to sunlight.

The generalized manifestations of the systemic disease are referable to involvement of various organs, including the kidney and heart. In the kidney, fibrinoid thickening of glomerular capillaries occurs, producing the characteristic "wire loops," which may be sufficient to result in renal insufficiency. The heart may suffer from an atypical endocarditis involving the valves, as well as fibrinoid degeneration of the epicardium and myocardium. The widespread tissue involvement and the nature of the lesions have led to the inclusion of this disease in that group known as the "collagen diseases," which also includes rheumatic fever, rheumatoid arthritis, polyarteritis nodosa, scleroderma and dermatomyositis.

Discoid lupus erythematosus is a relatively common disease which, like the systemic form, occurs predominantly in the third and fourth decades. It is also considerably more common in women than in men. Although any skin area may be involved by the discoid form of lupus erythematosus, the most common sites are the face, oral mucous membranes, chest, back and extremities.

The typical cutaneous lesions are slightly elevated red or purple macules that are often covered by gray or yellow adherent scales. Forceful removal of the scale reveals numerous "carpet tack" extensions which had dipped into enlarged pilosebaceous canals. The lesions increase in size by peripheral growth, this feature partially characterizing the disease. The periphery of the lesion appears pink or red, while the center exhibits an atrophic, scarred appearance indicative of the long-standing nature of the disease with characteristic central healing. The discoid form of the disease may also assume a typical "butterfly" distribution on the malar regions and across the bridge of the nose. Since this is not a constant feature of the disease and since a similar distribution of lesions may occur in certain other diseases, its diagnostic significance should not be overemphasized.

Epidermoid carcinoma and, less commonly, basal cell carcinoma have been reported developing in healed scars of discoid lupus. This is only an occasional finding, reportedly between 0.5 and 3.6 per cent of patients, and is thought to occur only in cases of 20 years' duration or more.

Oral Manifestations. Oral mucous membrane involvement is reported in 20 to 50 per cent of cases of discoid lupus erythematosus, and slightly more frequently in the systemic form of the disease, according to Andreasen. With the oral mucous membranes affected in such a high percentage of cases, the dentist must be aware of this problem. The oral mucosa reportedly may be involved either prior to or following the development of skin lesions or even in the absence of skin manifestations.

The oral lesions in the *discoid* form begin as erythematous areas, sometimes slightly elevated but more often depressed, usually without induration and typically with white spots. Occasionally, superficial, painful ulceration may occur with crusting or bleeding but no actual scale formation as is seen on the skin (Figs. 16–29; 16–30). The margins of the lesions are not sharply demarcated but frequently show the formation of a narrow zone of keratinization. Often, fine white striae radiate out from the margins. Central healing may result in depressed scarring. These lesions, which were symptomatic in 75 per cent of a group of 32 patients with oral manifestation described by Schiödt and his associates, are most common on the buccal mucosa, palate and tongue. In the case of the tongue, atrophy of the papillae and severe fissuring are also seen. The vermilion border of the lips, particularly the lower, is a very common site for these lesions. The erythematous, atrophic plaques, surrounded by a keratotic border, may involve the entire lip and extend onto the skin surface. Malignant transformation of these lip lesions occurs with some frequency, and the reported cases have been reviewed by Andreasen.

Oral lesions are also found in *systemic* lupus erythematosus. These are very similar to those found in discoid lupus except that hyperemia, edema and extension of the lesions is sometimes more pronounced, and there may be a greater tendency for bleeding, petechiae and superficial ulcerations which are surrounded by a red halo as a result of localized telangiectasis. Superimposed oral moniliasis as well as xerostomia have also been reported.

Sugarman pointed out that great variation in

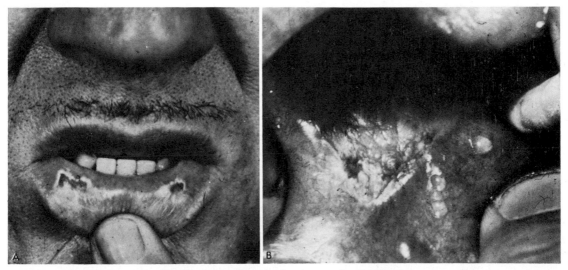

Figure 16–29. *Lupus erythematosus, chronic discoid.*
Typical lesions of the lip *(A)* and buccal mucosa *(B)*. (Courtesy of Dr. Boynton H. Booth.)

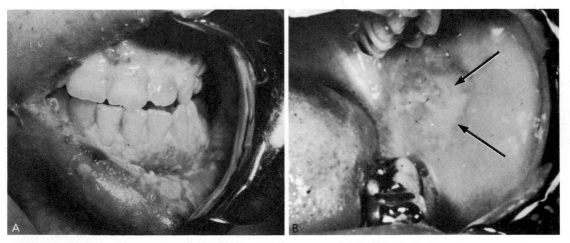

Figure 16–30. *Lupus erythematosus, chronic discoid.*
(*A*, Courtesy of Dr. Robert J. Gorlin and *B*, of Dr. Nathaniel H. Rowe.)

the oral lesions exists and that these frequently simulate other diseases, chiefly leukoplakia and lichen planus. For this reason, diagnosis based upon the clinical appearance of the oral lesions should not be encouraged. In fact, it has been stressed by Schiödt and his co-workers in a long-term follow-up study of 52 patients with discoid lupus erythematosus that those oral lesions which had undergone a transition into the leukoplakia-like lesions over a period of time even showed histopathologic and immunopathologic features similar to leukoplakia not preceded by lupus erythematosus.

Laboratory Findings. A specific test for the disease was established with the discovery of the "L.E." cell inclusion phenomenon by Hargraves and his associates. Although several techniques for this procedure have been described, the test consists essentially in the addition of the blood serum from a person under suspicion to the buffy coat of normal blood. If the patient is suffering from systemic lupus erythematosus, typical "L.E." cells will develop. This cell, or phenomenon, consists of a rosette of neutrophils surrounding a pale nuclear mass apparently derived from a lymphocyte. The basis of this phenomenon appears to lie in the gamma globulin of the serum from the patient. The significance of this test was described by Weiss and Swift, who pointed out the possibility of falsely positive reactions. On only rare occasions is the L.E. cell found in cases of discoid lupus erythematosus.

There is also an anemia, leukopenia, thrombocytopenia and elevated sedimentation rate, as well as an elevated serum gamma globulin level and a positive Coombs test, in a significant percentage of patients with either systemic or discoid disease. In addition, antinuclear antibodies can be demonstrated in patients with both forms of the disease, but these are far more common in those with systemic lupus.

Histologic Features. The histologic appearance of both forms of lupus erythematosus is similar, differing only in the degree of certain of the findings. According to Lever, discoid lupus erythematosus of the skin is characterized by hyperkeratosis with keratotic plugging, atrophy of the rete pegs, liquefaction degeneration of the basal layer of cells, perivascular infiltration of lymphocytes and their collection about dermal appendages, and basophilic degeneration of collagen and elastic fibers, with hyalinization, edema and fibrinoid change, particularly prominent immediately beneath the epithelium. Not all features are invariably present in

each case, however. In the systemic form of the disease the cutaneous lesions are similar in appearance, although the degenerative features and collagen disturbance are usually more prominent and the inflammatory features less severe. The histologic appearance of the tissue from a cutaneous lesion of any type of lupus erythematosus is not pathognomonic of the disease, but is certainly suggestive.

The histologic findings in oral lesions of both discoid and systemic lupus erythematosus have been described in detail by Andreasen and Poulsen. Shklar and McCarthy have also discussed the histopathology of the oral lesions in 25 cases and concluded that it is sufficiently characteristic that a definitive diagnosis can be made. In the *discoid* form, the lesions exhibit hyperorthokeratosis and/or hyperparakeratosis alternating with areas of epithelial atrophy. In the majority of cases, keratotic plugging down into the spinous layer, acanthosis and pseudoepitheliomatous hyperplasia are present. Hydropic degeneration and liquefaction necrosis of the basal cell layer also invariably occurs as well as subepithelial vesiculation or ulceration. In most cases, a thickening of the basement membrane can be demonstrated as a homogeneous, broad, eosinophilic and PAS-positive acellular band. Finally, there is a diffuse infiltrate of lymphocytes with smaller numbers of plasma cells and occasional polymorphonuclear leukocytes in superficial and deep connective tissue. This is quite reminiscent of that seen in lichen planus. Small focal perivascular collections of lymphocytes are found also, as well as degeneration and disintegration of collagen.

The systemic form of lupus exhibits histologic changes in the oral lesions that are virtually identical to those in the discoid type with the possible exception of the absence of keratinization.

Direct immunofluorescent testing is often used to confirm a suspected diagnosis of lupus erythematosus. It is basically a test used to detect the presence of immunoglobulins (IgG, IgM and IgA) at the epidermal-dermal junction or basement membrane zone of skin or oral mucosa of patients with the disease by incubating a biopsy specimen (either frozen section or one specially fixed in Michel solution) with a fluorescein-conjugated antiglobulin. The appearance of the immunoglobulins deposited in this location in discoid lupus generally is the "particulate" (or "speckled") pattern. These immunoglobulins were present at this specific histologic location in oral lesions in all patients with the systemic form and in nearly 75 per cent of patients with the discoid form in a series of 52 patients with lupus erythematosus reported by Schiödt and his associates in 1981. They also found a high incidence of complement C3 and of fibrinogen at this same zone utilizing appropriate conjugates. Interestingly, these immunoglobulins may also be demonstrated in the uninvolved skin and mucosa of a significant percentage of patients with systemic lupus, as well as in lesional skin or mucosa, but almost never in normal or uninvolved skin or mucosa of discoid patients. In a retrospective study of 130 cases of oral mucosal disease by direct immunofluorescence technique, Daniels and Quadra-White have concluded that this can provide a valuable criterion in diagnosing chronic ulcerative or erosive disease of the oral mucosa if the biopsy specimens are taken from appropriate sites and have attached epithelium.

Treatment. The majority of cases of systemic lupus erythematosus at one time terminated fatally. However, most of the cases can be aborted now and the patients kept in remission by corticosteroid therapy and/or antimalarial drugs. The discoid form may be slowly progressive over a period of many years. Occasionally spontaneous remission occurs or, in some instances, the systemic form of the disease develops superimposed on discoid lupus erythematosus. This happens in less than 5 per cent of cases, however.

SYSTEMIC SCLEROSIS

(Scleroderma; Dermatosclerosis; Hidebound Disease)

Progressive systemic sclerosis, a newer and more appropriate designation of the disease formerly called "scleroderma," is characterized by progressive fibrosis of skin and multiple organs and by vascular insufficiency through abnormalities in arterioles and capillaries. At one time, the disease was subclassified into two chief forms: (1) diffuse systemic and (2) the localized or morphea type including the circumscribed and the linear. Today, some investigators prefer to separate out the localized form, considering it neither to have any relationship to progressive systemic sclerosis nor to eventuate in the latter.

Raynaud's phenomenon is nearly always present in progressive systemic sclerosis; the hands and face are involved, but the feet are seldom affected. The term acrosclerosis is applied to those cases of the disease characterized by Raynaud's disease with sclerosis of the distal parts of the extremities, especially of the digits (sclerodactyly) and of the neck and face, particularly the nose.

Clinical Features. Progressive systemic sclerosis is a disease characterized by the ultimate induration of the skin and fixation of the epidermis to the deeper subcutaneous tissues. It may begin in children or young adults, although the greatest incidence is between 30 and 50 years of age, and exhibits a definite sex predilection, females being affected approximately twice as frequently as males.

Systemic sclerosis usually begins on the face, hands or trunk. Simultaneously with the development of the early typical indurated edema of the skin, neuralgia and paresthesia may occur as well as arthritis or simply vague joint pain. Erythema usually accompanies this cutaneous change. The disease progresses at a variable rate, but eventually much, if not all, of the body surface becomes involved. The skin takes on a yellow, gray or ivory-white waxy appearance. Brown pigmentation of the skin may also occur, but this is usually a late manifestation of the disease. Sometimes deposition of calcium in affected areas is also found. The skin becomes hardened and atrophic and cannot be wrinkled or picked up because of its firm fixation to the deep connective tissue. This contracture of the skin gives a masklike appearance to the face and a clawlike appearance to the hands.

Progressive diffuse systemic sclerosis may ultimately involve many internal organs by fibrosis, loss of smooth muscle and loss of visceral function. Those organs most frequently involved are the gastrointestinal tract, lungs, cardiovascular-renal system, musculoskeletal system and central nervous system.

One variant of systemic sclerosis is the CREST syndrome, an acronym of the five major findings: calcinosis cutis, Raynaud's phenomenon, esophageal dysfunction, sclerodactyly and telangiectasia. This form of the disease is sometimes not as severe as the usual systemic type.

The *etiology* of this disease is still unsettled, although several theories have been advanced supported by clinical and experimental data. These include: (1) an endocrine dysfunction, with features suggestive of both a thyroid and a parathyroid disturbance; (2) vascular disease, basically an endarteritis obliterans resulting in a decreased vascular bed; (3) a nervous disorder, since the skin lesions often follow the distribution of nerves or nerve roots and paresthetic disturbances are common; (4) toxic or infectious agents such as shock or pneumonia, influenza, diphtheria and exanthematous diseases; (5) an antigen-antibody allergic type of reaction or more specifically an autoimmune mechanism; and (6) a disease of adaptation. Onset following severe emotional shock is rather frequent also. The pathogenesis of the disease has been discussed by Winkelmann.

Circumscribed scleroderma, commonly termed *morphea*, is manifested by the appearance of one or more well-defined, slightly elevated or depressed cutaneous patches, which are white or yellowish and are surrounded by a violaceous halo. The plaques are varied in both size and shape. The lesions commonly occur on the sides of the chest and the thighs.

Occasionally the lesions occur as linear bands or ribbons on the face, particularly the forehead, on the chest and trunk or on an extremity. This has been termed *linear scleroderma*. Such a band, made up of a furrow with an elevated ridge on one side, is often termed a *coup de sabre*, since it resembles the mark produced by the blow of a saber. The circumscribed lesions eventually become stiff and hard. It has been reported that facial hemiatrophy is associated with this form of the disease occurring in children. The lesions are generally asymptomatic, although prickling, tingling and itching sensations have been described. The disease may persist for several months to many years, but, in this form, causes no deaths.

Oral Manifestations. The tongue, soft palate and larynx are the intraoral structures usually involved in progressive systemic sclerosis. Early mild edema of these structures is gradually followed by atrophy and induration of mucosal and muscular tissues. The tongue often becomes stiff and boardlike, causing the patient difficulty in eating and speaking. The gingival tissues are pale and unusually firm. The lips become thin, rigid and partially fixed, producing microstomia. Dysphagia, a choking sensation, inability to open and close the mouth and difficulty in beathing also occur. The reduced opening of the mouth and fixation of the jaw are a result of involvement of the peritemporomandibular joint tissues, and make dental care very difficult. Limitation of mouth opening was found in 80 per cent of a series of these patients by Marmary and his co-workers. Both Smith and Wade also have reviewed this disease with particular emphasis on the oral manifestations.

In addition, Alarcon-Segovia and his co-workers, studying 25 patients with progressive systemic sclerosis, found that all had pathologic changes in the minor salivary glands characteristic of Sjögren's disease: lymphocyte infiltration, duct cell proliferation and collagen infiltration. Weisman and Calcaterra also reported evidence of alterations of salivary gland function characteristic of the sicca syndrome in 12 per cent of 71 patients with scleroderma.

Roentgenographic Features. Extreme widening of the periodontal ligament, two to four times normal thickness, has been reported originally by Stafne and Austin as characteristic of scleroderma (Fig. 16–31). This may be so striking that, once the association is recognized, the occurrence of the periodontal disturbance as found on routine dental roentgenograms may be sufficient to establish a tentative diagnosis of systemic sclerosis. This has been confirmed by many studies such as those of White and his co-workers and of Marmary and his associates.

Bone resorption of the angle of the mandibular ramus, usually bilaterally, has also been reported by numerous investigators as occurring frequently in this disease. One additional roentgenographic feature reported has been

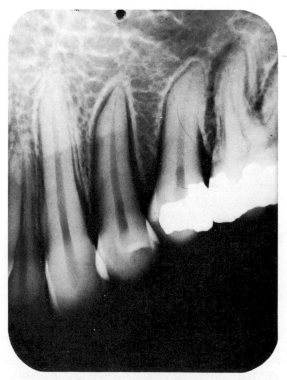

Figure 16–31. *Systemic sclerosis.*
The extreme widening of the periodontal ligament is obvious in the dental roentgenogram. (Courtesy of Dr. Edward C. Stafne.)

partial or complete resorption of condyles and/or coronoid processes of the mandible.

Histologic Features. Diffuse systemic sclerosis is characterized microscopically by thickening and hyalinization of the collagen fibers in the skin, the loss of dermal appendages, particularly the sweat glands, and atrophy of the epithelium with loss of rete pegs and increased melanin pigmentation. There is an increase in PAS-positive, diastase-resistant material present in the areas of the homogeneous collagen. Subcutaneous fat disappears, and the walls of the blood vessels become sclerotic. Mucous membrane changes are similar to those occurring in the skin.

The microscopic changes in the periodontal ligament consist of a widening due to an increase of collagen and oxytalan fibers as well as an appearance of hyalinization and sclerosis of collagen with a diminution in the number of connective tissue cells usually found. These changes have been described by Fullmer and Witte.

Treatment and Prognosis. There is no adequate treatment for progressive diffuse systemic sclerosis, although partial remissions have been reported following cortisone therapy. Circumscribed scleroderma has an excellent prognosis, since spontaneous remission usually occurs.

EHLERS-DANLOS SYNDROME

(Cutis Hyperelastica)

Ehlers-Danlos syndrome is a group of hereditary disorders of connective tissue which can be differentiated on clinical grounds by their mode of inheritance, the ultrastructural histology of the dermis and the biochemical findings. At least eight forms of the disease are now recognized (EDS I through VIII) with EDS I, EDS II and EDS III being the most common. These three are inherited as an autosomal dominant disease, but the biochemical bases are unknown although the collagen in each is abnormal. EDS IV is a clinically and genetically heterogeneous group in which there is an abnormality of type III collagen. EDS V is similar to EDS II but has an X-linked inheritance pattern. EDS VI is an autosomal recessive and characterized by a lysyl hydroxylase deficiency, so that the hydroxylysine content of skin is practically nil. EDS VII exists in two forms, one dominant and one recessive, that are identified biochemically as a result of different pro-

collagen enzyme abnormalities. EDS VIII appears to represent EDS II occurring in association with severe periodontitis. The molecular pathology in this disorder of collagen metabolism has been discussed by Byers and his associates.

Ehlers-Danlos syndrome appears closely related to and must be differentiated from Marfan syndrome, osteogenesis imperfecta, dentinogenesis imperfecta and pseudoxanthoma elasticum.

Clinical Features. The characteristic clinical features of this disease are the hyperelasticity of skin, hyperextensibility of the joints and fragility of the skin and blood vessels resulting in excessive bruising as well as defective healing of skin wounds. However, there may be considerable variation in the clinical manifestations depending upon the type of the syndrome present in the patient. For example, hyperextensibility of skin and joints is striking in EDS I and EDS III but very limited in EDS II and EDS IV. EDS IV is often called the *ecchymotic* type, since rupture of even large arteries as well as the intestine often occurs, producing a life-threatening situation. In instances in which the skin extensibility is pronounced, the patient has become known as the circus "rubber man." The facies are frequently distinctive with hypertelorism, a wide nasal bridge and epicanthic folds being common features. Protruding ears and frontal bossing are often present. Freely movable subcutaneous nodules are frequently found, and these appear to represent fibrosed lobules of fat. The scarring of the skin following wound healing in these patients is unusual inasmuch as the scars tend to spread rather than contract in time.

Oral Manifestations. The oral manifestations of this disease have been described in detail by Barabas and Barabas. In their series of cases, they found that the oral mucosa was of normal color but was excessively fragile and bruised easily. Although the mucosa did not hold sutures satisfactorily, healing was only slightly retarded and there was no defective scar formation. No remarkable hyperextensibility of mucous membrane could be demonstrated, and the patients had no difficulty in wearing dentures. The gingival tissues appeared fragile and bled after toothbrushing. Tooth mobility was not increased. Hypermobility of the temporomandibular joint, resulting in repeated dislocations of the jaw, has been reported.

Alterations in the structure of the teeth have also been reported by Barabas and these consist of a lack of normal scalloping of the dentino-enamel junction, the passage of many dentinal tubules into the enamel, the formation of much irregular dentin and an increased tendency to form pulp stones. Hypoplastic changes in the enamel have also been reported, while Hoff has further emphasized the dental changes.

Several families have also been reported with apparent Ehlers-Danlos syndrome with extensive periodontal destruction. This has been reviewed by Linch and Acton, who described an additional case.

Histologic Features. Histologic study of skin and connective tissues by routine techniques generally fails to reveal any characteristic or diagnostic abnormality. Ultrastructural changes in collagen have been reported in some forms of the disease, according to Byers and his associates.

Laboratory Findings. Blood clotting is normal but the capillary fragility test is usually positive.

Treatment. There is no known treatment for the disease. Surgical procedures should be carried out with care because difficulty in suturing and healing problems may exist.

FOCAL DERMAL HYPOPLASIA SYNDROME

(Goltz-Gorlin Syndrome)

The focal dermal hypoplasia syndrome is a disease transmitted as an autosomal dominant characteristic with incomplete penetrance which shows marked predilection for occurrence in females. Because of the widespread defects, it is usually characterized as a mesoectodermal dysplasia.

Clinical Features. The syndrome is characterized by relative focal absence of the dermis associated with herniation of the subcutaneous fat into the defects; skin atrophy, streaky pigmentation and telangiectasia; multiple papillomas of the mucosa and/or skin; anomalies of the extremities including syndactyly, polydactyly and adactyly; an asymmetrical face with pointed chin and notched nasal alae; asymmetrical ears; sunken eyes with sparse eyebrows and scalp hair; eye anomalies, most frequently iris and choroid colobomata and strabismus; and dental and oral anomalies.

Mental retardation is often present as is some retardation of physical growth. In addition, many other anomalies have also been reported with varying frequency.

Oral Manifestations. Papillomas of the lips have been a striking feature in a number of these patients as well as papillomas of the buccal mucosa or gingiva. In addition, the teeth are commonly defective in size, shape or structure. Microdontia is a common finding as is enamel hypoplasia. Cleft lips/cleft palate has also been described in several cases. Details of the disease have been discussed by Gorlin and his associates.

Treatment. There is no treatment for the disease.

SOLAR ELASTOSIS

(Senile Elastosis; Actinic Elastosis)

Solar elastosis is a dermatologic disease which is essentially a degenerative condition of skin associated with the general process of aging which itself may be influenced by hereditary factors including skin coloration or pigmentation or its absence, and exposure to the elements, especially sunlight and wind. Such skin, damaged by prolonged exposure to elements of the weather, has often been termed *sailor's skin* or *farmer's skin*. It is interesting that this disease, though common, has not been widely reported.

Clinical Features. This disturbance seldom occurs on the oral mucous membranes, but does involve the lip with considerable frequency. Although not confined to elderly patients, it is most common in this age group. The affected skin is wrinkled and appears dry, atrophic and flaccid. On the lip there may be mild keratosis and subtle blending of the vermilion with the skin surface.

Histologic Features. The chief microscopic characteristic is the apparent increase in the amount of elastic connective tissue fibers, a phenomenon that is best observed by special stains. In routine hematoxylin and eosin stained sections, the connective tissue may appear hyalinized, but it stains with hematoxylin rather than with eosin and this has been termed basophilic degeneration.

Treatment. There is no treatment for solar elastosis any more than for approaching old age in general.

REFERENCES

Abbey, L., and Shklar, G.: A histochemical study of oral lichen planus. Oral Surg., *31*:226, 1971.

Ackerman, A. B.: Focal acantholytic dyskeratosis. Arch. Dermatol., *106*:702, 1972.

Acosta, A. E., Hietanen, J., and Ivanyi, L.: Direct immunofluorescence on cytological smears in oral pemphigus. Br. J. Dermatol., 105:645, 1981.

Alarcon-Segovia, D., Ibanez, G., Hernandez-Ortiz, J., Velasquez-Forero, F., and Gonzalez-Jimenez, Y.: Sjogren's syndrome in progressive systemic sclerosis (scleroderma). Am. J. Med., 57:78, 1974.

Allen, A. C.: The Skin: A Clinocopathologic Treatise. 2nd ed. New York, Grune & Stratton, 1967.

Altman, J., and Perry, H. O.: The variations and course of lichen planus. Arch. Dermatol., 84:179, 1961.

Andreasen, J. O.: Oral lichen planus. I. A clinical evaluation of 115 cases. Oral Surg., 25:31, 1968.

Andreasen, J. O.: Oral lichen planus. II. A histologic evaluation of ninety-seven cases. Oral Surg., 25:158, 1968.

Andreasen, J. O.: Oral manifestations in discoid and systemic lupus erythematosus. I. Clinical investigation. Acta Odontol. Scand., 22:295, 1964.

Andreasen, J. O., Hjørting-Hansen, E., and Ulmansky, M.: Milia formation in oral lesions in epidermolysis bullosa. Acta Pathol. Microbiol. Scand. [A], 63:37, 1965.

Andreasen, J. O., and Poulsen, H. E.: Oral manifestations in discoid and systemic lupus erythematosus. II. Histologic investigation. Acta Odontol. Scand., 22:389, 1964.

Archard, H. O., Roebuck, N. F., and Stanley, H. R., Jr.: Oral manifestations of chronic discoid lupus erythematosus. Report of a case. Oral Surg., 16:696, 1963.

Arwill, T., Bergenholtz, A., and Olsson, O.: Epidermolysis bullosa hereditaria. III. A histologic study of changes in teeth in the polydysplastic dystrophic and lethal forms. Oral Surg., 19:723, 1965.

Baden, H. P.: Familial Schamberg's disease. Arch. Dermatol., 90:400, 1964.

Bang, G.: Acanthosis nigricans maligna. Oral Surg., 29:370, 1970.

Bánóczy, J., Sugár, L., and Frithiof, L.: White sponge nevus: Leukoedema exfoliativum mucosae oris. A report on forty-five cases. Swed. Dent. J., 66:481, 1973.

Barabas, G. M.: The Ehlers-Danlos syndrome. Abnormalities of the enamel, dentine, cementum and the dental pulp: an histological examination of 13 teeth from 6 patients. Br. Dent. J., 126:509, 1969.

Barabas, G. M., and Barabas, A. P.: The Ehlers-Danlos syndrome. A report of the oral and haematological findings in nine cases. Br. Dent. J., 123:473, 1967.

Bean, S. F., Alt, T. H., and Katz, H. I.: Oral pemphigus and bullous pemphigoid. J.A.M.A., 216:673, 1971.

Bennett, C. G., Shulman, S. T., and Baughman, R. A.: Prepubertal oral pemphigus vulgaris. J. Am. Dent. Assoc., 100:64, 1980.

Bernier, J. L., and Reynolds, M. C.: The relationship of senile elastosis to actinic radiation and to squamous cell carcinoma of the lip. Milit. Med., 117:209, 1955.

Bernier, J. L., and Tiecke, R. W.: Pemphigus, J. Oral Surg., 9:253, 1951.

Besserman-Nielsen, M.: Hypohidrotisk ektodermal dysplasi. Tandlaegebladet. 75:1057, 1971.

Brayshaw, H. A., and Orban, B.: Psoriasis gingivae. J. Periodontol., 24:156, 1953.

Brodie, A. G., and Sarnat, B. G.: Ectodermal dysplasia (anhidrotic type) with complete anodontia. Am. J. Dis. Child., 64:1046, 1942.

Brown, J., and Winkelmann, R. K.: Acanthosis nigricans: a study of 90 cases. Medicine (Baltimore), 47:33, 1968.

Buchner, A., and Begleiter, A.: Oral lesions in psoriatic patients. Oral Surg., 41:327, 1976.

Buchner, A., Lozada, F., and Silverman, S., Jr.: Histopathologic spectrum of oral erythema multiforme. Oral Surg., 49:221, 1980.

Burlakow, P., Medak, II., McGraw, E.A., and Tiecke, R.: The cytology of vesicular conditions affecting the oral mucosa. Part 2. Keratosis follicularis. Acta Cytol. (Baltimore), 13:407, 1969.

Burns, R. A., Reed, W. B., Swatek, F. E., and Omieczynski, D. T.: Familial benign chronic pemphigus. Arch. Dermatol., 96:254, 1967.

Butterworth, T., and Stream, L. P.: Clinical Genodermatology. Baltimore, Williams & Wilkins Company, 1962.

Byers, P. H., Barsh, G. S., and Holbrook, K. A.: Molecular pathology in inherited disorders of collagen metabolism. Hum. Pathol., 13:89, 1982.

Cannell, H.: Dyskeratosis congenita. Br. J. Oral Surg., 9:8, 1971.

Cannon, A. B.: White nevus of the mucosa (naevus spongiosus albus mucosae). Arch. Dermatol. Syph., 31:365, 1935.

Carney, R. G., Jr.: Incontinentia pigmenti (review of world literature). Arch. Dermatol., 112:535, 1976.

Carney, R. G., and Carney, R. G., Jr.: Incontinentia pigmenti. Arch. Dermatol., 102:157, 1970.

Carr, R. D., Heisel, E. B., and Stevenson, T. D.: CRST syndrome: a benign variant of scleroderma. Arch. Dermatol., 92:519, 1965.

Cawley, E. P., and Kerr, D. A.: Lichen planus. Oral Surg., 5:1069, 1952.

Chipps, J. E.: Erythema multiforme exudativum. Oral Surg., 4:345, 1951.

Christensen, E., Holmstrup, P., Wiberg-Jørgensen, F., Neumann-Jensen, B., and Pindborg, J. J.: Arterial blood pressure in patients with oral lichen planus. J. Oral Path., 6:139, 1977.

Christensen, E., Holmstrup, P., Wiberg-Jørgensen, F., Neumann-Jensen, B., and Pindborg, J. J.: Glucose tolerance in patients with oral lichen planus. J. Oral Path., 6:143, 1977.

Cohenour, W., and Gamble, J. W.: Acanthosis nigricans: review of literature and report of case. J. Oral Surg., 29:48, 1971.

Cook, T. J.: Hereditary ectodermal dysplasia of anhidrotic type. Am. J. Orthod. Oral Surg., 25:1008, 1939.

Cooke, B. E. D.: The diagnosis of bullous lesions affecting the oral mucosa. Br. Dent. J., 109:83, 131, 1960.

Idem: The oral manifestations of lichen planus: 50 cases. Br. Dent. J., 96:1, 1954.

Coursin, D. B.: Stevens-Johnson syndrome: nonspecific parasensitivity reaction? J.A.M.A., 198:113, 1966.

Crawford, E. G., Jr., Burkes, E. J., Jr., and Briggaman, R. A.: Hereditary epidermolysis bullosa: oral manifestations and dental therapy. Oral Surg., 42:490, 1976.

Curth, H. O.: Classification of acanthosis nigricans. Int. J. Dermatol., 15:592, 1976.

Curtis, A. C., and Slaughter, J. C.: The clinical diagnosis of dermatological lesions of the face and oral cavity. Am. J. Orthod. Oral Surg., 33:218, 1947.

Danbolt, N.: Acrodermatitis enteropathica. Acta Derm. Venereol. (Stockh), 36:275, 1956.

Danforth, R. A., and Green, T. L.: Oral warty dyskeratoma. Oral Surg., 49:523, 1980.

Daniels, T. E., and Quadra-White, C.: Direct immunofluorescence in oral mucosal disease: A diagnostic analysis of 130 cases. Oral Surg., 51:38, 1981.

Darling, A. I., and Crabb, H. S. M.: Lichen planus. Oral Surg., 7:1276, 1954.

Idem: Lichen planus of the mouth with associated ulceration. Oral Surg., 8:47, 1955.

Davis, R. K., Baer, P. N., Archard, H. O., and Palmer, J. H.: Tuberous sclerosis with oral manifestations. Report of two cases. Oral Surg., *17*:395, 1964.

Director, W.: Pemphigus vulgaris: a clinicopathologic study. Arch. Dermatol. Syph., *65*:155, 1952.

Domonkos, A. N., Arnold, H. L., Jr., and Odom, R. B.: Andrews' Diseases of the Skin. 7th ed. Philadelphia, W. B. Saunders Company, 1982.

Drury, R. E., and Prieto, A.: Epidermolysis bullosa dystrophica. Oral Surg., *18*:544, 1964.

Elkins, L., and Gruber, I. E.: Senile elastosis. Oral Surg., *4*:1007, 1951.

El-Labban, N. G., and Kramer, I. R. H.: Civatte bodies and the actively dividing epithelial cells in oral lichen planus. Br. J. Dermatol., *90*:13, 1974.

Idem: Light and electron microscopic study of liquefaction degeneration in oral lichen planus. Arch. Oral Biol., *20*:653, 1975.

Everett, E. D.: Mucocutaneous lymph node syndrome (Kawasaki disease) in adults. J.A.M.A., *242*:542, 1979.

Fischman, S. L., Barnett, M. L., and Nisengard, R. J.: Histopathologic, ultrastructural, and immunologic findings in an oral psoriatic lesion. Oral Surg., *44*:253, 1977.

Foster, M. E., and Nally, F. F.: Benign mucous membrane pemphigoid (cicatricial mucosal pemphigoid): a reconsideration. Oral Surg., *44*:697, 1977.

Foster, S. C., and Album, M. M.: Incontinentia pigmenti: Bloch-Sulzburger, Bloch-Seimens disease. Oral Surg., *29*:837, 1970.

Freedman, P. D., Lumerman, H., and Kerpel, S. M.: Oral focal acantholytic dyskeratosis. Oral Surg., *52*:66, 1981.

Frithiof, L., and Bánóczy, J.: White sponge nevus (leukoedema exfoliativum mucosae oris): ultrastructural observations. Oral Surg., *41*:607, 1976.

Fullmer, H. M., and Witte, W. E.: Periodontal membrane affected by scleroderma. Arch. Pathol., *73*:184, 1962.

Gardner, N. G., and Hudson, C. D.: The disturbances in odontogenesis in epidermolysis bullosa hereditaria letalis. Oral Surg., *40*:483, 1975.

Getzler, N. A., and Flint, A.: Keratosis follicularis: a study of one family. Arch. Dermatol., *93*:545, 1966.

Giallorenzi, A. F., and Goldstein, B. H.: Acute (toxic) epidermal necrolysis. Oral Surg., *40*:611, 1975.

Giansanti, J. S., Long, S. M., and Rankin, J. L.: The "tooth and nail" type of autosomal dominant ectodermal dysplasia. Oral Surg., *37*:576, 1974.

Goldman, H. M., and Bloom, J.: Oral manifestations of psoriasis: case reports. Oral Surg., *4*:48, 1951.

Goldman, H. M., Bloom, J., and Cogen, D. W.: Bullous lichen ruber planus. Oral Surg., *12*:1468, 1959.

Gorlin, R. J.: Epidermolysis bullosa. Oral Surg., *32*:760, 1971.

Gorlin, R. J., and Anderson, J. A.: The characteristic dentition of incontinentia pigmenti. J. Pediatr., *57*:78, 1960.

Gorlin, R. J., and Chaudhry, A. P.: The oral manifestation of keratosis follicularis. Oral Surg., *12*:1468, 1959.

Idem: Oral lesions accompanying pachyonchia congenita. Oral Surg., *11*:541, 1958.

Gorlin, R. J., Meskin, L. H., Peterson, W. C., Jr., and Goltz, R. W.: Focal dermal hypoplasia syndrome. Acta Dermatol., *43*:421, 1963.

Gorlin, R. J., and Pindborg, J. J.: Syndromes of the Head and Neck. New York, McGraw-Hill, 1964.

Graham, J. H., Johnson, W. C., and Helwig, E. B. (eds.): Dermal Pathology. Hagerstown, Harper and Row, 1972.

Greenbaum, S. S.: Oral lesions in pityriasis rosea. Arch. Dermatol. Syph., *44*:55, 1941.

Griffin, C. J., Jolly, M., and Smythe, J. D.: The fine structure of epithelial cells in normal and pathological buccal mucosa. II. Colloid body formation. Aust. Dent. J., *25*:12, 1980.

Griffith, M., Kaufman, H. S., and Silverman, S., Jr.: Studies on oral lichen planus: I. Serum immunoglobulins and complement. J. Dent. Res., *53*:623, 1974.

Grinspan, D., Villapol, L. O., Diaz, J., Bellver, B., Schneiderman, J., Palese, D., and Berdichesky, R.: Liquen rojo plano erosive de la mucosa bucal. Su asociacion con diabetes. Actes Finales del V Congreso Ibero Latino Americano de Dermatologia, 1963, p. 1243.

Grinspan, D., Diaz, J., Villapol, L. O., Schneiderman, J., Berdichesky, R., Palese, D., and Faerman, J.: Lichen ruber planus de la muqueuse buccale. Son association a un diabete. Bull. Soc. Fr. Dermatol. Syphiligr., *73*:898, 1966.

Grupper, C., and Avril, J.: Lichen erosif buccal diabete et hypertension (Syndrome de Grinspan). Bull. Soc. Fr. Dermatol Syphiligr., *72*:721, 1965.

Guequierre, J. P., and Wright, C. S.: Pityriasis rosea with lesions on mucous membranes. Arch. Dermatol. Syph., *43*:1000, 1941.

Guilhou, J.-J., Clot, J., Meynadier, J., and Lapinski, H.: Immunological aspects of psoriasis. I. Immunoglobulins and anti-IgG factors. Br. J. Dermatol., *94*:501, 1976.

Hansen, E. R., and Hjørting-Hansen, E.: Det Kroniske Slimhindepemfigoid med saerligt henblik paorale manifestationer. Tandlaegebladet, *67*:49, 1963.

Hargraves, M. M.: Discovery of the LE cell and its morphology. Mayo Clin. Proc., *44*:579, 1969.

Hargraves, M. M., Richmond, H., and Morton, R.: Presentation of two bone marrow elements: the "tart" cell and the "L.E." cell. Proc. Staff Meet., Mayo Clin., *23*:25, 1948.

Harrist, T. J., Murphy, G. F., and Mihm, M. C., Jr.: Oral warty dyskeratoma. Arch. Dermatol. *116*:929, 1980.

Hitchin, A. D., and Hall, D. C.: Incontinentia pigmenti (Bloch-Sulzberger syndrome) and its dental manifestations. Br. Dent. J., *116*:239, 1964.

Hoff, M.: Dental manifestations in Ehlers-Danlos syndrome. Oral Surg., *44*:864, 1977.

Holden, J. D., and Akers, W. A.: Goltz's syndrome: focal dermal hypoplasia. A combined mesoectodermal dysplasia. Am. J. Dis. Child., *114*:292, 1967.

Howell, J. B.: Nevus angiolipomatosus vs. focal dermal hypoplasia. Arch. Dermatol., *92*:238, 1965.

Hurt, W. C.: Observation on pemphigus vegetans. Oral Surg., *20*:481, 1965.

Jacobs, J. C.: Systemic lupus erythematosus in childhood. Pediatrics, *32*:257, 1963.

Jadinski, J. J., and Shklar, G.: Lichen planus of the gingiva. J. Periodontol., *47*:724, 1976.

Katz, S. I.: Dermatitis herpetiformis: the skin and the gut. Ann. Int. Med., *93*:857, 1980.

Klaus, S. N., and Winkelmann, R. K.: The clinical spectrum of urticaria pigmentosa. Mayo Clin. Proc., *40*:923, 1965.

Koszewski, B. J., and Hubbard, T. F.: Congenital anemia in hereditary ectodermal dysplasia. Arch. Dermatol., *74*:159, 1956.

Kövesi, G., and Bánóczy, J.: Follow-up studies in oral lichen planus. Int. J. Oral Surg., 2:13, 1973.

Krutchkoff, D. J., Cutler, L., and Laskowski, S.: Oral lichen planus: the evidence regarding potential malignant transformation. J. Oral Path., 7:1, 1978.

Kushnick, T., Paya, K., and Mamunes, P.: Chondroectodermal dysplasia. Am. J. Dis. Child., 103:77, 1962.

Laskaris, G.: Oral pemphigus vulgaris: An immunofluorescent study of fifty-eight cases. Oral Surg., 51:626, 1981.

Laskaris, G., and Angelopoulos, A.: Cicatricial pemphigoid: direct and indirect immunofluorescent studies. Oral Surg., 51:48, 1981.

Laskaris, G., and Nicolis, G.: Immunopathology of oral mucosa in bullous pemphigoid. Oral Surg., 50:340, 1980.

Laskaris, G., Sklavounou, A., and Bovopoulou, O.: Juvenile pemphigus vulgaris. Oral Surg., 51:415, 1981.

Lever, W. F.: Oral lesions in pemphigus. Am. J. Orthod. Oral Surg., 28:569, 1942.

Lever, W. F., and Schaumberg-Lever, G.: Histopathology of the Skin. 5th ed. Philadelphia, J. B. Lippincott Company, 1975.

Levin, H. L.: Psoriasis of the hard palate. Oral Surg., 7:280, 1954.

Idem: Oral manifestations and treatment of pemphigus vegetans. Oral Surg., 9:742, 1956.

Lewis, I. C., Stevens, E. M., and Farquhar, J. W.: Epidermolysis bullosa in the newborn. Arch. Dis. Child., 30:277, 1955.

Linch, D. C., and Acton, C. H. C.: Ehlers-Danlos syndrome presenting with juvenile destructive periodontitis. Br. Dent. J., 147:95, 1979.

Looby, J. P., and Burket, L. W.: Scleroderma of the face with involvement of the alveolar process. Am. J. Orthod. Oral Surg., 28:493, 1942.

Lowe, L. B., Jr.: Hereditary epidermolysis bullosa. Arch. Dermatol., 95:587, 1967.

Lozada, F., and Silverman, S., Jr.: Erythema multiforme. Oral Surg., 46:628, 1978.

Lyell, A.: Toxic epidermal necrolysis, an eruption resembling scalding of the skin. Br. J. Dermatol., 68:355, 1956.

MacCauley, F. J.: Incontinentia pigmenti (Bloch-Sulzberger syndrome): a case report. Br. Dent. J., 125:169, 1968.

Marmary, Y., Glaiss, R., and Pisanty, S.: Scleroderma: oral manifestations. Oral Surg., 52:32, 1981.

Maser, E. D.: Oral manifestations of pachyonychia congenita. Report of a case. Oral Surg., 43:373, 1977.

McCarthy, P. L., and Shklar, G.: Benign mucous-membrane pemphigus. N. Engl. J. Med., 258:726, 1958.

McCarthy, P. L., and Shklar, G.: Diseases of the Oral Mucosa. 2nd ed. Philadelphia, Lea & Febiger, 1980.

McClatchey, K. D., Silverman, S., Jr., and Hansen, L. S.: Studies on oral lichen planus: III. Clinical and histologic correlations in 213 patients. Oral Surg., 39:122, 1975.

McDaniel, W. H.: Epidermolysis bullosa. Arch. Dis. Child., 29:334, 1954.

McGinnis, J. P., Jr., and Turner, J. E.: Ultrastructure of the white sponge nevus. Oral Surg., 40:644, 1975.

McKusick, V. A.: Hereditary Disorders of Connective Tissue. 4th ed. St. Louis, C. V. Mosby Company, 1972.

McKusick, V. A., Egeland, J. A., Eldridge, R., and Krusen, D. E.: Dwarfism in the Amish. I. The Ellis-van Creveld syndrome. Bull. Hopkins Hosp., 115:306, 1964.

McMichael, A. J., Morhenn, V., Payne, R., Sasazuki, T., and Farber, E. M.: HLA C and D antigens associated with psoriasis. Br. J. Dermatol., 98:287, 1978.

Medak, H., Burlakow, P., McGrew, E. A., and Tiecke, R.: The cytology of vesicular conditions affecting the oral mucosa: pemphigus vulgaris. Acta Cytol. (Baltimore), 14:11, 1970.

Melish, M. E., Hicks, R. M., and Larson, E. J.: Mucocutaneous lymph node syndrome in the United States. Am. J. Dis. Child. 130:599, 1976.

Miller, R. L., Bernstein, M. L., and Arm, R. N.: Darier's disease of the oral mucosa: clinical case report with ultrastructural evaluation. J. Oral Path., 11:79, 1982.

Mitchell, R. D., and Smith, N. H. H.: Cicatricial pemphigoid: a review of eleven cases. Aust. Dent. J., 4:260, 1979.

Morales, A., Livingood, C. S., and Hu, F.: Familial benign chronic pemphigus. Arch. Dermatol., 93:324, 1966.

Morgan, J. D.: Incontinentia pigmenti (Bloch-Sulzberger syndrome). A report of four additional cases. Am. J. Dis. Child., 122:294, 1971.

Nisengard, R. J., Jablonska, S., Beutner, E. H., Shu, S., Chorzelski, T. P., Jarzabek, M., Blaszczyk, M. and Rzesa, G.: Diagnostic importance of immunofluorescence in oral bullous diseases and lupus erythematosus. Oral Surg., 40:365, 1975.

Patibanda, R.: Warty dyskeratoma of oral mucosa. Oral Surg., 52:422, 1981.

Perry, H. O., and Brunsting, L. A.: Pemphigus foliaceus: further observations. Arch. Dermatol., 91:10, 1965.

Person, J. R., and Rogers, R. S., III: Bullous and cicatricial pemphigoid. Clinical, histopathologic, and immunopathologic correlations. Mayo Clin. Proc., 52:54, 1977.

Pindborg, J. J., and Gorlin, R. J.: Oral changes in acanthosis nigricans (juvenile type). Acta Derm. Venereol. (Stockh) 42:63, 1962.

Pisanti, S., and Ship, I. I.: Oral psoriasis. Oral Surg., 30:351, 1970.

Pisanti, S., Sharav, Y., Kaufman, E., and Posner, L. N.: Pemphigus vulgaris: incidence in Jews of different ethnic groups, according to age, sex, and initial lesion. Oral Surg., 38:382, 1973.

Prindiville, D. E., and Stern, D.: Oral manifestations of Darier's disease. J. Oral Surg., 34:1001, 1976.

Pullon, P. A.: Ultrastructure of oral lichen planus. Oral Surg., 28:365, 1969.

Quinn, J. H.: Acute pemphigus vulgaris: dental significance. Oral Surg., 1:751, 1948.

Ramanathan, K., Omar-Ahmad, U. D., Kutty, M. K., Ching, L. K., and Dutt, A. K.: Porokeratosis Mibelli: report of a case. Br. Dent. J., 126:31, 1969.

Reed, R. J., and Leone, P.: Porokeratosis: a mutant clonal keratosis of the epidermis. I. Histogenesis. Arch. Dermatol., 101:340, 1970.

Reed, W. B., Lopez, D. A., and Landing, B.: Clinical spectrum of anhidrotic ectodermal dysplasia. Arch. Dermatol., 102:134, 1970.

Rees, T. D., Wood-Smith, D., and Converse, J. M.: The Ehlers-Danlos syndrome: with a report of three cases. Plast. Reconstr. Surg., 32:39, 1963.

Rice, J. S., Hurt, W. C., and Rovin, S.: Pemphigus vegetans. Report of an unusual case. Oral Surg., 16:1383, 1963.

Richter, B. J., and McNutt, N. S.: The spectrum of epidermolysis bullosa acquisita. Arch. Dermatol., 115:1325, 1979.

Robinson, H. M., Jr., and McCrumb, F. R., Jr.: Comparative analysis of the mucocutaneous-ocular syndromes. Arch. Dermatol. Syph., 61:539, 1950.

Robison, J. W., and Odom, R. B.: Bullous pemphigoid in children. Arch. Dermatol., 114:899, 1978.

Roenigk, H. H., Jr., Ryan, J. G., and Bergfeld, W. F.: Epidermolysis bullosa acquisita. Report of three cases and review of all published cases. Arch. Dermatol., 103:1, 1971.

Rook, A., Wilkinson, D. S., and Ebling, F. J. G. (eds.): Textbook of Dermatology. 3rd ed. Oxford, Blackwell Scientific Publications, 1979.

Rosenthal, I. H.: Generalized scleroderma (hidebound disease), its relation to the oral cavity, with case history and dental restoration). Oral Surg., 1:1019, 1948.

Russell, D. L., and Finn, S. B.: Incontinentia pigmenti (Bloch-Sulzberger syndrome): a case report with emphasis on dental manifestations. J. Dent. Child., 34:494, 1967.

Russotto, S. B., and Ship, I. I.: Oral manifestations of dermatitis herpetiformis. Oral Surg., 31:42, 1971.

Sadeghi, E. M., and Witkop, C.J.: Ultrastructural study of hereditary benign intraepithelial dyskeratosis. Oral Surg., 44:567, 1977.

Salmon, T. N., Robertson, G. R., Jr., Tracy, N. H., Jr., and Hiatt, W. R.: Oral psoriasis. Oral Surg., 38:48, 1974.

Schiödt, M., Andersen, L., Shear, M., and Smith, L. J.: Leukoplakia-like lesions developing in patients with oral discoid lupus erythematosus. Acta Odontol. Scand., 39:209, 1981.

Schiödt, M., Dabelsteen, E., Ullman, S., and Halberg, P.: Deposits of immunoglobulins and complement in oral lupus erythematosus. Scand. J. Dent. Res., 82:603, 1974.

Schiödt, M., Halberg, P., and Hentzer, B.: A clinical study of 32 patients with oral discoid lupus erythematosus. Int. J. Oral Surg., 7:85, 1978.

Schiödt, M., Holmstrup, P., Dabelsteen, E., and Ullman, S.: Deposits of immunoglobulins, complement, and fibrinogen in oral lupus erythematosus, lichen planus, and leukoplakia. Oral Surg., 51:603, 1981.

Sedano, H. O., Sauk, J. J., Jr., and Gorlin, R. J.: Oral Manifestations of Inherited Disorders. Boston, Butterworths, 1977.

Shelly, W. B.: Herpes simplex virus as a cause of erythema multiforme. J.A.M.A., 201:153, 1967.

Shklar, G.: Erosive and bullous oral lesions of lichen planus: histologic studies. Arch. Dermatol., 97:411, 1968.

Idem: Oral lesions of erythema multiforme: histologic and histochemical observations. Arch. Dermatol., 92:495, 1965.

Idem: The oral lesions of pemphigus vulgaris. Histochemical observations. Oral Surg., 23:629, 1967.

Shklar, G., and Cataldo, E.: Histopathology and cytology of oral lesions of pemphigus. Arch. Dermatol., 101:635, 1970.

Shklar, G., and McCarthy, P. L.: Oral manifestations of benign mucous membrane pemphigus (mucous membrane pemphigoid). Oral Surg., 12:950, 1959.

Idem: The oral lesions of lichen planus. Oral Surg., 14:164, 1961.

Idem: Histopathology of oral lesions of discoid lupus erythematosus. Arch. Dermatol., 114:1031, 1978.

Shklar, G., Frim, S., and Flynn, E.: Gingival lesions of pemphigus. J. Periodontol., 49:428, 1978.

Shklar, G., Meyer, I., and Zacarian, S. A.: Oral lesions in bullous pemphigoid. Arch. Dermatol., 99:663, 1969.

Silverman, S., Jr., and Griffith, M.: Studies on oral lichen planus: II. Follow-up on 200 patients, clinical characteristics, and associated malignancy. Oral Surg., 37:705, 1974.

Smith, D. B.: Scleroderma: its oral manifestations. Oral Surg., 11:865, 1958.

Sorrow, J. M., Jr., and Hitch, J. M.: Dyskeratosis congenita. Arch. Dermatol., 88:340, 1963.

Spouge, J. D., Trott, J. R., and Chesko, G.: Darier-White's disease: a cause of white lesions of the mucosa. Report of four cases. Oral Surg., 21:441, 1966.

Stafne, E. C., and Austin, L. T.: A characteristic dental finding in acrosclerosis and diffuse scleroderma. Am. J. Orthod. Oral Surg., 30:25, 1944.

Stern, L., Jr.: The diagnosis of pemphigus by its oral signs. Oral Surg., 2:1443, 1949.

Stillman, M. A., Bart, R. S., and Kopf, A. W.: Squamous cell carcinoma occurring in oral lichen planus. Cutis, 11:486, 1973.

Sugarman, M. M.: Lupus erythematosus. Oral Surg., 6:836, 1953.

Tanaka, N., Sekimoto, K., and Naoe, S.: Kawasaki disease: relationship with infantile periarteritis nodosa. Arch. Pathol. Lab. Med., 100:81, 1976.

Tanay, A., and Mehregan, A. H.: Warty dyskeratoma. Dermatologica, 138:155, 1969.

Taylor, M. H., and Peterson, D. S.: Kawasaki's disease. J. Am. Dent. Assoc., 104:44, 1982.

Terezhalmy, G. T.: Mucocutaneous lymph node syndrome. Oral Surg., 47:26, 1979.

Theodore, F. H.: Ocular-oral syndromes. Oral Surg., 5:259, 1952.

Tomich, C. E., and Burkes, E. J.: Warty dyskeratoma. Oral Surg., 31:798, 1971.

Tuffanelli, D. L., Kay, D., and Fukuyama, K.: Dermal-epidermal junction in lupus erythematosus. Arch. Dermatol., 99:652, 1969.

von Bülow, F. A., Hjörting-Hansen, E., and Ulmansky, M.: An electronmicroscopic study of oral mucosal lesions in erythema multiforme exudativum. Acta Pathol. Microbiol. Scand. [A], 66:145, 1966.

Voorhees, J. J., Stawiski, M., and Duell, E. A.: Increased cyclic GMP and decreased cyclic AMP levels in the hyperplastic, abnormally differentiated epidermis of psoriasis. Life Sci., 13:639, 1973.

Wade, G. W.: Scleroderma. Dent. Progr., 3:236, 1963.

Wald, C.., and Diner, H.: Dyskeratosis congenita with associated periodontal disease. Oral Surg., 37:736, 1974.

Walker, D. M.: Immunological processes involving the oral mucosa in lichen planus. Proc. Roy. Soc. Med., 69:7, 1976.

Walls, W. L., Altman, D. H., and Winslow, O. P.: Chondroectodermal dysplasia (Ellis-Van Creveld syndrome). A.M.A.J. Dis. Child., 98:242, 1959.

Weathers, D. R., and Driscoll, R. M.: Darier's disease of the oral mucosa. Oral Surg., 37:711, 1974.

Weathers, D. R., Baker, G., Archard, H. O., and Burkes, E. J., Jr.: Psoriasiform lesions of the oral mucosa (with emphasis on "ectopic geographic tongue"). Oral Surg., 37:872, 1974.

Weathers, D. R., Olansky, S., and Sharpe, L. O.: Darier's disease with mucous membrane involvement: a case report. Arch. Dermatol., 100:50, 1969.

Weisman, R. A., and Calcaterra, T. C.: Head and neck manifestations of scleroderma. Ann. Otol., 87:332, 1978.

Weiss, R. S., and Swift, S.: The significance of a positive L.E. phenomenon. Arch. Dermatol. Syph., 72:103, 1955.

Whinston, G. J.: Oral lesions of erythema multiforme. Oral Surg., 5:1207, 1952.

White, D. K., Leis, H. J., and Miller, A. S.: Intraoral psoriasis associated with widespread dermal psoriasis. Oral Surg., 41:174, 1976.

White, S. C., Frey, N. W., Blaschke, D. D., Ross, M. D., Clements, P. J., Furst, D. E., and Paulus, H. E.: Oral radiographic changes in patients with progressive systemic sclerosis (scleroderma). J. Am. Dent. Assoc., 94:1178, 1977.

Whitten, J. B.: The electron microscopic examination of congenital keratoses of the oral mucous membranes. I. White sponge nevus. Oral Surg., 29:69, 1970.

Idem: Intraoral lichen planus simplex: an ultrastructure study. J. Periodontol., 41:261, 1970.

Wiesenfeld, D., Martin, A., Scully, C., and Thomson, J.: Oral manifestations in linear IgA disease. Br. Dent. J., 153:398, 1982.

Winkelmann, R. K.: Classification and pathogenesis of scleroderma. Mayo Clin. Proc., 46:83, 1971.

Winter, G. B., and Geddes, M.: Oral manifestations of chondroectodermal dysplasia (Ellis-van Creveld syndrome). Report of a case. Br. Dent. J., 122:103, 1967.

Witkop, C. J., Jr.: Genetics and dentistry. Eugenics Q., 5:15, 1958.

Witkop, C. J., Jr. (ed.): Genetics and Dental Health. New York, McGraw-Hill, 1962.

Witkop, C. J., Jr., and Gorlin, R. J.: Four hereditary mucosal syndromes. Arch. Dermatol., 84:762, 1961.

Witkop, C. J., Jr., Shenkle, C. H., Graham, J. B., Murray, M. R., Rucknagel, D. L., and Byerly, B. H.: Hereditary benign intraepithelial dyskeratosis. II. Oral manifestations and hereditary transmission. Arch. Pathol., 70:696, 1960.

Wooten, J. W., Tarsitano, J. J., and LaVere, A. M.: Oral psoriasiform lesions: a possible prosthodontic complication. J. Prosthet. Dent., 24:145, 1970.

Wright, R. K., Mandy, S. H., Halprin, K. M., and Hsia, S. L.: Defects and deficiency of adenyl cyclase in psoriatic skin. Arch. Dermatol., 107:47, 1973.

Young, L. L., and Lenox, J. A.: Pachyonychia congenita. A long-term evaluation of associated oral and dermal lesions. Oral Surg., 36:663, 1973.

Zegarelli, D. J., and Zegarelli, E. V.: Intraoral pemphigus vulgaris. Oral Surg., 44:384, 1977.

Zegarelli, E. V., Everett, F. G., Kutscher, A. H., Gorman, J., and Kupferberg, N.: Familial white folded dysplasia of the mucous membranes. Arch. Dermatol., 80:59, 1959.

CHAPTER 17

Diseases of the Nerves and Muscles

DISEASES OF THE NERVES

One of the responsibilities of the dentist is the diagnosis and treatment of pain involving oral or paraoral structures. Although many of the cases of pain that confront him are directly associated with the teeth, others arise from diseases of nerves themselves and thus are not closely connected with the teeth. A comprehensive understanding of the disorders affecting the nerve pathways and the nerve supply of the various anatomic sites and structures associated with the oral cavity is essential for the dentist if he is to determine successfully the true nature of the pain and take appropriate measures to effect its relief.

DISTURBANCES OF THE FIFTH CRANIAL NERVE

Trigeminal Neuralgia

(Tic Douloureux; Trifacial Neuralgia; Fothergill's Disease)

Trigeminal neuralgia, often classified as a major neuralgia, is a disease involving the nerves which supply the teeth, jaws, face, and associated structures.

Etiology. The etiology of trigeminal neuralgia is as much a mystery today as it has been for several centuries. The proximity of the teeth to the site of the pain and particularly to the nerves involved suggested long ago that the teeth might be the source of the difficulty. When, however, the extraction of countless teeth in an effort to cure the disease failed to accomplish that purpose, the conclusion was finally reached that trigeminal neuralgia is most likely not dental in origin. Periodontal disease and traumatogenic occlusion have also been suggested

as causes, but with little foundation in fact. A further suggestion, also with negligible support, has been made that the disease might be related in some way to the degeneration of nerves of the deciduous teeth and the subsequent innervation of the permanent teeth.

A possible relation to circulatory insufficiency, either a direct cranial one or a reflex vasoconstriction from afferent stimuli of the vascular supply of the gasserian ganglion, has been suggested, since attacks may be provoked by vasoconstrictor drugs and may be decreased in severity and frequency by vasodilators. This theory is compatible with the predominant occurrence of the disease in elderly persons, who are the frequent victims of arteriosclerotic changes.

It is also recognized that trigeminal neuralgia occurs with some frequency in multiple sclerosis. According to Henderson, about 1 per cent of patients with multiple sclerosis have trigeminal neuralgia.

Clinical Features. Older adults are more commonly affected by trigeminal neuralgia than young persons, the disease seldom occurring before the age of 35 years. It is a well-established fact, but a completely unexplained one, that the right side of the face is affected in more patients than the left by a ratio of about 1.7 to 1.

The pain itself is of a searing, stabbing, or lancinating type which many times is initiated when the patient touches a "trigger zone" on the face. The term "tic douloureux" is properly applied only when the patient suffers from spasmodic contractions of the facial muscles although, through custom, this term is often used interchangeably with "trigeminal neuralgia." In the early stages of the disease the pain is relatively mild, but as the attacks progress over a period of months or years, they become

854

more severe and tend to occur at more frequent intervals. The early pain has been termed "pretrigeminal neuralgia" by Mitchell and is sometimes described as dull, aching or burning or resembling a sharp toothache. Later, the pain may be so severe that the patient lives in constant fear of an attack, and many sufferers have attempted suicide to put an end to their torment. Each attack of excruciating pain persists for only a few seconds to several minutes and characteristically disappears as promptly as it arises. As the attack occurs, the patient may clutch his face as if in terror of the dreaded pain. The patient is free of symptoms between the attacks, but unfortunately the frequency of occurrence of the painful seizures cannot be predicted.

The "trigger zones," which precipitate an attack when touched, are common on the vermilion border of the lips, the alae of the nose, the cheeks, and around the eyes. Usually any given patient manifests only a single trigger zone. The patient learns to avoid touching the skin over the trigger area and frequently goes unwashed or unshaven to forestall any possible triggering of an attack. In some cases it is not necessary that the skin actually be touched to initiate the painful seizure; exposure to a strong breeze or simply the act of eating or smiling has been known to precipitate it.

Any portion of the face may be involved by the pain, depending upon which branches of the fifth nerve are affected. The mandibular and maxillary divisions are more commonly involved than the ophthalmic; in some instances two divisions may be simultaneously affected. The disease is unilateral in nearly all cases, and seldom, if ever, does the pain cross the midline.

Differential Diagnosis. The unusual clinical nature of the disease—the presence of a "trigger zone," the fleeting but severe type of pain occasioned and the location of the pain—usually provides the key for establishing the diagnosis of trigeminal neuralgia. There are, however, a variety of diseases and conditions which may mimic this disease and which must be considered in the differential diagnosis.

One of the more common conditions mistaken for trigeminal neuralgia is migraine or migrainous neuralgia (Horton's syndrome, histamine headache, histamine cephalgia), but this severe type of periodic headache is persistent, at least over a period of hours, and has no "trigger zone." Sinusitis on occasion also has been confused with this disease so completely that radical sinus operations have been performed in the full expectancy of curing the patient of the "neuralgia." Again, the various clinical aspects of trigeminal neuralgia should exclude this diagnosis. The so-called Costen syndrome has also been reported to produce symptoms suggestive of trigeminal neuralgia.

Tumors of the nasopharynx can produce a similar type of pain, generally manifested in the lower jaw, tongue and side of the head with an associated middle ear deafness. This symptom complex, caused by a nasopharyngeal tumor, has been called *Trotter's syndrome* and was found to occur in 30 per cent of a series of patients with this type of neoplasm reported by Olivier. These patients also exhibit asymmetry and defective mobility of the soft palate and affected side. As the tumor progresses, trismus of the internal pterygoid muscle develops, and the patient is unable to open his mouth. The actual cause of the neuralgic pain in Trotter's syndrome is involvement of the mandibular nerve in the foramen ovale through which the tumor invades the calvarium.

A condition clinically similar to trigeminal neuralgia often occurs after attacks of herpes zoster of the fifth nerve. Termed *postherpetic neuralgia*, the pain usually involves the ophthalmic division of the fifth cranial nerve, but commonly regresses within two to three weeks. It may persist, however, particularly in elderly patients. The history of skin lesions prior to the onset of the neuralgia usually aids in the diagnosis.

Trigeminal neuritis or *trigeminal neuropathy* is a poorly understood condition which has a variety of presumed causes: (1) some dental surgical procedure, (2) pressure of a denture on the dental nerve, (3) surgical (other than dental) or mechanical trauma, (4) the therapeutic use of hydroxystilbamadine isethionate, (5) tumors of the head and neck, and (6) intracranial aneurysms. Some cases are idiopathic. It differs from trigeminal neuralgia by being described more often as an ache, variously stated as a burning, boring, pulling, drawing or pressure sensation. This continues over a period of hours, days or weeks rather than the instantaneous jolt of pain in trigeminal neuralgia. A series of patients with trigeminal neuritis has been studied by Goldstein and his co-workers who have emphasized the dental causes of the disease.

Finally, pain of dental origin may be of such a localized or referred nature that it simulates this disease. By careful observation and questioning of the patient, however, one can usually establish the correct diagnosis. However, an extremely diligent search is sometimes necessary to establish the dental origin of pain, particularly in cases of a split tooth or an interradicular periodontal abscess.

Treatment. The treatment of trigeminal neuralgia has been extremely varied over the years, and the degree of success which has resulted has not been outstanding. Each of the many types of treatment suggested has its advocates, but none is successful in all cases.

One of the earliest forms of treatment was peripheral neurectomy—sectioning of the nerve at the mental foramen, or at the supraorbital or infraorbital foramen. Since any relief afforded is temporary, this form of treatment has not been extensively used in recent years.

The injection of alcohol either into a peripheral nerve area or centrally into the gasserian ganglion has had many proponents throughout the years, despite its temporary benefit and attendant dangers. The patient may experience respite from all symptoms for a period of six months to several years after alcohol injection.

The inhalation of trichlorethylene, used because of its reported unusual effect in producing selective trigeminal anesthesia, is no longer extensively used.

The injection of boiling water into the gasserian ganglion has also been reported to be beneficial in causing respite from pain.

Surgical sectioning of the trigeminal sensory root by any of a number of techniques has come to be recognized by many surgeons as the treatment of choice when attempting to obtain a permanent cure.

In the past few years the use of phenytoin (Dilantin) in the management of trigeminal neuralgia has been found to be efficacious in some cases. Many reports of its use have now been published, and, though not uniformly successful, it does appear to afford good control of the neuralgia in early cases as well as in some advanced cases. The use of the drug must be continuous, since most reports indicate that cessation of its use is followed by return of pain. In case of failure to obtain relief with this drug, carbamazepine is often used. In fact, this drug is frequently used as a therapeutic challenge to the diagnosis of trigeminal neuralgia. Thus, if a patient who is presumed to have this disease does not respond rapidly to carbamazepine in 24 to 48 hours, then the diagnosis is seriously in doubt, according to Dalessio. Since the diagnosis of the disease is based on history alone, it has been pointed out that some patients are simply not good observers of their own symptoms.

One of the newest procedures for the management of trigeminal neuralgia is microsurgical decompression of the trigeminal root. This treatment is based on the observation that many patients with this disease have a tortuous vessel, usually one of the cerebellar arteries, looped against the trigeminal root near the brainstem. There is no ready explanation for the mechanism of how this might produce the paroxysmal pain. Still, microsurgical decompression has been reported by Voorhies and Patterson, as well as others, to produce good results, i.e., relief from pain for follow-up periods of up to 40 months.

Paratrigeminal Syndrome

(Raeder's Syndrome)

The paratrigeminal syndrome is a disease characterized by severe headache or pain in the area of the trigeminal distribution with signs of ocular sympathetic paralysis. The sympathetic symptoms and homolateral pain in the head or eye occur without vasomotor or trophic disturbances. These signs and symptoms usually appear suddenly. The disease appears to be most common in males, chiefly those of middle age.

Paratrigeminal syndrome presents some of the signs of Horner's syndrome (q.v.), but can be differentiated from it by the presence of pain and little or no change in sweating activity on the affected side of the face. The cause of the disease in unknown, but in the case reported by Lucchesi and Topazian, dramatic improvement occurred after elimination of dental infection. This may have been a fortuitous finding.

Sphenopalatine Neuralgia

(Sphenopalatine Ganglion Neuralgia; Lower-Half Headache; Sluder's Headache; Vidian Nerve Neuralgia; Atypical Facial Neuralgia; Histamine Cephalgia; Horton's Syndrome; Cluster Headache; Periodic Migrainous Neuralgia)

Sphenopalatine neuralgia is a pain syndrome originally described by Sluder as a symptom-complex referable to the nasal ganglion. Subsequently Vial described a similar syndrome, but believed that it involved the vidian nerve and concluded that the condition reported by Sluder should be termed "vidian neuralgia." In recent years, the term "periodic migrainous neuralgia" has been used to describe this clinical syndrome, and Eggleston has helped clarify some of the confusion surrounding the disorder.

At the present time, it is considered by most investigators to represent a variant of migraine.

Etiology. Sluder suggested that sphenopalatine ganglion neuralgia was due to vasoconstriction of vessels supplying the nasal mucosa. This view has been discarded, since there is no evidence to indicate that pain in this area accompanies vascular alteration. The theory of deviation of the nasal septum or of a septal spur causing irritation of the sphenopalatine ganglion has also been questioned. Irritation or inflammation of the vidian nerve in the vidian canal, secondary to sphenoid sinus infection, has been proposed as a cause of this form of neuralgia, but certain features of the disease, such as extended periods of freedom between attacks, cannot be explained on this basis. Finally, the most widely accepted evidence currently indicates that this syndrome is caused by vasodilatation involving the internal maxillary artery, a branch of the external carotid, particularly that portion supplying the sphenopalatine region. Because of the similarity in certain clinical features, Gilbert has suggested that the basic mechanism underlying this disease and Ménière's syndrome (q.v.) may be the same.

Clinical Features. Sphenopalatine ganglion neuralgia, or periodic migrainous neuralgia, is characterized by unilateral paroxysms of intense pain in the region of the eyes, the maxilla, the ear and mastoid, base of the nose, and beneath the zygoma. Sometimes the pain extends into the occipital area as well. These paroxysms of pain have a rapid onset, persist for about 15 minutes to several hours, and then disappear as rapidly as they began. There is no "trigger zone." In a series of 35 cases reported by Brooke, over 50 per cent of the patients described their pain as a toothache. Unfortunately, the attacks develop regularly, usually at least once a day, over a prolonged period of time. Interestingly, in some patients the onset of the paroxysm occurs at exactly the same time of day and, for this reason, the disease has been referred to as "alarm clock" headache. After some weeks or months, the attacks disappear completely and this period of freedom may persist for months or even years. However, all too frequently there is subsequent recurrence of paroxysms.

In addition to the pain sensation experienced by the patient, a number of other complaints may be noted as an accompaniment of this disease. Sneezing, swelling of the nasal mucosa and severe nasal discharge often appear simultaneously with the painful attacks, as well as epiphora, or watering of the eyes, and bloodshot eyes. Paresthetic sensations of the skin over the lower half of the face also are reported. It has been noted by many investigators that attacks are precipitated in some patients by either emotional stress or injudicious intake of alcohol.

Men are affected more commonly than women and the majority of patients experience their first manifestations of the disease before the age of 40 years.

Treatment. Numerous methods of treatment of the sphenopalatine ganglion syndrome have been proposed, none of which is successful in every instance. One of the most widely used of these has been cocainization of the sphenopalatine ganglion or alcohol injection of this structure. Resection of the ganglion has been carried out in some instances, as well as surgical correction of septal defects.

It has been found that ergotamine will often produce immediate and complete relief of symptoms. In those cases where it is not totally effective, combining it with methysergide, an antiserotonin agent, appears to produce a synergistic action usually providing total relief. However, both drugs carry some risk of serious side effects if given in large doses or over a prolonged period.

Orolingual Paresthesia

(Glossodynia or Painful Tongue; Glossopyrosis or "Burning" Tongue)

Paresthesia of the oral mucous membrane is a common clinical occurrence. It presents a great problem to the dentist because he is frequently unable to discover a cause for the complaint. The condition undoubtedly represents a symptom rather than a disease entity, but because of its clinical frequency and the specific nature of the complaint it is included in this section on diseases of the nerves and nervous system.

Etiology. A great variety of local and systemic disorders have been implicated in the cause of orolingual paresthesia. These have been reviewed by Karshan and his associates and include the following: (1) deficiency states such as pernicious anemia and pellagra, (2) diabetes, (3) gastric disturbances such as hyperacidity or hypoacidity, (4) psychogenic factors, (5) trigeminal neuralgia, (6) periodontal disease, (7) xerostomia, (8) hypothyroidism, (9) referred pain from abscessed teeth or tonsils, (10) angioneurotic edema, (11) mercurialism, (12) Moeller's glossitis, (13) oral habits such as excessive use of tobacco, spices, and the like, (14) antibiotic therapy, and (15) local dental causes such as dentures, irritating clasps or new fixed bridges. In addition, Schaffer pointed out two other possible etiologic factors: an electrogalvanic discharge occurring between dissimilar metallic dental restorations, and temporomandibular joint disturbances.

A great number of cases of orolingual paresthesia are undoubtedly based on psychogenic factors, the most common being emotional conflict, sexual maladjustment and cancerophobia. A considerable series of patients were reviewed by Ziskin and Moulton, who emphasized this nervous background, but nevertheless applied the term "idiopathic orolingual pain" to the disease.

Clinical Features. The tongue is most frequently the site of the paresthetic sensations, thus the origin of the terms "glossodynia" and "glossopyrosis"; however, any site in the oral cavity may be affected by these varying symptoms. The sensations most commonly encountered are pain, burning, itching and stinging of the mucous membranes. It is significant that the appearance of the tissues is usually normal; there are no apparent lesions to explain the untoward complaints.

The disease most frequently occurs in women past the menopause, although men are occasionally seen with this paresthesia. It is rare in children.

Treatment. A vast variety of therapeutic agents have been used in an attempt to relieve the symptoms of this disease. Kutscher and his co-workers reported the results of nearly 50 different drugs of various types, including topical anesthetics, analgesics, smooth- and skeletal-muscle relaxants, sedatives, antibacterial and antifungal agents, antihistamines, vitamins, enzyme digestants, central nervous system stimulants, salivary stimulants, vasodilators and sex hormones. They concluded that, except in occasional instances, permanent remission of the condition cannot be expected after drug therapy.

Auriculotemporal Syndrome

(Frey's Syndrome; Gustatory Sweating)

The auriculotemporal syndrome is an unusual phenomenon which arises as a result of damage to the auriculotemporal nerve and subsequent reinnervation of sweat glands by parasympathetic salivary fibers.

Etiology. The syndrome follows some surgical operation such as removal of a parotid tumor or the ramus of the mandible, or a parotitis of some type that has damaged the auriculotemporal nerve. After a considerable amount of time following surgery, during which the damaged nerve regenerates, the parasympathetic salivary nerve supply develops, innervating the sweat glands, which then function after salivary, gustatory or psychic stimulation. Some cases of gustatory sweating appear to be due to transaxonal excitation rather than to actual anatomic misdirection of fibers.

Clinical Features. The patient typically exhibits flushing and sweating of the involved side of the face, chiefly in the temporal area, during eating. The severity of this sweating may often be increased by tart foods. Of further interest is the fact that profuse sweating may be evoked by the parenteral administration of pilocarpine or eliminated by the administration of atropine or by a procaine block of the auriculotemporal nerve.

There is a form of gustatory sweating which occurs in otherwise normal individuals when they are eating certain foods, particularly spicy or sour ones. This consists of diffuse facial sweating, not simply a perioral sweating, and may even be on a hereditary basis, as suggested by Mailander.

There is a somewhat similar condition known as "crocodile tears" in which patients exhibit profuse lacrimation when food is eaten, particularly hot or spicy foods. It generally follows facial paralysis, either of Bell's palsy type or the result of herpes zoster, head injury or intracranial operative trauma. According to Golding-Wood, whenever an autonomic nerve degenerates, from injury or disease, any closely adjacent normal autonomic fibers will give out sprouts which can connect up with appropriate cholinergic or adrenergic endings; thus, a salivary-lacrimal reflex arc is established resulting in "crocodile tears."

The auriculotemporal syndrome is not a common condition. Nevertheless the possibility of its occurrence must always be considered after surgical procedures in the area supplied by the ninth cranial nerve. The syndrome is a possible complication not only of parotitis, parotid abscess, parotid tumor and ramus resection, but also of mandibular resection for correction of prognathism, as in the case of Chisa and his associates. It has been reported as a complication in as high as 80 per cent of cases following parotidectomy. In a study reported by McGibbon and Paletta, it was found that 14 per cent of a series of 70 patients who had had a radical neck dissection during the treatment of a tumor later had manifestations of gustatory sweating when eating. A review of the affected patients indicated that all had had the tail of the parotid gland excised.

Treatment. Treatment of the auriculotemporal syndrome by intracranial division of the auriculotemporal nerve has been reported to be successful.

DISTURBANCES OF THE SEVENTH CRANIAL NERVE

Bell's Palsy

(Seventh Nerve Paralysis; Facial Paralysis)

Bell's palsy is a disease which occasionally is encountered by the dentist and which, in some instances, has arisen after certain dental procedures.

Etiology. The cause of Bell's palsy is unknown. Although some cases reportedly have occurred after exposure to cold, this is considered by many workers to be a chance finding and not a cause. The disease does not appear to result from specific infection, but has been reported to arise in cases of both local and systemic disease. The occurrence of occasional cases following the extraction of teeth has suggested a possible relation to trauma, although the role of the injection of the local anesthetic might also be considered in the etiology of the disease. Some evidence indicates that the disease may be caused by ischemia of the nerve near the stylomastoid foramen, resulting in edema of the nerve, its compression in the bony canal and, finally, paralysis.

It is obvious that facial paralysis may result from trauma or a surgical procedure, such as removal of a parotid gland tumor, in which the facial nerve is sectioned.

Clinical Features. Bell's palsy begins abruptly as a paralysis of the facial musculature, usually unilaterally. Familial occurrence of Bell's palsy has been reported on a number of occasions, such as the case of Burzynski and Weisskopf, and hereditary factors may play a role in the etiology of the disease. Women are affected more commonly than men, and the middle-aged are most susceptible, although no age group is exempt. The disease arises more frequently in the spring and fall than at other times of the year. It may develop within a few hours or be present when the patient awakens in the morning. In some cases it is preceded by pain on the side of the face which is ulti-

mately involved, particularly within the ear, in the temple or mastoid area, or at the angle of the jaw.

The muscular paralysis manifests itself by the drooping of the corner of the mouth, from which saliva may run, the watering of the eye, and the inability to close or wink the eye, which may lead to infection. When the patient smiles, the paralysis becomes obvious, since the corner of the mouth does not rise nor does the skin of the forehead wrinkle or the eyebrow raise (Fig. 17–1). The patient has a typical masklike or expressionless appearance. Speech and eating usually become difficult, and occasionally the taste sensation on the anterior portion of the tongue is lost or altered.

In many cases of a mild nature the disease regresses spontaneously within several weeks to a month. Any residual manifestation of the disease which persists for over one year is apt to represent a permanent alteration.

Recurrent attacks of facial paralysis, identical with Bell's palsy, associated with multiple episodes of non-pitting, non-inflammatory painless edema of the face, cheilitis granulomatosa, and fissured tongue or lingua plicata is known as the *Melkersson-Rosenthal syndrome*. The

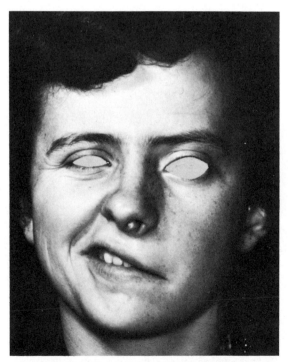

Figure 17–1. *Bell's palsy due to facial nerve paralysis.* The patient demonstrates the typical unilateral paralysis of the facial musculature with inability to smile or close the eye on the affected side. (Courtesy of Dr. Wilbur C. Moorman.)

facial edema resembles angioneurotic edema and involves the upper lip, occasionally the lower, and sometimes the nose, tongue or maxillary alveolar process. The fissured or scrotal tongue has been reported to be present in only about 25 to 40 per cent of cases with the other manifestations. An excellent review and a discussion of this syndrome have been presented by Vistnes and Kernahan.

Treatment. There is no specific treatment for Bell's palsy, since the etiology of the disease is unknown. The use of vasodilator drugs, e.g., histamine, has proved beneficial in some cases. Administration of physiologic flushing doses of nicotinic acid has produced excellent results in a series of cases reported by Kime, when treatment was instituted within a week after onset of the disease. In permanent paralysis surgical anastomosis of nerves has been carried out with some success. An attempt should be made to prevent infection of the involved eye, but other special precautions are seldom necessary.

DISTURBANCES OF THE NINTH CRANIAL NERVE

Glossopharyngeal Neuralgia

Pain similar to that of trigeminal neuralgia may arise from the glossopharyngeal nerve. This condition is not as common as trigeminal neuralgia, but when it occurs, the pain may be as severe and excruciating. The condition has been reviewed by Bohm and Strang.

Clinical Features. This neuralgia occurs without sex predilection in middle-aged or older persons and manifests itself as a sharp, shooting pain in the ear, the pharynx, the nasopharynx, the tonsil or the posterior portion of the tongue. It is almost invariably unilateral, and the paroxysmal, rapidly subsiding type of pain characteristic of trigeminal neuralgia is also a feature here. Numerous mild attacks may be interspersed by occasional severe ones.

The patient usually has a "trigger zone" in the posterior oropharynx or tonsillar fossa. These zones are difficult to localize but can be found by careful probing. Because of the location of these trigger zones, certain actions are recognized as inciting the episodes of pain. These include such simple acts as swallowing, talking, yawning or coughing.

The etiology of glossopharyngeal neuralgia is unknown. Neural ischemia has been suggested, but without conclusive evidence.

Treatment. The treatment of glossopharyngeal neuralgia has generally consisted in resection of the extracranial portion of the nerve or intracranial section. The injection of alcohol into the glossopharyngeal nerve has not been as widely accepted as has similar treatment in the case of trigeminal neuralgia. Periods of remission with subsequent recurrence are common in this disease.

MISCELLANEOUS DISTURBANCES OF NERVES

Motor System Disease

(Motor Neuron Disease; The Amyotrophies)

Motor system disease constitutes a group of closely related conditions of unknown etiology which occur in three clinically variant forms usually referred to as (1) progressive muscular atrophy, (2) amyotrophic lateral sclerosis, and (3) progressive bulbar palsy. They are called the motor system disease, since they all manifest corticospinal and anterior horn cell degeneration and exhibit either bulbar (tongue, pharyngeal, laryngeal) or limb muscle involvement.

Clinical Features. *Progressive muscular atrophy* is characterized by progressive weakness of the limbs with associated muscular atrophy, reflex loss and sensory disturbances. It shows a strong hereditary pattern, affects males more frequently than females and tends to occur in childhood. The initial symptoms usually consist of difficulty in walking, with leg pain and paresthesia. Atrophy of the foot, leg and hand muscles ultimately occurs with the appearance of a typical foot-drop, steppage gait and stork-legs.

Amyotrophic lateral sclerosis generally occurs between the ages of 40 and 50 years and affects males more frequently. Precipitating factors in the appearance of the disease have often been described, and these include fatigue, alcohol intoxication, trauma and certain infections such as syphilis, influenza, typhus and epidemic encephalitis. A genetically determined form of the disease is known to occur in Guam and the Pacific Islands but a hereditary type in the Western world has yet to be proven. Nevertheless, Fleck and Zurrow have reported familial amyotrophic lateral sclerosis in which four of five siblings in a family were involved. The initial symptoms consist of weakness and spasticity of the limbs, difficulty in swallowing and talking with indistinct speech and hoarseness.

Atrophy and fasciculations of the tongue with impairment or loss of palatal movements may also occur. The oral findings have been discussed by Roller and his co-workers.

Progressive bulbar palsy is characterized by difficulties in swallowing and phonation, hoarseness, facial weakness and weakness of mastication. It generally occurs in patients in the fifth and sixth decades of life with a familial pattern in some instances. The initial symptoms are gradual in onset and consist of difficulty in articulation, with impairment and finally loss of swallowing. Chewing is difficult as the facial muscles become weakened. These patients exhibit atrophy of the face, masseter and temporal muscles, and tongue with fasciculations of the face and tongue. There is also impairment of the palate and vocal cords.

Pseudobulbar palsy is a disease unrelated to the "motor system disease." It results from loss or disturbance of the cortical innervation of the bulbar nuclei, usually seen in patients with multiple cerebral thrombi as a result of cerebral arteriosclerosis. The typical patient with pseudobulbar palsy has suffered a cerebrovascular accident with paralysis of one arm and leg but no swallowing difficulty. A subsequent "stroke," however, may result in paralysis of the opposite limbs with impairment of swallowing and talking, associated with loss of emotional control. In this disease there is hypertonia and failure of voluntary muscle control rather than spasticity.

Treatment and Prognosis. There is no specific treatment for motor system disease. In most instances the disease is fatal, although temporary remissions sometimes occur.

Multiple Sclerosis

(Disseminated Sclerosis)

Multiple sclerosis is an acute or chronic, remittent or progressive disease of unknown etiology, but usually classified as one of the "demyelinating diseases," affecting chiefly the white matter of the central nervous system. Although numerous theories about the cause of the disease have been advanced, the most logical of these suggest that (1) the lesions are allergic hypersensitivity manifestations of the nervous tissue due to antigen-antibody reactions; (2) the lesions are due to scattered venous thromboses in the nervous system associated with altered coagulation of blood; and (3) the lesions are due to repeated, transitory, localized vasoconstriction in various portions of the nervous system, precipitated by emotional disturbances or fatigue. Many patients with multiple sclerosis have an increased gamma globulin concentration in the cerebrospinal fluid. Some also have an increase in serum gamma globulin, although the full significance of these findings is not known.

Clinical Features. Multiple sclerosis occurs chiefly in the younger age groups with onset of symptoms most frequently between the ages of 20 and 40 years. There is no consistent sex predilection, and a familial incidence is often observed.

The disease is characterized by: (1) a variety of ocular disturbances, including visual impairment as a manifestation of retrobulbar neuritis, nystagmus and diplopia, (2) fatigability, weakness and stiffness of extremities with ataxia or gait difficulty involving one or both legs, (3) superficial or deep paresthesia, (4) personality and mood deviation toward friendliness and cheerfulness, and (5) autonomic effector derangements, such as bladder and/or rectal retention or incontinence. Charcot's triad is a well-known diagnostic triad characteristic of multiple sclerosis but not invariably present. It consists of intention tremor, nystagmus and dysarthria or scanning speech, an imperfect speech articulation.

Facial and jaw weakness occurs in some patients, and a staccato type of speech has been described. In addition, both Bell's palsy and trigeminal neuralgia have been reported in some patients with multiple sclerosis, but these are not common and the findings may be fortuitous.

Treatment and Prognosis. There is no treatment for multiple sclerosis. Although remissions of the disease frequently occur, patients usually follow an ingravescent course leading to death, often from supervening infection.

Orofacial Dyskinesia

Orofacial dyskinesia is a condition thought to result from either an extrapyramidal disorder or a complication of phenothiazine therapy. However, a similar situation has been reported as a result of disruption of dental proprioception. Thus, Sutcher and his associates have reported a group of edentulous patients wearing full upper and lower dentures in gross malocclusion, who exhibited the involuntary movements typical of orofacial dyskinesia but in somewhat less severe form. These patients showed either a marked diminution or total disappearance of symptoms when dentures with proper physiologic craniomandibular relationships were constructed.

Clinical Features. This disorder occurs more frequently in persons over the age of 60 years than in the young. It is characterized by severe, involuntary, dystonic movements of the facial, oral and cervical musculature. Thus, irregular and involuntary movements such as lip-smacking and lip-licking, protrusion of the lips as in pouting, protrusion of the tongue and mandible with uncoordinated movements, and grimacing are all typical manifestations. The dyskinesia may occur alone or in association with torticollis or generalized dystonia.

Treatment. Surgical operations similar to those carried out in the treatment of Parkinson's disease generally cause improvement in the symptoms of the disease, although antiparkinsonian drug therapy has met with only limited success. It has also been suggested that correction of denture occlusion may be an effective therapeutic procedure.

Ménière's Disease

Ménière's disease is a symptom complex of unknown etiology.

Clinical Features. This disease is characterized by deafness, tinnitus and vertigo usually beginning in middle age and, if untreated, persisting indefinitely with occasional periods of remission. It commences with tinnitus and deafness which are unilateral in approximately 90 per cent of the cases. The low-pitched tinnitus has been described as a roar or hum or, in some cases, as a hissing sound, while the deafness has been described as an inner-ear deafness of the conductive type which fluctuates in degree. Vertigo is often a late symptom of the disease and many times is accompanied by attacks of nausea and vomiting which may be incapacitating. The vertigo usually has a sudden explosive onset and persists for several minutes to several hours. Some patients can foretell an attack by alteration in the pitch or intensity of the tinnitus.

These same signs and symptoms commonly occur in cases of cardiovascular disorders or with cerebral arteriosclerosis. True Ménière's disease, however, has specific histopathologic changes in the labyrinth, which were originally described in 1938 by Hallpike and Cairns. The nonspecific term "Ménière's syndrome" is often used to describe conditions characterized by labyrinthine vertigo not necessarily associated with the changes reported by these investigators. In true Ménière's disease there is dilatation of the endolymphatic spaces of the labyrinth with absence of an inflammatory reaction. The increased endolymphatic fluid pressure appears to diminish and distort the response to stimulation of the end-organs of the labyrinth and cochlea.

The basis of the endolymphatic dilatation is unknown. It has been suggested that the basic cause of this disorder is either an autonomic vasomotor dysfunction or an intrinsic allergy. The suggestion of a nutritional deficiency does not seem valid in view of the typical unilateral occurrence.

Treatment. No treatment of Ménière's disease is wholly effective. Management by drugs is generally unsuccessful, although some patients react favorably to vasodilators such as histamine or niacin. When conservative treatment fails, surgical intervention may be considered to relieve the vertigo. This consists in section of the eighth nerve or destructive labyrinthotomy, both of which appear equally effective in eliminating acute attacks of vertigo.

Migraine

(Migraine Syndrome)

Migraine is a syndrome presenting manifestations of diffuse disturbances in body function occurring during or after stress, characterized by severe periodic headache, irritability, and nausea. The cause of the disease is unknown, but has been postulated to be a discharge of autonomic centers in the forebrain, leading to constriction in portions of the cerebral arterial tree. In susceptible patients this may become manifest in the preheadache phenomenon. Then, as part of an attempt to maintain cranial homeostasis, there is a decrease in constrictor tone in certain other cranial arteries, particularly branches of the external carotid. These secondary effects, possibly hormonal as well as neurogenic in origin, are the source of the headache.

Clinical Features. Migraine usually begins during the second decade of life and is especially common in professional persons. The frequency of attacks is extremely variable. They may occur at frequent intervals over a period of years or on only a few occasions during the lifetime of the patient.

A prodromal stage (preheadache phenomenon) is noted by some patients, consisting of lethargy and dejection several hours before the headache. Visual phenomena such as scintillations, hallucinations or scotomas are often described. Other less common prodromal phenomena include vertigo, aphasia, confusion, unilateral paresthesia or facial weakness.

The headache phase consists in severe pain in the temporal, frontal and retro-orbital areas, although other sites such as parietal, postauricular, occipital or suboccipital are also occasionally involved. The pain is usually unilateral, but may become bilateral and generalized. The pain is not necessarily confined to the same side of the head in successive attacks. The pain is usually described as a deep, aching, throbbing type.

At the time of the headache the patient may appear extremely ill. The face is usually pale, sallow, and sweaty. He is irritable and fatigued, and his memory and concentration are impaired. Anorexia and vomiting may occur, as well as a variety of visual disturbances. Prolonged and painful contraction of head and neck muscles is found in some patients.

Treatment and Prognosis. The treatment of migraine includes a wide variety of drugs ranging from acetylsalicylic acid and codeine to ergotamine, methysergide and norepinephrine. The prognosis of the disease is good, since the condition is not dangerous and may undergo complete and permanent remission.

Temporal Arteritis
(Giant Cell Arteritis)

Temporal arteritis is a cause of headache which is frequently diagnosed erroneously as "atypical migraine." It is a relatively uncommon condition, as is any arteritis or periarteritis of cranial arteries.

It is basically a focal granulomatous inflammation of arteries, especially the cranial vessels, although in severe cases arteries throughout the body may be involved. The temporal arteries are particularly prone to develop these lesions. Occasionally, similar lesions are found throughout the skeletal muscles related to their vasculature, and this condition has been termed "polymyalgia arteritica."

The disease is of unknown etiology, although there is evidence that it is an immunologic reaction to some component of the arterial wall, possibly the elastic lamina. The disease has been reviewed in detail by Healey and Wilske and by Huston and his associates, and it has been discussed under the term "carotid system arteritis" by Troiano and Gaston.

Clinical Features. Temporal arteritis occurs most frequently in older persons usually between the ages of 55 and 80 years. It affects women far more frequently than men.

The onset of the disease may be slow and insidious, or the disease may develop suddenly with a headache or a burning, throbbing type of pain, sometimes beginning elsewhere than over the course of the temporal artery. A general malaise, chills and fever and weight loss with anorexia, nausea, and vomiting may precede any manifestations of pain. These are sometimes followed by aching and stiffness of the muscles of the shoulders and hips, which is often termed "polymyalgia rheumatica."

The pain frequently may be localized first in the teeth, temporomandibular joint, scalp, or occiput. Nearly one-half of patients complain of tiredness, fatigue and pain on repetitive chewing. This jaw claudication probably represents an external insufficiency of the carotid artery and musculature ischemia. Ultimately, however, there is localized inflammation or cellulitis over the swollen, nodular, tortuous artery.

Eye pain, photophobia, diplopia and even blindness may accompany the temporal symptoms. According to Sandok, permanent visual loss occurs in 25 to 50 per cent of patients.

The erythrocyte sedimentation rate is markedly elevated in the majority of these patients and a mild leukocytosis may also be found. These are non-specific findings, however, and do not establish the diagnosis.

Treatment and Prognosis. The response of temporal arteritis to corticosteroid therapy is excellent, and clinical manifestations subside within a few days. In occasional cases in which there is widespread systemic vascular involvement, the course of the disease may be progressively downhill and may terminate fatally.

Causalgia

Causalgia is a term applied to severe pain which arises after injury to or sectioning of a peripheral sensory nerve. Although few reports of this condition exist in the dental literature, cases do occur after the extraction of teeth.

Clinical Features. Causalgia may develop in patients of any age. It usually follows extraction of a multirooted tooth, particularly when the extraction is difficult or traumatic. The pain arises within a few days to several weeks after the extraction and has a typical burning quality from which the condition derives its name. The pain itself develops locally at the site of the injury and is evoked by contact or by application of heat or cold. It is an interesting feature of the disease that an attack may be elicited not only by actual touch stimulation but also by emotional disturbances.

Behrman reported 10 cases of causalgia following tooth extraction, while Elfenbaum reported 30 cases following similar surgical procedures. In both series it was reported that the pain was intensified by the application of heat, by ingestion of alcohol, during the menstrual periods, or at times when the patient became frustrated or upset.

It is surprising, considering the great numbers of teeth extracted, that far more cases of causalgia have not been reported. Possibly the condition has not been recognized as such, but rather has been ascribed simply to the patient's imagination or to the trauma occurring during the surgical procedure. Behrman suggested that the manifestation of causalgia in some patients but not in others may be due to an abnormality in the nerves of individual patients rather than to a peculiarity in the nature of the lesion per se.

Treatment. The treatment of intraoral causalgia is indeed a difficult one. The injection of procaine, alcohol nerve block, phenol cauterization and surgical curettement of bone in the involved area have generally proved ineffective. In some instances resection of the nerves in the retrogasserian region has afforded relief. Unfortunately, the typical history in these cases reveals that the patient submits to numerous procedures, but still continues to suffer from the severe pain.

Differential Diagnosis. Causalgia should be differentiated from local pain due to simple traumatic injury to soft tissue or bone during the extraction procedure. In addition, there is another interesting disease which typically produces referred pain in the posterior portion of the mandible: *subacute thyroiditis*. The etiology of subacute thyroiditis is unknown, although its incidence of occurrence appears to be increasing. The mechanism for referral of pain to the jaw in this disease is not clear, but has been reported to occur in over 35 per cent of patients with thyroiditis, according to the report by Tolman and his associates. Since patients may seek dental treatment for relief of their symptoms, the possibility of the thyroid condition

must be remembered. Treatment of the thyroiditis almost invariably results in subsidence of the jaw pain.

Atypical Facial Pain

(*Atypical Facial Neuralgia; Facial Causalgia*)

Atypical facial pain constitutes a group of conditions in which there is a vague, deep, poorly localized pain in the regions supplied by the fifth and ninth cranial nerves and the second and third cervical nerves. The pain is not associated with trigeminal neuralgia, glossopharyngeal neuralgia, postherpetic neuralgia, or with diseases of the teeth, throat, nose, sinuses, eyes or ears. The distribution of this pain is unanatomic, since it involves portions of the sensory supply of two or more nerves and may cross the midline. This pain, which lacks a trigger zone, is constant and persists for weeks, months or even years.

The difficult problem of atypical facial pain has been reviewed by Rushton and his associates, who suggested that designation by this term should be reserved for only those cases in which a definite diagnosis is not possible and in which there is realization that surgical treatment holds little promise of aiding the patients. A large group of the series of patients presented by Rushton and his co-workers were classified as psychogenic with regard to possible origin of the neuralgia, although many other patients showed no reliable cause for their condition.

One condition which must always be considered in the differential diagnosis of any vague or atypical orofacial pain is *Eagle's syndrome*. This syndrome consists of either elongation of the styloid process or ossification of the stylohyoid ligament causing dysphagia, sore throat, otalgia, glossodynia, headache, vague orofacial pain or pain along the distribution of the internal and external carotid arteries. Probably the most consistent symptom is pharyngeal pain. It is common for the difficulty to arise following tonsillectomy, presumably from fibrous tissue that forms and is stretched and rubbed over the elongated styloid process. However, many cases are not preceded by tonsillectomy, and this is especially true of the form known as the *carotid artery syndrome*, in which pressure exerted by either a deviant styloid process or an ossified ligament causes impingement on the internal or external carotid arteries between which the styloid process normally lies. This entire problem has been reviewed in detail by Ettinger and Hanson, by Russell, by Sanders and Weiner and by Baddour and his associates.

Horner's Syndrome

(Sympathetic Ophthalmoplegia)

Horner's syndrome is a condition characterized by: (1) miosis, or contraction of the pupil of the eye due to paresis of the dilator of the pupil, (2) ptosis, or drooping of the eyelid due to paresis of the smooth muscle elevator of the upper lid, and (3) anhidrosis and vasodilatation over the face due to interruption of sudomotor and vasomotor control. Its chief significance lies in the fact that it indicates the presence of a primary disease. The exact features of the syndrome depend upon the degree of damage of sympathetic pathways to the head and the site of this damage. Thus lesions in the brain stem, chiefly tumors or infections, or in the cervical or high thoracic cord occasionally will produce this syndrome. Preganglionic fibers in the anterior spinal roots to the sympathetic chain in the low cervical and high thoracic area are rather commonly involved by infection, trauma or pressure as by aneurysm or tumor to produce Horner's syndrome. Finally, involvement of the carotid sympathetic plexus by lesions of the gasserian ganglion or an aneurysm of the internal carotid artery may produce the typical facial sweating defect as well as facial pain and sensory loss.

Jaw-Winking Syndrome

Marcus Gunn Phenomenon; Pterygoid-Levator Synkinesis)

This interesting condition consists of congenital unilateral ptosis, with rapid elevation of the ptotic eyelid occurring on movement of the mandible to the contralateral side. It is commonly recognized in the infant by the mother when, on breast-feeding her baby, she notices one of its eyelids shoot up, as in the case reported by Smith and Gans.

At least some cases are hereditary, although it is reported that the phenomenon may begin in later life following an injury or disease. From reported cases, it appears that males are affected more frequently than females, and the left upper eyelid is involved more frequently than the right. It is also thought that about 2 per cent of all cases of congenital ptosis are due to this condition.

There are numerous theories concerning the etiology of the disease and these have been reviewed by Simpson. The most widely accepted is that the levator palpebrae muscle is connected, not only with the third nucleus, but also with the external pterygoid portion of the fifth nucleus. However, there is some evidence of supranuclear involvement.

An interesting condition known as the *Marin Amat syndrome* or *inverted Marcus Gunn phenomenon* is usually seen after peripheral facial paralysis. In this condition, the eye closes automatically when the patient opens his mouth forcefully and fully, as in chewing, and tears may flow.

Specific Infections of Nerves

Several specific infections may affect the nerves supplying the oral cavity and adjacent structures. For a discussion of these infections, see Chapter 6.

Specific Tumors of Nerves

The tumors derived from nerve tissue are discussed in the chapters on tumors of the oral cavity in Section I.

DISEASES OF THE MUSCLES

Diseases of the skeletal muscles of the face and oral cavity occur with sufficient frequency to be of considerable concern to the dentist. Many of these primary diseases manifest a generalized muscular involvement so that facial and oral manifestations constitute only a minor portion of the clinical problem. In other instances the facial or oral manifestations represent a major feature of the disease, and these may present serious functional problems that must be met and solved. Secondary diseases of muscle are seen with somewhat greater frequency, and they also present difficulties in diagnosis and clinical management.

Little attention was directed to diseases and dysfunctions of the muscular system by the dental profession until recent years, when the physiologic and pathologic function of muscle became an obviously important clinical responsibility. Thus, the specialty practices of orthodontics, prosthodontics and periodontics, among others, are especially allied in their interests in muscle diseases.

Remarkable advancements have been made

in recent years in the development and application of new techniques to the study of muscle physiology and pathology. One such technique, electromyography, has found extensive clinical application to dental problems, and though such investigations are still preliminary, the technique offers great promise in our ultimate understanding of some of the clinical problems in dentistry.

There is no satisfactory classification of the various diseases of muscles, owing in part to their obscure etiology in many instances and our often fragmentary knowledge of the disease processes. The classification proposed by Lilienthal, based chiefly on etiology of the diseases, is of practical use even though it has certain disadvantages. In a modified form, it is presented below.

Classification of Diseases of Muscle
I. Primary myopathies, limited to or predominant in muscle
   A. Dystrophies
   B. Myotonias (dystrophic, congenital, acquired)
   C. Hypotonias
   D. Myasthenias
   E. Myositis (including dermatomyositis and myositis ossificans)
   F. Metabolic defects (glycolytic, myoglobinuria)
   G. Miscellaneous (amyoplasias, contractures, degenerations)
II. Secondary myopathies, representing muscular reaction to primarily extramuscular disease
   A. Atrophy (traumatic, neuropathic secondary to metabolic, vascular, nutritional, infectious and toxic processes)
     1. Denervation
     2. Disuse and fixation
     3. Aging and cachexia
   B. Hypertrophy
     1. Developmental
     2. Functional
   C. Endocrine
   D. Internal environment
     1. Chemical
     2. Vascular
   E. Infection
     1. Specific (Trichinella, Toxoplasma, Coxsackie virus)
     2. General (rickettsial, typhoid, pneumococcal pneumonia)
     3. Postinfectious asthenia

No attempt will be made in this chapter to discuss all diseases of muscles shown in the foregoing classification. Instead, only those conditions which have been reported to present facial or oral manifestations will be considered. Furthermore, specific tumors of muscle and certain infections which may involve muscle are

not included in the classification and will not be considered in this section, since they are discussed in other chapters.

DYSTROPHIES

Muscular dystrophy is a primary, progressively degenerative disease of skeletal muscle. The basic disorder lies within the muscle fiber itself, since the muscular nerves and nerve endings at the neuromuscular junction are normal. Actually, a number of different diseases fall within this category, all characterized by (1) symmetric distribution of muscular atrophy, (2) retention of faradic excitability in proportion to the remaining power of contraction, (3) intact sensibility and preservation of cutaneous reflexes, (4) liability to heredofamilial incidence, and (5) unknown etiology.

The important forms of muscular dystrophy include: (1) severe generalized familial muscular dystrophy, (2) mild restricted muscular dystrophy, (3) myotonic dystrophy, (4) ophthalmoplegic dystrophy, and (5) late distal muscular dystrophy. Only the first two will be discussed here, since they present prominent orofacial findings. Myotonic dystrophy will be discussed under the section on myotonias. Zundel and Tyler have published an excellent review of all the muscular dystrophies.

Severe Generalized Familial Muscular Dystrophy

(Pseudohypertrophic Muscular Dystrophy of Duchenne)

This disease is best described as a rapidly progressive muscle disease usually beginning in early childhood, presenting strong familial transmission usually through unaffected females, and occurring predominantly in males, with or without pseudohypertrophy. It is the most common form of muscular dystrophy.

Clinical Features. Severe generalized familial muscular dystrophy begins in childhood, usually before the age of 6 years and rarely after 15 years. The earliest signs are inability to walk or run, the children falling readily, with muscular enlargement and weakness. The muscles of the extremities are generally those first affected, but even the facial muscles may be involved. This muscular enlargement ultimately proceeds to atrophy, however, and the limbs appear flaccid. Atrophy from the onset of the disease is apparent in certain groups of muscles, chiefly those of the pelvis, lumbosacral spine and shoulder girdle. It is this atrophy which is responsible for the postural and ambulatory defects, such as the waddling gait.

The muscles of mastication, facial and ocular muscles, and laryngeal and pharyngeal muscles are usually involved only late in the course of the disease.

Histologic Features. There is gradual disappearance of muscle fibers as the disease progresses, until ultimately no fibers may be recognized, being replaced entirely by connective tissue and fat. Persistent fibers show variation in size in earlier stages of the disease, some being hypertrophic, but others atrophic.

Laboratory Findings. The serum creatine phosphokinase level is elevated in all males affected by this disease and in about 70 per cent of the female carriers as well. It is significant that this CPK elevation occurs prior to the clinical manifestations of the disease in the males.

Treatment and Prognosis. There is no treatment for this disease, and patients seldom live beyond the age of 20 years.

Mild Restricted Muscular Dystrophy

(Facioscapulohumeral Dystrophy of Landouzy and Déjerine)

Mild restricted muscular dystrophy is a slowly progressive proximal myopathy which primarily involves the muscles of the shoulder and face and has a weak familial incidence. It frequently presents long remissions and sometimes complete arrest. One variant of this disease is a slowly progressive one without facial weakness.

Clinical Features. This disease begins at any age, from 2 years to 60 years, although the onset in the majority of cases is in the first two decades of life. There is no sex predilection for occurrence of the disease. Frequently no familial history can be found, but some cases appear to be transmitted as an autosomal dominant trait.

The earliest signs of the condition may be inability to raise the arms above the head and inability to close the eyes even during sleep as a result of weakness of facial muscles. The lips develop a characteristic looseness and protrusion which have been described as "tapir-lips," a part of the "myopathic facies," and the patients are unable to whistle or smile. The scapular muscles become atrophic and weak, with

subsequent alteration in posture, as do the muscles of the upper arm.

Cardiac abnormalities, including cardiomegaly and tachycardia, are often present, and many patients die of sudden cardiac failure.

Histologic Features. No specific microscopic findings are found in this disease. There is some variation in size of muscle fibers and moderate infiltration of fiber bundles by connective tissue. Individual fibers ultimately become atrophic.

Treatment and Prognosis. There is no treatment for the disease. Some patients undergo temporary periods of remission or even complete arrest. There may be mild disability. The possibility of cardiac failure is always present, however.

MYOTONIAS

Myotonia is a failure of muscle relaxation after cessation of voluntary contraction. It occurs in three chief forms: (1) dystrophic, (2) congenital, and (3) acquired myotonia, and though each presents the same basic defect, there are sufficient differences between the three types to warrant their separation. Paramyotonia is a disorder related to the other myotonias, but differing from them in several important aspects.

Dystrophic Myotonia

(Myotonic Dystrophy; Dystrophia Myotonica)

Dystrophic myotonia has been described by Adams and his associates as a steadily progressive, familial, distal myopathy with associated weakness of the muscles of the face, jaw and neck, and levators of the eyelids, a tendency for myotonic persistence of contraction in the affected parts, and testicular atrophy. It is inherited as an autosomal dominant characteristic.

Clinical Features. Atrophy of muscles is a characteristic feature of this disease, generally manifested first in the muscles of the hands and forearms. This muscular wasting does not appear usually until the third decade of life, but may be seen earlier, even in childhood.

Alterations in the facial muscles are one of the prominent features of the disease. These consist of ptosis of the eyelids and atrophy of the masseter and sternocleidomastoid muscles. The masseteric atrophy produces a narrowing of the lower half of the face which, with the ptosis and generalized weakness of the facial musculature, gives the patient a characteristic "myopathic facies" and "swan neck." In addition, the muscles of the tongue commonly show myotonia but seldom atrophy. Thus it is obvious that myotonia and atrophy, although frequently associated, are not necessarily related.

Pharyngeal and laryngeal muscles in patients with dystrophic myotonia also exhibit weakness manifested by a weak, monotonous, nasal type of voice and subsequent dysphagia. Recurrent dislocation of the jaw is also reported to be common in this disease.

Other clinical features frequently associated with dystrophic myotonia include testicular atrophy, which is so common as to be considered an integral part of the syndrome; cataracts, even in a high percentage of young patients; hypothyroidism with coldness of extremities, slow pulse and loss of hair; and functional cardiac changes.

Histologic Features. Enlargement of scattered muscle fibers and the presence of centrally placed muscle nuclei in long rows have been described as being characteristic of dystrophic myotonia and may be found in muscles without clinical evidence of atrophy. True hypertrophy of some fibers is almost invariably found, as well as isolated fibers which show extreme degenerative changes, including nuclear proliferation, intense basophilic cytoplasmic staining and phagocytosis. In advanced muscular atrophy, fibers appear small, and there may be interstitial fatty infiltration.

Treatment and Prognosis. There is no treatment for this disease. It progresses inevitably over a period of many years, producing disability and ultimately death.

Congenital Myotonia

(Thomsen's Disease; Myotonia Congenita)

Congenital myotonia is an anomaly of muscular contraction in which an inheritance pattern has been established in about 25 per cent of the reported cases. Thus, it is an autosomal dominant trait but with incomplete penetrance in some families. The characteristic feature of the disease is myotonia associated with muscular hypertrophy.

Clinical Features. Congenital myotonia commences early in childhood and may be first noticed because of difficulties in learning to stand and walk. The degree of myotonia varies, but is generally severe and affects all skeletal muscles, especially those of the lower limbs.

Muscular contraction induces severe, painless muscular spasms, actually a delay in relaxation. Electrical or physical stimulation of a muscle produces characteristic prolonged contraction or "percussion contraction."

The muscles are large, and patients with this disease are described as presenting a Herculean appearance. The muscles of the thighs, forearms and shoulders are especially affected, as well as the muscles of the neck and the masseter muscles of the face. The muscles of the tongue are not reported to be affected by the hypertrophy, although they may be involved by the myotonia.

Blinking with strong closure of the eyes will sometimes produce a prolonged contraction of the lids. Spasms of the extraocular muscles may lead to convergent strabismus. Interestingly, a sudden movement such as sneezing often produces a prolonged spasm of the muscles of the face, tongue, larynx, neck and chest, and there may be respiratory embarrassment.

A subjective increase in disability following exposure to cold has been described by many patients with this disease.

Histologic Features. Muscle biopsy reveals no alterations from normal except for hypertrophy of all muscle fibers.

Treatment and Prognosis. There is no specific treatment of the disease, but the prognosis is good. In fact, some regression of the disease occurs in occasional patients.

Acquired Myotonia

Acquired myotonia, as described here, refers to spasms of muscles, although such spasms are generally considered to be more intense than those occurring in typical myotonia. Nevertheless, the similarity in physiologic response of muscle in true myotonia and in muscular spasm justifies its inclusion here as a form of myotonia. If these spasms are intermittent, the condition is called *clonus* (myoclonic contractions); if constant, the term *trismus* is applied (myotonic contractions). All gradations in degree of spasmodic contraction occur, ranging from slight muscular twitches to severe, painful, prolonged muscular cramps.

Spasm involving the facial muscles is seen in a variety of situations such as epilepsy, diseases of the central nervous system and tetany. Such spasms on a local basis are far more common, however, and these occur in a variety of conditions such as (1) pericoronal infection, especially of third molars, (2) infectious myositis, and (3) hysteria (hysterical trismus).

The spasms, which are usually painful, may be transitory or may persist for a period of several days or until the cause of the disease is treated.

Hemifacial Spasm

Hemifacial spasm is a disease characterized by repeated, rapid, painless, irregular, non-rhythmic, uncontrollable, unilateral contractures of the facial muscles in adults, chiefly women. The cause of this condition is unknown, but appears to be a peripheral facial nerve lesion. Some studies indicate that there may be compression of the facial nerve in the facial canal adjacent to the stylomastoid foramen.

Clinical Features. Hemifacial spasm usually begins in the periorbital muscles, but soon spreads to the entire half-face. It is first manifested as a brief transitory twitching, but may progress to sustained spasms. These spasms are often triggered by fatigue, tension or facial activity and are of brief duration, usually only a few seconds. Interestingly, they may continue through sleep and even awaken the patient.

In cases of long-standing hemifacial spasm, mild facial contracture may occur, as well as lid closure and lip pursing.

Hemifacial spasm must be differentiated from emotional tics and focal convulsive seizures, but this is usually not difficult.

Treatment and Prognosis. There is no treatment for this disease, but decompression of the facial nerve in its canal has offered relief in some cases. The prognosis is good despite remissions and recurrences over a period of years.

Paramyotonia

Paramyotonia is a nonprogressive myotonia inherited as an autosomal dominant characteristic that is not associated with muscular wasting. Characteristically, the cramping attacks are precipitated by exposure to cold.

Clinical Features. Paramyotonia is manifested by cramping, stiffness and weakness of the muscles of the face and neck, fingers and hands upon exposure to cold. The eyelids are closed, and the face assumes a masklike appearance. The tongue may exhibit a similar cramping after drinking cold liquids, and the speech becomes blurred. In many cases myotonia of the tongue may be induced by percussion, although this is not true of other muscles. Although the muscular cramping may disappear within an hour, the weakness may persist for several days.

Histologic Features. Reports of microscopic study of muscles from patients with paramyotonia are almost entirely lacking. Information available indicates that there are no significant histologic changes in muscle fibers.

Treatment and Prognosis. There is no specific treatment for paramyotonia, but the prognosis is excellent with frequent improvement during adult life.

HYPOTONIAS

Hypotonia is a reduction or complete absence of tonus in muscles. There are many causes of hypotonia and delay in motor development in infants, so that this condition should be regarded only as a symptom which may be found in many diseases. Certain congenital diseases may result in hypotonia, such as (1) diseases of the central nervous system (e.g., atonic diplegia), (2) lipoid and glycogen storage diseases (e.g., Tay-Sachs disease), (3) mongolism, (4) cretinism, and (5) achondrodysplasia. Hypotonia also may result from strictly neuromuscular diseases, however, including (1) infantile muscular atrophy, (2) infantile muscular dystrophy, (3) amyotonia congenita, (4) congenital nonprogressive myopathy, and (5) neonatal myasthenia gravis.

Many of these latter diseases, all occurring in infancy, have certain features in common, including hypotonia, reduced tendon reflexes and muscular weakness. Because of the difficulty encountered in their separation, the term "floppy infant syndrome" has sometimes been applied to describe the chief clinical manifestation of these unfortunate children. As the term would imply, these infants have a generalized weakness so that their bodies hang limply with inability to sit, stand or walk. The hypotonia involves the muscles of the face and tongue as well, but these findings are secondary to the generalized condition. For this reason this particular group of diseases warrants no detailed consideration.

MYASTHENIAS

Myasthenia is an abnormal weakness and fatigue in muscle following activity. The myasthenias constitute a group of diseases in which there is a basic disorder of muscle excitability and contractility and include (1) myasthenia gravis, (2) familial periodic paralysis, and (3) aldosteronism. The rarity of the latter two diseases and their lack of clinical manifestations of significant interest to the dentist preclude their discussion here.

Myasthenia Gravis

Myasthenia gravis is a chronic disease characterized by progressive weakness of skeletal muscles, particularly those innervated by the cranial nerves. The disease does not affect smooth or cardiac muscle.

Etiology. The basic lesion in myasthenia gravis is a defect in neuromuscular transmission which bears amazing resemblance to that abnormality which occurs after the administration of curare. It appears that the fault is in the acetylcholine mechanism, the motor end-organ being normal.

Many investigators have attempted to relate myasthenia gravis to the endocrine system because of the great number of cases of thymic hyperplasia or tumors of the thymus associated with the disease. It is reported that in as many as 70 per cent of cases of myasthenia gravis, the thymus gland exhibits lymphoid follicular hyperplasia. In an additional 10 to 15 per cent of cases, a thymoma is present. Conversely, it is reported that about 75 per cent of patients with a thymoma exhibit manifestations of myasthenia gravis. It is thought by some investigators that the thymic hyperplasia may be a reflection of the production of antimuscle antibodies.

Classically, the disease has also been related to pregnancy, menstruation, and hyperthyroidism, but these associations may be more apparent than real. There is no evidence that the disease is hereditary, although a transitory neonatal myasthenia gravis may occur in infants of affected mothers.

Clinical Features. Myasthenia gravis occurs chiefly in adults in the middle-age group, with a predilection for women, and is characterized by a rapidly developing weakness in voluntary muscles following even minor activity. Of interest to the dentist is the fact that the muscles of mastication and facial expression are involved by this disease, frequently before any other muscle group. The patient's chief complaints may be difficulty in mastication and in deglutition, and dropping of the jaw. Speech is often slow and slurred. Disturbances in taste sensation occur in some patients.

Diplopia and ptosis, along with drooping of the face, lend a sorrowful appearance to the patient. The neck muscles may be so weak that the head cannot be held up without support. Patients with this disease rapidly become exhausted, lose weight, become further weakened and may eventually become bedfast. Death frequently occurs from respiratory failure.

The clinical course of patients with myasthenia gravis is extremely variable. Some patients enter an acute exacerbation of their disease and succumb very shortly, but others live for many years with only the slightest evidence of disability. On this basis, two forms of the disease are now recognized: one, a steadily progressive type; the other, a remitting, relapsing type.

Histologic Features. There are usually no demonstrable changes in the muscle. Occasionally, focal collections of small lymphocytes, or "lymphorrhages," are found surrounding small blood vessels in the interstitial tissue of affected muscles. In a few cases foci of atrophy or necrosis of muscle fibers have been described. There are no pathognomonic features, however.

Treatment and Prognosis. It is interesting that the drug of choice used in treatment of myasthenia gravis provides such remarkable relief of symptoms in such a short time that it is commonly used as the diagnostic test for the disease. Physostigmine, an anticholinesterase, administered intramuscularly, improves the strength of the affected muscles in a matter of minutes, although the remission is only temporary. No "cure" for the disease is known, even though the prognosis is good in the relapsing type.

MYOSITIS

Myositis refers to an inflammation of muscle tissue and is entirely nonspecific, since a great many bacterial, viral, fungal or parasitic infections, as well as certain physical and chemical injuries, may give rise to the condition. In addition, a variety of diseases of unknown etiology may produce or at least be associated with myositis. Since the various diseases resulting in myositis are discussed elsewhere in this text, only four specific forms of myositis will be considered here: (1) dermatomyositis, (2) myositis ossificans, generalized and traumatic, (3) proliferative myositis, and (4) focal myositis.

Dermatomyositis

(Polymyositis; Neuromyositis; Dermatomucosomyositis)

Dermatomyositis in an acute or chronic disease of unknown etiology, but is classified as one of the "collagen diseases," related particularly to scleroderma and lupus erythematosus. It is characterized by a gradual onset with vague and indefinite prodromata followed by edema, dermatitis, myositis, and sometimes neuritis and mucositis. The universally present component of this disease with its varied expressions is the myositis.

Clinical Features. Dermatomyositis may occur in patients of any age from very young children to elderly adults, but the majority of cases occur in the fifth decade of life. There is no sex predilection in its occurrence.

The more acute form of the disease, seen more commonly in children, begins with an erythematous skin eruption, edema, tenderness, swelling and weakness of the proximal muscles of the limbs. Accompanying these manifestations are fever and leukocytosis. The skin lesions frequently calcify and form calcium carbonate nodules with a foreign body reaction. This is known as *calcinosis cutis*, whereas the term *calcinosis universalis* is applied when these calcified masses are found generalized throughout the soft tissues.

The chronic form of the disease is similar, but may not show dermal involvement (polymyositis only), although all gradations are present between the two extremes. In some cases a long interval may supervene between the appearance of the dermal lesions and the muscle dysfunction. In addition, Raynaud's phenomenon or paroxysmal digital cyanosis may be an early manifestation. The muscular stiffness and weakness are often symmetric in distribution.

The cutaneous lesions usually consist of a diffuse erythema with desquamation, although other types of rashes have been described. This rash is most frequently seen on the face, eyelids, ears, anterior neck and overlying articulations.

Oral Manifestations. The oral lesions, consisting of diffuse stomatitis and pharyngitis, are extremely common. Telangiectatic lesions of the vermilion border of the lips and cheeks may also occur. In addition, involvement of the muscles of the jaws, tongue and pharynx may pose problems in eating and phonation. A detailed discussion of the oral and facial manifestations of dermatomyositis has been presented by Sanger and Kirby.

Histologic Features. The muscle fibers in dermatomyositis exhibit widespread degeneration and hyalinization. In advanced cases the muscle fibers disappear, leaving only the fibrous stroma. Many fibers show vacuolization, granulation and fragmentation with phagocytosis of disintegrating fibers. Diffuse leukocytic infiltration is also frequently pronounced.

Laboratory Findings. Patients with this disease sometimes manifest a mild anemia or leukocytosis. In addition, creatinuria is a constant finding, as well as elevated levels of serum transaminase and aldolase.

Treatment and Prognosis. There is no specific treatment for the disease, although symptomatic treatment may be of considerable benefit to the patient. In the more acute forms of the disease, death may occur rapidly. In other cases there may be recovery, sometimes with a residual disability.

Generalized Myositis Ossificans

(Progressive Myositis Ossificans; Interstitial Ossifying Myositis)

Generalized myositis ossificans is a disease of unknown etiology which affects the interstitial tissues of muscle as well as tendons, ligaments, fascia, aponeuroses and even the skin. Basically, masses of fibrous tissue and bone occur within these structures with secondary atrophy and destruction of the associated muscles due to pressure and inactivity.

Clinical Features. Generalized myositis ossificans usually occurs in young children or adolescents with the development of soft, fluctuant or firm nodular swellings anywhere on the body but frequently on the neck or back. These masses may develop spontaneously or after minor trauma. They vary considerably in size and shape and may disappear or become transformed into bony nodules. These are usually painless and are covered by a reddened skin which may ulcerate as a result of pressure from the underlying mass.

Any skeletal muscle may be affected, but those of the trunk and proximal limbs are most frequently involved. Interestingly, certain muscles tend to escape involvement: the tongue, larynx, diaphragm and perineal muscles. Ultimately, entire groups of muscles become transformed into bone with resulting limitation of movement. The masseter muscle is often involved so that fixation of the jaw occurs. The patient becomes transformed into a rigid organism sometimes encountered in circuses as the "petrified man."

Histologic Features. The muscle in this disease is gradually replaced by connective tissue which undergoes osteoid formation and subsequently ossification. In some cases cartilage formation may also be evident. Characteristically, intact muscle fibers may be found within the bony tissue.

Treatment and Prognosis. There is no treatment for the disease. It is progressive until death results, usually from a pulmonary infection secondary to the respiratory difficulties arising from involvement of the intercostal muscles.

Traumatic Myositis Ossificans

(Myositis Ossificans Circumscripta; Traumatic Ossifying Myositis; Ossifying Hematoma)

Traumatic myositis ossificans is a disease characterized by ossification in muscle following either a single acute traumatic episode or a series of minor traumatic injuries to muscles. It is interesting that ossification of solitary muscles may occur as an occupational disease. For example, horseback riders and jockeys develop "rider's bone" in the thigh adductors; cavalrymen may develop an osseous plate on the outer surface of the thigh due to repeated trauma by their sabres; infantrymen develop a "drill or exercise bone" in the deltoid or pectoral muscle from repeated impact during firing their rifles; and fencers and baseball pitchers develop ossification in the biceps and brachial muscles due to overextension of the arm. In addition, athletes in certain contact sports may develop myositis ossificans after acute traumatic injury to any muscle.

The exact mechanism of the ossification is not entirely clear. Several possible theories have been reviewed by Carey: (1) traumatization of the periosteum of an adjacent bone with the displacement of osteoblasts into the muscle and subsequent formation of bone, (2) activation of periosteal implants already present in muscle by trauma or hemorrhage, (3) metaplasia of the pluripotential intermuscular connective tissue into bone, and (4) metaplasia of fibrocartilage, a normal constituent of many muscle tendons, into bone. It is of significance that the attempts of Tweeddale and his associates to induce myositis ossificans experimentally in animals by traumatic injury to muscle and periosteum and injection of blood into muscle have met with uniform failure. Therefore some unknown factors favoring ossification must also be present, particularly since so few muscle injuries actually do ossify.

It is recognized that this typical ossifying lesion can occur in superficial tissue away from muscle. This has been discussed by Kwittken

and Branche, who have proposed the term "fasciitis ossificans" for such cases.

Clinical Features. Myositis ossificans developing after a single acute traumatic injury usually manifests as a firm, painful mass in the injured muscle within one to four weeks. In some cases motion is limited by the lesion. Chronic cases of myositis ossificans are usually asymptomatic and may be discovered accidentally. In some cases there is a mild discomfort associated with a progressive limitation of motion.

Oral Manifestations. Myositis ossificans involving the muscles of the face, particularly the masseter and temporal muscles, has been reported on numerous occasions, usually following a single acute traumatic injury. Goodsell, as well as Plezia and his associates, has reviewed the literature dealing with myositis ossificans of the masseter muscle and found that, in most reported cases, growth of the calcified lesion has been rapid, maximum size obtained, and then the lesion remained static or even diminished in size. Some difficulty in opening the mouth may be experienced by patients with myositis ossificans of the masseter muscle.

Roentgenographic Features. The roentgenographic pattern of myositis ossificans may appear either as a feathery type of calcification in muscle, following ossification of a hematoma which dissected along muscle bundles, or as a solitary irregular calcified mass occurring in a simple hematoma. The radiopaque calcification may be first seen within two to three weeks of the traumatic experience and show a progressive increase in radiodensity (Fig. 17–2).

Histologic Features. Traumatic myositis ossificans exhibits varying stages from hemorrhage, degeneration of muscle and connective tissue hyperplasia to chondrification and ossification. The osteoid and bone trabeculae formed often trap viable muscle fibers, but these may ultimately disappear. The trabecular pattern is often extremely bizarre and, with the cartilage and myxomatous tissue present may resemble callus formation. The more mature tissue is usually found on the periphery of the lesion.

The rapidly proliferating bony tissue often produces a sufficiently atypical microscopic picture to confuse the lesion with osteosarcoma, and this mistake has been made on numerous occasions in the past (Fig. 17–3). Ackerman carefully described the problems in microscopic differential diagnosis between these two diseases. The term "pseudomalignant myositis ossificans" has even been applied by Lagier and

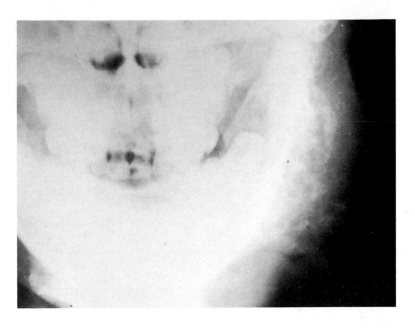

Figure 17–2. *Traumatic myositis ossificans involving masseter muscle.*

Cox to emphasize their similarities. Although some reports in the literature have described transformation of myositis ossificans into osteosarcoma, this probably does not occur.

Treatment and Prognosis. Treatment of myositis ossificans is essentially surgical excision. Recurrence has been reported in some cases, but this is not characteristic. The prognosis is good, since the lesion is a localized, inflammatory one.

Proliferative Myositis

Proliferative myositis has been defined by Enzinger and Dulcey as a pseudosarcomatous process of muscle characterized by an ill-defined proliferation of basophilic giant cells and fibroblasts chiefly involving the perimysium, epimysium and neighboring fascia. It is sometimes mistaken for a sarcoma because of its rapidity of growth and, histologically, its cellularity and the presence of giant cells. While mechanical trauma may play a role in the development of proliferative myositis, there may be other causes as well. It was first described by Kern in 1960.

Clinical Features. Patients afflicted by this condition have ranged in age from the early 20s to the early 80s, with a median age of 50 years. There is a slight predilection for occurrence in males. The lesion is manifested as a firm solitary nodule that is deep-seated and not attached to overlying skin. It grows rapidly but is seldom tender or painful. Four of the 33 cases reported

by Enzinger and Dulcey occurred in the head and neck area.

Histologic Features. Proliferative myositis is characterized by a poorly demarcated fibroblastic proliferation involving the epimysium, perimysium and endomysium and by the presence of large, basophilic giant cells resembling ganglion cells or rhabdomyoblasts. The process affects primarily stromal tissue and leaves muscle fibers virtually uninvolved. There is never complete replacement of muscle tissue over a large circumscribed area as in nodular fasciitis or myositis ossificans, from which proliferative myositis must be differentiated. It must also be separated from proliferative fasciitis, described by Chung and Enzinger, which is very similar to proliferative myositis, especially microscopically, except that the lesion is superficial and does not involve muscle.

Treatment. Proliferative myositis is treated by simple local excision and has no tendency to recur.

Focal Myositis

Focal myositis is a benign inflammatory pseudotumor of skeletal muscle first described by Heffner and his associates in 1977 as a new and distinct clinicopathologic entity. The actual etiology is unknown but, even though a history of trauma is absent in most cases, it is speculated that a subclinical injury, such as a muscle tear, might initiate the condition.

Clinical Features. Focal myositis presents as

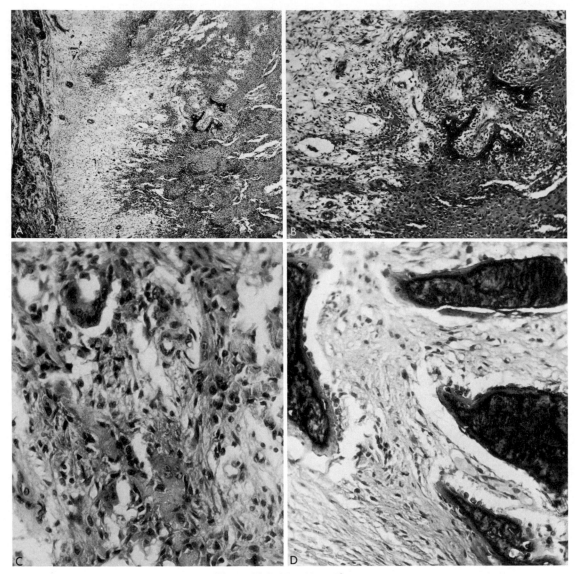

Figure 17–3. *Myositis ossificans.*
The characteristic features of connective tissue hyperplasia, myxomatous tissue, osteoid and bone are well demonstrated. (Courtesy of Dr. William G. Sprague.)

a rapidly enlarging mass within a single skeletal muscle. The most common sites reported are the lower leg, thorax, abdomen, and forearm; however, involvement of perioral musculature and submandibular and buccal mucosa has been reported by Ellis and Brannon.

There is no apparent sex predilection and the age range has been from 10 to over 65 years of age, with a mean of nearly 40 years of age. While lesions have a duration of only a few weeks, some lesions are present a year or longer. Some cases are asymptomatic; others

are characterized by a dull, aching pain. There are no other local or systemic manifestations of disease present.

Histologic Features. There are microscopic changes in random muscle fibers, rather than grouped bundles, consisting of atrophy, hypertrophy, necrosis with phagocytosis, and regeneration. Lymphocytic infiltration is usually present in the interstitial tissue, as is an increase in fibrous connective tissue in endomysial and perimysial locations. It should be stressed that a careful consideration of both clinical and histologic findings is essential in order to establish a definitive diagnosis of focal myositis.

Treatment. The lesion should be excised; it does not recur.

Differential Diagnosis. A variety of conditions, especially from the clinical aspect, must be considered in the differential diagnosis. These include a benign or malignant neoplasm within muscle, nodular fasciitis, proliferative myositis, myositis ossificans, polymyositis and, in the oral region, a salivary gland lesion.

MISCELLANEOUS MYOPATHIES

Congenital Facial Diplegia

(Möbius Syndrome)

Congenital facial diplegia is a nonfamilial deficient development of cranial muscles consisting of facial diplegia with bilateral paralysis of the ocular muscles, particularly the abducens. The cause of the disease is now recognized as being a primary muscle defect with secondary degeneration of the sixth and seventh cranial nerve nuclei, although it was originally thought to be a primary nuclear hypoplasia with secondary muscle atrophy.

Clinical Features. Congenital facial diplegia is usually manifested in infancy during the first few days of life by failure to close the eyes during sleep. Because of the partial or complete facial paralysis, the infant exhibits no change in facial expression even when crying or laughing. The prominent lips are often everted, and the mouth may remain partially opened.

There is difficulty in mastication; saliva frequently drools from the corners of the mouth, and speech is severely impaired.

The majority of patients have other associated congenital deformities, including external ophthalmoplegia, deformity of the external ears, deafness, defects of the pectoral muscles, paresis of the tongue, soft palate or jaw muscles, clubfoot, mental defects and epilepsy.

Histologic Features. There are no conclusive microscopic studies of muscle in patients with congenital facial diplegia.

Treatment and Prognosis. There is no treatment for the disease, but the prognosis appears to be good, barring complications.

Atrophy of Muscle

Atrophy of muscle refers to a decrease in the size of individual muscle fibers which were once normal. The condition is entirely nonspecific, since it occurs in many situations, some of which have been previously described. A partial listing of some of the recognized causes of muscle atrophy is given below.

1. Disuse and fixation
2. Aging and cachexia
3. Denervation
4. Muscular dystrophies
5. Nutritional disturbances
6. Infections and toxins
7. Muscular hypotonias
8. Metabolic disturbances
9. Vascular changes

Atrophy of muscle has been confused occasionally with aplasia or agenesis of muscles. Thus, some diseases are a result of muscular aplasia, or actually hypoplasia, rather than an actual decrease in size of normal fibers. One form of muscle atrophy, facial hemiatrophy (q.v.), has been discussed in Chapter 1.

Hypertrophy of Muscle

Hypertrophy of muscle refers to an increase in size of individual muscle fibers. This should be separated from pseudohypertrophy, in which the over-all increase in the size of a muscle is due to an increase in interstitial connective tissue.

The causes of muscular hypertrophy are also nonspecific and occur in a variety of situations listed below.

1. Developmental defects
2. Functional disturbances
3. Inflammations and infections
4. Metabolic changes
5. Neoplasms

Two forms of muscular hypertrophy are of interest to the dentist: (1) macroglossia, which has been discussed previously in Chapter 1, and (2) hypertrophy of the masseter muscle.

Masseteric hypertrophy occurs usually in two situations: (1) congenital facial hemihypertrophy (q.v.) and (2) functional hypertrophy as a result of unusual muscle function through habit or necessity after certain surgical procedures involving the jaws. This condition has been reviewed by Bloem and Van Hoof.

Specific Tumors of Muscles

Those tumors derived from muscle tissue are discussed in the chapter on tumors of the oral cavity in Section I.

REFERENCES

Ackerman, L. V.: Extra-osseous localized non-neoplastic bone and cartilage formation (so-called myositis ossificans). Clinical and pathological confusion with malignant neoplasms. J. Bone Joint Surg., 40:279, 1958.

Adams, R. D., Denny-Brown, D., and Pearson, C. M.: Diseases of Muscle. A Study in Pathology. 2nd ed. New York, Harper and Bros., 1962.

Afonsky, D.: The trigeminal nerve. Oral Surg., 5:913, 1952.

Baddour, H. M., McAnear, J. T., and Tilson, H. B.: Eagle's syndrome. Oral Surg., 46:486, 1978.

Baker, A. B. (ed.): Clinical Neurology. New York, Paul B. Hoeber, Inc., 1955, Vols. I–III.

Behrman, S.: Facial neuralgias. Br. Dent. J., 86:197, 1949.

Bloem, J. J., and Van Hoof, R. F.: Hypertrophy of the masseter muscle. Plast. Reconstr. Surg., 47:138, 1971.

Bohn, E., and Strang, R. R.: Glossopharyngeal neuralgia. Brain, 85:371, 1962.

Bourgoyne, J. R.: Trifacial neuralgia: treatments, history and observations. Oral Surg., 1:689, 1948.

Bourne, G. N.: The Structure and Function of Muscle. 2nd ed. New York, Academic Press, Inc., 1974, Vols. I–IV.

Brooke, R. I.: Periodic migrainous neuralgia: a cause of dental pain. Oral Surg., 46:511, 1978.

Brunner, H.: Present status of diagnosis and management of Ménière's syndrome. Arch. Otolaryngol., 40:38, 1944.

Burzynski, N. J., and Weisskopf, B.: Familial occurrence of Bell's palsy. Oral Surg., 36:504, 1973.

Caldwell, J. B., and Hughes, K. W.: Hypertrophy of the masseter muscles and mandible. J. Oral Surg., 15:329, 1957.

Carey, E. J.: Multiple bilateral traumatic parosteal bone and callus formation of the femurs and left innominate bone. Arch. Surg., 8:592, 1924.

Chisa, N., Mendelson, C. G., and Darnley, J. D.: Auriculotemporal syndrome. Arch. Dermatol., 90:457, 1964.

Chung, E. B., and Enzinger, F. M.: Proliferative fasciitis. Cancer, 36:1450, 1975.

Coburn, D. F., and Shofstall, C. K.: Glossopharyngeal neuralgia. Arch. Otolaryngol., 33:663, 1941.

Couch, C. D., Jr.: Facial pain. J. Oral Surg., 14:216, 1956.

Dalessio, D. J.: Treatment of trigeminal neuralgia. J.A.M.A., 245:2519, 1981.

Day, K. M.: Ménière's disease: present concepts of diagnosis and management. Ann. Otol. Rhinol. Laryngol., 59:966, 1950.

Dencer, D.: Bilateral idiopathic masseter hypertrophy. Br. J. Plast. Surg., 14:149, 1961.

Douglas, B. L., and Huebsch, R. F.: Atypical facial neuralgia resulting from fractured styloid process of the temporal bone. Oral Surg., 6:1199, 1953.

Dysart, B. R.: Modern view of neuralgia referable to Meckel's ganglion. Arch. Otolaryngol., 40:29, 1944.

Eggleston, D. J.: Periodic migrainous neuralgia. Oral Surg., 29:524, 1970.

Elfenbaum, A.: Causalgia in dentistry: an abandoned pain syndrome. Oral Surg., 7:594, 1954.

Ellis, G. L., and Brannon, R. B.: Focal myositis of the perioral musculature. Oral Surg., 48:337, 1979.

Enzinger, F. M., and Dulcey, F.: Proliferative myositis. Report of thirty-three cases. Cancer, 20:2213, 1967.

Ettinger, R. L., and Hanson, J. G.: The styloid or "Eagle" syndrome: an unexpected consequence. Oral Surg., 40:336, 1975.

Fleck, H., and Zurrow, H. B.: Familial amyotrophic lateral sclerosis. N.Y. State J. Med., 67:2368, 1967.

Flynn, J. E., and Graham, J. H.: Myositis ossificans. Surg. Gynecol. Obstet., 118:1001, 1964.

Ford, F. R.: Diseases of the Nervous System in Infancy. Childhood and Adolescence. 6th ed. Springfield, Ill., Charles C Thomas, 1973.

Gardner, D. G., and Zeman, W.: Biopsy of the dental pulp in the diagnosis of metachromatic leucodystrophy. Dev. Med. Child. Neurol., 7:620, 1965.

Gilbert, G. J.: Ménière's syndrome and cluster headaches: recurrent paroxysmal focal vasodilatation. J.A.M.A., 191:691, 1965.

Golding-Wood, P. H.: Crocodile tears. Br. Med. J., 1:1518, 1963.

Goldstein, N. P., Gibilisco, J. A., and Rushton, J. G.: Trigeminal neuropathy and neuritis: a study of etiology with emphasis on dental causes. J.A.M.A., 183:458, 1963.

Goodsell, J. O.: Traumatic myositis ossificans of the masseter muscle: review of the literature and report of a case. J. Oral Surg., 20:116, 1962.

Gurney, C. E.: Chronic bilateral benign hypertrophy of masseter muscles. Am. J. Surg., 73:137, 1947.

Hallpike, C. S., and Cairns, H.: Observations on the pathology of Ménière's syndrome. Proc. R. Soc. Med., 31:1317, 1938.

Hardman, R.: The floppy infant. Am. J. Dis. Child., 101:525, 1961.

Harrigan, W. F.: Facial pain. Oral Surg., 5:563, 1952.

Healey, C. A., and Wilske, K. R.: Temporal arteritis. Med. Clin. North. Am., 61:261, 1977.

Heffner, R. R., Jr., Armbrustmacher, V. W., and Earle, K. M.: Focal myositis. Cancer, 40:301, 1977.

Henderson, W R.: Trigeminal neuralgia: pain and treatment. Br. Med. J., 1:7, 1967.

Hollenhorst, R. W., Brown, J. R., Wagener, H. P., and Shick, R. M.: Neurologic aspects of temporal arteritis. Neurology, 10:490, 1960.

Huston, K. A., Hunder, G. G., Lie, J. T., Kennedy, R. H., and Elveback, L. R.: Temporal arteritis: a 25-year epidemiologic, clinical and pathologic study. Ann. Intern. Med., 88:162, 1978.

Ivers, R. R., and Goldstein, N. P.: Multiple sclerosis: a current appraisal of symptoms and signs. Mayo Clin. Proc., 38:457, 1963.

Jaeger, R.: A method for controlling pain of the face and jaws caused by tic douloureux. Science, 120:466, 1954.

Karshan, M., Kutscher, A. H., Silver, H. F., Stein, G., and Ziskin, D. E.: Studies in the etiology of idiopathic orolingual paresthesias. Am. J. Dig. Dis., 19:341, 1952.

Keeling, C. W.: Myasthenia gravis. J. Oral Surg., 9:224, 1951.

Kern, W. H.: Proliferative myositis; a pseudosarcomatous reaction to injury. A report of seven cases. Arch. Pathol., 69:209, 1960.

Kettel, K.: Bell's palsy. Arch. Otolaryngol., 46:427, 1947.

Kime, C. E.: Bell's palsy: a new syndrome associated with treatment by nicotinic acid. A.M.A. Arch. Otolaryngol., 68:28, 1958.

Kutscher, A. H., Silver, H. F., Stein, G., Ziskin, D. E., and Karshan, M.: Therapy of idiopathic orolingual paresthesias. N.Y. State J. Med., 52:1401, 1952.

Kwittken, J., and Branche, M.: Fasciitis ossificans. Am. J. Clin. Pathol., 51:251, 1969.

Lagier, R., and Cox, J. N.: Pseudomalignant myositis ossificans. A pathological study of eight cases. Hum. Pathol., 6:653, 1975.

Lilienthal, J. L., Jr.: Diseases of the Muscles; in R. L. Cecil and R. F. Loeb, eds.: Textbook of Medicine. 9th ed. Philadelphia, W. B. Saunders Company, 1955.

Loomis, B. E.: Trifacial neuralgia. J. Am. Dent. Assoc., 24:50, 1937.

Lucchesi, F. J., and Topazian, D. S.: Raeder's syndrome. Oral Surg., 15:923, 1962.

Mailander, J. C.: Hereditary gustatory sweating. J.A.M.A., 201:203, 1967.

McDougal, J. J.: Möbius syndrome: a congenital facial diplegia syndrome. J. Conn. State Dent. Assoc., 34:21, 1960.

McGibbon, B. M., and Paletta, F. X.: Further concepts in gustatory sweating. Plast. Reconstr. Surg., 49:639, 1972.

Meyers, C. E.: Diagnosis of neurological disease. Oral Surg., 1:480, 1948.

Mitchell, R. G.: Pre-trigeminal neuralgia. Br. Dent. J., 149:167, 1980.

Mulder, D. W.: The clinical syndrome of amyotrophic lateral sclerosis. Proc. Staff Meet., Mayo Clin., 32:427, 1957.

Nable, D. S.: Migrainous neuralgia (Horton's syndrome). Oral Surg., 15:927, 1962.

Olivier, R. M.: Trotter's syndrome. Report of a case. Oral Surg., 15:527, 1962.

Plezia, R. A., Mintz, S. M., and Calligaro, P.: Myositis ossificans traumatica of the masseter muscle. Report of a case. Oral Surg., 44:351, 1977.

Richards, R. N.: The Möbius syndrome. J. Bone Joint Surg., 35A:437, 1953.

Roller, N. W., Garfunkel, A., Nichols, C., and Ship, I. I.: Amyotrophic lateral sclerosis. Oral Surg., 37:46, 1974.

Rowland, L. P.: Diseases of muscles and neuromuscular junction; in P. B. Beeson, W. McDermott, and Wyngaarden, J. B. (eds.): Cecil Textbook of Medicine. 15th ed. Philadelphia, W. B. Saunders Company, 1979.

Rushton, J. G.: Cranial nerve neuralgias. Med. Clin. North Am., 44:.69, 1960.

Rushton, J. G., Gibilisco, J. A., and Goldstein, N. P.: Atypical facial pain. J.A.M.A., 171:545, 1959.

Russell, T. E.: Eagle's syndrome: diagnostic considerations and report of case. J. Am. Dent. Assoc., 94:548, 1977.

Sanders, B., and Weiner, J.: Eagle's syndrome. J. Oral Med., 32:44, 1977.

Sandok, B. A.: Temporal arteritis. J.A.M.A., 222:1405, 1972.

Sanger, R. G., and Kirby, J. W.: The oral and facial manifestations of dermatomyositis with calcinosis. Oral Surg., 35:476, 1973.

Schaffer, J.: Clinical pathology of the tongue. Oral Surg., 4:1287, 1951; 5:87, 1952.

Shapiro, H. H.: Differential diagnosis of dental pain. Oral Surg., 4:1353, 1951.

Sicher, H.: Problems of pain in dentistry. Oral Surg., 7:149, 1954.

Simpson, D. G.: Marcus Gunn phenomenon following squint and ptosis surgery: definition and review. Arch. Ophthalmol., 56 743, 1956.

Skinner, D. A.: The treatment of Bell's palsy with histamine. Ann. Otol., Rhinol. Laryngol., 59:197, 1950.

Sluder, G.: Five unusual cases of nasal (sphenopalatine) ganglion neurosis. South. Med. J., 11:312, 1918.

Smith, E. E., and Gans, M. E.: Jaw-winking (Marcus Gunn phenomenon). J. Pediatr., 50:52, 1957.

Stones, H. H.: Facial pain: review of aetiological factors. Proc. R. Soc. Med., 49 39, 1956.

Stoy, P. J., and Gregg, G.: Bell's palsy following local anaesthesia. Br. Dent. J., 91:292, 1951.

Streeto, J. M., and Watters, F. B.: Melkersson's syndrome: multiple recurrences of Bell's palsy and episodic facial edema. N. Engl. J. Med., 271:308, 1964.

Stuteville, O. H., and Levignac, J.: The neuralgias and vascular algias of the face. Oral Surg., 6:1413, 1953.

Sutcher, H. D., Underwood, R. B., Beatty, R. A., and Sugar, O.: Orofacial dyskinesia: a dental dimension. J.A.M.A., 216:1459, 1971.

Thoma, K. H.: Trismus hystericus. Oral Surg., 6:449, 1953.

Tolman, D. E., Gibilisco, J. A., and McConahey, W. M.: Subacute thyroiditis: a diagnostic possibility for the dentist. Oral Surg., 15:293, 1962.

Troiano, M. F., and Gaston, G. W.: Carotid system arteritis: an overlooked and misdiagnosed syndrome. J. Am. Dent. Assoc., 91:589, 1975.

Tweeddale, D. N., Higgins, G. M., and Wakim, K. G.: Attempts to produce myositis ossificans in the rat. Lab. Invest., 6:346, 1957.

Vernale, C. A.: Traumatic myositis ossificans of the masseter muscle. Oral Surg., 26:8, 1968.

Vistnes, L. M., and Kernahan, D. A.: The Melkersson-Rosenthal syndrome. Plast. Reconstr. Surg., 48:126, 1971.

Voorhies, R., and Patterson, R. H.: Management of trigeminal neuralgia (tic douloureux). J.A.M.A., 245:2521, 1981.

Wade, G. W., Galiber, F. A., and Thomas, A. L.: Transitory unilateral facial paralysis (Bell's palsy). Oral Surg., 8:719, 1955.

Wagener, H. P., and Hollenhorst, R. W.: The ocular lesions of temporal arteritis. Am. J. Ophthalmol., 45:617, 1958.

Wartenberg, R.: Progressive facial hemiatrophy. Arch. Neurol. Psychiat., 54:75, 1945.

Idem: Hemifacial Spasm. A Clinical and Pathophysiologic Study. New York, Oxford University Press, 1952.

Weisengreen, H. H., and Winters, S. E.: Pathways of referred pain, with special reference to head and neck. Oral Surg., 5:500, 1952.

Wolff, H. G.: Headache and Other Head Pain. 4th ed. New York, Oxford University Press, 1980.

Woolsey, R. D.: Trigeminal neuralgia treatment of surgical decompression of posterior root. J.A.M.A., 159:1713, 1955.

Wyngaarden, J. B., and Smith, L. H.: Cecil Textbook of Medicine. 16th ed. Philadelphia, W. B. Saunders Company, 1982.

Ziskin, D. E., and Moulton, R.: Glossodynia: a study of idiopathic orolingual pain. J. Am. Dent. Assoc., 33:1422, 1946.

Zundel, W. S. and Tyler, F. H.: The muscular dystrophies. N. Engl. J. Med., 273:537, 1965.

APPENDIX

TABLES OF NORMAL VALUES

Appendix Table I. Normal Laboratory Values

TEST	MATERIAL USED AND COMMENTS	NORMAL*
Albumin	Serum. See *Protein*	
Amino acid nitrogen	Serum	3.5–6.0
Amylase	Serum or plasma	80–150 units (Somogyi). (1 unit is 1 mg. of reducing sugar liberated as glucose per 100 ml. of serum)
Ascorbic acid	Serum or plasma	0.7–2.0
Basal metabolic rate ..... (B.M.R.)		Minus 15% to plus 15%
Bilirubin (van den Bergh)	Serum	Direct: 0–0.2 Total: 0.1–1.0
Bromide	Serum or plasma	Less than 50
Bromsulphalein test ...... (B.S.P.)	Serum. Liver function test. Method is valueless in patients with obvious jaundice	Less than 10% retained in 30 min.
Calcium, diffusible	Serum, consists of ionized and non-ionized calcium	4.5–5.0
Calcium, nondiffusible	Serum, nonionized calcium. Contains protein-bound calcium fraction	4.5–6.0
Calcium, total	Serum. Total calcium equals diffusible plus nondiffusible	9.0–11.5 (4.5–5.5 mEq./liter)
Calcium, total	Feces, 24-hour specimen	70–90% of ingested calcium eliminated in feces
Calcium, total	Urine, 24-hour specimen	10–30% of ingested calcium eliminated in urine
Carbon dioxide-combining power (CO$_2$ capacity) ..	Serum or plasma. Normal milliequivalent values expressed as bicarbonate or carbonic acid	Adults: 55–70 vols. % (25–35 mEq./liter) Children: 40–55 vols. % (18–25 mEq./liter)
Carotenoids	Serum	80–400 μg./100 ml.
Cephalin flocculation	Serum. Liver function test	Below 2+ in 48 hours
Chloride	Serum or plasma	570–620 (as NaCl) 340–370 (as Cl) (96–105 mEq./liter as Cl)
Chloride	Spinal fluid	720–750
Chloride	Urine, 24-hour specimen	10–16 gm./24 hr.
Cholesterol, esters	Serum or plasma	80–200
Cholesterol, total	Serum or plasma	120–260
Congo red test	Serum or plasma. Test for amyloidosis and nephrosis	10–30% eliminated from blood in 1 hr.
Copper	Serum	100–200 μg./100 ml.
Creatine	Whole blood	3–7
Creatine	Urine, 24-hour specimen	Adults: 0–200/24 hr. Children: 10–15/24 hr.
Creatinine	Serum	0.6–1.3
Creatinine	Urine, 24-hour specimen	1–1.8 gm./24 hr.
Fatty acids, total	Serum	250–500
Fibrin	Plasma	0.3–0.6 gm./100 ml.
Glucose	Whole blood Serum Postprandial	60–90 70–105 Less than 140
Glucose	Spinal fluid	40–60
Hippuric acid	Urine. Liver function test	
Oral		3 gm. benzoic acid excreted/4 hr.
Intravenous		0.7–0.95 gm. benzoic acid excreted/1 hr.

Appendix Table I. Normal Laboratory Values (Continued)

TEST	MATERIAL USED AND COMMENTS	NORMAL*
Hydrogen ion concentration	Whole blood, serum or plasma	7.3–7.5 units
Icteric index	Serum	4–6 units
Iodine, protein-bound	Serum	3–8 micrograms/100 ml.
Lecithin	Serum or plasma	225–250
Lipase	Serum	0.8–1.5 units (Alper) 0.2–1.5 units (Cherry-Crandall)
Lipids, total	Serum	470–750
Nitrogen, nonprotein	Whole blood	25–35
Nitrogen, urea	Whole blood	9–17
pH	Whole blood, serum or plasma	7.3–7.5 units
Phenolsulfonphthalein ... (P.S.P.)	Urine. Renal function test	40–60% 1st hour 20–25% 2nd hour
Phosphatase, acid	Serum	0–2.5 units (King-Armstrong) 0–1.5 phenol units
Phosphatase, alkaline	Serum	Adults: 1.5–5.0 units (Bodansky) 5–10 units (King-Armstrong) 1.0–3.5 phenol units Children: 5–14 units (Bodansky) 15–20 units (King-Armstrong) 4–12 phenol units
Phospholipids	Serum	150–350
Phosphorus, inorganic	Serum	Adults: 3.0–4.5 Children: 4.5–6.0
Potassium	Serum	16–22 (4.1–5.6 mEq./liter)
Protein, total	Serum	6–8 gm./100 ml.
Albumin		3.2–4.1 gm./100 ml.
Alpha globulin		0.7–1.5 gm./100 ml.
Beta globulin		0.7–1.3 gm./100 ml.
Gamma globulin		0.7–1.3 gm./100 ml.
Total globulin		2.6–3.8 gm./100 ml.
Albumin–globulin ratio . (A/G ratio)		1.5–2.5:1
Protein, total	Spinal fluid	20–40
Sodium	Serum	315–340 (137–147 mEq./liter)
Sulfates	Serum	2.5–5.0
Thymol turbidity	Serum. Liver function test	0–4 units
Uric acid	Whole blood	2–4
Urobilinogen	Feces, 4-day specimen	150–300
Urobilinogen	Urine, 24-hour specimen	8 or less
Vitamin A	**Serum**	15–60 μg./ml.
Vitamin C	Serum or plasma	0.7–2.0
Volume, blood	Whole blood and plasma	70–100 cc. blood/kg. 35–50 cc. plasma/kg.
Zinc turbidity	Serum. Liver function test	2–8 units

* All values expressed as milligrams per 100 ml. unless otherwise specified.

Appendix Table II. Normal Red Blood Cell Values

AGE	RED CELL COUNT (MILLIONS PER CU. MM. BLOOD)	HEMOGLOBIN* (GM. PER 100 ML.)	HEMATOCRIT (VOL. PACKED CELLS PER 100 ML.)	SEDIMENTATION RATE IN 1 HR. (WINTROBE METHOD)	RETICULO-CYTES (% OF ERYTHRO-CYTES)
Children					
First year	6.1–4.5 (Values decrease with increasing age; high at birth)	25–11.2	64–35	0–2 mm. (At birth)	2–6 (at birth) 0.5–1.5 (2–5 days after birth)
2–10 years	4.6–4.7	11.5–12.9	35.3–37.5	3–13 mm.	0.5–1.5
11–15 years	4.8	13.4	39		0.5–1.5
Adults					
Females	4.2–5.4	12–16	37–47	0–15 mm.	0.5–1.5
Males	4.6–6.2	14–18	40–54	0–6.5 mm.	

* Hemoglobin values by oxygen capacity method.

Appendix Table III. Normal White Blood Cell Values

TOTAL WHITE CELL COUNT PER CU. MM. BLOOD
Infants: 8,000–16,500
4– 7 years: 6,000–15,000 (average 10,700)
8–18 years: 4,500–13,500 (average 8,300)
Adults: 5,000–10,000 (average 7,000)

RELATIVE (DIFFERENTIAL) AND ABSOLUTE VALUES FOR LEUKOCYTE COUNTS IN NORMAL ADULTS PER CU. MM. BLOOD*

TYPE OF CELL	PER CENT	ABSOLUTE NUMBER		
		AVERAGE	MINIMUM	MAXIMUM
Total leukocytes		7000	5000	10,000
Myelocytes	0	0	0	0
Juvenile neutrophils	3–5	300	150	400
Segmented neutrophils	54–62	4000	3000	5800
Eosinophils	1–3	200	50	250
Basophils	0–0.75	25	15	50
Lymphocytes	25–33	2100	1500	3000
Monocytes	3–7	375	285	500

*From M. M. Wintrobe: Clinical Hematology. 6th ed. Philadelphia, Lea & Febiger, 1967.

Appendix Table IV. Normal Blood Platelet Values and Associated Phenomena

Total number of platelets: 150,000–400,000 per cu. mm. blood

Bleeding time: Under 5 minutes (Duke's method)

Clotting time: 1–7 minutes (capillary tube method)
2.5–5 minutes (Kruse and Moses method)
5–10 minutes (Lee and White method)

Prothrombin time: 10–20 seconds (Quick method)

Clot retraction time:
Qualitative begins 1–6 hours; complete at 24 hours
Quantitative 80–90%

Capillary fragility (tourniquet test):
More than 10 petechiae per 1 inch circle—positive

Heterophile antibodies (sheep cell agglutination):
Below 1:56 dilution

Incidence of blood groups in normal population:

Group O —40%
A —45
B —12
AB— 4

Rh positive—85%
negative—15

Appendix Table V. Normal Average Values of Urine

Physical characteristics
Volume, 24-hour specimen .... 1500 ml.
Specific gravity 1.015–1.025
Turbidity .... None
Color .... Amber

Chemical characteristics
pH .... Slightly acid
Total acidity .... 25–40 ml. N/10
NaOH to neutralize
100 ml. urine

Water .... 95% of total urine

Inorganic constituents
Chloride (as NaCl) .... 9.0 gm./liter
Phosphorus (as P_2O_5) .... 2.0 gm./liter
Total sulfur (as SO_3) .... 1.5 gm./liter
Sodium (as Na_2O) .... 4.0 gm./liter
Potassium (as K_2O) .... 2.0 gm./liter
Calcium (as CaO) .... 0.2 gm./liter
Magnesium (as MgO) .... 0.2 gm./liter
Iron .... 0.003 gm./liter

Organic constituents
Urea .... 15–25 gm./liter
Uric acid .... 0.4–0.6 gm./liter
Creatinine .... 0.8–1.5 gm./liter
Ammonia .... 0.6 gm./liter
Undetermined N .... 0.6 gm./liter

Traces of other substances

Appendix Table VI.   Normal Chronologic Development of Deciduous Teeth

	CALCIFICATION BEGINS (MOS. IN UTERO)	CROWN COMPLETED (MOS.)	ERUPTION (MOS.)	ROOT COMPLETED (YRS.)	ROOT RE- SORPTION BEGINS (YRS.)	TOOTH SHED (YRS.)
Central incisor	4–5	2– 4	6– 9	1½–2	5–6	7– 8
Lateral incisor	4–5	2– 5	7–10	1½–2	5–6	7– 9
Cuspid	5	9	16–20	2½–3	6–7	10–12
First molar	5	6	12–16	2 –2½	4–5	9–11
Second molar	6	10–12	20–30	3	4–5	10–12

Adapted from original data of Logan and Kronfeld.

Appendix Table VII.   Normal Chronologic Development of Permanent Teeth

	CALCIFICATION BEGINS	CROWN COMPLETED (YRS.)	ERUPTION (YRS.)	ROOT COMPLETED (YRS.)
Maxilla				
Central incisor	3–4 mos.	4 – 5	7– 8	10
Lateral incisor	1 yr.	4 – 5	8– 9	11
Cuspid	4–5 mos.	6 – 7	11–12	13–15
First bicuspid	1½–1¾ yrs.	5 – 6	10–11	12–13
Second bicuspid	2–2½ yrs.	6 – 7	10–12	12–14
First molar	Birth	2½– 3	6– 7	9–10
Second molar	2½–3 yrs.	7 – 8	12–13	14–16
Third molar	7–9 yrs.	12 –16	17–25	18–25
Mandible				
Central incisor	3–4 mos.	4 – 5	6– 7	9
Lateral incisor	3–4 mos.	4 – 5	7– 8	10
Cuspid	4–5 mos.	6 – 7	9–11	12–14
First bicuspid	1¾–2 yrs.	5 – 6	10–12	12–13
Second bicuspid	2¼–2½ yrs.	6 – 7	11–12	13–14
First molar	Birth	2½– 3	6– 7	9–10
Second molar	2½–3 yrs.	7 – 8	11–13	14–15
Third molar	8–10 yrs.	12 –16	17–25	18–25

Adapted from original data of Logan and Kronfeld.

INDEX